5 ISSUE

JUNE 2001

clinical evidence

The international source of the
best available evidence for
effective health care

BMJ
Publishing
Group

Editorial Office
BMJ Publishing Group, BMA House, Tavistock Square, London, WC1H 9JR, United Kingdom. Tel: +44 (0)20 7387 4499; Fax: +44 (0)20 7383 6242 www.bmjpg.com

Subscription prices
Clinical Evidence is published six monthly (June/December) by BMJ Publishing Group in print, online, and CD-ROM formats. The annual subscription rates for Issues 5 and 6 (June 2001 and December 2001) are:

Individual: £75 • US$110 • Can$160
Institutional: £160 • US$240 • Can$345
Student: £55 • US$80 • Can$120

The above rates include print or CD-ROM format, with online access at no additional cost for individuals and students. The institutional rate is for print/CD-ROM only. Institutions may purchase online site licenses separately. For further information, visit the subscription pages of our website www.clinicalevidence.org or contact Miranda Lonsdale, Sales Manager at clinicalevidence@bmjgroup.com

All subscriptions from countries outside the Americas to be directed to BMJ Publishing Group, PO Box 299, London, WC1H 9TD, UK.
Tel: +44 (0)20 7383 6270 • Fax: +44 (0)20 7383 6402• Email: subscriptions@bmjgroup.com
All subscriptions from countries in the Americas to BMJ-Clinical Evidence, PO Box 512, Annapolis Jct, MD 20701-0512, USA.
Tel: 1-800-373-2897/1-240-646-700 • Fax: 1-240-646-7005 • Email: clinevide@pmds.com
Alternatively, you can visit our website to order online www.clinicalevidence.org

Bulk subscriptions for societies and organisations
The Publishers offer discounts for any society or organisation buying bulk quantities for their members/ specific groups. Please contact Miranda Lonsdale, Sales Manager at mlonsdale@bmjgroup.com

Contributors
If you are interested in becoming a contributor to *Clinical Evidence* please contact us at clinicalevidence@bmjgroup.com

Clinical Evidence CD-ROM
This is a new addition this issue to the *Clinical Evidence* product range. It can be purchased to complement the print edition, and online access is included at no additional cost to individual and student CD-ROM subscribers. For further information see the subscription card at the back of this book or visit www.clinicalevidence.org

Rights
For information on translation rights, please contact Daniel Raymond-Barker at clinicalevidence@bmjgroup.com

Printed by Quebecor World, Hawkins, Tennessee
Designed by Pete Wilder, The Designers Collective Limited, London UK

Acknowledgements

We thank the following people and organisations for their advice and support: The Cochrane Collaboration, and especially Iain Chalmers, Mike Clarke, Phil Alderson, and Carol Lefebvre; the NHS Centre for Reviews and Dissemination, and especially Jos Kleijnen and Julie Glanville; the NHS Executive, and especially Andrew Burnett, Chris Henshall, and Tom Mann; the British National Formulary, and especially Dinesh Mehta; the Health Information Research Unit at McMaster University, and especially Brian Haynes and Ann McKibbon; the Sowerby Centre for Health Informatics at Newcastle, especially Nick Booth, Peter Johnson, and Neill Jones; and the clinicians, epidemiologists, and members of patient support groups who have acted as peer reviewers. We are grateful to the clinicians and patients who spare time to take part in focus groups, which are crucial to the development of *Clinical Evidence*. Finally, we would like to acknowledge the readers who have taken the time to send us their comments and suggestions.

Contents

Welcome to Issue 5

Welcome to Issue 5 of *Clinical Evidence*, the six monthly, updated compendium of evidence on the effects of clinical interventions. *Clinical Evidence* summarises the current state of knowledge and uncertainty about the prevention and treatment of clinical conditions, based on thorough searches and appraisal of the literature. It is not a textbook of medicine nor a book of guidelines. It describes the best available evidence, and if there is no good evidence, it says so.

RESPONSE TO ISSUE 4

The printed Issue 4 of *Clinical Evidence* was received by around 600 000 people around the world, including 500 000 physicians, nurses, and medical students in the USA, and 50 000 people in the UK (mainly general practitioners in England). Translations are now available in French[1] and in German,[2] and are received by another 11 000 health carers. Each day, a further 50 people register on the Internet. *Clinical Evidence* is also available in England via the NHS National Electronic Library for Health.[3]

We continue to be encouraged by the positive messages from people receiving *Clinical Evidence* for the first time. We also receive many specific requests for information. We are often asked how *Clinical Evidence* should be used, and whether it is designed to be read topic by topic, or whether it should be used for specific problems. The central concept is that *Clinical Evidence* is designed to save the time, effort, and frustration of trying to keep up to date with the literature.

Our hope is that *Clinical Evidence* will improve patient care.[4] A recent independent survey[5] indicates that doctors already rank *Clinical Evidence* in their top three favourite sources of information. A questionnaire of 389 GP principals and consultants in two English Health Authorities assessed how useful *Clinical Evidence* had been in their clinical practice, and how it compared with other sources of evidence. Of these, 95 respondents (24%) already identified *Clinical Evidence* as one of their three favourite sources of information. When asked about frequency of use, 1% said they used it daily, 28% weekly, and 43% monthly. *Clinical Evidence* was used in or after a consultation by 59%. The book, rather than the online version, was preferred by 61% of the doctors, but 64% were interested in using a combination of media.

Evidence from the new website gives a few clues about how *Clinical Evidence* is being used. Soon after registering, many users browse through most sections—seeing what is there and how far the links go. Later, the frequency of contacts varies, ranging from 1–112 contacts a month (mean 2.4 contacts/month/user). Most sessions are brief (4 minutes) and involve only a few content pages (5 pages). Each content page is examined for around a minute. The current "top 10" topics (chapters) are listed in the table (p xi); they are major cardiovascular and respiratory topics, and back pain. Popular options receive more hits, but the time spent per page is about the same. We think this is consistent with *Clinical Evidence* being used like a telephone directory—most users dropping in repeatedly for specific items, rather than reading large tracts in one go.

We have had many requests to provide PowerPoint™ slides of the content that can be adapted for presentations to do with education or research. These are now available for the "top 10" topics and, if they are useful, we will provide PowerPoint™ presentations for all topics.

Another common request has been for a CD-ROM version of *Clinical Evidence*. This is now available. You can find out more about it on the website.

WHAT'S NEW IN ISSUE 5?

There are 14 new topics (including Influenza, Acute atrial fibrillation, Colonic diverticular disease, *Helicobacter pylori* eradication, Meniere's disease, Trigeminal neuralgia, and Lyme disease). All the new topics are labelled on the contents page. Secondly, 20 topics have been expanded, including Asthma, Schizophrenia, Alzheimer's disease, Breast cancer (non-metastatic), and Unstable angina. The new interventions are labelled on the summary page for each topic. Thirdly, 96 of the 120 topics from Issue 4 have been updated and re-edited. This has involved performing a *Clinical Evidence* search from the date of the previous search, appraising any new studies that were identified, and incorporating the new evidence into the *Clinical Evidence* review (for example, that angiotensin II receptor blockers reduce mortality from heart failure, and that paracetamol is likely to be beneficial in reducing pain from acute otitis media).

UPDATING

Medical knowledge is fluid and rapidly changing. The biggest challenge facing *Clinical Evidence* is to produce high quality updates for a large number of topics at regular intervals. The delays in producing a quality paper publication are appreciable, and an inevitable trade-off exists between speed of updating and time for quality control. Issue 5 will be distributed in June 2001. It will have been printed during May. Authoring, peer review, clinical editing, and quality control checks ended in early April. Literature searches for the updated topics in this issue were performed between Summer 2000 and January 2001. The lag from search to publication is 5 to 9 months, and by the time the next issue is published, the unavoidable lag is 11 to 15 months. We are now stating the search date under the title of every topic.

We have redesigned the *Clinical Evidence* website so that, from the launch of Issue 5, all updated and corrected topics will be posted directly and regularly to the web. This will reduce the search to publication time by 2 to 8 months. We aim to ensure that topics on the website are within 12 months of their search dates.

ERRORS

New research is the main reason for updating the evidence, but changes also arise because of the need to correct errors. Error correction arises when previously published research is amended,[6] is withdrawn because of proven or suspected fraud,[7] or when simple errors have arisen during editing or preparation for press. These corrections need to be available quickly. Readers who want to ensure that the information they use is current should either check the website periodically for updates and corrections, or should register on the website to receive e-mail alerts about all important updates. The specific procedures we have devised for dealing with corrections are listed on page xviii. Errors from previous issues are detailed there.

THE FUTURE

We have firm plans for *Clinical Evidence* to include more topics, but to provide a thinner book that fits in a pocket. A concise paper version, which can be used in conjunction with a larger book, CD-ROM, or online version of *Clinical Evidence* will be piloted with issue 6 and, if successful, will be made available for issue 7 (June 2002). The concise version will contain "smart" summaries of the questions and key messages. Our aim is to use the available space to hold the most useful evidence we can identify. More detail will be presented for frequently accessed topics. Specialist versions will allow tailoring of the content to meet particular needs. We will include questions about diagnosis in Issue 7.

Your views are very important to us. Requests from readers are now one of the most important factors in identifying the questions that need answering in *Clinical Evidence*. You can influence the development of *Clinical Evidence* by letting us know your views on what we are doing and how we could do it better.

	Mean viewing time per page (minutes)	Hits (relative to mean for all topics)
TABLE **The 10 most frequently visited topics on the website.**		
Heart failure	1.38	5.5
Primary prevention	1.51	5.3
Secondary prevention of ischaemic cardiac events	1.33	5.2
Acute myocardial infarction	1.32	5.2
DVT and pulmonary embolism	1.10	4.2
Stroke management	1.36	3.9
Unstable angina	1.10	3.6
Low back pain	1.59	3.5
Asthma	1.31	2.9
Gastro-oesophageal reflux	1.13	2.8

Figures for March 2001 showing the time spent viewing individual web pages by individual viewers during a single session, and the number of hits (relative to the mean for all topics).

REFERENCES

1. Décider pour traiter. *Clinical Evidence* (édition Française). Meudon, France; RanD, 2001.
2. Clinical Evidence: die besten Studien für die beste klinische Praxis. Bern; Verlag Hans Huber, 2000.
3. http://nww.nelh.nhs.uk (via NHSnet) or http://www.nelh.nhs.uk (via Internet).
4. Barton S. Using clinical evidence. *BMJ* 2001;322:503–504.
5. Sue Gordon. A survey of use of *Clinical Evidence* in Northumberland & Gateshead & South Tyneside Health Authorities. http://bmj.com, 7 Mar 2001 http://www.bmj.com/cgi/content/full/322/7285/503#responses.
6. Schrier RW, Estacio RO. Additional follow-up from the ABCD trial in patients with type 2 diabetes and hypertension. *N Engl J Med* 2000;343:1969.
7. Rennie D, Evans I, Farthing MJG, et al. Dealing with research misconduct in the United Kingdom. *BMJ* 1998;316: 1726–1733.

About Clinical Evidence

The inspiration for *Clinical Evidence* came in a phone call in 1995. Tom Mann and his colleagues at the NHS Executive asked the BMJ Publishing Group to explore the possibility of developing an evidence "formulary" along the lines of the *British National Formulary*. They recognised that clinicians were under increasing pressure to keep up to date and to base their practice more firmly on evidence, but that few had the necessary time or skills to do this. Their idea was to provide a pocket book containing concise and regularly updated summaries of the best available evidence on clinical interventions. However, they didn't think that the NHS could develop such a formulary itself. "It would be marvellous", said Tom Mann, "if somebody would just do it." A small team at the BMJ set to work to produce a pilot version of what was then called the *Clinical Effectiveness Directory*.

Since that pilot, a great deal has changed. In collaboration with the American College of Physicians–American Society of Internal Medicine, we convened an international advisory board, held focus groups of clinicians, talked to patient support groups, and adopted countless good ideas from early drafts by our contributors. Throughout we have kept in mind an equation set out by Slawson et al.[1] This states that the usefulness of any source of information is equal to its relevance, multiplied by its validity, divided by the work required to extract the information. In order to be as useful as possible, we aimed for high relevance, high validity, and low work in terms of the reader's time and effort. We also kept in mind principles of transparency and explicitness. Readers needed to understand where our information came from and how it was assembled.

A UNIQUE RESOURCE

Clinical Evidence joins a growing number of sources of evidence based information for clinicians. But it has several features that, we think, make it unique.

- Its contents are driven by questions rather than by the availability of research evidence. Rather than start with the evidence and summarise what is there, we have tried to identify important clinical questions, and then to search for and summarise the best available evidence to answer them.
- It identifies but does not try to fill important gaps in the evidence. In a phrase used by Jerry Osheroff, who has led much of the recent research on clinicians' information needs,[2] *Clinical Evidence* presents the dark as well as the light side of the moon. We feel that it will be helpful for clinicians to know when their uncertainty stems from gaps in the evidence rather than gaps in their own knowledge.
- It is updated every six months. This means that you can rely on it to keep you up to date in the areas that are covered.
- It specifically aims not to make recommendations. This is because we feel that simply summarising the evidence will make it more widely useful. The experience of the clinical practice guideline movement has shown that it is nearly impossible to make recommendations that are appropriate in every situation. Differences in individual patients' baseline risks and preferences, and in the local availability of interventions, will always mean that the evidence must be individually interpreted rather than applied across the board. *Clinical Evidence* provides the raw material for developing locally applicable clinical practice guidelines, and for clinicians and patients to make up their own minds on the best course of action. We supply the evidence, you make the decisions.

COMPLEMENTARY BUT DIFFERENT

We are often asked how *Clinical Evidence* differs from two other high quality sources of evidence based information: The Cochrane Library; and the evidence based journals *ACP Journal Club, Evidence Based Medicine, Evidence Based Mental Health,* and *Evidence Based Nursing.*

Clinical Evidence is complementary to but different from the work of the Cochrane Collaboration, which produces and publishes high quality systematic reviews of controlled trials.[3] *Clinical Evidence* has been called the friendly front end of the Cochrane Library, since it takes this, and other, high quality information, and pulls it together in one place in a concise format. Many of our advisors and contributors are active members of the Cochrane Collaboration, and we are exploring closer ties between *Clinical Evidence* and the Collaboration in the way the evidence is searched for, summarised, and accessed by users.

Clinical Evidence is also complementary to but different from the evidence based journals, which select and abstract the best and most clinically relevant articles as they appear in the world's medical literature. Together these journals form a growing archive of high quality abstracts of individual articles, many of which are now pooled on the *Best Evidence* CD. *Clinical Evidence* takes a different approach. It begins not with the journals but with clinical questions. It is able to answer some. For others it simply reports that no good evidence was found.

A WORK IN PROGRESS
Clinical Evidence is an evolving project. We knew before we started that we were undertaking an enormous task, but the more we worked the more we realised its enormity. We recognise that there is some mismatch between what we aim eventually to achieve and what we have achieved so far. While we have made every effort to ensure that the searches were thorough and that the appraisals of studies were objective (see p xvii), we will inevitably have missed some important studies. In order not to make unjustified claims about the accuracy of the information, we use phrases such as "we found no systematic review" rather than "there is no systematic review". In order to be as explicit as possible about the methods used for each contribution, we have asked each set of contributors to provide a brief methods section, describing the searches that were performed and how individual studies were selected.

UPDATING AND EXPANDING CLINICAL EVIDENCE
Our expectation is that *Clinical Evidence* will evolve rapidly in its early years. Indeed, it is already becoming a family of products, appearing in different formats and languages for different audiences: German and French editions have just been published, and Italian and Japanese language versions are already in development. In particular, *Clinical Evidence* will evolve in response to the needs of clinicians. We have tried hard to anticipate those needs (not least by involving clinicians at every stage), but it is only when people begin to use *Clinical Evidence* in daily practice that we can know how best to develop it. That's why your feedback is so important to us, and we are arranging for various ways to evaluate the product.

REFERENCES
1. Slawson DC, Shaughnessy AF, Bennett JH. Becoming a medical information master: feeling good about not knowing everything. *J Fam Pract* 1994;38:505–513.
2. Ely JW, Osheroff JA, Ebell MJ, et al. Analysis of questions asked by family doctors regarding patient care. *BMJ* 1999; 319:358–361.
3. http://hiru.mcmaster.ca/cochrane/default.htm

A guide to the text

The summary page for each topic presents the questions addressed, some key messages, and a list of the interventions covered, categorised according to whether they have been found to be effective or not. We have developed the categories of effectiveness from one of the Cochrane Collaboration's first and most popular products, *A guide to effective care in pregnancy and childbirth*.[1] The categories we now use are explained in the table below.

Fitting interventions into these categories is not always straightforward. For one thing, the categories represent a mix of several hierarchies: the level of benefit (or harm), the level of evidence (RCT or observational data), and the level of certainty around the finding (represented by the confidence interval). Another problem is that much of the evidence that is most relevant to clinical decisions relates to comparisons between different interventions rather than to comparison with placebo or no intervention. Where necessary, we have indicated the comparisons in brackets. A third problem is that interventions may have been tested, or found to be effective, in only one group of people, such as those at high risk of an outcome. Again, we have indicated this where possible. But perhaps most difficult of all has been to trying to maintain consistency across different topics. We are working on refining the criteria for putting interventions under each category.

Interventions that cannot be tested in an RCT (perhaps because of ethical or practical reasons) are sometimes cited in the categorisation table, but they are always identified clearly with an asterix (for example, oxygen in severe acute asthma).

TABLE	Categorisation of treatment effects in *Clinical Evidence*.
Beneficial	Interventions whose effectiveness has been demonstrated by clear evidence from randomised controlled trials, and expectation of harms that is small compared with the benefits.
Likely to be beneficial	Interventions for which effectiveness is less well established than for those listed under "beneficial".
Trade off between benefits and harms	Interventions for which clinicians and patients should weigh up the beneficial and harmful effects according to individual circumstances and priorities.
Unknown effectiveness	Interventions for which there are currently insufficient data or data of inadequate quality.
Unlikely to be beneficial	Interventions for which lack of effectiveness is less well established than for those listed under "likely to be ineffective or harmful".
Likely to be ineffective or harmful	Interventions whose ineffectiveness or harmfulness has been demonstrated by clear evidence.

NEGATIVE FINDINGS

A surprisingly hard aspect to get right has been the reporting of negative findings. As we have had to keep reminding ourselves, saying that there is no good evidence that a treatment works is not the same as saying that the treatment doesn't work. In trying to get this right, we may have erred too much on the side of caution; when in doubt we have changed summary phrases from, for example, "the review found no difference", to "the review found no evidence of a difference". We recognise that to get this right, we need a better handle on the power of individual systematic reviews and trials to demonstrate statistically significant differences between groups, and better information on what constitutes clinically important differences in the major outcomes for each intervention. In the meantime, we hope that the text makes a clear distinction between lack of benefit and lack of evidence of benefit.

OUTCOMES

Clinical Evidence focuses on outcomes that matter to patients, meaning those that patients themselves are aware of, such as symptom severity, quality of life, survival, disability, walking distance, and live birth rate. We are less interested in proxy outcomes such as blood lipid concentrations, blood pressure, or ovulation rates. Each topic includes a list of the main patient oriented outcomes, and where possible describes how these are measured. We have for the moment decided not to address the vexed question of what constitutes a clinically important change in an outcome, but we would welcome any suggestions.

EFFECTS, NOT EFFECTIVENESS

A key aim of *Clinical Evidence* is to emphasise the important trade offs between advantages and disadvantages of different treatment options. We therefore talk about the effects of interventions, both positive and negative, rather than the effectiveness, and for each question or intervention option we present data on benefits and harms under separate headings.

HARMS

"Harms" include adverse effects of treatment and inconvenience to the patient. Finding good evidence on harms of treatments is not easy. Ideally these would come from RCTs, but many trials are not sufficiently large or long term to capture rarer or more distant events, and many do not adequately report adverse effects. We have asked contributors to keep the negative effects of interventions in mind at all times. Where good evidence is available, we indicate the frequency of adverse effects. However, because RCTs are not reliable sources of evidence about harms, and because of the principle that a physician should strive to do no harm, we also include weaker forms of evidence about harms.

DRUG INFORMATION

We make no systematic attempt to provide information on drug dosages, formulations, indications, and contraindications. For this information, we refer readers to their national drug formularies. Drug dosages are included when a question explores the relative effects of different doses.

INFORMATION ON COST

We have decided not to include information on the cost or cost effectiveness of interventions. This is not because we believe cost to be unimportant, but because the question of what constitutes good evidence on cost is much disputed and because costs vary greatly both within and between countries. However, we believe that it will become increasingly untenable for clinicians to act without paying attention to resources. Future companion publications of *Clinical Evidence* may provide relevant information on costs.

NUMERICAL DATA

Whenever possible, data are presented in the same form as in the original studies. However, sometimes we have changed the units or type of information in an attempt to present the results in a systematic and easily interpretable form.

AN INTERNATIONAL APPROACH TO THE EVIDENCE

Clinical Evidence takes an international approach to the evidence. This means including drugs that are not licensed in some countries. It also means keeping in mind the practicalities of treating people in rich as well as poorer countries, by covering interventions even if they have been superceded (for example, single drug treatment for HIV infection as opposed to three drug treatment).

COMPETING INTERESTS

In line with the *BMJ*'s policy,[2] our aim is not to try to eliminate conflicts of interest but to make them explicit, so that readers can judge for themselves what influence if any these may have had on the contributors' interpretation of the evidence. We therefore ask all contributors to let us know about any potential competing interests, and we append any that are declared to the end of the contribution. Where the contributor gives no competing interests, we record "none declared".

CHANGES SINCE THE LAST ISSUE

The text has been edited and updated. Substantive changes since the last issue are listed at the end of each topic. These are defined as:

- Presentation of additional evidence that either confirms or alters the conclusions
- Re-evaluation of the evidence
- Correction of an important error

HOW TO USE THE INFORMATION IN CLINICAL EVIDENCE

The type of information contained in *Clinical Evidence* is necessary but not sufficient for the provision of effective, high quality health care. It is intended as an aid to clinical decision making, to be used in conjunction with other important sources of information. These other sources include estimates of people's baseline risk of a condition or outcome based on history, physical examination, and clinical investigations; individual preferences; economic arguments; availability of treatments; and local expertise.

Some guidance on how to apply research evidence in practice is available on our website (www.clinicalevidence.org) and in appendix 3 in this issue.

REFERENCES

1. Enkin M, Keirse M, Renfrew M, et al. *A guide to effective care in pregnancy and childbirth*. Oxford: Oxford University Press, 1998.
2. Smith R. Beyond conflict of interest. *BMJ* 1998;317:219–292.

How Clinical Evidence is put together

The summaries in *Clinical Evidence* result from a rigorous process aimed at ensuring that the information they contain is both reliable and relevant to clinical practice.

SELECTING TOPICS
Clinical Evidence aims to cover common or important clinical conditions seen in primary and hospital care. To decide which conditions to cover in the first few issues, we reviewed national data on consultation rates, morbidity, and mortality, and took advice from generalist clinicians and patient groups. See our website (www.clinicalevidence.org) for a list of conditions that we are planning to cover in future issues. Further suggestions are welcome.

SELECTING THE QUESTIONS
The questions in *Clinical Evidence* concern the benefits and harms of preventative and therapeutic interventions, with emphasis on outcomes that matter to patients. Questions are selected for their relevance to clinical practice by section advisors and contributors, in collaboration with primary care clinicians and patient groups. Each new issue of *Clinical Evidence* will include new questions as well as updates of existing questions. Readers can suggest new clinical questions using the feedback slips to be found at the back of the book and on the *Clinical Evidence* website (www.clinicalevidence.org), or by writing directly to *Clinical Evidence*.

SEARCHING AND APPRAISING THE LITERATURE
For each question, the literature is searched using the Cochrane Library, Medline, Embase and, occasionally, other electronic databases, looking first for good systematic reviews of RCTs; then for good RCTs published since the search date of the review. Where we find no good recent systematic reviews, we search for individual RCTs. The date of the search is recorded in the methods section for each topic. Of the studies that are identified in the search, we select and summarise only a small proportion. The selection is done by critically appraising the abstracts of the studies identified in the search, a task performed independently by two information scientists using validated criteria similar to those of Sackett, et al[1] and Jadad.[2,3] Where the search identifies more than one or two good reviews or trials, we select those we judge to be the most robust or relevant, using the full text of the article. Where we identify few or no good reviews or trials, we include other studies but highlight their limitations. Contributors, who are chosen for their expertise in the field and their skills in epidemiology, are asked to review our selection of studies, and to justify any additions or exclusions they wish to make.

Our search strategy and critical appraisal criteria are available on our website (www.clinicalevidence.org).

SUMMARISING THE EVIDENCE, PEER REVIEW, AND EDITING
The contributors summarise the evidence relating to each question. Each topic is then peer reviewed by the section advisors, and by at least three external expert clinicians. The revised text is then extensively edited by editors with clinical and epidemiological training, and data are checked against the original study reports.

REFERENCES
1. Sackett DL, Haynes RB, Guyatt GH, Tugwell P. *Clinical Epidemiology: A basic science for clinical medicine.* 2nd ed. Boston: Little Brown, 1991.
2. Jadad A. Assessing the quality of RCTs: Why, what, how and by whom? In: Jadad A. *Randomised Controlled Trials.* London: BMJ Books, 1998:45–60.
3. Jadad AR, Moore RA, Carroll D, Jenkinson C, et al. Assessing the quality of reports of randomized clinical trials: is blinding necessary? *Control Clin Trials* 1996;17:1–12.

Feedback and Error Correction

Despite the extensive peer review and quality checks, we expect that the text will contain some errors and inconsistencies. Please let us know if you find any errors, either by using the comment card at the back of the book or by emailing us at CEfeedback@bmjgroup.com.

Errors are graded as minor, moderate, and major based on an assessment of their potential impact. All errors are corrected in the next printed issue of *Clinical Evidence*. Anything other than a minor error is immediately corrected in the text displayed on our website (http://www.clinicalevidence.org) and a list of errors corrected is available there. Any major errors are highlighted on the log in page of the website.

If you wish to be notified automatically by e-mail of any corrections and updates, then register for the *Clinical Evidence* alerting service on our website. If you are using the information in *Clinical Evidence* to guide your clinical practice then it is essential to register so that you can be remain as up to date as possible. Typographical errors in Issue 4 are listed below.

TABLE	Issue 4 typographical errors and corrections.		
Topic	**Page**	**Error**	**Correction**
Obesity	328	Dexfenfluramine, fenfluramine, and fenfluramine plus phentermine are incorrectly labelled as *Likely to be beneficial.*	The correct categorisation is *Likely to be ineffective or harmful*. The rest of the text to support the categorisation is correct.
Opportunistic infections and HIV	411	Clofazimine of high dose clarithromycin (for MAC in people with previous MAC), and Valaciclovir (CMV) are incorrectly labelled as *Likely to be beneficial.*	The correct categorisation is *Likely to be ineffective or harmful*. The rest of the text to support the categorisation is correct.

Absolute risk (AR) This is the probability that an individual will experience the specified outcome during a specified period. It lies in the range 0 to 1, or is expressed as a percentage. In contrast to common usage, the word "risk" may refer to adverse events (such as myocardial infarction), or desirable events (such as cure).

Absolute risk reduction (ARR) The absolute difference in risk between the experimental and control groups in a trial. It is used when the risk in the control group exceeds the risk in the experimental group, and is calculated by subtracting the AR in the experimental group from the AR in the control group. This figure does not give any idea of the proportional reduction between the two groups; for this, relative risk reduction (RRR) is needed (see below).

Absolute risk increase (ARI) The absolute difference in risk between the experimental and control groups in a trial. It is used when the risk in the experimental group exceeds the risk in the control group, and is calculated by subtracting the AR in the control group from the AR in the experimental group. This figure does not give any idea of the proportional increase between the two groups; for this, relative risk increase (RRI) is needed (see below).

Bias Systematic deviation of study results from the true results, due to the way(s) in which the study is conducted.

Case control study A study design that examines a group of people who have experienced an event (usually an adverse event) and a group of people who have not experienced the same event, and looks at how exposure to suspect (usually noxious) agents differed between the two groups. This type of study design is most useful for trying to ascertain the cause of rare events, such as rare cancers.

Clinically significant A finding that is clinically important. Here, "significant" takes its everyday meaning of "important" (compared with statistically significant, see below). Where the word "significant" or "significance" is used without qualification in the text, it is being used in its statistical sense.

Cohort study A non-experimental study design that follows a group of people (a cohort), and then looks at how events differ among people within the group. A study that examines a cohort, who differ in respect to exposure to some suspected risk factor (e.g. smoking), is useful for trying to ascertain whether exposure is likely to cause specified events (e.g. lung cancer). Prospective cohort studies (which track participants forward in time) are more reliable than retrospective cohort studies.

Completer analysis Analysis of data from only those participants who remained at the end of the study. Compare with intention to treat analysis, which uses data from all participants who enrolled (see below).

Confidence interval (CI) The 95% confidence interval (or 95% confidence limits) would include 95% of results from studies of the same size and design in the same population. This is close but not identical to saying that the true size of the effect (never exactly known) has a 95% chance of falling within the confidence interval. If the 95% confidence interval for a relative risk or an odds ratio crosses 1, then this is taken as no evidence of an effect. The practical advantages of a confidence interval (rather than a P value) is that they present the range of likely effects.

Controls in a randomised controlled trial refer to the participants in its comparison group. They are allocated either to placebo, no treatment, or a standard treatment.

Crossover randomised trial A trial in which participants receive one treatment and have outcomes measured, and then receive an alternative treatment and have outcomes measured again. The order of treatments is randomly assigned. Sometimes a period of no treatment is used before the trial starts and in between the treatments (washout periods) to minimise interference between the treatments (carry over effects). Interpretation of the results from crossover RCTs can be complex.

Cross sectional study A study design that involves surveying a population about an exposure, or condition, or both, at one point in time. It can be used for assessing prevalence of a condition in the population.

Effect size Many methods are used to quantify the size of an effect. For dichotomous outcomes, relative risk and odds ratio are examples. Typically, the term effect size is used for continuous variables (such as pain scores or height), where the standardised mean difference or weighted mean difference (see below) are commonly used.

Event The occurrence of a dichotomous outcome that is being sought in the study (such as myocardial infarction, death, or a four point improvement in pain score).

Experimental study A study in which the investigator studies the effect of intentionally altering one or more factors under controlled conditions.

False negative A person with the target condition (defined by the gold standard) who has a negative test result.

False positive A person without the target condition (defined by the gold standard) who has a positive test result.

Hazard ratio (HR) This is broadly equivalent to relative risk, but is useful when the risk is not constant with respect to time. It uses information collected at different times. The term is typically used in the context of survival over time. If the hazard ratio is 0.5 then the relative risk of dying in one group is half the risk of dying in the other group.

Heterogeneity In the context of meta-analysis, heterogeneity means dissimilarity between studies. It can be due to use of different statistical methods (statistical heterogeneity), or evaluation of people with different characteristics, treatments or outcomes (clinical heterogeneity). Heterogeneity may render pooling of data in meta-analysis unreliable or inappropriate.

Homogeneity Similarity (see heterogeneity).

Incidence The number of new cases of a condition occurring in a population over a specified period of time.

Intention to treat analysis Analysis of data for all participants based on the group to which they were randomised and not based on the actual treatment they received.

Likelihood ratio The ratio of the probability that an individual with the target condition has a specified test result to the probability that an individual without the target condition has the same specified test result.

Meta-analysis A statistical technique that summarises the results of several studies in a single weighted estimate, in which more weight is given to results of studies with more events and somethines to studies of higher quality.

Morbidity Rate of illness but not death.

Mortality Rate of death.

Negative likelihood ratio (LR–) The ratio of the probability that an individual with the target condition has a negative test result to the probability that an individual without the target condition has a negative test result. This is the same as the ratio of number of the false negatives to the number of true negatives, and the same as the ratio (1-sensitivity/specificity).

Negative predictive value (NPV) The chance of not having a disease given a negative test result (not to be confused with specificity, which is the other way round; see below)

NS See Not significant.

Not significant/Non-significant (NS) In *Clinical Evidence*, not significant means that the observed difference, or a larger difference, could have arisen by chance with a probability of more than one in 20 (i.e. 5%), assuming that there is no underlying difference. This is not the same as saying there is no effect, just that this experiment does not provide convincing evidence of an effect. This could be because the trial was not powered to detect an effect that does exist, because there was no effect, or because of the play of chance.

Number needed to harm (NNH) One measure of treatment harm. It is the number of people you would need to treat with a specific intervention for a given period of time to cause one additional adverse outcome. NNH can be calculated as 1/ARI. In *Clinical Evidence*, these are usually rounded downwards.

Number needed to treat (NNT) One measure of treatment effectiveness. It is the number of people you would need to treat with a specific intervention for a given period of time to prevent one additional adverse outcome or achieve one additional beneficial outcome. NNT can be calculated as 1/ARR (see appendix 2). In *Clinical Evidence*, NNTs are usually rounded upwards.

Odds The odds of an event happening is defined as the probability that an event will occur, expressed as a proportion of the probability that the event will not occur.

Odds ratio (OR) One measure of treatment effectiveness. It is the odds of an event happening in the experimental group, expressed as a proportion of the odds of an event happening in the control group. The closer the OR is to one, the smaller the difference in effect between the experimental intervention and the control intervention. If the OR is greater (or less) than one, then the effects of the treatment are more (or less) than those of the control treatment. Note that the effects being measured may be adverse (e.g. death or disability) or desirable (e.g. survival). When events are rare, the OR is analagous to the relative risk (RR), but as event rates increase, the OR and RR diverge.

Odds reduction The complement of odds ratio (1-OR), similar to the relative risk reduction (RRR) when events are rare.

P value The probability that an observed difference, or a greater difference occurred by chance, if it is assumed that there is in fact no real difference between the effects of the interventions. If this probability is less than 1 in 20 (which is when the P value is less than 0.05), then the result is conventionally regarded as being "statistically significant".

Placebo A substance given in the control group of a clinical trial, which is ideally identical in appearance and taste or feel to the experimental treatment and without any disease specific effects. The term is sometimes applied in the context of non-pharmacological interventions.

Positive likelihood ratio (LR+) The ratio of the probability that an individual with the target condition has a positive test result to the probability that an individual without the target condition has a positive test result. This is the same as the ratio of number of the false negatives to the number of true negatives, and the same as the ratio (1-sensitivity/specificity).

Positive predictive value (PPV) The chance of having a disease given a positive test result (not to be confused with sensitivity, which is the other way round; see below).

Power A study has adequate power if it can reliably detect a clinically important difference (i.e. between two treatments) if one actually exists. The power of a study is increased when it includes more events or when its measurement of outcomes is more precise.

Pragmatic study An RCT designed to provide results that are directly applicable to normal practice (compared with explanatory trials that are intended to clarify efficacy under ideal conditions). Pragmatic RCTs recruit a population that is representative of those who are normally treated, allow normal compliance with instructions (by avoiding incentives and by using oral instructions with advice to follow manufacturers instructions), and analyse results by "intention to treat" rather than by "on treatment" methods.

Prevalence The proportion of people with a finding or disease in a given population at a given time.

Publication bias is when a likelihood of a study being published varies with the results it finds. Usually, this occurs when studies that find a significant effect are more likely to be published than studies that do not find a significant effect, so making it appear from surveys of the published literature that treatments are more effective than is truly the case.

Randomised controlled trial (RCT) Typically a trial in which participants are randomly assigned to two groups: one (the experimental group) receiving the intervention that is being tested, and the other (the comparison or control group) receiving an alternative treatment or placebo. This design allows assessment of the relative effects of interventions. Sometimes, RCTs have more than one experimental group.

Regression analysis Given data on a dependent variable and one or more independent variables, regression analysis involves finding the "best" mathematical model to describe or predict the dependent variable as a function of the independent variable(s). There are several regression models that suit different needs. Common forms are linear, logistic, and proportional hazards.

Relative risk (RR) The number of times more likely (RR greater than 1) or less likely (RR less than 1) an event is likely to happen in one group compared with another. It is the ratio of the absolute risk for each group. It is analogous to the odds ratio (OR) when events are rare.

Relative risk increase (RRI) The proportional increase in risk between experimental and control participants in a trial.

Relative risk reduction (RRR) The proportional reduction in risk between experimental and control participants in a trial. It is the complement of the relative risk (1-RR).

Sensitivity The chance of having a positive test result given that you have a disease (not to be confused with positive predictive value [PPV], which is the other way around; see above).

Significant By convention taken to mean statistically significant at the 5% level (see statistically significant). This is the same as a 95% confidence interval not including the value corresponding to no effect.

Specificity The chance of having a negative test result given that you do not have a disease (not to be confused with negative predictive value [NPV], which is the other way around; see above).

Standardised mean difference (SMD) A measure of effect size used when outcomes are continuous (such as height, weight, or symptom scores) rather than dichotomous (such as death or myocardial infarction). The mean differences in outcome between the groups being studied are standardised to account for differences in scoring methods (such as pain scores). The measure is a ratio, and therefore has no units.

Statistically significant means that the findings of a study are unlikely to be due to chance. Significance at the commonly cited 5% level ($P < 0.05$) means that the observed difference or greater difference would occur by chance in only one in 20 similar studies. Where the word "significant" or "significance" is used without qualification in the text, it is being used in this statistical sense.

Systematic review A review in which specified and appropriate methods have been used to identify, appraise, and summarise studies addressing a defined question. It can, but need not, involve meta-analysis. In *Clinical Evidence*, the term systematic review refers to a systematic review of RCTs unless specified otherwise.

True negative A person without the target condition (defined by the gold standard) who has a negative test result.

True positive A person with the target condition (defined by the gold standard) who also has a positive test result.

Validity The soundness or rigour of a study. A study is internally valid if the way it is designed and carried out means that the results are unbiased and give you an accurate estimate of the effect that is being measured. A study is externally valid if its results are applicable to people encountered in regular clinical practice.

Weighted mean difference (WMD) A measure of effect size used when outcomes are continuous (such as symptom scores or height) rather than dichotomous (such as death or myocardial infarction). The mean differences in outcome between the groups being studied are weighted to account for different sample sizes and differing precision between studies. The WMD is an absolute figure, and so takes the units of the original outcome measure.

Search date January 2001: new for this issue

Gregory YH Lip and Sridhar Kamath

QUESTIONS

INTERVENTIONS

Likely to be beneficial

**To be covered in future issues of
Clinical Evidence**
DC cardioversion
Class Ia antiarrhythmic drugs
(quinidine, procainamide,
disopyramide)
Class Ic antiarrhythmic drugs
(flecainide, propafenone)
Class III antiarrhythmic drugs
(amiodarone, sotalol, ibutilide,
dofeltilide)
Effects of antithrombotic therapy
Acute atrial fibrillation following
cardiac surgery

Key Messages

- We found little direct evidence from RCTs that included people solely with acute atrial fibrillation. Most of the available evidence is extrapolated from RCTs that include people with other types of atrial fibrillation.
- We found limited evidence from two small RCTs that β blockers increase the chance of returning to sinus rhythm compared with verapamil.
- We found three small RCTs of rate limiting calcium antagonists versus placebo. One RCT found that verapamil was much less effective than amiodarone at restoring sinus rhythm.
- Three RCTs have found good evidence that digoxin is no better than placebo at restoring sinus rhythm in people with acute atrial fibrillation, but digoxin lowered the ventricular rate in the short term more than placebo.

Acute atrial fibrillation

DEFINITION Acute atrial fibrillation refers to the sudden onset of rapid, irregular and chaotic atrial activity, and the 48 hours after that onset. It includes both the first symptomatic onset of persistent atrial fibrillation and episodes of paroxysmal atrial fibrillation. It is sometimes difficult to distinguish episodes of new onset atrial fibrillation from newly diagnosed atrial fibrillation. Atrial fibrillation within 72 hours of onset is sometimes called recent onset atrial fibrillation. In this review, we have excluded episodes of atrial fibrillation that arise during or soon after cardiac surgery.

INCIDENCE/ PREVALENCE We found limited evidence of the incidence or prevalence of acute atrial fibrillation. Extrapolation from the Framingham study[1] suggests an incidence in men of 3 per 1000 person years at age 55 years, rising to 38 per 1000 person years at 94 years. In women, the incidence was 2 per 1000 person years at age 55 years, and 32.5 per 1000 person years at 94 years. The prevalence of atrial fibrillation ranged from 0.5% for people aged 50–59 years to 8.8% in people aged 80–89 years. Among acute emergency medical admissions in the UK, 3–6% have atrial fibrillation, and about 40% were newly diagnosed.[2,3] Among acute hospital admissions in New Zealand, 10.4% (95% CI 8.6% to 11.5%) had documented atrial fibrillation.[4]

AETIOLOGY/ RISK FACTORS Paroxysms of atrial fibrillation are more common in athletes.[5] Age increases the risk of developing acute atrial fibrillation. Men are more likely to develop atrial fibrillation than women (38 year follow up from the Framingham Study, RR after adjustment for age and known predisposing conditions 1.5).[6] Atrial fibrillation can occur in association with underlying disease (both cardiac and non-cardiac) or can arise in the absence of any other condition. Epidemiological surveys have found that risk factors for the development of acute atrial fibrillation include ischaemic heart disease, hypertension, heart failure, valve disease, diabetes, alcohol abuse, thyroid disorders, and disorders of the lung and pleura.[1] In a UK survey of acute hospital admissions with atrial fibrillation, a history of ischaemic heart disease was present in 33%, heart failure in 24%, hypertension in 26%, and rheumatic heart disease in 7%.[3] In some populations, the acute effects of alcohol explain a large proportion of the incidence of acute atrial fibrillation.

PROGNOSIS We found no evidence about the proportion of people with acute atrial fibrillation who develop more chronic forms of atrial fibrillation (e.g. paroxysmal, persistent, or permanent atrial fibrillation). Observational studies and placebo arms of RCTs have found that over 50% of people with acute atrial fibrillation revert spontaneously within 24–48 hours, especially atrial fibrillation associated with an identifiable precipitant such as alcohol or myocardial infarction. We found little evidence about the effects on mortality and morbidity of acute atrial fibrillation where no underlying cause is found. Acute atrial fibrillation during myocardial infarction is an independent predictor of both short term and long term mortality.[7] Onset of atrial fibrillation reduces cardiac output by 10–20% irrespective of the underlying ventricular rate[8,9] and can contribute to heart failure. People with acute atrial fibrillation who present with heart failure have worse prognosis. Acute atrial fibrillation is associated with a risk of imminent stroke.[10–13] One case series used trans-oesophageal echocardiography in people who had developed acute atrial fibrillation within the preceding 48 hours; it found that 15% had atrial thrombi.[14] An ischaemic stroke associated with atrial fibrillation is more likely to be fatal, have a recurrence, and leave a serious functional deficit among survivors, than a stroke not associated with atrial fibrillation.[15]

AIMS To reduce symptoms, morbidity and mortality, with minimum adverse effects.

OUTCOMES Major outcomes include measures of symptoms, recurrent stroke or transient ischaemic attack, thromboembolism, death, and major bleeding. Proxy measures include heart rhythm, ventricular rate, timing to restoration of sinus rhythm. Frequent spontaneous reversion to sinus rhythm makes it difficult to interpret short term studies of rhythm; treatments may accelerate restoration of sinus rhythm without increasing the proportion of people who eventually convert. The clinical importance of changes in mean heart rate is also unclear.

METHODS *Clinical Evidence* search and appraisal January 2001. Current Contents, textbooks, review articles and recent abstracts were reviewed. Many studies were not solely in people with acute atrial fibrillation. The text indicates where results have been extrapolated from studies of paroxysmal, persistent, or permanent atrial fibrillation. Atrial fibrillation that follows coronary surgery has been excluded.

QUESTION **What are the effects of treatments for acute atrial fibrillation?**

OPTION **β BLOCKERS**

One small RCT found that timolol versus placebo reduced ventricular rate. A small comparative RCT found that esmolol versus verapamil increased the chance of returning to sinus rhythm.

Benefits: We found no systematic review. **Versus placebo:** We found one RCT (61 people with atrial fibrillation of unspecified duration, ventricular rate > 120/minute), which compared intravenous timolol (1 mg) versus intravenous placebo given immediately and repeated twice at 20 minute intervals if sinus rhythm was not achieved.[16] It found that 20 minutes after the last injection, intravenous timolol versus placebo significantly increased the proportion of people who had a ventricular rate below 100 a minute (41% with timolol *v* 3% with placebo; P < 0.01), and increased the proportion of people who converted to sinus rhythm, although the increase was not significant (5/29 [17%] *v* 2/32 [6%], P = 0.18). **Versus verapamil:** We found one RCT (31 people with onset of atrial fibrillation or atrial flutter [see glossary, p 6] within the previous 48 hours), which found that esmolol versus verapamil increased the proportion of people who returned to sinus rhythm (50% *v* 12%; P < 0.03) but had no significant effect on the final ventricular rate (100/minute with esmolol *v* 98/minute with verapamil).[17]

Harms: β Blockers may exacerbate heart failure and hypotension in acute atrial fibrillation. β Blockers plus rate limiting calcium channel blockers (diltiazem, verapamil) may increase the risk of asystole and sinus arrest.[18–20] β Blockers can precipitate bronchospasm.[21] In the RCT, both esmolol and verapamil were associated with mild hypotension.

Comment: Esmolol is a rapidly acting intravenous β blocker. In addition to the evidence from people with acute atrial fibrillation, we found one systematic review of β blockers versus placebo in people with either acute or chronic atrial fibrillation.[22] It found that in seven of 12 comparisons at rest and in all during exercise, β blockers reduced ventricular rate compared with placebo. We found no RCTs that reported quality of life, functional capacity, or mortality.

OPTION	RATE LIMITING CALCIUM CHANNEL ANTAGONISTS (VERAPAMIL AND DILTIAZEM)

We found three small RCTs of rate limiting calcium antagonists versus placebo. One RCT found that verapamil was much less effective than amiodarone at restoring sinus rhythm.

Benefits: We found no systematic review in people with acute atrial fibrillation. **Versus placebo:** We found three RCTs.[23–25] The first RCT (21 men with atrial fibrillation and a rapid ventricular rate, age 37–70 years) was a crossover comparison of intravenous verapamil versus saline.[23] It found that intravenous verapamil versus saline reduced ventricular rate within 10 minutes (reduction > 15% of the initial rate: 17/20 [85%] with verapamil v 2/14 [14%] with saline). It also found that three people converted to sinus rhythm, but it is not clear from the results whether these effects can be attributed to verapamil or saline. The second RCT (double blind crossover study of 20 people with atrial fibrillation or atrial flutter [see glossary, p 6] for 2 hours to 2 years) compared intravenous low dose verapamil versus placebo.[24] A positive response was defined as conversion to sinus rhythm or a decrease of the ventricular response to less than 100 a minute, or by more than 20% of the initial rate. If a positive response did not occur within 10 minutes, then a second bolus injection was given (placebo for people who initially received verapamil, verapamil for people who initially received placebo). The response rate was not significantly different between low dose verapamil and placebo arms. With the first bolus injection, verapamil versus placebo significantly reduced ventricular rate (mean heart rate 118/minute with verapamil arm v 138/minute with placebo), and more people converted to sinus rhythm within 30 minutes but the difference was not significant (3/20 with verapamil v 0/15 with placebo, P = 0.12). The third RCT (113 people with either acute or chronic atrial fibrillation or flutter, mean age 64, 83% male, ventricular rate > 120/minute) found that intravenous diltiazem versus placebo significantly improved the proportion of people who achieved the combined outcome of conversion to sinus rhythm or ventricular rate less than 100 a minute or ventricular rate reduced by more than 20% of the initial rate (93% v 12%, P < 0.001).[25] **Versus amiodarone:** We found one RCT (24 consecutive people with acute paroxysms of atrial fibrillation lasting 20 minutes to 48 hours, 15 male, mean age 71 years, mean ventricular rate 125/minute) of intravenous verapamil versus intravenous amiodarone.[26] It found that amiodarone converted more people to sinus rhythm than verapamil in the 3 hours after the injection (77% with amiodarone v 0% with verapamil; P < 0.001). **Versus digoxin:** We found one RCT (30 consecutive people, 10 male, mean age 72 years, 26 with acute atrial fibrillation, 4 with atrial flutter, unspecified duration) comparing intravenous diltiazem versus intravenous digoxin versus both.[27] It found significant reductions of ventricular rate by diltiazem within 5 minutes, and by digoxin only after 3 hours. No additional benefit was found with the combination of digoxin and diltiazem. **Versus other calcium channel blockers:** We found no systematic reviews or large RCTs. We found one double blind crossover RCT (7 people with acute atrial fibrillation and 2 with atrial flutter),[28] which compared intravenous diltiazem versus verapamil, and found no significant differences in rate control or measures of systolic function.

Harms: Rate limiting calcium antagonists may exacerbate heart failure and hypotension. In people with Wolff Parkinson White syndrome (see glossary, p 6), verapamil may increase the ventricular rate and can cause ventricular arrhythmias.[29]

Comment: The evidence suggests that rate limiting calcium channel blockers such as verapamil and diltiazem reduce ventricular rate in acute or recent onset atrial fibrillation, but they are probably no better than placebo in restoring sinus rhythm. We found no studies of the effect of rate limiting calcium channel blockers on exercise tolerance in people with acute or recent onset atrial fibrillation, but studies in people with chronic atrial fibrillation have found improved exercise tolerance.

OPTION	DIGOXIN

Three RCTs have found that digoxin is no better than placebo at restoring sinus rhythm in people with acute atrial fibrillation, but digoxin lowered the ventricular rate in the short term more than placebo.

Benefits: **Versus placebo:** We found no systematic review of digoxin for acute atrial fibrillation but found three RCTs.[30–32] The first RCT (239 people with atrial fibrillation within 7 days of onset, mean age 66 years, mean ventricular rate 122/minute)[30] found that intravenous digoxin (mean 0.88 mg) versus placebo did not increase the restoration of sinus rhythm by 16 hours (51% with digoxin v 46% with placebo). It found a rapid and clinically important reduction in ventricular rate at 2 hours (to 105/minute with digoxin v 117/minute with placebo; P = 0.0001). Similar findings were reported in two smaller RCTs.[31,32] One RCT (40 people within 7 days of the onset of atrial fibrillation, mean age 64 years, 23 male) compared high dose intravenous digoxin (1.25 mg) versus placebo. Restoration to sinus rhythm was not significantly different (9/19 [47%] with digoxin v 8/20 [40%] with placebo, P = 0.6). The ventricular rate after 30 minutes was significantly lower compared with placebo (P < 0.02).[31] The second RCT (36 people within 7 days of the onset of atrial fibrillation) compared oral digoxin versus placebo.

Acute atrial fibrillation

Conversion to sinus rhythm by 18 hours was not significantly different (50% with digoxin v 44% with placebo; ARR +6%, 95% CI −11% to +22%).[32]

Harms: Digoxin at toxic doses may result in visual, gastrointestinal and neurological symptoms, heart block, and arrhythmias.

Comment: The peak action of digoxin is delayed, taking 6–12 hours to reduce mean ventricular rate below 100 a minute. We found one systematic review and RCTs of digoxin versus placebo in people with chronic atrial fibrillation, which found that control of the ventricular rate control during exercise was poor unless a β blocker or rate limiting calcium antagonist (verapamil or diltiazem) was used in combination.[22,33,34] The evidence suggests that digoxin is no better than placebo at restoring sinus rhythm in people with recent onset atrial fibrillation.

GLOSSARY

Atrial flutter A similar arrhythmia to atrial fibrillation but the atrial electrical activity is less chaotic and has a characteristic saw tooth appearance on an electrocardiogram.

Wolff Parkinson White syndrome Occurs when an additional electrical pathway exists between the atria and the ventricles as a result of anomalous embryonic development. The extra pathway may cause rapid arrhythmias. Worldwide it affects about 0.2% of the general population. In people with Wolff Parkinson White syndrome, β blockers, calcium channel blockers, and digoxin can increase the ventricular rate and cause ventricular arrhthmias.

REFERENCES

1. Benjamin EJ, Wolf PA, Kannel WA. The epidemiology of atrial fibrillation. In: Falk RH, Podrid P, eds. *Atrial fibrillation: mechanisms and management.* 2nd ed. Philadelphia; Lippincott-Raven Publishers, 1997:1–22.

2. Lip GYH, Tean KN, Dunn FG. Treatment of atrial fibrillation in a district general hospital. *Br Heart J* 1994;71:92–95.

3. Zarifis J, Beevers DG, Lip GYH. Acute admissions with atrial fibrillation in a British multiracial hospital population. *Br J Clin Pract* 1997;51:91–96.

4. Stewart FM, Singh Y, Persson S, Gamble GD, Braatvedt GD. Atrial fibrillation: prevalence and management in an acute general unit. *Aust N Z J Med* 1999;29:51–58.

5. Furlanello F, Bertoldi A, Dallago M, et al. Atrial fibrillation in elite athletes. *J Cardiovasc Electrophysiol* 1998;9(8 suppl):63–68.

6. Kannel WB, Wolf PA, Benjamin EJ, Levy D. Prevalence, incidence, prognosis, and predisposing conditions for atrial fibrillation: population-based estimates. *Am J Cardiol* 1998; 82:2N–9N.

7. Pedersen OD, Bagger H, Kober L, Torp-Pedersen C. The occurrence and prognostic significance of atrial fibrillation/flutter following acute myocardial infarction. TRACE Study group. TRAndolapril Cardiac Evalution. *Eur Heart J* 1999;20:748–754.

8. Clark DM, Plumb VJ, Epstein AE, Kay GN. Hemodynamic effects of an irregular sequence of ventricular cycle lengths during atrial fibrillation. *J Am Coll Cardiol* 1997;30:1039–1045.

9. Schumacher B, Luderitz B. Rate issues in atrial fibrillation: consequences of tachycardia and therapy for rate control. *Am J Cardiol* 1998;82: 29N–36N.

10. Peterson P, Godfredson J. Embolic complications in paroxysmal atrial fibrillation. *Stroke* 1986;17: 622–626.

11. Sherman DG, Goldman L, Whiting RB, Jurgensen K, Kaste M, Easton JD. Thromboembolism in patients with atrial fibrillation. *Arch Neurol* 1984; 41:708–710.

12. Wolf PA, Kannel WB, McGee DL, Meeks SL, Bharucha NE, McNamara PM. Duration of atrial fibrillation and imminence of stroke: the Framingham study. *Stroke* 1983;14:664–667.

13. Corbalan R, Arriagada D, Braun S, et al. Risk factors for systemic embolism in patients with paroxysmal atrial fibrillation. *Am Heart J* 1992; 124:149–153.

14. Stoddard ME, Dawkins PR, Prince CR, Ammash NM. Left atrial appendage thrombus is not uncommon in patients with acute atrial fibrillation and a recent embolic event: a transesophageal echocardiographic study. *J Am Coll Cardiol* 1995; 25:452–459.

15. Lin HJ, Wolf PA, Kelly-Hayes M, et al. Stroke severity in atrial fibrillation. The Framingham Study. *Stroke* 1996;27:1760–1764.

16. Sweany AE, Moncloa F, Vickers FF, Zupkis RV, Rahway NJ. Antiarrhythmic effects of intravenous timolol in supraventricular arrhythmias. *Clin Pharmacol Ther* 1985;37:124–127.

17. Platia EV, Michelson EL, Porterfield JK, Das G. Esmolol versus verapamil in the acute treatment of atrial fibrillation or atrial flutter. *Am J Cardiol* 1989;63:925–929.

18. Lee TH, Salomon DR, Rayment CM, Antman EM. Hypotension and sinus arrest with exercise-induced hyperkalemia and combined verapamil/propranolol therapy. *Am J Med* 1986;80:1203–1204.

19. Misra M, Thakur R, Bhandari K. Sinus arrest caused by atenolol-verapamil combination. *Clin Cardiol* 1987;10:365–367.
20. Yeh SJ, Yamamoto T, Lin FC, Wang CC, Wu D. Repetitive sinoatrial exit block as the major mechanism of drug-provoked long sinus or atrial pause. *J Am Coll Cardiol* 1991;18:587–595.
21. Doshan HD, Rosenthal RR, Brown R, Slutsky A, Applin WJ, Caruso FS. Celiprolol, atenolol and propranolol: a comparison of pulmonary effects in asthmatic patients. *J Cardiovasc Pharmacol* 1986; 8(suppl 4):105–108.
22. Segal JB, McNamara RL, Miller MR, et al. The evidence regarding the drugs used for ventricular rate control. *J Fam Pract* 2000;49:47–59.
23. Aronow WS, Ferlinz J. Verapamil versus placebo in atrial fibrillation and atrial flutter. *Clin Invest Med* 1980;3:35–39.
24. Waxman HL, Myerburg RJ, Appel R, Sung RJ. Verapamil for control of ventricular rate in paroxysmal supraventricular tachycardia and atrial fibrillation or flutter: a double-blind randomized cross-over study. *Ann Intern Med* 1981;94:1–6
25. Salerno DM, Dias VC, Kleiger RE, et al. Efficacy and safety of intravenous diltiazem for treatment of atrial fibrillation and atrial flutter: the Diltiazem-Atrial Fibrillation/Flutter Study Group. *Am J Cardiol* 1989;63:1046–1051.
26. Noc M, Stajer D, Horvat M. Intravenous amiodarone versus verapamil for acute conversion of paroxysmal atrial fibrillation to sinus rhythm. *Am J Cardiol* 1990;65:679–680.
27. Schreck DM, Rivera AR, Tricarico VJ. Emergency management of atrial fibrillation and flutter: intravenous diltiazem versus intravenous digoxin *Ann Emerg Med* 1997;29:135–140.
28. Phillips BG, Gandhi AJ, Sanoski CA, Just VL, Bauman JL. Comparison of intravenous diltiazem and verapamil for the acute treatment of atrial fibrillation and atrial flutter. *Pharmacotherapy* 1997;17:1238–1245.
29. Strasberg B, Sagie A, Rechavia E, et al. Deleterious effects of intravenous verapamil in Wolff-Parkinson-White patients and atrial fibrillation. *Cardiovasc Drugs Ther* 1989;2:801–806.
30. DAAF trial group. Intravenous digoxin in acute atrial fibrillation. Results of a randomized, placebo-controlled multicentre trial in 239 patients. The Digitalis in Acute AF (DAAF) Trial Group. *Eur Heart J* 1997;18:649–654.
31. Jordaens L, Trouerbach J, Calle P, et al. Conversion of atrial fibrillation to sinus rhythm and rate control by digoxin in comparison to placebo. *Eur Heart J* 1997;18:643–648.
32. Falk RH, Knowlton AA, Bernard SA, Gotlieb NE, Battinelli NJ. Digoxin for converting recent-onset atrial fibrillation to sinus rhythm. *Ann Intern Med* 1987;106:503–506.
33. Farshi R, Kistner D, Sarma JS, Longmate JA, Singh BN. Ventricular rate control in chronic atrial fibrillation during daily activity and programmed exercise: a crossover open-label study of five drug regimens. *J Am Coll Cardiol* 1999;33:304–310.
34. Klein HO, Pauzner H, Di Segni E, David D, Kaplinsky E. The beneficial effects of verapamil in chronic atrial fibrillation. *Arch Intern Med* 1979; 139:747–749.

Gregory YH Lip

Sridhar Kamath

Haemostasis Thrombosis
and Vascular Biology Unit
University Department of Medicine
City Hospital
Birmingham
UK

Competing interests: GL is UK principal investigator for the ERAFT Trial (Knoll) and has been reimbursed by various pharmaceutical companies for attending several conferences, and running educational programmes and research projects. SK, none declared.

Acute myocardial infarction

Search date November 2000

Shamir Mehta

QUESTIONS

INTERVENTIONS

Key Messages

- Good evidence from systematic reviews supports the following interventions in people presenting with symptoms of acute myocardial infarction:
  - Aspirin (at least 160 mg chewed and swallowed immediately and continued daily for at least a few years and perhaps lifelong).
  - Thrombolytic treatment (streptokinase ± intravenous/subcutaneous heparin or tissue plasminogen activator [tPA] + intravenous heparin) in people with ST elevation on their presenting electrocardiogram (ECG).
  - β Blocker (started intravenously within hours of infarction and continued orally for several years) in people without contraindications.
  - Angiotensin converting enzyme (ACE) inhibitor (started within 24 hours of infarction and continued daily) for about a month in people at low risk of death, and for several months in people with heart failure at any time during hospital admission or with a left ventricular ejection fraction less than 40%.
  - Nitrates (shown to be safe for symptomatic relief in this setting, but to have at most a modest effect on mortality).
  - In high risk people who present early (< 4 hours after onset of symptoms) and have ST elevation, primary percutaneous transluminal coronary angioplasty (PTCA) is more effective than thrombolytic treatment, provided it can be performed quickly (< 90 minutes after hospital arrival) by an experienced operator and staff in a high volume centre.
- Systematic reviews have found no evidence of mortality benefit from calcium channel blockers during or after acute myocardial infarction; there is potential for increased mortality in people with heart failure.

© *Clinical Evidence* 2001;5:8–23.

DEFINITION	Acute myocardial infarction (AMI) is the sudden occlusion of a coronary artery leading to myocardial death.
INCIDENCE/ PREVALENCE	AMI is one of the most common causes of mortality in both developed and developing nations. In 1990, ischaemic heart disease was the leading cause of death worldwide, accounting for about 6.3 million deaths. The age standardised incidence varies among and within countries.[1] Each year, about 900 000 people in the USA experience an AMI, and about 225 000 of them die. About half of these people die within 1 hour of symptoms and before reaching a hospital emergency room.[2] Event rates increase with age for both sexes and are higher in men than women, and in poorer than richer people at all ages. The incidence of death from AMI has fallen in many Western countries over the past 20 years.
AETIOLOGY/ RISK FACTORS	The immediate mechanism of AMI is rupture of an atheromatous plaque causing thrombosis and occlusion of coronary arteries and myocardial death. Factors that may convert a stable plaque into an unstable plaque (the "active plaque") have yet to be fully elucidated; however, shear stresses, inflammation, and autoimmunity have been proposed. The changing rates of coronary heart disease in different populations are only partly explained by changes in the standard risk factors for ischaemic heart disease (particularly fall in blood pressure and smoking).
PROGNOSIS	AMI may lead to a host of mechanical and electrical complications, including death, ventricular dysfunction, congestive heart failure, cardiogenic shock, fatal and non-fatal arrhythmia, valvular dysfunction, or myocardial rupture.
AIMS	To relieve pain; to restore blood supply to heart muscle; to reduce incidence of complications (such as congestive heart failure, myocardial rupture, valvular dysfunction, fatal and non-fatal arrhythmia); to prevent recurrent ischaemia and infarction; and to decrease mortality.
OUTCOMES	**Efficacy outcomes:** Rates of major cardiovascular events, including death, recurrent AMI, refractory ischaemia, and stroke. **Safety outcomes:** Rates of major bleeding and intracranial haemorrhage.
METHODS	*Clinical Evidence* update search and appraisal November 2000.

QUESTION   Which treatments improve outcomes in acute myocardial infarction?

OPTION   ASPIRIN

One systematic review of RCTs has found that, in people with AMI, aspirin reduces mortality (one life saved per 40 people treated during the acute phase), reinfarction (one fewer non-fatal reinfarction per 100 people treated), and stroke (one fewer non-fatal stroke per 300 people treated). The evidence suggests an optimal dose of aspirin of 160–325 mg acutely, followed by long term treatment with at least 75 mg/day indefinitely.

Benefits: **Aspirin versus placebo:** We found one systematic review (search date 1990, 9 RCTs, 18 773 people), which compared antiplatelet agents versus placebo soon after the onset of AMI and for a period of at least 1 month afterwards.[3] The absolute and relative benefits found in the systematic review are shown in figure 1, p 22. The largest of the RCTs (17 187 people with suspected AMI) compared placebo versus aspirin (162.6 mg) chewed and swallowed on the day of AMI and continued daily for 1 month.[4] In subsequent long term follow up, the mortality benefit was maintained for up to 4 years.[5] In the systematic review, the most widely tested aspirin regimens were 75–325 mg/day.[3] Doses throughout this range seemed similarly effective, with no evidence that "higher" doses were more effective (500–1500 mg/day: odds reduction compared with placebo 21%, 95% CI 14% to 27%) than "medium" doses (160–325 mg/day: odds reduction 28%, 95% CI 22% to 33%) or "lower" doses (75–160 mg/day: odds reduction 26%, 95% CI 5% to 42%). There was insufficient evidence for efficacy of doses below 75 mg/day. One study found that administering a loading dose of 160–325 mg/day achieved a prompt antiplatelet effect.[6]

Harms: In the largest trial, there was no significant increase in rates of cerebral haemorrhage or bleeds requiring transfusion (0.4% on aspirin and placebo).[4] There was a small absolute excess of "minor" bleeding (ARI 0.6%, 95% CI not available, P < 0.01).

Comment: None.

OPTION	THROMBOLYSIS

Systematic reviews of RCTs have found that prompt thrombolytic treatment (within 6 hours and perhaps up to 12 hours and longer after the onset of symptoms) reduces mortality in people with AMI and ST elevation or bundle branch block on their presenting ECG. Fifty six people would need treatment in the acute phase to prevent one additional death. Strokes, intracranial haemorrhage, and major bleeds are more common in people given thrombolysis; with one additional stroke for every 250 people treated and one additional major bleed for every 143 people treated. The reviews have found that intracranial haemorrhage is more common in people of advanced age and low body weight, those with hypertension on admission, and those given tPA rather than another thrombolytic agent.

Benefits: **Versus placebo:** We found one overview (9 large RCTs, 58 600 people with suspected AMI) comparing thrombolysis versus placebo.[7] Baseline ECGs showed ST segment elevation in 68% of people, and ST segment depression, T wave abnormalities, or no abnormality in the rest. Thrombolysis versus placebo reduced short term mortality (9.6% with thrombolysis v 11.5% with placebo; ARR 1.9%; RR 0.82, 95% CI 0.77 to 0.87; NNT 56). Greatest benefit was found in the large group of people presenting with ST elevation (RR 0.79) or bundle branch block (RR 0.75). Reduced rates of death were seen in people with all types of infarct, but the benefit was several times greater in those with anterior infarction (ARR 3.7%) compared with those with inferior infarction (ARR 0.8%) or infarctions in other zones (ARR 2.7%). Long term follow up of one of the RCTs found that the benefit of thrombolysis versus placebo on mortality persists at 12 years (36/107 [34%] dead with thrombolysis v 55/112 [49%] with placebo; ARR 15%, 95% CI 2.4% to 29%;

RR 0.69, 95% CI 0.49 to 0.95; NNT 7).[8] **Timing of treatment:** The earlier systematic review found that the thrombolytic treatment was given, the greater the absolute benefit (see figure 2, p 23). For each hour of delay, the absolute risk reduction for death decreased by 0.16% (ARR for death if given within 6 hours of symptoms 3%; ARR for death if given 7–12 hours after onset of symptoms 2%).[9] Too few people in the systematic review received treatment more than 12 hours after the onset of symptoms to determine whether the benefits of thrombolytic treatment given after 12 hours would outweigh the risks. Extrapolation of the data (see figure 2, p 23) suggests that, at least for people with ST elevation, there may be some net benefit of treatment between 12 and 18 hours after symptom onset (ARR for death 1%). **Streptokinase versus tPA:** We found one non-systematic review[9] (3 large RCTs, see table 1, p 20[10–12]), comparing streptokinase versus tPA. The first RCT was unblinded and in people with ST elevation and symptoms of AMI for less than 6 hours. Participants were first randomised to intravenous tPA 100 mg over 3 hours or streptokinase 1.5 MU over 1 hour, and then further randomised to subcutaneous heparin 12 500 U twice daily beginning 12 hours later, or no heparin. It found heparin added no significant benefit (AR of death in hospital 8.5% v 8.9% on no heparin; RRR 0.05, 95% CI –0.04 to +0.14).[10] In the second RCT, people with suspected AMI presenting within 24 hours of symptoms were randomised to receive either streptokinase 1.5 MU over 1 hour, tPA 0.6 MU/kg every 4 hours, or anisoylated plasminogen streptokinase activator complex (APSAC) 30 U/3 minutes, and then further randomised to subcutaneous heparin 12 500 U starting at 7 hours and continued for 7 days, or no heparin. All received aspirin on admission. At 35 days, mortality was similar among the three regimens (streptokinase 10.6%, APSAC 10.5%, tPA 10.3%), and the addition of heparin provided no significant benefit (AR of death 10.3% v 10.6% on no heparin).[11] The third RCT was unblinded and in people with ST segment elevation presenting within 6 hours of symptom onset. Participants were randomised to one of four regimens: streptokinase 1.5 MU over 1 hour plus subcutaneous heparin 12 500 U twice daily starting 4 hours after thrombolytic treatment; streptokinase 1.5 MU over 1 hour plus intravenous heparin 5000 U bolus followed by 1000 U/hour; accelerated tPA 15 mg bolus then 0.75 mg/kg over 30 minutes followed by 0.50 mg/kg over 60 minutes, plus intravenous heparin 5000 U bolus then 1000 U/hour; or tPA 1.0 mg/kg over 60 minutes, 10% given as a bolus, plus streptokinase 1.0 MU over 60 minutes.[12] Meta-analysis of the three trials, weighted by sample size, found no significant difference in the combined outcome of any stroke or death (ARs 9.4% for streptokinase only regimens v 9.2% for tPA based regimens, including the combined tPA and streptokinase arm in the third trial; ARR for tPA v streptokinase 0.2%, 95% CI –0.2% to +0.5%; RRR 2.1%).[9] **Comparison of other thrombolytic agents:** These comparisons will be considered in a future issue of *Clinical Evidence*.

Harms: **Stroke/intracerebral haemorrhage:** The risk of stroke was increased by thrombolytic treatment given in the acute phase (ARI compared with placebo 0.4%, 95% CI 0.2% to 0.5%; NNH 250).[7] In the third trial comparing different thrombolytic treatments, the overall incidence of intracerebral haemorrhage was 0.7% and of stroke 1.4%, of which 31% were severely disabling and 50% were intracerebral haemorrhages. The risk of haemorrhagic stroke was higher with tPA (AR 0.72%) than with streptokinase and subcutaneous heparin (AR 0.49%) or with streptokinase and intravenous heparin (AR 0.54%, P = 0.03 for tPA compared with combined streptokinase arms).[12] **Predictive factors for stroke/intracranial haemorrhage:** Multivariate analysis of data from a large database of people who experienced intracerebral haemorrhage after thrombolytic treatment identified four independent predictors of increased risk of intracerebral haemorrhage: age ≥65 years (OR 2.2, 95% CI 1.4 to 3.5), weight < 70 kg (OR 2.1, 95% CI 1.3 to 3.2), hypertension on admission (OR 2.0, 95% CI 1.2 to 3.2), and use of tPA rather than another thrombolytic agent (OR 1.6, 95% CI 1.0 to 2.5). Absolute risk of intracranial haemorrhage was 0.26% on streptokinase in the absence of risk factors, and 0.96%, 1.32%, and 2.17% in people with one, two, or three risk factors.[13] Analysis of 592 strokes in 41 021 people from the trials found seven factors to be predictors of intracerebral haemorrhage: advanced age, lower weight, history of cerebrovascular disease, history of hypertension, higher systolic or diastolic pressure on presentation, and use of tPA rather than streptokinase.[14,15] **Major bleeding:** The risk of major bleeding was increased by thrombolytic treatment given in the acute phase (ARI compared with placebo 0.7%; 95% CI 0.6% to 0.9%; NNH 143).[7] Bleeding was most common in people undergoing procedures (coronary artery bypass grafting or PTCA). Spontaneous bleeds were observed most often in the gastrointestinal tract.[12]

Comment: The evidence suggests that it is far more important to administer prompt thrombolytic treatment than to debate which thrombolytic agent should be used. A strategy of rapid use of any thrombolytic in a broad population is likely to lead to the greatest impact on mortality. When the results of RCTs are taken together, tPA based regimens do not seem to confer a significant advantage in the combined outcome of any stroke and death (unrelated to stroke) over streptokinase. The legitimacy of combining the results of the three trials can be questioned, as the selection criteria and protocols differed in important aspects (see review for arguments to justify combining the results of these trials despite their apparent differences).[9]

OPTION   β BLOCKERS

Systematic reviews of RCTs have found that oral β blockers given within hours of infarction reduce both mortality and reinfarction in people with AMI. Adding β blockers to thrombolytic treatment confers additional benefit. Most benefit is obtained from long term use of β blockers.

Benefits: **Given within hours of infarction:** We found three systematic reviews (search date 1997,[16] search date not stated,[17] search date 1987[18]) of early use of β blockers. The older reviews identified 27 RCTs and found that, within 1 week of treatment, β blockers significantly reduced the risk of death and major vascular events (RR for the combined outcome of death, non-fatal cardiac arrest, or non-fatal reinfarction 0.84, 1110 events v 1298 events, 95% CI not available, P < 0.001). The largest of the RCTs (16 027 people with AMI) compared intravenous atenolol 5–10 mg given immediately followed by 100 mg orally given daily for 7 days versus standard treatment (no β blocker).[19] After 7 days, atenolol reduced vascular mortality compared with control (3.9% with atenolol v 4.6% with control; ARR 0.7%; RR 0.85, 95% CI 0.73 to 0.88; NNT 147). The RCT found more benefit in people with ECG evidence of AMI at entry (in people with ECG suggesting anterior infarction, inferior infarction, both, or bundle branch block, AR of death 5.33% on atenolol, 6.49% for controls; ARR 1.16%; NNT 86, 95% CI not available). People older than 65 years and those with large infarcts had the most benefit.[19] The recent systematic review (search date 1997, 82 RCTs, 54 234 people)[16] separately analysed 51 short term RCTs (up to 6 weeks after the onset of pain) and 31 long term RCTs. Most of the RCTs did not include thrombolysis. In the short term studies seven RCTs reported no deaths, and many reported only a few. Meta-analysis of the RCTs that reported at least one death found that β blockers versus placebo reduced mortality, but the reduction was not significant in the short term (ARR 0.4%, OR 0.96, 95% CI 0.85 to 1.08). In the longer term RCTs, β blockers versus placebo significantly reduced mortality over 6 months to 4 years (OR 0.77, 95% CI 0.69 to 0.85). About 84 people would need treatment for 1 year to avoid one death. No significant difference in effectiveness was found between different types of β blocker (based on cardioselectivity or intrinsic sympathomimetic activity). Most evidence was obtained with propranolol, timolol, and metoprolol. **In people receiving thrombolytic treatment:** We found one RCT (1434 people with AMI), which compared early versus delayed metoprolol in people who had been given thrombolysis (tPA).[20] Early treatment began on day 1 (intravenous then oral) and delayed treatment on day 6 (oral). At 6 days, people receiving early treatment had significantly lower rates of reinfarction (AR 2.7% early v 5.1% delayed, 95% CI not available, P = 0.02) and recurrent chest pain (AR 18.8% v 24.1%, P < 0.02). There were no early (6 days) or late (1 year) differences observed in mortality or left ventricular ejection fraction between the two groups. **Long term use:** See β blockers under secondary prevention of ischaemic cardiac events, p 95.

Harms: People with asthma or severe congestive cardiac failure were excluded from most trials. Many of the early trials tended to enrol people at low risk of death soon after AMI. In people given immediate rather than delayed β blockers following tPA, there was a non-significantly increased frequency of heart failure during the initial admission to hospital (15.3% v 12.2%, P = 0.10).[20] The presence of first degree heart block and bundle branch block was associated with an increased frequency of adverse events.

Comment: β Blockers may reduce rates of cardiac rupture and ventricular fibrillation. This may explain why people older than 65 years and those with large infarcts benefited most, as they also have higher rates of these complications. The trials were mostly conducted in the prethrombolytic era. The trial comparing early versus delayed β blockade following thrombolysis was too small to rule out an effect on mortality of β blockers when added to thrombolysis.[20]

Acute myocardial infarction

OPTION	ANGIOTENSIN CONVERTING ENZYME (ACE) INHIBITORS

One systematic review of four large RCTs has found that ACE inhibitors used within 24 hours of onset of symptoms reduce mortality in people with AMI. The question of whether ACE inhibitors should be offered to everyone presenting with AMI or only to people with signs of heart failure remains unresolved.

Benefits: **In all people after an AMI:** We found one overview[21] and one systematic review[22] of ACE inhibitors versus placebo after myocardial infarction. The overview (4 large RCTs, 98 496 people) compared ACE inhibitors versus placebo given to all people irrespective of clinical heart failure or left ventricular dysfunction, within 36 hours of the onset of symptoms of AMI.[21] After 30 days, ACE inhibitors versus placebo reduced mortality (7.1% with ACE inhibitors v 7.6% with placebo; RR 0.93, 95% CI 0.89 to 0.98; NNT 200). Most of this benefit was in the first 7 days after AMI. The absolute benefit was larger in some high risk groups: people in Killip class 2–3 (clinically moderate to severe heart failure at first presentation; RR 0.91; NNT 71, 99% CI 36 to 10 000), people with heart rates > 100 beats/minute at entry (RR 0.86; NNT 44, 99% CI 25 to 185), and people with an anterior AMI (RR 0.87; NNT 94, 99% CI 56 to 303). ACE inhibitors also reduced the incidence of non-fatal cardiac failure (AR 14.6% v 15.2%, 95% CI not available; P = 0.01). The second systematic review (search date 1997, 15 RCTs, 15 104 people) found similar results.[22] **In selected people after an AMI:** A selective strategy was tested in three trials.[23–25] Treatment was restricted to people with clinical heart failure, objective evidence of left ventricular dysfunction, or both, and was started a few days after AMI (about 6000 people). These trials found consistently that long term treatment with ACE inhibitors in this selected population was associated with a significant reduction in mortality and reinfarction (RRRs from one trial:[21] for cardiovascular death 21%, 95% CI 5% to 35%; for development of severe heart failure 37%, 95% CI 20% to 50%; for congestive heart failure requiring admission to hospital 22%, 95% CI 4% to 37%; and for recurrent AMI 25%, 95% CI 5% to 40%).

Harms: The systematic review found an excess of persistent hypotension (AR 17.6% v 9.3%, 95% CI for difference not available; P < 0.01) and renal dysfunction (AR 1.3% v 0.6%; P < 0.01) in people given ACE inhibitors.[21] The relative and absolute risks of these adverse effects were uniformly distributed across both the high and lower cardiovascular risk groups.

Comment: The largest benefits of ACE inhibitors in AMI are seen when treatment is started within 24 hours. The evidence does not answer the question of which people with an AMI should be offered ACE inhibitors, and for how long after AMI it remains beneficial to start treatment with an ACE inhibitor. We found one systematic review (based on individual data from about 100 000 people in RCTs of ACE inhibitors), which found that people receiving both aspirin and ACE inhibitors had the same relative risk reduction as those receiving ACE inhibitors alone (i.e. there was no evidence of a clinically relevant interaction between ACE inhibitors and aspirin).[26]

OPTION	NITRATES

RCTs performed before and during the thrombolytic era have found that intravenous nitrates are safe in the acute management of symptoms in people with AMI, but may reduce mortality only slightly.

Benefits: **Without thrombolysis:** We found one systematic review (search date not stated, 10 RCTs comparing intravenous nitroglycerine or nitroprusside v placebo, 2000 people with AMI).[27] The trials were all conducted in the prethrombolytic era. Nitrates reduced the relative risk of death by 35% (95% CI 16% to 55%). The observed benefit of nitrates seemed to be mostly during the acute hospitalisation period, with modest or little long term survival benefit. **With aspirin/ thrombolysis:** During the thrombolytic era, two large RCTs compared nitrates given acutely versus placebo in 58 050 and 17 817 people with AMI (90% received aspirin and about 70% received thrombolytic treatment).[28,29] In one RCT, people received oral controlled release mononitrate 30–60 mg/day.[28] In the other RCT, people received intravenous nitroglycerine for 24 hours followed by transdermal nitroglycerine 10 mg daily.[29] Neither trial found a significant improvement in survival, either in the total sample or in subgroups of people at different risk of death. Nitrates were a useful adjunctive treatment to help control symptoms in people with AMI.

Harms: The systematic review and the large trials found no significant harm associated with routine use of nitrates in people with AMI.[27–29]

Comment: The two large trials had features that may have caused them to not find a benefit even if one exists: a large proportion of people took nitrates outside the study; there was a high rate of concurrent use of other hypotensive agents; people were relatively low risk; and nitrates were not titrated to blood pressure and heart rate.[28,29]

OPTION	CALCIUM CHANNEL BLOCKERS

RCTs have found that calcium channel blockers given to people within the first few days of an AMI do not reduce deaths, and may increase deaths in people with reduced left ventricular function.

Benefits: **Dihydropyridine calcium channel blockers:** We found one non-systematic review (search date not stated, 2 large RCTs)[30] comparing short acting nifedipine versus placebo in people treated within the first few days of AMI.[31,32] Neither found evidence of benefit and both found trends towards increased mortality on nifedipine. One trial was terminated prematurely because of lack of efficacy. It found a 33% increase in mortality on nifedipine that did not reach significance.[32] We found insufficient data on sustained release nifedipine, amlodipine, or felodipine in this setting. **Verapamil:** We found one systematic review, (search date 1997, 7 RCTs, 6527 people),[33] which found that verapamil versus placebo in acute myocardial infarction had no significant effect on mortality (RR 0.86, 95% CI 0.71 to 1.04).

Harms: Two systematic reviews of trials of any kind of calcium channel blockers in people with AMI found a non-significant increase in mortality of about 4% and 6%.[34,35] One trial in 2466 people with

AMI compared diltiazem 60 mg orally four times daily started 3–15 days after AMI versus placebo.[36] Overall there was no effect on total mortality or reinfarction between the two groups, but subgroup analysis found a 41% increase in death or reinfarction in people with congestive heart failure (RRI 1.41, 95% CI 1.01 to 1.96).

Comment: None.

OPTION   PRIMARY PERCUTANEOUS TRANSLUMINAL CORONARY ANGIOPLASTY (PTCA) VERSUS THROMBOLYSIS

One systematic review of RCTs has found that, in the short term, primary PTCA is at least as effective as (and possibly superior to) thrombolysis in the treatment of AMI, in terms of reducing mortality, reinfarction, and haemorrhagic stroke. However, the trials were conducted mainly in high volume, specialist centres. The effectiveness of PTCA compared with thrombolysis in less specialist centres remains to be defined.

Benefits: We found two systematic reviews[37,38] of primary PTCA v primary thrombolysis in people with AMI. **Death and reinfarction:** The first systematic review (search date 1996, 10 RCTs, 2606 people) found that primary PTCA versus primary thrombolysis reduced mortality at 30 days after intervention (4.4% for primary PTCA v 6.5% for primary thrombolysis; ARR 2.1%; OR 0.66, 95% CI 0.46 to 0.94; NNT 48).[37] The effect was similar regardless of which thrombolysis regimen was used. There was significant reduction in the combined end point of death and reinfarction with PTCA (OR 0.58, 95% CI 0.44 to 0.76). The largest single RCT (1138 people, ST elevation on ECG, within 12 hours of symptom onset) found less favourable results. It compared primary PTCA versus accelerated tPA.[39] At 30 days, there was no significant difference in mortality between the two groups (AR 5.7% v 7.0%), but primary PTCA significantly reduced the primary end point of death, non-fatal AMI, or non-fatal disabling stroke (AR 9.6% v 13.7% on tPA; OR 0.67, 95% CI 0.47 to 0.97). This effect was substantially attenuated by 6 months. One of the included studies has reported long term follow up: it found that primary PTCA versus primary thrombolysis improves mortality over 5 years (25/194 [13%] with angioplasty v 48/201 [24%] with streptokinase; RR 0.54, 95% CI 0.36 to 0.87).[40] The second systematic review (search date 1998, 10 RCTs, 2573 people) found overall similar results, with significant reductions in mortality and in reinfarction.[38]

Harms: **Stroke:** The review found that PTCA was associated with a significant reduction in the risk of all types of stroke (AR 0.7% v 2.0%) and haemorrhagic stroke (AR 0.1% v 1.1%).[36] In the largest trial, the collective rate of haemorrhagic stroke in people given thrombolysis was 1.1%, substantially higher than that observed in trials comparing thrombolysis with placebo.[39] This may have been because the trials summarised above were in older people and used tPA. However, the lower rates of haemorrhagic stroke with primary PTCA were consistent across almost all trials, and this may be the major advantage of PTCA over thrombolysis.

Comment: Although collectively the trials found an overall short term reduction in deaths with PTCA compared with thrombolysis, there were several pitfalls common to individual trials, most of which may have inflated the benefit of PTCA.[41] Trials comparing PTCA with thrombolysis could not be easily blinded, and ascertainment of end points that required some judgement, such as reinfarction or stroke, may have been influenced by the investigators' knowledge of the treatment allocation (only one trial had a blinded adjudication events committee). Also, people allocated to PTCA were discharged 1–2 days earlier than those allocated to thrombolysis, which favoured PTCA by reducing the time for detection of in hospital events. In addition, the trials conducted before the largest trial[39] should be viewed as hypothesis generating, in that the composite outcome (death, reinfarction, and stroke) was not prospectively defined, and attention was only placed on these end points after there seemed to be some benefit on post hoc analysis. The results are also based on short term outcomes only and do not provide information on collective long term benefit. For example, in the largest trial, the composite end point was significant at 30 days, but with a wide degree of uncertainty, and this was substantially attenuated to a non-significant difference by 6 months.[39] The lower mortality and reinfarction rates reported with primary PTCA are promising but not conclusive, and the real benefits may well be smaller. Only in a minority of centres that perform a high volume of PTCA, and in the hands of experienced interventionalists, may primary PTCA be clearly superior to thrombolytic treatment. Elsewhere, primary PTCA may be of greatest benefit in people with contraindications to thrombolysis, in people in cardiogenic shock, or in people where the mortality reduction with thrombolysis is modest and the risk of intracranial haemorrhage is increased, for example, elderly people.[42] The value of PTCA over thrombolysis in people presenting to hospital more than 12 hours after onset of chest pain remains to be tested.

Substantive changes since last issue

Thrombolysis Long term follow up of one RCT of thrombolysis versus placebo;[8] conclusion unchanged.

ACE inhibitors New systematic review;[26] found no interaction between ACE inhibitors and aspirin.

REFERENCES

1. Murray C, Lopez A. Mortality by cause for eight regions of the world: global burden of disease study. *Lancet* 1997;349:1269–1276.

2. National Heart, Lung, and Blood Institute. *Morbidity and mortality: chartbook on cardiovascular, lung, and blood diseases.* Bethesda, Maryland: US Department of Health and Human Services, Public Health Service, National Institutes of Health; May 1992.

3. Antiplatelet Trialists' Collaboration. Collaborative overview of randomised trials of antiplatelet therapy I: prevention of death, myocardial infarction, and stroke by prolonged antiplatelet therapy in various categories of people. *BMJ* 1994;308:81–106. Search date March 1990; primary sources Medline, Current Contents.

4. Second International Study of Infarct Survival (ISIS-2) Collaborative Group. Randomized trial of intravenous streptokinase, oral aspirin, both or

neither among 17–187 cases of suspected acute myocardial infarction. *Lancet* 1988;ii:349–360.

5. Baigent BM, Collins R. ISIS-2: four year mortality of 17187 patients after fibrinolytic and antiplatelet therapy in suspected acute myocardial infarction study [abstract]. *Circulation* 1993;(suppl I):I-291.

6. Patrignani P, Filabozzi P, Patrono C. Selective cumulative inhibition of platelet thromboxane production by low-dose aspirin in healthy subjects. *J Clin Invest* 1982;69:1366–1372.

7. Fibrinolytic Therapy Trialists' (FTT) Collaborative Group. Indications for fibrinolytic therapy in suspected acute myocardial infarction: collaborative overview of early mortality and major morbidity results of all randomized trials of more than 1000 patients. *Lancet* 1994;343:311–322.

8. French JK, Hyde TA, Patel H, et al. Survival 12 years after randomization to streptokinase: the influence of thrombolysis in myocardial infarction

flow at three to four weeks. *J Am Coll Cardiol* 1999;34:62–69.

9. Collins R, Peto R, Baigent BM, Sleight DM. Aspirin, heparin and fibrinolytic therapy in suspected acute myocardial infarction. *N Engl J Med* 1997;336:847–860.

10. Gruppo Italiano per lo studio della streptochinasi nell'infarto miocardico (GISSI). GISSI-2: a factorial randomised trial of alteplase versus streptokinase and heparin versus no heparin among 12–490 patients with acute myocardial infarction. *Lancet* 1990;336:65–71.

11. Third International Study of Infarct Survival (ISIS-3) Collaborative Group. ISIS-3: a randomised comparison of streptokinase vs tissue plasminogen activator vs anistreplase and of aspirin plus heparin vs aspirin alone among 41–299 cases of suspected acute myocardial infarction. *Lancet* 1992;339:753–770.

12. The GUSTO Investigators. An international randomized trial comparing four thrombolytic strategies for acute myocardial infarction. *N Engl J Med* 1993;329:673–682.

13. Simoons MI, Maggioni AP, Knatterud G, et al. Individual risk assessment for intracranial hemorrhage during thrombolytic therapy. *Lancet* 1993;342:523–528.

14. Gore JM, Granger CB, Simoons MI, et al. Stroke after thrombolysis: mortality and functional outcomes in the GUSTO-1 trial. *Circulation* 1995; 92:2811–2818.

15. Berkowitz SD, Granger CB, Pieper KS, et al. Incidence and predictors of bleeding after contemporary thrombolytic therapy for myocardial infarction. *Circulation* 1997;95:2508–2516.

16. Freemantle N, Cleland J, Young P, Mason J, Harrison J. Beta blockade after myocardial infarction: systematic review and meta regression analysis. *BMJ* 1999;318:1730–1737. Search date 1997; primary sources Medline, Embase, Biosis, Healthstar, Sigle, IHTA, Derwent drug file, dissertation abstracts, Pascal, international pharmaceutical abstracts, science citation index, and handsearch of reference lists.

17. Yusuf S, Peto R, Lewis S, et al. Beta-blockade during and after myocardial infarction: an overview of the randomized trials. *Prog Cardiovasc Dis* 1985;27:355–371. Search date not stated; primary sources computer-aided search of the literature; manual search of reference lists; and enquiries to colleagues about relevant papers.

18. Sleight P for the ISIS Study Group. Beta blockade early in acute myocardial infarction. *Am J Cardiol* 1987;60:6A–12A.

19. First International Study of Infarct Survival (ISIS-1). Randomised trial of intravenous atenolol among 16–027 cases of suspected acute myocardial infarction. *Lancet* 1986;ii:57–66.

20. Roberts R, Rogers WJ, Mueller HS, et al. Immediate versus deferred beta-blockade following thrombolytic therapy in patients with acute myocardial infarction: results of the thrombolysis in myocardial infarction (TIMI) II-B study. *Circulation* 1991;83:422–437.

21. ACE inhibitor Myocardial Infarction Collaborative Group. Indications for ACE Inhibitors in the early treatment of acute myocardial infarction: systematic overview of individual data from 100 000 patients in randomised trials. *Circulation* 1998;97:2202–2212. Search date not stated; primary source collaboration group of principal investigators of all randomized trials who collated individual patient data.

22. Domanski MJ, Exner DV, Borkowf CB, Geller NL, Rosenberg Y, Pfeffer MA. Effect of angiotensin converting enzyme inhibition on sudden cardiac death in patients following acute myocardial infarction. A meta-analysis of randomized clinical trials. *J Am Coll Cardiol* 1999;33:598–604. Search date August 1997; primary sources Medline, and handsearches of reference lists.

23. Pfeffer MA, Braunwald E, Moye LA, et al. Effect of captopril on mortality and morbidity in patients with left ventricular dysfunction after myocardial infarction. *N Engl J Med* 1992;327:669–677.

24. The Acute Infarction Ramipril Efficacy (AIRE) Study Investigators. Effect of ramipril on mortality and morbidity of survivors of acute myocardial infarction with clinical evidence of heart failure. *Lancet* 1993;342:821–828.

25. The Trandolapril Cardiac Evaluation (TRACE) Study Group. A clinical trial of the angiotensin-converting-enzyme inhibitor trandolapril in patients with left ventricular dysfunction after myocardial infarction. *N Engl J Med* 1995;333:1670–1676.

26. Latini R, Tognoni G, Maggioni AP, et al. Clinical effects of early angiotensin-converting enzyme inhibitor treatment for acute myocardial infarction are similar in the presence and absence of aspirin. Systematic overciew of individual data from 96,712 randomized patients. *J Am Coll Cardiol* 2000;35:1801–1807. Search date not stated; primary sources individual patient data on all trials involving more than 1000 patients.

27. Yusuf S, Collins R, MacMahon S, Peto R. Effect of intravenous nitrates on mortality in acute myocardial infarction: an overview of the randomised trials. *Lancet* 1988;1:1088–1092. Search date not stated; primary sources literature, colleagues, investigators, and pharmaceutical companies.

28. Fourth International Study of Infarct Survival (ISIS-4) Collaborative Group. ISIS-4: a randomised factorial trial assessing early oral captopril, oral mononitrate, and intravenous magnesium sulphate in 58 050 patients with suspected acute myocardial infarction. *Lancet* 1995;345:669–685.

29. Gruppo Italiano per lo studio della streptochinasi nell'infarto miocardico (GISSI). GISSI-3: effects of lisinopril and transdermal glyceryl trinitrate singly and together on 6-week mortality and ventricular function after acute myocardial infarction. *Lancet* 1994;343:1115–1122.

30. Opie LH, Yusuf S, Kubler W. Current status of safety and efficacy of calcium channel blockers in cardiovascular diseases: a critical analysis based on 100 studies. *Prog Cardiovasc Dis* 2000;43: 171–196.

31. Wilcox RG, Hampton JR, Banks DC, et al. Early nifedipine in acute myocardial infarction: the TRENT study. *BMJ* 1986;293:1204–1208.

32. Goldbourt U, Behar S, Reicher-Reiss H, et al. Early administration of nifedipine in suspected acute myocardial infarction: the secondary prevention reinfarction Israel nifedipine trial 2 study. *Arch Intern Med* 1993;153:345–353.

33. Pepine CJ, Faich G, Makuch R. Verapamil use in patients with cardiovascular disease: an overview of randomized trials. *Clin Cardiol* 1998;21:633–641. Search date 1997; primary Medline, Science Citation Index, Current Contents, and handsearches of reference lists.

34. Yusuf S, Furberg CD. Effects of calcium channel blockers on survival after myocardial infarction. *Cardiovasc Drugs Ther* 1987;1:343–344. Search dates and primary sources not stated.

35. Teo KK, Yusuf S, Furberg CD. Effects of prophylactic antiarrhythmic drug therapy in acute myocardial infarction: an overview of results from randomized controlled trials. *JAMA* 1993;270: 1589–1595. Search date not stated; primary sources Medline and correspondence with investigators and pharmaceutical companies.

36. The Multicenter Diltiazem Post Infarction Trial Research Group. The effect of diltiazem on mortality and reinfarction after myocardial infarction. *N Engl J Med* 1988;319:385–392.
37. Weaver WD, Simes RJ, Betriu A, et al. Comparison of primary coronary angioplasty and intravenous thrombolytic therapy for acute myocardial infarction: a quantitative review. *JAMA* 1997;278: 2093–2098. Search date March 1996; primary sources Medline and scientific session abstracts of stated journals.
38. Cucherat M, Bonnefoy E, Tremeau G. Primary angioplasty versus intravenous thrombolysis for acute myocardial infarction. In: The Cochrane Library, Issue 1, 2001. Oxford: Update Software. Search date January 1998; primary sources The Cochrane Library, Medline, references from reviews, and experts.
39. The GUSTO IIb Angioplasty Substudy Investigators. A clinical trial comparing primary coronary angioplasty with tissue plasminogen activator for acute myocardial infarction. *N Engl J Med* 1997; 336:1621–1628.
40. Zijlstra F, Hoorntje JC, de Boer MJ, et al. Long-term benefit of primary angioplasty as compared with thrombolytic therapy for acute myocardial infarction. *N Engl J Med* 1999 341:1413–1419.
41. Yusuf S, Pogue J. Primary angioplasty compared to thrombolytic therapy for acute myocardial infarction [editorial]. *JAMA* 1997;278:2110–2111.
42. Van de Werf F, Topol EJ, Lee KL, et al. Variations in patient management and outcomes for acute myocardial infarction in the United States and other countries: results from the GUSTO trial. *JAMA* 1995;273:1586–1591.

Shamir Mehta
Assistant Professor of Medicine
Faculty of Health Sciences
McMaster University
Hamilton, Ontario
Canada

Competing interests: The author has received a fee for speaking at symposia.

TABLE 1 Direct randomised comparisons of the standard streptokinase regimen with various tPA based fibrinolytic regimens in patients with suspected AMI in the GISSI-2, ISIS-3, and GUSTO-1 trials (see text, p 11).[10-12]

Trial and treatment	Number of participants randomised	Any stroke Absolute number (%)	Any death Absolute number (%)	Death not related to stroke* Absolute number (%)	Stroke or death Absolute number (%)
GISSI-2†					
Streptokinase	10396	98 (0.9)	958 (9.2)	916 (8.8)	1014 (9.8)
t-PA	10372	136 (1.3)	993 (9.6)	931 (9.0)	1067 (10.3)
Effect/1000 people treated with t-PA instead of streptokinase		3.7 ± 1.5 more	3.6 ± 4.0 more	1.7 ± 4.0 more	5.3 ± 4.2 more
ISIS-3‡					
Streptokinase	13 780	141 (1.0)	1455 (10.6)	1389 (10.1)	1530 (11.1)
t-PA	13 746	188 (1.4)	1418 (10.3)	1325 (9.6)	1513 (11.0)
Effect/1000 people treated with t-PA instead of streptokinase		3.5 ± 1.3 more	2.4 ± 3.7 fewer	4.4 ± 3.6 fewer	1.0 ± 3.8 fewer
GUSTO-1§					
Streptokinase (subcutaneous heparin)	9841	117 (1.2)	712 (7.3)	666 (6.8)	783 (8.0)
Streptokinase (intravenous heparin)	10 410	144 (1.4)	763 (7.4)	709 (6.8)	853 (8.2)
t-PA alone	10 396	161 (1.6)	653 (6.3)	585 (5.6)	746 (7.2)
t-PA plus streptokinase	10 374	170 (1.6)	723 (7.0)	647 (6.2)	817 (7.9)
Effect/1000 people treated with t-PA-based regimens instead of streptinokinase		3.0 ± 1.2 more	6.6 ± 2.5 fewer	8.6 ± 2.4 fewer	5.5 ± 2.6 fewer

TABLE 1 continued

χ²/2 heterogeneity of effects between 3 trials	0.7	5.6	7.0	5.4
P value	0.3	0.06	0.03	0.07
Weighted average of all 3 trials¶				
Effect/1000 patient treated with t-PA-based regimens instead of streptokinase	3.3±0.8 more	2.9±1.9 fewer	4.9±1.8 fewer	1.6±1.9 fewer
P value	<0.001	>0.1	0.01	0.4

Values are numbers (%). This table should not be used to make direct non-randomised comparisons between the absolute event rates in different trials, because the patient populations may have differed substantially in age and other characteristics. Deaths recorded throughout the first 35 days are included for GISSI-2 and ISIS-3 and throughout the first 30 days for GUSTO-1. Numbers randomised and numbers with follow up are from the ISIS-3 report[11] and GUSTO-1[12] (supplemented with revised GUSTO-1 data from the National Auxiliary Publications Service), and numbers with events and the percentages (based on participants with follow up) are from the ISIS-3 report[11] and Van de Werf, et al.[42] Plus-minus values are ± SD. In all three trials, streptokinase was given in an intravenous infusions of 1.5 million units over a period of 1 hour.

*Death not related to stroke was defined as death without recorded stroke.

†In the GISSI-2 trial, the t-PA regimen involved an initial bolus of 10 mg, followed by 50 mg in the first hour and 20 mg in each of the second and third hours.

‡In the ISIS-3 trial, the t-PA regimen involved 40 000 clot-lysis units per kilogram of body weight as an initial bolus, followed by 360 000 units per kilogram in the first hour and 67 000 units per kilogram in each of the next 3 hours.

§In the GUSTO-1 trial, the t-PA alone regimen involved an initial bolus of 15 mg, followed by 0.75 mg per kilogram (up to 50 mg) in the first 30 minutes and 0.5 mg per kilogram (up to 35 mg) in the next hour; in the GUSTO-1 trial the other t-PA based regimen involved 0.1 mg of t-PA per kilogram (up to 9 mg) as an initial bolus and 0.9 mg per kilogram (up to 81 mg) in the remainder of the first hour, plus 1 million units of streptokinase in the first hour.

¶The weights are proportional to the sample sizes of the trials, so this average gives most weight to the GUSTO-1 trial and least to the GISSI-2 trials.[9]

Reproduced from Collins R, Peto R, Baigent BM, Sleight DM. Aspirin, heparin and fibrinolytic therapy in suspected AMI. *N Engl J Med* 1997;336:847–860, with permission of the publisher.

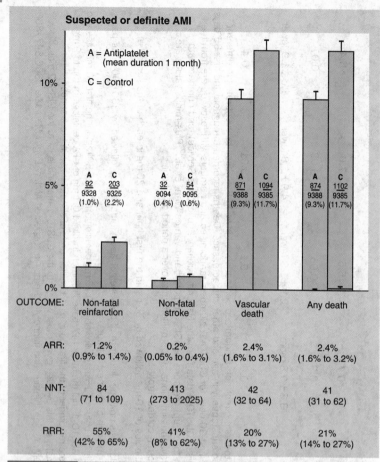

Suspected or definite AMI

A = Antiplatelet (mean duration 1 month)
C = Control

OUTCOME:	Non-fatal reinfarction	Non-fatal stroke	Vascular death	Any death
A	92 / 9328 (1.0%)	32 / 9094 (0.4%)	871 / 9388 (9.3%)	874 / 9388 (9.3%)
C	203 / 9325 (2.2%)	54 / 9095 (0.6%)	1094 / 9385 (11.7%)	1102 / 9385 (11.7%)
ARR:	1.2% (0.9% to 1.4%)	0.2% (0.05% to 0.4%)	2.4% (1.6% to 3.1%)	2.4% (1.6% to 3.2%)
NNT:	84 (71 to 109)	413 (273 to 2025)	42 (32 to 64)	41 (31 to 62)
RRR:	55% (42% to 65%)	41% (8% to 62%)	20% (13% to 27%)	21% (14% to 27%)

FIGURE 1 Absolute effects of antiplatelet treatment on various outcomes in people with a prior suspected or definite acute myocardial infarction.[3] The columns show the absolute risks over 1 month for each category; the error bars are the upper 95% confidence interval. In "any death" column non-vascular deaths are represented by lower horizontal lines. The table displays for each outcome the absolute risk reduction (ARR), the number of people needing treatment for 1 month to avoid one additional event (NNT), and the relative risk reduction (RRR), with their 95% CIs (see text, p 9). Published with permission.[3]

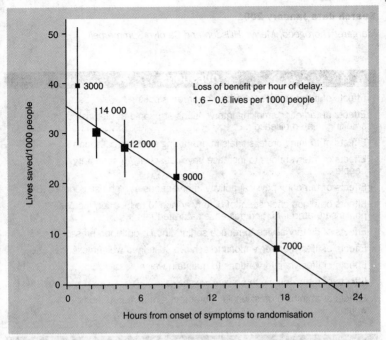

FIGURE 2 Absolute number of lives saved at 1 month per 1000 people receiving thrombolytic treatment plotted against the time from the onset of symptoms to randomisation among 45 000 people with ST segment elevation or bundle branch block.[7] Numbers along the curve are the number of people treated at different times (see text, p 11). Published with permission.[9]

Cardiovascular disorders

Search date January 2001

Margaret Thorogood, Melvyn Hillsdon and Carolyn Summerbell

© *Clinical Evidence* 2001;5:24–42.

Key Messages

Smoking

- Systematic reviews of RCTs have found that simple, one off, advice from a physician during a routine consultation is associated with 2% of smokers quitting smoking and not relapsing for 1 year. Additional encouragement or support may increase (by a further 3%) the effectiveness of the advice. Individual advice from a psychologist achieves a similar quit rate (3%), and advice from trained nurse counsellors, or from trained counsellors who are neither doctors nor nurses, increases quit rates compared with minimal intervention.

- One systematic review of RCTs and one subsequent RCT have found that nicotine replacement is an effective additional component of cessation strategies in smokers who smoke at least 10 cigarettes daily. We found no clear evidence that any method of delivery of nicotine is more effective than others. We found limited evidence from three RCTs with follow up of 2–6 years that the additional benefit of nicotine replacement therapy on quit rates reduces with time.

- One systematic review of RCTs found no evidence that acupuncture increased rates of smoking cessation at 12 months.

- One systematic review of RCTs found very limited evidence that exercise might increase smoking cessation.

- One systematic review of antidepressants used as part of a smoking cessation programme has found that buproprion increases quit rates. Moclobemide and anxiolytics did not significantly increase quit rates.

- Two systematic reviews have found that, in pregnant women, antismoking interventions increase abstinence rates and reduce the risk of low birthweight babies. Interventions without nicotine replacement were as effective as nicotine replacement in men and healthy non-pregnant women.

- One systematic review and two subsequent RCTs found that antismoking advice improves smoking cessation in people at higher risk of smoking related disease.

- One systematic review has found that training health professionals to give antismoking advice increases the frequency of antismoking interventions being offered, but found no good evidence that the effectiveness of the interventions is increased.

Physical activity and diet

- We found weak evidence from systematic reviews and subsequent RCTs that counselling sedentary people increases physical activity compared with no intervention. Limited evidence from RCTs suggests that consultation with an exercise specialist versus a physician may increase physical activity at 1 year.

- One RCT found that, in women over 80 years, exercise advice delivered in the home by physiotherapists increased physical activity and reduced their risk of falling.

- Systematic reviews have found that advice on cholesterol lowering diet (that is, advice to lower fat intake or increase the ratio of polyunsaturated to saturated fatty acid) leads to a small reduction in blood cholesterol concentrations in the long term (6 months or more).

- Systematic reviews and one RCT have found that salt restriction significantly reduces blood pressure in people with hypertension, and found limited evidence that salt restriction was effective in preventing hypertension. The RCT found limited evidence that advice on restricting salt intake was less effective than advice on weight reduction in preventing hypertension.

Changing behaviour

- Systematic reviews found that a combination of advice on diet and exercise supported by behaviour therapy was probably more effective than either diet or exercise advice alone in the treatment of obesity, and might lead to sustained weight loss.

DEFINITION	Cigarette smoking, diet, and level of physical activity are important in the aetiology of many chronic diseases. Individual change in behaviour has the potential to decrease the burden of chronic disease, particularly cardiovascular disease.
INCIDENCE/ PREVALENCE	In the developed world, the decline in smoking has slowed and the prevalence of regular smoking is increasing in young people. A sedentary lifestyle is becoming increasingly common and the prevalence of obesity is increasing rapidly.
AIMS	To encourage individuals to reduce or abandon unhealthy behaviours and to take up healthy behaviours; to support the maintenance of these changes in the long term.
OUTCOMES	Ideally the outcomes considered would be clinical, and would relate to the underlying conditions (longevity, quality of life, rate of stroke, or myocardial infarction). However, most studies report proxy outcomes, such as the proportion of people changing behaviour (e.g. stopping smoking) in a specified period.
METHODS	*Clinical Evidence* update search and appraisal January 2001.

QUESTION   Which interventions reduce cigarette smoking?

OPTION   COUNSELLING

Systematic reviews of RCTs have found that simple, one off advice from a physician during a routine consultation is associated with 2% of smokers quitting smoking and not relapsing for 1 year. Additional encouragement or support may increase (by a further 3%) the effectiveness of the advice. Individual advice from a psychologist achieves a similar quit rate (3%), and advice from trained nurse counsellors, or from trained counsellors who are neither doctors nor nurses, increases quit rates compared with minimal intervention.

Benefits:	We found four systematic reviews.[1–4] The first (search date not stated, 17 RCTs, 14 438 smokers) evaluated simple advice from physicians. The advice was typically of less than 5 minutes duration. It found that 1.9% of smokers (95% CI 0.1% to 2.8%) stopped smoking as a direct result of the advice and did not relapse for at least 1 year.[1] Rates of cessation in the control groups ranged from 1.1% to 14.1%, and in the intervention groups from 1.5% to 14.5%. The results were similar when the analysis was confined to the six trials in which cessation was confirmed by biochemical markers. Ten RCTs assessed the effect of additional support, such as additional visits and encouragement or demonstrations of exhaled carbon monoxide in the person's breath. There was a high degree of heterogeneity (with rates of cessation ranging from −0.5% to +29%), but the overall estimate of smokers quitting for 1 year was 5% (95% CI 1% to 8%). Five trials of individual sessions with a psychologist found that the number of smokers quitting at 1 year as

a result of advice was 2.8% (95% CI 1.3% to 4.2%). The second systematic review (search date 1998, 11 RCTs) of interventions provided by counsellors trained in smoking cessation (other than doctors and nurses) used a broad definition of counselling including all contacts with a smoker that lasted at least 10 minutes. Six of the RCTs had follow up for at least 1 year, whereas the rest had a minimum follow up of 6 months. The review found that counselling increased the rate of quitting (263/1381 [14%] quit with counselling v 194/1899 [10%] with control; OR of quitting 1.55, 95% CI 1.27 to 1.90).[2] The third review (search date 1999, 19 RCTs, 4 with follow up for < 1 year) considered the effectiveness of smoking interventions delivered by a nurse. It found that advice from a nurse increased the rate of quitting (621/4689 [13.2%] quit with advice v 402/3223 [12.5%] with control; OR 1.43, 95% CI 1.24 to 1.6).[3] The final systematic review (search date 1995) identified 23 trials of smoking advice in general practice.[4] In 20 of the trials, a general practitioner gave advice, although nurses or counsellors were also involved in four of these trials. In three trials, the advice was given solely by a nurse or health visitor. Smoking cessation was measured for between 6 months and 2 years. There was significant heterogeneity because of the inclusion of two trials (both involving only general practitioners) with notably larger effects. When these two trials were excluded, the review found that advice significantly increased the odds of smoking cessation (935/9361 [9.7%] quit with advice v 513/7952 [6.8%] with control; OR 1.32, 95% CI 1.18 to 1.48). The review found that (by indirect comparisons) intensive advice was more effective than brief advice (616/7651 [8%] quit with brief advice v 391/6486 [6%] with control; OR for quitting after brief advice 1.27, 95% CI 1.11 to 1.45; with intensive advice 319/2070 [15.4%] quit v 122/1106 [11.0%]; OR after intensive advice 1.46, 95% CI 1.18 to 1.80). Fifty smokers would need to be given brief advice (or 25 smokers given intensive advice) for one additional person to quit for at least 6 months.[4]

Harms: We found no evidence of harm.

Comment: The effects of advice may be considered disappointingly small, but a year on year reduction of 2% in the number of smokers would represent a significant public health gain (see smoking cessation under primary prevention, p 63).

OPTION NICOTINE REPLACEMENT

One systematic review and one subsequent RCT have found that nicotine replacement is an effective component of cessation strategies in smokers who smoke at least 10 cigarettes a day. Fifteen such smokers would have to be treated with nicotine replacement to produce one extra non-smoker at 12 months, but this overestimates effectiveness, because relapse will continue after 12 months. Higher dose (4 mg) gum is more effective than lower dose (2 mg) gum in very dependent smokers. We found no clear evidence that any one method of delivery of nicotine is more effective, or evidence of further benefit after 8 weeks' treatment with patches. Long term relapse may occur in people who quit, but the review found that the rate of relapse was not greater in those who quit with the aid of nicotine replacement. Abstinence after 1 week is a strong predictor of 12 month abstinence.

Changing behaviour

Benefits: **Abstinence at 12 months:** We found one systematic review and one subsequent RCT.[5,6] The systematic review (search date 2000) identified 48 trials of nicotine gum, 30 trials of nicotine transdermal patches, four of nicotine intranasal spray, four of inhaled nicotine, and two of sublingual tablet.[5] All forms of nicotine replacement were more effective than placebo. When the abstinence rates for all trials were pooled according to the longest duration of follow up available, the odds of abstinence were increased by 71% (95% CI 60% to 82%) with nicotine replacement compared with placebo. Seventeen per cent of smokers allocated to nicotine replacement successfully quit, compared with 10% in the control group. The review found no significant difference in benefit between different forms of nicotine replacement (OR for abstinence 1.63 for nicotine gum v 2.27 for nicotine nasal spray). In trials that directly compared 4 mg with 2 mg nicotine gum, the higher dose improved abstinence in highly dependent smokers (pooled OR of abstinence 2.67, 95% CI 1.69 to 4.22). Pooled analysis of six trials, which compared high dose versus standard dose patches, found that high dose may slightly increase abstinence (OR 1.21, 95% CI 1.03 to 1.42). The review found no evidence of a difference in effectiveness for 16 hour patches versus 24 hour patches, and no difference in effect in trials where the dose was tapered compared with those where the patches were withdrawn abruptly. Use of the patch for 8 weeks was as effective as longer use, and there was very weak evidence in favour of nicotine replacement in relapsed smokers. The subsequent RCT (3585 people) found that abstinence at 1 week was a strong predictor of 12 month abstinence (25% of those abstinent at 1 week were abstinent at 12 months v 2.7% of those not abstinent at 1 week).[6] One meta-analysis of relapse rates in nicotine replacement trials found that nicotine replacement increased abstinence at 12 months, but that the addition of nicotine replacement did not significantly affect relapse rates between 6 weeks and 12 months.[7]

Longer term abstinence: We found three RCTs,[8–10] which found that nicotine replacement does not affect long term abstinence. In one RCT, which compared nicotine spray versus placebo, 47 people abstinent at 1 year were followed for up to a further 2 years and 5 months, after which there was still a significant, although smaller, difference in abstinence (in longer term 15.4% abstinent with nicotine spray v 9.3% with placebo; NNT for 1 extra person to abstain 7 at 1 year v 11 at 3.5 years).[8] The second RCT compared 5 months of nicotine patches plus nicotine spray versus the same patches plus a placebo spray. It found no significant difference between treatments after 6 years (16.2% abstinent with nicotine spray v 8.5% with placebo spray, P = 0.08).[9] The third trial compared patches delivering different nicotine doses versus placebo patches. The trial followed everyone that quit at 6 weeks for a further 4 to 5 years, and found no significant difference in relapse between the groups. Overall, 73% of people who quit at 6 weeks relapsed.[10]

Harms: Nicotine gum has been associated with hiccups, gastrointestinal disturbances, jaw pain, and orodental problems. Nicotine transdermal patches have been associated with skin sensitivity and irritation. Nicotine inhalers and nasal spray have been associated with local irritation at the site of administration. Nicotine sublingual tablets have been reported to cause hiccups, burning, and smarting sensations in the mouth, sore throat, coughing, dry lips, and mouth ulcers.[11]

Comment: Nicotine replacement may not represent an "easy cure" for nicotine addiction, but it does improve the cessation rate. The evidence suggests that the majority of smokers attempting cessation fail at any one attempt, or relapse over the next 5 years. Multiple attempts may be needed.

OPTION   ACUPUNCTURE

One systematic review found no evidence that acupuncture increases rates of smoking cessation at 12 months.

Benefits: We found one systematic review (search date 1999, 18 RCTs, 3772 people) comparing acupuncture with sham acupuncture, other treatment, or no treatment. Only five trials (2535 people) reported abstinence after at least 12 months.[12] The review found that acupuncture versus control treatment produced no significant reduction in smoking cessation at 12 months (OR 1.02, 95% CI 0.72 to 1.43).

Harms: None were documented.

Comment: None.

OPTION   PHYSICAL EXERCISE

One systematic review of RCTs found limited evidence that exercise might increase smoking cessation.

Benefits: We found one systematic review (search date 1999, 8 RCTs)[13] of exercise compared with control interventions. Four small RCTs in the review reported point prevalence of non-smoking at 12 months and found no significant benefit from exercise, but these studies were insufficiently powered to exclude a clinically important effect. One RCT (281 women) found that three exercise sessions a week for 12 weeks plus a cognitive behaviour programme (see glossary, p 39) improved continuous abstinence from smoking at 12 months compared with the behaviour programme alone (16/134 [12%] with exercise v 8/147 [5%] with control; ARR +6.5%, 95% CI −19% to +0.0%; RR 2.2, 95% CI 0.98 to 4.5).[14]

Harms: None were documented.

Comment: None.

OPTION   ANTIDEPRESSANT AND ANXIOLYTIC TREATMENT

Systematic reviews have found that quit rates are significantly increased by buprorion, but not by moclobemide or anxiolytics.

Benefits: **Antidepressants:** We found one systematic review of antidepressants (search date 2000, 12 RCTs).[15] Eight of the RCTs (3230 people) reported 12 month cessation rates. It found that buprorion 300 mg daily increased cessation at 12 months compared with control treatment (4 RCTs; AR quitting 21% with buprorion v 8%

with control; OR 2.73, 95% CI 1.90 to 3.94; NNT 8).[15] Another RCT in the review found that combined buproprion plus a nicotine patch was more efficacious than a patch alone (OR 2.65, 95% CI 1.58 to 4.45), but not more effective than buproprion alone. In two included trials (1 with 6 month and 1 with 12 month follow up), nortriptyline improved long term (6–12 month) abstinence rates compared with placebo (OR 2.83, 95% CI 1.59 to 5.03). One RCT of moclobemide found no significant difference in abstinence at 12 months. **Anxiolytics:** We found one systematic review of anxiolytics (search date 2000, 6 RCTs).[16] Four of the RCTs (626 people) reporting 12 month cessation rates found no significant increase in abstinence with anxiolytics versus control treatment.[16]

Harms: Headache, insomnia, and dry mouth were reported in people using buproprion.[15] Nortriptyline can cause sedation and urinary retention, and can be dangerous in overdose. The largest RCT found that discontinuation rates caused by adverse events were 3.8% with placebo, 6.6% for nicotine replacement therapy, 11.9% for buproprion, and 11.4% for buproprion plus nicotine replacement therapy.[17] Anxiolytics may cause dependence and withdrawal problems, tolerance, paradoxical effects, and impair driving ability.

Comment: None.

| QUESTION | Are smoking cessation interventions more effective in people at high risk of smoking related disease? |

| OPTION | IN PREGNANT WOMEN |

Two systematic reviews of RCTs have found that the effect of antismoking interventions in pregnant women increases abstinence rates and decreases the risk of giving birth to low birthweight babies. The increase in abstinence with non-nicotine replacement interventions was similar to the increase found in trials of nicotine replacement in men and non-pregnant women. One RCT found no evidence that nicotine patches increased quit rates in pregnant women compared with placebo, although birthweight was greater in babies born to mothers given active patches.

Benefits: We found two systematic reviews[1,18] and one additional RCT.[19] The most recent review (search date 1999, 34 RCTs) assessed smoking cessation interventions in pregnancy. It found that smoking cessation programmes improved abstinence (OR of abstinence in late pregnancy with antismoking programmes v no programmes 0.53, 95% 0.47 to 0.60).[18] The findings were similar if the analysis was restricted to trials in which abstinence was confirmed by means other than self reporting. The review also found that antismoking programmes reduced the risk of low birthweight babies, but found no evidence of an effect on the rates of very low birthweight babies or perinatal mortality, although the power to detect such effects was low (OR for low birthweight babies 0.80, 95% CI 0.69 to 0.99). The review calculated that of 100 smokers attending a first antenatal visit, 10 stopped spontaneously and a further six to seven stopped as the result of a smoking cessation programme. Five included trials examined the effects of interventions to prevent relapse in 800 women who had quit smoking. Collectively, these trials found no evidence that the interventions reduced relapse rate.[18] One earlier systematic review (search date not stated, 10 RCTs, 4815 pregnant women) of antismoking interventions[1] included one trial of physician advice, one trial of advice by a health educator, one trial of group sessions, and seven trials of behaviour therapy based on self help manuals. Cessation rates among trials ranged from 1.9–16.7% in the control groups and from 7.1–36.1% in the intervention groups. The review found that antismoking interventions significantly increased the rate of quitting (ARI with intervention v no intervention 7.6%, 95% CI 4.3% to 10.8%).[1] The additional RCT found that nicotine patches did not significantly alter quit rates in pregnant women compared with placebo. However, active patches were associated with greater birthweight in babies born to treated mothers (mean difference in birthweight with nicotine v placebo 186 g, 95% CI 35 g to 336 g).[19]

Harms: None documented.

Comment: The recent review found that some women quit smoking before their first antenatal visit, and the majority of these will remain abstinent.[18]

OPTION	IN PEOPLE AT HIGH RISK OF DISEASE

One systematic review of RCTs and two subsequent RCTs have found that antismoking advice improves smoking cessation in people at high risk of smoking related disease.

Benefits: We found no trials in which the same intervention was used in high and low risk people. We found one systematic review (search date not stated, 4 RCTs, 13 208 healthy men at high risk of heart disease)[1] and two subsequent RCTs.[20,21] The review found that antismoking advice improved smoking cessation rates compared with control interventions (ARI of smoking cessation 21%, 95% CI 10% to 31%; NNT 5, 95% CI 4 to 10).[1] One early trial (223 men), which was included in the review, used non-random allocation after myocardial infarction. The intervention group was given intensive advice by the therapeutic team while in the coronary care unit. The trial found that the self reported cessation rate at 1 year or more was higher in the intervention group than the control group (63% quit in the intervention group v 28% in the control group; ARI of quitting 36%, 95% CI 23% to 48%).[22] The first subsequent RCT compared postal advice on smoking cessation versus no intervention in men aged 30–45 years with either a history of asbestos exposure, or forced expiratory volume in 1 second (FEV_1) in the lowest quartile for their age. Postal advice increased the self reported sustained cessation rate at 1 year compared with no intervention (5.6% with postal advice v 3.5%; P < 0.05; NNT 48).[20] The second RCT (100 people) compared minimal advice versus a 6 month programme of bedside counselling plus seven brief telephone counselling sessions after myocardial infarction. It found that the more intensive programme increased reported abstinence at 12 months compared with minimal counselling (AR of abstinence 55% with programme v 34% with minimal advice, P = 0.05).[21]

Harms: None were documented.

Comment: There was heterogeneity in the four trials included in the review, partly because of a less intense intervention in one trial and the recording of a change from cigarettes to other forms of tobacco as success in another. One of the included trials was weakened by use of self reported smoking cessation as an outcome and non-random allocation to the intervention.[22]

QUESTION **Does training of professionals increase the effectiveness of smoking cessation interventions?**

One systematic review has found that training professionals increases the frequency of antismoking interventions being offered, but found no good evidence that antismoking interventions are more effective if the health professionals delivering the interventions received training.

Benefits: We found one systematic review (search date 2000, 9 RCTs),[23] which included eight RCTs of training medical practitioners and one RCT of training dental practitioners to give antismoking advice. All the trials took place in the USA. The training was provided on a group basis, and variously included lectures, videotapes, role plays, and discussion. The importance of setting quit dates and offering follow up was emphasised in most of the training programmes. The review found no good evidence that training professionals leads to higher quit rates in people receiving antismoking interventions from those professionals, although training increased the frequency with which such interventions were offered. Three of the trials used prompts and reminders to practitioners to deploy smoking cessation techniques, and found that prompts increased the frequency of health professional interventions.[23]

Harms: None were documented.

Comment: The results of the systematic review should be interpreted with caution because there were variations in the way the analysis allowed for the unit of randomisation.

QUESTION **Which interventions increase physical activity in sedentary people?**

OPTION COUNSELLING

We found weak evidence from systematic reviews and subsequent RCTs that sedentary people can be encouraged to increase their physical activity. Interventions that encourage moderate rather than vigorous exercise, and do not require attendance at a special facility, may be more successful. Increases in walking in previously sedentary women can be sustained over at least 10 years. Brief advice from a physician is probably not effective in increasing physical activity. We found limited evidence from RCTs that primary care consultation with an exercise specialist may increase physical activity at 1 year compared with no advice.

Benefits: We found two systematic reviews[24,25] and seven subsequent RCTs.[26–32] The first review (search date 1996, 11 RCTs based in the USA, 1699 people) assessed single factor physical activity promotion.[24] Seven trials evaluated advice to undertake exercise from home (mainly walking, but including jogging and swimming), and six evaluated advice to undertake facility based exercise (including jogging and walking on sports tracks, endurance exercise, games, swimming, and exercise to music classes). An increase in activity in the intervention groups was seen in trials in which home based moderate exercise was encouraged and regular brief follow up of participants was provided. In most of the trials, participants were self selected volunteers, so the effects of the interventions may have been exaggerated. The second systematic review (search date not stated, 3 RCTs, 420 people) compared "lifestyle" physical activity interventions with either standard exercise treatment or a control group.[25] Lifestyle interventions were defined as those concerned with the daily accumulation of moderate or vigorous exercise as part of everyday life. The first RCT (60 adults, 65–85 years old) found significantly more self reported physical activity in the lifestyle group than a standard exercise group. The second RCT (235 people, 35–60 years old) found no significant difference in physical activity between the groups. The third RCT (125 women, 23–54 years old) of encouraging walking found no significant difference in walking levels at 30 months' follow up between people receiving an 8 week behavioural intervention and those receiving a 5 minute telephone call and written information about the benefits of exercise, although both groups increased walking. Six of the additional trials involved primary care delivered interventions.[26–28,30–32] The two trials, in which advice was delivered by an exercise specialist rather than a physician, found significant improvement in self reported physical activity at long term (> 6 months) follow up compared with controls.[30,31] Short term improvement was found in two further trials, but not maintained at 9 months or 1 year.[27,28] One quasi-randomised trial (776 people in a primary care setting) tested the effect of brief physician advice plus a mailed leaflet on physical activity. It found short term improvement in self-reported activity with the intervention versus control, although after 12 months no significant difference was maintained.[29] One RCT (229 women) of encouraging women to increase walking found significantly increased walking in the intervention group. Ten year follow up of 86% of the original women in the trial found that women who had been encouraged to walk reported significantly more walking (median estimated calorie expenditure from self reported amount of walking 1344 kcal/week in women given encouragement v 924 kcal/week in women not encouraged to walk, $P = 0.01$).[33]

Harms: None of the reviews, or the trials, reported any incidences of harm from taking up exercise.

Comment: Self reporting of effects by people in a trial, especially where blinding to interventions is not possible (as is the case with advice or encouragement), is a potential source of bias. Several trials are in progress, including one in the UK, in which people in primary care have been randomised to two different methods of encouragement to increase walking, or to a no intervention arm. One ongoing multisite trial in the USA has randomised 874 people to one of three experimental counselling interventions.[34]

| QUESTION | What are effects of exercise advice in high risk people? |

| OPTION | IN WOMEN AGED OVER 80 YEARS |

One RCT found exercise advice increased physical activity in women aged over 80 years and decreased the risk of falling.

Benefits: We found no systematic review. One RCT (233 women > 80 years old, conducted in New Zealand) compared four visits from a physiotherapist who advised a course of 30 minutes of home based exercises three times a week that was appropriate for the individual, versus a similar number of social visits.[35] After 1 year, women who had received physiotherapist visits were significantly more active than women in the control group, and 42% were still completing the recommended exercise programme at least three times a week. The mean annual rate of falls in the intervention group was 0.87 compared with 1.34 in the control group, a difference of 0.47 falls a year (95% CI 0.04 to 0.90).

Harms: No additional harms in the intervention group were reported.

Comment: None.

| QUESTION | What are the effects on blood cholesterol of dietary advice to reduce fat, increase polyunsaturated fats, and decrease saturated fats? |

| OPTION | COUNSELLING |

Systematic reviews have found that advice on eating a cholesterol lowering diet (that is, advice to reduce fat intake or increase the polyunsaturated to saturated fatty acid ratio in the diet) leads to a small reduction in blood cholesterol concentrations in the long term (6 months or more). We found evidence of a dose response, in that dietary advice recommending more stringent reduction in fat and cholesterol intake lowered blood cholesterol more than less stringent advice. We found no evidence to support the effectiveness of such advice in primary care.

Benefits: **Effects on blood cholesterol:** We found three systematic reviews[11,36,37] and one subsequent RCT, which reported biochemical rather than clinical end points.[38] None of these systematic reviews included evidence after 1996. One review (search date 1993) identified five trials of cholesterol lowering dietary advice (principally advice from nutritionists or specially trained counsellors) with follow up for 9–18 months.[36] It found a reduction in blood cholesterol concentration in the intervention group of 0.22 mmol/litre (95% CI 0.05 to 0.39 mmol/l) compared with the control group. However, there was significant heterogeneity (P < 0.02), with two outlying studies — one showing no effect and one showing a larger effect. This review excluded trials in people at high risk of heart disease. Another systematic review (search date 1996) identified 13 trials of more than 6 months' duration and included people at high risk of heart disease.[11] It found that dietary advice reduced blood cholesterol (mean reduction in blood cholesterol concentration with advice 4.5%, 95% CI 3.9% to 5.1%; given a mean baseline cholesterol of 6.3 mmol/litre, mean absolute reduction about 0.3 mmol/l). The third systematic review (search date 1995, 1 trial,[39] 76 people) found no significant difference between brief versus intensive advice from a general practitioner and dietician on blood cholesterol at 1 year.[37] The subsequent RCT (186 men and women at high risk of coronary heart disease) compared advice on healthy eating versus no intervention. At 1 year, it found no significant differences between groups in total and low density lipoprotein cholesterol concentrations for either sex, even though the reported percentage of energy from fat consumed by both women and men in the advice group decreased significantly compared with that reported by the women and men in the control group.[38] These results may reflect bias caused by self-reporting of dietary intake. **Effects on clinical outcomes:** We found two systematic reviews, which reported on morbidity and mortality.[11,40] The first (search date 1996) compared 13 separate and single dietary interventions.[11] It found no significant effect of dietary interventions on total mortality (OR 0.93, 95% CI 0.84 to 1.03) or coronary heart disease mortality (OR 0.93, 95% CI 0.82 to 1.06), but found a reduction in non-fatal myocardial infarction (OR 0.77, 95% CI 0.67 to 0.90). The second review (search date 1999, 27 studies including 40 intervention arms, 30 901 person years) found dietary advice to reduce or modify dietary fat versus no dietary advice had no significant effect on total mortality (HR 0.98, 95% CI 0.86 to 1.12) or cardiovascular disease mortality (HR 0.98, 95% CI 0.77 to 1.07), but significantly reduced cardiovascular disease events (HR 0.84, 95% CI 0.72 to 0.99).[40] RCTs in which people were followed for more than 2 years showed significant reductions in the rate of cardiovascular disease events. The relative protection from cardiovascular disease events was similar in both high and low risk groups, but was significant only in high risk groups.

Harms: We found no evidence about harms.

Comment: The finding of a 0.2–0.3 mmol/litre reduction in blood cholesterol in the two systematic reviews accords with the findings of a meta-analysis of the plasma lipid response to changes in dietary fat and cholesterol.[41] The analysis included data from 244 published studies (trial duration 1 day to 6 years), and concluded that adherence to dietary recommendations (30% energy from fat, < 10% saturated fat, and < 300 mg cholesterol per day) compared with average US dietary intake would reduce blood cholesterol by about 5%.

QUESTION **Does dietary advice to reduce sodium intake lead to a sustained fall in blood pressure?**

Systematic reviews and RCTs have found that salt restriction reduces blood pressure in people with normal blood pressure, and in people with hypertension. The effect was more pronounced in older people. We found no evidence of effects on morbidity and mortality.

Benefits: We found three systematic reviews[36,42,43] and one additional RCT[44] about the long term effects of advice to restrict salt. The first systematic review (search date 1993, 5 trials with follow up for 9–18 months) compared dietary advice (mainly from nutritionists or specially trained counsellors) with control treatment. It found that the advice slightly reduced systolic blood pressure (change in blood pressure: −1.9 mm Hg systolic, 95% CI −3.0 to −0.8 mm Hg), but not diastolic blood pressure (−1.2 mm Hg, 95% CI −2.6 to +0.2 mm Hg).[36] The second review (8 RCTs in adults over 44 years with and without hypertension) found no clearly significant systolic blood pressure changes after at least 6 months' follow up with advice on salt restriction versus no dietary advice either in people with hypertension (−2.9 mm Hg, 95% CI −5.8 to 0.0 mm Hg) or in people without hypertension (−1.3 mm Hg, 95% CI −2.7 to +0.1 mm Hg). Small but significant changes in mean diastolic blood pressure were found in people with hypertension (+2.1 mm Hg, 95% CI −4.0 to −0.1 mm Hg) but not in people without hypertension (−0.8 mm Hg, 95% CI −1.8 to +0.2 mm Hg).[42] The definitions of hypertension varied between the trials. The third review (search date 1996, 30 RCTs) found that in people aged over 44 years defined as having hypertension, a reduction in sodium intake of 100 mmol a day resulted in a decrease of 6.3 mm Hg in systolic blood pressure and 2.2 mm Hg in diastolic pressure.[43] For younger people with hypertension, the systolic fall was 2.4 mm Hg and the diastolic fall was negligible. Three RCTs of salt restriction followed people without hypertension for over 12 months, and found conflicting results. One RCT (181 people) found that advice to restrict salt was less effective in preventing hypertension in overweight people than advice on weight reduction at 7 years.[45] One RCT (585 people) found that advice to restrict salt was as effective as advice to reduce weight for reducing blood pressure in overweight people with hypertension at 15–36 months.[44]

Harms: None reported.

Comment: None.

QUESTION   What are the effects of lifestyle interventions to achieve sustained weight loss?

Systematic reviews and subsequent RCTs have found that a combination of advice on diet and exercise, supported by behaviour therapy, is probably more effective in achieving weight loss than either diet or exercise advice alone. A low energy, low fat diet is the most effective lifestyle intervention for weight loss. RCTs have found no significant differences in weight loss between interventions to promote physical activity. Weight regain is likely, but weight loss of 2–6 kg may be sustained over at least 2 years.

Benefits: We found three systematic reviews,[46–48] and 12 additional RCTs.[49–60] One systematic review (search date 1995) identified 99 studies, including some that tested either dietary or physical activity interventions with or without a behaviour intervention component. The combination of diet and exercise in conjunction with behavioural therapy produced greater weight loss than diet alone. However, this finding was based on the results of one RCT in which a mean weight loss of 3.8 kg at 1 year was observed in a group receiving diet guidelines and behaviour intervention compared with a significantly different mean loss of 7.9 kg in a group receiving the same intervention plus a programme of walking.[46] The second systematic review of the detection, prevention, and treatment of obesity (search date 1999, 11 RCTs and additional prospective cohort studies) included eight RCTs comparing dietary prescriptions with exercise, counselling, or behavioural therapy for the treatment of obesity, and three RCTs comparing dietary counselling alone with no intervention. In both comparisons, initial weight loss was followed by gradual weight regain once treatment had stopped (mean difference in weight change at least 2 years after baseline: 2–6 kg for dietary prescription trials, and 2–4 kg for dietary counselling trials).[47] The third systematic review of RCTs and observational studies found similar results; it found that a combination of diet and exercise, supported by behaviour therapy, was more effective than any one or two of these individual interventions.[48] One additional RCT compared advice on an energy restricted diet to advice on a fat restricted diet.[53] Weight loss was greater on an energy restricted diet than on the fat restricted diet at 6 months (−11.2 kg v −6.1 kg, $P < 0.001$) and at 18 months (−7.5 kg v −1.8 kg, $P < 0.001$). Seven RCTs focused on physical activity.[49–51,55–57,60] The heterogeneity of interventions makes pooling of data inappropriate, but no major differences were found between the various behaviour therapies and exercise regimes. One RCT[52] found behavioural choice treatment (see glossary, p 39) versus standard behaviour therapy (see glossary, p 39) resulted in greater weight loss at 12 months (−10.1 kg v −4.3 kg, $P < 0.01$). One RCT (166 people) compared standard behaviour therapy plus support from friends with standard behaviour therapy without support. It found no additional weight loss at 16 months with social support from friends (−4.7 kg v −3.0 kg, $P < 0.3$).[54] A further RCT (62 women) found that 1 year weight loss was greater in women following a standard versus a modified cognitive behaviour programme (−3.6 kg v 2.0 kg, $P = 0.02$).[59]

Harms: The systematic reviews and RCTs provided no evidence about harms resulting from diet or exercise for weight loss.

Comment: None.

QUESTION What are the effects of lifestyle interventions to maintain weight loss?

One systematic review and additional RCTs have found that most types of maintenance strategy result in smaller weight gains or greater weight losses compared with no contact. Strategies that involve personal contact with a therapist, family support, walking training programmes, multiple interventions, or are weight focused appear most effective.

Benefits: We found one systematic review[46] and six additional RCTs.[61–66] The systematic review (search date 1995, 21 studies) compared different types and combinations of interventions. It found that increased contact with a therapist in the long term produced smaller weight gain or greater weight loss, and that additional self help peer groups, self management techniques, or involvement of the family or spouse may increase weight loss. The largest weight loss was seen in programmes using multiple strategies. Two additional small RCTs (102 people[61] and 100 people in two trials[65]) assessed simple strategies without face to face contact with a therapist. Frequent phone contacts, optional food provision, continued self monitoring, urge control, or relapse prevention did not reduce the rate of weight regain. One small RCT (117 people) found that phone contacts plus house visits did reduce the rate of weight regain compared with no intervention (3.65 kg v 6.42 kg, P = 0.048).[62] One RCT (82 women) compared two walking programmes (4.2 MJ/week or 8.4 MJ/week) plus diet counselling versus diet counselling alone following a 12 week intensive weight reduction programme.[66] Both walking programmes reduced weight regain at 1 year (reduction in weight gain compared with dietary counselling alone 2.7 kg, 95% CI 0.2 kg to 5.2 kg with low intensity programme and 2.6 kg, 95% CI 0.0 kg to 5.1 kg with high intensity programme). At 2 years, weight regain was not significantly different between high intensity programme and control, but was reduced in the low intensity group (reduction in weight gain 3.5 kg, 95% CI 0.2 kg to 6.8 kg with low intensity programme and 0.2 kg, 95% CI –3.1 kg to +3.6 kg). One additional small RCT (67 people) found that people on a weight focused programme maintained weight loss better than those on an exercise focused programme (0.8 kg v 4.4 kg, P < 0.01).[63] One 5 year RCT (489 menopausal women) compared behavioural intervention in two phases aimed at lifestyle changes in diet and physical activity with lifestyle assessment. People in the intervention group were encouraged to lose weight during the first 6 months (phase I), and thereafter maintain this weight loss for a further 12 months (phase II). The intervention resulted in weight loss compared to control during the first 6 months (–8.9 lb v –0.8 lb, P < 0.05), most of which was sustained over phase II (–6.7 lb v +0.6 lb, P < 0.05).[64]

Harms: We found no direct evidence that interventions designed to maintain weight loss are harmful.

Comment: Weight regain is common. The resource implication of providing long term maintenance of any weight loss may be a barrier to the routine implementation of maintenance programmes.

QUESTION What are the effects of lifestyle advice to prevent weight gain?

One small RCT found that low intensity education increased weight loss. An extension of this RCT found no significant effect on weight gain from a mailed newsletter with or without a linked financial incentive.

Benefits: We found three systematic reviews,[46,47,67] which included the same two RCTs.[68,69] The second RCT was an extension of the first. The first RCT (219 people) compared low intensity education with a financial incentive to maintain weight versus an untreated control group. It found significantly greater average weight loss in the intervention group than in the control group (–2.1 lb v –0.3 lb, P = 0.03).[68] The second RCT (228 men and 998 women) compared a monthly newsletter versus the newsletter plus a lottery incentive versus no contact. There was no significance difference in weight gain after 3 years between the groups (1.6 kg v 1.5 kg v 1.8 kg).[60]

Harms: None reported.

Comment: None.

QUESTION	What are the effects of training professionals in promoting reduction of body weight?

One systematic review of poor quality RCTs found little evidence on the sustained effect of interventions to improve health professionals' management of obesity. One subsequent small RCT found limited evidence that training for primary care doctors in nutrition counselling plus a support programme reduced body weight of the people in their care over 1 year.

Benefits: We found one systematic review (search date 1998, 12 RCTs, 5 with follow up > 1 year)[70] and one subsequent RCT.[71] The studies in the review were heterogeneous and poor quality. The subsequent RCT (45 people) compared nutrition counselling training plus a support programme for primary care doctors versus usual care.[71] The nutrition supported intervention compared with usual care increased weight loss at 1 year (additional weight loss 2.3 kg, P < 0.001).

Harms: None reported.

Comment: The doctors were randomly allocated to treatment but the analysis of results was based on the people in the care of those doctors. No allowance was made for cluster bias. This increases the likelihood that the additional weight loss could have occurred by chance.

GLOSSARY

Behavioural choice treatment A cognitive behavioural intervention based on a decision making model of women's food choice. This relates situation specific eating behaviour to outcomes and goals using decision theory. The outcomes and goals governing food choice extend beyond food related factors to include self esteem and social acceptance.

Cognitive behaviour programme Traditional cognitive behavioural topics (e.g. self-monitoring, stimulus control, coping with cravings and high risk situations, stress management, and relaxation techniques) along with topics of particular importance to women (e.g. healthy eating, weight management, mood management, and managing work and family).

Standard behaviour therapy A behavioural weight management programme that incorporates moderate calorie restriction to promote weight loss.

Substantive changes since last issue

Maintaining weight loss New RCT;[66] conclusion unchanged.

Advice to reduce sodium intake New RCT;[44] conclusions unchanged.

Lifestyle interventions for sustained weight loss Four new RCTs;[57–60] conclusions unchanged.

Counselling and physical activity Two additional RCTs.[31,32]

Nicotine replacement Systematic review updated;[5] conclusions unchanged.

Antidepressants and anxiolytics for smoking cessation Systematic review of antidepressants updated[15] and additional systematic review of anxiolytics identified;[16] conclusions unchanged.

Antismoking interventions in pregnant women New RCT;[19] conclusions unchanged.

Antismoking interventions in people at high risk of disease New RCT;[21] conclusions unchanged.

Training professionals to increase effectiveness of smoking cessation interventions Systematic review updated;[23] conclusion changed. Now finds no good evidence that training professionals increases effectiveness of interventions, although frequency of interventions is increased.

REFERENCES

1. Law M, Tang JL. An analysis of the effectiveness of interventions intended to help people stop smoking. Arch Intern Med 1995;155:1933–1941. Search date not specified but before 1995; primary sources Medline and Index Medicus; dates not given, but selected trials range from 1967 to 1993.

2. Lancaster T, Stead LF. Individual behavioural counselling for smoking cessation. In: The Cochrane Library, Issue 4, 2000. Oxford: Update Software. Search date October 1998; primary sources Cochrane Tobacco Addiction Group Trials Register to October 1998.

3. Rice VH, Stead LF. Nursing interventions for smoking cessation. In: The Cochrane Library, Issue 1, 2000. Oxford: Update Software. Search date May 1999; primary sources Cochrane Tobacco Addiction Group Trials Register to May 1999, and Cinahl 1983 to May 1999.

4. Ashenden R, Silagy C, Weller D. A systematic review of the effectiveness of promoting lifestyle change in general practice. Family Practice 1997; 14:160–176. Search date May 1995; primary sources Medline, Psychlit, Sociofile, Cinahl, Embase, and Drug; all searched from the year of their inception up to May 1995.

5. Silagy C, Mant D, Fowler G, Lancaster T. Nicotine replacement therapy for smoking cessation. In: The Cochrane Library, Issue 4, 2000. Oxford: Update Software. Search date April 2000; primary sources Cochrane Tobacco Addiction Group Trials Register.

6. Tonneson P, Paoletti P, Gustavsson G, et al. Higher dose nicotine patches increase one year smoking cessation rates: results from the European CEASE trial. Eur Respir J 1999;13:238–246.

7. Stapleton J. Cigarette smoking prevalence, cessation and relapse. Stat Methods Med Res 1998;7:187–203. Search date and primary sources not given.

8. Stapleton JA, Sutherland G, Russell MA. How much does relapse after one year erode effectiveness of smoking cessation treatments? Long term follow up of a randomised trial of nicotine nasal spray. BMJ 1998;316:830–831.

9. Blondal T, Gudmundsson J, Olafsdottir I, et al. Nicotine nasal spray with nicotine patch for smoking cessation: randomised trial with six years follow up. BMJ 1999;318:285–289.

10. Daughton DM, Fortmann SP, Glover ED, et al. The smoking cessation efficacy of varying doses of nicotine patch delivery systems 4 to 5 years post-quit day. Prev Med 1999;28:113–118.

11. Ebrahim S, Davey Smith G. Health promotion in older people for the prevention of coronary heart disease and stroke. Health promotion effectiveness reviews series, No 1. London: Health Education Authority, 1996. Search date December 1994; primary sources Medline, hand searches of reference lists, and citation search on BIDS for Eastern European trials.

12. White AR, Rampes H, Ernst E. Acupuncture for smoking cessation. In: The Cochrane Library, Issue 4, 2000. Oxford: Update Software. Search date 1999; primary sources Cochrane Tobacco Addiction Group Register, Medline, Psychlit, Dissertation Abstracts, Health Planning and Administration, SocialSciSearch, Smoking and Health, Embase, Biological Abstracts and Drug.

13. Ussher MH, Taylor AH, West R, McEwen A. Does exercise aid smoking cessation? Addiction 2000; 95:199–208.

14. Marcus BH, Albrecht AE, King TK, et al. The efficacy of exercise as an aid for smoking cessation in women. Arch Intern Med 1999;159: 1229–1234.

15. Hughes JR, Stead LF, Lancaster T. Antidepressants for smoking cessation. In: The Cochrane Library, Issue 4, 2000. Oxford Update Software. Search date July 2000; primary sources Cochrane Tobacco Addiction Group trials register.

16. Hughes JR, Stead LF, Lancaster T. Anxiolytics for smoking cessation. In: The Cochrane Library, Issue 4, 2000. Oxford Update Software. Search date July 2000; primary sources Cochrane Tobacco Addiction Group trials register.

17. Jorenby DE, Leischow SJ, Nides MA, et al. A controlled trial of sustained-release buprorion. A nicotine patch, or both for smoking cessation. N Engl J Med 1999;340:685–691.

18. Lumley J, Oliver S, Waters E. Interventions for promoting smoking cessation during pregnancy. In: The Cochrane Library, Issue 4, 2000. Oxford: Update Software. Search date October 1998; primary sources Cochrane Tobacco Addiction Group Trials Register to October 1998.

19. Wisborg K, Henriksen TB, Jespersen LB, Secher NJ. Nicotine patches for pregnant smokers: A randomized controlled study. Obstet Gynecol 2000;96:967–971.

20. Humerfelt S, Eide GE, Kvale G, et al. Effectiveness of postal smoking cessation advice: a randomized controlled trial in young men with reduced FEV_1 and asbestos exposure. Eur Respir J 1998;11: 284–290.

21. Dornelas EA, Sampson RA, Gray JF, Waters D, Thompson PD. A randomized controlled trial of smoking cessation counselling after myocardial infarction. Prev Med 2000;30:261–268.

22. Burt A, Thornley P, Illingworth D, et al. Stopping smoking after myocardial infarction. Lancet 1974; 1:304–306.

23. Lancaster T, Silagy C, Fowler G, Spiers I. Training health professionals in smoking cessation. In: The Cochrane Library, Issue 4, 2000. Oxford: Update Software. Search date 2000; primary sources Specialised Register of the Cochrane Tobacco Addiction Group.

24. Hillsdon M, Thorogood M. A systematic review of physical activity promotion strategies. Br J Sports Med 1996;30:84–89. Search date 1996; primary sources Medline, Excerpta Medica, Sport, SCISearch 1966 to 1996, and hand search of reference lists.

25. Dunn AL, Anderson RE, Jakicic JM. Lifestyle physical activity interventions. History, short- and long-term effects and recommendations. Am J Prev Med 1998;15:398–412. Search date not given; primary sources Medline, Current Contents, Biological Abstracts, The Johns Hopkins Medical Institutions Catalog, Sport Discus, and Grateful Med.

26. Goldstein MG, Pinto BM, Marcus BH, et al. Physician-based physical activity counseling for middle-aged and older adults: a randomised trial. Ann Behaviour Med 1999;1:40–47.

27. Harland J, White M, Drinkwater C, et al. The Newcastle exercise project: a randomised

controlled trial of methods to promote physical activity in primary care. *BMJ* 1999;319:828–832.

28. Taylor, A, Doust, J, Webborn, N. Randomised controlled trial to examine the effects of a GP exercise referral programme in Hailsham, East Sussex, on modifiable coronary heart disease risk factors. *J Epidemiol Community Health* 1998;52: 595–601.

29. Bull F, Jamorozik K. Advice on exercise from a family physician can help sedentary patients to become active. *Am J Prev Med* 1998;15:85–94.

30. Stevens W, Hillsdon M, Thorogood M, McArdle D. Cost-effectiveness of a primary care based physical activity intervention in 45–74 year old men and women; a randomised controlled trial. *Br J Sports Med* 1998;32:236–241.

31. Halbert JA, Silagy CA, Finucane PM, Withers RT, Hamdorf PA. Physical activity and cardiovascular risk factors: effect of advice from an exercise specialist in Australian general practice. *Med J Aust* 2000;173:84–87.

32. Norris SL, Grothaus LC, Buchner DM, Pratt M. Effectiveness of physician-based assessment and counseling for exercise in a staff model HMO. *Prev Med* 2000;30:513–523.

33. Pereira MA, Kriska AN, Day RD, et al. A randomized walking trial in postmenopausal women. *Arch Intern Med* 1998;158:1695–1701.

34. King A, Sallis JF, Dunn AL, et al. Overview of the activity counselling trial (ACT) intervention for promoting physical activity in primary health care settings. *Med Sci Sports Exerc* 1998;30:1086–1096.

35. Campbell AJ, Robertson MC, Gardner MM, et al. Randomised controlled trial of a general practice programme of home based exercise to prevent falls in elderly women. *BMJ* 1997;315:1065–1069.

36. Brunner E, White I, Thorogood M, et al. Can dietary interventions change diet and cardiovascular risk factors? A meta-analysis of randomised controlled trials. *Am J Public Health* 1997;87:1415–1422. Search date July 1993; primary sources computer and manual searches of databases and journals. No further details given.

37. Tang JL, Armitage JM, Lancaster T, et al. Systematic review of dietary intervention trials to lower blood total cholesterol in free living subjects. *BMJ* 1998;316:1213–1220. Search date 1996; primary sources Medline, Human Nutrition, Embase, and Allied and Alternative Health 1966 to 1995; hand search of *Am J Clin Nutr*, and reference list checks.

38. Stefanick ML, Mackey S, Sheehan M, et al. Effects of diet and exercise in men and postmenopausal women with low levels of HDL cholesterol and high levels of LDL cholesterol. *N Engl J Med* 1998;339:12–20.

39. Tomson Y, Johannesson M, Aberg H. The costs and effects of two different lipid intervention programmes in primary health care. *J Intern Med* 1995;237:13–17.

40. Hooper L, Summerbell C, Higgins J, et al. Dietary advice, modification or supplementation aimed at lipid lowering for prevention of cardiovascular disease in patients with and without ischaemic heart disease. In: The Cochrane Library, Issue 4, 2000. Oxford: Update Software. Search date 1999, primary sources Cochrane Library, Medline, Embase, CAB Abstracts, CVRCT registry, related Cochrane groups' trial registers, trials known to experts in the field, and biographies.

41. Howell WH, McNamara JD, Tosca MA, et al. Plasma lipid and lipoprotein responses to dietary fat and cholesterol: a meta-analysis. *Am J Clin Nutr* 1997;65:1747–1764. Search date 1994; primary source Medline 1966 to February 1994,

hand search of selected review publications and bibliographies.

42. Ebrahim S, Davey Smith G. Lowering blood pressure: a systematic review of sustained effects of non-pharmacological interventions. *J Public Health* 1998;2:441–448. Search date April 1998; primary sources Medline and hand searches of reference lists.

43. Fodor JG, Whitmore B, Leenen F, Larochelle P. Recommendations on dietary salt. *Can Med Assoc J* 1999;160(suppl 9):29–34. Search date 1996; primary sources Medline, hand searches of reference lists, personal files, and contact with experts.

44. Whelton PK, Appel LJ, Espeland MA, et al. Sodium reduction and weight loss in the treatment of hypertension in older persons. A randomized controlled Trial of Nonpharmacologic Interventions in the Elderly (TONE). *JAMA* 1998;279:839–846.

45. He J, Whelton PK, Appel LJ, et al. Long-term effects of weight loss and dietary sodium reduction on incidence of hypertension. *Hypertension* 2000;35:544–549.

46. Glenny A-M, O'Meara S, Melville A, Shelton T, Wilson C. The treatment and prevention of obesity: a systematic review of the literature. *Int J Obesity* 1887:21;715–737. Published in full as NHS CRD report 1997, No10. *Systematic review of interventions in the treatment and prevention of obesity*. http://ww.york.ac.uk/inst/crd/obesity.htm. Search date 1995; primary sources Medline; Embase; DHSS data; Current Research in UK; Science citation index; Social science citation index; Conference Proceedings index; SIGLE; Dissertation Abstracts; Sport; Drug Info; AMED (Allied and alternative medicine; ASSI (abstracts and indexes); CAB; NTIS (national technical information dB); Directory of Published Proceedings (Interdoc); Purchasing Innovations database; Health promotion database; S.S.R.U.; DARE (CRD, database of systematic reviews; NEED (CRD, database of health economic reviews); all databases searched from starting date to the end of 1995.

47. Douketis JD, Feightner JW, Attia J, Feldman WF. Periodic health examination, 1999 update. Detection, prevention and treatment of obesity. Canadian Task Force on Preventive Health Care. *Can Med Assoc J* 1999;160:513–525. Search date 1999; primary sources Medline (1996 to April 1998); Current Contents (1966 to 1999); and hand search of references.

48. The National Heart, Lung, and Blood Institute. Clinical guidelines on the identification, evaluation, and treatment of overweight and obesity in adults. Bethesda Maryland: National Institutes of Health, 1998; website http://www.nhlbi.nih.gov/nhlbi/guidelns/ob_home.htm

49. Wing RR, Polley BA, Venditti E, et al. Lifestyle intervention in overweight individuals with a family history of diabetes. *Diabetes Care* 1998;21:350–359.

50. Anderson RE, Wadden TA, Barlett SJ, et al. Effects of lifestyle activity v structured aerobic exercise in obese women. *JAMA* 1999;281:335–340.

51. Jakicic JM, Winters C, Lang W, Wing RR. Effects of intermittent exercise and use of home exercise equipment on adherence, weight loss, and fitness in overweight women. *JAMA* 1999;282:1554–1560.

52. Sbrocco T, Nedegaard RC, Stone JM, Lewis EL. Behavioural choice treatment promotes continuing weight loss. *J Consult Clin Psychol* 1999;67:260–266.

53. Harvey-Berino J. Calorie restriction is more effective for obesity treatment than dietary fat restriction. *Ann Behav Med* 1999;21:35–39.

54. Wing RR, Jeffery RW. Benefits of recruiting participants with friends and increasing social support for weight loss and maintenance. *J Consult Clin Psychol* 1999;67:132–138.

55. Jeffery RW, Wing RR, Thorson C, Burton LR. Use of personal trainers and financial incentives to increase exercise in a behavioural weight loss program. *J Consult Clin Psychol* 1998;66:777–783.

56. Craighead LW, Blum MD. Supervised exercise in behavioural treatment for moderate obesity. *Behav Ther* 1989;20:49–59.

57. Donnelly JE, Jacobsen DJ, Heelan KS, Seip R, Smith S. The effects of 18 months of intermittent vs. continuous exercise on aerobic capacity, body weight and composition, and metabolic fitness in previously sedentary, moderately obese females. *Int J Obesity* 2000;24:566,–572.

58. Kunz K, Kreimel K, Gurdet C, Lenhart P, Wirth B, Irsigler, K. Comparison of behaviour modification and conventional dietary advice in a long-term weight reduction programme for obese women [abstract]. *Diabetologia* 1982;23:181.

59. Rapoport L, Clark M, Wardle J. Evaluation of a modified cognitive-behavioural programme for weight management. *Int J Obesity* 2000;24:1726–1737.

60. Wing R, Epstein LH, Paternostro-Bayles M, et al. Exercise in a behavioural weight control program for obese patients with type 2 (non insulin dependent) diabetes. *Diabetologica* 1988;31:902–909.

61. Bonato DP, Boland FJ. A comparison of specific strategies for long-term maintenance following a behavioural treatment program for obese women. *Int J Eat Disord* 1986;5:949–958.

62. Hillebrand TH, Wirth A. Evaluation of an outpatient care program for obese patients after an inpatient treatment. *Prav Rehab* 1996;8:83–87.

63. Leermakers EA, Perri MG, Shigaki CL, Fuller PR. Effects of exercise-focused versus weight-focused maintenance programs on the management of obesity. *Addict Behav* 1999;24:219–227.

64. Simkin-Silverman LR, Wing RR, Boraz MA, Meilan EN, Kuller LH. Maintenance of cardiovascular risk factor changes among middle-aged women in a lifestyle intervention trial. *Women's Health: Research on Gender, Behaviour, and Policy* 1998; 4:255–271.

65. Wing RR, Jeffery RW, Hellerstedt WL, Burton LR. Effect of frequent phone contacts and optional food provision on maintenance of weight loss. *Ann Behav Med* 1996;18:172–176.

66. Fogelholm M, Kukkonen-Harjula K, Nenonen A, Pasanen M. Effects of walking training on weight maintenance after a very-low-energy diet in premenopausal obese women: a randomized controlled trial. *Arch Intern Med* 2000;160:2177–2184.

67. Hardeman W, Griffin S, Johnston M, et al. Interventions to prevent weight gain: a systematic review of psychological models and behaviour change methods. *Int J Obesity* 2000;4:131–143. Search date not stated; primary sources Medline, Embase, Psychlit, The Cochrane Library, Current Contents, ERIC, HealthStar, Social Science Citation Index, and hand searches of reference lists.

68. Forster JL, Jeffery RW, Schmid TL, Kramer FM. Preventing weight gain in adults: a pound of prevention. *Health Psychol* 1988;7:515–525.

69. Jeffery RW, French SA. Preventing weight gain in adults: the pound of prevention study. *Am J Public Health* 1999;89:747–751.

70. Harvey EL, Glenny A, Kirk SFL, Summerbell CD. Improving health professionals' management and the organisation of care for overweight and obese people. In: The Cochrane Library, Issue 4, 2000. Oxford: Update Software. Search date January 1998; primary sources specialised registers of the Cochrane Effective Practice and Organisation of Care Group May 1997; The Cochrane Depression, Anxiety and Neurosis Group August 1997; The Cochrane Diabetes Group August 1997; The Cochrane Controlled Trials Register September 1997; medline 1966 to January 1998; Embase 1988 to December 1997; Cinahl 1982 to November 1997; Psychlit 1974 to December 1997; Sigle 1980 to November 1997; Sociofile 1974 to October 1997; Dissertation Abstracts 1861 to January 1998; Conference Papers Index 1973 to January 1998; Resource Database in Continuing Medical Education; hand searches of seven key journals; and contacts with experts in the field.

71. Ockene IS, Hebert JR, Ockene JK, et al. Effect of physician-delivered nutrition counseling training and an office-support program on saturated fat intake, weight, and serum lipid measurements in a hyperlipidemic population: Worcester area trial for counseling in hyperlipidemia (WATCH). *Arch Intern Med* 1999;159:725–731.

Margaret Thorogood
Reader in Public Health
and Preventative Medicine

Melvyn Hillsdon
Lecturer in Health Promotion

London School of Hygiene
and Tropical Medicine
University of London
London
UK

Carolyn Summerbell
Reader in Human Nutrition
School of Health
University of Teesside
Middlesborough
UK
Competing interests: None declared.

Search date October 2000: expanded this issue

Robert McKelvie

INTERVENTIONS

Key Messages

Non-drug treatments

- We found conflicting evidence about multidisciplinary care. One systematic review has found that multidisciplinary approaches to nutrition, patient counselling, and education reduce hospital admissions, may improve quality of life, and enhance patient knowledge. However, the review excluded one large RCT that found that multidisciplinary follow up increased re-admission rates.
- RCTs have found that prescribed exercise training improves functional capacity and quality of life, and reduces the rate of adverse cardiac events.

Drug and invasive treatments

- Two systematic reviews and recent RCTs have found that angiotensin converting enzyme (ACE) inhibitors reduce mortality, admission to hospital for heart failure, and ischaemic events in people with heart failure. Relative benefits are similar in different groups of people, but absolute benefits are greater in people with severe heart failure.
- One systematic review and one recent RCT found no evidence of a difference between angiotensin II receptor blockers and ACE inhibitors in their effects on mortality, or on functional capacity and symptoms.

Cardiovascular disorders

- RCTs have found that positive inotropic drugs improve symptoms but do not reduce mortality. Many of the non-digoxin positive inotropic drugs may increase mortality. Only digoxin has been found to improve morbidity in people already receiving diuretics and ACE inhibitors.

- Systematic reviews found strong evidence that adding a β blocker to ACE inhibitors decreases the rate of death and admission to hospital. The reviews found less robust evidence that β blockers improve exercise capacity and reduce mortality.

- We found no evidence supporting the use of calcium channel blockers in heart failure.

- One RCT has found that, in people with severe heart failure, adding an aldosterone receptor antagonist to ACE inhibitor treatment reduces mortality compared with ACE inhibitors alone.

- Systematic reviews found weak evidence suggesting that amiodarone may reduce mortality in people with heart failure.

- Evidence extrapolated from one systematic review in people treated after a myocardial infarction suggests that non-amiodarone antiarrhythmic drugs may increase mortality in people with heart failure.

- One systematic review has found good evidence that an implantable cardiac defibrillator (ICD) reduces mortality in people with heart failure who have experienced a cardiac arrest. The review found conflicting evidence for prophylactic implantation of ICDs in people at high risk of arrhythmia.

- We found no RCTs of anticoagulation in people with heart failure. We found conflicting evidence from two large retrospective cohort studies.

- We found no RCTs of antiplatelet agents versus placebo in people with heart failure. Retrospective analyses have included too few events to establish or exclude a clinically important effect of antiplatelet agents in people with heart failure.

- RCTs have found good evidence that, in people with asymptomatic left ventricular systolic dysfunction, ACE inhibitors delay the onset of symptomatic heart failure and reduce cardiovascular events.

DEFINITION Heart failure occurs when abnormality of cardiac function causes failure of the heart to pump blood at a rate sufficient for metabolic requirements, or maintains cardiac output only with a raised filling pressure. It is characterised clinically by breathlessness, effort intolerance, fluid retention, and poor survival. It can be caused by systolic or diastolic dysfunction and is associated with neurohormonal changes.[1] Left ventricular systolic dysfunction (LVSD) is defined as a left ventricular ejection fraction (LVEF) below 0.40. It can be symptomatic or asymptomatic. Defining and diagnosing diastolic heart failure can be difficult. Recently proposed criteria include: (1) clinical evidence of heart failure; (2) normal or mildly abnormal left ventricular systolic function; and (3) evidence of abnormal left ventricular relaxation, filling, diastolic distensibility, or diastolic stiffness.[2] The clinical utility of these criteria is limited by difficulty in standardising assessment of the last criterion.

INCIDENCE/ Both the incidence and prevalence of heart failure increase with
PREVALENCE age. Under 65 years of age the incidence is 1/1000 men a year and 0.4/1000 women a year. Over 65 years, incidence is 11/1000 men a year and 5/1000 women a year. Under 65 years the prevalence of heart failure is 1/1000 men and 1/1000 women; over 65 years the

prevalence is 40/1000 men and 30/1000 women.[3] The prevalence of asymptomatic LVSD is 3% in the general population.[4-6] The mean age of people with asymptomatic LVSD is lower than that for symptomatic individuals. Both heart failure and asymptomatic LVSD are more common in men.[4-6] The prevalence of diastolic heart failure in the community is unknown. The prevalence of heart failure with preserved systolic function in people in hospital with clinical heart failure varies from 13% to 74%.[7,8] Less than 15% of people with heart failure under 65 years have normal systolic function, whereas the prevalence is about 40% in people over 65 years.[7]

AETIOLOGY/ RISK FACTORS Coronary artery disease is the most common cause of heart failure.[3] Other common causes include hypertension and idiopathic dilated congestive cardiomyopathy. After adjustment for hypertension, the presence of left ventricular hypertrophy remains a risk factor for the development of heart failure. Other risk factors include cigarette smoking, hyperlipidaemia, and diabetes mellitus.[4] The common causes of left ventricular diastolic dysfunction are coronary artery disease and systemic hypertension. Other causes are hypertrophic cardiomyopathy, restrictive or infiltrative cardiomyopathies, and valvular heart disease.[8]

PROGNOSIS The prognosis of heart failure is poor, with 5 year mortality ranging from 26-75%.[3] Up to 16% of people are re-admitted with heart failure within 6 months of first admission. In the USA it is the leading cause of hospital admission among people over 65 years old.[3] In people with heart failure, a new myocardial infarction increases the risk of death (RR 7.8, 95% CI 6.9 to 8.8); 34% of all deaths in people with heart failure are preceded by a major ischaemic event.[9] Sudden death, mainly caused by ventricular arrhythmias, is responsible for 25-50% of all deaths, and is the most common cause of death in people with heart failure.[10] The presence of asymptomatic LVSD increases an individual's risk of having a cardiovascular event. One large prevention trial found that, for a 5% reduction in ejection fraction, the risk ratio for mortality was 1.20 (95% CI 1.13 to 1.29), for hospital admission for heart failure it was 1.28 (95% CI 1.18 to 1.38), and for development of heart failure it was 1.20 (95% CI 1.13 to 1.26).[4] The annual mortality of patients with diastolic heart failure varies in observational studies (1.3-17.5%).[7] Reasons for this variation include age, the presence of coronary artery disease, and variation in the partition value used to define abnormal ventricular systolic function. The annual mortality for left ventricular diastolic dysfunction is lower than found in patients with systolic dysfunction.[11]

AIMS To relieve symptoms; to improve quality of life; to reduce morbidity and mortality, with minimum adverse effects.

OUTCOMES Functional capacity (assessed by the New York Heart Association [NYHA] functional classification or more objectively by using standardised exercise testing or the 6 minute walk test);[12] quality of life (assessed with questionnaires);[13] mortality; adverse effects of treatment. Proxy measures of clinical outcome (e.g. LVEF, hospital re-admission rates) are used here only when clinical outcomes are unavailable.

METHODS *Clinical Evidence* update search and appraisal October 2000.

QUESTION What are the effects of non-drug treatments?

OPTION MULTIDISCIPLINARY INTERVENTIONS

We found conflicting evidence. One systematic review has found that multidisciplinary approaches to nutrition, patient counselling, and education reduce hospital admissions, may improve quality of life, and enhance patient knowledge. However, the review excluded a large RCT, which found that multidisciplinary follow up increased re-admission rates.

Benefits: We found one systematic review (search date 1998, 7 RCTs, 1164 people with heart failure), which compared treatment for 1–6 months in a multidisciplinary programme versus conventional care alone.[14] The multidisciplinary programme included non-drug treatments such as nutrition advice, counselling, patient education, and exercise training. Six of the RCTs (666 people) were chosen for analysis in the systematic review. The RCTs found that multidisciplinary programmes reduced hospital use, and improved quality of life, functional capacity, patient satisfaction, and compliance with diet and medication compared with conventional care. The four RCTs (543 people) that reported hospital re-admissions over 1–6 months found significant reductions with the intervention (89/286 [31%] with intervention v 116/257 [45%] with control; ARR 14%, 95% CI 6% to 21%; RRR 31%, 95% CI 13% to 47%; NNT 7, 95% CI 5 to 17). The seventh RCT was excluded from analysis in the systematic review but it is not clear how this study differs from those included, apart from its findings. The seventh study included 504 men with heart failure who received conventional follow up or an intensive follow up with their primary care physician and a nurse. This RCT found an increased hospital re-admission rate over 6 months in the intervention group compared with controls (130/249 [52%] for intervention v 106/255 [42%] for control; ARI 11%, 95% CI 2% to 19%; RRI 26%, 95% CI 5% to 46%). Combination of the results of this study with the others found that the intervention had no definite effect compared with control (219/535 [41%] for intervention v 222/512 [43%] for control; ARR +2.4%, 95% CI –3.6% to +8.2%; RRR +5.6%, 95% CI –8% to +19%).

Harms: We found no reports of harm associated with multidisciplinary management.[14]

Comment: Studies were small, involved highly selected patient populations, and were usually performed in academic centres so results may not generalise to smaller community centres. The systematic review excluded, without a priori exclusion criteria, a seventh RCT that found different effects. Interventions varied among studies, and relative merits of each strategy are unknown. Studies generally lasted less than 6 months, and it is not known how well people adhere to treatment over the longer term. Larger studies are needed to define the effects on mortality and morbidity of longer term multidisciplinary interventions.

OPTION	EXERCISE

RCTs have found that prescribed exercise training improves functional capacity and quality of life. One recent RCT has also found that exercise significantly reduces adverse cardiac events.

Benefits: We found one non-systematic review,[15] two systematic reviews,[16,17] one overview of RCTs from a collaborative group,[18] and one subsequent RCT[19] of exercise training in people with heart failure. The reviews and overview identified 20 small RCTs, which reported only proxy outcomes (maximum exercise time [see glossary, p 60], oxygen uptake, various biochemical measures, and unvalidated symptom scores) in a small number of people over a few weeks. No significant adverse effects were found. The subsequent RCT (99 people with heart failure, 88 men) compared 12 months of exercise training versus a control group with no exercise.[19] After 12 months, exercise compared with control improved quality of life ($P < 0.001$), fatal or non-fatal cardiac events (17/50 [34%] with training v 37/49 [76%] with control; ARR 42%, 95% CI 20% to 58%; RRR 55%, 95% CI 27% to 77%; NNT 2), mortality (9/50 [18%] v 20/49 [41%]; RRR 56%, 95% CI 13% to 80%; NNT 4), and hospital re-admission for heart failure (5/50 [10%] v 14/49 [29%]; ARR 19%, 95% CI 3% to 25%; RRR 65%, 95% CI 12% to 88%; NNT 5).[19]

Harms: The reviews and overview reported no important adverse effects associated with prescribed exercise training.[15,16,18]

Comment: The studies were small, involved highly selected patient populations, and were performed in well resourced academic centres. The results may not generalise to smaller community centres. The specific form of exercise training varied among studies and the relative merits of each strategy are unknown. The studies generally lasted less than 1 year and long term effects are unknown. Larger studies over a longer period are needed.

QUESTION	What are the effects of drug treatments in heart failure?

OPTION	ANGIOTENSIN CONVERTING ENZYME (ACE) INHIBITORS

Two systematic reviews and recent RCTs have found that ACE inhibitors reduce mortality, admission to hospital for heart failure, and ischaemic events in people with heart failure. Relative benefits are similar in different groups of people, but absolute benefits are greater in people with severe heart failure.

Benefits: We found two systematic reviews of ACE inhibitors versus placebo in heart failure.[20,21] The first systematic review (search date 1994, 32 RCTs, duration 3–42 months, 7105 people, NYHA class II or worse [see glossary, p 60])[20] found that ACE inhibitors versus placebo reduced mortality (611/3870 [16%] with ACE inhibitors v 709/3235 [22%] with placebo; ARR 6%, 95% CI 4% to 8%; OR 0.77, 95% CI 0.67 to 0.88; NNT 16). Relative reductions in mortality were similar in different subgroups (stratified by age, sex, cause of heart failure, and NYHA class). The second systematic overview (search date not stated, 5 RCTs, 12 763 people with left ventricular dysfunction or heart failure, mean duration 35 months) analysed results from individuals in long term and large RCTs that compared ACE inhibitors versus placebo.[21] Three RCTs were in people for 1 year after myocardial infarction. In these three post infarction trials (5966 people), ACE inhibitor versus placebo significantly reduced mortality (702/2995 [23.4%] v 866/2971 [29.1%]; OR 0.74, 95% CI 0.66 to 0.83), re-admission for heart failure (355/2995 [11.9%] v 460/2971 [15.5%]; OR 0.73, 95% CI 0.63 to 0.85), and reinfarction (324/2995 [10.8%] v 391/2971 [13.2%]; OR 0.80, 95% CI 0.69 to 0.94]). For all five trials, ACE inhibitors versus placebo reduced mortality (1467/6391 [23.0%] v 1710/6372 [26.8%]; OR 0.80, 95% CI 0.74 to 0.87), reinfarction (571/6391 [8.9%] v 703/6372 [11.0%]; OR 0.79, 95% CI 0.70 to 0.89), and re-admission for heart failure (876/6391 [13.7%] v 1202/6372 [18.9%]; OR 0.67, 95% CI 0.61 to 0.74). The benefits began soon after the start of therapy, persisted long term, were independent of age, sex, and baseline use of diuretics, aspirin, and β blockers. Although there was a trend towards greater relative reduction in mortality or re-admission for heart failure in people with lower ejection fractions, benefit was apparent over the range examined. **Other ischaemic events:** Individual RCTs that studied high risk groups found that ACE inhibitors significantly reduced some ischaemic event rates. One RCT in people with left ventricular dysfunction found that, compared with placebo, ACE inhibitors reduced myocardial infarction (combined fatal or non-fatal myocardial infarction: 9.9% v 12.3%; RRR 23%, 95% CI 2% to 39%), hospital admission for angina (15% v 19%; RRR 27%, 95% CI 12% to 40%), and the combined end point of cardiac death, non-fatal myocardial infarction, or hospital admission for angina (43% v 51%; RRR 23%, 95% CI 14% to 32%).[9] Effects on hospital re-admissions were observed shortly after starting ACE inhibitor treatment, although effects on ischaemic events were not apparent for at least 6 months and peaked at 36 months. **Dosage:** We found one large RCT (3164 people with NYHA class II–IV heart failure), which compared low dose lisinopril (2.5 mg or 5.0 mg daily) versus high dose lisinopril (32.5 mg or 35 mg daily).[22] It found no significant difference in mortality (717/1596 [44.9%] with low dose v 666/1568 [42.5%] with high dose; ARR 8%, 95% CI not given; hazard ratio 0.92, 95% CI 0.80 to 1.03; P = 0.128), but found that high dose lisinopril reduced the combined outcome of death or hospital admission for any reason (1338 events with low dose [83.8%] v 1250 events with high dose [79.7%]; ARR 12%; hazard ratio 0.88, 95% CI 0.82–0.96; P = 0.002) and reduced admissions for heart failure (1576 admissions with low dose v 1199 admissions with high dose; ARR 24%; P = 0.002). **Comparison of different ACE inhibitors:** The first systematic review found similar benefits with different ACE inhibitors.[20]

Harms:

We found no systematic review. The main adverse effects documented in large trials were cough, hypotension, hyperkalaemia, and renal dysfunction. Compared with placebo, ACE inhibitors increased the incidence of cough (37% v 31%; ARI 7%, 95% CI 3% to 11%; RRI 23%, 95% CI 11% to 35%; NNH 14), dizziness or fainting (57%

v 50%; ARI 7%, 95% CI 3% to 11%; RRI 14%, 95% CI 6% to 21%; NNH 14), increased creatinine concentrations above 177 µmol/litre (10.7% v 7.7%; ARI 3%, 95% CI 0.6% to 6%; RRI 38%, 95% CI 9% to 67%; NNH 34), and increased potassium concentrations above 5.5 mmol/litre (ARs 6.4% v 2.5%; ARI 4%, 95% CI 2% to 7%; RRI 156%, 95% CI 92% to 220%; NNH 26).[23] Angioedema was not found to be more common with ACE inhibitors than placebo (3.8% taking enalapril v 4.1% taking placebo; ARI +0.3%, 95% CI −1.4% to +1.5%).[23] The trial comparing low and high doses of lisinopril found that most adverse effects were more common with high dose (no P value reported; dizziness: 12% with low dose v 19% with high dose; hypotension: 7% with low dose v 11% with high dose; worsening renal function: 7% with low dose v 10% with high dose; significant change in serum potassium concentration: 7% with low dose v 7% with high dose), although there was no difference in withdrawal rates between groups (17% discontinued with high dose v 18% with low dose). The trial found that cough was less commonly experienced with high dose compared with low dose lisinopril (cough: 13% with low dose v 11% with high dose).

Comment: The relative beneficial effects of ACE inhibitors were similar in different subgroups of people with heart failure. Most RCTs evaluated left ventricular function by assessing LVEF, but some studies defined heart failure clinically, without measurement of left ventricular function in people at high risk of developing heart failure (soon after myocardial infarction). It is unclear whether there are additional benefits from adding ACE inhibitor therapy to people with heart failure who are already taking antiplatelet therapy, and of adding antiplatelet therapy to people with heart failure who are already taking an ACE inhibitor (see antiplatelet agents, p 57).

OPTION	ANGIOTENSIN II RECEPTOR BLOCKERS

One RCT has found that angiotensin II receptor antagonists improve symptom indices compared with placebo. RCTs found no evidence that angiotensin II receptor blockers altered functional capacity or symptoms compared with ACE inhibitors, but the trials were too small to rule out clinically important differences. We found moderate evidence from one RCT that angiotensin II receptor blockers are as effective as ACE inhibitors in reducing all cause mortality.

Benefits: **Versus placebo:** We found one overview[24] and one additional RCT.[18] The overview (3 RCTs, all 12 weeks' duration, 890 people with heart failure NYHA class II and III) found that losartan versus placebo significantly reduced mortality (11/616 [1.8%] with losartan v 13/274 [4.7%] with placebo; OR 0.34, 95% CI 0.14 to 0.80).[24] The RCT (844 people with heart failure NYHA class II and III) compared 12 weeks of candesartan cilexetil (4 mg daily, 208 people v 8 mg daily, 212 people v 16 mg daily, 213 people) versus placebo (211 people).[25] It found that 16 mg candesartan cilexetil daily versus placebo improved exercise time in a standardised symptom limited bicycle ergonometry exercise (47.2 v 30.8 seconds, P = 0.0463). All doses of candesartan cilexetil compared with placebo significantly improved the dyspnoea fatigue index (see glossary, p 60) score (P < 0.001). **Versus ACE inhibitors:**

We found one overview (3 RCTs, 1004 people)[24] and one subsequent RCT.[26] Two of the RCTs in the overview (116 people, NYHA class II and III, duration 8 weeks; and 166 people, NYHA class III and IV, duration 12 weeks) compared losartan versus enalapril. The third RCT in the overview (722 people, NYHA class II and III, duration 48 weeks) compared losartan versus captopril. The overview combined the results of these RCTs and found no significant reduction in mortality for losartan versus ACE inhibitors (25/538 [4.6%] with losartan v 34/466 [7.3%] with ACE inhibitors; OR 0.60, 95% CI 0.34 to 1.04). The subsequent RCT (3152 people, aged ≥60 years, NYHA class II–IV, LVEF ≤40%) found losartan (titrated to 50 mg once daily) versus captopril (titrated to 50 mg three times daily) produced no significant differences in mortality after a median of 555 days (280/1578 [17.7%] with losartan v 250/1574 [15.9%] with captopril; HR 1.13, 95% CI 0.95 to 1.35; P = 0.16). There was also no significant difference in sudden death or resuscitated cardiac arrest (142/1578 [9.0%] v 115/1574 [7.3%]; HR 1.25, 95% CI 0.98 to 1.60; P = 0.08).[26] Significantly fewer patients in the losartan group discontinued study treatment because of adverse effects (9.7% v 14.7%; P < 0.001), including cough (0.3% v 2.7%).

Harms: We found no systematic review. The RCT comparing different doses of candesartan cilexetil versus placebo found no evidence of a difference among groups for serious adverse events (placebo 4.7%; 4 mg 1.4%; 8 mg 5.7%; 16 mg 5.6%) or withdrawal because of adverse events (placebo 4.3%; 4 mg 1.9%; 8 mg 4.7%; 16 mg 5.6%).[25]

Comment: The overview of losartan was company sponsored and included all clinical studies in their evaluation programme.[24] None of the trials of an angiotensin II receptor blocker compared with an ACE inhibitor have been designed with mortality as the primary end point. In people who are truly intolerant of an ACE inhibitor the evidence supports the use of an angiotensin II receptor blocker with the expectation, at the very least, of symptomatic improvement of the heart failure. Pilot studies have examined the efficacy, tolerability, and safety of combining angiotensin II receptor blockers and ACE inhibitors in people with symptomatic heart failure.[27,28] Larger studies are in progress.

OPTION   POSITIVE INOTROPIC AGENTS

We found no evidence that positive inotropic drugs other than digoxin reduce mortality and morbidity in people with heart failure, and most RCTs found that they increased mortality. One well designed RCT found that digoxin decreased the rate of hospital admissions and cointervention for worsening heart failure in people already receiving diuretics and ACE inhibitors, although it found no evidence of an effect on mortality.

Benefits: **Digoxin:** We found one systematic review (search date 1992, 13 RCTs, duration 3–24 weeks, 1138 people with heart failure and sinus rhythm)[29] and one recent large RCT.[30] The systematic review found that six of the 13 RCTs enrolled people without assessment of ventricular function and may have included some people with mild or no heart failure. Other limitations of the older trials included crossover designs and small sample sizes. In people who were in sinus rhythm with heart failure, the systematic review found fewer people with clinical worsening of heart failure (52/628 [8.3%] with digoxin v 131/631 [20.8%] with placebo; ARR 12.5%, 95% CI 9.5% to 14.7%; RRR 60%, 95% CI 46% to 71%) but did not find a definite effect on mortality (16/628 [2.5%] with digoxin v 15/631 [2.4%] with placebo; ARR −0.2%, 95% CI −2.6% to +1.1%; RRR −7%, 95% CI −113% to +47%). The subsequent large RCT randomised 6800 people (88% male, mean age 64 years, NYHA class I–III, 94% already taking ACE inhibitors, 82% taking diuretics) to blinded additional treatment with either digoxin or placebo for a mean of 37 months.[30] Digoxin did not reduce all cause mortality compared with placebo (1181/3397 [34.8%] with digoxin v 1194/3403 [35.1%] with placebo; ARR +0.3%, 95% CI −2.0% to +2.6%; RRR 0.9%, 95% CI −6% to +7%). The number of people admitted to hospital for worsening heart failure was substantially reduced in the digoxin group over 37 months (910/3397 [27%] for digoxin v 1180/3403 [35%] for placebo; ARR 8%, 95% CI 6% to 10%; RRR 23%, 95% CI 17% to 28%; NNT 13) as was the combined outcome of death or hospital admission caused by worsening heart failure (1041/3397 [31%] for digoxin v 1291/3403 [38%] for placebo; ARR 7.3%, 95% CI 5.1% to 9.4%; RRR 19%, 95% CI 13% to 25%; NNT 14). **Other inotropic agents:** Non-digitalis inotropic agents have been evaluated in RCTs, including up to 3600 people. Some of these studies found improved functional capacity and quality of life but not consistently across all studies. We found no evidence that positive inotropic agents decrease mortality; most RCTs found increased risk of death (see harms below).

Harms: We found no systematic review. **Digoxin:** The RCT (6800 people) found that more participants had suspected digoxin toxicity in the digoxin group versus placebo (11.9% v 7.9%; ARI 4%, 95% CI 2.4% to 5.8%; RRI 50%, 95% CI 30% to 73%; NNH 25).[30] The trial found no evidence that digoxin increased the risk of ventricular fibrillation or tachycardia compared with placebo (37/3397 [1.1%] with digoxin v 27/3403 [0.8%] with placebo; ARI +0.3%, 95% CI −0.1% to +1.0%; RRI 37%, 95% CI −16% to +124%). Digoxin compared with placebo increased rates of supraventricular arrhythmia (2.5% with digoxin v 1.2% with placebo; ARI 1.3%, 95% CI 0.5% to 2.4%; RRI 108%, 95% CI 44% to 199%; NNH 77) and second or third degree atrioventricular block (1.2% v 0.4%; ARI 0.8%, 95% CI 0.2% to 1.8%; RRI 193%, 95% CI 61% to 434%; NNH 126). **Other inotropic agents:** RCTs found that non-digitalis positive inotropic agents increase mortality compared with placebo.[10] One RCT (1088 people with heart failure) found milrinone versus placebo increased mortality over 6 months (168/561 [30%] v 127/527 [24%] for placebo; ARI 6%, 95% CI 0.5% to 12%; RRI 24%, 95% CI 2% to 49%; NNH 17).[31] Another RCT (3833 people with heart failure) found increased mortality with 60 mg vesnarinone a day versus placebo for 9 months (292/1275 [23%] for 60 mg vesnarinone v 242/1280 [19%] for placebo; ARI 4%, 95% CI 1% to 8%; RRI 21%, 95% CI 4% to 40%; NNH 25).[10]

Comment: None.

OPTION	β BLOCKERS

We found strong evidence from systematic reviews of RCTs that adding β blockers to standard treatment with ACE inhibitors in people with moderate heart failure reduces the rate of death or hospital admission. The reviews found less robust evidence that β blockers improve exercise capacity.

Benefits: We found one recent systematic review[32] and two subsequent large RCTs[29,30] of the effects of β blockers in heart failure. The systematic review (search date not stated, 18 RCTs of β blockers versus placebo, 1.5–44 months, 3023 people with heart failure) obtained details of outcomes directly from trial investigators.[32] The participants had idiopathic dilated cardiomyopathy (1718 people) or ischaemic heart disease (1513 people). Trials in people after an acute myocardial infarction were excluded. Most participants had NYHA class II or III symptoms. The systematic review found strong evidence that β blockers reduced the combined outcome of death or admission to hospital (239/1486 [16%] on β blockers v 293/1155 [25%] on placebo; ARR 9%, 95% CI 7% to 12%; RRR 37%, 95% CI 26% to 46%; NNT 11). The result was robust to the addition of neutral results from further trials. The review also found that addition of β blockers reduced total mortality compared with placebo (130/1718 [8%] for β blockers v 156/1305 [12%] for placebo; ARR 4%, 95% CI 2% to 6%; RRR 37%, 95% CI 21% to 50%; NNT 23) and improved NYHA class. These results were less robust (the conclusion could be altered by addition or removal of only one moderate sized study). The two subsequent RCTs[33,34] found stronger evidence of reduced mortality from the additional use of β blockers compared with placebo in heart failure. The first RCT (2647 people, NYHA class III–IV) compared additional bisoprolol versus placebo.[33] The RCT was stopped early because of significant reduction in the bisoprolol group after 1.3 years in all cause mortality (156/1327 [11.8%] for bisoprolol v 228/1320 [17.3%] for placebo; ARR 5.5%, 95% CI 3.0% to 7.6%; RRR 32%, 95% CI 18% to 44%; NNT 18) and sudden deaths (48/1327 [3.6%] for bisoprolol v 83/1320 [6.3%] for placebo; ARR 2.7%, 95% CI 1.2% to 3.7%; RRR 42%, 95% CI 19% to 60%; NNT 37). The second RCT (3991 people, NYHA class II–IV) compared additional controlled release metoprolol versus placebo.[34] It was stopped early because of significant reduction in the metoprolol group of mortality after 1 year (145/1990 [7.3%] for metoprolol v 217/2001 [10.8%] for placebo; ARR 3.6%, 95% CI 1.9% to 4.9%; RRR 33%, 95% CI 18% to 45%; NNT 28), sudden death and deaths from worsening heart failure.

Harms: Fears that β blockers may cause excessive problems with worsening heart failure, bradyarrhythmias, or hypotension have not been confirmed. In one RCT, the overall drug discontinuation rate for adverse reactions was 7.8% in the placebo group and 5.7% in the carvedilol group.[32] The findings from the RCT of metoprolol were similar, with the study drug discontinued in 13.9% of the controlled release metoprolol group and in 15.3% of the placebo group (RR 0.91, 95% CI 0.78 to 1.06).[34]

Comment: Good evidence was found for the use of β blockers in people with moderate symptoms (NYHA class II–III) receiving standard treatment, including ACE inhibitors. The value of β blockers needs clarification in NYHA class IV, in heart failure with preserved ejection fraction, in asymptomatic LVSD, and in heart failure after an acute myocardial infarction. The RCTs of β blockers have consistently found a mortality benefit, but it is not clear whether or not the benefit is a class effect. One recent small RCT (150 people) of metoprolol versus carvedilol found some differences in surrogate outcomes, but both drugs produced similar improvements in symptoms, submaximal exercise tolerance, and quality of life.[35] An RCT is comparing the effect of metoprolol versus carvedilol on survival.[35]

OPTION   CALCIUM CHANNEL BLOCKERS

We found no evidence that calcium channel blockers are of benefit in people with heart failure.

Benefits: **After myocardial infarction:** See calcium channel blockers under acute myocardial infarction, p 8. **Other heart failure:** We found one non-systematic review (3 RCTs, 1790 people with heart failure)[10] and one subsequent RCT.[10] One RCT (1153 people, NYHA class III–IV, LVEF < 0.30, using diuretics digoxin and ACE inhibitors) found that amlodipine versus placebo had no significant effect on the primary combined end point of all cause mortality and hospital admission for cardiovascular events over 14 months (222/571 [39%] for amlodipine v 246/582 [42%] for placebo; ARR +3.4%, 95% CI −2.3% to +8.8%; RRR 8%, 95% CI −6% to +21%).[36] Subgroup analysis of people with primary cardiomyopathy found a reduction in mortality (45/209 [22%] for amlodipine v 74/212 [35%] for placebo; ARR 13%, 95% CI 5% to 20%; RRR 38%, 95% CI 15% to 57%; NNT 7). There was no significant difference in the group with heart failure caused by coronary artery disease. The subsequent RCT (186 people, idiopathic dilated cardiomyopathy, NYHA class I–III) compared diltiazem versus placebo.[10] It found no evidence of a difference in survival with diltiazem versus placebo in those who did not have a heart transplant, although people on diltiazem had improved cardiac function, exercise capacity, and subjective quality of life. A third RCT (451 people with mild heart failure, NYHA class II–III) compared felodipine versus placebo.[10] No significant adverse or beneficial effect was found.

Harms: Calcium channel blockers have been found to exacerbate symptoms of heart failure or increase mortality in people with pulmonary congestion after myocardial infarct or ejection fraction less than 0.40 (see calcium channel blockers under acute myocardial infarction, p 8).[10]

Comment: Many of the RCTs were underpowered and had wide confidence intervals. An RCT is in progress to test the hypothesis that amlodipine decreases mortality in people with primary dilated cardiomyopathy.

OPTION	ALDOSTERONE RECEPTOR ANTAGONISTS

One recent large RCT of people with severe heart failure (on usual treatment including ACE inhibitor) has found that adding an aldosterone receptor antagonist (spironolactone) further decreases mortality.

Benefits: We found no systematic review. We found one RCT of spironolactone (25 mg daily) versus placebo in 1663 people with heart failure (NYHA class III–IV, LVEF < 0.35, all taking ACE inhibitors and loop diuretics, and most taking digoxin).[37] The trial was stopped early because of a significant reduction in the primary end point of all cause mortality for spironolactone versus placebo after 2 years (mortality 284/822 [35%] for spironolactone v 386/841 [46%] for placebo; ARR 11%, 95% CI 7% to 16%; RRR 25%, 95% CI 15% to 34%; NNT 9).

Harms: The trial found no evidence that spironolactone in combination with an ACE inhibitor may result in an increased incidence of clinically significant hyperkalaemia. Gynaecomastia or breast pain was reported in 10% of men given spironolactone and 1% of men given placebo.[37]

Comment: The RCT was large and well designed. As only NYHA functional class III–IV patients were randomised into the study, these data cannot necessarily be generalised to people with milder heart failure.

OPTION	ANTIARRHYTHMIC DRUG TREATMENT

Systematic reviews found weak evidence that amiodarone reduces total mortality in people with heart failure. Other antiarrhythmic agents may increase mortality in people with heart failure.

Benefits: **Amiodarone:** We found two systematic reviews of the effects of amiodarone versus placebo in heart failure.[38,39] The most recent review (10 RCTs, 4766 people) included people with a wide range of conditions (symptomatic and asymptomatic heart failure, ventricular arrhythmia, recent myocardial infarction, and recent cardiac arrest).[38] Eight of these studies reported the number of deaths. The review found that treatment with amiodarone over 3–24 months reduced the risk of death from any cause compared with placebo or conventional treatment (436/2262 [19%] for amiodarone v 507/2263 [22%] for control; ARR 3%, 95% CI 0.8% to 5.3%; RRR 14%, 95% CI 4% to 24%; NNT 32). This review did not perform any subgroup analyses to reveal the effect of amiodarone on people with heart failure. The earlier systematic review found eight RCTs (5101 people after myocardial infarction) of prophylactic amiodarone versus placebo or usual care and five RCTs (1452 people with heart failure).[39] Mean follow up was 16 months. Analysis of data from all 13 RCTs found a lower total mortality with amiodarone than control (10.9% v 12.3% dead per year). The effect was significant with some methods of calculation (fixed effects model: OR 0.87, 95% CI 0.78 to 0.99) but not with others (random effects model: OR 0.85, 95% CI 0.71 to 1.02). The effect of amiodarone was significantly greater in RCTs that compared amiodarone versus usual care than in placebo controlled RCTs. Deaths classified as arrhythmic death or sudden death were significantly reduced by amiodarone compared with placebo (OR 0.71, 95% CI 0.59 to 0.85). Subgroup analysis found a significant effect of amiodarone in the five heart failure RCTs (19.9% deaths per year v 24.3% in the placebo group; OR 0.83, 95% CI 0.70 to 0.99). **Other antiarrhythmics:** Apart from β blockers, other antiarrhythmic drugs seem to increase mortality in people at high risk (see antiarrhythmics under secondary prevention of ischaemic cardiac events, p 95).

Harms: **Amiodarone:** Amiodarone was not found to increase the non-arrhythmic death rate (OR 1.02, 95% CI 0.87 to 1.19).[39] In placebo controlled RCTs, after 2 years 41% of people in the amiodarone group and 27% in the placebo group had permanently discontinued study medication.[34] In 10 RCTs of amiodarone versus placebo, amiodarone increased the odds of reporting adverse drug reactions compared with placebo (OR 2.22, 95% CI 1.83 to 2.68). Nausea was the most common adverse effect. Hypothyroidism was the most common serious adverse effect (7.0% of amiodarone treated group versus 1.1% of controls). Hyperthyroidism (1.4% v 0.5%), peripheral neuropathy (0.5% v 0.2%), lung infiltrates (1.6% v 0.5%), bradycardia (2.4% v 0.8%), and liver dysfunction (1.0% v 0.4%) were all more common in the amiodarone group.[39] **Other antiarrhythmics:** These agents (particularly class I antiarrhythmics) may increase mortality (see antiarrhythmics under secondary prevention of ischaemic cardiac events, p 95).

Comment: **Amiodarone:** RCTs of amiodarone versus usual treatment found larger effects than placebo controlled trials.[39] These findings suggest bias; unblinded follow up may be associated with reduced usual care or improved adherence with amiodarone. Further studies are required to assess the effects of amiodarone treatment on mortality and morbidity in people with heart failure.

OPTION	IMPLANTABLE CARDIAC DEFIBRILLATORS

Three RCTs have found good evidence that the ICD reduces mortality in people with heart failure who have experienced a cardiac arrest. The review found conflicting evidence for prophylactic implantation of ICDs in people at risk of arrhythmia.

Benefits: We found no systematic review. We found three RCTs examining the effects of ICDs in people with left ventricular dysfunction.[40–42] The first RCT (1016 people resuscitated after ventricular arrhythmia plus either syncope or other serious cardiac symptom plus left ventricular ejection fraction ≤ 0.40) compared an ICD versus an antiarrhythmic drug (mainly amiodarone).[40] ICDs versus an antiarrhythmic drug improved survival at 1, 2, and 3 years (1 year survival: 89.3% with ICD v 82.3% with antiarrhythmic; 2 year survival 81.6% v 73.7%; 3 year survival 75.4% v 64.1%). The second RCT included 196 people with NYHA class I–III heart failure and previous myocardial infarction, a left ventricular ejection fraction ≤ 0.35, a documented episode of asymptomatic unsustained ventricular tachycardia, and inducible non-suppressible ventricular tachyarrhythmia on electrophysiologic study.[41] Ninety five people received an implantable defibrillator and 101 received conventional medical treatment. The trial found that ICDs compared with conventional treatment reduced mortality over a mean of 27 months (deaths: 15/95 [16%] with ICD [11 from cardiac cause] v 39/101 [39%] with conventional therapy [27 from cardiac cause]; HR 0.46, 95% CI 0.26 to 0.82). The third RCT included 1055 people aged under 80 years who were scheduled for coronary artery bypass surgery, had a left ventricular ejection less than 0.36, and had electrocardiographic abnormalities. It found that ICD (446 people) at the time of bypass surgery versus no ICD (454 people) produced no significant difference in mortality over a mean of 32 months (deaths: 101/446 [23%] with ICD [71 from cardiac causes] v 95/454 [21%] with control [72 from cardiac causes]; HR 1.07, 95% CI 0.81 to 1.42; P = 0.64).[42]

Harms: The three RCTs found that the main adverse effects of ICDs were infection (about 5%), pneumothorax (about 2%), bleeding requiring further operation (about 1%), serious haematomas (about 3%), cardiac perforation (about 0.2%), problems with defibrillator lead (about 7%), and malfunction of defibrillator generator (about 3%).[40–42]

Comment: The RCTs were all in people with previous ventricular arrhythmias. It is uncertain whether asymptomatic ventricular arrhythmia is in itself a predictor of sudden death in people with moderate or severe heart failure.[43] The role of ICDs in other groups of people with heart failure awaits evaluation. Several RCTs of prophylactic ICD treatment are ongoing in people with heart failure and in survivors of acute myocardial infarction.[44]

| OPTION | ANTICOAGULATION | New |

We found no RCTs of anticoagulation in people with heart failure. We found conflicting evidence from two large retrospective cohort studies.

Benefits: We found no RCTs of anticoagulation in people with heart failure. We found conflicting evidence from two large retrospective cohort studies.[45,46] The first retrospective analysis (2 RCTs) assessed the effect of anticoagulants used at the discretion of individual investigators on the incidence of stroke, peripheral arterial embolism, and pulmonary embolism.[45] One RCT (642 men with chronic heart failure) compared hydralazine and isosorbide dinitrate versus prazosin versus placebo. The other RCT (804 men with chronic heart failure) compared enalapril plus isosorbide dinitrate versus hydralazine plus isosorbide dinitrate. All people were given digoxin and diuretics. The retrospective analysis found that without treatment the incidence of all thromboembolic events was low (2.7 per 100 patient years in the first RCT, 2.1 per 100 patient years in the second RCT) and that anticoagulation did not reduce the incidence of thromboembolic events (2.9 per 100 patient years in the first RCT, 4.8 per 100 patient years in the second RCT). In this group of people, atrial fibrillation was not found to be associated with a higher risk of thromboembolic events. The second retrospective analysis included two large RCTs, which compared enalapril versus placebo in 2569 people with symptomatic and asymptomatic left ventricular dysfunction.[46] The analysis found that people treated with warfarin at baseline had significantly lower risk of death during follow up (hazards ratio adjusted for baseline differences 0.76, 95% CI 0.65 to 0.89). Warfarin use was associated with a reduction in the combined outcome of death plus hospitalisation for heart failure (adjusted HR 0.82, 95% CI 0.72 to 0.93). The benefit with warfarin use was not significantly influenced by the presence or absence of symptoms, randomisation to enalapril or placebo, gender, presence or absence of atrial fibrillation, age, ejection fraction, NYHA classification, or cause of heart failure. Warfarin reduced cardiac mortality, specifically deaths that were sudden, associated with heart failure, or associated with myocardial infarction.

Harms: Neither cohort study reported harms of anticoagulation.

Comment: Neither of the retrospective studies were designed to determine the incidence of thromboembolic events in heart failure or the effects of treatment. Neither study included information about the intensity of anticoagulation or warfarin use. We found several additional cohort studies, which showed a reduction in thromboembolic events with anticoagulation, but they all reported results for groups of people that were too small to provide useful data. An RCT is needed to compare anticoagulation versus no anticoagulation in people with heart failure.

| OPTION | ANTIPLATELET AGENTS | New |

We found no RCTs. Retrospective analyses have included two few events to establish or exclude a clinically important effect of antiplatelet agents in people with heart failure. In people not taking ACE inhibitors we found limited evidence from one retrospective cohort analysis that the incidence of thromboembolic events in people with heart failure was low and not significantly improved with antiplatelet therapy. It is unclear from limited evidence from two retrospective cohort analyses whether there are additional reductions in the incidence of thromboembolic events from adding ACE inhibitor therapy to antiplatelet therapy in people with heart failure. It is unclear whether adding antiplatelet therapy to ACE inhibitor treatment in people with heart failure is beneficial.

Benefits: **In people not taking ACE inhibitors:** We found no systematic review and no RCTs. We found one retrospective cohort analysis of one RCT in 642 men with heart failure.[45] The RCT compared hydralazine plus isosorbide dinitrate versus prazosin versus placebo in men receiving digoxin and diuretics. Aspirin, dipyridamole, or both, were used at the discretion of the investigators. The number of thromboembolic events was low in both groups (only 1 stroke and no pulmonary or peripheral emboli in 184 patient years of treatment with antiplatelet drugs v 21 strokes, 4 peripheral and 4 pulmonary emboli in 1068 patient years of treatment without antiplatelet drugs; 0.5 events per 100 patient years with antiplatelet agents v 2.0 events per 100 patient years without antiplatelet agents; P = 0.07). **In people taking ACE inhibitors:** We found no RCTs. We found two large retrospective cohort studies.[45,47] The first retrospective analysis (1 RCT) assessed the effect of antiplatelet agents used at the discretion of individual investigators on the incidence of stroke, peripheral arterial embolism, and pulmonary embolism.[45] The RCT (804 men with chronic heart failure) compared enalapril plus isosorbide dinitrate versus hydralazine plus isosorbide dinitrate. It found that the incidence of all thromboembolic events was low without antiplatelet treatment and, although antiplatelet agents reduced the thromboembolic rate, the difference was not significant (2.1 events per 100 patient years with no antiplatelet agent v 1.6 per 100 patient years with antiplatelet agents; P = 0.48). The second cohort analysis included two large RCTs, which compared enalapril versus placebo (2569 people with symptomatic and asymptomatic left ventricular dysfunction). It found that people treated with antiplatelet agents at baseline had a significantly lower risk of death (HR adjusted for baseline differences 0.82, 95% CI 0.73 to 0.92).[47] Subgroup analysis suggested that an effect of antiplatelet agents might be present in people who were randomised to placebo (mortality HR for antiplatelet treatment at baseline v no antiplatelet treatment at baseline 0.68, 95% CI 0.58 to 0.80), but not in people randomised to enalapril (mortality HR for antiplatelet treatment v no antiplatelet treatment 1.00, 95% CI 0.85 to 1.17).

Harms: Neither study reported harms of treatment.

Comment: Both retrospective studies have limitations common to studies with a retrospective cohort design. One study did not report on the proportions of people taking aspirin and other antiplatelet agents.[45] The other study noted that more than 95% of people took aspirin, but the dosage and consistency of antiplatelet use was not noted.[47] One retrospective overview (4 RCTs, 96 712 people, search date not stated) provided additional evidence about the effect of aspirin on the benefits of early ACE inhibitors in heart failure.[48] It found a similar reduction in 30 day mortality with ACE inhibitor versus control for those people not taking aspirin compared to those taking aspirin (no aspirin: OR 0.90, 95% CI 0.81 to 1.01; aspirin: OR 0.94, 95% CI 0.89 to 0.99). However, the analysis may not be valid because the group of people who did not receive aspirin were older and had a worse baseline prognosis than those taking aspirin. The effects of antiplatelet therapy in combination with ACE inhibitors in people with heart failure requires further research.

QUESTION **What are the effects of ACE inhibitors in people at high risk of heart failure?**

RCTs have found good evidence that ACE inhibitors can delay development of symptomatic heart failure and reduce the frequency of cardiovascular events in people with asymptomatic LVSD, and in people with other cardiovascular risk factors for heart failure.

Benefits: **In people with asymptomatic LVSD:** We found no systematic review but found two RCTs. One large RCT examined ACE inhibitors versus placebo over 40 months in people with asymptomatic LVSD (LVEF < 0.35).[49] It found no evidence that ACE inhibitors significantly decreased total mortality and cardiovascular mortality compared with placebo (all cause mortality: 313/2111 [14.8%] for ACE inhibitor v 334/2117 [15.8%] for placebo; ARR 0.9%, 95% CI −1.3% to +2.9%; RRR 6%, 95% CI −8% to +19%; cardiovascular mortality: 265/2111 [12.6%] for ACE inhibitor v 298/2117 [14.1%] for placebo; ARR +1.5%, 95% CI −0.6% to +3.3%; RRR

11%, 95% CI −4% to +24%). During the study, more people assigned to the placebo than to the enalapril group received digoxin, diuretics, or ACE inhibitor that were not part of the study protocol, which may have contributed to the lack of significant difference in mortality between the two groups. Compared with placebo, ACE inhibitors reduced symptomatic heart failure, reduced hospital admission for heart failure, and reduced fatal or non-fatal myocardial infarction (symptomatic heart failure: 438/2111 [21%] for ACE inhibitor v 640/2117 [30%] for placebo; ARR 9.5%, 95% CI 7% to 12%; RRR 31%, 95% CI 23% to 39%; NNT 11; admission for heart failure: 306/2111 [15%] for ACE inhibitor v 454/2117 [21%] for placebo; ARR 7%, 95% CI 5% to 9%; RRR 32%, 95% CI 23% to 41%; NNT 14; fatal or non-fatal myocardial infarction: 7.6% for ACE inhibitor v 9.6% for placebo; ARR 2%, 95% CI 0.4% to 3.4%; RRR 21%, 95% CI 4% to 35%).[9,49] A second trial in asymptomatic people after myocardial infarction with documented LVSD found that ACE inhibitors (captopril) reduced mortality and reduced risk of ischaemic events compared with placebo.[50] **In people with other risk factors:** We found one large RCT comparing ramipril 10 mg daily versus placebo in 9297 high risk people (people with vascular disease or diabetes plus one other cardiovascular risk factor) who were not known to have LVSD or heart failure, for a mean of 5 years.[51] It found that ramipril reduced the risk of heart failure (9.0% with ramipril v 11.5% with placebo, RR 0.77, 95% CI 0.67 to 0.87, P < 0.001). Ramipril also reduced the combined risk of myocardial infarction or stroke or cardiovascular death, reduced the risk of these outcomes separately, and reduced all cause mortality (see ACE inhibitors in people at high risk under secondary prevention of ischaemic cardiac events, p 95). During the trial, 496 people underwent echocardiography; 2.6% of these people were found to have ejection fraction less than 0.40. Retrospective review of charts found that left ventricular function had been documented in 5193 people; 8.1% had a reduced ejection fraction.

Harms: We found no systematic review. The first RCT over 40 months found that a high proportion of people in both groups reported adverse effects (76% in the enalapril group v 72% in the placebo group).[49] Dizziness or fainting (46% v 33%) and cough (34% v 27%) were reported more often in the enalapril group (no P value reported). The incidence of angioedema was the same (1.4%) in both groups. Study medication was permanently discontinued by 8% of the participants in the enalapril group versus 5% in the placebo group (no P value reported).

Comment: Asymptomatic LVSD is prognostically important, but we found no prospective studies that have assessed the usefulness of screening to detect its presence.

QUESTION	What are the effects of treatments for diastolic heart failure? New

We found no randomised controlled trials in people with diastolic heart failure.

Benefits: We found no systematic review or RCTs in people with diastolic heart failure.

Cardiovascular disorders

Harms: We found no evidence on the harms of treatments for diastolic heart failure.

Comment: The causes of diastolic dysfunction vary among people with diastolic heart failure. Current treatment is empirical, based on the results of small clinical studies, and consists of treating the underlying cause and coexistent conditions with interventions optimised for individuals.[6,52,53] RCTs with clinically relevant outcome measures are needed to determine the benefits and harms of treatment in diastolic heart failure.

GLOSSARY

Dyspnoea fatigue index Measures impact of breathlessness on ability to carry out activities of daily living, with a scale from 0 to 12.

Exercise time This is the total time in seconds that a person is able to pedal in a standardised symptom limited bicycle ergonometry exercise test.

NYHA class Classification of severity by symptoms. Class I: no limitation of physical activity; ordinary physical activity does not cause undue fatigue or dysponea. Class II: slight limitation of physical activity; comfortable at rest, but ordinary physical activity results in fatigue or dyspnoea. Class III: limitation of physical activity; comfortable at rest, but less than ordinary activity causes fatigue or dyspnoea. Class IV: unable to carry on any physical activity without symptoms; symptoms are present even at rest; if any physical activity is undertaken, symptoms are increased.

Substantive changes since last issue

Angiotensin II receptor blockers One new overview found improvement in mortality with angiotensin II receptor blockers similar to ACE inhibitors.[24] One new RCT found no significant effect on mortality and morbidity with losartan versus captopril.[26] Categorisation of angiotensin II receptor blockers moved from "unknown" to "beneficial".

REFERENCES

1. Poole-Wilson PA. History, definition, and classification of heart failure. In: Poole-Wilson PA, Colucci WS, Massie BM, Chatterjee K, Coats AJS, eds. *Heart failure. Scientific principles and clinical practice.* London: Churchill Livingston, 1997:269–277.

2. Working Group Report. How to diagnose diastolic heart failure: European Study Group on Diastolic Heart Failure. *Eur Heart J* 1998;19:990–1003.

3. Cowie MR, Mosterd A, Wood DA, et al. The epidemiology of heart failure. *Eur Heart J* 1997; 18:208–225.

4. McKelvie RS, Benedict CR, Yusuf S. Prevention of congestive heart failure and management of asymptomatic left ventricular dysfunction. *BMJ* 1999;318:1400–1402.

5. Bröckel U, Hense HW, Museholl M, Döring A, Riegger GA, Schunkert H. Prevalence of left ventricular dysfunction in the general population [abstract]. *J Am Coll Cardiol* 1996;27(suppl A):25.

6. Mosterd A, deBruijne MC, Hoes A, Deckers JW, Hofman A, Grobbee DE. Usefulness of echocardiography in detecting left ventricular dysfunction in population-based studies (the Rotterdam study). *Am J Cardiol* 1997;79:103–104.

7. Vasan RS, Benjamin EJ, Levy D. Congestive heart failure with normal left ventricular systolic function. *Arch Intern Med* 1996;156:146–157.

8. Davie AP, Francis CM, Caruana L, Sutherland GR, McMurray JV. The prevalence of left ventricular diastolic filling abnormalities in patients with suspected heart failure. *Eur Heart J* 1997;18: 981–984.

9. Yusuf S, Pepine CJ, Garces C, et al. Effect of enalapril on myocardial infarction and unstable angina in patients with low ejection fractions. *Lancet* 1992;340:1173–1178.

10. Gheorghiade M, Benatar D, Konstam MA, Stoukides CA, Bonow RO. Pharmacotherapy for systolic dysfunction: a review of randomized clinical trials. *Am J Cardiol* 1997;80(suppl 8B): 14–27H.

11. Gaasch WH. Diagnosis and treatment of heart failure based on LV systolic or diastolic dysfunction. *JAMA* 1994;271:1276–1280.

12. Bittner V, Weiner DH, Yusuf S, et al, for the SOLVD Investigators. Prediction of mortality and morbidity with a 6-minute walk test in patients with left ventricular dysfunction. *JAMA* 1993;270:1702–1707.

13. Rogers WJ, Johnstone DE, Yusuf S, et al, for the SOLVD Investigators. Quality of life among 5 025 patients with left ventricular dysfunction randomized between placebo and enalapril. The studies of left ventricular dysfunction. *J Am Coll Cardiol* 1994;23:393–400.

14. Rich MW. Heart failure disease management: a critical review. *J Cardiac Fail* 1999;5:64–75. Search dates 1983 to 1998; primary sources Medline; references in published articles.

15. Miller TD, Balady GJ, Fletcher GF. Exercise and its role in the prevention and rehabilitation of cardiovascular disease. *Ann Behav Med* 1997;19: 220–229.

16. Dracup K, Baker DW, Dunbar SB, et al. Management of heart failure. II. Counseling, education and lifestyle modifications. *JAMA* 1994; 272:1442–1446. Search date 1993; primary sources Medline; Embase.

17. Piepoli MF, Flater M, Coats AJS. Overview of studies of exercise training in chronic heart failure: the need for a prospective randomized multi-centre European trial. *Eur Heart J* 1998;19:830–841. Search date and primary sources not stated; computed-aided search performed.

18. European Heart Failure Training Group. Experience from controlled trials of physical training in chronic heart failure. Protocol and patient factors in effectiveness in the improvement in exercise tolerance. *Eur Heart J* 1998;19:466–475.

19. Belardinelli R, Georgiou D, Cianci G, Purcaro A. Randomized, controlled trial of long-term moderate exercise training in chronic heart failure. Effects on functional capacity, quality of life, and clinical outcomes. *Circulation* 1999;99:1173–1182.

20. Garg R, Yusuf S, for the Collaborative Group on ACE Inhibitor Trials. Overview of randomized trials of angiotensin-converting enzyme inhibitors on mortality and morbidity in patients with heart failure. *JAMA* 1995;273:1450–1456. Search date 1994; primary sources Medline; correspondence with investigators and pharmaceutical firms.

21. Flather M, Yusuf S, Køber L, et al, for the ACE-Inhibitor Myocardial Infarction Collaborative Group. Long-term ACE-inhibitor therapy in patients with heart failure or left-ventricular dysfunction: a systematic overview of data from individual patients. *Lancet* 2000;355:1575–1581. Search date not stated; primary sources Medline; Ovid; and hand searches of reference lists and personal contact with researchers, colleagues and principal investigators of the trials identified.

22. Packer M, Poole-Wilson PA, Armstrong PW, et al, on behalf of the ATLAS Study Group. Comparative effects of low and high doses of the angiotensin-converting enzyme inhibitor, lisinopril, on morbidity and mortality in chronic heart failure. *Circulation* 1999;100:2312–2318.

23. SOLVD Investigators. Effect of enalapril on survival in patients with reduced left ventricular ejection fractions and congestive heart failure. *N Engl J Med* 1991;325:293–302.

24. Sharma D, Buyse M, Pitt B, Rucinska EJ, and the Losartan Heart Failure Mortality Meta-analysis Study Group. Meta-analysis of observed mortality data from all-controlled, double-blind, multiple-dose studies of losartan in heart failure. *Am J Cardiol* 2000;85:187–192.

25. Riegger GAJ, Bouzo H, Petr P, et al, for the Symptom, Tolerability, Response to Exercise Trial of Candesartan Cilexetil in Heart Failure (STRETCH) Investigators. Improvement in exercise tolerance and symptoms of congestive heart failure during treatment with candesartan cilexetil. *Circulation* 1999;100:2224–2230.

26. Pitt B, Poole-Wilson PA, Segal R, et al, on behalf of the ELITE II investigators. Effect of losartan compared with captopril on mortality in patients with symptomatic heart failure: randomised trial. *Lancet* 2000;355:1582–1587.

27. McKelvie R, Yusuf S, Pericak D, Lindgren E, Held P, for the RESOLVD Investigators. Comparison of candesartan, enalapril, and their combination in congestive heart failure: randomized evaluation of strategies for left ventricular dysfunction (RESOLVD pilot study). *Circulation* 1999;100:1056–1064.

28. Hamroff G, Katz SD, Mancini D, et al. Addition of angiotensin II receptor blockade to maximal angiotensin-converting enzyme inhibition improves exercise capacity in patients with severe congestive heart failure. *Circulation* 1999;99:990–992.

29. Kraus F, Rudolph C, Rudolph W. Wirksamkeit von Digitalis bei Patienten mit chronischer Herzinsuffizienz und Sinusrhythmus. *Herz* 1993; 18:95–117. Search date 1992; primary source Medline.

30. Digitalis Investigation Group. The effect of digoxin on mortality and morbidity in patients with heart failure. *N Engl J Med* 1997;336:525–533.

31. Packer M, Carver JR, Rodeheffer RJ, et al, for the PROMISE Study Research Group. Effect of oral milrinone on mortality in severe chronic heart failure. *N Engl J Med* 1991;325:1468–1475.

32. Lechat P, Packer M, Chalon S, Cucherat M, Arab T, Boissel J-P. Clinical effects of β-adrenergic blockade in chronic heart failure. A meta-analysis of double-blind, placebo-controlled, randomized trials. *Circulation* 1998;98:1184–1191. Search date not stated; primary sources Medline; reference lists; colleagues; pharmaceutical industry.

33. CIBIS-II Investigators and Committees. The cardiac insufficiency bisoprolol study II (CIBIS-II): a randomised study. *Lancet* 1999;353:9–13.

34. MERIT-HF Study Group. Effect of metoprolol CR/XL in chronic heart failure: metoprolol CR/XL randomised intervention trial in congestive heart failure. *Lancet* 1999;353:2001–2007.

35. Metra M, Giubbini R, Nodari S, Boldi E, Modena MG, Cas LD. Differential effects of β-blockers in patients with heart failure: a prospective, randomized, double-blind comparison of the long-term effects of metoprolol versus carvedilol. *Circulation* 2000;102:546–551.

36. Packer M, O'Connor CM, Ghali JK, et al, for the Prospective Randomized Amlodipine Survival Evaluation Study Group. Effect of amlodipine on morbidity and mortality in severe chronic heart failure. *N Engl J Med* 1996;335:1107–1114.

37. Pitt B, Zannad F, Remme WJ, et al, for the Randomized Aldactone Evaluation Study Investigators. The effects of spironolactone on morbidity and mortality in patients with severe heart failure. *N Engl J Med* 1999;341:709–717.

38. Piepoli M, Villani GQ, Ponikowski P, Wright A, Flather MD, Coats AJ. Overview and meta-analysis of randomised trials of amiodarone in chronic heart failure. *Int J Cardiol* 1998;66:1–10. Search date 1997; primary sources unspecified computerised literature database.

39. Amiodarone Trials Meta-Analysis Investigators. Effect of prophylactic amiodarone on mortality after acute myocardial infarction and in congestive heart failure: meta-analysis of individual data from 6500 patients in randomised trials. *Lancet* 1997; 350:1417–1424. Search date not stated; primary sources literature review, computerised literature review, and discussion with colleagues.

40. The Antiarrhythmic versus Implantable Defibrillators (AVID) Investigators. A comparison of antiarrhythmic-drug therapy with implantable defibrillators I patients resuscitated from near-fatal ventricular arrhythmias. *N Engl J Med* 1997;337: 1576–1583.

41. Moss AJ, Hall WJ, Cannom DS, et al. Improved survival with an implanted defibrillator in patients with coronary disease at high risk for ventricular arrhythmia. *N Engl J Med* 1996;335:1933–1940.

42. Bigger JT for The Coronary Artery Bypass Graft (CABG) Patch Trial Investigators. Prophylactic use of implanted cardiac defibrillators in patients at high risk for ventricular arrhythmias after coronary-artery bypass graft surgery. *N Engl J Med* 1997; 337:1569–1575.

43. Teerlink JR, Jalaluddin M, Anderson S, et al. Ambulatory ventricular arrhythmias in patients with

heart failure do not specifically predict an increased risk of sudden death. *Circulation* 2000; 101:40–46.

44. Connolly SJ. Prophylactic antiarrhythmic therapy for the prevention of sudden death in high-risk patients: drugs and devices. *Eur Heart J* 1999(suppl C):31–35.

45. Dunkman WB, Johnson GR, Carson PE, Bhat G, Farrell L et al, for the V-HeFT Cooperative Studies Group. Incidence of thromboembolic events in congestive heart failure. *Circulation* 1993;87:94–101.

46. Al-Khadra AS, Salem DN, Rand WM, et al. Warfarin anticoagulation and survival: A cohort analysis from the studies of left ventricular dysfunction. *J Am Coll Cardiol* 1998;31:749–753.

47. Al-Khadra AS, Salem DN, Rand WM, Udelson JE, Smith JJ, et al. Antiplatelet agents and survival: A cohort analysis from the studies of left ventricular dysfunction (SOLVD) Trial. *J Am Coll Cardiol* 1998; 31:419–425.

48. Latini R, Tognoni G, Maggioni AP, Baigent C, Braunwald E, et al, on behalf of the Angiotensin-converting Enzyme Inhibitor Myocardial Infarction Collaborative Group. Clinical effects of early angiotensin-converting enzyme inhibitor treatment for acute myocardial infarction are similar in the presence and absence of aspirin. Systematic overview of individual data from 96 712 randomized patients. *J Am Coll Cardiol* 2000;35: 1801–1807.

49. SOLVD Investigators. Effect of enalapril on mortality and the development of heart failure in asymptomatic patients with reduced left ventricular ejection fractions. *N Engl J Med* 1992; 327:685–691.

50. Rutherford JD, Pfeffer MA, Moyé LA, et al. Effects of captopril on ischaemic events after myocardial infarction. *Circulation* 1994;90:1731–1738.

51. The Heart Outcome Prevention Evaluation Study Investigators. Effects of an angiotensin-converting-enzyme inhibitor, ramipril, on cardiovascular events in high-risk patients. *N Engl J Med* 2000; 342:145–153.

52. The Task Force of the Working Group on Heart Failure of the European Society of Cardiology: The treatment of heart failure. *Eur Heart J* 1997;18: 736–753.

53. Tendera M. Ageing and heart failure: the place of ACE inhibitors in heart failure with preserved systolic function. *Eur Heart J* 2000;2(suppl I):I8–I14.

Robert McKelvie
Associate Professor of Medicine
McMaster University
Hamilton, Ontario
Canada

Competing interests: None declared.

Cardiovascular disorders

Search date December 2000

Clinical Evidence writers on primary prevention

INTERVENTIONS

Likely to be beneficial
Physical activity 66
Eating more fruit and
   vegetables. 68
Smoking cessation 70

Trade off between benefits and harms
Antiplatelet treatment (aspirin) . .82
Anticoagulant treatment
   (warfarin) 83

Likely to be ineffective or harmful
β Carotene 69

SPECIFIC INTERVENTIONS FOR LOWERING BLOOD PRESSURE
Beneficial
Diuretics in high risk people 79
β Blockers in high risk people. . .79

Likely to be beneficial
Physical activity. 72
Low fat, high fruit and vegetable
   diet. 73
Reduced alcohol consumption . .74
Dietary salt restriction 74
Smoking cessation 75

Weight loss. 75
Potassium supplementation 76
Fish oil supplementation 76
Other antihypertensive drugs in
   high risk people 77

Trade off between benefits and harms
Calcium channel blockers 78
Drug treatment in low risk
   people 82

Unknown effectiveness
Calcium supplementation 77
Magnesium supplementation . . .77

SPECIFIC INTERVENTIONS FOR LOWERING CHOLESTEROL CONCENTRATIONS
Likely to be beneficial
Cholesterol reduction in high
   risk people 80
Low fat diet 81

Covered elsewhere in this issue
See cardiovascular disease in
   diabetes, p 376

Cardiovascular disorders

Exercise

- Observational studies have found that moderate to high physical activity reduces coronary heart disease (CHD) and stroke. They also found that sudden death after strenuous exercise was rare, more common in sedentary people, and did not outweigh the benefits.

Diet

- Observational studies have found that consumption of fruit and vegetables is associated with reduced ischaemic vascular disease.
- RCTs found no evidence that β carotene supplements are effective and have found that they may be harmful.
- We found insufficient evidence to support antioxidant supplements in healthy people.

Smoking

- Observational studies have found a strong association between smoking and overall mortality and ischaemic vascular disease.
- Several large cohort studies have found that the increased risk associated with smoking falls after stopping smoking.

SPECIFIC INTERVENTIONS

In people with raised blood pressure

- We found prospective evidence that lifestyle interventions reduce blood pressure but insufficient evidence that these interventions reduce mortality or morbidity.
- Systematic reviews have found good evidence that drug treatment reduces blood pressure.
- Trials of drug treatment have found a greater reduction in blood pressure compared with trials of lifestyle changes, although we found no head to head comparisons.
- Systematic reviews have found that the main determinant of benefit of treatment for hypertension is the pretreatment absolute cardiovascular disease risk.
- The evidence of beneficial effects on mortality and morbidity is strongest for diuretics, β blockers, and ACE inhibitors.
- We found no direct evidence on effects of lowering blood pressure beyond 140/80 mmHg.
- Systematic reviews have found that, in people over age 60 years with systolic blood pressures greater than 160 mmHg, lowering systolic blood pressure decreased total mortality and fatal and non-fatal cardiovascular events.

Antithrombotic drugs

- We found insufficient evidence to identify which asymptomatic individuals would benefit overall and which would be harmed by regular treatment with aspirin.
- One RCT found that the benefits and harms of oral anticoagulation among individuals without symptoms of cardiovascular disease were finely balanced and that net effects were uncertain.

To lower cholesterol

- Systematic reviews have found that reducing cholesterol concentration in asymptomatic people lowers the rate of cardiovascular events but found no evidence that cholesterol reduction by any method reduces overall death rate in people at low baseline risk of cardiovascular events.

■ Systematic reviews and RCTs have found that combined use of cholesterol lowering diet and lipid lowering drugs reduces cholesterol concentration more than lifestyle interventions alone.

DEFINITION	Primary prevention in this context is the long term management of people at increased risk but with no evidence of cardiovascular disease. Clinically overt ischaemic vascular disease includes acute myocardial infarction (AMI), angina, stroke, and peripheral vascular disease. Many adults have no symptoms or obvious signs of vascular disease, even though they have atheroma and are at increased risk of ischaemic vascular events because of one or more risk factors (see aetiology below).
INCIDENCE/ PREVALENCE	In the USA, about 42% of all deaths are from vascular disease. AMI and its sequelae remain the most common single cause of death.
AETIOLOGY/ RISK FACTORS	Identified major risk factors for ischaemic vascular disease include increasing age, male sex, raised low density lipoprotein cholesterol, reduced high density lipoprotein cholesterol, raised blood pressure, smoking, diabetes, family history of cardiovascular disease, obesity, and sedentary lifestyle. For many of these risk factors, observational studies show a continuous gradient of increasing risk of cardiovascular disease with increasing levels of the risk factor, with no obvious threshold level. Although by definition event rates are higher in high risk people, of all ischaemic vascular events that occur in the population, most occur in people with intermediate levels of absolute risk because there are many more of them than there are people at high risk; see appendix 1.[1]
PROGNOSIS	About half of people who suffer an AMI die within 28 days, and two thirds of AMIs occur before the person reaches hospital.[2] The benefits of intervention in unselected people with no evidence of cardiovascular disease (primary prevention) are small because in such people the baseline risk is small. However, absolute risk of ischaemic vascular events varies dramatically, even among people with similar levels of blood pressure or cholesterol. Estimates of absolute risk can be based on simple risk equations or tables (see appendix 1).[3,4]
AIMS	To reduce mortality and morbidity from cardiovascular disease, with minimum adverse effects.
OUTCOMES	Incidence of fatal and non-fatal cardiovascular events (including coronary, cerebrovascular, renal, and eye disease, and heart failure). Surrogate outcomes include changes in levels of individual risk factors, such as blood pressure.
METHODS	*Clinical Evidence* update search and appraisal December 2000.

QUESTION	Does physical activity reduce the risk of vascular events in asymptomatic people?

Charles Foster and Michael Murphy

We found strong observational evidence that moderate to high levels of physical activity reduce the risk of non-fatal and fatal CHD and stroke. People who are physically active (those who undertake moderate levels of activity daily or almost daily) typically experience 30–50% reductions in relative risk of CHD compared with people who are sedentary, after adjustment for other risk factors. The absolute risk of sudden death after strenuous activity is small (although greatest in people who are habitually sedentary) and does not outweigh observed benefits.

Benefits:
Effects of physical activity on CHD: We found no RCTs. Three systematic reviews (search date 1995,[5] and not stated[6,7]) evaluated observational studies and found increased risk of CHD in sedentary compared with active people. Since 1992, 17 large, well conducted prospective, non-randomised studies, with follow up periods ranging from 18 months to 29 years, have specifically examined the association between physical activity and risk of non-fatal or fatal CHD.[8–24] The studies found that risk declined with increasing levels of physical activity (for examples of activity levels see table 1, p 90) (AR for CHD death in people with sedentary lives [rare or no physical activity] 70 per 10 000 person years v 40 per 10 000 person years in people with the highest level of activity [> 3500 kcal per week], absolute benefit of high levels of physical activity 30 lives saved per 10 000 person years). **Effects of physical fitness on CHD:** We found no RCTs. One systematic review (search date not stated) identified seven large, well designed prospective, non-randomised studies of the effects of physical fitness on CHD.[25] All used reproducible measures of physical fitness. Five studies adjusted for other CHD risk factors. These found an increased risk of death from CHD in people with low levels of physical fitness compared with those with high levels (RR of death lowest quartile v highest quartile ranged from 1.2 to 4.0). Most studies reported only baseline measures of physical fitness, thus not accounting for changes in fitness. One recent large follow up study found lower risk among people who increased their fitness level (RR for CVD death compared with those whose level of fitness did not change 0.48, 95% CI 0.31 to 0.74).[26] **Effects of physical activity on stroke:** We found no RCTs and no systematic review of observational studies. We found 12 observational studies (published between 1990 and 1999), based on 3680 strokes among North American, Japanese, and European populations.[27–40] Most of these found that moderate activity was associated with reduced risk of stroke compared with inactivity (RR of stroke, moderate activity v inactivity about 0.5). One cohort study from Japan found that "heavy" physical activity reduced the risk of stroke compared with "moderate" activity (RR of stroke, "heavy" v "moderate" activity about 0.3; P < 0.05).[38] In most studies, the benefits were greater in older people and in men. Most studies were conducted in white men in late middle age, which potentially limits their applicability to other groups of people. The results usually persisted after

adjustment for other known risk factors for stroke (blood pressure, blood lipids, body mass index, and smoking) and after exclusion of people with pre-existing diseases that might limit physical activity and increase risk of stroke. The more recent studies found maximum reduction in the risk of stroke with moderate as opposed to high levels of physical exercise levels.

Harms: No direct evidence of harm was reported in the studies described. We found two studies in people who had experienced non-fatal myocardial infarction, conducted in the USA and Germany. Each involved more than 1000 events and found that 4–7% of these events occurred within 1 hour of strenuous physical activity.[41–43] Strenuous activity was estimated to have raised the relative risk of AMI between two and sixfold in the hour after activity, with risks returning to baseline after that. However, the absolute risk remained low, variously estimated at six deaths per 100 000 middle aged men a year[44] or 0.3 to 2.7 events per 10 000 person hours of exercise.[45] Both studies found that the relative risk of AMI after strenuous activity was much higher in people who were habitually sedentary (RR 107, 95% CI 67 to 171) compared with the relative risk in those who engaged in heavy physical exertion on five or more occasions per week (RR 2.4, 95% CI 1.5 to 3.7).[41] Injury is likely to be the most common adverse event, but we found too few population data to quantify its risk.

Comment: Findings from these observational studies should be interpreted with caution. The studies varied in definitions of levels of activity and fitness. The level of activity or fitness experienced by each participant was not experimentally assigned by an investigator (as in an RCT) but resulted from self selection. Active (or fit) participants are likely to differ from inactive (or unfit) participants in other ways that also influence their risk of cardiovascular disease. Confounding of this type can be partially controlled by adjustment for other known risk factors (such as age, smoking status, and body mass index), but it is likely that some residual confounding will remain, which could overestimate the effect of exercise. The studies have found that the absolute risk of sudden death during or immediately after physical activity is small and does not outweigh the observed benefits.

QUESTION **What intensity and frequency of physical activity improves fitness?**

Charles Foster and Michael Murphy

Small RCTs have found that at least moderate intensity exercise (equivalent to brisk walking) is necessary to improve fitness. We found insufficient evidence on the effects of short bouts of exercise several times a day compared with longer daily bouts.

Benefits: **Intensity:** We found no systematic review. Numerous small RCTs of varying quality have been conducted in different subpopulations. In general, these found that over a period of 6–12 months, low intensity activity programmes produced no measurable changes in maximum oxygen consumption (Vo_2max), whereas moderate intensity activity programmes (equivalent to brisk walking) typically produced improvements, of 20% in oxygen consumption in sedentary people. Table 1, p 90, gives the intensity of effort required for a range of physical activities. Two recent RCTs compared structured aerobic exercise (such as step classes and aerobics classes) with lifestyle activity programmes (such as regular walking and using stairs instead of elevators) among obese women[46] and sedentary men and women.[47] Both studies reported similar, significant changes in measures of cardiovascular fitness and blood pressure with each intervention, and these changes were sustained for at least 2 years after intervention. One prospective follow up study of women previously involved in a randomised trial of physical activity found that women who start a programme of regular walking maintain higher levels of physical activity 10 years after the intervention.[48] **Frequency:** We found no systematic review. One RCT (36 men) compared 8 weeks of a single daily session of 30 minutes of exercise versus three daily sessions of 10 minutes each.[49] It found no significant difference in fitness benefit between groups.

Harms: None reported.

Comment: None.

QUESTION **What are the effects of dietary interventions on the risk of heart attack and stroke in asymptomatic people?**

Andy Ness

OPTION **EATING MORE FRUIT AND VEGETABLES**

Cohort studies have found that eating more fruit and vegetables reduces the risk of heart attack and stroke. The size and nature of any real protective effect is uncertain.

Benefits: **Ischaemic heart disease:** We found no RCTs. We found three systematic reviews of observational studies.[50–52] With addition of recently published studies[53–60] to those reported in the first review,[50] a protective association was observed for ischaemic heart disease in 13 of 24 cohort studies. In the second review, the authors calculated a summary measure of the protective association of 15% between those above the 90th centile and those below the 10th centile for fruit and vegetable consumption.[51] In the third review the authors estimated that increased intake of fruit and vegetables of about 150 g a day was associated with a reduced risk of CHD of between 20–40%.[52] The validity of these estimates has been questioned. One large, high quality cohort study found that eating more vegetables was associated with decreased coronary mortality (≥ 117 g vegetables per day v < 61 g vegetables per day RRR 34%, 95% CI 4% to 54%); for fruit, the association was more modest and not significant (≥ 159 g fruit per day v < 75 g fruit per day RRR +23, 95% CI −12% to +46%).[61] **Stroke:** We found no RCTs but we found two systematic reviews examining the evidence from observational studies for stroke.[50,52] With addition of recently published studies[53,58,62–67] to those reported in the first review,[50] a protective association was observed in 10 of 16 cohort studies for stroke. In the second review the authors estimated that increased intake of fruit and vegetables of about 150 g a day was associated with a reduced risk of stroke of 0–25%.[52] The basis for this estimate is not clear. One large, high quality cohort study in US health professionals found that increased fruit and vegetable intake was associated with a decreased risk of ischaemic stroke (RRR per daily serving of fruit and vegetables 6%, 95% CI 1% to 10%; RRR in the fifth of the population eating the most fruit and vegetables v the fifth eating the least 31%, 95% CI 8% to 48%).[68]

Harms: None were identified.

Comment: Lack of trial evidence and deficiencies in the data available from observational studies mean that the size and nature of any real protective effect is uncertain.[69,70] The observed associations could be the result of confounding as people who eat more fruit and vegetables often come from higher socioeconomic groups and adopt other healthy lifestyles.[71]

OPTION   ANTIOXIDANTS

We found no evidence of benefit from β carotene supplements, and RCTs suggest that they may be harmful. Other antioxidant supplements may be beneficial, but we found insufficient trial evidence to support their use.

Benefits: **β Carotene:** We found one systematic review of prospective studies and RCTs (search date not stated, published in 1997), which did not pool data because of heterogeneity among studies.[72] Most prospective cohort studies of β carotene found a modest protective association with increased intake,[72–75] although several large trials of β carotene supplementation found no evidence of benefit.[75,76]
Vitamin C: We found two systematic reviews,[72,77] which mostly included the same studies, and seven subsequent prospective studies.[57,63,67,69,78–80] Three of 14 cohort studies found a significant protective association between vitamin C and CHD, and two of 11 studies found a protective association between vitamin C and stroke. We found no large trials of vitamin C supplementation alone. Two large trials of multivitamin supplements have been carried out in Linxian, China.[72,81–83] One trial (that was included in the reviews) was carried out in 29 584 participants drawn from the general population who were randomised by using a factorial design to one of four arms: arm A–retinol (10 000 IU) and zinc (22.5 mg); arm B–riboflavin (5.2 mg) and niacin (40 mg); arm C–ascorbic acid (120 mg) and molybdenum (30 µg); arm D–carotene (15 mg), selenium (50 µg), and vitamin E (30 mg). After 6 years the trial found that the treatment assigned to people in arm D reduced all cause mortality and death due to stroke (RRR for death from any cause arm D v other arms 9%, 95% CI 1% to 16%). It found no reduction in stroke or all cause mortality among the other arms.[72] The other trial (subsequent to the reviews) included 3318 people with oesophageal dysplasia who were randomised to placebo or a multivitamin supplement that contained 14 vitamins and 12 minerals, including vitamin C (180 mg), vitamin E (60 IU [1 IU = 0.67 mg]), β carotene (15 mg), and selenium (50 µg). After 6 years it found that the supplement did not significantly reduce

stroke or death from all causes (RRR for all cause mortality 7%, 95% CI −16% to +25%; RRR for stroke 33%, 95% CI −7% to +63%).[81,82] **Vitamin E:** We found one systematic review and additional prospective studies.[72] Eight large cohort studies (5 of which were included in the review) have examined the association between vitamin E intake and ischaemic heart disease. Six found a significant protective association,[72,78,84] whereas two found no significant association.[57,85] In three studies the protective association was with dietary vitamin E.[72,82] In the others it was either wholly or mainly with vitamin E supplements.[72,85] In the review, the largest RCT of vitamin E alone versus placebo (in 29 133 Finnish smokers) found that vitamin E did not significantly reduce mortality compared with placebo (RRR for death 2%, 95% CI −9% to +5%) after 5–8 years. (See above for the results of the Linxian trials.)[72,81–83] Four cohort studies found no association between vitamin E intake and stroke.[67,79,80,86] **Antioxidant minerals:** We found little epidemiological evidence about the cardioprotective effect of copper, zinc, or manganese on the heart.[87] Cohort studies reported an increased risk of ischaemic heart disease in people with low blood selenium concentrations.[86] Most of these were carried out in Finland, a country with low intakes of antioxidants.[89] (See also the results of the Linxian trials.)[71,79–81] **Flavonoids:** We found no systematic review. We found five cohort studies,[65,89–92] three of which reported a reduced risk of ischaemic heart disease with increased flavonoid intake.[65,89,90] One of four observational studies reported a reduced risk of stroke with increased flavonoid intake.[65–67,86]

Harms: Several large trials found that β carotene supplements may increase cardiovascular mortality (pooled data from four RCTs, RRI for cardiovascular death 12%, 95% CI 4% to 22%).[75] Explanations for these results include use of the wrong isomer, the wrong dose, or a detrimental effect on other carotenoid levels.[93,94]

Comment: Trials of antioxidants such as β carotene and vitamin E have not produced any evidence of benefit. Routine use of antioxidant supplements is not justified by the currently available evidence. More trials of antioxidant supplementation are under way.[95]

QUESTION By how much does smoking cessation, or avoidance of starting smoking, reduce risk?

Julian J Nicholas and Thomas Kottke

Observational studies have found that cigarette smoking is strongly related to overall mortality. We found evidence from both observational and randomised studies that cigarette smoking increases the risk of CHD and stroke. The evidence is strongest for stroke.

Benefits: Several large cohort studies examining the effects of smoking have been extensively reviewed by the US surgeon general[96] and the UK Royal College of Physicians.[97] The reviews concluded that cigarette smoking was causally related to disease and that smoking cessation substantially reduced the risk of cancer, respiratory disease, CHD, and stroke. **Death from all causes:** The longest prospective cohort study, in 34 439 male British doctors whose smoking habits were periodically assessed over 40 years (1951–1991), found a strong association between smoking and increased mortality. It found that smokers were about three times more likely to die in middle age (45–64 years) and twice as likely to die in older age (65–84 years) compared with lifelong non-smokers (95% CIs not given).[98] The prospective nurses' health study followed 117 001 middle aged female nurses for 12 years. It found that the total mortality in current smokers was nearly twice that in lifelong non-smokers (RR of death 1.87, 95% CI 1.65 to 2.13).[99] **CHD:** One review (published in 1990) identified 10 cohort studies, involving 20 million person years of observation.[96] All studies found a higher incidence of CHD among smokers (pooled RR of death from CHD compared with non-smokers 1.7, 95% CI not available).[96] People smoking more than 20 cigarettes a day were more likely to have a coronary event (RR 2.5, 95% CI not given).[97] Middle aged smokers were more likely to experience a first non-fatal AMI compared with people who had never smoked (RR in men 2.9, 95% CI 2.4 to 3.4; RR in women 3.6, 95% CI 3.0 to 4.4).[100,101] One RCT of advice encouraging smoking cessation in 1445 men aged 40–59 years found that more men given advice to stop smoking gave up cigarettes (mean absolute reduction in men continuing to smoke after advice v control 53%). The trial found no evidence that men given advice to stop had a significantly lower mortality from CHD (RRR 18%, 95% CI −18% to +43%).[102] The wide confidence intervals mean that there could have been anything from a 43% decrease to an 18% increase in rates of CHD death in men given advice to quit, regardless of whether they actually gave up smoking. **Stroke:** One systematic review (published in 1989) found 32 studies (17 cohort studies with concurrent or historical controls, 14 case control studies, and one hypertension intervention trial). It found good evidence that smoking was associated with an increased risk of stroke (RR of stroke in cigarette smokers v non-smokers 1.5, 95% CI 1.4 to 1.6).[103] Smoking was associated with an increased risk of cerebral infarction (RR 1.92, 95% CI 1.71 to 2.16) and subarachnoid haemorrhage (RR 2.93, 95% CI 2.48 to 3.46), but no increased risk of intracerebral haemorrhage (RR 0.74, 95% CI 0.56 to 0.98). The relative risk of stroke in smokers versus non-smokers was highest in those aged under 55 years (RR 2.9, 95% CI 2.40 to 3.59) and lowest in those aged over 74 years (RR 1.11, 95% CI 0.96 to 1.28).

Harms: We found no evidence that stopping smoking increases mortality in any subgroup of smokers.

Comment: We found no evidence of publication or other overt bias that may explain the observed association between smoking and stroke. There was a dose-response curve between the number of cigarettes smoked and the relative risk for stroke, consistent with a causal relation. The absolute risk reduction from stopping smoking will be highest for those with the highest absolute risk of vascular events.

QUESTION How quickly do risks diminish when smokers stop smoking?

Julian J Nicholas and Thomas Kottke

Observational studies have found that the risk of death and cardiovascular events falls when people stop smoking. The risk can take many years to approach that of non-smokers, particularly in those with a history of heavy smoking.

Benefits:
Death from all causes: In people who stopped smoking, observational studies found that death rates fell gradually to lie between those of lifelong smokers and people who had never smoked. Estimates for the time required for former smokers to bring their risk of death in line with people who had never smoked varied among studies but may be longer than 15 years.[104] Actuarial projections from one study among British doctors predicted that life expectancy would improve even among people who stopped smoking in later life (65 years and over).[98] **CHD:** Observational studies found that, in both male and female ex-smokers, the risk of coronary events rapidly declined to a level comparable with that of people who had never smoked after 2–3 years and was independent of the number of cigarettes smoked before quitting.[96] **Stroke:** The US surgeon general's review of observational studies found that the risk of stroke decreased in ex-smokers compared with smokers (RR of stroke, smokers v ex-smokers 1.2, 95% CI not available) but remained raised for 5–10 years after cessation compared with those who had never smoked (RR of stroke ex-smokers v never smokers 1.5, 95% CI not available).[96] One recent study in 7735 middle aged British men found that 5 years after smoking cessation the risk of stroke in previously light smokers (< 20 cigarettes per day) was identical to that of lifelong non-smokers, but the risk in previously heavy smokers (> 21 cigarettes per day) was still raised compared with lifelong non-smokers (RR of stroke, previously heavy smokers v never smokers 2.2, 95% CI 1.1 to 4.3).[105] One observational study in 117 001 middle aged female nurses also found a fall in risk on stopping smoking and found no difference between previously light and previously heavy smokers (RR in all former smokers 2–4 years after stopping smoking 1.17, 95% CI 0.49 to 2.23).[99]

Harms:
We found no evidence that stopping smoking increases mortality in any subgroup of smokers.

Comment:
For a review of the evidence on methods of changing smoking behaviour, see secondary prevention of ischaemic cardiac events, p 95.

QUESTION What are the effects of lifestyle changes in asymptomatic people with primary hypertension?

Cindy Mulrow

OPTION PHYSICAL ACTIVITY

One systematic review of RCTs has found that aerobic exercise reduces blood pressure (see table 2, p 91).

Benefits: We found no RCTs examining the effects of exercise on morbidity, mortality, or quality of life. One systematic review (search date 1996, 29 RCTs, 1533 sedentary adults with normal blood pressure, age 18–79 years) examined the effects on blood pressure of at least 4 weeks of regular aerobic exercise versus no exercise.[106] Exercise regimens included walking, jogging, cycling, or both, often lasting 45–60 minutes a session, for 3 days a week (mean exercise intensity about 60–70% of Vo_2max). Compared with non-exercising control groups, groups randomised to aerobic exercise reduced their systolic blood pressure by 4.7 mm Hg (95% CI 4.4 to 5.0 mm Hg) and diastolic blood pressure by 3.1 mm Hg (95% CI 3.0 to 3.3 mm Hg). Greater reductions were seen in people with higher initial blood pressures. Trials with interventions lasting longer than 6 months' duration in adults aged 45 years or over with hypertension found smaller mean reductions in blood pressure but with wide confidence intervals (systolic reduction 0.8 mm Hg, 95% CI 5.9 mm Hg reduction to 4.2 mm Hg increase).[107]

Harms: Musculoskeletal injuries may occur, but their frequency was not documented.

Comment: Many adults find aerobic exercise programmes difficult to sustain. The clinical significance of the observed reductions in blood pressure is uncertain. The type and amount of exercise most likely to result in benefits are unclear, with some recent studies showing some benefits with simple increases in lifestyle activity. One cohort study in 173 men with hypertension found that "regular heavy activity several times weekly" compared with no or limited spare time physical activity reduced all cause and cardiovascular mortality (all cause mortality RR 0.43, 95% CI 0.22 to 0.82; cardiovascular mortality RR 0.33, 95% CI 0.11 to 0.94).[108]

| OPTION | LOW FAT, HIGH FRUIT AND VEGETABLE DIET |

One RCT has found that a low fat, high fruit and vegetable diet modestly reduced blood pressure (see table 2, p 91).

Benefits: We found no systematic review and no RCTs examining the effects of low fat, high fruit and vegetable diet on morbidity or mortality in people with primary hypertension. For evidence from cohort studies in asymptomatic people in general see, p 68. One RCT (459 adults with systolic blood pressures of < 160 mm Hg and diastolic blood pressures of 80–90 mm Hg) compared effects on blood pressure of three diets (control diet low in both magnesium and potassium v fruit and vegetable diet high in both potassium and magnesium v combination of the fruit and vegetable diet with a low fat diet high in both calcium and protein).[109] After 8 weeks the fruit and vegetable diet reduced systolic and diastolic blood pressure compared with the control diet (mean change in systolic blood pressure −2.8 mm Hg, 97.5% CI −4.7 to −0.9 mm Hg; mean change in diastolic blood pressure −1.1 mm Hg, 97.5% CI −2.4 mm Hg to +0.3 mm Hg). The combination diet also reduced systolic and diastolic blood pressure compared with the control diet (mean change in systolic blood pressure −5.5 mm Hg, 97.5% CI −7.4 mm Hg to −3.7 mm Hg; mean change in diastolic blood pressure −3.0 mm Hg, 97.5% CI −4.3 to −1.6 mm Hg).

Cardiovascular disorders

Harms: We found no direct evidence that a low fat, high fruit and vegetable diet is harmful.

Comment: The trial was of short duration and participants were supplied with food during the intervention period.[109] Other studies have found that long term maintenance of particular diets is difficult for many people, although low fat, high fruit and vegetable diets may have multiple benefits (see changing behaviour, p 24).

OPTION   REDUCED ALCOHOL CONSUMPTION

One systematic review of RCTs found inconclusive evidence regarding effects of alcohol reduction on blood pressure.

Benefits: We found no RCTs examining the effects of reducing alcohol consumption on morbidity or mortality. Over 60 population studies have reported associations between alcohol consumption and blood pressure; the relation was found to be generally linear, although several studies reported a threshold effect at about two to three standard drinks a day.[110] Any adverse effect of up to two drinks a day on blood pressure was found to be either small or non-existent. One systematic review of seven trials in 751 people with hypertension (mainly men) found that data were inconclusive on the benefits of reducing alcohol among moderate to heavy drinkers (25–50 drinks weekly).[111]

Harms: We found no direct evidence that reducing alcohol intake to as few as two drinks a day was harmful.

Comment: Most data were from observational studies. RCTs were small and lacked reliable information about adherence. Substantial reductions in alcohol use in both control and intervention groups were observed, with limited ability to detect differences between groups.

OPTION   SALT RESTRICTION

One systematic review of RCTs has found that salt restriction may lead to modest reductions in blood pressure, with more benefit in people older than 45 years than in younger people (see table 2, p 91).

Benefits: We found no RCT examining the effects of salt restriction on morbidity or mortality. We found one systematic review (search date 1997, 58 trials, 2161 people with hypertension, age 23–73 years)[112] and one subsequent RCT (875 men and women with hypertension, age 60–80 years, duration 30 months),[113] which examined the effects of salt restriction on blood pressure. Interventions were low salt diets, with or without weight reduction. People in the control groups took their usual diet. Changes in salt intake varied among trials in the systematic review; a mean reduction in sodium intake of 118 mmol (6.7 g) a day for 28 days led to reductions of 3.9 mm Hg (95% CI 3.0 to 4.8 mm Hg) in systolic blood pressure and 1.9 mm Hg (95% CI 1.3 to 2.5 mm Hg) in diastolic blood pressure.[112] The subsequent RCT in elderly people found that a mean decrease in salt intake of about 40 mmol (2.35 g) a day reduced systolic blood pressure by 2.6 mm Hg (95% CI 0.4 to 4.8 mm Hg) and diastolic blood pressure by 1.1 mm Hg

(95% CI 0.3 mm Hg rise in diastolic to 2.5 mm Hg fall). An earlier systematic review (search date 1994) identified 28 RCTs in 1131 people with hypertension. It found that lesser reductions of 60 mmol per day led to smaller reductions in systolic/diastolic blood pressure of 2.2 mm Hg/0.5 mm Hg and found greater effects in trials, in which mean age was over 45 years (6.3/2.2 mm Hg).[114]

Harms: We found no direct evidence that low salt diets may increase morbidity or mortality. Epidemiological data conflict, with one observational study suggesting that very low salt intakes may be associated with increased incidence of myocardial infarction in middle aged men.[115]

Comment: Small trials tended to report larger reductions in systolic and diastolic blood pressure than larger trials. This is consistent with publication bias or less rigorous methodology in small trials.[114]

| OPTION | SMOKING CESSATION |

Epidemiological data clearly identify that smoking is a significant risk factor for cardiovascular disease (see question, p 70). We found no direct evidence that stopping smoking decreases blood pressure in people with hypertension.

Benefits: We found no direct evidence that stopping smoking reduces blood pressure in people with hypertension, although we found good evidence that, in general, smoking cessation reduces risk of cardiovascular disease (see question, p 70).

Harms: We found insufficient evidence in this context.

Comment: None.

| OPTION | WEIGHT LOSS |

One systematic review and additional RCTs have found that modest weight reductions of 3–9% of body weight are achievable in motivated middle aged and older adults, and may lead to modest reductions in blood pressure in obese people with hypertension. Many adults find it difficult to maintain weight loss (see table 2, p 91).

Benefits: We found no RCTs examining the effects of weight loss on morbidity and mortality. We found one systematic review (published in 1998, 18 RCTs, 2611 middle aged people, mean age 50 years, mean weight 85 kg, mean blood pressure 152/98 mm Hg, 55% men) and two subsequent RCTs[116,117] that examined the effects of weight loss on blood pressure.[118] In the systematic review, caloric intakes ranged from 450 to 1500 kcal a day; most diets led to weight reductions of 3–9% of body weight. Combined data from the six trials that did not vary antihypertensive regimens during the intervention period found that reducing weight reduced systolic and diastolic blood pressures (mean reduction in systolic pressure, weight loss v no weight loss 3 mm Hg, 95% CI 0.7 to 6.8 mm Hg; mean reduction in diastolic blood pressure 2.9 mm Hg diastolic, 95% CI 0.1 to 5.7 mm Hg). Trials that allowed adjustment of antihypertensive regimens found that lower doses and fewer antihypertensive drugs were needed in the weight reduction groups

Cardiovascular disorders

compared with control groups. The two subsequent RCTs found that sustained weight reduction of 2–4 kg significantly reduced systolic blood pressure at 1–3 years by about 1 mmHg.[116,117]

Harms: We found no direct evidence that intentional gradual weight loss of less than 10% of body weight is harmful in obese adults with hypertension.

Comment: None.

| OPTION | POTASSIUM SUPPLEMENTATION |

One systematic review of RCTs has found that a daily potassium supplementation of about 60 mmol (2 g, which is about the amount contained in 5 bananas) is feasible for many adults and reduces blood pressure a little (see table 3, p 91).

Benefits: We found no RCTs examining the effects of potassium supplementation on morbidity or mortality. One systematic review (search date 1995, 21 RCTs, 1560 adults with hypertension, age 19–79 years) compared the effects on blood pressure of potassium supplements (60–100 mmol potassium chloride daily) versus placebo or no supplement.[119] It found that, compared with the control interventions, potassium supplements reduced systolic and diastolic blood pressures (mean decrease in systolic blood pressure with potassium supplements 4.4 mm Hg systolic, 95% CI 2.2 to 6.6 mm Hg; mean decrease in diastolic blood pressure 2.5 mm Hg diastolic, 95% CI 0.1 to 4.9 mm Hg).

Harms: We found no direct evidence of harm in people without kidney failure and in people not taking drugs that increase serum potassium concentration. Gastrointestinal adverse effects such as belching, flatulence, diarrhoea, or abdominal discomfort occurred in 2–10% of people.[119]

Comment: None.

| OPTION | FISH OIL SUPPLEMENTATION |

One systematic review of RCTs has found that fish oil supplementation in large doses of 3 g a day modestly lowers blood pressure (see table 3, p 91).

Benefits: We found no RCTs examining the effects of fish oil supplementation on morbidity or mortality. One systematic review (search date not stated, 7 brief RCTs, 339 people with hypertension—mainly middle aged white men, mean age 50 years) compared effects on blood pressure of fish oil (usually 3 g daily as capsules) versus no supplements or "placebo".[120] The contents of placebo capsules varied among trials. Some used oil mixtures containing omega-3 polyunsaturated fatty acids, some without. The review found that fish oil supplements reduced blood pressure compared with control interventions (mean decrease in blood pressure in treatment group v control group 4.5 mm Hg systolic, 95% CI 1.2 to 7.8 mm Hg, and 2.5 mm Hg diastolic, 95% CI 0.6 to 4.4 mm Hg).

Harms: Belching, bad breath, fishy taste, and abdominal pain occurred in about a third of people taking high doses of fish oil.[120]

Comment: The trials were of short duration and used high doses of fish oil. Such high intake may be difficult to maintain. We found no evidence of beneficial effect on blood pressure at lower intakes.

OPTION CALCIUM SUPPLEMENTATION

We found insufficient evidence on the effects of calcium supplementation specifically in people with hypertension. One systematic review of RCTs in people both with and without hypertension found that calcium supplementation may reduce systolic blood pressure by small amounts (see table 3, p 91).

Benefits: We found no RCTs examining the effects of calcium supplementation on morbidity or mortality. One systematic review (search date 1994, 42 RCTs, 4560 middle aged adults) compared the effects on blood pressure of calcium supplementation (500–2000 mg daily) versus placebo or no supplements.[121] It found that calcium supplements reduced blood pressure by a small amount (mean systolic blood pressure reduction, supplement v control 1.4 mm Hg, 95% CI 0.7 to 2.2 mm Hg; mean diastolic reduction 0.8 mm Hg, 95% CI 0.2 to 1.4 mm Hg).

Harms: Adverse gastrointestinal effects, such as abdominal pain, were generally mild and varied among particular preparations.

Comment: Data relating specifically to people with hypertension are limited by few studies with small sample sizes and short durations.

OPTION MAGNESIUM SUPPLEMENTATION

We found limited and conflicting evidence on the effect of magnesium supplementation on blood pressure in people with hypertension and normal magnesium concentrations.

Benefits: We found no RCTs examining the effects of magnesium supplementation on morbidity or mortality. A few small, short term RCTs found mixed results on effects on blood pressure reduction (see table 3, p 91).

Harms: We found insufficient evidence.

Comment: None.

QUESTION What are the effects of drug treatment in primary hypertension?

Cindy Mulrow and Rod Jackson

OPTION ANTIHYPERTENSIVE DRUGS VERSUS PLACEBO

Many systematic reviews of RCTs have found that drug treatment decreases the risk of fatal and non-fatal stroke, cardiac events, and total mortality in specific populations of people. The biggest benefit is seen in people with highest baseline risk of cardiovascular disease.

Benefits: We found many systematic reviews. One review (search date 1997, 17 RCTs with morbidity and mortality outcomes, duration > 1 year, 37 000 people) found that antihypertensive drugs versus placebo produced variable reductions of systolic/diastolic blood pressure that averaged around 12–16/5–10 mm Hg.[122] It found evidence of benefit in total death rate, cardiovascular death rate, stroke, major coronary events, and congestive cardiac failure, but the absolute results depended on age and the severity of the hypertension (see below). The biggest benefit was seen in those with the highest baseline risk. The trials mainly compared placebo versus diuretics (usually thiazides with the addition of amiloride or triamterene) and versus β blockers (usually atenolol or metoprolol) in a stepped care approach. One systematic review (search date 1999, 8 RCTs, 15 693 people) found that, in people over 60 years old with systolic hypertension, treatment of systolic pressures greater than 160 mm Hg decreased total mortality and fatal and non-fatal cardiovascular events. Absolute benefits were greater in men than women, in people aged over 70, and in those with prior cardiovascular events or wider pulse pressure. The relative hazard rates associated with a 10 mm Hg higher initial systolic blood pressure were 1.26 (P = 0.0001) for total mortality, 1.22 (P = 0.02) for stroke, but only 1.07 (P = 0.37) for coronary events. Active treatment reduced total mortality (RR 0.87, 95% CI 0.78 to 0.98, P = 0.02).[123] **Target diastolic blood pressure:** We found one RCT (18 790 people, mean age 62 years, diastolic blood pressures between 100–115 mm Hg), which aimed to evaluate the effects on cardiovascular risk of target diastolic blood pressures of 90, 85, and 80 mm Hg.[124] However, mean achieved diastolic blood pressures were 85, 83, and 81 mm Hg, which limited power to detect differences among groups. There were no significant differences in major cardiovascular events among the three groups.

Harms: **Mortality and major morbidity:** One systematic review of RCTs comparing diuretics and β blockers versus placebo found no increase in non-cardiovascular mortality in treated people.[122] One systematic review (9 case control and 3 cohort studies) found that long term diuretic use may be associated with an increased risk of renal cell carcinoma (OR in case control studies 1.55, 95% CI 1.4 to 1.7).[125] Absolute risks cannot be calculated from these studies, but renal cell carcinoma is rare, so the absolute risk increase of any real effect would be correspondingly small. Renal cell carcinoma can cause hypertension; this fact may have confounded the results of these studies. **Quality of life and tolerability:** One systematic review and several recent trials found that quality of life was not adversely affected and may be improved in those who remain on treatment.[126,127]

Comment: Trials included people who were healthier than the general population, with lower rates of cardiovascular risk factors, cardiovascular disease, and comorbidity. People with higher cardiovascular risk can expect greater short term absolute risk reduction than seen in the trials, whereas people with major competing risks such as terminal cancer or end stage Alzheimer's disease can expect smaller risk reduction. In the systematic review,[122] five of the trials were in middle aged adults with mild to moderate hypertension. Seven of the trials were in people older than 60 years. On average, every 1000 person years of treatment in older adults prevented five strokes (95% CI 2 to 8), three coronary events (95% CI 1 to 4), and four cardiovascular deaths (95% CI 1 to 8). Drug treatment in middle aged adults prevented one stroke (95% CI 0 to 2) for every 1000 person years of treatment and did not significantly affect coronary events or mortality.

| OPTION | COMPARING ANTIHYPERTENSIVE DRUG TREATMENTS |

Two systematic reviews have found that initial treatment with diuretics, ACE inhibitors, or β blockers reduces mortality and morbidity, with minimal adverse effects. RCTs found no significant morbidity or mortality differences among these agents. We found limited evidence from one systematic review of RCTs that diuretics, β blockers, and ACE inhibitors reduced coronary heart disease and heart failure more than calcium channel antagonists. One RCT has found that a thiazide diuretic is superior to an α blocker in reducing cardiovascular events, particularly congestive heart failure.

Benefits: **β Blockers versus diuretics:** One systematic review (search date 1995, > 48 000 people) identified RCTs comparing effects of high and low dose diuretics versus β blockers.[128] A second systematic review (search date 1998) was limited to 10 RCTs in 16 164 elderly people.[129] These reviews did not summarise direct comparisons of diuretics versus β blockers but compared results of trials that used diuretics as first line agents versus results of trials that used β blockers as first line agents. The reviews found no significant difference between diuretics and β blockers for lowering blood pressure. They found that diuretics reduced coronary events, but found no evidence that β blockers reduced coronary events. **β Blockers versus ACE inhibitors:** One single blind RCT (10 985 people, aged 25–66 years) found that an ACE inhibitor (captopril) was no more effective than conventional treatment (diuretics or β blockers) in reducing cardiovascular morbidity or mortality. Captopril increased the risk of stroke compared with β blockers (125 people would need to be treated with ACE inhibitor rather than β blocker for one extra stroke to occur, 95% CI 69 to 651 people). However, the methods of the trial may limit the validity of results (see comment below).[130] **Comparison of β blockers, diuretics, ACE inhibitors, and calcium channel antagonists:** One unblinded RCT (6600 people, aged 70–84 years) compared diuretics, β blockers, or both, versus calcium channel antagonists (felodipine or isradipine) versus ACE inhibitors (enalapril or lisinopril). It found no significant difference in blood pressure control or cardiovascular morbidity or mortality.[131] One systematic review (search date 2000, 8 RCTs) compared different antihypertensive regimens, and found no significant differences in outcome among people initially treated with β blockers, diuretics, or ACE inhibitors.[132] However, it found that β blockers or diuretics decreased coronary events compared with calcium channel antagonists, and increased stroke rate, although there was no significant difference for all cause mortality (OR for mortality, β blockers or diuretics v calcium antagonists 1.01, 95% CI 0.92 to 1.11). ACE inhibitors did not significantly alter all cause mortality or stroke rate compared with calcium channel antagonists, but decreased coronary events (OR for ACE inhibitor v calcium antagonist 1.03, 95% CI 0.91 to 1.18 for all cause mortality; 1.02, 95% CI 0.85 to 1.21 for stroke; 0.81, 95% CI 0.68 to 0.97 for coronary events).[132] **Comparison of α blockers and diuretics:** A double blind RCT (335 high risk people with hypertension) found no differences in coronary heart disease outcomes between doxazosin, an α blocker, compared with chlorthalidone. However, doxazosin compared with chlorthalidone increased the total number of cardiovascular events (4 year rate 25% v 22%; HR 1.25, 95% CI 1.17 to 1.33) and, in particular, increased congestive heart failure (4 year rate 8% v 4%; HR 2.04,, 95% CI 1.79 to 2.32).[133] **Drug treatment in people with diabetes:** See cardiovascular disease in diabetes, p 376.

Harms: **Quality of life and tolerability:** In the three long term, double blind comparisons of low dose diuretics, β blockers, ACE inhibitors, and calcium channel blockers, tolerability and overall quality of life indicators tended to be more favourable for diuretics and β blockers than for newer drugs.[134–136] One systematic review (search date 1998) of RCTs comparing thiazides versus β blockers found that thiazides were associated with fewer withdrawals because of adverse effects (RR 0.69, 95% CI 0.63 to 0.76).[137] Adverse effects are agent specific. The recent unblinded RCT comparing diuretics, β blockers, calcium channel antagonists, and ACE inhibitors found that after 5 years of follow up, 26% of people receiving felodipine or isradipine reported ankle oedema, 30% receiving enalapril or lisonopril reported cough, and 9% receiving diuretics and/or β blockers reported cold hands and feet.[131] **Major harm controversies:** Case control, cohort, and randomised studies suggest that short and intermediate acting dihydropyridine calcium channel blockers, such as nifedipine and isradipine, may increase cardiovascular morbidity and mortality.[138]

Comment: Results of the large ACE inhibitor trial reported above warrant cautious interpretation because a flaw in the randomisation process resulted in unbalanced groups.[130]

QUESTION **What are the effects of lowering cholesterol concentration in asymptomatic people?**

Michael Pignone

Systematic reviews have found that, in people with a high baseline risk, cholesterol reduction reduces non-fatal myocardial infarction (see cholesterol reduction under secondary prevention of ischaemic cardiac events, p 95). RCTs have found that benefit is related to an individual's baseline risk of cardiovascular events and to the degree of cholesterol lowering rather than to the individual's absolute cholesterol concentration (see figure 1, p 94).

Benefits: We found many reviews of the effects of cholesterol lowering on cardiovascular event rates, CHD mortality, and total mortality in people with no previous history of cardiovascular disease. Most concluded that cholesterol reduction lowered cardiovascular events but that there was insufficient evidence that cholesterol reduction lowers overall mortality when used in people with no existing cardiovascular symptoms (primary prevention).[144–148] **Statins:** We found four systematic reviews that considered the effect of HMG-CoA reductase inhibitors (statins) versus placebo on clinical outcomes in people given long term (≥ 6 months) treatment.[144–148] All included the two large primary prevention trials using statins (13 200 people). All found similar results. After 4–6 years of treatment for primary prevention, statins compared with placebo did not significantly reduce all cause mortality (OR 0.87, 95% CI 0.71 to 1.06) or CHD mortality (OR 0.73, 95% CI 0.51 to 1.05), but did reduce major coronary events (OR 0.66, 95% CI 0.57 to 0.76) and cardiovascular mortality (OR 0.68, 95% CI 0.50 to 0.93).[149] The absolute risk reduction for CHD events, CHD mortality, and total mortality varied with the baseline risk in the placebo group of each trial (see figure 1, p 94).[147] **Other treatments:** We found no systematic review specifically in people with low baseline risk (< 0.5% annual risk of CHD events). We found two systematic reviews that looked at statins and non-statin treatments together versus placebo or no treatment, specifically for primary prevention. Both found similar results. The most recent review found four RCTs (2 with statins, one with fibrates, and one with cholestyramine, 21 087 people).[147] It found that cholesterol reduction therapy versus placebo significantly reduced CHD events and CHD mortality, but found no significant effect on overall mortality (OR for therapy v placebo; 0.70, 95% CI 0.62 to 0.79 for CHD events; 0.71, 95% CI 0.56 to 0.91 for CHD mortality; 0.94, 95% CI 0.81 to 1.09 for overall mortality). **Low fat diet:** See changing behaviour, p 24.

Harms: Specific harms of statins are discussed under secondary prevention of ischaemic cardiac events, p 95.

Comment: The CHD event rate in the placebo group of the two large primary prevention trials using statins was 0.6%[139] and 1.5 %[143] a year. If the 17% relative reduction in total mortality observed in the higher risk West of Scotland trial is real, then about 110 high risk people without known CHD would need to be treated for 5 years to save one life. We found no RCTs evaluating the effect of statins in asymptomatic people aged over 75 years. Several large studies are under way.[150] We found one systematic review (search date 1996, 59 RCTs, 173 160 people receiving drug treatments, dietary intervention, or ileal bypass), which did not differentiate primary and secondary prevention and included RCTs of any cholesterol lowering intervention, irrespective of duration, as long as mortality data were reported.[151] Overall, baseline risk was similar in people allocated to all interventions. Among non-surgical treatments, the review found that only statins reduced CHD mortality (RR v control: 0.69, 95% CI 0.59 to 0.80 for statins; 0.44, 95% CI 0.18 to 1.07 for n–3 fatty acids; 0.98, 95% CI 0.78 to 1.24 for fibrates; 0.71, 95% CI 0.51 to 0.99 for resins; 1.04, 95% CI 0.93 to 1.17 for hormones; 0.95, 95% CI 0.83 to 1.10 for niacin; 0.91, 95% CI 0.82 to 1.01 for diet), and that only statins and n–3 fatty acids reduced all cause mortality (RR v control: 0.79, 95% CI 0.71 to 0.89 for statins; 0.68, 95% CI 0.53 to 0.88 for n–3 fatty acids; 1.06, 95% CI 0.78 to 1.46 for fibrates; 0.85, 95% CI 0.66 to 1.08 for resins; 1.09, 95% CI 1.00 to 1.20 for hormones; 0.96, 95% CI 0.86 to 1.08 for niacin; 0.97, 95% CI 0.81 to 1.15 for diet).

Cardiovascular disorders

Cathie Sudlow

OPTION ANTIPLATELET TREATMENT

We found the role of antiplatelet treatment in individuals without symptoms of cardiovascular disease to be uncertain. We found insufficient evidence from RCTs to identify which individuals would benefit overall and which would be harmed by regular treatment with aspirin (see tables 4 and 5, pp 92, 93)

Benefits: We found two systematic reviews[155,156] and one subsequent RCT.[157] We have included this trial in our own meta-analysis, which pools data from the five large RCTs that we have found to date, comparing aspirin versus control in a total of about 55 000 low risk individuals with or without identifiable risk factors (see tables 4 and 5, pp 92, 93).[124,152–154,157] The first systematic review of RCTs of antiplatelet treatment (search date 1990) included about 30 000 people.[155] Most were involved in two large trials of aspirin versus control among male doctors in the UK (aspirin dose 500 mg daily) and the USA (aspirin dose 325 mg every other day).[152,153] We found three RCTs published after the review, in asymptomatic individuals with identifiable risk factors for vascular events. All three had a factorial design. Results are summarised in tables 4 and 5, pp 92, 93. The first compared aspirin (75 mg daily) versus placebo, and low intensity warfarin (target international normalised ratio [INR] 1.5) versus placebo in 5000 middle-aged men with CHD score in the top 20–25% of the population distribution.[154] The second RCT compared aspirin (75 mg daily) versus placebo in three groups with different intensities of blood pressure reduction in a total of about 19 000 people with hypertension, most of whom had no history of vascular disease.[124] The third RCT compared aspirin (100 mg daily) versus placebo, and vitamin E versus placebo in about 4500 people aged > 50 years, recruited from general practices. Participants had at least one major cardiovascular risk factor (hypertension, hypercholesterolaemia, diabetes, obesity, family history of premature myocardial infarction, or age ≥65 years).[157] Our meta-analysis also included these three RCTs, and found that, overall, aspirin reduced myocardial infarction, slightly reduced vascular events (ARR 1/1000 people per year), but had an uncertain effect on stroke (see table 4, p 92). The second systematic review (published 2000) found similar results, but did not include the most recently published RCT.[157] It included one RCT (among about 3000 individuals with diabetes), who were at substantially higher risk of vascular events (about 4% per year) than the low risk individuals in the primary prevention trials included in our meta-analysis (see table 4, p 92).

Harms: Serious, potentially life threatening bleeding is the most important adverse effect of antiplatelet treatment. Intracranial bleeds are uncommon, but they are often fatal and usually cause substantial disability in survivors. Major extracranial bleeds occur mainly in the gastrointestinal tract and may require hospital admission or blood transfusion but do not generally result in permanent disability and are rarely fatal. Table 5 shows the approximate excess annual rates for intracranial and major extracranial bleeds (see table 5, p 93).

Comment: Individuals in primary prevention trials were at much lower risk of vascular events (average 1% per year in the control group) than the high risk people with clinical manifestations of cardiovascular disease that were included in the first overview (average 9% per year in the control group).[155] The absolute benefit of aspirin was therefore small and, as it was of similar magnitude to the risks of bleeding, the net effects were statistically uncertain. The size and direction of the effects of aspirin in particular individuals may well depend on specific factors, such as age, blood pressure, smoking status, or history of diabetes mellitus. At present there is insufficient information to identify which individuals would benefit overall and which would be harmed by regular treatment with aspirin. Futher information will soon be available from a detailed overview of individual participant data from the completed primary prevention trials (Baigent C, personal communication, 2001); from the Women's Health Study, comparing aspirin 100 mg daily versus placebo among 40 000 healthy postmenopausal women;[158] and from the Aspirin in Asymptomatic Atherosclerosis trial, comparing low dose aspirin versus placebo among 3 300 middle-aged participants with asymptomatic atherosclerosis, identified by an ankle brachial pressure index of ≥ 0.9 (Fowkes G, personal communication, 2000).

OPTION ANTICOAGULANT TREATMENT

We found evidence from one RCT that the benefits and risks of low intensity oral anticoagulation among individuals without evidence of cardiovascular disease are finely balanced, and the net effects are uncertain.

Benefits: We found no systematic review. We found one RCT assessing anticoagulation (with a low target INR of 1.5) among people without evidence of cardiovascular disease.[154] It found that the proportional effects of warfarin were similar among people allocated aspirin or placebo, and overall warfarin non-significantly reduced the odds of a vascular event over about 6.5 years compared with placebo (253 events in 2762 people allocated to warfarin, AR 9.2% v 288 events in 2737 people allocated to placebo, AR 10.5%; mean ARR warfarin v placebo about 2 events per 1000 individuals per year; reduction in odds of vascular event warfarin v placebo 14%, 95% CI −2% to +28%). Compared with placebo, warfarin reduced the rate of all ischaemic heart disease by 21% (95% CI 4% to 35%), but had no significant effect on the rate of stroke (increase in AR 15%, 95% CI −22% to +68%) or other causes of vascular death.

Harms: Allocation to warfarin was associated with a non-significant excess of about 0.4 intracranial bleeds per 1000 individuals a year (14/2762 [0.5%] warfarin v 7/2737 [0.3%] placebo) and a non-significant excess of extracranial bleeds of about 0.5 per 1000 individuals a year (21/2545 [0.8%] warfarin v 12/2540 [0.5%] placebo).

Cardiovascular disorders

Comment: As is the case for aspirin, the benefits and risks of low intensity oral anticoagulation among people without evidence of cardiovascular disease are finely balanced. The number of individuals randomised to date is only about 10% of the number included in primary prevention trials of aspirin (see above), and so the reliable identification of those who may benefit from such treatment will require further large scale randomised evidence.

Substantive changes since last issue

Fruit and vegetables Additional cohort study examining effect on stroke risk;[67] conclusions unchanged.

Antioxidants Two additional cohort studies examining effect on stroke risk;[67,80] conclusions unchanged.

Weight loss Two additional RCTs;[116,117] conclusions unchanged.

Antihypertensive drug treatments New systematic review comparing different antihypertensive regimens.[132] It found no consistent differences between diuretics, β blockers, and ACE inhibitors, but found that compared with these agents, calcium channel antagonists increase coronary events but decrease stroke rate. Compared with ACE inhibitors, calcium channel antagonists did not alter stroke rate but increased coronary events.

Cholesterol lowering treatment, statins Two additional systematic reviews;[147,148] conclusions unchanged.

Cholesterol lowering treatment, other treatments Two additional meta-analyses;[147,148] conclusions unchanged.

Aspirin Additional RCT updates author's meta-analysis;[157] benefits section restructured; conclusions unchanged.

REFERENCES

1. Heller RF, Chinn S, Pedoe HD, Rose G. How well can we predict coronary heart disease? Findings of the United Kingdom heart disease prevention project. *BMJ* 1984;288:1409–1411.

2. Tunstall-Pedoe H, Morrison C, Woodward M, Fitzpatrick B, Watt G. Sex differences in myocardial infarction and coronary deaths in the Scottish MONICA population of Glasgow 1985 to 1991: presentation, diagnosis, treatment, and 28-day case fatality of 3991 events in men and 1551 events in women. *Circulation* 1996;93: 1981–1992.

3. Anderson KV, Odell PM, Wilson PWF, Kannel WB. Cardiovascular disease risk profiles. *Am Heart J* 1991;121:293–298.

4. National Health Committee. Guidelines for the management of mildly raised blood pressure in New Zealand. Wellington Ministry of Health, 1993. http://www.nzgg.org.nz/library/gl_complete/ bloodpressure/table1.cfm

5. Powell KE, Thompson PD, Caspersen CJ, Kendrick JS. Physical activity and the incidence of coronary heart disease. *Ann Rev Public Health* 1987;8: 253–287. Search date 1995; primary sources computerised searches of personal files, *J Chronic Dis* 1983–1985 and *Am J Epidemiol* 1984–1985.

6. Berlin JA, Colditz GA. A meta-analysis of physical activity in the prevention of coronary heart disease. *Am J Epidemiol* 1990;132:612–628. Search date not stated; primary sources review articles and Medline.

7. Eaton CB. Relation of physical activity and cardiovascular fitness to coronary heart disease. Part I: A meta-analysis of the independent relation of physical activity and coronary heart disease. *J Am Board Fam Pract* 1992;5:31–42. Search date not stated; primary source Medline.

8. Fraser GE, Strahan TM, Sabate J, Beeson WL, Kissinger D. Effects of traditional coronary risk factors on rates of incident coronary events in a low-risk population: the Adventist health study. *Circulation* 1992;86:406–413.

9. Lindsted KD, Tonstad S, Kuzma JW. Self-report of physical activity and patterns of mortality in Seventh-Day Adventist men. *J Clin Epidemiol* 1991;44:355–364.

10. Folsom AR, Arnett DK, Hutchinson RG, Liao F, Clegg LX, Cooper LS. Physical activity and incidence of coronary heart disease in middle-aged women and men. *Med Sci Sports Exerc* 1997;29:901–909.

11. Jensen G, Nyboe J, Appleyard M, Schnohr P. Risk factors for acute myocardial infarction in Copenhagen, II: Smoking, alcohol intake, physical activity, obesity, oral contraception, diabetes, lipids, and blood pressure. *Eur Heart J* 1991;12:298–308.

12. Simonsick EM, Lafferty ME, Phillips CL, et al. Risk due to inactivity in physically capable older adults. *Am J Public Health* 1993;83:1443–1450.

13. Haapanen N, Miilunpalo S, Vuori I, Oja P, Pasanen M. Association of leisure time physical activity with the risk of coronary heart disease, hypertension and diabetes in middle-aged men and women. *Int J Epidemiol* 1997;26:739–747.

14. Sherman SE, D'Agostino RB, Cobb JL, Kannel WB. Does exercise reduce mortality rates in the elderly? Experience from the Framingham heart study. *Am Heart J* 1994;128:965–672.

15. Rodriguez BL, Curb JD, Burchfiel CM, et al. Physical activity and 23-year incidence of coronary heart disease morbidity and mortality among middle-aged men: the Honolulu heart program. *Circulation* 1994;89:2540–2544.

16. Eaton CB, Medalie JH, Flocke SA, Zyzanski SJ, Yaari S, Goldbourt U. Self-reported physical activity

predicts long-term coronary heart disease and all-cause mortalities: 21-year follow-up of the Israeli ischemic heart disease study. *Arch Fam Med* 1995;4:323–329.

17. Stender M, Hense HW, Doring A, Keil U. Physical activity at work and cardiovascular disease risk: results from the MONICA Augsburg study. *Int J Epidemiol* 1993;22:644–650.

18. Leon AS, Myers MJ, Connett J. Leisure time physical activity and the 16-year risks of mortality from coronary heart disease and all-causes in the multiple risk factor intervention trial (MRFIT). *Int J Sports Med* 1997;18(suppl 3):208–315.

19. Rosolova H, Simon J, Sefrna F. Impact of cardiovascular risk factors on morbidity and mortality in Czech middle-aged men: Pilsen longitudinal study. *Cardiology* 1994;85:61–68.

20. Luoto R, Prattala R, Uutela A, Puska P. Impact of unhealthy behaviors on cardiovascular mortality in Finland, 1978–1993. *Prev Med* 1998;27:93–100.

21. Woo J, Ho SC, Yuen YK, Yu LM, Lau J. Cardiovascular risk factors and 18-month mortality and morbidity in an elderly Chinese population aged 70 years and over. *Gerontology* 1998;44:51–55.

22. Gartside PS, Wang P, Glueck CJ. Prospective assessment of coronary heart disease risk factors: The NHANES I epidemiologic follow-up study (NHEFS) 16-year follow-up. *J Am Coll Nutr* 1998;17:263–269.

23. Dorn JP, Cerny FJ, Epstein LH, Naughton J, et al. Work and leisure time physical activity and mortality in men and women from a general population sample. *Ann Epidemiol* 1999;9:366–373.

24. Hakim AA, Curb JD, Petrovitch H, et al. Effects of walking on coronary heart disease in elderly men: the Honolulu heart program. *Circulation* 1999;100:9–13.

25. Eaton CB. Relation of physical activity and cardiovascular fitness to coronary heart disease, part II: cardiovascular fitness and the safety and efficacy of physical activity prescription. *J Am Board Fam Pract* 1992;5:157–165. Search date not stated; primary sources Medline and hand searches.

26. Blair SN, Kohl HW 3rd, Barlow CE, Paffenbarger RS Jr, Gibbons LW, Macera CA. Changes in physical fitness and all-cause mortality: a prospective study of healthy and unhealthy men. *JAMA* 1995;273:1093–1098.

27. Sacco RL, Gan R, Boden-Albala B, et al. Leisure-time physical activity and ischemic stroke risk: the Northern Manhattan stroke study. *Stroke* 1998; 29:380–387.

28. Shinton R. Lifelong exposures and the potential for stroke prevention: the contribution of cigarette smoking, exercise, and body fat. *J Epidemiol Community Health* 1997;51:138–143.

29. Gillum RF, Mussolino ME, Ingram DD. Physical activity and stroke incidence in women and men. The NHANES I epidemiologic follow-up study. *Am J Epidemiol* 1996;143:860–869.

30. Kiely DK, Wolf PA, Cupples LA, Beiser AS, Kannel WB. Physical activity and stroke risk: the Framingham study [correction appears in *Am J Epidemiol* 1995;141:178]. *Am J Epidemiol* 1994; 140:608–620.

31. Abbott RD, Rodriguez BL, Burchfiel CM, Curb JD. Physical activity in older middle-aged men and reduced risk of stroke: the Honolulu heart program. *Am J Epidemiol* 1994;139:881–893.

32. Haheim LL, Holme I, Hjermann I, Leren P. Risk factors of stroke incidence and mortality: a 12-year follow-up of the Oslo study. *Stroke* 1993; 24:1484–1489.

33. Wannamethee G, Shaper AG. Physical activity and stroke in British middle aged men. *BMJ* 1992; 304:597–601.

34. Menotti A, Keys A, Blackburn H, et al. Twenty-year stroke mortality and prediction in twelve cohorts of the seven countries study. *Int J Epidemiol* 1990; 19:309–315.

35. Lindenstrom E, Boysen G, Nyboe J. Risk factors for stroke in Copenhagen, Denmark. II. Lifestyle factors. *Neuroepidemiology* 1993;12:43–50.

36. Lindenstrom E, Boysen G, Nyboe J. Lifestyle factors and risk of cerebrovascular disease in women: the Copenhagen City heart study. *Stroke* 1993;24:1468–1472.

37. Folsom AR, Prineas RJ, Kaye SA, Munger RG. Incidence of hypertension and stroke in relation to body fat distribution and other risk factors in older women. *Stroke* 1990;21:701–706.

38. Nakayama T, Date C, Yokoyama T, Yoshiike N, Yamaguchi M, Tanaka H. A 15.5-year follow-up study of stroke in a Japanese provincial city: the Shibata study. *Stroke* 1997;28:45–52.

39. Lee IM, Hennekens CH, Berger K, Buring JE, Manson JE. Exercise and risk of stroke in male physicians. *Stroke* 1999;30:1–6.

40. Evenson KR, Rosamond WD, Cai J, et al. Physical activity and ischemic stroke risk: the atherosclerosis in communities study. *Stroke* 1999;30:1333–1339.

41. Mittleman MA, Maclure M, Tofler GH, Sherwood JB, Goldberg RJ, Muller JE. Triggering of acute myocardial infarction by heavy physical exertion. Protection against triggering by regular exertion: determinants of myocardial infarction onset study investigators. *N Engl J Med* 1993;329:1677–1683.

42. Willich SN, Lewis M, Lowel H, Arntz HR, Schubert F, Schroder R. Physical exertion as a trigger of acute myocardial infarction: triggers and mechanisms of myocardial infarction study group. *N Engl J Med* 1993;329:1684–1690.

43. Pate RR, Pratt M, Blair SN, et al. Physical activity and public health. A recommendation from the Centers for Disease Control and Prevention and the American College of Sports Medicine. *JAMA* 1995;273:402–407.

44. Thompson PD. The cardiovascular complications of vigorous physical activity. *Arch Intern Med* 1996;156:2297–2302.

45. Oberman A. Exercise and the primary prevention of cardiovascular disease. *Am J Cardiol* 1985;55:10–20.

46. Andersen RE, Wadden TA, Bartlett SJ, Zemel B, Verde TJ, Franckowiak SC. Effects of lifestyle activity vs structured aerobic exercise in obese women: a randomized trial. *JAMA* 1999;281:335–340.

47. Dunn AL, Marcus BH, Kampert JB, Garcia ME, Kohl HW, Blair SN. Comparison of lifestyle and structured interventions to increase physical activity and cardiorespiratory fitness: a randomized trial. *JAMA* 1999;281:327–434.

48. Pereira MA, Kriska AM, Day RD, Cauley JA, LaPorte RE, Kuller LH. A randomized walking trial in postmenopausal women: effects on physical activity and health 10 years later. *Arch Intern Med* 1998;158:1695–1701.

49. DeBusk RF, Stenestrand U, Sheehan M, Haskell WL. Training effects of long versus short bouts of exercise in healthy subjects. *Am J Cardiol* 1990; 65:1010–1013.

50. Ness AR, Powles JW. Fruit and vegetables and cardiovascular disease: a review. *Int J Epidemiol* 1997;26:1–13. Search date 1995; primary sources Medline, Embase, and hand searches of personal bibliographies, books, reviews, and citations in located reports.

51. Law MR, Morris JK. By how much does fruit and vegetable consumption reduce the risk of ischaemic heart disease? *Eur J Clin Nutr* 1998; 52:549–556. Search date not stated; primary sources Medline, Science Citation Index, and hand searches of review articles.

52. Klerk M, Jansen MCJF, van't Veer P, Kok FJ. *Fruits and vegetables in chronic disease prevention.* Wageningen: Grafisch Bedrijf Ponsen and Looijen, 1998. Search date 1998; primary sources Medline, Current Contents, and Toxline.

53. Key TJA, Thorogood M, Appleby PN, Burr ML. Dietary habits and mortality in 11 000 vegetarians and health conscious people: results of a 17 year follow up. *BMJ* 1996;313:775–779.

54. Pietinen P, Rimm EB, Korhonen P, et al. Intake of dietary fibre and risk of coronary heart disease in a cohort of Finnish men. *Circulation* 1996;94: 2720–2727.

55. Mann JI, Appleby PN, Key TJA, Thorogood M. Dietary determinants of ischaemic heart disease in health conscious individuals. *Heart* 1997;78:450–455.

56. Geleijnse M. Consumptie van groente en fruit in het risico op myocardinfarct 1997. Basisrapportage. Rotterdam: Erasmus Universiteit (cited in appendix XIII of review by Klerk).

57. Todd S, Woodward M, Tunstall-Pedoe H, Bolton-Smith C. Dietary antioxidant vitamins and fiber in the etiology of cardiovascular disease and all-cause mortality: results from the Scottish heart health study. *Am J Epidemiol* 1999;150:1073–1080.

58. Bazzano L, Ogden LG, Vupputuri S, Loria C, Myers L, Whelton PK. Fruit and vegetable intake reduces cardiovascular mortality: results from the NHANES I epidemiologic follow-up study (NHEFS). 40th Annual Conference Cardiovascular Epidemiology and Prevention [abstract]. *Circulation* 2000;8–8.

59. Lui S, Manson JE, Cole SR, Willett WC, Buring JE. Fruit and vegetable intake and risk of cardiovascular disease. 40th Annual Conference Cardiovascular Epidemiology and Prevention [abstract]. *Circulation* 2000;30–31.

60. Lui S, Manson JE, Lee I-M, et al. Fruit and vegetable intake and risk of cardiovascular disease: the Women's Health Study. *Am J Clin Nutr* 2000;72:922–928.

61. Knekt P, Reunanen A, Jarvinen R, Heliovaara M, Aromaa A. Antioxidant vitamin intake and coronary mortality in a longitudinal population study. *Am J Epidemiol* 1994;139:1180–1189.

62. Keli SO, Hertog MGL, Feskens EJM, Kromhout D. Dietary flavonoids, antioxidant vitamins, and incidence of stroke. *Arch Intern Med* 1996;156: 637–642.

63. Daviglus ML, Orencia AJ, Dyer AR, et al. Dietary vitamin C, beta-carotene and 30-year risk of stroke: results from the Western Electric study. *Neuroepidemiology* 1997;16:69–77.

64. Ascherio A, Rimm EB, Hernan MA, et al. Prospective study of potassium intake and risk of stroke among US men. *Can J Cardiol* 1997;13: 44B.

65. Yochum L, Kushi LH, Meyer K, Folsom AR. Dietary flavonoid intake and risk of cardiovascular disease in postmenopausal women. *Am J Epidemiol* 1999; 149:943–949.

66. Knekt P, Isotupa S, Rissanen H, et al. Quercetin intake and the incidence of cerebrovascular disease. *Eur J Clin Nutr* 2000;54:415–417.

67. Hirvonen T, Virtamo J, Korhonen P, Albanes D, Pietinen P. Intake of flavonoids, carotenoids, vitamin C and E, and risk of stroke in male smokers. *Stroke* 2000;31:2301–2306.

68. Joshipura KJ, Ascherio A, Manson JE, et al. Fruit and vegetable intake in relation to risk of ischemic stroke. *JAMA* 1999;282:1233–1239.

69. Ness AR, Powles JW. Does eating fruit and vegetables protect against heart attack and stroke? *Chem Indus* 1996;792–794.

70. Ness AR, Powles JW. Dietary habits and mortality in vegetarians and health conscious people: several uncertainties exist. *BMJ* 1997;314:148.

71. Serdula MK, Byers T, Mokhad AH, Simoes E, Mendleim JM, Coates RJ. The association between fruit and vegetable intake and chronic disease risk factors. *Epidemiology* 1996;7:161–165.

72. Lonn EM, Yusuf S. Is there a role for antioxidant vitamins in the prevention of cardiovascular disease? An update on epidemiological and clinical trials data. *Can J Cardiol* 1997;13:957–965. Search date not stated; primary sources Medline, science citation index, handsearching.

73. Jha P, Flather M, Lonn E, Farkouh M, Yusuf S. The antioxidant vitamins and cardiovascular disease: a critical review of epidemiologic and clinical trial data. *Ann Intern Med* 1995;123:860–872.

74. Roxrode KM, Manson JE. Antioxidants and coronary heart disease: observational studies. *J Cardiovasc Risk* 1996;3:363–367.

75. Egger M, Schneider M, Davey Smith G. Spurious precision? Meta-analysis of observational studies. *BMJ* 1998;316:140–144.

76. Gaziano JM. Randomized trials of dietary antioxidants in cardiovascular disease prevention and treatment. *J Cardiovasc Risk* 1996;3:368–371.

77. Ness AR, Powles JW, Khaw KT. Vitamin C and cardiovascular disease — a systematic review. *J Cardiovasc Risk* 1997;3:513–521. Search date 1996; primary sources Medline, Embase, and hand searches of personal bibliographies, books, reviews and citations in located reports.

78. Klipstein-Grobusch K, Geleijnse JM, den Breeijen JH, et al. Dietary antioxidants and risk of myocardial infarction in the elderly: the Rotterdam study. *Am J Clin Nutr* 1999;69:261–266.

79. Ascherio A, Rimm EB, Hernan MA, et al. Relation of consumption of vitamin E, vitamin C, and carotenoids to risk for stroke among men in the United States. *Ann Intern Med* 1999;130:963–970.

80. Yochum L, Folsom AR, Kushi LH. Intake of antioxidant vitamins and risk of death from stroke in postmenopausal women. *Am J Clin Nutr* 2000; 72:476–483.

81. Li J, Taylor PR, Li B, et al. Nutrition intervention trials in Linxian, China: multiple vitamin/mineral supplementation, cancer incidence, and disease-specific mortality among adults with esophageal dysplasia. *J Natl Cancer Inst* 1993;85:1492–1498.

82. Mark SD, Wang W, Fraumeni JF, et al. Lowered risks of hypertension and cerebrovascular disease after vitamin/mineral supplementation. *Am J Epidemiol* 1996;143:658–664.

83. Mark SD, Wang W, Fraumeni JFJ, et al. Do nutritional supplements lower the risk of stroke or hypertension? *Epidemiology* 1998;9:9–15.

84. Losonczy KG, Harris TB, Havlik RJ. Vitamin E and vitamin C supplement use and risk of all-cause and coronary mortality in older persons: the established populations for epidemiologic studies of the elderly. *Am J Clin Nutr* 1996;64:190–196.

85. Sahyoun NR, Jacques PF, Russell RM. Carotenoids, vitamin C and E, and mortality in an elderly population. *Am J Epidemiol* 1996;144: 501–511.

86. Keli SO, Hertog MGL, Feskens EJM, Kromhout D. Dietary flavonoids, antioxidant vitamins, and incidence of stroke. *Arch Intern Med* 1996;156: 637–642.

87. Houtman JP. Trace elements and cardiovascular disease. *J Cardiovasc Risk* 1996;3:18–25.

88. Nève J. Selenium as a risk factor for cardiovascular disease. *J Cardiovasc Risk* 1996;3: 42–47.

89. Hertog MGL, Feskens EJM, Holliman PCH, Katan MB, Kromhout D. Dietary antioxidant flavonoids and risk of coronary heart disease: the Zutphen elderly study. *Lancet* 1993;342:1007–1011.

90. Knekt P, Jarvinen R, Reunanen A, Maatela J. Flavonoid intake and coronary mortality in Finland: a cohort study. *BMJ* 1996;312:478–481.

91. Rimm EB, Katan MB, Ascherio A, Stampfer MJ, Willett WC. Relation between intake of flavonoids and risk for coronary heart disease in male health professionals. *Ann Intern Med* 1996;125:384–389.

92. Hertog MGL, Sweetnam PM, Fehily AM. Antioxidant flavonols and ischemic heart disease in a Welsh population of men: the Caerphilly study. *Am J Clin Nutr* 1997;65:1489–1494.

93. Doering WV. Antioxidant vitamins, cancer, and cardiovascular disease. *N Engl J Med* 1996;335: 1065.

94. Pietrzik K. Antioxidant vitamins, cancer, and cardiovascular disease. *N Engl J Med* 1996;335: 1065–1066.

95. Hennekens CH, Gaziano JM, Manson JE, Buring JE. Antioxidant vitamin cardiovascular disease hypothesis is still promising, but still unproven: the need for randomised trials. *Am J Clin Nutr* 1995; 62(suppl):1377–1380.

96. US Department of Health and Human Services. *The health benefits of smoking cessation: a report of the Surgeon General.* Rockville, Maryland: US Department of Health and Human Services, Public Health Service, Centers for Disease Control, 1990. DHHS Publication (CDC) 90–8416.

97. Royal College of Physicians. *Smoking and health now.* London: Pitman Medical and Scientific Publishing, 1971.

98. Doll R, Peto R, Wheatley K, Gray R, Sutherland I. Mortality in relation to smoking: 40 years' observations on male British doctors. *BMJ* 1994; 309:901–911.

99. Kawachi I, Colditz GA, Stampfer MJ, et al. Smoking cessation in relation to total mortality rates in women: a prospective cohort study. *Ann Intern Med* 1993;119:992–1000.

100. Rosenberg L, Kaufman DW, Helmrich SP, Shapiro S. The risk of myocardial infarction after quitting smoking in men under 55 years of age. *N Engl J Med* 1985;313:1511–1514.

101. Rosenberg L, Palmer JR, Shapiro S. Decline in the risk of myocardial infarction among women who stop smoking. *N Engl J Med* 1990;322: 213–217.

102. Rose G, Hamilton PJ, Colwell L, Shipley MJ. A randomised controlled trial of anti-smoking advice: 10-year results. *J Epidemiol Community Health* 1982;36:102–108.

103. Shinton R, Beevers G. Meta-analysis of relation between cigarette smoking and stroke. *BMJ* 1989;298:789–794. Search date 1988; primary source index references from three studies on cigarette smoking and stroke on medicine 1965–1988.

104. Rogot E, Murray JL. Smoking and causes of death among US veterans: 16 years of observation. *Public Health Rep* 1980;95:213–222.

105. Wannamethee SG, Shaper AG, Ebrahim S. History of parental death from stroke or heart trouble and the risk of stroke in middle-aged men. *Stroke* 1996;27:1492–1498.

106. Halbert JA, Silagy CA, Finucane P, Withers RT, Hamdorf PA. The effectiveness of exercise training in lowering blood pressure: a meta-analysis of randomised controlled trials of 4 weeks or longer. *J Hum Hypertens* 1997;11: 641–649. Search date 1996; primary sources Medline, Embase, Science Citation Index.

107. Ebrahim S, Davey Smith G. Lowering blood pressure: a systematic review of sustained non-pharmacological interventions. *J Public Health Med* 1998;20:441–448. Search date 1995; primary source Medline.

108. Engstom G, Hedblad B, Janzon L. Hypertensive men who exercise regularly have lower rate of cardiovascular mortality. *J Hypertens* 1999;17: 737–742.

109. Appel LJ, Moore TJ, Obarzanek E, et al. A clinical trial of the effects of dietary patterns on blood pressure. *N Engl J Med* 1997;336:1117–1124.

110. Beilin LJ, Puddey IB, Burke V. Alcohol and hypertension: kill or cure? *J Hum Hypertens* 1996;10(suppl 2):1–5.

111. Campbell NRC, Ashley MJ, Carruthers SG, et al. Recommendations on alcohol consumption. *Can Med Assoc J* 1999;(suppl 9):13–20. Search date 1996; primary source Medline.

112. Graudal NA, Galloe AM, Garred P. Effects of sodium restriction on blood pressure, renin, aldosterone, catecholamines, cholesterols, and triglyceride. *JAMA* 1998;279:1383–1391. Search date 1997; primary source Medline.

113. Whelton PK, Appel LJ, Espelland MA, et al. Sodium reduction and weight loss in the treatment of hypertension in older persons: a randomized controlled trial of non pharmacologic interventions in the elderly (TONE). *JAMA* 1998; 279:839–846.

114. Midgley JP, Matthew AG, Greenwood CMT, Logan AG. Effect of reduced dietary sodium on blood pressure. *JAMA* 1996;275:1590–1597. Search date 1994; primary sources Medline, Current Contents.

115. Alderman MH, Madhavan S, Cohen H, Sealey JE, Laragh JH. Low urinary sodium associated with greater risk of myocardial infarction among treated hypertensive men. *Hypertension* 1995; 25:1144–1152.

116. Stevens VJ, Obarzanek E, Cook NR, et al. Long-term weight loss and changes in blood pressure: results of the trials of hypertension prevention, phase 11. *Ann Intern Med* 2001;134:1–11.

117. Metz JA, Stern JS, Kris-Etherton P, et al. A randomized trial of improved weight loss with a prepared meal plan in overweight and obese patients. *Arch Intern Med* 2000;160:2150–2158.

118. Brand MB, Mulrow CD, Chiquette E, et al. Weight-reducing diets for control of hypertension in adults. In: The Cochrane Library, Issue 4, 1998 Oxford: Update Software. Search date 1997; primary source Cochrane Library, Medline.

119. Whelton PK, He J, Cutler JA, et al. Effects of oral potassium on blood pressure: meta-analysis of randomized controlled clinical trials. *JAMA* 1997; 277:1624–1632. Search date 1995; primary source Medline.

120. Morris MC, Sacks F, Rosner B. Does fish oil lower blood pressure? A meta-analysis of controlled clinical trials. *Circulation* 1993;88:523–533. Search date not given; primary source Index Medicus.

121. Griffith LE, Guyatt GH, Cook RJ, et al. The influence of dietary and nondietary calcium supplementation on blood pressure. *Am J Hypertens* 1999;12:84–92. Search date 1994; primary sources Medline, Embase.

122. Gueyffier F, Froment A, Gouton M. New meta-analysis of treatment trials of hypertension: improving the estimate of therapeutic benefit. *J*

Hum Hypertens 1996;10:1–8. Search date 1997; primary source Medline.

123. Staessen JA, Gasowski J, Wang JG, et al. Risks of untreated and treated isolated systolic hypertension in the elderly: meta-analysis of outcome trials. *Lancet* 2000;355:865–872. Search date 1999; primary sources other systematic reviews and reports from collaborative trialists.

124. Hansson L, Zanchetti AZ, Carruthers SG, et al. Effects of intensive blood pressure lowering and low-dose aspirin in patients with hypertension: principal results of the hypertension optimal treatment (HOT) trial. *Lancet* 1998;351:1755–1762.

125. Grossman E, Messerli FH, Goldbourt U. Does diuretic therapy increase the risk of renal cell carcinoma? *Am J Cardiol* 1999;83:1090–1093. Search dates 1966 to 1998; primary sources Medline.

126. Beto JA, Bansal VK. Quality of life in treatment of hypertension: a meta-analysis of clinical trials. *Am J Hypertens* 1992;5:125–133. Search date 1990; primary sources Medline, ERIC.

127. Croog SH, Levine S, Testa MA. The effects of antihypertensive therapy on quality of life. *N Engl J Med* 1986;314:1657–1664.

128. Psaty BM, Smith NS, Siscovick DS, et al. Health outcomes associated with antihypertensive therapies used as first line agents: a systematic review and meta-analysis. *JAMA* 1997;277:739–745. Search date 1995; primary source Medline.

129. Messerli FH, Grossman E, Goldbourt. Are beta blockers efficacious as first-line therapy for hypertension in the elderly? A systematic review. *JAMA* 1998;279:1903–1907. Search date 1998; primary source Medline.

130. Hansson L, Lindholm LH, Niskanen L, et al. Effect of angiotensin-converting-enzyme inhibition compared with conventional therapy on cardiovascular morbidity and mortality in hypertension: the captopril prevention project (CAPP) randomised trial. *Lancet* 1999;353:611–616.

131. Hansson L, Lindholm L, Ekbom T, et al. Randomised trial of old and new antihypertensive drugs in elderly patients: cardiovascular mortality and morbidity in the Swedish trial in old patients with hypertension-2 study. *Lancet* 1999;354:1751–1756.

132. Blood Pressure Lowering Treatment Trialists' Collaboration. Effects of ACE inhibitors, calcium antagonists, and other blood-pressure-lowering drugs: results of prospectively designed overviews of trials. *Lancet* 2000;356:1955–1964. Search date July 2000; primary sources WHO-International Society of Hypertension registry of randomised trials; trials were sought that had not been published or presented their results before July 1995.

133. The ALLHAT Officers and Coordinators for the ALLHAT Collaborative Research Group. Major cardiovascular events in hypertensive patients randomized to doxazosin vs chlorthalidone: the antihypertensive and lipid-lowering treatment to prevent heart attack trial (ALLHAT). *JAMA* 2000; 283:1967–1975.

134. Neaton JD, Grimm RH, Prineas RJ, et al. Treatment of mild hypertension study: final results. *JAMA* 1993;270:713–724.

135. Materson BJ, Reda DJ, Cushman WC, et al. Single drug therapy for hypertension in men. *N Engl J Med* 1993;328:914–921.

136. Philipp T, Anlauf M, Distler A, Holzgreve H, Michaelis J, Wellek S. Randomised, double blind, multicentre comparison of hydrochlorothiazide, atenolol, nitrendipine, and enalapril in antihypertensive treatment: results of the HANE study. *BMJ* 1997;315:154–159.

137. Wright JM, Lee CH, Chambers CK. Systematic review of antihypertensive therapies: does the evidence assist in choosing a first line drug? *Can Med Assoc J* 1999;161:25–32. Search date 1998; primary sources Medline 1996 to 1997, Cochrane Library to 1998.

138. Cutler JA. Calcium channel blockers for hypertension — uncertainty continues. *N Engl J Med* 1998;338:679–680.

139. Downs JR, Clearfield M, Weis S, et al. Primary prevention of acute coronary events with lovastatin in men and women with average cholesterol levels: results of the AFCAPS/TexCAPS. *JAMA* 1998;279:1615–1622.

140. Scandinavian Simvastatin Survival Study Group. Randomized trial of cholesterol lowering in 4444 patients with coronary heart disease: the Scandinavian simvastatin survival study (4S). *Lancet* 1995;344:1383–1389.

141. Long-term Intervention with Pravastatin in Ischemic Disease (LIPID) Study Program. Prevention of cardiovascular events and death with pravastatin in patients with coronary heart disease and a broad range of initial cholesterol levels. *N Engl J Med* 1998;339:1349–1357.

142. Sacks FM, Pfeffer MA, Moye LA, et al, for the Cholesterol and Recurrent Events Trial Investigators. Effect of pravastatin on coronary events after myocardial infarction in patients with average cholesterol levels. *N Engl J Med* 1996; 335:1001–1009.

143. Shepherd J, Cobbe SM, Ford I, et al, for the West of Scotland Coronary Prevention Study Group. Prevention of coronary heart disease with pravastatin in men with hypercholesterolemia. *N Engl J Med* 1995;333:1301–1307.

144. Katerndahl DA, Lawler WR. Variability in meta-analytic results concerning the value of cholesterol reduction in coronary heart disease: a meta-meta-analysis. *Am J Epidemiol* 1999; 149:429–441. Search date 1995; primary sources Medline and meta-analysis bibliographies.

145. Froom J, Froom P, Benjamin M, Benjamin BJ. Measurement and management of hyperlipidemia for the primary prevention of coronary heart disease. *J Am Board Fam Pract* 1998;11:12–22.

146. Ebrahim S, Davey Smith G, McCabe CCC, et al. What role for statins? A review and economic model. *Health Technology Assessment* 1999;3: 19;1–91. Search dates 1997; primary sources Medline, Cochrane Controlled Trials Register, and personal contact with investigators working in the field of cholesterol lowering.

147. Pignone M, Phillips C, Mulrow C. Use of lipid lowering drugs for primary prevention of coronary heart disease: meta-analysis of randomised trials. *BMJ* 2000;321(7267):983–986. Search date 1999; primary sources Medline, Cochrane Library, and hand searches of bibliographies of systematic reviews and clinical practice guidelines.

148. Cucherat M, Lievre M, Gueyffier F. Clinical benefits of cholesterol lowering treatments. Meta-analysis of randomized therapeutic trials. *Presse Med* 2000 May 13;29:965–976. Search date and primary sources not stated.

149. LaRosa JC, He J, Vupputuri S. Effect of statins on risk of coronary disease: a meta-analysis of randomized controlled trials. *JAMA* 1999;282: 2340–2346. Search date 1998; primary sources Medline, bibliographies and authors' reference files.

150. Carlsson CM, Carnes M, McBride PE, Stein JH. Managing dyslipidaemia in older adults. *J Am Geriatr Society* 1999;47:1458–1465.

151. Bucher HC, Griffith LE, Guyatt G. Systematic review on the risk and benefit of different cholesterol-lowering interventions. *Arterioscler Thromb Vasc Biol* 1999:19;187–195. Search date October 1996; primary sources Medline, Embase, and hand searches of bibliographies.

152. Peto R, Gray R, Collins R, et al. Randomised trial of prophylactic daily aspirin in British male doctors. *BMJ* 1988;296:313–316.

153. Steering Committee of the Physicians' Health Study Research Group. Final report on the aspirin component of the ongoing physicians' health study. *N Engl J Med* 1989;321:129–135.

154. Medical Research Council's General Practice Research Framework. Thrombosis prevention trial: randomised trial of low-intensity anticoagulation with warfarin and low dose aspirin in the primary prevention of ischaemic heart disease in men at increased risk. *Lancet* 1998;351:233–241.

155. Antiplatelet Trialists' Collaboration. Collaborative overview of randomised trials of antiplatelet therapy — I: prevention of death, myocardial infarction, and stroke by prolonged antiplatelet therapy in various categories of patients. *BMJ* 1994;308:81–106. Search date 1990; primary sources Medline, Current Contents, hand searches of reference lists of trials and review articles, journal abstracts and meeting proceedings, trial register of the International Committee on Thrombosis and Haemostasis, and personal contacts with colleagues and antiplatelet manufacturers.

156. Hart RG, Halperin JL, McBride R, Benavente O, Man-Son-Hing M, Kronmal RA. Aspirin for the primary prevention of stroke and other major vascular events. Meta-analysis and hypotheses. *Arch Neurol* 2000;57:326–332. Search date 1998; primary sources unspecified computerised medical databases 1980 to 1998, Cochrane Collaboration registry 1998, and hand searched references of Antiplatelet Trialists' Collaboration publications.

157. Collaborative group of the Primary Prevention Project (PPP). Low-dose aspirin and vitamin E in people at cardiovascular risk: a randomised trial in general practice. *Lancet* 2001;357:89–95.

158. Buring JE, Hennekens CH for the Women's Health Study Group. Women's health study: summary of the study design. *J Myocard Ischemia* 1992;4:27–29

Michael Murphy
Director, ICRF General Practice
Research Group

Charles Foster
British Heart Foundation Scientist

Cathie Sudlow
Specialist Registrar in Neurology
Department of Neurology
Derriford Hospital
Plymouth
UK

Julian Nicholas
Resident Physician
Mayo Clinic
Rochester, MN
USA

Cindy Mulrow
Professor of Medicine
University of Texas
Health Science Center
San Antonio, TX
USA

Andy Ness
Senior Lecturer in Epidemiology
University of Bristol
Bristol
UK

Michael Pignone
Assistant Professor of Medicine
Division of General Internal Medicine,
University of North Carolina
Chapel Hill, NC
USA

Competing interests: CM has participated in multicentre research trials evaluating antihypertensive agents that were funded by industry; other authors, none declared.

| TABLE 1 | Examples of common physical activities by intensity of effort required in multiples of the resting rate of oxygen consumption during physical activity. Based on table from Pate et al (see text, p 66).[43] |

Activity type	Light activity (< 3.0 METs)	Moderate activity (3.0–6.0 METs)	Vigorous activity (> 6.0 METs)
Walking	Slowly (1–2 mph)	Briskly (3–4 mph)	Briskly uphill or with a load
Swimming	Treading slowly	Moderate effort	Fast treading or swimming
Cycling	–	For pleasure or transport (≤ 10 mph)	Fast or racing (> 10 mph)
Golf	Power cart	Pulling cart or carrying clubs	–
Boating	Power boat	Canoeing leisurely	Canoeing rapidly (> 4 mph)
Home care	Carpet sweeping	General cleaning	Moving furniture
Mowing lawn	Riding mower	Power mower	Hand mower
Home repair	Carpentry	Painting	–

mph, miles per hour; METs, work metabolic rate/resting metabolic rate; 1 MET represents the rate of oxygen consumption of a seated adult at rest.

TABLE 2 Effectiveness of lifestyle interventions for lowering blood pressure in people with primary hypertension: results of RCTs (see text, pp 72–75).

Intervention	Mean decrease in syst/diast BP (mmHg)	Number of RCTs (people)	Participants	Duration (weeks)	Mean change in targeted factor
Exercise	5/3	29 (1533)	80% male, age 28–72	> 4	50 mins aerobic 3 x a week
Low fat high fruit and vegetable diet	5.5/3*	1 (459)	50% male, mean age 44	8	
Weight loss	3/3	18 (2611)	55% male, mean age 50	2–52	3–9% of body weight
Salt restriction	4/2	58 (2161)	Mean age 49	1–52	118 mmol/day
	2/0.5	28 (1131)	Mean age 47	4	60 mmol/day

* Data presented for 459 people with systolic BP below 160 mmHg and diastolic BP 80–95 mmHg; for the subgroup of 133 people with systolic BP ≥140 mmHg or diastolic BP ≥90 mmHg, the mean decrease of BP was 11.4/5.5; syst/diast BP, systolic/diastolic blood pressure.

TABLE 3 Effectiveness of dietary supplementation for lowering blood pressure in people with primary hypertension: results of RCTs (see text, pp 76, 77).

Intervention	Decrease in syst/diast BP (mmHg)	Number of RCTs (people)	Participants	Duration	Change in targeted factor
Potassium supplement	4.4/2.5	21 (1560)	Age 19–79	1–24 weeks	60–100 mmol/day
Fish oil supplement	4.5/2.5	7 (339)	Mean age 50	Mean 8 weeks	3 g/day or more
Calcium supplement	2/0	12 (383)	Not clear	8 weeks median	800–1500 mg/day

Cardiovascular disorders

TABLE 4 Effects of antiplatelet treatment (mainly aspirin) on vascular events (non-fatal myocardial infarction, non-fatal stroke, or vascular death) among individuals without evidence of cardiovascular disease (see text, p 82).

Trials (duration)	Annual risk of vascular event (control)	Vascular events Antiplatelet, Control and Odds ratio*(CI†)	Avoided events (1000 person years)	Myocardial infarction Antiplatelet, Control and Odds ratio*(CI†)	Stroke Antiplatelet, Control and Odds ratio*(CI†)
UK doctors[152] (70 months)	1.5%	288/3429, 280/3420‡ 1.03 (0.6 to 2.3)	−0.4	169/3429, 176/3420‡ 0.96 (0.7 to 1.4)	91/3429, 78/3420‡ 1.16 (0.7 to 1.9)
US physicians[153] (60 months)	0.7%	321/11037, 387/11034 0.82 (0.7 to 1.0)	1.2	139/11037, 239/11034 0.58 (0.5 to 0.8)	119/11037, 98/11034 1.22 (0.9 to 1.7)
TPT[154] (76 months)	1.8%	239/2545, 270/2540 0.87 (0.7 to 1.1)	2.0	154/2545, 190/2540 0.80 (0.7 to 1.1)	47/2545, 48/2540 0.98 (0.6 to 1.7)
HOT[124] (46 months)	1.0%	315/9399, 368/9391 0.85 (0.7 to 1.0)	1.5	82/9399, 127/9391 0.65 (0.5 to 0.9)	146/9399, 148/9391 0.99 (0.7 to 1.3)
PPP[157] (44 months)	0.8%	45/2226, 64/2269 0.71 (0.4 to 1.2)	2.2	19/2226, 28/2269 0.69 (0.3 to 1.5)	16/2226, 24/2269 0.68 (0.3 to 1.6)
All trials (56 months)	1.0%	1208/28636 (4.2%), 1369/28654 (4.8%) 0.86§ (0.8 to 0.9)	1.2	563/28636 (2.0%), 760/28654 (2.4%) 0.71§ (0.6 to 0.8)	419/28636 (1.5%), 396/28654 (1.4%) 1.05§ (0.9 to 1.2)

Data from individual trial publications and from the APT overview (1994).[155] The effects of aspirin were similar in the absence or presence of warfarin, so the data presented are not stratified by warfarin allocation. * Odds ratios calculated using the "observed minus expected" method.[155] † 99% CI for individual trials, 95% CI for "All trials". ‡ Number of patients in control group was 1710 (randomisation ratio 2 : 1); numerator and denominator multiplied by 2 to calculate totals for absolute differences between antiplatelet and control group event rates; actual numbers of events used to calculate odds ratios and confidence intervals. ¶ Weighted by study size. § Heterogeneity of odds ratios between 5 trials not significant (P > 0.05).

TABLE 5 Effects of aspirin on intracranial bleeds and major extracranial bleeds in RCTs among individuals without evidence of cardiovascular disease (see text, p 82).

Trials	Antiplatelet	Control	Summary odds ratio* (95% CI)	Excess bleeds per 1000 people treated per year
Intracranial bleeds				
UK doctors[152]	13/3429	12/3420†		
US physicians[153]	23/11037	12/11034		
TPT[154]	12/2545	6/2540		
HOT[124]	14/9399	15/9391		
PPP[157]	2/2226	3/2269		
All trials	64/28 636 (0.22%)	48/28654 (0.17%)	1.4(0.9 to 2.0)	0.1 (P = 0.1)
Major extracranial bleeds				
UK Doctors[152]	21/3429	20/3420†		
US Physicians[153]	48/1 037	28/11 034		
TPT[154]	20/2545	13/2540		
HOT[124]	122/9399	63/9391		
All trials	211/26 410 (0.8%)	134/28 095 (0.5%)	1.7(1.4 to 2.1)	0.7 (P < 0.00001)

Data from individual trial publications. * Odds ratios calculated using the "observed minus expected" method.[155] † Number of patients in control group was 1710 (randomisation ratio 2 : 1); numerator and denominator multiplied by 2 to calculate differences between antiplatelet and control group event rates; actual numbers of events used to calculate odds ratios and confidence intervals.

Primary prevention

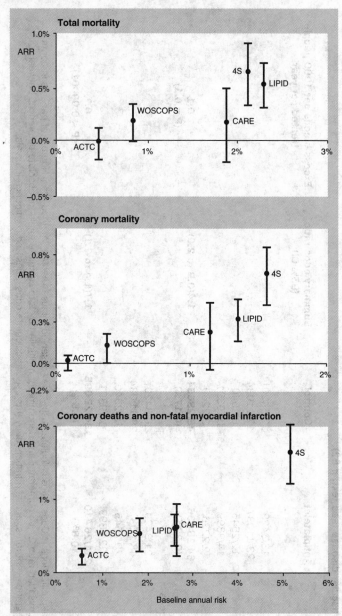

FIGURE 1 Effects of cholesterol lowering: relation between the ARR (for annual total mortality, coronary heart disease mortality, coronary deaths, and non-fatal myocardial infarction) and the baseline risk of those events in the placebo group for 5 large statin trials (ACTC = AFCAPS/TexCAPS,[139] 4S,[140] LIPID,[141] CARE,[142] WOSCOPS[143]) (see text, p 80).

Search date November 2000

Clinical Evidence writers on secondary prevention of ischaemic cardiac events

QUESTIONS

INTERVENTIONS

Key Messages

Antithrombotic treatment

- One collaborative overview and subsequent RCTs have found that antiplatelet treatment reduces the risk of serious vascular events, and suggests that aspirin 75 mg daily is as effective as higher doses. We found no clear evidence that any other antiplatelet regimen is definitely superior to medium dose aspirin (75–325 mg daily) in the prevention of vascular events. One systematic review has found that clopidogrel is a safe and effective alternative to aspirin.

- One systematic review has found that anticoagulants produce a similar reduction in the risk of serious vascular events to that produced by aspirin. However, aspirin versus oral anticoagulants causes fewer haemorrhages. The systematic review has found no clear evidence that the addition of oral anticoagulants to aspirin produced additional benefit.

Other drug treatments

- Systematic reviews have found that:
  - β Blockers reduce all cause mortality, coronary mortality, recurrent non-fatal myocardial infarction (MI), and sudden death in people after MI.
  - In people who have had an MI with or without left ventricular dysfunction, angiotensin converting enzyme (ACE) inhibitors reduce rates of death, hospitalisation for congestive heart failure, and recurrent non-fatal MI.
  - Using class I antiarrhythmic agents after MI increases the risk of cardiovascular mortality and sudden death.
  - Amiodarone reduces the risk of sudden death and marginally reduces overall mortality in people at high risk of death after MI. We found limited evidence that sotalol may be harmful rather than beneficial in people after MI.
  - Calcium channel blockers do not reduce mortality in people after MI or with chronic coronary heart disease. Diltiazem and verapamil may reduce rates of reinfarction and refractory angina in people after MI who do not have heart failure.

- One large well designed RCT of hormone replacement therapy (HRT) versus placebo found no reduction of major cardiovascular events in postmenopausal women with established coronary artery disease, despite strong evidence from RCTs that HRT improves some cardiovascular risk factors.

Cholesterol reduction

- One systematic review has found that lowering cholesterol with statins substantially reduces the risk of cardiovascular mortality and morbidity with no evidence of an increase in non-cardiovascular mortality.

Blood pressure reduction

- We found no direct evidence of the effects of lowering blood pressure in people with established coronary heart disease. Observational studies and extrapolation from trials of blood pressure reduction in people with no history of ischaemic cardiac events support the lowering of blood pressure in those with concomitant risk factors that put them at higher risk. The evidence for benefit is strongest for β blockers.

Non-drug treatments

- The role of vitamin E, β carotene, and vitamin C remains unclear.

- RCTs found that advising people with coronary artery disease to eat more fish (particularly fatty fish) or more fruit and vegetables, bread, pasta, potatoes, olive oil, and rapeseed margarine (a more Mediterranean diet) may result in a substantial survival benefit. We found no strong evidence from RCTs of a beneficial effect of low fat or high fibre diets on major non-fatal coronary heart disease events or coronary heart disease mortality.

■ Systematic reviews have found that cardiac rehabilitation improves coronary risk factors and reduces the risk of major cardiac events in people after MI. The role of exercise alone in reducing the risk of adverse cardiovascular outcomes is not clear.

■ We found no RCTs of the effects of smoking cessation on cardiovascular events in people with coronary heart disease. Epidemiological studies have found that people with coronary heart disease who stop smoking rapidly reduce their risk of recurrent coronary events or death. The use of nicotine patches seems safe in people with coronary heart disease.

■ One systematic review of mainly poor quality RCTs found that psychological and stress management may decrease rates of MI or cardiac death in people with coronary heart disease.

Surgical treatments

■ RCTs performed up to the mid 1980s have found that, compared with medical treatment, coronary artery bypass grafting (CABG) carries a greater risk of death in the first year but reduces the risk of death from coronary artery disease at 5 and 10 years. Greatest benefit occurrs in people with more severe disease (multivessel disease, left ventricular dysfunction, or MI). We found no evidence of increased protection against subsequent MI. One more recent RCT, using modern techniques and with optimal background medical treatment, has found even greater superiority of surgical revascularisation over non-invasive treatment.

■ RCTs have found that, in comparison with percutaneous transluminal coronary angioplasty (PTA), intracoronary stents affords superior acute and long term clinical and angiographic results.

DEFINITION	Secondary prevention in this context is the long term management of people with a prior acute MI, and of people at high risk of ischaemic cardiac events for other reasons, such as a history of angina or coronary surgical procedures.
INCIDENCE/ PREVALENCE	Coronary artery disease is the leading cause of death in developed countries and is becoming a major cause of mortality and morbidity in developing countries. There are pronounced international, regional, and temporal differences in death rates. In the USA, the prevalence of overt coronary artery disease approaches 4%.[1]
AETIOLOGY/ RISK FACTORS	Most ischaemic cardiac events are associated with atheromatous plaques that can cause acute obstruction of coronary vessels. Atheroma is more likely in elderly people, in those with established coronary artery disease, and in those with risk factors (such as smoking, hypertension, high cholesterol, diabetes mellitus).
PROGNOSIS	Almost half of those who suffer an acute MI die before they reach hospital. Of those hospitalised, 7–15% die in hospital and another 7–15% die during the following year. People who survive the acute stage of MI fall into three prognostic groups, based on their baseline risk (see table 1, p 125):[2–4] high (20% of all survivors), moderate (55%), and low (25%) risk. Long term prognosis depends on the degree of left ventricular dysfunction, the presence of residual ischaemia, and the extent of any electrical instability. Further risk stratification procedures include evaluation of left ventricular

Cardiovascular disorders

function (by echocardiography or nuclear ventriculography) and of myocardial ischaemia (by non-invasive stress testing).[4–8] Those with low left ventricular ejection fraction, ischaemia, or poor functional status may be evaluated further by cardiac catheterisation.[9]

AIMS   To improve long term survival and quality of life; to prevent (recurrent) MI, unstable angina, left ventricular dysfunction, heart failure, and sudden cardiac death; and to restore and maintain normal activities.

OUTCOMES   Mortality (total, cardiovascular, coronary, sudden death, noncardiovascular); morbidity (MI, severe angina, and stroke); or quality of life.

METHODS   *Clinical Evidence* update search and appraisal November 2000.

QUESTION   What are the effects of antithrombotic treatment?

Cathie Sudlow

OPTION   ANTIPLATELET TREATMENT

One collaborative overview has found that prolonged antiplatelet treatment reduces the risk of serious vascular events in people at high risk of ischaemic cardiac events. Along with subsequent RCTs, it found that, for prolonged use, aspirin 75 mg daily is as effective as higher doses. We found no clear evidence that any other antiplatelet regimen is superior to medium dose aspirin (i.e. 75–325 mg daily) to prevent vascular events, although one RCT has found that clopidogrel appears to be a safe and effective alternative.

Benefits: **Antiplatelet treatment versus control:** One collaborative overview (search date not stated) found that a month or more of antiplatelet treatment significantly reduced the odds of a vascular event (non-fatal MI, non-fatal stroke, or vascular death) by about a quarter compared with control, among about 70 000 people at high risk of occlusive arterial disease (odds reduction 27%, 95% CI 24% to 30%).[10] Most of these people were at high risk of ischaemic cardiac events, and some people (including those with a history of MI, those with stable angina, and those who had undergone coronary revascularisation procedures) were at particularly high risk. Among the 20 000 people with a prior MI, antiplatelet treatment prevented 18 non-fatal recurrent MIs, six non-fatal strokes, and 13 vascular deaths per 1000 people treated for about 2 years. The review also found that antiplatelet treatment reduced all cause mortality (see figure 1, p 126). **Different daily doses of aspirin:** About two thirds of the RCTs in the overview involved an aspirin regimen, and medium dose aspirin (75–325 mg daily) was the most widely tested of these. Indirect comparisons found that daily doses of less than 160 mg (mostly 75–150 mg), 160–325 mg, and 500–1500 mg prevented similar proportions of vascular events among high risk people, whereas direct comparisons also showed that daily aspirin doses of 75–325 mg or 500–1500 mg were similarly effective.[10] One additional recent RCT (almost 3000 people at high risk of cardiovascular events) directly compared lower doses of aspirin (81 mg or 325 mg daily) versus higher doses (650 mg or 1300 mg daily). It found that lower doses produced a slightly lower rate of stroke, MI, or death than higher doses (AR 6.2% with lower doses v AR 8.4 % with higher doses; P = 0.03).[11] The review found only limited evidence for the effectiveness of daily doses of aspirin of less than 160 mg. One subsequent RCT (2000 people with stable angina) compared aspirin 75 mg daily with placebo.[12] It found that a daily dose of aspirin 75 mg reduced the composite outcome of MI or sudden death compared with placebo (RRR 34%, 95% CI 24% to 49%). **Alternative antiplatelet regimens to aspirin:** The 1994 review found no evidence that any antiplatelet regimen was more effective than medium dose aspirin alone in the prevention of vascular events.[10] One systematic review of randomised trials (search date 1999), comparing either ticlopidine or clopidogrel with aspirin, found four trials among 22 656 people at high risk of vascular disease (including 6000 presenting with recent MI).[13] Most of these people were included in a large trial of clopidogrel (75 mg daily) versus aspirin (325 mg daily).[14] Compared with aspirin, the thienopyridines reduced the odds of a vascular event by 9% (OR 0.91, 95% CI 0.84 to 0.98; P = 0.01), but there was substantial uncertainty about the size of any additional benefit (11 events prevented per 1000 people treated for about 2 years [95% CI 2 to 19 events]).[13]

Harms: Bleeding is the most important adverse effect of antiplatelet treatment. The 1994 overview found that the excess risk of intracranial bleeding with antiplatelet treatment was small (at most 1 or 2 bleeds per 1000 people per year) in trials of long term treatment.[10] Antiplatelet treatment produced a small but significant excess of non-fatal major extracranial bleeds (3 bleeds per 1000 people), but there was no clear excess of fatal extracranial bleeds.[10] In one RCT directly comparing two different doses of aspirin, 1200 mg daily was associated with more gastrointestinal bleeding than 325 mg daily,[15] although we found no good evidence for a variation in gastrointestinal bleeding risk in the range 75–325 mg daily. The systematic review of randomised trials of the thienopyridine derivatives versus aspirin found that the thienopyridines produced significantly less gastrointestinal haemorrhage and upper gastrointestinal upset than aspirin. However, they increased the odds of skin rash and of diarrhoea: ticlopidine by about twofold and clopidogrel by about a third. Ticlopidine (but not clopidogrel) increased the odds of neutropenia.[13] Observational studies have also found that ticlopidine is associated with thrombocytopenia and thrombotic thrombocytopenic purpura.[16,17] However, we found no clear evidence of an excess of haematological adverse side effects with clopidogrel.[18,19] The results of two RCTs (about 1700 people undergoing coronary artery stenting) of clopidogrel plus aspirin versus ticlopidine plus aspirin suggested clopidogrel to be superior to ticlopidine in terms of safety and tolerability.[20,21]

Comment: Among people at high risk of cardiac events, the large absolute reductions in serious vascular events far outweighed any absolute risks.

ORAL ANTICOAGULANTS IN THE ABSENCE OF
ANTIPLATELET TREATMENT

One systematic review has found that high or moderate intensity oral anticoagulants given alone reduce the risk of serious vascular events in people with coronary artery disease, but were associated with substantial risks of bleeding. Oral anticoagulants require regular monitoring for intensity of anticoagulant effect.

Benefits: One systematic overview (search date 1999) of the effects of oral anticoagulation in people with coronary artery disease found 16 trials of high intensity anticoagulation (international normalised ratio [INR] > 2.8 — see glossary, p 120) versus control in 10 056 people, and four trials of moderate intensity anticoagulation (INR 2–3) versus control in 1365 people. Antiplatelet therapy was not routinely given in any of these 20 trials. The review found that high intensity anti-coagulation reduced the odds of the combined outcome of death, MI, or stroke compared with control (odds reduction 43%, 95% CI 37% to 49%; about 98 events avoided per 1000 people treated). Compared with control, moderate intensity anti-coagulation reduced these odds by a somewhat smaller, non-significant amount.[22] In direct comparisons of high or moderate intensity oral anticoagulation with aspirin, the effects on death, MI, or stroke were similar (OR 1.04, 95% CI 0.80 to 1.34).[22]

Harms: Compared with control, high intensity anticoagulation increased the odds of major (mainly extracranial) bleeding about sixfold (OR 6.0, 95% CI 4.4 to 8.2; absolute increase of 39 events per 1000 people treated), and moderate intensity anticoagulation also increased the odds of major bleeding about eightfold (OR 7.7, 95% CI 3.3 to 17.6).[22] Compared with aspirin, high or moderate intensity oral anticoagulation increased the odds of major bleeding more than twofold (OR 2.4, 95% CI 1.6 to 3.6).[22]

Comment: Oral anticoagulants provide substantial protection against vascular events in the absence of antiplatelet therapy, but the risks of serious bleeding are higher than for antiplatelet treatment and regular monitoring is required. Medium dose aspirin provides similar protection, but is safer and easier to use; see antiplatelet treatment below.

ORAL ANTICOAGULANTS IN ADDITION TO ANTIPLATELET
TREATMENT

One systematic review found no evidence that the addition of low intensity oral anticoagulation (target INR < 1.5) to aspirin produces additional benefit. The effects of adding a more intensive anticoagulant regimen (target INR 2–3) are uncertain.

Benefits: One systematic overview (search date 1999) found six RCTs that examined the effects of adding an oral anticoagulant regimen to aspirin in 8915 people with coronary artery disease. Three of these trials assessed the addition of a low intensity (target INR < 1.5) regimen to aspirin in a total of 8435 people, and found no significant reduction in the odds of death, MI, or stroke (OR 0.91, 95% CI 0.79 to 1.06).[22] Trials assessing the addition of a moderate intensity (INR 2–3) oral anticoagulant regimen to aspirin were too small (480 people) to produce reliable estimates of efficacy and safety.[22]

Harms: Too few major bleeds have been recorded in RCTs to quantify reliably the effects of adding oral anticoagulants to aspirin. The review found a non-significant excess of major bleeds produced by the addition of low intensity oral anticoagulation to aspirin (OR 1.29, 95% CI 0.96 to 1.75), as well as by the addition of more intense anticoagulation (OR 1.88, 95% CI 0.59 to 6.00).[22]

Comment: The issue of whether adding a moderately intense oral anticoagulant regimen to aspirin provides additional net benefit to people at high risk of ischaemic cardiac events is being assessed in several ongoing RCTs.

| QUESTION | What are the effects of other drug treatments? |

Eva Lonn

| OPTION | β BLOCKERS |

We found strong evidence from systematic reviews of RCTs that β blockers reduce the risk of all cause mortality, coronary mortality, recurrent non-fatal MI, and sudden death in people after MI. Most benefit was seen in those at highest risk of death after an MI (> 50 years old; previous MI, angina pectoris, hypertension, or treatment with digitalis; transient mechanical or electrical failure; higher heart rate at study entry). About a quarter of people suffered adverse effects.

Benefits: **Survival and reinfarction:** One systematic review (search date 1993, 26 RCTs, over 24 000 people) compared oral β blockers versus placebo within days or weeks of an acute MI (late intervention trials) and continued for between 6 weeks to 3 years. Most RCTs followed participants for 1 year. The review found improved survival in people given β blockers (RRR 23%, 95% CI 14% to 30%).[23] One prior systematic review (search date not stated, 24 RCTs) found that long term use of β blockers versus placebo after MI reduced total mortality (RRR about 20%; NNT 48), sudden death (RRR about 30%; NNT 63), and non-fatal reinfarction (RRR about 25%; NNT 56).[24] **Anginal symptoms:** We found no good RCTs evaluating the antianginal effects of β blockers in people after MI. One trial found atenolol more effective than placebo in people with chronic stable effort angina or silent ischaemia.[25] **Different types of β blockers:** The earlier review found no differences between β blockers with and without cardioselectivity or membrane stabilising properties, but it raised concerns about the lack of efficacy of β blockers with intrinsic sympathomimetic activity in long term management after MI.[24] One RCT (607 people after MI) found that acebutolol, a β blocker with moderate partial agonist activity, decreased 1 year mortality compared with placebo (AR of death: 11% with placebo, 6% with acebutolol; RRR 48%, 95% CI 9% to 71%).[26] **Effects in different subgroups:** One systematic review (search date 1983, 9 RCTs) compared β blockers versus placebo started more than 24 hours after onset of symptoms of acute MI and continued for 9–24 months.[27] Pooled analysis of individual data (13 679 people) found that the benefits of β blockers versus placebo on mortality seemed comparable in men and women. The highest absolute benefit from β blockers was found in subgroups with the highest baseline risks (that is, those with the highest mortality on placebo): those over 50 years of age; those with a history of previous MI, angina pectoris, hypertension, or treatment with digitalis; those with transient signs or symptoms of mechanical or electrical failure in the early phases of MI; and those with a higher heart rate at study entry. Low risk subgroups had smaller mean absolute benefit.

Harms: Adverse effects include shortness of breath, bronchospasm, bradycardia, hypotension, heart block, cold hands and feet, diarrhoea, fatigue, reduced sexual activity, depression, nightmares, faintness, insomnia, blacking out, and hallucinations. Rates vary in different studies. One RCT reported an absolute risk increase for any adverse effect on propranolol compared with placebo of 24% (95% CI not available). Serious adverse effects were uncommon and only a small proportion of people withdrew as a result.[28]

Comment: Continued benefit has been reported from the use of β blockers up to 6 years after MI (ARR for mortality 5.9%, 95% CI not available; P = 0.003; RRR 18%). However, the study was not blinded after 33 months.

OPTION   ANGIOTENSIN CONVERTING ENZYME (ACE) INHIBITORS

In people who have had an MI and have left ventricular dysfunction, there is strong evidence from a systematic review of RCTs that ACE inhibitors versus placebo reduce rates of death, hospitalisation for congestive heart failure, and recurrent non-fatal MI. The effects of ACE inhibitors in people who have had an MI but do not have left ventricular dysfunction have not yet been adequately evaluated.

Benefits: **In people with low left ventricular ejection fraction:** One systematic review (search date not stated, 3 RCTs)[29] compared ACE inhibitors (captopril, ramipril, or trandolapril) versus placebo started 3–16 days after acute MI and continued for 15–42 months. It analysed individual data from 5966 people with a recent MI and with clinical manifestations of congestive heart failure or moderate left ventricular dysfunction (left ventricular ejection fraction ≥35–40%). ACE inhibitors versus placebo significantly reduced rates of death (RRR 26%, 95% CI 17% to 34%; NNT 17 people treated for about 2 years to prevent 1 death), hospitalisation for congestive heart failure (RRR 27%, 95% CI 15% to 37%; NNT 28), and recurrent non-fatal MI (RRR 20%, 95% CI 6% to 31%; NNT 43).
In people without impaired ventricular function or evidence of congestive heart failure: We found no systematic review but found one large RCT (9297 people at high risk of cardiovascular events), which found that the ACE inhibitor ramipril (10 mg/day) versus placebo reduced the composite primary outcome of cardiovascular death, stroke, or MI over an average of 4.7 years (RRR for composite outcome: 22%, NNT 26; RRR for cardiovascular death: 26%, NNT 50; RRR for MI: 20%, NNT 42; RRR for stroke: 32%, NNT

67; RRR for death from all causes: 16%, NNT 56). The RCT found that ramipril reduced the need for revascularisation procedures and reduced heart failure related outcomes (need for revascularisation: RRR 15%, no CI provided; heart failure related outcomes: RRR 23%, no CI provided). Ramipril versus placebo produced benefit in subgroups examined, including women and men; people aged over and under 65 years; those with and without a history of coronary artery disease; hypertension; diabetes; peripheral vascular disease; cerebrovascular disease; and those with and without microalbuminuria at study entry.[30] **In people with diabetes:** See antihypertensive treatment under cardiovascular disease in diabetes, p 376.[31]

Harms: The major adverse effects reported in these trials were cough (ARI versus placebo of 5–10%), dizziness, hypotension (5–10%), renal failure (< 3%), hyperkalaemia (< 3%), angina, syncope, diarrhoea (2%), and, for captopril, alteration in taste (2% of captopril users).[29]

Comment: There are several other ongoing large RCTs evaluating the use of ACE inhibitors in people without clinical manifestations of heart failure and with no or with mild impairment in left ventricular systolic function. These include one trial of trandolapril in 8000 people with coronary artery disease, and one trial of perindopril in 10 500 people with stable coronary artery disease.[32]

OPTION CLASS I ANTIARRHYTHMIC AGENTS (QUINIDINE, PROCAINAMIDE, DISOPYRIMIDE, ENCAINIDE, FLECAINIDE, MORACIZINE)

One systematic review of RCTs has found that the use of class I antiarrhythmic agents after MI increases the risk of cardiovascular mortality and sudden death.

Benefits: None (see harms below).

Harms: One systematic review (search date 1993, 51 RCTs, 23 229 people) compared class I antiarrhythmic drugs versus placebo; given acutely and later in the management of MI.[23] The review found that the antiarrhythmic agents increased mortality (AR of death 5.6% v 5.0% with placebo; OR 1.14, 95% CI 1.01 to 1.28). One RCT (1498 people with MI and asymptomatic or mildly symptomatic ventricular arrhythmia) found that encainide or flecainide versus placebo increased the risk of death or cardiac arrest after 10 months (RR 2.38, 95% CI 1.59 to 3.57; NNH 17).[33]

Comment: The evidence implies that class I antiarrhythmics should not be used in people after MI or with significant coronary artery disease.

OPTION CLASS III ANTIARRHYTHMIC AGENTS (AMIODARONE, SOTALOL)

Two systematic reviews of RCTs have found that amiodarone versus placebo reduces the risk of sudden death and marginally reduces mortality in people at high risk of death after MI. Limited evidence on the effects of sotalol suggests that it may be harmful rather than beneficial in this setting.

Benefits: We found two systematic reviews.[34,35] The first systematic review (search date not stated, individual data from 6553 high risk people in 13 RCTs) compared amiodarone versus control treatments. Participants were selected with a recent MI and a high risk of death from cardiac arrhythmia (based on low left ventricular ejection fraction, frequent ventricular premature depolarisations or non-sustained ventricular tachycardia, but no history of sustained symptomatic ventricular tachycardia or ventricular fibrillation); 78% from eight RCTs had a recent MI, and 22% from five RCTs had congestive heart failure.[34] Most trials were placebo controlled with a mean follow up of about 1.5 years. The people with congestive heart failure were symptomatic but stable and did not have a recent MI, although in most cases the heart failure was ischaemic in origin. All RCTs used a loading dose of amiodarone (400 mg/day for 28 days or 800 mg/day for 14 days) followed by a maintenance dose (200–400 mg/day). Amiodarone versus placebo significantly reduced total mortality (ARs 10.9% per year with amiodarone v 12.3% per year with placebo; RRR 13%, 95% CI 1% to 22%; NNT 71 per year to avoid 1 additional death), and rates of sudden cardiac death (RRR 29%, 95% CI 15% to 41%; NNT 59). Amiodarone had similar effects in the post MI and congestive heart failure studies. The second systematic review (search date 1997, 5864 people with MI, congestive heart failure, left ventricular dysfunction, or cardiac arrest) found similar results.[35]

Harms: Adverse events leading to discontinuation of amiodarone were hypothyroidism (expressed per 100 person years: 7.0 v 1.1 on placebo; OR 7.3), hyperthyroidism (1.4 v 0.5; OR 2.5), peripheral neuropathy (0.5 v 0.2; OR 2.8), lung infiltrates (1.6 v 0.5; OR 3.1), bradycardia (2.4 v 0.8; OR 2.6), and liver dysfunction (1.0 v 0.4; OR 2.7).[34]

Comment: The reviews' conclusions are probably specific to amiodarone.[34,35] One RCT found increased mortality with the class III antiarrhythmic agent sotalol compared with placebo in 3121 people with MI and left ventricular dysfunction (ARs for death 5% v 3.1%; RR 1.65, 95% CI 1.15 to 2.36). The trial was terminated prematurely after less than 1 year of follow up.[36] The two largest RCTs of amiodarone after MI found a favourable interaction between β blockers and amiodarone, with additional reduction in cardiac mortality.[37,38]

| OPTION | CALCIUM CHANNEL BLOCKERS |

One systematic review of RCTs found no benefit from calcium channel blockers in people after MI or with chronic coronary heart disease. Diltiazem and verapamil may reduce rates of reinfarction and refractory angina in people after MI who do not have heart failure.

Benefits: One systematic review (search date 1993, 24 RCTs) compared calcium channel blockers (including dihydropyridines, diltiazem, and verapamil) versus placebo administered early or late during the course of acute MI or unstable angina and continued in the intermediate or long term.[23] Two of the RCTs used angiographic regression of coronary stenosis as an outcome in people with stable coronary heart disease treated with calcium channel blockers. The review found no significant difference in the absolute risk of death compared with placebo (AR 9.7% v 9.3%; ARI on calcium channel blockers compared with placebo 0.4%, 95% CI −0.4% to +1.2%; OR 1.04, 95% CI 0.95 to 1.14). **Diltiazem and verapamil:** The review found no significant effect compared with placebo (OR 0.95, 95% CI 0.82 to 1.09).[23] Three RCTs comparing diltiazem or verapamil versus placebo found decreased rates of recurrent infarction and refractory angina with active treatment but only for those people without signs or symptoms of heart failure. For those with clinical manifestations of heart failure, the trends were towards harm.[39–41] **Dihydropyridines:** The review found no significant effect compared with placebo (OR 1.16, 95% CI 0.99 to 1.35). Several individual RCTs of dihydropyridines found increased mortality, particularly when these agents were started early in the course of acute MI and in the absence of β blockers.

Harms: Adverse effects reported of verapamil and diltiazem include atrioventricular block, atrial bradycardia, new onset heart failure, hypotension, dizziness, oedema, rash, constipation, and pruritus.

Comment: Newer generation dihydropyridines, such as amlodipine and felodipine, have not been well studied in people after MI but have been found to be safe in people with heart failure, including heart failure of ischaemic origin.

OPTION	HORMONE REPLACEMENT THERAPY

We found no clear evidence from RCTs that HRT reduces major cardiovascular events in postmenopausal women with established coronary artery disease, despite strong evidence from RCTs that HRT improves some cardiovascular risk factors.

Benefits: **Combined oestrogen and progestins:** We found no systematic review. One large RCT (2763 postmenopausal women with coronary heart disease) found that conjugated equine oestrogen (0.625 mg/day) plus medroxyprogesterone acetate (2.5 mg/day) versus placebo for an average of 4.1 years produced no significant difference in the risk of non-fatal MI plus deaths caused by coronary heart disease (172/1380 [12.5%] with HRT v 176/1383 [12.7%] with placebo; ARR +0.2%, 95% CI −2.2% to +2.7%; RRR +1%, 95% CI −2.2% to +2.0%).[42] It also found no significant difference in secondary cardiovascular outcomes (coronary revascularisation, unstable angina, congestive heart failure, resuscitated cardiac arrest, stroke or transient ischaemic attack, and peripheral arterial disease) or in all cause mortality. **Oestrogen alone:** We found no good RCTs of oestrogen alone (without progestins) in the secondary prevention of coronary heart disease in postmenopausal women. One RCT found that high dose oestrogen (5 mg conjugated equine oestrogen/day) increased the risk of MI and thromboembolic events in men with pre-existing coronary heart disease.[43]

Harms: Pooled estimates from observational studies found an increased risk of endometrial cancer (RR > 8) and of breast cancer (RR 1.25 to 1.46) when oestrogen was used for over 8 years. In most observational studies, the addition of progestins prevented endometrial cancer but not breast cancer. The risk of venous thromboembolism, including pulmonary embolism and deep vein thrombosis, was three to four times higher with HRT than without. However, because the incidence of venous thromboembolism is low in postmenopausal women, the absolute increase in risk was only about one to two additional cases of venous thromboembolism in 5000 users a year.[44] In the RCT described above,[42] more women in the HRT than in the placebo group experienced venous thromboembolism (34/1380 v 12/1383; OR 2.65, 95% CI 1.48 to 4.75) and gall bladder disease (84/1380 v 62/1383; OR 1.38, 95% CI 0.99 to 1.92).

Comment: Many observational studies have found reduced rates of clinical events caused by coronary heart disease in postmenopausal women using HRT, especially in women with pre-existing coronary heart disease. Hormone users experienced 35–80% fewer recurrent events than non-users.[45,46] Meanwhile, several RCTs have found that HRT improves cardiovascular risk factors.[47] It is not known whether studies longer than 4 years would show a benefit.

QUESTION What are the effects of cholesterol reduction?

Michael Pignone

Systematic reviews and large subsequent RCTs have found that lowering cholesterol in people at high risk of ischaemic coronary events substantially reduces the risk of overall mortality, cardiovascular mortality, and non-fatal cardiovascular events. One systematic review of primary and secondary prevention trials has found that statins constitute the single most effective type of treatment for reducing cholesterol and reducing cardiovascular risk. The absolute benefits increased as baseline risk increased, but were not additionally influenced by the individual's absolute cholesterol concentration. We found no direct evidence for effects in people aged over 75 years, or for effects of combined treatments to reduce cholesterol and other cardiovascular risk factors.

Benefits: **Statins:** We found one systematic review (search date 1998, 5 RCTs, 30 817 people) that compared long term (≥ 4 years) treatment with statins versus placebo.[48] Combining the three secondary prevention trials, the review found that statins reduced coronary heart disease mortality, cardiovascular mortality, and all cause mortality compared with control over a mean of 5.4 years (coronary heart disease mortality: OR 0.71, 95% CI 0.63 to 0.80; cardiovascular mortality: OR 0.73, 95% CI 0.66 to 0.82; all cause mortality: OR 0.77, 95% CI 0.70 to 0.85). Combining primary and secondary prevention, it found that statins compared with control reduced major coronary events (RRR 31%, 95% CI 26% to 35%; ARR 3.6%, 95% CI 2.9% to 4.3%; NNT 28, 95% CI 23 to 34) and all cause mortality (RRR 21%, 95% CI 14% to 28%; ARR 16%, 95% CI 11% to 22%; NNT 61, 95% CI 45 to 95). Absolute risk reduction increased as baseline risk increased in primary prevention (see figure 1 in primary prevention, p 63). Differences between the baseline cholesterol concentration seemed to play no role in determining the results of the trials, in the ranges studied to date. **Effects of statins in different groups of people:** Combining results from primary and secondary prevention trials, the review found that, compared with placebo, statins reduced coronary events by a similar proportional amount in men (reduction in OR 31%, 95% CI 26% to 35%; ARR 3.7%, 95% CI 2.9% to 4.4%), in women (reduction in OR 29%, 95% CI 31% to 42%; ARR 3.3%, 95% CI 1.3% to 5.2%), in people under 65 years (reduction in OR 31%, 95% CI 24% to 36%; ARR 3.2%, 95% CI 2.4% to 4.0%), and in people over 65 years (reduction in OR 32%, 95% CI 23% to 39%; ARR 4.4%, 95% CI 3.0% to 5.8%). The reduction of coronary heart disease events in women involved more non-fatal and fewer fatal events than in men. One large RCT found no significant increase in mortality with statins versus placebo for the subgroup of women, but the confidence interval was wide (RR 1.16, 95% CI 0.68 to 1.99).[48] Other RCTs have not yet reported mortality results for women. **Intensity of statin treatment:** We found one RCT (1351 people with a history of saphenous vein coronary artery bypass graft) that compared aggressive reduction of cholesterol with lovastatin and, if necessary, cholestyramine (aiming for target low density lipoprotein cholesterol 1.6–2.2 mmol/l [60–85 mg/dl]) with more moderate reduction (target low density lipoprotein cholesterol 3.4–3.7 mmol/l [130–140 mg/dl]) with the same drugs. The trial found that aggressive treatment reduced the risk of needing repeat revascularisation at 4 years (6.5% with aggressive treatment v 9.2% with moderate treatment, P = 0.03).[49] After an additional 3 years, aggressive treatment reduced the risk of revascularisation and cardiovascular death compared with moderate treatment (AR of revascularisation 19% with aggressive treatment v 27% with moderate treatment, P = 0.0006; AR for cardiovascular death 7.4% with aggressive treatment v 11.3% with moderate treatment, P = 0.03).[50] **Fibrates:** We found one systematic review[51] and two additional RCTs.[52,53] The systematic review (search date 1999, 4 RCTs) compared fibrates versus placebo in people with known coronary heart disease. The review identified one RCT (2531 men with coronary heart disease and a level of high density lipoprotein cholesterol below 1 mmol/l) that found gemfibrozil versus placebo reduced the composite outcome of non-fatal MI plus death from coronary heart disease after a median of 5.1 years (AR 219/1264 [17%] for gemfibrozil v 275/1267 [22%] for placebo; ARR 4.4%, 95% CI 1.4% to 7%; RRR 20%, 95% CI 6% to 32%; NNT 23, 95% CI 14 to 73). The review identified three trials comparing clofibrate versus placebo, which found no consistent difference between groups. The two additional RCTs[52,53] both compared bezafibrate versus placebo. The larger RCT (3090 people selected with previous MI or stable angina, high density lipoprotein cholesterol < 45 mg/dl, and low density lipoprotein cholesterol < 180 mg/dl) found that bezafibrate versus placebo did not significantly reduce all cause mortality or the composite end point of MI plus sudden death (AR for MI or sudden death 13.6% with bezafibrate v 15.0% with placebo; cumulative ARR at 6.2 years 7.3%, P = 0.24).[52] The smaller RCT (92 young male survivors of MI) found that bezafibrate versus placebo significantly reduced the combined outcome of death, reinfarction, plus revascularisation (26% with bezafibrate v 7% with placebo, P = 0.019).[53] **Other treatments:** We found one systematic review (search date 1996, 59 RCTs, 173 160 people), which did not differentiate primary and secondary prevention, and included RCTs of any cholesterol lowering intervention, irrespective of duration, as long as mortality data were reported. It included drug treatments (statins, n–3 fatty acids, fibrates, resins, hormones, or niacin), dietary intervention alone, or surgery (ileal bypass) alone.[54] Overall, baseline risk was similar among all intervention groups. Among non-surgical treatments, the review found that only statins reduced coronary heart disease mortality, and that only statins and n–3 fatty acids reduced all cause mortality (RR of coronary heart disease mortality, treatment v control 0.69, 95% CI 0.59 to 0.80 for statins; 0.44, 95% CI 0.18 to 1.07 for n–3 fatty acids; 0.98, 95% CI 0.78 to 1.24 for fibrates; 0.71, 95% CI 0.51 to 0.99 for resins; 1.04, 95% CI 0.93 to 1.17 for hormones; 0.95, 95% CI 0.83 to 1.10 for niacin; 0.91, 95% CI 0.82 to 1.01 for diet. RR of all cause mortality, treatment v control 0.79, 95% CI 0.71 to 0.89 for statins; 0.68, 95% CI 0.53 to 0.88 for n–3 fatty acids; 1.06, 95% CI 0.78 to 1.46 for fibrates; 0.85, 95% CI 0.66 to 1.08 for resins; 1.09, 95% CI 1.00 to 1.20 for hormones; 0.96, 95% CI 0.86 to 1.08 for niacin; 0.97, 95% CI 0.81 to 1.15 for diet). **Cholesterol lowering versus angioplasty:** We found no systematic review. One RCT found that aggressive lipid lowering treatment was as effective as PTA for reducing ischaemic events, although anginal symptoms were reduced more by PTA (see PTA versus medical treatment, p 116).

Harms: Total non-cardiovascular events, total and tissue specific cancers, and accident and violent deaths have been reported in statin trials. However, the systematic review of long term statin trials found no significant difference between statins and placebo in terms of non-cardiovascular mortality, cancer incidence, asymptomatic elevation of creatinine kinase (> 10 times upper reference limit), or elevation of transaminases (> 3 times upper reference limit) during a mean of 5.4 years of treatment (OR of event, statin v placebo 0.93, 95% CI 0.81 to 1.07 for non-cardiovascular mortality; 0.99, 95% CI 0.90 to 1.08 for cancer; 1.25, 95% CI 0.83 to 1.89 for creatinine kinase rise; 1.13, 95% CI 0.95 to 1.33 for transaminase rise).[48] We found no evidence of additional harm associated with cholesterol lowering in elderly people, or in people following acute MI.

Comment: The evidence indicates that, in a wide range of clinical contexts, the relative risk reduction depends on the size of the fall in cholesterol and is not otherwise dependent on the method by which cholesterol is lowered. The absolute benefit over several years of lowering cholesterol will therefore be greatest in people with the highest baseline risk of an ischaemic cardiac event. Even if the relative risk reduction attenuates at older age, the absolute reduction risk for ischaemic cardiac events may be higher in elderly people than in younger individuals. However, long term benefit for cholesterol lowering has not yet been directly shown in those older than 75 years. Additional information may be provided by the Heart Protection Study (20 000 participants, completion 2000, simvastatin),[55] the Women's Health Initiative (48 000 participants, completion 2007, diet, up to age 79 years),[56] and the Antihypertensive and Lipid Lowering Treatment to Prevent Heart Disease Trial (10 000 participants, completion 2002, pravastatin, no upper age limit).[57] It is not known whether cholesterol reduction will provide benefit for those with initial cholesterol concentrations lower than those selected in the published trials. We found no evidence to indicate whether starting statin treatment immediately after acute infarction provides additional benefits. We found no large direct comparisons of cholesterol modifying drugs; it remains unclear whether any one drug has advantages over others in subgroups of high risk people with particular lipid abnormalities. Because the main aim of treatment is to reduce absolute risk (rather than to reduce the cholesterol to any particular concentration), treatments aimed at lowering cholesterol need evaluating for effectiveness in comparison and in combination with other possible risk factor interventions in each individual.

| QUESTION | What are the effects of blood pressure reduction? |

Eva Lonn

We found no direct evidence of the effects of blood pressure lowering in people with established coronary heart disease. Observational studies, and extrapolation of primary prevention trials of blood pressure reduction, support the lowering of blood pressure in those at high risk of ischaemic coronary events. The evidence for benefit is strongest for β blockers, although not specifically in people with raised blood pressure. The target blood pressure in these people is not clear.

Benefits: We found no systematic review and no RCTs designed specifically to examine blood pressure reduction in those with established coronary heart disease. Prospective epidemiological studies have established that blood pressure continues to be a risk factor for cardiovascular events in people who have already experienced MI. Prospective follow up of 5362 men who reported prior MI during screening for one large RCT found no detectable association between systolic blood pressure and coronary heart disease mortality, and increased coronary heart disease mortality for those with lowest diastolic blood pressure in the first 2 years of follow up.[58] After 15 years there were highly significant linear associations between both systolic and diastolic blood pressure and increased risk of coronary heart disease mortality (stronger relation for systolic blood pressure), with apparent benefit for men with blood pressure maintained at levels lower than the arbitrarily defined "normal" levels. Experimental evidence of benefit from lowering of blood pressure in those with coronary heart disease requires extrapolation from primary prevention trials, because trials of antihypertensive treatment in elderly people[59-61] are likely to have included people with preclinical coronary heart disease. Mortality benefit has been established for β blockers after MI (see option, p 101), for verapamil and diltiazem after MI in those without heart failure (see calcium channel blockers, p 104), and for ACE inhibitors after MI, especially in those with heart failure (see ACE inhibitors, p 102).

Harms: Some observational studies have found increased mortality among those with low diastolic blood pressure.[62] Trials in elderly people of blood pressure lowering for hypertension or while treating heart failure[63] found no evidence of a J shaped relation between blood pressure and death.

Secondary prevention of ischaemic cardiac events

Comment: Without specific studies comparing different antihypertensive treatments, the available evidence is strongest for a beneficial effect of β blockers when treating survivors of an MI who have raised blood pressure. We found no specific evidence about the target level of blood pressure.

QUESTION What are the effects of non-drug treatments?

Andy Ness and Eva Lonn

OPTION DIETARY INTERVENTIONS

RCTs have found that advising people with coronary heart disease to eat more fish (particularly oily fish), more fruit and vegetables, bread, pasta, potatoes, olive oil, and rapeseed margarine (a more Mediterranean diet) may result in a substantial survival benefit. We found no strong evidence from RCTs for a beneficial effect of low fat or high fibre diets on major non-fatal coronary heart disease events or coronary heart disease mortality.

Benefits: **Low fat diets:** One systematic review (search date not stated) found no evidence that allocation to a low fat diet reduced mortality from coronary heart disease in people after MI (RR 0.94, 95% CI 0.84 to 1.06).[64] One large RCT (2033 middle aged men with a recent MI) compared three dietary options: fat advice (to eat less fat); fibre advice (to eat more cereal fibre); and fish advice (to eat at least two portions of fatty fish a week).[65] Advice to reduce fat was complicated and, though fat intake reduced only slightly in the fat advice group, fruit and vegetable intake increased by about 40 g a day.[66] However, there was no clear reduction in mortality (unadjusted RR at 2 years for death from any cause 0.97, 95% CI 0.75 to 1.27). **High fibre diets:** In the trial, people advised to eat more fibre doubled their intake, but survival was non-significantly worse (unadjusted RR at 2 years for death from any cause 1.23, 95% CI 0.95 to 1.60). **High fish diets:** In the trial, those advised to eat more fish ate three times as much fish, although about 14% could not tolerate the fish and were given fish oil capsules. Those given fish advice were significantly less likely to die within 2 years (RRR 29%, 95% CI 7% to 46%; NNT 30). In a second trial, 11 324 people who had survived a recent MI were randomised to receive 1 g daily of n-3 PUFA (fish oil) or no fish oil. Those given fish oil were less likely to die within 3.5 years (RRR 0.14, 95% CI 0.03 to 0.24).[67] **Mediterranean diet:** One RCT (605 middle aged people with a recent MI) compared advice to eat a Mediterranean diet (more bread, more vegetables, more fruit, more fish, and less meat, and to replace butter and cream with rapeseed margarine) versus usual dietary advice.[68] There were several dietary differences between the groups. Fruit intake, for example, was about 50 g/day higher in the intervention group than the control group. After 27 months the trial was stopped prematurely because of better outcomes in the intervention group. There were 20 deaths in the control group and eight in the intervention group (adjusted RRR of death 70%, 95% CI 18% to 89%; NNT 25 over 2 years).

Harms: No major adverse effects have been reported.

Comment: Diets low in saturated fat and cholesterol can lead to 10–15% reductions in cholesterol concentrations in highly controlled settings, such as in metabolic wards.[69] In people in the community, the effects are more modest: 3–5% reductions in cholesterol concentrations in general population studies and 9% reductions in people after MI.[64,70–72] Several RCTs of intensive dietary intervention in conjunction with multifactorial risk reduction treatment found decreased progression of anatomic extent of coronary heart disease on angiography.[73] A trial of advice to eat more fruit and vegetables in men with angina is under way (M Burr, personal communication). **Effect on cardiovascular risk factors:** Other studies have investigated the effects of dietary interventions on cardiovascular risk factors rather than the effect on cardiovascular morbidity and mortality. One systematic review (search date 1992) suggested that garlic may reduce cholesterol by about 10%.[74] Some trials in this review had methodological flaws. More recent reports (published in 1998) found no effects of garlic powder or garlic oil on cholesterol concentrations.[75,76] One systematic review (search date 1991) reported modest reductions in cholesterol levels of 2–5% from oats and psyllium enriched cereals (high fibre diets), although we found no evidence that high fibre diets reduce mortality in people with coronary heart disease.[73] One systematic review of soy protein also reported modest reductions in cholesterol concentrations.[77]

| OPTION | ANTIOXIDANT VITAMINS (VITAMIN E, β CAROTENE, VITAMIN C) |

The role of vitamin E, β carotene, and vitamin C in the long term management of people at high risk for ischaemic cardiac events remains unclear.

Benefits: We found no systematic review of RCTs. **Vitamin E and β carotene:** Four large RCTs have looked at vitamin E in people with coronary artery disease.[67,78–80] The first RCT (2002 people with angiographically proven ischaemic heart disease)[78] used a high dose of vitamin E (400 IU or 800 IU) and follow up was brief (median 510 days). The RCT found that vitamin E reduced non-fatal coronary events (RRR 77%, 95% CI 53% to 89%), but also found a non-significant increase in coronary death (RRI +18%, 95% CI –0.4% to +127%), and all cause mortality. The second RCT (29 133 male Finnish smokers) compared β carotene and vitamin E supplements with placebo. The dose of vitamin E (50 mg/day) was smaller than that used in the first trial. In the subgroup analysis of data from the 1862 men with prior MI, the trial found that vitamin E reduced non-fatal MI (RRR 38%, 95% CI 4% to 59%), but non-significantly increased coronary death (RRI +33%, 95% CI –14% to +105%).[79] There were significantly more deaths from coronary heart disease on β carotene than placebo. The third RCT (11 324 people)[67] used a factorial design to compare vitamin E (300 mg) daily versus no vitamin E (as well as fish oil versus no fish oil). After 3.5 years there was a small and non-significant reduction in the risk of cardiovascular death and deaths from all causes in those who received vitamin E compared with those who did not (RRR all cause mortality

0.92%, 95% CI 0.82% to 1.04%). There was no significant change in the rate of non-fatal coronary events in those who received vitamin E (RRI 4%, 95% CI –12% to +22%).[67] The fourth RCT (9541 people at high cardiovascular risk, 80% with prior clinical coronary artery disease, remainder with other atherosclerotic disease or diabetes with ≥1 additional cardiovascular risk factor) compared natural source vitamin E (D-alpha tocopherol acetate) 400 IU/day versus placebo and followed participants for an average of 4.7 years.[80] It found no significant differences in any cardiovascular outcomes between vitamin E and placebo (AR for major fatal or non-fatal cardiovascular event 16.2% with vitamin E v 15.5% with placebo, P = NS; AR for cardiovascular death 7.2% with vitamin E v 6.9% with placebo, P = NS; AR for non-fatal MI 11.2% v 11.0% with placebo, P = NS; AR for stroke 4.4% with vitamin E v 3.8% with placebo, P = NS; AR for death from any cause 11.2% with vitamin E v 11.2% with placebo, P = NS). Pooled analysis from all four of these major RCTs found no evidence that vitamin E altered cardiovascular events and all cause mortality compared with placebo when given for 1.3–4.5 years. One additional smaller RCT (196 people on haemodialysis, aged 40–75 years) compared high dose vitamin E (800 IU/day) versus placebo.[81] After a median of 519 days, it found that vitamin E reduced the rate of combined cardiovascular end points but found no significant effect for all cause mortality (RRR for cardiovascular end points, vitamin E v placebo 46%, 95% CI 11% to 77%; mortality, vitamin E v placebo RRI 9%, 95% CI RRR 30% to RRI 70%).[81] **Vitamin C:** We found three small RCTs comparing vitamin C with placebo. The first RCT (538 people admitted to an acute geriatric unit) compared vitamin C (200 mg daily) versus placebo for 6 months.[82] The second RCT (297 elderly people with low vitamin C levels) compared vitamin C (150 mg daily for 12 weeks, then 50 mg daily) versus placebo for 2 years.[83] The third RCT (199 elderly people) compared vitamin C (200 mg daily) versus placebo for 6 months.[84] The three RCTs were small and brief, and their combined results provide no evidence of any substantial early benefit of vitamin C supplementation (RRI for mortality for vitamin v placebo +8%, 95% CI –7% to +26%).

Harms: Two of the trials of vitamin E found non-significant increases in the risk of coronary death (see benefits above).[78,79] Four large RCTs of β carotene supplementation in primary prevention found no cardiovascular benefits, and two of the trials raised concerns about increased mortality (RRI for cardiovascular death, β carotene v placebo 12%, 95% CI 4% to 22%) and cancer rates.[85]

Comment: One systematic review of epidemiological studies found consistent associations between increased dietary or supplemental intake of vitamin E, or both, and lower cardiovascular risk and less consistent associations for β carotene and vitamin C.[85] Most observational studies of antioxidants have excluded people with pre-existing disease.[86,87] The results of the trial in people on haemodialysis raises the possibility that high dose vitamin E supplementation may be beneficial in those at high absolute risk of coronary events.[81] Further trials in such groups are required to confirm or refute this finding.

OPTION   **CARDIAC REHABILITATION INCLUDING EXERCISE**

Systematic reviews of RCTs have found that cardiac rehabilitation improves coronary risk factors and reduces the risk of major cardiac events in people after MI. The role of exercise alone in reducing the risk of adverse cardiovascular outcomes is not clear.

Benefits: **Cardiac rehabilitation:** Three systematic reviews identified RCTs of cardiac rehabilitation, including exercise in people after MI.[88–90] Rehabilitation included medical evaluation, prescribed exercise, cardiac risk factor modification, education, and counselling. The reviews found 20–25% reductions in cardiovascular deaths in the treatment groups. One review (22 RCTs, 4554 people with a recent MI) found, after a mean of 3 years, significant reductions in total mortality (RRR 20%, no CI given), cardiovascular mortality (RRR 22%, no CI given), and fatal reinfarction (RRR 25%, no CI given), but no significant difference in non-fatal reinfarction.[89] **Exercise alone:** One more recent qualitative systematic review (search date not stated) found that rehabilitation with exercise alone had little effect on rates of non-fatal MI or overall mortality but a small beneficial effect on angina.[91]

Harms: No study documented an increased risk of reinfarction or other adverse cardiovascular outcomes for exercise rehabilitation compared with control. Rates of adverse cardiovascular outcomes (syncope, arrhythmia, MI, or sudden death) were low (2–3/100 000 person hours) in supervised rehabilitation programmes, and rates of fatal cardiac events during or immediately after exercise training were reported in two older surveys as ranging from one in 116 400 to one in 784 000 person hours.[91]

Comment: The three reviews included RCTs performed before the widespread use of thrombolytic agents and β blockers after MI. Most participants were men under 70 years of age. Other interventions aimed at risk factor modification were often provided in the intervention groups (including nutritional education, counselling in behavioural modification, and, in some trials, lipid lowering medications). We found no strong evidence that exercise training and cardiac rehabilitation programmes increased the proportion of people returning to work after MI.

OPTION   **SMOKING CESSATION**

We found no RCTs of the effects of smoking cessation on cardiovascular events in people with coronary heart disease. Moderate evidence from epidemiological studies indicates that people with coronary heart disease who stop smoking rapidly reduce their risk of recurrent coronary events or death. The use of nicotine patches seems safe in people with coronary heart disease.

Benefits: We found no RCTs evaluating the effects of smoking cessation on coronary mortality and morbidity. Many observational studies found that people with coronary heart disease who stop smoking rapidly reduce their risk of cardiac death and MI (RRR about 50% for recurrent coronary events or premature death compared with continuing smokers)[92] (see smoking cessation under primary prevention, p 63). The

Cardiovascular disorders

studies found that about half of the benefits occur in the first year of stopping smoking, followed by a more gradual decrease in risk, reaching the risk of never smokers after several years of abstinence.[92] Among people with peripheral arterial disease and stroke, smoking cessation has been shown in observational studies to be associated with improved exercise tolerance, decreased risk of amputation, improved survival, and reduced risk of recurrent stroke.

Harms: Two recent RCTs found no evidence that nicotine replacement using transdermal patches in people with stable coronary heart disease increased cardiovascular events.[93,94]

Comment: One RCT compared the impact of firm and detailed advice to stop smoking in 125 survivors of acute MI versus conventional advice in 85 people.[95] Allocation to the intervention or control group was determined by day of admission. At follow up over 1 year after admission, 62% of the intervention group and 28% of the control group were non-smokers. Mortality and morbidity were not reported.

| OPTION | PSYCHOLOGICAL AND STRESS MANAGEMENT INTERVENTIONS |

One systematic review of mainly poor quality RCTs found that psychological and stress management may decrease rates of MI or cardiac death in people with coronary heart disease.

Benefits: One systematic review (search date not stated, 23 RCTs, 3180 people with coronary artery disease) compared a diverse range of psychosocial treatments (2024 people) versus usual treatment (1156 people).[96] Mortality results were available in only 12 RCTs. Psychosocial interventions versus control interventions significantly reduced mortality (RRR for death 41%; OR survival 1.70, 95% CI 1.09 to 2.64) and non-fatal events in the first 2 years of follow up after MI (RRR 46%; OR for no event 1.84, 95% CI 1.12 to 2.99).[96]

Harms: No specific harms were reported.

Comment: These results should be interpreted with caution because of the methodological limitations of the individual RCTs and the use of a diverse range of interventions (relaxation, stress management, counselling). The RCTs were generally small, with short follow up, and used non-uniform outcome measures. Methods of concealment allocation were not assessed. The authors of the review acknowledged the strong possibility of publication bias but made no attempt to quantify it. The results were inconsistent across trials.[97] Several observational studies have found that depression and social isolation (lack of social and emotional support) are independent predictors of mortality and non-fatal coronary heart disease events in people after MI.[98]

QUESTION   What are the effects of surgical treatments?

Charanjit Rihal

OPTION   CORONARY ARTERY BYPASS GRAFTING (CABG) VERSUS MEDICAL TREATMENT

RCTs performed up to the mid 1980s have found that, in comparison with medical treatment, CABG carried a greater risk of death in the first year but reduced the risk of death from coronary artery disease at 5 and 10 years. Greatest benefit occurred in people with more severe disease (multivessel disease, left ventricular dysfunction, or MI). There was no evidence of increased protection against subsequent MI. A more recent RCT, using modern techniques and with optimal background medical treatment, found even greater superiority of revascularisation.

Benefits: One systematic review (search date not stated, 7 RCTs, individual results from 2649 people with coronary heart disease) compared CABG with medical treatment.[99] Most participants were middle aged men with multivessel disease but good left ventricular function who were enrolled from 1972 to 1984 (97% were male; 82% 41–60 years old; 80% with ejection fraction > 50%; 60% with prior MI; and 83% with two or three vessel disease).[99] Participants assigned to CABG also received medical treatment, and 40% initially assigned to medical treatment underwent CABG in the following 10 years. One subsequent RCT (558 people with asymptomatic ischaemia with positive exercise test or ambulatory electrocardiogram) compared medical treatment versus revascularisation (CABG or PTA).[100] **Mortality and MI:** The systematic review found that CABG versus medical treatment reduced mortality at 5 years (intention to treat analysis: RRR 39%, 95% CI 23% to 52%), 7 years (RRR 32%, 95% CI 17% to 44%), and 10 years (RRR 17%, 95% CI 2% to 30%).[99] In the subsequent RCT, mortality at 2 years was significantly lower after routine revascularisation (AR of death 1.1% v 6.6% and 4.4% in the two medical groups, P < 0.02).[100] No impact of CABG on subsequent infarction was found either in individual trials or in the systematic review, possibly because those assigned to surgery had increased rates of infarction in the perioperative period (see harms below). In the RCT, revascularisation reduced rates of death or MI compared with medical treatment (AR of MI or death 4.7% with revascularisation v 8.8% and 12.1% with medical treatment, P < 0.04).[100] **Other non-fatal end points:** Most trials did not prospectively collect data on re-admission rates, recurrent angina, or quality of life. **Effects in different people:** The systematic review found that the relative benefits were similar in participants with different baseline risk (OR for death 0.61 if left ventricular function normal and 0.59 if abnormal). The absolute benefit of CABG was greatest in people with an abnormal ejection fraction, because the baseline risk of death was twice as high in this group (ejection fraction > 50%: ARR of death over 5 years 5%; ejection fraction < 50%: ARR 10%). Both absolute and relative mortality benefits were higher in people with a greater number of diseased coronary arteries, especially those with three vessel disease (OR of death 0.58, P < 0.001), and those with left main coronary artery disease (OR 0.32, P = 0.004) or any involvement of the left anterior descending coronary artery (OR 0.58), even if only one or two vessels were involved.[99]

Harms: **Perioperative complications:** In the systematic review, of the 1240 participants who underwent CABG, 40 (3.2%) died and 7.1% had documented non-fatal MI within 30 days of the procedure. At 1 year, the estimated incidence of death or MI was 11.6% with CABG and 8% with medical treatment (RRI 45%, 95% CI 18% to 103%).[99] The diagnosis of MI after CABG is difficult, and its true incidence may be higher. In the recent RCT, those assigned to routine revascularisation had significantly lower rates of death or MI after 2 years (AR for death 1.1% v 6.6% and 4.4% for the 2 medical groups, P < 0.02; AR for death or MI 4.7% v 12.1% and 8.8% in the 2 medical groups, P < 0.04).[100]

Comment: The results of the systematic review may not be generaliseable to current practice. Participants were 65 years or younger, but over half of CABG procedures are now performed on people over 65 years. Almost all participants were male. High risk people, such as those with severe angina and left main coronary artery stenosis, were under represented. Internal thoracic artery grafts were used in less than 5% of participants. Lipid lowering agents (particularly statins) and aspirin were used infrequently (aspirin used in 3% of participants at enrolment). Only about half of participants were taking β blockers. The systematic review may underestimate the real benefits of CABG in comparison with medical treatment alone becuase medical and surgical treatment for coronary artery disease were not mutually exclusive; by 5 years, 25% of people receiving medical treatment had undergone CABG surgery and by 10 years, 41% had undergone CABG surgery. The underestimate of effect would be greatest among people at high risk. People with previous CABG have not been studied in RCTs, although they now represent a growing proportion of those undergoing CABG.

| OPTION | CORONARY PERCUTANEOUS TRANSLUMINAL ANGIOPLASTY (PTA) VERSUS MEDICAL TREATMENT FOR STABLE CORONARY ARTERY DISEASE |

One systematic review has found that in people with stable coronary artery disease, in comparison with medical treatment, coronary PTA is more effective for alleviating angina pectoris and improving exercise tolerance, but is associated with a higher rate of CABG. The review found no evidence that PTA reduces mortality, MI, or need for later angioplasty. RCTs have found that PTA is associated with increased risk of emergency CABG and of MI during and soon after the procedure.

Benefits: We found one systematic review (search date 1998, 6 RCTs, 1904 people with stable coronary artery disease) comparing balloon angioplasty versus balloon PTA.[101] Follow up varied from 6–57 months. **Mortality, MI, angina, and subsequent intervention:** The review found that PTA significantly reduced the rate of angina, but increased the rate of CABG compared with medical treatment (RR for angina: PTA v medical treatment 0.70, 95% CI 0.50 to 0.98; RR for CABG: PTA v medical treatment 1.59, 95% CI 1.09 to 2.32). The review found no significant difference between PTA and medical treatment for death (RR 1.32, 95% CI 0.65 to 2.70), for MI (RR 1.42, 95% CI 0.90 to 2.25), or in the need for later PTA (RR 1.29, 95% CI 0.72 to 3.36). The review found significant heterogeneity among trials. **Quality of life:** The largest RCT identified by the review (1018 people) found that PTA improved physical functioning, vitality, and general health compared with medical treatment at 3 months and 1 year (measured with SF-36 instrument at 1 year: 33% of people treated with PTA rated their health as "much improved" v 22% with medical therapy, P = 0.008), but found no significant difference at 3 years. The improvements were related to breathlessness, angina, and treadmill tolerance. High transfer (27%) from the medical to PTA group may partly explain the lack of difference between groups at 3 years.[102] **Effects in different people:** One of the RCTs in the systematic review found that antianginal benefit from PTA was limited to people with moderate to severe (grade 2 or worse) angina (20% lower incidence of angina and 1 minute longer treadmill exercise times compared with medical treatment).[103] People with mild symptoms at enrolment derived no significant improvement in symptoms.

Harms: Procedural death and MI, as well as repeat procedures for restenosis, are the main hazards of PTA. Four RCTs included in the review reported complications of PTA. In the first RCT, two (1.9%) emergency CABG operations and five (4.8%) MIs occurred at the time of the procedure. By 6 months, the PTA group had higher rates of CABG surgery (7% v 0%) and non-protocol PTA (15.2% v 10.3%).[104,105] In the second RCT, the higher rate of death or MI with PTA was attributable to one death and seven procedure related MIs.[103] The third RCT found a procedure related CABG rate and MI rate of 2.8% each, and the fourth found rates of 2% for CABG and 3% for MI.[101]

Comment: We found good evidence that PTA treats the symptoms of angina pectoris, but we found no evidence that it reduces the overall incidence of death or MI in people with stable angina. This may be because of the risk of complications during and soon after the procedure, and because most PTAs are performed for single vessel disease.

OPTION **CORONARY PTA VERSUS CABG FOR MULTIVESSEL DISEASE**

One systematic review has found that, in low to medium risk people, PTA versus CABG has no significant effect on mortality, the risk of MI, and the quality of life. PTA is less invasive but increases the number of repeat procedures. The relevant RCTs were too small to exclude a 20–30% difference in mortality. The largest RCT has found that CABG versus PTA improves long term survival in people with diabetes who are treated with oral hypoglycaemic drugs or insulin and have multivessel coronary disease.

Benefits: We found two systematic reviews (search date not stated, 8 RCTs, 3371 people)[106,107] and one subsequent RCT.[108] **Angina pectoris:** One systematic review[105] found that the prevalence of moderate to severe angina pectoris (grade 2 or worse) was significantly higher after PTA than after CABG at 1 year (RR 1.6, 95% CI 1.3 to 1.9).

After 3 years this difference had decreased as rates of repeat revascularisation increased in the people allocated to PTA (RR 1.2, 95% CI 1.0 to 1.5). **Mortality:** The systematic review[106] found no significant difference in all cause mortality between groups (AR 7.3% after PTA v 6.8%; OR 1.09, 95% CI 0.88 to 1.35).[106] The smaller subsequent RCT (392 people) found no significant difference between CABG and PTA after 8 years of follow up, although the trial was too small to exclude a clinically important difference (AR for survival 83% with CABG v 79% with PTA, P = 0.40).[108] **Death or MI:** In all RCTs, the combined end point of death or MI was not significantly different between groups (AR 13.8% v 13.4%; OR 1.05, 95% CI 0.89 to 1.23).[107] The largest of these RCTs found that CABG versus PTA had no significant effect on death or MI after a mean follow up of 7.7 years (alive and no MI: 75.3% with CABG v 73.5% with PTA, P = 0.46).[109] **Repeat procedures:** In all RCTs, the need for repeat procedures was significantly higher in people allocated to PTA (AR 44% with PTA v 6.0% with CABG; OR 7.9, 95% CI 6.9 to 9.0).[110] **Quality of life:** Both PTA and CABG groups had significant improvements in quality of life measures and return to employment, but no difference was found between the PTA and CABG groups over 3–5 years of follow up.[111,112]

Harms: See harms of PTA versus medical treatment, p 117. CABG is more invasive than PTA, but PTA is associated with a greater need for repeat procedures.

Comment: **In people with diabetes:** Subgroup analysis of the largest RCT (1829 people) found that in people with diabetes (353 people), CABG reduced all cause mortality more than PTA both after 5 years (AR of death 19.4% with CABG v 34.5% with PTA; P = 0.003)[110] and after 7 years (AR of death with CABG 23.6% v 44.3% with PTA; P = 0.0011).[109] Such a difference was not observed among non-diabetics or any other subgroup (AR of death in people without diabetes 13.6% with CABG v 13.2% with PTA, P = 0.72).[109] **In all participants:** Although no major differences in death or MI were observed in the nine RCTs,[106–108] these trials enrolled people at relatively low risk of cardiac events. It is therefore premature to conclude that PTA and CABG are equivalent for all people with multivessel disease. Fewer than 20% of participants had left ventricular dysfunction, almost 70% had one or two vessel disease, and observed mortality was only 2.6% for the first year, and 1.1% a year thereafter. Participants enrolled in the largest trial more closely approximated to moderate risk people, but this was caused primarily by the higher proportion of participants with diabetes mellitus.[110] Even in that trial nearly 60% of participants had two vessel coronary artery disease. Finally, even though nine trials were included in the meta-analysis, the total enrolment of 5200 falls short of what would be needed to show mortality differences of 20–30% among people at low and moderate risk. Large mortality differences between the two procedures (40–50%) are unlikely. **Multivessel stenting versus multivessel CABG:** One RCT (unpublished as of December 2000) has compared multivessel CABG versus multivessel PTA in 1205 people with an ejection fraction greater than 30% (the ARTS Investigators, personal communication, 1999).

RCTs have found that, in comparison with coronary PTA, intracoronary stents afford superior acute and long term clinical and angiographic results.

Benefits:

We found no systematic review. **For disease of native coronary arteries:** We found four RCTs comparing elective stenting with PTA.[112–115] At 12 months, intracoronary stents significantly reduced the risk of recurrent angina (13% v 30%, P = 0.04) but not of death, MI, or need for CABG.[109] At 6 months, all four RCTs found a lower prevalence of angiographic restenosis (31% v 42%, P = 0.046; 22% v 32%, P = 0.02; 17% v 40%, P = 0.02; 18.2% v 24.9%, P = 0.055), and a lower rate of repeat PTA (13.5% v 23.3%; RR 0.58, 95% CI 0.40 to 0.85).[112–115] After 2 years of follow up, the fourth trial found that stenting reduced all clinical cardiac events compared with PTA (AR for death, MI, repeat PTA, or CABG 19.8% with stent v 27.5% with PTA, P = 0.048). The difference was accounted for almost entirely by lower rates of repeat target lesion revascularisation in the stent group (AR 17.2% with stent v 25.5% with PTA, P = 0.02).[115] **For saphenous vein graft lesions in people with prior CABG:** We found one RCT (220 people) comparing elective stents with standard balloon angioplasty.[114] Acute angiographic results were better with stents than balloon angioplasty. At 6 months, there was no significant difference in rates of restenosis (37% v 46%, P = 0.24), but the overall incidence of death, MI, CABG, or repeat PTA was lower in the stent group (27% v 42%, P = 0.03). **For treatment of chronic total occlusions:** Chronic occlusions of the coronary arteries are particularly prone to restenosis and reocclusion following PTA. We found three RCTs comparing PTA alone with PTA followed by insertion of stents.[116–118] One RCT (119 people with chronic total occlusion) found that stenting compared with PTA reduced angina (angina free at 6 months: 57% of stent group v 24% of PTA only group, 95% CI not available, P < 0.001) and angiographic restenosis (> 50% stenosis on follow up angiography: 74% with PTA v 32% with stent, P < 0.001). Repeat procedures were undertaken less often among people with a stent than among people receiving PTA (22% v 42%, P = 0.025).[117] In the second RCT (110 people) those treated with stents experienced less ischaemia (14% v 46%, P = 0.002), had less restenosis (32% v 68%, P < 0.001), and underwent fewer repeat procedures (5.3% v 22%, P = 0.038) by 9 months.[118] The third RCT (110 people) found that, at angiographic follow up after 4 months, those with stents experienced less restenosis (26% v 62%, P = 0.01), less reocclusion (2% v 1%, P = 0.05), and fewer repeat PTAs (24% v 55%, P = 0.05). No deaths or CABG operations occurred in either group. The incidence of MI was low in both groups (0% stent v 2% PTA, P = NS).[119] **For treatment of restenosis after initial PTA:** We found one RCT (383 people) of coronary stenting versus balloon angioplasty for treatment of restenosis. During 6 months of follow up, the stent group experienced fewer recurrent restenoses (18% v 32%, P = 0.03) and repeat procedures (10% v 27%, P = 0.001). Survival free of MI or repeat revascularisation was 84% in the stent group and 72% in the PTA group (P = 0.04).[120]

Harms: Initially, aggressive combination antithrombotic and anticoagulant regimens were used because of a high incidence of stent thrombosis and MI. These regimens led to a high incidence of arterial access site bleeding.[108] More recently, improved stent techniques and use of aspirin and ticlopidine have reduced both stent thrombosis and arterial access site bleeding.[115,120] Currently, the risk of stent thrombosis is less than 1%.[114,121,122] Haemorrhage (particularly femoral artery bleeding) was more frequent after stenting than PTA alone,[116] but occurred in less than 3% following stenting when antiplatelet drugs were used without long term anticoagulants.

Comment: It is unclear whether stenting influences the relative benefits and harms of percutaneous procedures compared with CABG.

GLOSSARY

International normalised ratio (INR) A value derived from a standardised laboratory test that measures the effect of an anticoagulant. The laboratory materials used in the test are calibrated against internationally accepted standard reference preparations, so that variability between laboratories and different reagents is minimised. Normal blood has an INR of 1. Therapeutic anticoagulation often aims to achieve an INR value of 2–3.5.

Substantive changes since last issue

PTA v medical treatment New systematic review replaces RCTs.[101] It found that angioplasty improved angina and was associated with increased rates of CABG, but found no evidence of effect for death, MI, or subsequent angioplasty.

PTA v medical treatment Follow up of an RCT included in the systematic review.[102] It found that PTA was associated with improved quality of life at 3 months and 1 year, but not at 3 years.

PTA v CABG Two new RCTs.[108,109] They found no significant difference between groups at 8 years.

PTA v CABG Unpublished RCT. It found similar results for event free survival in both groups.

PTA v stent Additional RCT;[116] results consistent with previous trials.

Antioxidant vitamins Additional RCT in people on haemodialysis;[81] conclusion unchanged.

Cholesterol reduction Long term follow up of an existing RCT;[50] conclusion unchanged.

Cholesterol reduction New systematic review[51] and two additional RCTs.[52,53] Conclusions for gemfibrozil unchanged. The trials found inconsistent results for bezafibrate versus placebo.

REFERENCES

1. Greaves EJ, Gillum BS. 1994 Summary: national hospital discharge survey. Advance data from Vital and Health Statistics, no. 278. Hyattsville, Maryland: National Center for Health Statistics, 1996.

2. Shaw LJ, Peterson ED, Kesler K, Hasselblad V, Califf RM. A meta-analysis of predischarge risk stratification after acute myocardial infarction with stress electrocardiographic, myocardial perfusion, and ventricular function imaging. Am J Cardiol 1996;78:1327–1337. Search date 1995; primary sources Medline, and hand search of bibliographies of review articles.

3. Kudenchuk PJ, Maynard C, Martin JS, et al. Comparison, presentation, treatment and outcome of acute myocardial infarction in men versus women (the myocardial infarction triage and intervention registry). Am J Cardiol 1996;78: 9–14.

4. The Task Force on the Management of Acute Myocardial Infarction of the European Society of Cardiology. Acute myocardial infarction: pre-hospital and in-hospital management. Eur Heart J 1996;17:43–63.

5. Peterson ED, Shaw LJ, Califf RM. Clinical guideline: part II. Risk stratification after myocardial infarction. Ann Intern Med 1997;126: 561–582.

6. The Multicenter Postinfarction Research Group. Risk stratification and survival after myocardial infarction. N Engl J Med 1983;309:331–336.

7. American College of Cardiology/American Heart Association Task Force on Practice Guidelines (Committee on Exercise Testing). ACC/AHA

guidelines for exercise testing. *J Am Coll Cardiol* 1997;30:260–315.

8. Fallen E, Cairns J, Dafoe W, et al. Management of the postmyocardial infarction patient: a consensus report – revision of the 1991 CCS guidelines. *Can J Cardiol* 1995;11:477–486.

9. Madsen JK, Grande P, Saunamaki, et al. Danish multicenter randomized study of invasive versus conservative treatment in patients with inducible ischemia after thrombolysis in acute myocardial infarction (DANAMI). *Circulation* 1997;96:748–755.

10. Antiplatelet Trialists' Collaboration. Collaborative overview of randomised trials of antiplatelet therapy – I: prevention of death, myocardial infarction, and stroke by prolonged antiplatelet therapy in various categories of patients. *BMJ* 1994;308:81–106. Search date March 1990; primary source Medline; Current Contents; hand search of journals, reference lists and conference proceedings; authors of trials and drug manufacturers.

11. Taylor DW, Barnett HJM, Haynes RB, et al, for the ASA and Carotid Endarterectomy (ACE) Trial Collaborators. Low-dose and high-dose acetylsalicylic acid for patients undergoing carotid endarterectomy: a randomised controlled trial. *Lancet* 1999;353:2179–2184.

12. Juul-Möller S, Edvardsson N, Jahnmatz B, Rosen A, Soreneson S, Omblus R, for the Swedish Angina Pectoris Aspirin Trial (SAPAT) Group. Double-blind trial of aspirin in primary prevention of myocardial infarction in patients with stable chronic angina pectoris. *Lancet* 1992;340:1421–1425.

13. Hankey GJ, Sudlow CLM, Dunbabin DW. Thienopyridine derivatives (ticlopidine, clopidogrel) versus aspirin for preventing stroke and other serious vascular events in high vascular risk patients. In: The Cochrane Library, Issue 2, 2000. Oxford: Update Software. Search date March/July 1999; primary sources Medline; Embase; Cochrane Stroke Group Register March 1999; Antithrombotics Trialists' database; authors of trials; and drug manufacturers.

14. CAPRIE Steering Committee. A randomised, blinded, trial of clopidogrel versus aspirin in patients at risk of ischaemic events. *Lancet* 1996; 348:1329–1339.

15. Farrell B, Godwin J, Richards S, Warlow C. The United Kingdom transient ischaemic attack (UK-TIA) aspirin trial: final results. *J Neurol Neurosurg Psychiatry* 1991;54:1044–1054.

16. Moloney BA. An analysis of the side effects of ticlopidine. In: Hass WK, Easton JD, eds. *Ticlopidine, Platelets and Vascular Disease*. New York: Springer, 1993:117–139.

17. Bennett CL, Davidson CJ, Raisch DW, Weinberg PD, Bennett RH, Feldman MD. Thrombotic thrombocytopenic purpura associated with ticlopidine in the setting of coronary artery stents and stroke prevention. *Arch Int Med* 1999;159: 2524–2528.

18. Bennett CL, Connors JM, Carwile JM, et al. Thrombotic thrombocytopenic purpura associated with clopidogrel. *N Engl J Med* 2000;342:1773–1777.

19. Hankey GJ. Clopidogrel and thrombotic thrombocytopenic purpura. *Lancet* 2000;356: 269–270.

20. Müller C, Büttner HJ, Petersen J, Roskamm H. A randomized comparison of clopidogrel and aspirin versus ticlopidine and aspirin after the placement of coronary-artery stents. *Circulation* 2000;101: 590–593.

21. Bertrand ME, Rupprecht H-J, Urban P, Gershlick AH, for the CLASSICS Investigators. Double-blind study of the safety of clopidogrel with and without a loading dose in combination with aspirin compared with ticlopidine in combination with aspirin after coronary stenting. The Clopidogrel Aspirin Stent International Cooperative Study (CLASSICS). *Circulation* 2000;102:624–629.

22. Anand SS, Yusuf S. Oral anticoagulant therapy in patients with coronary artery disease: a meta-analysis. *JAMA* 1999;282:2058–2067. Search date July 1999; primary sources Medline, Embase, Current Contents, hand searches of reference lists, experts, pharmaceutical companies.

23. Teo KK, Yusuf S, Furberg CD. Effects of prophylactic antiarrhythmic drug therapy in acute myocardial infarction. *JAMA* 1993;270:1589–1595. Search date 1993; primary sources Medline; hand search of reference lists; details of unpublished trials sought from pharmaceutical industry/other investigators.

24. Yusuf S, Peto R, Lewis J, Collins R, Sleight P. Beta blockade during and after myocardial infarction: An overview of the randomized trials. *Prog Cardiovasc Dis* 1985;27:335–371. No details of search date or primary sources given.

25. Pepine CJ, Cohn PF, Deedwania PC, et al for the ASIST Study Group. Effects of treatment on outcome in mildly symptomatic patients with ischemia during daily life: the atenolol silent ischemia study (ASIST). *Circulation* 1994;90:762–768.

26. Boissel J-P, Leizerovicz A, Picolet H, et al, for the APSI Investigators. Secondary prevention after high-risk acute myocardial infarction with low-dose acebutolol. *Am J Cardiol* 1990;66:251–260.

27. The Beta-Blocker Pooling Project Research Group. The beta-blocker pooling project (BBPP): subgroup findings from randomized trials in post infarction patients. *Eur Heart J* 1988;9:8–16. Search date placebo controlled trials published by December 1983; details of primary sources not given.

28. Beta-blocker Heart Attack Trial Research Group. A randomized trial of propranolol in patients with acute myocardial infarction: I. Mortality results. *JAMA* 1982;247:1707–1714.

29. Flather M, Kober L, Pfeffer MA, et al. Meta-analysis of individual patient data from trials of long-term ACE-inhibitor treatment after acute myocardial infarction (SAVE, AIRE, and TRACE studies). *Circulation* 1997;96(suppl 1;abs 3957): I–706. No details of search date or primary sources given.

30. The Heart Outcomes Prevention Evaluation (HOPE) Investigators. Effects of an angiotensin-converting enzyme inhibitor, ramipril, on cardiovascular events in high-risk patients. *N Engl J Med* 2000; 342;145–153.

31. Heart Outcomes Prevention Evaluation (HOPE) Investigators. Effects of ramipril on cardiovascular and microvascular outcomes on people with diabetes mellitus: results of the hope study and MICRO-HOPE substudy. *Lancet* 2000;355:253–259.

32. Yusuf S, Lonn E. Anti-ischaemic effects of ACE inhibitors: review of current clinical evidence and ongoing clinical trials. *Eur Heart J* 1998;19(suppl J):J36–44.

33. Echt DS, Liebson PR, Mitchell LB, et al. Mortality and morbidity in patients receiving encainide, flecainide, or placebo. *N Engl J Med* 1991;324: 781–788.

34. Amiodarone Trials Meta-Analysis Investigators. Effect of prophylactic amiodarone on mortality after acute myocardial infarction and in congestive heart failure: meta-analysis of individual data from 6500 patients in randomised trials. *Lancet* 1997; 350:1417–1424. No details of search date or primary sources given.

35. Sim I, McDonald KM, Lavori PW, Norbutas CM, Hlatky MA. Quantitative overview of randomized trials of amiodarone to prevent sudden cardiac death. Circulation 1997;96:2823–2829. Search date 1997; primary sources Medline, and Biosis.

36. Waldo AL, Camm AJ, de Ruyter H, et al, for the SWORD Investigators. Effect of d-sotalol on mortality in patients with left ventricular dysfunction after recent and remote myocardial infarction. Lancet 1996;348:7–12.

37. Cairns JA, Connolly SJ, Roberts R, Gent M, for the Canadian Amiodarone Myocardial Infarction Arrhythmia Trial Investigators. Randomized trial of outcome after myocardial infarction in patients with frequent or repetitive ventricular premature depolarisations: CAMIAT. Lancet 1997;349:675–682.

38. Julian DG, Camm AJ, Janse MJ, et al, for the European Myocardial Infarct Amiodarone Trial Investigators. Randomised trial of effect of amiodarone on mortality in patients with left-ventricular dysfunction after recent myocardial infarction: EMIAT. Lancet 1997;349:667–674.

39. Gibson R, Boden WE, Theroux P, et al. Diltiazem and reinfarction in patients with non-Q-wave myocardial infarction. N Engl J Med 1986;315:423–429.

40. The Multicenter Diltiazem Postinfarction Trial Research Group. The effect of diltiazem on mortality and reinfarction after myocardial infarction. N Engl J Med 1988;319:385–392.

41. The Danish Study Group on Verapamil in Myocardial Infarction. Effect of verapamil on mortality and major events after acute myocardial infarction: the Danish verapamil infarction trial II (DAVIT II). Am J Cardiol 1990;66:779–785.

42. Hulley S, Grady D, Bush T, et al. Randomized trial of estrogen plus progestin for secondary prevention of coronary heart disease in postmenopausal women. JAMA 1998;280:605–613.

43. Coronary Drug Research Project Research Group. The coronary drug project: initial findings leading to modifications of its research protocol. JAMA 1970;214:1303–1313.

44. Daly E, Vessey MP, Hawkins MM, Carson JL, Gough P, Marsh S. Risk of venous thromboembolism in users of hormone replacement therapy. Lancet 1996;348:977–980.

45. Newton KM, LaCroix AZ, McKnight B, et al. Estrogen replacement therapy and prognosis after first myocardial infarction. Am J Epidemiol 1997;145:269–277.

46. Sullivan JM, El-Zeky F, Vander Zwaag R, et al. Effect on survival of estrogen replacement therapy after coronary artery bypass grafting. Am J Cardiol 1997;79:847–850.

47. The Writing Group for the PEPI Trial. Effects of estrogen or estrogen/progestin regimens on heart disease risk factors in postmenopausal women. JAMA 1995;273:199–208.

48. Miettinen TA, Pyorala K, Olsson AG, Musliner TA, Cook TJ, et al. Cholesterol-lowering therapy in women and elderly patients with myocardial infarction or angina pectoris: findings from the Scandinavian Simvastatin Survival Study (4S). Circulation 1997;96:4211–4218.

49. LaRosa JC, He J, Vupputuri S. Effect of statins on risk of coronary disease: A meta-analysis of randomized controlled trials. JAMA 1999;282:2340–2346. Search date 1998; primary sources Medline, bibliographies, and authors' reference files.

50. Knatterud GL, Rosenberg Y, Campeau L, et al. Long-term effects on clinical outcomes of aggressive lowering of low-density lipoprotein cholesterol levels and low-dose anticoagulation in the post coronary artery bypass graft trial. Post CABG Investigators. Circulation 2000;102:157–165.

51. Montagne O, Vedel I, Durand-Zaleski I. Assessment of the impact of fibrates and diet on survival and their cost-effectiveness: evidence from randomized, controlled trials in coronary heart disease and health economic evaluations. Clin Ther 1999;21:2027–2035. Search date not stated; primary sources Medline, hand search of reference lists, and systematic reviews.

52. Anon. Secondary prevention by raising HDL cholesterol and reducing triglycerides in patients with coronary artery disease: the Bezafibrate Infarction Prevention (BIP) study. Circulation 2000;102:21–27.

53. Ericsson CG, Hamsten A, Nilsson J, Grip L, Svane B, de Faire U. Angiographic assessment of effects of bezafibrate on progression of coronary artery disease in young male postinfarction patients. Lancet 1996;347:849–853.

54. Bucher HC, Griffith LE, Guyatt G. Systematic review on the risk and benefit of different cholesterol-lowering interventions. Arterioscler Thromb Vasc Biol 1999;19:187–195. Search date October 1996; primary sources Medline, Embase, bibliographic searches.

55. Anon. MRC/BHF Heart Protection Study of cholesterol-lowering therapy and of antioxidant vitamin supplementation in a wide range of patients at increased risk of coronary heart disease death: early safety and efficacy experience. Eur Heart J 1999;20:725–741.

56. The Women's Health Initiative Study Group. Design of the women's health initiative clinical trial and observational study. Control Clin Trials 1998; 19:61–109.

57. Davis BR, Cutler JA Gordon DJ, et al, for the ALLHAT Research Group. Rationale and design for the antihypertensive and lipid lowering treatment to prevent heart attack trial (ALLHAT). Am J Hypertens 1996;9:342–360.

58. Flack JM, Neaton J, Grimm R, et al. Blood pressure and mortality among men with prior myocardial infarction. Circulation 1995;92:2437–2445.

59. Dahlof B, Lindholm LH, Hansson L, et al. Morbidity and mortality in the Swedish trial in old patients with hypertension (STOP-hypertension). Lancet 1991;338:1281–1285.

60. Medical Research Council Working Party. MRC trial on treatment of hypertension in older adults: principal results. BMJ 1992;304:405–412.

61. Systolic Hypertension in Elderly Patients (SHEP) Cooperative Research Group. Prevention of stroke by antihypertensive treatment in older persons with isolated systolic hypertension. JAMA 1991; 265:3255–3264.

62. D'Agostini RB, Belanger AJ, Kannel WB, et al. Relationship of low diastolic blood pressure to coronary heart disease death in presence of myocardial infarction: the Framingham study. BMJ 1991;303:385–389.

63. Pfeffer MA, Braunwald E, Moye LA, et al, on behalf of the SAVE investigators. Effect of captopril on mortality and morbidity in patients with left ventricular dysfunction after myocardial infarction: results of the survival and ventricular enlargement trial. N Engl J Med 1992;327:669–677.

64. NHS Centre for Reviews and Dissemination, University of York. Cholesterol and coronary heart disease: screening and treatment. Eff Health Care 1998;4:Number 1. Search date and primary sources not given.

65. Burr ML, Fehily AM, Gilbert JF, et al. Effects of changes in fat, fish, and fibre intakes on death and myocardial reinfarction: diet and reinfarction

trial (DART). *Lancet* 1989;2:757–761.

66. Fehily AM, Vaughan-Williams E, Shiels K, et al. The effect of dietary advice on nutrient intakes: evidence from the diet and reinfarction trial (DART). *J Hum Nutr Dietetics* 1989;2:225–235.

67. GISSI-Prevenzione Investigators. Dietary supplementation with n-3 polyunsaturated fatty acids and vitamin E after myocardial infarction: results of the GISSI-Prevenzione. *Lancet* 1999; 354:447–455.

68. De Lorgeril M, Renaud S, Mamelle N, et al. Mediterranean alpha-linolenic acid-rich diet in secondary prevention of coronary heart disease. *Lancet* 1994;343:1454–1459.

69. Clarke R, Frost C, Collins R, et al. Dietary lipids and blood cholesterol: quantitative meta-analysis of metabolic ward studies. *BMJ* 1997;314:112–117. Search date 1995; primary sources Medline 1960–1995, hand search of reference lists and nutrition journals.

70. Tang JL, Armitage JM, Lancaster T, et al. Systematic review of dietary intervention trials to lower blood total cholesterol in free-living subjects. *BMJ* 1998;316:1213–1220. Search date 1997; primary sources Medline, Human Nutrition, Embase, and Allied and Alternative Medicine 1966–1997, hand searching the *Am J Clin Nutr*, and references of review articles.

71. Brunner E, White I, Thorogood M, et al. Can dietary interventions change diet and cardiovascular risk factors? A meta-analysis of randomized controlled trials. *Am J Public Health* 1997;87:1415–1422. Search date 1993; primary sources Medline 1966 to July 1993, and manual search of selected journals.

72. Ebrahim S, Davey SG. *Health promotion in older people for the prevention of coronary heart disease and stroke.* London: Health Education Authority, 1996.

73. Waters D. Lessons from coronary atherosclerosis "regression" trials. *Cardiol Clin* 1996;14:31–50.

74. Silagy C, Neil A. Garlic as a lipid lowering agent: a meta-analysis. *J R Coll Physicians Lond* 1994;28:39–45. Search date July 1992; primary sources Medline 1966 to July 1992; Alternative Medicine database; authors of published studies; manufacturers; and hand searched references.

75. Isaacson JL, Moser M, Stein EA, et al. Garlic powder and plasma lipids and lipoproteins. *Arch Intern Med* 1998;158:1189–119.

76. Berthold HK, Sudhop T, von Bergmann K. Effect of a garlic oil preparation on serum lipoproteins and cholesterol metabolism. *JAMA* 1998;279:1900–1902.

77. Ripsin CM, Keenan JM, Jacobs DR Jr, et al. Oat products and lipid lowering: a meta-analysis. *JAMA* 1992;267:3317–3325. Search date 1991; primary sources Medline 1966–1991; unpublished trials solicited from all known investigators of lipid-oats association.

78. Stephens NG, Parsons A, Schofield PM, et al. Randomised controlled trial of vitamin E in patients with coronary disease: Cambridge heart antioxidant study (CHAOS). *Lancet* 1996;347:781–786.

79. Rapola JM, Virtamo J, Ripatti S, et al. Randomised trial of α-tocopherol and β-carotene supplements on incidence of major coronary events in men with previous myocardial infarction. *Lancet* 1997;349:1715–1720.

80. The Heart Outcomes Prevention Evaluation Study Investigators. Vitamin E supplementation and cardiovascular events in high-risk patients. The Heart Outcomes Prevention Evaluation Study Investigators. *N Engl J Med* 2000;342:154–160.

81. Boaz M, Smetana S, Weinstein T, et al. Secondary prevention with antioxidants of cardiovascular disease in endstage renal disease (SPACE): randomised placebo-controlled trial. *Lancet* 2000; 356:1213–18.

82. Wilson TS, Datta SB, Murrell JS, Andrews CT. Relation of vitamin C levels to mortality in a geriatric hospital: a study of the effect of vitamin C administration. *Age Aging* 1973;2:163–170.

83. Burr ML, Hurley RJ, Sweetnam PM. Vitamin C supplementation of old people with low blood levels. *Gerontol Clin* 1975;17:236–243.

84. Hunt C, Chakkravorty NK, Annan G. The clinical and biochemical effects of vitamin C supplementation in short-stay hospitalized geriatric patients. *Int J Vitam Nutr Res* 1984;54:65–74.

85. Lonn EM, Yusuf S. Is there a role for antioxidant vitamins in the prevention of cardiovascular diseases? An update on epidemiological and clinical trials data. *Can J Cardiol* 1997;13:957–965. Search date 1996; primary sources Medline 1965–1996; and one reference from 1997.

86. Jha P, Flather M, Lonn E, Farkouh M, Yusuf S. The antioxidant vitamins and cardiovascular disease: a critical review of epidemiologic and clinical trial data. *Ann Intern Med* 1995;123:860–872.

87. Ness AR, Powles JW, Khaw KT. Vitamin C and cardiovascular disease: a systematic review. *J Cardiovasc Risk* 1997;3:513–521. Search date not given; primary sources Medline, experts, and hand searched references.

88. Oldridge NB, Guyatt GH, Fisher MS, Rimm AA. Cardiac rehabilitation after myocardial infarction: combined experience of randomized clinical trials. *JAMA* 1988;260:945–950. Search date not specified; primary sources Medline.

89. O'Connor GT, Buring JE, Yusuf S, et al. An overview of randomized trials of rehabilitation with exercise after myocardial infarction. *Circulation* 1989;80:234–244. No details of search date or primary sources given.

90. Berlin JA, Colditz GA. A meta-analysis of physical activity in the prevention of coronary heart disease. *Am J Epidemiol* 1990;132:612–628. No details of search date or primary sources given.

91. Wenger NK, Froelicher NS, Smith LK, et al. *Cardiac rehabilitation and secondary prevention.* Rockville, Maryland: Agency for Health Care Policy and Research and National Heart, Lung and Blood Institute, 1995. Search date and primary source not given.

92. US Department of Health and Human Services. *The health benefits of smoking cessation: a report of the surgeon general.* Bethesda, Maryland: US DHSS, 1990.

93. Working Group for the Study of Transdermal Nicotine in Patients with Coronary Artery Disease. Nicotine replacement therapy for patients with coronary artery disease. *Arch Intern Med* 1994;154:989–995.

94. Joseph AM, Norman SM, Ferry LH, et al. The safety of transdermal nicotine as an aid to smoking cessation in patients with cardiac disease. *N Engl J Med* 1996;335:1792–1798.

95. Burt A, Thornley P, Illingworth D, White P, Shaw TRD, Turner R. Stopping smoking after myocardial infarction. *Lancet* 1974;1:304–306.

96. Linden W, Stossel C, Maurice J. Psychosocial interventions in patients with coronary artery disease: a meta-analysis. *Arch Intern Med* 1996;156:745–752. No details of search date or primary sources given.

97. US Department of Health and Human Services. Cardiac rehabilitation. AHCPR Publication No 96–0672, 1995;121–128.

98. Hemingway H, Marmot M. Psychosocial factors in the primary and secondary prevention of coronary heart disease: a systematic review. In: Yusuf S, Cairns JA, Camm AJ, Fallen EL, Gersh BJ, eds.

Cardiovascular disorders

Evidence based cardiology. London: BMJ Books, 1998. Search date 1996; primary sources Medline 1966–1996; manual searching of bibliographies of retrieved articles and review articles.

99. Yusuf S, Zucker D, Peduzzi P, et al. Effect of coronary artery bypass graft surgery on survival: overview of 10-year results from randomized trials by the coronary artery bypass graft surgery trialists collaboration. *Lancet* 1994;344:563–570. No search date or primary sources given.

100. Davies RF, Goldberg AD, Forman S, et al. Asymptomatic cardiac ischemia pilot (ACIP) study two-year follow-up: outcomes of patients randomized to initial strategies of medical therapy versus revascularization. *Circulation* 1997;95:2037–2043.

101. Bucher HC, Hengstler P, Schindler C, Guyatt GH. Percutaneous transluminal coronary angioplasty versus medical treatment for non-acute coronary heart disease: Meta-analysis of randomised controlled trials. *BMJ* 2000;321:73–77. Search date December 1998; primary sources Medline 1979 to December 1998; Embase 1979 to December 1998; Cochrane Database 1979 to December 1998; Biological Abstracts 1979 to December 1998; Health Periodicals Database 1979 to December 1998; PASCAL 1979 to December 1998; and hand searched references.

102. Pocock SJ, Henderson RA, Clayton T, Lyman GH, Chamberlain DA. Quality of life after coronary angioplasty or continued medical treatment for angina: three-year follow-up in the RITA-2 trial. *J Am Coll Cardiol* 2000;35:907–914.

103. RITA-2 Trial Participants. Coronary angioplasty versus medical therapy for angina: the second randomized intervention treatment of angina (RITA-2) trial. *Lancet* 1997;350:461–468.

104. Parisi AF, Folland ED, Hartigan P. A comparison of angioplasty with medical therapy in the treatment of single-vessel coronary artery disease. *N Engl J Med* 1992;326:10–16.

105. Morris KG, Folland ED, Hartigan PM, Parisi AF. Unstable angina in late follow-up of the ACME trial. *Circulation* 1995;92(supplement I):1–725.

106. Pocock SJ, Henderson RA, Rickards AF, et al. Meta-analysis of randomized trials comparing coronary angioplasty with bypass surgery. *Lancet* 1995;346:1184–1189. No details of search date or primary sources given.

107. Rihal CS, Gersh BJ, Yusuf S. Chronic coronary artery disease: coronary artery bypass surgery vs percutaneous transluminal coronary angioplasty vs medical therapy. In: Yusuf S, Cairns JA, Camm JA, Fallen EL, Gersh BJ, eds. *Evidence based cardiology.* London: BMJ Books, 1998.

108. King SB, Kosinski AS, Guyton RA, Lembo NJ, Weintraub WS. Eight-Year Mortality in the Emory Angioplasty Versus Surgery Trial (EAST). *J Am Coll Cardiol* 2000;35:1116–1121.

109. The BARI Investigators. Seven-Year Outcome in the Bypass Angioplasty Revascularization Investigation (BARI) By Treatment and Diabetic Status. *J Am Coll Cardiol* 2000;35:1122–1129.

110. Bypass Angioplasty Revascularization Investigation (BARI) Investigators. Comparison of coronary bypass surgery with angioplasty in patients with multivessel disease. *N Engl J Med* 1996;335:7–225.

111. Hlatky MA, Rogers WJ, Johnstone I, et al. Medical care costs and quality of life after randomization to coronary angioplasty or coronary bypass surgery. *N Engl J Med* 1997;336:92–99.

112. Wåhrborg P. Quality of life after coronary angioplasty or bypass surgery. *Eur Heart J* 1999;20:653–658.

113. Serruys PW, de Jaeger P, Kiemeneij F. A comparison of balloon-expandable-stent implantation with balloon angioplasty in patients with coronary artery disease. *N Engl J Med* 1994;33:489–495.

114. Versaci F, Gaspardone A, Tomai F, Crea F, Chiariello L, Gioffre PA. A comparison of coronary-artery stenting with angioplasty for isolated stenosis of the proximal left anterior descending coronary artery. *N Engl J Med* 1997;336:817–822.

115. Savage MP, Douglas JS, Fischman DL, et al. Stent placement compared with balloon angioplasty for obstructed coronary bypass grafts. *N Engl J Med* 1997;337:740–747.

116. Witkowski A, Ruzyllo W, Gil R, et al. A randomized comparison of elective high-pressure stenting with balloon angioplasty: six-month angiographic and two-year clinical follow-up. On behalf of AS (Angioplasty or Stent) trial investigators. *Am Heart J* 2000;140:264–271.

117. Sirnes P, Golf S, Yngvar M, et al. Stenting in chronic coronary occlusion (SICCO): a randomized controlled trial of adding stent implantation after successful angioplasty. *J Am Coll Cardiol* 1996;28:1444–1451.

118. Rubartelli P, Niccoli L, Verna E, et al. Stent implantation versus balloon angioplasty in chronic coronary occlusions: results from the GISSOC trial. *J Am Coll Cardiol* 1998;32:90–96.

119. Sievert H, Rohde S, Utech A, et al. Stent or angioplasty after recanalization of chronic coronary occlusions? (the SARECCO trial). *Am J Cardiol* 1999;84:386–390.

120. Erbel R, Haude M, Hopp HW, et al. Coronary artery stenting compared with balloon angioplasty for restenosis after initial balloon angioplasty. *N Engl J Med* 1998;23:1682–1688.

121. Schomig A, Neumann EF, Kastrati A, et al. A randomized comparison of antiplatelet and anticoagulation therapy after the placement of intracoronary stents. *N Engl J Med* 1996;334:1084–1089.

122. Leon MB, Baim DS, Gordon P, et al. Clinical and angiographic results from the stent anticoagulation regimen study (STARS). *Circulation* 1996;94(supplement I):1–685.

Cathie Sudlow
Specialist Registrar in Neurology
Department of Neurology
Derriford Hospital
Plymouth, UK

Eva Lonn
Associate Professor of Medicine
Hamilton General Hospital
Hamilton, Canada

Secondary prevention of ischaemic cardiac events

Michael Pignone
Division of General Internal Medicine
University of North Carolina
Chapel Hill, NC
USA

Andrew Ness
Senior Lecturer in Epidemiology
University of Bristol
Bristol
UK

Charanjit Rihal
Consultant Cardiologist
Mayo Clinic and Mayo Foundation
Rochester
USA

Competing interests: None declared.

TABLE 1 **Prognostic groups for people who survive the acute stage of MI (see text, p 97).**

Baseline risk	1 year mortality	Clinical markers[2–4]
High	10–50%	Older age; history or previous MI; reduced exercise tolerance (New York Heart Association functional classes II–IV) before admission; clinical signs of heart failure in the first 2 days (Killip classes IIb, III, and IV) or persistent heart failure on days 3–5 after infarction; early increased heart rate; persistent or early appearance of angina at rest or with minimal exertion; and multiple or complex ventricular arrhythmias during monitoring in hospital.
Moderate	10%	–
Low	2–5%	Younger age (< 55 years), no previous MI, an event free course during the first 5 days after MI.[2]

Secondary prevention of ischaemic cardiac events

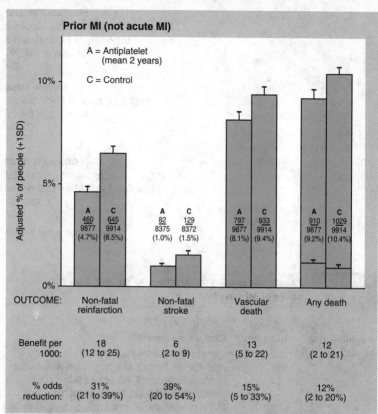

FIGURE 1 The absolute effects of antiplatelet treatment on various outcomes in people with prior MI: results of a systematic review.[10] The columns show the absolute risks over 2 years for each outcome. The error bars represent standard deviations. In the "any death" column, non-vascular deaths are represented by lower horizontal lines (see text, p 98).

Search date September 2000

Gord Gubitz and Peter Sandercock

QUESTIONS

INTERVENTIONS

ACUTE ISCHAEMIC STROKE
Beneficial

Trade off between benefits and harms

Unlikely to be beneficial

Likely to be ineffective or harmful

INTRACEREBRAL HAEMATOMAS
Unknown effectiveness

To be covered in future issues of *Clinical Evidence*
Other treatments for acute ischaemic stroke: corticosteroids, fibrinogen depleting agents, glycerol, haemodilution techniques. Prevention of deep venous thrombosis/pulmonary embolism in people with stroke.

See glossary, p 136

Key Messages

Systematic reviews of RCTs have found that:

- Stroke rehabilitation units reduce death and severe disability.

- Thrombolysis reduces the risk of dependency, but increases the risk of death (both from intracranial haemorrhage and from any cause).

- Early use of aspirin after an ischaemic stroke confirmed by computerised tomography (CT) scan reduces the chance of death and dependency and improves the chance of complete recovery. (We found indirect evidence that aspirin should not be delayed if a CT scan is not readily available within 48 hours. A combined prospective analysis of two large RCTs found that people given aspirin, who were subsequently found to have a haemorrhagic rather than an ischaemic stroke, had the same outcomes as people who were given placebo.)

- Blood pressure reduction soon after acute ischaemic stroke has not been adequately tested in large scale RCTs, and may be harmful.

- One RCT found no evidence that low molecular weight heparin is superior to aspirin alone for the treatment of acute ischemic stroke in people with atrial fibrillation.

Cardiovascular disorders

- We found no evidence that immediate systemic anticoagulation improves outcome after ischaemic stroke.
- RCTs found no evidence that calcium channel antagonists, lubeluzole, GABA agonists, glycine antagonists or N-methyl-D-aspartate (NMDA) antagonists improve clinical outcomes in people with acute ischaemic stroke.
- We found no evidence of benefit from surgical evacuation of cerebral or cerebellar haematomas.

DEFINITION   Stroke is characterised by rapidly developing clinical symptoms and signs of focal, and at times global, loss of cerebral function lasting more than 24 hours or leading to death, with no apparent cause other than that of vascular origin.[1] Ischaemic stroke is defined as stroke caused by vascular insufficiency (such as cerebrovascular thromboembolism) rather than haemorrhage.

INCIDENCE/   Stroke is the third most common cause of death in most developed
PREVALENCE countries.[2] It is a worldwide problem; about 4.5 million people die from stroke each year. Stroke can occur at any age, but half of all strokes occur in people over 70 years old.[3]

AETIOLOGY/   About 80% of all acute strokes are caused by cerebral infarction,
RISK FACTORS usually resulting from thrombotic or embolic occlusion of a cerebral artery.[4] The remainder are caused either by intracerebral or subarachnoid haemorrhage.

PROGNOSIS   About 10% of all people with acute ischaemic strokes will die within 30 days of stroke onset.[5] Of those who survive the acute event, about 50% will experience some level of disability after 6 months.[6]

AIMS   To minimise impairment, disability, and secondary complications, with minimal adverse effects from treatment.

OUTCOMES   Risk of death or dependency (generally assessed as the proportion of people dead or requiring physical assistance for transfers, mobility, dressing, feeding, or toileting 3–6 months after stroke onset[6]); quality of life.

METHODS   *Clinical Evidence* update search and appraisal September 2000.

QUESTION   **What are the effects of specialised care in people with stroke?**

One systematic review of RCTs has found that people with stroke who are managed in specialist stroke rehabilitation units are more likely to be alive and living at home a year after the stroke than those managed in general medical wards, and that stroke unit care reduces time spent in hospital. Observational studies have found that these results are reproducible in routine clinical settings.

Benefits: We found one systematic review (search date 1998, 20 RCTs, 3864 people with stroke) comparing specialised stroke rehabilitation units versus conventional care.[7] In most trials, the specialised stroke rehabilitation unit consisted of a designated area or ward, although some trials used a mobile "stroke team". Participants in these trials were usually transferred to stroke care within the first or second week following stroke onset. People cared for in a stroke rehabilitation unit had lower rates of death or dependency after a median follow up of 1 year (RRR 10%, 95% CI 5% to 15%; NNT 16,

95% CI 10 to 43) (see figure 1, p 139).[1] The length of stay was calculated differently for many of the trials, so the consequent heterogeneity between results limits generalisability. Overall, length of stay in the stroke unit group was reduced by about 2–11 days. Since the review, two of the included trials have published follow up results. One RCT (220 people) found that care in a combined acute and rehabilitation unit compared with care in general wards increased the proportion of people able to live at home 10 years after their stroke (ARI 11%, 95% CI 1.9% to 20%; NNT 9, 95% CI 5 to 52).[8] The second RCT (220 people) compared treatment in a 15 bed multidisciplinary stroke rehabilitation unit versus treatment in general medical wards.[9] Five years after the stroke, the risk of death or disability for people treated in the stroke unit was reduced (RR 0.91, 95% CI 0.83 to 0.99). We found one additional RCT,[10] which randomised 76 people 2–10 days after their stroke to either an integrated care pathway (see glossary, p 136) or to conventional multidisciplinary care on a stroke rehabilitation unit in the UK. All received similar occupational and physical therapy. Conventional treatment versus the integrated care pathway produced more improvement in the Barthel Index from 4–12 weeks (P < 0.01), and higher scores on the Euroquol (Quality of Life Scale) after 6 months (P < 0.05). It found no significant difference between the two treatments in mortality, length of hospital stay, or the proportion of people requiring long term institutional care.

Harms: No detrimental effects attributable to stroke units were reported.

Comment: Although the proportional reduction in death or dependency seems larger with thrombolysis, stroke unit care is applicable to most stroke people, whereas thrombolysis is applicable only to a small proportion. The systematic review did not provide data on which aspects of the multidisciplinary approach led to improved outcome, although one limited retrospective analysis of one of the RCTs found that several factors, including early mobilisation, increased use of oxygen, intravenous saline solutions, and antipyretics may have been responsible.[11] Most of the trials excluded the most mild and severe strokes. Following publication of the systematic review,[7] prospective observational data have been collected in one large series of over 14 000 people in 80 Swedish hospitals.[12] In this series, people admitted to stroke units had reduced dependence at 3 months (RRR 6%, 95% CI 1% to 11%). Although biases are inherent in such observational data, the findings suggest that the results of the meta-analysis may be reproducible in routine clinical settings.

QUESTION What are the effects of medical treatment in acute ischaemic stroke?

OPTION THROMBOLYSIS

We found little evidence on the balance between benefits and harms from thrombolysis in acute ischaemic stroke. One systematic review found that thrombolysis given soon after acute ischaemic stroke reduced overall risk of death and dependency in the long term, but that this benefit was achieved at the cost of an increased short term risk of fatal intracranial haemorrhage. It remains unclear which people are most likely to benefit or be harmed.

Cardiovascular disorders

Stroke management

Benefits: We found one systematic review (search date 1999, 17 RCTs, 5216 highly selected people) comparing thrombolysis versus placebo given soon after the onset of stroke.[13] All trials used computerised tomography (CT) or magnetic resonance scanning before randomisation to exclude intracranial haemorrhage or other non-stroke disorders. The systematic review included results for three different thrombolytic agents: streptokinase, urokinase, and recombinant tissue plasminogen activator (rt-PA), but direct comparison of different thrombolytic drugs was not possible. Two trials used intra-arterial administration and the rest used the intravenous route. Thrombolysis reduced the risk of death or dependency at the end of the studies (ARR 4.2%, 95% CI 1.2% to 7.2%; RRR 7%, 95% CI 3% to 12%; NNT 24, 95% CI 14 to 83) (see figures 1 and 2, p 139).[13] In the subset of trials assessing intravenous rt-PA, the findings were similar (ARR 5.7%, 95% CI 2.0% to 9.4%; RRR 10%, 95% CI 4% to 16%; NNT 18, 95% CI 11 to 50). Further meta-analysis (4 RCTs, individual results of 1292 people with acute ischaemic stroke treated with streptokinase or placebo) found that streptokinase versus placebo had no clear effect on the proportion of people dead or dependent at 3 months and included the possibility of both substantial benefit or substantial harm (RRR +1%, 95% CI −6% to +8%).[14] People allocated to streptokinase were more likely to be dead after 3 months (RRI 46%, 95% CI 24% to 73%). The combination of aspirin plus streptokinase significantly increased mortality at 3 months (P = 0.005), but this did not affect the combined risk of death or severe disability (95% CI not available; P = 0.28).

Harms: **Fatal intracranial haemorrhage:** In the systematic review, thrombolysis increased fatal intracranial haemorrhage compared with placebo (ARI 4.4%, 95% CI 3.4% to 5.4%; RRI 396%, 95% CI 220% to 668%; NNH 23, 95% CI 19 to 29).[13] In the subset of trials assessing intravenous rt-PA, the findings were similar (ARI 2.9%, 95% CI 1.7% to 4.1%; RRI 259%, 95% CI 102% to 536%; NNH 34, 95% CI 24 to 59). **Death:** In the systematic review, thrombolysis compared with placebo increased the risk of death by the end of the follow up (ARI 3.3%, 95% CI 1.2% to 5.4%; RRI 23%, 95% CI 10% to 38%; NNH 30, 95% CI 19 to 83).[13] This excess of deaths was offset by fewer people being alive but dependent 6 months after stroke onset. The net effect was a reduction in the number of people who were dead or dependent.

Comment: There was no significant heterogeneity of treatment effect overall, but heterogeneity of results was noted for the outcomes of death, and death or dependency at final follow up among the eight trials of intravenous rt-PA.[12] Explanations may include the combined use of antithrombotic agents (aspirin or heparin within the first 24 hours of thrombolysis), stroke severity, the presence of early ischaemic changes on CT scan, and the time from stroke onset to randomisation. A subgroup analysis suggested that thrombolysis may be more beneficial if given within 3 hours of symptom onset, but the duration of the "therapeutic time window" could not be determined reliably. Most of the trial results were of outcome at 3 months; only one trial reported 1 year outcome data.[15] We found little evidence about which people are most and least likely to benefit from thrombolysis. A number of trials of different thrombolytic regimens are underway.[16]

OPTION	ASPIRIN

One systematic review of RCTs has found that antiplatelet treatment with aspirin started within 48 hours of acute ischaemic stroke reduces the risk of death and dependence, as does the continued long term use of aspirin (see aspirin under stroke prevention, p 140). Most people included in the systematic review had a CT scan to exclude haemorrhage before treatment was started; in such people aspirin was beneficial. Subgroup analysis of two large RCTs found evidence that aspirin should not be delayed if a CT scan is not readily available within 48 hours: people given aspirin who were subsequently found to have a haemorrhagic rather than an ischaemic stroke had the same outcomes as people who were given placebo.

Benefits: **Early use of aspirin:** We found one systematic review (search date 1999, 8 RCTs, 41 325 people with definite or presumed ischaemic stroke),[17] which compared antiplatelet treatment started within 14 days of the stroke versus placebo. Ninety eight per cent of the data in the systematic review came from two large RCTs of aspirin 160–300 mg daily started within 48 hours of stroke onset.[18,19] Most people had an ischaemic stroke confirmed by CT scan before randomisation, but people who were conscious could be randomised before CT scan if the stroke was very likely to be ischaemic on clinical grounds. Treatment duration varied from 10–28 days. Aspirin started within the first 48 hours of acute ischaemic stroke reduced death or dependency at 6 months' follow up (RRR 3%, 95% CI 1% to 5%; NNT 77, 95% CI 43 to 333) (see figure 1, p 139) and increased the number of people making a complete recovery (NNT 91, 95% CI 50 to 500). A prospective combined analysis[20] of the two large RCTs[18,19] found a significant reduction in the outcome of further stroke or death with aspirin versus placebo (ARR 0.9%, 95% CI 0.75% to 1.85%; NNT 111, 95% CI 54 to 133). The effect was similar across subgroups (older v younger; male v female; impaired consciousness or not; atrial fibrillation or not; blood pressure; stroke subtype; timing of CT scanning). For the 773 people subsequently found to have had a hemorrhagic stroke rather than an ischaemic stroke, the subgroup analysis found no difference in the outcome of further stroke or death between those who were randomised to aspirin versus placebo (16% v 18%, ARR +2.0%, 95% CI–4.0% to +6.6%).[20] **Long term treatment (3 years):** See aspirin under stroke prevention, p 140.

Harms: Aspirin caused an excess of about two intracranial and four extracranial haemorrhages per 1000 people treated, but these small risks were more than offset by the reductions in death and disability from other causes both in the short term[17] and in the long term.[21] Common adverse effects of aspirin (such as dyspepsia and constipation) were dose related.[22]

Comment: We found no clear evidence that any one dose of aspirin is more effective than any other in the treatment of acute ischaemic stroke.

One recent meta-regression analysis of the dose response effect of aspirin on stroke found a uniform effect of aspirin in a range of doses from 50–1500 mg/day.[23] People unable to swallow safely after a stroke may be given aspirin as a suppository.

| OPTION | IMMEDIATE SYSTEMIC ANTICOAGULATION |

One systematic review of RCTs has found no short or long term improvement in acute ischaemic stroke with immediate systemic anticoagulants (unfractionated heparin, low molecular weight heparin, heparinoids, or specific thrombin inhibitors) versus usual care without systemic anticoagulants. Immediate systemic anticoagulants reduce the risk of deep venous thrombosis and pulmonary embolus, but this benefit is offset by a dose dependent risk of intracranial and extracranial haemorrhage. In people with acute ischaemic stroke and atrial fibrillation, one RCT has found no evidence that low molecular weight heparin is superior to aspirin alone.

Benefits: **Death or dependency:** We found one systematic review[24] and one subsequent RCT.[25] The systematic review (search date 1999, 21 RCTs, 23 427 people) compared unfractionated heparin, low molecular weight heparin, heparinoids, oral anticoagulants, or specific thrombin inhibitors versus usual care without systemic anticoagulants.[24] Over 80% of the data came from one trial, which randomised people with any severity of stroke to either subcutaneous heparin or placebo, usually after exclusion of haemorrhagic stroke by CT scan.[19] The systematic review found no significant difference in the proportion of people dead or dependent in the treatment and control groups at the end of follow up (3–6 months after the stroke: ARR +0.4%, 95% CI –0.9% to +1.7%; RRR 0%, 95% CI –2% to +3%).[24] There was no clear short or long term benefit of anticoagulants in any prespecified subgroups (stroke of presumed cardioembolic origin v others; different anticoagulants). The subsequent RCT (449 people with acute stroke and atrial fibrillation) found no significant difference between dalteparin (a low molecular weight heparin) versus aspirin for the primary outcome of recurrent ischaemic stroke during the first 14 days (ARI +1.0%, 95% CI –3.6% to +6.2%) or for secondary outcomes, including functional outcome at 3 months.[25] **Deep venous thrombosis and pulmonary embolism:** We found three systematic reviews.[24,26,27] The first systematic review included 10 small heterogeneous RCTs (22 000 people), which assessed anticoagulants in 916 people at high risk of deep venous thrombosis after their stroke.[24] Anticoagulation compared with control reduced the risk of deep vein thrombosis (ARR 29%, 95% CI 24% to 35%; RRR 64%, 95% CI 54% to 71%; NNT 3, 95% CI 2 to 4) and reduced symptomatic pulmonary embolism (ARR 0.3%, 95% CI 0.1% to 0.6%; RRR 38%, 95% CI 16% to 54%; NNT 333, 95% CI 167 to 1000).[24] No RCT performed investigations in all people to rule out silent events. The frequency of reported pulmonary emboli was low and varied among RCTs, so there may have been under-ascertainment. Two other systematic reviews (search dates 1999[26] and 1999,[27] same 5 RCTs in each review, 705 people with acute ischaemic stroke) found that low molecular weight heparins or heparinoids versus unfractionated heparin significantly reduced deep venous thrombosis (AR 13% with

LMWH or heparinoids v 22% with unfractionated heparin; ARR 9%, 95% CI 4.5% to 16%).[26,27] The number of events was too small to estimate the effects of low molecular weight heparins or heparinoids versus unfractionated heparin on death, intracranial haemorrhage, or functional outcome in survivors.

Harms: One systematic review found that anticoagulation slightly increased symptomatic intracranial haemorrhages within 14 days of starting treatment compared with control (ARI 0.93%, 95% CI 0.68% to 1.18%; RRI 163%, 95% CI 95% to 255%; NNH 108, 95% CI 85 to 147).[24] The large trial of subcutaneous heparin found that this effect was dose dependent (symptomatic intracranial haemorrhage by using medium dose compared with low dose heparin for 14 days, RRI 143%, 95% CI 82% to 204%; NNH 97, 95% CI 68 to 169).[19] The review also found a dose dependent increase in major extracranial haemorrhages after 14 days of treatment with anticoagulants (ARI 0.91%, 95% CI 0.67% to 1.15%; RRI 231%, 95% CI 136% to 365%; NNH 109, 95% CI 87 to 149).[24] The subsequent RCT of dalteparin versus aspirin for people with acute stroke and atrial fibrillation found no difference in adverse events, including symptomatic or asymptomatic intracerebral haemorrhage, progression of symptoms, or early or late death.[25]

Comment: Full publication is awaited of the results of a recently completed trial of the low molecular weight heparin tinzaparin.[28] Alternative treatments to prevent deep venous thrombosis and pulmonary embolism after acute ischaemic stroke include aspirin and compression stockings. The evidence relating to these will be reviewed in a future issue of *Clinical Evidence*.

OPTION	BLOOD PRESSURE REDUCTION

One systematic review of RCTs found no evidence that blood pressure reduction is of benefit in people with acute ischaemic stroke, but suggests that treatment may be harmful.

Benefits: We found one systematic review (search date 1997, 3 RCTs, 113 people with acute stroke) comparing blood pressure lowering treatment versus placebo.[29] Several different antihypertensive agents were used. The trials collected insufficient clinical data to allow an analysis of the relation between changes in blood pressure and clinical outcome.

Harms: Two placebo controlled RCTs have suggested that people treated with antihypertensive agents may have a worse clinical outcome and increased mortality. The first (295 people with acute ischaemic stroke) compared nimodipine (a calcium channel antagonist) versus placebo. The trial was stopped prematurely because of an excess of unfavourable neurological outcomes in the nimodipine treated group. Exploratory analyses confirmed that this negative correlation was related to reductions in mean arterial blood pressure ($P = 0.02$) and diastolic blood pressure ($P = 0.0005$).[30] The second RCT (302 people with acute ischaemic stroke) evaluated β blockers (atenolol or propranolol). There was a non-significant increase in death for people taking β blockers, and no difference in the proportion of people achieving a good outcome.[31] One systematic review (search date 1994, 9 RCTs, 3719 people with acute stroke) compared nimodipine versus placebo; no net benefit was found.[32] A second review (published in 1998, 24 RCTs, 6894 people) found a non-significant increase in the risk of death with calcium antagonists versus placebo (RRR 8%, 95% CI 1% reduction to 18% increase).[33] Although treatment with calcium antagonists in these trials was intended for neuroprotection, blood pressure was lower in the treatment group in several trials.

Comment: Population based studies suggest a direct and continuous association between blood pressure and the risk of recurrent stroke.[34] However, acute blood pressure lowering in acute ischaemic stroke may lead to increased cerebral ischaemia. The systematic review[30] identified several ongoing RCTs and we identified two additional ongoing RCTs not included in the systematic review.[35,36]

OPTION	NEUROPROTECTIVE AGENTS

Systematic reviews found no evidence that calcium channel blockers, GABA agonists, glycine antagonists, or NMDA antagonists improved clinical outcomes in people with acute ischaemic stroke. RCTs found no evidence that lubeluzole improved clinical outcomes in people with acute ischaemic stroke.

Benefits: We found no systematic reviews evaluating the general effectiveness of neuroprotective agents in acute ischaemic stroke. **Calcium channel antagonists:** We found one systematic review (search date 1999, 28 RCTs, 7521 people with acute ischaemic stroke) comparing calcium channel antagonists versus placebo.[37] It found that calcium channel antagonists did not significantly reduce the risk of poor outcome (including death) at the end of the follow up period compared with placebo (ARI of poor outcome +4.9%, 95% CI –2.5% to +7.3%; RRI +4%, 95% CI –2% to +9%). **GABA agonists:** We found one systematic review (search date 1999, 3 RCTs, 1002 people with acute ischaemic stroke), which found no significant difference between piracetam (a GABA agonist) and control groups for the number of people dead or dependent at the end of follow up (ARI +0.2%, 95% CI –6.0% to +6.4%; RRI 0%, 95% CI –11% to +9%).[38] We found one RCT (1360 people with acute stroke), which found no significant effect of clomethiazole (a GABA agonist) versus placebo on achievement of functional independence (ARR +1.5%, 95% CI –4.0% to +6.6%; RRR +3.0%, 95% CI –7% to +13%).[39] **Lubeluzole:** We found two RCTs assessing lubeluzole, an inhibitor of presynaptic glutamate release.[40,41] Intention to treat analysis of the first trial (721 people) found that lubeluzole did not significantly reduce mortality at 12 weeks (AR 20.7 % with lubeluzole v 25.2% with placebo; ARR 4.5%; P = NS; RRR +18%, 95% CI –7% to +37%). The second RCT (725 people; 365 randomised to lubeluzole, 360 to placebo) also found no significant difference in mortality at 12 weeks with lubeluzole versus placebo (intention to treat analysis: ARR +0.6%, 95% CI –4.8% to +7.4%; RRR +3%, 95% CI –22% to +29%). A third RCT has been completed, but full publication is awaited.[42] **Glycine antagonists:** We found two RCTs.[43,44] One RCT (1804 conscious people with limb weakness evaluated within 6 hours of stroke onset) found no significant difference between gavestinel (GV150526, a glycine antagonist) versus placebo in survival and outcome at 3 months as measured by the Barthel Index (ARR +1.0%, 95% CI –3.5% to +6.0%).[43] The second RCT (published only in abstract) also found no significant difference in functional outcome at the end of follow up.[44] **NMDA antagonists:** Two recent RCTs evaluating the NMDA antagonist CGS19775 (see glossary, p 136) found no significant difference in the proportion of people with a Barthel Index Score over 60, but data were limited as the trials were terminated because of adverse outcomes after only 31% of the total planned patient enrolment.[45]

Harms: In the systematic review of calcium antagonists, indirect and limited comparisons of intravenous versus oral administration of calcium antagonist found no significant difference in adverse events (ARI of adverse events, intravenous v oral +2.3%, 95% CI –0.9% to +3.7%; RRI +17%, 95% CI –3% to +41%).[37] In the systematic review of piracetam, there was a non-significant increase in death with piracetam versus placebo, which was no longer apparent after correction for imbalance in stroke severity.[38] Lubeluzole has also been noted to have adverse outcomes, especially at higher doses. One phase II trial of lubeluzole in 232 people was terminated prematurely because of an excess of deaths in the arm randomised to a higher dosage of drug.[46] This problem has not been noted with the lower drug dosages used in the published phase III studies.[40,41] The trials of CGS19775 were terminated after enrolling 567 people because of greater early mortality in the CGS19775 groups.[45]

Comment: A systematic review is being developed to assess all of the lubeluzole data.[47] Another systematic review[48] is being developed for tirilazad, a steroid derivative that has shown no evidence of clinical benefit in one major trial that was terminated prematurely on the advice of the independent monitoring committee.[49] The effects of the cell membrane precursor citicholine have been evaluated in a number of small trials, and a systematic review is in progress.[50] Systematic reviews are also being developed for antioxidants,[51] and for excitatory amino acid modulators.[51] Several RCTs are ongoing, including one trial of intravenous magnesium sulphate[52] and another assessing the role of diazepam (a GABA agonist).[53]

QUESTION What are the effects of surgical treatment for intracerebral haematomas?

OPTION EVACUATION

We found that the balance between benefits and harms has not been clearly established for the evacuation of supratentorial haematomas. We found no evidence from RCTs on the role of evacuation or ventricular shunting in people with infratentorial haematoma whose conscious level is declining.

Benefits: **For supratentorial haematomas:** We found one systematic review of RCTs (search date 1998),[54] as well as one systematic review (search date 1997) that also assessed information from case series.[55] Both systematic reviews assessed the same four

Cardiovascular disorders

RCTs (354 people with primary supratentorial intracerebral haemorrhage) comparing surgery (craniotomy in 3 trials and endoscopy in 1) versus best medical treatment. Neither review found any significant short or long term differences in death or disability for surgically treated people (ARI 3.3%, 95% CI −5.9% to +12.5%; RRI 5%, 95% CI −7% to +19%). **For infratentorial haematomas:** We found no evidence from systematic reviews or RCTs on the role of surgical evacuation or ventricular shunting.[56]

Harms: The systematic reviews[54,55] found that for the 254 people randomised to craniotomy rather than best medical treatment, there was increased death and disability (ARI 12%, 95% CI 1.8% to 22%; RRI 17%, 95% CI 2% to 34%; NNH 8, 95% CI 5 to 56). For the 100 people randomised to endoscopy rather than best medical practice, there was no significant effect on death and disability (RRR 24%, 95% CI −2% to +44%).

Comment: Current practice is based on the consensus opinion that people with infratentorial (cerebellar) haematomas whose conscious level is declining probably benefit from evacuation of the haematoma. The systematic reviews identified several ongoing RCTs assessing the evacuation of supratentorial haematomas.

GLOSSARY

Integrated care pathway A model of care that includes definition of therapeutic goals and specification of a timed plan designed to promote multidiciplinary care, improve discharge planning, and reduce the length of hospital stay.

NMDA antagonist Glutamate can bind to N-methyl-D-aspartate (NMDA) receptors on cell surfaces. One hypothesis proposed that glutamate released during a stroke can cause further harm to neurones by stimulating the NMDA receptors. NMDA antagonists block these receptors.

Substantive changes since last issue

Specialised care One new RCT comparing an integrated care pathway (see below) versus conventional multidisciplinary care on a stroke unit.[10] People receiving conventional care had greater improvement between 4–12 weeks, but there were no other differences between groups.

Thrombolysis One new meta-analysis comparing streptokinase with placebo;[14] conclusions unchanged.

Aspirin Analysis of two large RCTs found that people given aspirin who were subsequently found to have a haemorrhagic rather than an ischaemic stroke had the same outcomes as people who were given placebo.[20] New evidence suggesting that aspirin should not be delayed if a CT scan is not readily available within 48 hours.

Anticoagulation One RCT found no difference between low molecular weight heparin and aspirin for treatment of stroke in people with known atrial fibrillation.[25]

Anticoagulation Two systematic reviews of the same five RCTs found no difference between low molecular weight heparins or heparinoids and unfractionated heparins to prevent deep vein thrombosis in people with acute ischaemic stroke.[26,27]

Glycine antagonists One new RCT; conclusions unchanged.[43]

REFERENCES

1. Hatano S. Experience from a multicentre stroke register: a preliminary report. *Bull World Health Organ* 1976;54:541–553.

2. Bonita R. Epidemiology of stroke. *Lancet* 1992; 339:342–344.

3. Bamford J, Sandercock P, Dennis M, Warlow C, Jones L, McPherson K. A prospective study of acute cerebrovascular disease in the community: the Oxfordshire community stroke project, 1981–1986. 1. Methodology, demography and incident

cases of first ever stroke. *J Neurol Neurosurg Psychiatry* 1988;51:1373–1380.

4. Bamford J, Dennis M, Sandercock P, Burn J, Warlow C. A prospective study of acute cerebrovascular disease in the community: the Oxfordshire community stroke project, 1981– 1986. 2. Incidence, case fatality rates and overall outcome at one year of cerebral infarction, primary intracerebral and subarachnoid haemorrhage. *J Neurol Neurosurg Psychiatry* 1990;53:16–22.

5. Bamford J, Dennis M, Sandercock P, Burn J, Warlow C. The frequency, causes and timing of death within 30 days of a first stroke: the Oxfordshire community stroke project. *J Neurol Neurosurg Psychiatry* 1990;53:824–829.

6. Wade DT. Functional abilities after stroke: measurement, natural history and prognosis. *J Neurol Neurosurg Psychiatry* 1987;50:177–182.

7. Stroke Unit Trialists' Collaboration. Organised inpatient (stroke unit) care for stroke. In: The Cochrane Library, Issue 3, 2000. Oxford: Update Software. Search date June 1998; primary sources Cochrane Collaboration Stroke Group, hand searches of reference lists of relevant articles, preliminary findings publicised at stroke conferences, and personal contact with colleagues.

8. Indredavik B, Bakke RPT, Slordahl SA, Rokseth R, Haheim LL. Stroke unit treatment. 10-year follow-up. *Stroke* 1999;30:1524–1527.

9. Lincoln NB, Husbands S, Trescoli C, Drummond AER, Gladman JRF, Berman P. Five year follow up of a randomised controlled trial of a stroke rehabilitation unit. *BMJ* 2000;320:549.

10. Sulch D, Perez I, Melbourn A, Kalra L. Randomized controlled trial of integrated (managed) care pathway for stroke rehabilitation. *Stroke* 2000;31: 1929–1934.

11. Indredavik B, Bakke RPT, Slordahl SA, Rokseth R, Haheim LL. Treatment in a combined acute and rehabilitation stroke unit. Which aspects are most important. *Stroke* 1999;30:917–923.

12. Stegmayr B, Asplund K, Hulter-Asberg K, et al. Stroke units in their natural habitat: can results of randomized trials be reproduced in routine clinical practice? For the risk-stroke collaboration. *Stroke* 1999;30:709–714.

13. Wardlaw JM, del Zoppo G, Yamaguchi T. Thrombolysis for acute ischaemic stroke. In: The Cochrane Library, Issue 3, 2000. Oxford: Update Software. Search date March 1999; primary sources Cochrane Collaboration Stroke Group, Medline, Embase, the Ottawa Stroke Trials Registry, hand searches of references quoted in thrombolysis papers, published abstracts of neurological and cerebrovascular symposia, direct contact with principal investigators of trials, colleagues and pharmaceutical companies.

14. Cornu C, Boutitie F, Candelise L, et al. Streptokinase in acute ischemic stroke: an individual patient data meta-analysis: the thrombolysis in acute stroke pooling project. *Stroke* 2000;31:1555–1560.

15. Kwiatkowski T, Libman R, Frankel M, et al. Effects of tissue plasminogen activator for acute ischemic stroke at one year. National Institute of Neurological Disorders and stroke recombinant tissue plasminogen activator stroke study group. *N Engl J Med* 1999;340:1781–1787.

16. University of Washington Stroke Centre website: http://stroke.wustl.edu/trials

17. Gubitz G, Sandercock P, Counsell C. Antiplatelet therapy for acute ischaemic stroke. In: The Cochrane Library, Issue 3, 2000. Oxford: Update Software. Search date March 1999; primary sources Cochrane Collaboration Stroke Group,

Register of the Antiplatelet Trialists Collaboration, MedStrategy, and contact with pharmaceutical companies marketing antiplatelet agents.

18. CAST. Randomised placebo-controlled trial of early aspirin use in 20 000 patients with acute ischaemic stroke. CAST (Chinese Acute Stroke Trial) collaborative group. *Lancet* 1997;349: 1641–1649.

19. International Stroke Trial Collaborative Group. The international stroke trial (IST): a randomised trial of aspirin, heparin, both or neither among 19 435 patients with acute ischaemic stroke. *Lancet* 1997;349:1569–1581.

20. Chen Z, Sandercock P, Pan H, et al. Indications for early aspirin use in acute ischemic stroke: a combined analysis of 40 000 randomized patients from the Chinese Acute Stroke Trial and the International Stroke Trial. *Stroke* 2000;31:1240– 1249.

21. Antiplatelet Trialists' Collaboration. Collaborative overview of randomised trials of antiplatelet therapy I: prevention of death, myocardial infarction and stroke by prolonged antiplatelet therapy in various categories of patients. *BMJ* 1994;308:81–106. Search date 1990; primary sources Medline and Current Contents.

22. Slattery J, Warlow CP, Shorrock CJ, Langman MJS. Risks of gastrointestinal bleeding during secondary prevention of vascular events with aspirin – analysis of gastrointestinal bleeding during the UK-TIA trial. *Gut* 1995;37:509–511.

23. Johnson ES, Lanes SF, Wentworth CE, Satterfield MH, Abebe BL, Dicker LW. A metaregression analysis of the dose-response effect of aspirin on stroke. *Arch Intern Med* 1999;159:1248–1253.

24. Gubitz G, Sandercock P, Counsell C, Signorini D. Anticoagulants for acute ischaemic stroke. In: The Cochrane Library, Issue 3, 2000. Oxford: Update Software. Search date March 1999; primary sources Cochrane Collaboration Stroke Group, MedStrategy, Antithrombotic Therapy Trialists' Collaboration Trials Register, and contact with manufacturers of anticoagulants.

25. Berge E, Abdelnoor M, Nakstad P, Sandset P. Low-molecular-weight heparin versus aspirin in people with acute ischaemic stroke and atrial fibrillation: a double-blind randomised study. HAEST Study Group. Heparin in Acute Embolic Stroke Trial. *Lancet* 2000;355:1205–1210.

26. Counsell C, Sandercock P. Low-molecular-weight heparins or heparinoids versus standard unfractionated heparin for acute ischaemic stroke. In: The Cochrane Library, Issue 3, 2000. Oxford: Update Software. Search date August 1999; primary sources Cochrane Collaboration Stroke Group, MedStrategy, Antithrombotic Therapy Trialists' Collaboration Trials Register, and contact with manufacturers of anticoagulants.

27. Bath P, Iddenden R, Bath F. Low-molecular-weight heparins and heparinoids in acute ischemic stroke: a meta-analysis of randomized controlled trials. *Stroke* 2000;31:1770–1778. Search date 1999; primary sources Cochrane Stroke Group Database of Trials in Acute Stroke, Cochrane Library, and hand searches of reference lists of identified publications.

28. Bath P for the TAIST Investigators. Tinzaparin in acute ischaemic stroke trial (TAIST). *Cerebrovasc Dis* 2000;10(suppl 2):81.

29. Blood Pressure in Acute Stroke Collaboration (BASC). Interventions for deliberately altering blood pressure in acute stroke. In: The Cochrane Library, Issue 3, 2000. Oxford: Update Software. Search date May 1997; primary sources Cochrane Stroke Group Trials Register, Ottawa Stroke Trials Registry, Medline, Embase, ISI, handsearches of existing review articles, and personal contact with

Cardiovascular disorders

researchers in the field and pharmaceutical companies.

30. Wahlgren NG, MacMahon DG, DeKeyser J, Ingredavik B, Ryman, T. Intravenous nimodipine west European stroke trial (INWEST) of nimodipine in the treatment of acute ischaemic stroke. Cerebrovasc Dis 1994;4:204–210.

31. Barer DH, Cruickshank JM, Ebrahim SB, Mitchell JRA. Low dose beta blockade in acute stroke (BEST trial): an evaluation. BMJ 1988;296:737–741.

32. Mohr JP, Orgogozo JM, Harrison MJG, et al. Meta-analysis of oral nimodipine trials in acute ischaemic stroke. Cerebrovasc Dis 1994;4:197–203. Search date 1994; primary source Bayer database.

33. Horn J, Orgogozo JM, Limburg M. Review on calcium antagonists in ischaemic stroke; mortality data. Cerebrovasc Dis 1998;8(suppl 4):27.

34. Rodgers A, MacMahon S, Gamble G. Blood pressure and risk of stroke patients with cerebrovascular disease. BMJ 1996;313:147.

35. Schrader J, Rothemeyer M, Luders S, Kollmann K. Hypertension and stroke – rationale behind the ACCESS trial. Basic Res Cardiol 1998;93(suppl 2):69–78.

36. Bath P, Bath F for the ENOS Investigators. Efficacy of Nitric Oxide in Stroke (ENOS) Trial – A prospective large randomised controlled trial in acute stroke [abstract]. Cerebrovasc Dis 2000;10(suppl 2):8.

37. Horn J, Limburg M. Calcium antagonists for acute ischemic stroke. In: The Cochrane Library, Issue 3, 2000. Oxford: Update Software. Search date March 1999; primary source Cochrane Stroke Review Group Trials Register.

38. Ricci S, Celani MG, Cantisani AT, Righetti E. Piracetam for acute ischaemic stroke. In: The Cochrane Library, Issue 3, 2000. Oxford: Update Software. Search date January 1999; primary sources Cochrane Stroke Review Group Trials Register, Medline, Embase, BIDIS ISI, handsearches of 15 journals, and contact with manufacturers.

39. Wahlgren NG, Ranasinha KW, Rosolacci T, et al. Clomethiazole acute stroke study (CLASS): results of a randomised, controlled trial of clomethiazole versus placebo in 1360 acute stroke patients. Stroke 1999;30:21–28.

40. Grotta J, for the US and Canadian Lubeluzole Stroke Study Group. Lubeluzole treatment for acute ischaemic stroke. Stroke 1997;28:2338–2346.

41. Diener HC. Multinational randomised controlled trail of lubeluzole in acute ischaemic stroke. Cerebrovasc Dis 1998;8:172–181.

42. Wessel TC. Determinants of outcome in the lubeluzole clinical trial [abstract]. In: Proceedings of the Seventh Annual Conference on ischemic stroke. Advances in novel therapeutic development. Washington DC. November 19–20, 1998. IBC USA Conferences Inc, Southborough, MA.

43. Lees K, Asplund K, Carolei A, et al. Glycine antagonist (gavestinel) in neuroprotection (GAIN International) in people with acute stroke: a randomised controlled trial. Lancet 2000;355;1949–1954.

44. Sacco R for the GAIN Americas Collaborative Group. GV150526 in the treatment of acute stroke: Results of the GAIN Americas Trial. Cerebrovasc Dis 2000;10(suppl 2):106.

45. Davis S, Lees K, Albers G, et al for the ASSIST Investigators. Selfotel in acute ischemic stroke. Possible neurotoxic effects of an NMDA antagonist. Stroke 2000;31:347–354.

46. Wahlgren NG, MacMahon DG, De Keyser J, Indredavik B, Ryman T for the INWEST Study Group. Intravenous nimodipine west European stroke trial (INWEST) of nimodipine in the treatment of acute ischaemic stroke. Cerebrovasc Dis 1994;4:204–210.

47. Gandolfo C, Conti M. Lubeluzole for acute ischemic stroke [Protocol]. In: The Cochrane Library, Issue 3, 2000. Oxford: Update Software.

48. Bath P for the Tirilazad International Steering Committee. Tirilazad for acute ischaemic stroke [Protocol]. In: The Cochrane Library, Issue 3, 2000. Oxford: Update Software.

49. The RANTTAS Investigators. A randomized trial of tirilazad mesylate in patients with acute stroke (RANTTAS). Stroke 1996;27:1453–1458.

50. Saver JL, Wilterdink J. Choline precursors for acute and subacute ischemic and hemorrhagic stroke [Protocol]. In: The Cochrane Library, Issue 3, 2000. Oxford: Update Software.

51. Cochrane Stroke Review Group. Department of Clinical Neurosciences, Western General Hospital, Crewe Road, Edinburgh, UK EH4 2XU. URL: http://www.dcn.ed.ac.uk/csrg.

52. Muir KW, Lees KR. IMAGES. Intravenous magnesium efficacy in stroke trial [abstract]. Cerebrovasc Dis 1996;6:75P383.

53. Lodder, J, van Raak L, Kessels F, Hilton A. Early GABA-ergic activation study in stroke (EGASIS). Cerebrovasc Dis 2000;10(suppl 2):80.

54. Prasad K , Shrivastava A. Surgery for primary supratentorial intracerebral haemorrhage. In: The Cochrane Library, Issue 3, 2000. Oxford: Update Software. Search date August 1998; primary sources Cochrane Collaboration Stroke Group, handsearches of reference lists of all identified trials, specialist journals and monographs.

55. Hankey G, Hon C. Surgery for primary intracerebral hemorrhage: is it safe and effective? A systematic review of case series and randomised trials. Stroke 1997;28:2126–2132. Search date June 1997; primary sources Medline, and hand searches of reference lists of identified articles , published epidemiological studies, and reviews.

56. Warlow CP, Dennis MS, van Gijn J, et al, eds. Treatment of primary intracerebral haemorrhage. In: Stroke: a practical guide to management. Oxford: Blackwell Science,1996:430–437.

Gord Gubitz

Assistant Professor, Division of Neurology, Dalhousie University, Halifax, Canada

Peter Sandercock

Professor of Neurology

Neurosciences Trials Unit, University of Edinburgh, Edinburgh, UK

Competing interests: GG none declared. PS has given lectures and symposia and received lecture fees and travel expenses from Boehringer Ingelheim, Sanofi, BMJ Publishing Group, and a variety of other companies. PS has also received support from Boehringer Ingelheim and Glaxo Wellcome for trials and research.

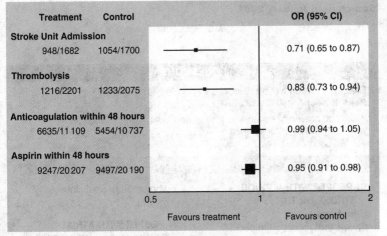

FIGURE 1 Proportional effects on "death or dependency" at the end of scheduled follow up: results of systematic reviews.[7,13,18,19] Data refer only to benefits and not to harms (see text, p 128).

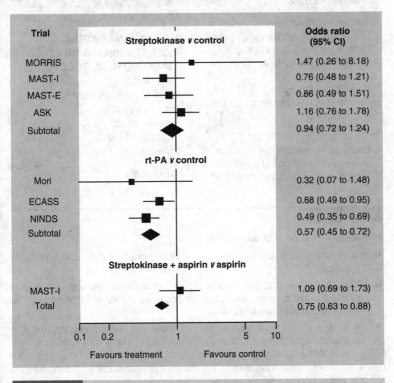

FIGURE 2 Effect of thrombolysis on death and dependency at end of trial: results of review (see text, p 130).[13]

Cardiovascular disorders

Search date January 2001

Clinical Evidence writers on secondary prevention of stroke

INTERVENTIONS

Key Messages

In people with a prior stroke or TIA

- We found insufficient evidence from RCTs about routine blood pressure reduction.
- RCTs have found that statins may prevent stroke in people with a history of coronary heart disease. We found inconclusive evidence in those with no history of coronary heart disease.
- RCTs have found that routine use of prolonged antiplatelet treatment is beneficial unless there is a clear contraindication, and that aspirin 75 mg daily is as effective as higher doses. We found no good evidence that any other antiplatelet regimen is superior to medium dose aspirin (75–325 mg daily) in the prevention of vascular events.
- RCTs have found that clopidogrel or the combination of aspirin and dipyridamole are safe and effective alternatives to medium dose aspirin.

- One systematic review has found that ticlopidine or clopidogrel reduces the odds of a vascular event compared with aspirin but there was substantial uncertainty about the size of any additional benefit.
- One systematic review found no evidence of benefit from anticoagulation in people in sinus rhythm, but an increased risk of serious bleeding.
- One systematic review has found that carotid endarterectomy reduces the risk of major stroke in people with moderate and severe carotid stenosis provided the risks of imaging and surgery are small.
- We found that the role of percutaneous transluminal angioplasty (PTA) has not been adequately evaluated.

In people with atrial fibrillation and a prior stroke or TIA

- Systematic reviews and RCTs have found that anticoagulants reduce the risk of stroke, provided there is a low risk of bleeding and careful monitoring. Aspirin reduces the risk of stroke, but less effectively than anticoagulants. These findings support the use of aspirin in people with atrial fibrillation and contraindications to anticoagulants.

In people with atrial fibrillation but no other major risk factors for stroke

- Systematic reviews and RCTs have found that anticoagulants are of net benefit, provided there is a low risk of bleeding and careful monitoring. Aspirin is a reasonable alternative in people with contraindications to anticoagulants.

DEFINITION	Prevention in this context is the long term management of people with a prior stroke or transient ischaemic attack (TIA), and of people at high risk of stroke for other reasons such as atrial fibrillation. **Stroke:** See definition under stroke management, p 127. **TIA:** Similar to a mild ischaemic stroke except that symptoms last for less than 24 hours.[1]
INCIDENCE/ PREVALENCE	See incidence/prevalence under stroke management, p 127.
AETIOLOGY/ RISK FACTORS	See aetiology under stroke management, p 127. Risk factors for stroke include prior stroke or TIA, increasing age, hypertension, diabetes, cigarette smoking, and emboli associated with atrial fibrillation, artificial heart valves, or myocardial infarction. The relation with cholesterol is less clear; an overview of prospective studies among healthy middle aged individuals found no association between total cholesterol and overall stroke risk.[2] However, one review of prospective observational studies in eastern Asian people found that cholesterol was positively associated with ischaemic stroke but negatively associated with haemorrhagic stroke.[3]
PROGNOSIS	People with a history of stroke or TIA are at high risk of all vascular events, such as myocardial infarction, but are at particular risk of subsequent stroke (about 10% in the first year and about 5% per year thereafter); see figure 1, p 157, and figure 1, in secondary prevention of ischaemic cardiac events, p 95.[4,5] People with intermittent atrial fibrillation treated with aspirin should be considered at similar risk of stroke, compared to people with sustained atrial fibrillation treated with aspirin (rate of ischaemic stroke per year, intermittent v sustained, 3.2% v 3.3%).[6]
AIMS	To prevent death or disabling stroke, as well as other serious non-fatal outcomes, especially myocardial infarction, with minimal adverse effects from treatment.

Cardiovascular disorders

OUTCOMES	Rates of death; dependency; myocardial infarction; and stroke.
METHODS	*Clinical Evidence* update search and appraisal January 2001.

QUESTION What are the effects of interventions in people with prior stroke or TIA?

OPTION BLOOD PRESSURE REDUCTION

Cathie Sudlow

We found insufficient evidence for routine blood pressure reduction among people with a prior stroke or TIA, but a large, ongoing RCT will provide further information.

Benefits: We found two overviews[7,8] and three subsequent RCTs.[9–11] One overview of RCTs of antihypertensive treatment (usually comprising a diuretic, a β-blocker, or both), in about 48 000 people with hypertension, most of whom had no history of vascular disease, found that a reduction of about 10–12/5–6 mmHg in systolic/diastolic blood pressure over 2–3 years reduced the risk of stroke (OR 0.62, 95% CI 0.55 to 0.69).[7] A subsequent RCT (4695 elderly people with systolic hypertension) found similar results with a calcium channel antagonist (nitrendipine) versus placebo: a reduction of about 10/5 mmHg over 2 years reduced the risk of stroke (RRR 42%, 95% CI 17% to 60%).[9] In the overview, the proportional effects of treatment on stroke were similar among people with differing degrees of hypertension, among middle aged and elderly people, and among people with or without a prior stroke or TIA.[7] Two of the RCTs (about 500 people) specifically examined blood pressure reduction in people with both hypertension and a prior stroke or TIA. These two RCTs were included in another overview of antihypertensive treatment versus placebo (4 RCTs, about 3000 people with prior stroke or TIA with or without hypertension).[8] Similar, but statistically uncertain, results were obtained: an average diastolic blood pressure reduction of 3 mmHg for about 3 years non-significantly reduced the risk of stroke (OR 0.81, 95% CI 0.61 to 1.01). An unconfirmed preliminary report from a further RCT in China (5665 people with a prior stroke or TIA) comparing a diuretic (indapamide) versus placebo found that reducing diastolic blood pressure by about 2 mm Hg over 2 years significantly reduced stroke incidence (RRR 29%, 95% CI 12% to 42%).[10] We found one large subsequent RCT (9297 people at high risk of vascular disease, including 1000 with prior stroke or TIA, about half had hypertension). It found that about 5 years of ramipril (an angiotensin converting enzyme [ACE] inhibitor) versus placebo reduced the diastolic blood pressure by an average of 2 mm Hg, reduced the risk of stroke (RRR 31%, 95% CI 16% to 44%), and reduced the risk of combined outcome of stroke, myocardial infarction, or cardiovascular death (RRR 22%, 95% CI 14% to 30%). The relative risk reduction was similar among those with or without a prior stroke or TIA, and among those with or without hypertension.[11]

Harms: In people with a history of stroke, reports of an apparently J-shaped relationship between blood pressure and subsequent stroke have led to concerns that blood pressure reduction may actually increase the risk of recurrent stroke, perhaps because of reduced cerebral perfusion.[12] However, preliminary analyses of data from over 15 000 people with a history of cerebrovascular or coronary events included in trials in the overview found a positive relation between diastolic blood pressure and the subsequent risk of stroke; for every 5 mmHg decrease in diastolic blood pressure there was about a 15% proportional reduction in stroke risk. These analyses found no evidence of any threshold below which a lower diastolic blood pressure was not associated with a lower stroke risk.[12,13] The RCTs found no evidence that reducing diastolic blood pressure was hazardous, at least down to about 80 mmHg.[7]

Comment: There is persisting uncertainty about the net effects of blood pressure reduction among people with a previous cerebrovascular event. Further information will be provided by a large RCT that is currently assessing the balance of benefits and risks of treatment with the ACE inhibitor perindopril among 6000 people with a history of stroke or TIA.[8]

OPTION	CHOLESTEROL REDUCTION

We found insufficient evidence about the effects of routinely reducing cholesterol in people with a prior stroke or TIA. Evidence from large RCTs suggests benefit from reducing cholesterol with a statin in people with prior stroke or TIA who also have a definite history of coronary heart disease (see table 1, p 156).

Benefits: **Effects of cholesterol lowering on stroke:** Large RCTs have assessed the effects of reducing cholesterol on coronary heart disease risk, in many thousands of people, both in those with a history of coronary heart disease and in healthy people. These trials did not specifically aim to include people with a prior stroke or TIA, but many reported on stroke as an outcome.[14–16] We found several overviews of these trials, reporting similar findings, and three of these include all of the relevant data.[14,15,17] The overviews found no evidence that reducing mean total cholesterol by about 11% with a fibrate, resin, or dietary regimen significantly altered stroke, but found that reducing mean total cholesterol by about 21% with a statin reduced the relative odds of stroke by 24% (and reduced the relative odds of coronary heart disease by a third) (see table 1, p 156).[14–16] One subsequent, large RCT assessed the effects of treatment designed to raise high density lipoprotein (HDL) cholesterol and lower triglycerides. The RCT (2531 men with coronary heart disease and low HDL cholesterol) compared gemfibrozil versus placebo, given over about 5 years. It found that gemfibrozil increased HDL cholesterol (by about 6%), reduced triglycerides, did not change low density lipoprotein (LDL) cholesterol, and reduced total cholesterol (by about 4%). Compared with placebo, gemfibrozil produced a significant reduction in coronary heart disease (RRR 22%, 95% CI 7% to 35%), but a non-significant reduction in stroke (RRR +25%, 95% CI –6% to +47%).[18] **Effects of cholesterol reduction in people with a prior stroke or TIA:** We found only two small, early RCTs that directly assessed effects of reducing cholesterol in people with a prior stroke or TIA. The drug used (clofibrate in both cases) produced only a small fall in the mean cholesterol, and the results were inconclusive.[19,20]

Harms: The overviews found uncertain effects of statins on fatal stroke (RR 95% CI ranging from an increase of about a half to one third reduction) (see table 1, p 156),[14] possibly because lowering cholesterol may slightly increase the risk of haemorrhagic stroke, which is more likely than ischaemic stroke to be fatal.[3] Only two large scale statin trials reported haemorrhagic stroke separately, and there were too few events (10 events) to draw any conclusions.[21,22]

Comment: A planned prospective overview of individual participant data from all RCTs of cholesterol reduction aims to summarise the effects of reducing cholesterol among different groups of people, including those with a prior stroke or TIA.[23]

OPTION   ANTIPLATELET TREATMENT

RCTs have found that prolonged antiplatelet treatment is beneficial for people with a prior (presumed ischaemic) stroke or TIA, unless there is a clear contraindication. We found no clear evidence that any other antiplatelet regimen is superior to medium dose aspirin (75–325 mg daily) in the prevention of vascular events. Aspirin 75 mg daily is as effective as higher doses in the long term prevention of vascular events, but it remains unclear whether doses lower than 75 mg daily are sufficient. RCTs have found that clopidogrel or the combination of aspirin and dipyridamole are safe and effective alternatives to medium dose aspirin.

Benefits: **Antiplatelet treatment versus no antiplatelet treatment:** One systematic review (search date 1990, 70 000 people at high risk of occlusive arterial disease)[5] found that, compared with no antiplatelet treatment, 1 month or more of antiplatelet treatment reduced the risk of a non-fatal myocardial infarction, non-fatal stroke, or vascular death (OR 0.73, 95% CI 0.70 to 0.76). The review included about 10 000 people with a prior (presumed ischaemic) stroke or TIA, among whom about 20 non-fatal strokes, nine non-fatal myocardial infarctions, and 11 vascular deaths were prevented per 1000 people treated with antiplatelet treatment for about 3 years. There was also a clear reduction in all cause mortality (see figure 1, p 157).[5] Subsequent, large RCTs of antiplatelet treatment versus control among several thousand patients with a prior stroke or TIA found similar results.[24–26] **Different daily doses of aspirin:** About two thirds of the RCTs in the systematic review involved an aspirin regimen, and medium dose aspirin (75–325 mg daily) was the most widely tested. Direct comparisons among 2425 high risk people found the effects on vascular events of daily doses of 75–325 mg or 500–1500 mg to be similar.[5] One subsequent RCT (2849 people undergoing carotid endarterectomy) found that lower doses of 81 mg or 325 mg produced a slightly lower rate of stroke, myocardial infarction, or death than higher doses of 650 mg or 1300 mg daily (AR 6.2% with lower doses v AR 8.4 % with higher doses; P = 0.03).[27] Indirect comparisons in the systematic review found that daily doses of less than 160 mg (mostly 75–150 mg), 160–325 mg, and 500–1500 mg had similar effects in preventing vascular events.[5] The inclusion of data from two subsequent large

RCTs among high risk people (one of them including almost 1400 people with a prior ischaemic stroke or TIA)[24] assessing a daily dose of exactly 75 mg versus control,[24,28] found that this aspirin dose significantly reduced vascular events (OR 0.71, 95% CI 0.61 to 0.83).[5] We found more limited evidence for effects of doses under 75 mg daily. One RCT (about 6000 people with prior stroke or TIA) found that, compared with placebo, aspirin 50 mg daily reduced the combined outcome of stroke or death (RRR 13%, 95% CI 1% to 25%).[25] A second RCT (about 3000 people with recent TIA or minor ischaemic stroke) directly compared aspirin 30 mg daily versus 283 mg daily, and found no evidence of a difference in effect, although the trial could not rule out a clinically important difference.[29] **Dipyridamole and aspirin:** The systematic review found no clear evidence that any regimen was more effective than medium dose aspirin alone in the prevention of vascular events. It found that adding dipyridamole to aspirin did not seem to produce a reduction in vascular events compared with aspirin alone, but the possibility of a small additional benefit was not excluded.[5] One more recent RCT found that, although adding dipyridamole to aspirin 50 mg daily significantly reduced stroke (RRR about 23%), the combination did not significantly reduce the combined risk of stroke or death (RRR 13%, P = NS).[25] A detailed review of all trials that have assessed the addition of dipyridamole to aspirin is underway.[30] **Thienopyridines (clopidogrel and ticlopidine):** We found one systematic review of RCTs comparing either ticlopidine or clopidogrel with aspirin (search date 1999, 4 RCTs, 22 656 people at high risk of vascular disease, including 9840 with a TIA or ischaemic stroke).[31] Most people were included in a large trial of clopidogrel (75 mg daily) versus aspirin (325 mg daily).[32] Compared with aspirin, the thienopyridines reduced the odds of a vascular event by 9% (OR 0.91, 95% CI 0.84 to 0.98), but there was substantial uncertainty about the size of any additional benefit (11 events prevented per 1000 people treated for about 2 years, 95% CI 2 to 19 events).[31]

Harms: Potentially life threatening bleeding is the most important adverse effect of antiplatelet treatment. **Intracranial haemorrhages:** These are uncommon, but often fatal, and usually cause significant disability in survivors. The systematic review found that any excess risk of intracranial bleeding with antiplatelet treatment was small, at most one or two per 1000 people a year in trials of long term treatment.[5] **Extracranial haemorrhages:** Unlike intracranial events, extracranial bleeds are much less likely to cause permanent disability or death. The 1994 review found that antiplatelet treatment was significantly associated with a small excess of three per 1000 non-fatal major extracranial bleeds, but no clear excess of fatal extracranial bleeds.[5] **Different doses of aspirin:** In a direct randomised comparison, aspirin 1200 mg daily was associated with more gastrointestinal bleeding than 325 mg daily.[33] We found no definite evidence for any clinically relevant variation in gastrointestinal bleeding risk in the range 75–325 mg daily. However, it seems reasonable to choose the lowest conveniently available dose in this range. **Adverse effects of thienopyridines:** The systematic review of thienopyridines versus aspirin found that the thienopyridines caused significantly less gastrointestinal haemorrhage and upper gastrointestinal upset than aspirin. However, they increased the

Cardiovascular disorders

incidence of skin rash and of diarrhoea (ticlopidine by about twofold and clopidogrel by about a third). Ticlopidine (but not clopidogrel) increased the incidence of neutropenia.[31] Observational studies have also found that ticlopidine is associated with thrombocytopenia and thrombotic thrombocytopenic purpura.[34,35] However, we found no definite evidence of an excess of haematological adverse effects with clopidogrel.[36,37] The results of two RCTs of clopidogrel plus aspirin versus ticlopidine plus aspirin in about 1700 people undergoing coronary artery stenting suggested clopidogrel to be superior to ticlopidine in terms of safety and tolerability.[38,39]

Comment: In people with a prior stroke or TIA, the large absolute reductions in serious vascular events produced by antiplatelet treatment far outweighed any absolute hazards.

| OPTION | LONG TERM ORAL ANTICOAGULATION FOR PEOPLE IN NORMAL SINUS RHYTHM |

Gord Gubitz and Peter Sandercock

One systematic review comparing oral anticoagulants versus placebo found no significant difference in the risk of stroke recurrence after presumed ischaemic stroke in people in normal sinus rhythm. Risk of fatal intracranial and extracranial haemorrhage was increased.

Benefits: We found one systematic review (search date not stated, 9 small RCTs, mean duration 1.8 years) comparing oral anticoagulants (warfarin, dicoumarol, phenindione) versus placebo.[40] The review included 1214 people in normal sinus rhythm with previous non-embolic presumed ischaemic stroke or TIA, and found no clear benefit of anticoagulation on death or dependency (ARR +4%, 95% CI −6% to +14%; RRR +5%, 95% CI −9% to +18%), or on mortality or recurrent stroke.

Harms: By the end of the RCTs, the review found a significantly increased risk of fatal intracranial haemorrhage (ARI 2%, 95% CI 0.4% to 3.6%; RR 2.51, 95% CI 1.12 to 5.60; NNH 49 people treated with anticoagulants over 1.8 years for one additional non-fatal extracranial haemorrhage, 95% CI 27 to 240).[31] The risk of fatal and non-fatal extracranial haemorrhage was also increased by anticoagulants compared with placebo (ARI 5.1%, 95% CI 3.0% to 7.2%; RR 5.86, 95% CI 2.39 to 14.3; NNH 20, 95% CI 14 to 33).
Warfarin versus aspirin: One RCT (1316 people) compared aspirin versus oral anticoagulant (target international normalised ratio [INR] 3.0 to 4.5 — see glossary, p 152) for about 14 months after TIA or non-disabling stroke.[41] The trial was stopped early because of an excess number of poor outcomes (almost exclusively related to cerebral haemorrhage) in the anticoagulant group compared with control (AR 12.4% anticoagulant v 5.4% control; ARI 7%, 95% CI 4% to 10%; NNH 14, 95% CI 10 to 25).

Comment: The trials in the systematic review all had major problems with their methods, including poor monitoring of anticoagulation.[40] All were completed before introducing routine computerised tomography (CT) scanning, which means that people with primary haemorrhagic strokes could have been included. The systematic review could not therefore provide a reliable and precise overall estimate of the balance of risk and benefit regarding death or dependency. Most people in the trial comparing warfarin and aspirin did have a CT scan, but an adverse outcome was still seen with anticoagulants. Two further RCTs are in progress: one compares a lower intensity of adjusted dose warfarin (to maintain an INR of 1.4–2.8) with aspirin 325 mg four times daily within 30 days after stroke and treated for at least 2 years,[42] whereas the other assesses warfarin (to maintain an INR of 2.0 to 3.0) versus aspirin (any dose between 30–325 mg) versus aspirin plus dipyridamole (400 mg daily).[43]

OPTION	CAROTID ENDARTERECTOMY FOR PEOPLE WITH RECENT CAROTID TERRITORY ISCHAEMIA

One systematic review has found that carotid endarterectomy reduces the risk of major stroke and death in people with a recent carotid territory TIA or non-disabling ischaemic stroke who have moderate or severe symptomatic stenosis of the ipsilateral carotid artery. People with milder degrees of stenosis do not benefit from endarterectomy. Evidence from two other systematic reviews suggest a possible benefit in people with asymptomatic but severe stenosis, but the results of a new large scale trial are awaited.

Benefits: **People with symptomatic stenosis:** We found one systematic review (search date 1999, 3 RCTs, 6143 people with a recent neurological event in the territory of a stenosed ipsilateral carotid artery) comparing carotid surgery versus control treatment.[44] Ninety six per cent of these data came from two large RCTs.[45,46] Participants were randomised within 4 and 6 months of the onset of vascular symptoms. The trials used different methods to measure degree of stenosis. The trials included 1247 people with severe stenosis (70–99%,[46] 80–99%[45]), 1259 people with moderate stenosis (50–69%,[46] 70–79%[45]), and 3397 people with mild stenosis (< 50%,[46] < 70%[45]). The degree of benefit from surgery was related to the degree of stenosis. For people with severe stenosis, there was a significant decrease in the subsequent risk of major stroke or death (ARR 6.7%, 95% CI 3.2% to 10.0%; RR 0.52, 95% CI 0.37 to 0.73; NNT 15, 95% CI 10 to 31). People with moderate stenosis also benefited (ARR 4.7%, 95% CI 0.8% to 8.7%; RR 0.73, 95% CI 0.56 to 0.95; NNT 21, 95% CI 11 to 125). People with mild stenosis did not benefit from surgery but had an increased risk of stroke (RR 0.80, 95% CI 0.56 to 1.0). In the trial with longer follow up, the annual risk of stroke after 3 years was not significantly different between people who had had surgery and those who had not.[45] In the other trial, people with severe stenosis had a benefit from endarterectomy at 8 years follow up.[47] **People with asymptomatic stenosis:** We found two systematic reviews (search dates both 1998) evaluating carotid endarterectomy for asymptomatic carotid stenosis (no carotid territory TIA or minor stroke within the past few months).[48,49] One review included results from five RCTs (2440 people).[48] The other review included results from 2203 people from four of these five RCTs, after excluding the fifth RCT because of weak methods.[49] Both reviews found similar results. Carotid endarterectomy reduced the risk of perioperative stroke or death or subsequent ipsilateral stroke (for the review of 4 RCTs:[49] AR 4.9% over 3 years in the surgical group v 6.8% in the medical group; ARR 1.9%, 95% CI 0.1% to 3.9%; NNT 52, 95% CI 26 to 1000; for the review of 5 RCTs:[48] 4.7% over 3 years in the surgical group v 7.4% in the medical group; ARR 2.7%, 95% CI 0.8% to 4.6%; NNT 37, 95% CI 22 to 125). Although the risk of perioperative stroke or death from carotid surgery for people with asymptomatic stenosis seems to be lower than in people with symptomatic stenosis, the risk of stroke or death without surgery in asymptomatic people is relatively low and so, for most people, the balance of risk and benefit from surgery remains unclear.[48,49]

Harms: **People with symptomatic stenosis:** The systematic review of endarterectomy for symptomatic stenosis found that carotid surgery was associated with a definite risk of recurrent stroke or death.[44] The relative risk of disabling stroke or death within 30 days of randomisation was 2.5 (95% CI 1.6 to 3.8). A second systematic review (search date 1996, 36 studies) identified several risk factors for operative stroke and death from carotid endarterectomy, including female sex, occlusion of the contralateral internal carotid artery, stenosis of the ipsilateral external carotid artery, and systolic blood pressure greater than 180 mmHg.[50] Endarterectomy is also associated with other postoperative complications, including wound infection (3%), wound haematoma (5%), and lower cranial nerve injury (5–7%). **People with asymptomatic stenosis:** Given the low prevalence of severe carotid stenosis in the general population, there is concern that screening and surgical intervention in asymptomatic people may result in more strokes than it prevents.[51]

Comment: **People with symptomatic stenosis:** The two RCTs contributing most of the data to the systematic review[38,39] used different techniques to measure the degree of carotid stenosis, but conversion charts are available and were used in the systematic review.[44] The trials, as well as observational studies,[4] found that risk of recurrent stroke was highest about the time of the symptomatic event. **People with asymptomatic stenosis:** A large scale trial is ongoing.[52]

| OPTION | CAROTID PERCUTANEOUS TRANSLUMINAL ANGIOPLASTY |

We found that carotid PTA has not been adequately assessed in people with a recent carotid territory TIA or non-disabling ischaemic stroke who have severe stenosis of the ipsilateral carotid artery.

Benefits: We found no systematic review or placebo controlled RCTs. **Carotid PTA:** One RCT (504 people with a recent carotid territory TIA or non-disabling ischaemic stroke with stenosis of the ipsilateral carotid artery) compared "best medical treatment" plus carotid PTA versus "best medical treatment" plus carotid endarterectomy.[53] Too few people were randomised to provide reliable estimates of efficacy. Preliminary results have been published in abstract form, suggesting that rates of stroke or death at 30 days were similar in endarterectomy and PTA groups. Three year outcome results have also been published in abstract form,[54] finding that although there was a significant increase in restenosis in people undergoing PTA (21% v 5% of people undergoing endarterectomy, P < 0.0001), there was no difference between the two groups in rates of disabling stroke or death, or ipsilateral stroke. **Vertebral artery PTA:** The RCT randomised only

16 people between vertebral PTA and best medical treatment. This did not provide enough data for reliable estimates of efficacy.[53]

Harms: We found insufficient randomised data upon which to comment. Analysis of the safety data of the RCT has not yet been published.[53]

Comment: Two ongoing RCTs are comparing carotid endarterectomy versus primary stenting in people with recently symptomatic severe carotid stenosis.[55,56]

QUESTION What are the effects of anticoagulant and antiplatelet treatment in people with atrial fibrillation?

Gord Gubitz, Peter Sandercock, and Gregory Lip

Systematic reviews have found that people with atrial fibrillation at high risk of stroke (see glossary, p 152) and with no contraindications benefit from anticoagulation. Antiplatelet agents are less effective than warfarin, and are associated with a lower bleeding risk, but are a reasonable alternative if warfarin is contraindicated or if risk of ischaemic stroke is low. The best time to begin anticoagulation after an ischaemic stroke is unclear.

Benefits: Three risk strata have been identified based on evidence derived from one overview of five RCTs,[57] and one subsequent RCT.[58] **People with atrial fibrillation at high risk of stroke, adjusted dose warfarin versus placebo:** We found one overview[50] and two systematic reviews[59,60] examining the effect of warfarin in different groups of people with atrial fibrillation at high risk of stroke. The overview (5 RCTs, 2461 elderly people with atrial fibrillation and a variety of stroke risks) compared warfarin versus placebo.[51] The review found that anticoagulation reduced the risk of stroke over a mean of 5 years (ARR 4.4%, 95% CI 2.8% to 6.0%; RR 0.32, 95% CI 0.21 to 0.5; NNT 23 over 1 year, 95% CI 17 to 36). The first systematic review (search date not stated) identified two RCTs comparing warfarin with placebo in 1053 people with chronic non-rheumatic atrial fibrillation and a history of prior stroke or TIA.[59] Most people (98%) came from one double blind RCT (669 people within 3 months of a minor stroke or TIA),[61] which compared anticoagulant (target INR 2.5 to 4.0) versus aspirin versus placebo. It found that anticoagulants reduced the risk of recurrent stroke over about 2 years (ARR 13.7%, 95% CI 7.3% to 20.1%; RR 0.39, 95% CI 0.25 to 0.63; NNT 7 over 1 year, 95% CI 5 to 14). The second systematic review (search date 1999, 16 RCTs, 9874 people) included six RCTs (2900 people) of adjusted dose warfarin versus placebo (5 RCTs) or versus control (1 RCT) in high risk people (45% had hypertension, 20% had experienced a previous stroke or TIA).[60] These six RCTs included five primary prevention RCTs and one secondary prevention RCT.[62] Target INR varied among RCTs (2.0–2.6 in primary prevention RCTs and 2.9 in the secondary prevention RCT). The results of this systematic review were similar to the others. The meta-analysis found that adjusted dose warfarin reduced the risk of stroke (5 primary prevention RCTs: ARR 4.0%, 95% CI 2.3% to 5.7%; NNT 25, 95% CI 18 to 43. One secondary prevention RCT: ARR 14.5%, 95% CI 7.7% to 21.3%; NNT 7, 95% CI 5 to 13. Combined primary and secondary prevention RCTs: ARR

5.5%, 95% CI 3.7% to 7.3%; NNT 18, 95% CI 14 to 27). **Adjusted dose warfarin versus minidose warfarin:** We found no systematic review or RCTs of low dose warfarin regimens in people with atrial fibrillation and a recent transient ischaemic attack or acute stroke. We found one RCT (1044 people with atrial fibrillation at high risk of stroke), which compared low, fixed dose warfarin (target INR 1.2–1.5) plus aspirin (325 mg per day) with standard adjusted dose warfarin treatment (target INR 2.0–3.0).[58] Adjusted dose warfarin significantly reduced the combined rate of ischaemic stroke or systemic embolism (ARR 6.0%, 95% CI 3.4% to 8.6%; NNT 17, 95% CI 12 to 29) and of disabling or fatal stroke (ARR 3.9%, 95% CI 1.6% to 6.1%; NNT 26, 95% CI 16 to 63). We found three additional RCTs,[63–65] which aimed to evaluate adjusted dose warfarin versus low dose warfarin and aspirin, but were stopped prematurely when the results of the earlier trial[58] were published. Analyses of the optimal anticoagulation intensity for stroke prevention in atrial fibrillation found that stroke risk was substantially increased at INR levels below 2.[62,66] **Adjusted dose warfarin versus aspirin:** We found two systematic reviews of warfarin versus different antiplatelet regimens in people at higher risk of stroke.[60,67] The first systematic review (search date not stated, 1 RCT)[62] found that, in elderly people with atrial fibrillation and a prior history of stroke or TIA, warfarin (target INR 2.5–4.0) versus aspirin (300 mg) reduced the risk of stroke (AR 22.6% for aspirin v 8.9% for warfarin; ARR 14%, 95% CI 7% to 20%; RR 0.39, 95% CI 0.24 to 0.64; NNT 7, 95% CI 5 to 14).[67] The second systematic review (search date 1999, 16 RCTs, 9874 people) included five RCTs (4 primary prevention RCTs and 1 secondary prevention RCT; 2837 people) of adjusted dose warfarin versus aspirin in high risk people (45% had hypertension, 20% had experienced a previous stroke or TIA).[60] Target INR varied among RCTs (2.0–4.5 in primary prevention RCTs, 2.5–4.0 in the secondary prevention RCT). Adjusted dose warfarin versus aspirin reduced the overall risk of stroke (ARR 2.9%, 95% CI 0.9% to 4.8%; NNT 34, 95% CI 21 to 111). The effect varied widely among the five RCTs, none of which were blinded. **Adjusted dose warfarin versus other antiplatelet treatment:** One systematic review (search date 1999) compared adjusted dose warfarin versus other antiplatelet agents such as indobufen.[60] One RCT included in the review (916 people within 15 days of stroke onset) compared warfarin (INR 2.0–3.5) with indobufen.[68] It found no significant difference in the rate of recurrent stroke between the two groups (AR 5% for indobufen v 4% for warfarin; ARR +1.0%, 95% CI −1.7% to +3.7%). **Aspirin versus placebo:** We found one non-systematic review,[69] which included one RCT of people with atrial fibrillation and prior stroke or TIA. Aspirin reduced the risk of stroke, although the confidence interval included the possibility of no benefit (RRR 21%, 95% CI 0% to 38%). **In people with atrial fibrillation at moderate risk of stroke:** See glossary, p 152. We found no RCT that considered this group specifically. **In people with atrial fibrillation at low risk of stroke, anticoagulants:** See glossary, p 152. We found one systematic review and one overview comparing warfarin with placebo in people with atrial fibrillation and a variety of stroke risks.[57,70] Both reviews included the same five RCTs. The overview (2461 people) found that, for people younger than 65 years with atrial fibrillation (but no history of either hypertension, stroke, TIA, or diabetes), the annual stroke rate was the same with warfarin or placebo (1% per year).[57] The systematic review (search date 1999, 2313 people, mean age 69 years, 20% aged over 75 years; 45% had hypertension, 15% diabetes, and 15% a prior history of myocardial infarction) found that warfarin (INR 2.0–2.6) versus placebo reduced fatal and non-fatal ischaemic stroke (ARR 4.0%, 95% CI 2.4% to 5.6%; NNT 25, 95% CI 18 to 42), reduced all ischaemic strokes or intracranial haemorrhage (ARR 4.5%, 95% CI 2.8% to 6.2%; NNT 22, 95% CI 16 to 36), and reduced the combined outcome of disabling or fatal ischaemic stroke or intracranial hemorrhage (ARR 1.8%, 95% CI 0.5% to 3.1%; NNT 56, 95% CI 32 to 200). **Antiplatelet treatment:** We found two systematic reviews.[60,71] The first (search date 1999, 2 RCTs, 1680 people with either paroxysmal or sustained non-valvular atrial fibrillation confirmed by electrocardiogram but without previous stroke or TIA, 30% age > 75 years) compared aspirin with placebo.[71] In primary prevention, aspirin did not significantly reduce ischaemic stroke (OR 0.71, 95% CI 0.46 to 1.10; ARR +1.6%, 95% CI –0.5% to +3.7%), all stroke (OR 0.70, 95% CI 0.45 to 1.08; ARR +1.8%; 95% CI –0.5% to +3.9%), all disabling or fatal stroke (OR 0.88, 95% CI 0.48 to 1.58; ARR +0.4%, 95% CI –1.2% to +2.0%), or the composite end point of stroke, myocardial infarction, or vascular death (OR 0.76, 95% CI 0.54 to 1.05; ARR +2.3%, 95% CI –0.4% to +5.0%). The second systematic review (search date 1999)[60] included three RCTs of primary prevention. The average rate of stroke among people taking placebo was 5.2%. Meta-analysis of the three RCTs found that antiplatelet agents versus placebo reduced the risk of stroke (ARR 2.2%, 95% CI 0.3% to 4.1%; NNT 45, 95% CI 24 to 333).

Harms: The major risk of anticoagulants and antiplatelet agents was haemorrhage. In the overview evaluating elderly people with variable risk factors for stroke, the absolute risk of major bleeding was 1% for placebo, 1% for aspirin, and 1.3% for warfarin.[57] Another systematic review,[60] found the absolute risk of intracranial haemorrhage increased from 0.1% a year with control to 0.3% a year with warfarin, but the difference was not statistically significant. The absolute risks were three times higher in people who had bled previously. Both bleeding and haemorrhagic stroke were more common in people aged over 75 years. The risk of death after a major bleed ranged from 13–33%, and risk of subsequent morbidity in those who survived a major bleed was 15%. The risk of bleeding was associated with an INR greater than 3, fluctuating INRs, and uncontrolled hypertension. In the systematic review evaluating people with prior stroke or TIA, major extracranial bleeding was more frequent with anticoagulation than with placebo (ARI 4.9%, 95% CI 1.6% to 8.2%; RR 6.2, 95% CI 1.4 to 27.1; NNH 20, 95% CI 12 to 63).[59] The studies were too small to define the rate of intracranial haemorrhage (none occurred in the 2 RCTs). In a systematic review comparing anticoagulants and antiplatelet agents, major extracranial bleeding was more frequent with anticoagulation (ARI 4.9%, 95% CI 1.6% to 8.2%; RR 6.4, 95% CI 1.5 to 28.1; NNH 20, 95% CI 12 to 63).[67] The studies were too small to define the rate of intracranial haemorrhage (in one RCT, none of the people on anticoagulant and one person on aspirin had an intracranial bleed). In the systematic review of oral anticoagulants versus placebo in low risk people,[70] the number of intracranial haemorrhages was small (5 in the treatment group and 2 in the control group), with a non-significant increase in the treatment group. Likewise, in the systematic review assessing antiplatelet therapy in low risk people with atrial fibrillation,[71] too few haemorrhages occurred to characterise the effects of aspirin.

Comment: As well as the trade offs between benefits and harms, each person's treatment preferences should be considered when deciding how to treat.[72–77] We found net benefit of anticoagulation for people in atrial fibrillation who have had a TIA or stroke, or who are over 75 years of age and at a high risk of stroke. We found less clear cut evidence for those aged 65–75 years at high risk, and for those with moderate risk (that is, over age 65 not in a high risk group; those under 65 years of age with clinical risk factors), or for those at low risk (under 65 years of age with no other risk factors). The benefits of warfarin in the RCTs may not translate into effectiveness in clinical practice.[78,79] In the RCTs, most strokes in people randomised to warfarin occurred while they were not in fact taking warfarin, or were significantly underanticoagulated at the time of the event. People in the RCTs were highly selected (< 10%, range 3–40% of eligible people were randomised); many were excluded after assessments for the absence of contraindications and physicians' refusal to enter them into the study. Many of the studies were not double blinded and in some there was poor agreement between raters for "soft" neurological end points. The frequent monitoring of warfarin treatment under trial conditions and motivation of people/ investigators was probably more than that seen in usual clinical practice. The best time to start anticoagulation after an ischaemic stroke is unclear. The evidence supports the need to identify the baseline risk of individuals and to use antithrombotic therapy judiciously.

GLOSSARY

International normalised ratio (INR) A value derived from a standardised laboratory test that measures the effect of an anticoagulant like warfarin. The laboratory materials used in the test are calibrated against internationally accepted standard reference preparations, so that variability between laboratories and different reagents is minimised. Normal blood has an INR of 1. Therapeutic anticoagulation often aims to achieve an INR value of 2–3.5.

People at high risk of stroke People of any age with a previous TIA or stroke, or a history of rheumatic vascular disease, coronary artery disease, congestive heart failure, and/or impaired left ventricular function or echocardiography; and people aged 75 years and over with hypertension, diabetes, or both.

People at moderate risk of stroke People over 65 years of age who are not in the high risk group; and people under 65 years of age with clinical risk factors, including diabetes, hypertension, peripheral arterial disease, and ischaemic heart disease.

People at low risk of stroke All other people under 65 years of age with no history of stroke, TIA, embolism, hypertension, diabetes, or other clinical risk factors.

Substantive changes since last issue

Carotid endarterectomy New systematic review;[49] conclusions unchanged.

REFERENCES

1. Hankey GJ, Warlow CP. *Transient ischaemic attacks of the brain and eye*. London: WB Saunders, 1994.
2. Prospective Studies Collaboration. Cholesterol, diastolic blood pressure, and stroke: 13 000 strokes in 450 000 people in 45 prospective cohorts. *Lancet* 1995;346:1647–1653.
3. Eastern Stroke and Coronary Heart Disease Collaborative Research Group. Blood pressure, cholesterol, and stroke in eastern Asia. *Lancet* 1998;352:1801–1807.
4. Warlow CP, Dennis MS, van Gijn J, et al. Predicting recurrent stroke and other serious vascular events. In: *Stroke. A practical guide to management*. Oxford: Blackwell Science, 1996:545–552.
5. Antiplatelet Trialists' Collaboration. Collaborative overview of randomised trials of antiplatelet therapy – I: prevention of death, myocardial infarction, and stroke by prolonged antiplatelet therapy in various categories of patients. *BMJ* 1994;308:81–106. Search date March 1990; primary sources Medline; Current Contents; hand searches of journals, reference lists, and conference proceeedings; and contact with authors of trials and manufacturers.
6. Hart RG, Pearce LA, Rothbart RM, McAnulty JH, Asinger RW, Halperin JL. Stroke with intermittent atrial fibrillation: incidence and predictors during aspirin therapy. Stroke Prevention in Atrial fibrillation Investigators. *J Am Coll Cardiol* 2000; 35:183–187.
7. Collins R, MacMahon S. Blood pressure, antihypertensive drug treatment and the risks of stroke and of coronary heart disease. *Br Med Bull* 1994;50:272–298.
8. PROGRESS Management Committee. Blood pressure lowering for the secondary prevention of stroke: rationale and design of PROGRESS. *J Hypertension* 1996;14(suppl 2):41–46.
9. Staessen JA, Fagard R, Thijs L, et al for the Systolic Hypertension in Europe (Syst–Eur) Trial Investigators. Randomised double-blind comparison of placebo and active treatment for older patients with isolated systolic hypertension. *Lancet* 1997;350:757–764.
10. PATS Collaborating Group. Post-stroke antihypertensive treatment study: a preliminary result. *Chinese Med J* 1995;108:710–717.
11. The Heart Outcomes Prevention Evaluation Study Investigators. Effects of an angiotensin-converting-enzyme inhibitor, ramipril, on death from cardiovascular causes, myocardial infarction, and stroke in high-risk patients. *N Engl J Med* 2000; 342:145–153.
12. Rodgers A, MacMahon S, Gamble G, Slattery J, Sandercock P, Warlow C, for the United Kingdom Transient Ischaemic Attack Collaborative Group. Blood pressure and risk of stroke in patients with cerebrovascular disease. *BMJ* 1996;313:147.
13. Neal B, Clark T, MacMahon S, Rodgers A, Baigent C, Collins R, on behalf of the Antithrombotic Trialists' Collaboration. Blood pressure and the risk of recurrent vascular disease. *Am J Hypertension* 1998;11:25A–26A.
14. Hebert PR, Gaziano M, Hennekens CH. An overview of trials of cholesterol lowering and risk of stroke. *Arch Intern Med* 1995;155:50–55.
15. Hebert PR, Gaziano JM, Chan KS, Hennekens CH. Cholesterol lowering with statin drugs, risk of stroke, and total mortality: an overview of randomized trials. *JAMA* 1997;278:313–321. Search date 1995; primary sources not specified, Cholesterol and Current Events (CARE) data added in October 1996.
16. The long-term intervention with pravastatin in ischaemic disease (LIPID) study group. Prevention of cardiovascular events and death with pravastatin in patients with coronary heart disease and a broad range of initial cholesterol levels. *N Engl J Med* 1998;339:1349–1357.
17. Acheson J, Hutchinson EC. Controlled trial of clofibrate in cerebral vascular disease. *Atherosclerosis* 1972;15:177–183.
18. Anonymous. The treatment of cerebrovascular disease with clofibrate. Final report of the Veterans' Administration Cooperative Study of Atherosclerosis, neurology section. *Stroke* 1973; 4:684–693
19. Di Mascio R, Marchioli R, Tognoni G. Cholesterol reduction and stroke occurrence: an overview of randomized clinical trials. *Cerebrovasc Dis* 2000; 10:85–92.
20. Rubins HB, Robins SJ, Collins D, et al. Gemfibrozil for the secondary prevention of coronary heart disease in men with low levels of high-density lipoprotein cholesterol. *N Engl J Med* 1999;341: 410–418.
21. Plehn JF, Davis BR, Sacks FM, et al for the CARE Investigators. Reduction of stroke incidence after myocardial infarction with pravastatin: the cholesterol and recurrent events (CARE) study. *Circulation* 1999;99:216–223.
22. Scandinavian Simvastatin Survival Study Group. Randomised trial of cholesterol lowering in 4444 patients with coronary heart disease: the Scandinavian simvastatin survival study (4S). *Lancet* 1994;344:1383–1389.
23. Cholesterol Treatment Trialists' Collaboration. Protocol for a prospective collaborative overview of all current and planned randomized trials of cholesterol treatment regimens. *Am J Cardiol* 1995;75:1130–1134.
24. SALT Collaborative Group. Swedish aspirin low-dose trial (SALT) of 75 mg aspirin as secondary prophylaxis after cerebrovascular ischaemic events. *Lancet* 1991;338:1345–1349.
25. Diener HC, Cunha L, Forbes C, Sivenius J, Smets P, Lowenthal A. European secondary prevention study 2: dipyridamole and acetylsalicylic acid in the secondary prevention of stroke. *J Neurol Sci* 1996;143:1–13.
26. Gotoh F, Tohgi H, Hirai S, Terashi A, Fukuuchi Y, Otomo E, et al. Cilostazol Stroke Prevention Study: a placebo-controlled double-blind trial for secondary prevention of cerebral infarction. *J Stroke Cerebrovasc Dis* 2000;9:147:157
27. Taylor DW, Barnett HJM, Haynes RB, et al, for the ASA and Carotid Endarterectomy (ACE) Trial Collaborators. Low-dose and high-dose acetylsalicylic acid for patients undergoing carotid endarterectomy: a randomised controlled trial. *Lancet* 1999;353:2179–2184.
28. Juul-Möller S, Edvardsson N, Jahnmatz B, Rosen A, Soreneson S, Omblus R, for the Swedish Angina Pectoris Aspirin Trial (SAPAT) Group. Double-blind trial of aspirin in primary prevention of myocardial infarction in patients with stable chronic angina pectoris. *Lancet* 1992;340:1421–1425.
29. The Dutch TIA Study Group. A comparison of two doses of aspirin (30 mg vs 283 mg a day) in patients after a transient ischaemic attack or minor ischaemic stroke. *N Engl J Med* 1991;325: 1261–1266.
30. Sudlow C, Baigent C, on behalf of the Antithrombotic Trialists' Collaboration. Different antiplatelet regimens in the prevention of vascular events among patients at high risk of stroke: new evidence from the antithrombotic trialists' collaboration. Seventh European Stroke

Conference, Edinburgh, May, 1998. *Cerebrovasc Dis* 1998;8(suppl 4):68.

31. Hankey GJ, Sudlow CLM, Dunbabin DW. Thienopyridine derivatives (ticlopidine, clopidogrel) versus aspirin for preventing stroke and other serious vascular events in high vascular risk patients. In: The Cochrane Library, Issue 1, 2001. Oxford: Update Software. Search date March 1999; primary sources Cochrane Stroke Group Trials Register, Antithrombotic Trialists' database, and personal contact with Sanofi pharmacological company.

32. CAPRIE Steering Committee. A randomised, blinded, trial of clopidogrel versus aspirin in patients at risk of ischaemic events. *Lancet* 1996; 348:1329–1339.

33. Farrell B, Godwin J, Richards S, Warlow C. The United Kingdom transient ischaemic attack (UK-TIA) aspirin trial: final results. *J Neurol Neurosurg Psychiatry* 1991;54:1044–1054.

34. Moloney BA. An analysis of the side effects of ticlopidine. In: Hass WK, Easton JD, eds. *Ticlopidine, Platelets and Vascular Disease.* New York: Springer, 1993:117–139.

35. Bennett CL, Davidson CJ, Raisch DW, Weinberg PD, Bennett RH, Feldman MD. Thrombotic thrombocytopenic purpura assoicated with ticlopidine in the setting of coronary artery stents and stroke prevention. *Arch Int Med* 1999;159: 2524–2528.

36. Bennett CL, Connors JM, Carwile JM, et al. Thrombotic thrombocytopenic purpura associated with clopidogrel. *N Engl J Med* 2000;342:1773–1777.

37. Hankey GJ. Clopidogrel and thrombotic thrombocytopenic purpura. *Lancet* 2000;356: 269–270.

38. Müller C, Büttner HJ, Petersen J, Roskamm H. A randomized comparison of clopidogrel and aspirin versus ticlopidine and aspirin after the placement of coronary-artery stents. *Circulation* 2000;101: 590–593.

39. Bertrand ME, Rupprecht H-J, Urban P, Gershlick AH, for the CLASSICS Investigators. Double-blind study of the safety of clopidogrel with and without a loading dose in combination with aspirin compared with ticlopidine in combination with aspirin after coronary stenting. The Clopidogrel Aspirin Stent International Cooperative Study (CLASSICS). *Circulation* 2000;102:624–629.

40. Liu M, Counsell C, Sandercock P. Anticoagulants for preventing recurrence following ischaemic stroke or transient ischaemic attack. In: The Cochrane Library, Issue 1, 2001. Oxford: Update Software. Search date not stated; primary sources Cochrane Stroke Group Trials Register, and contact with companies marketing anticoagulant agents.

41. The Stroke Prevention in Reversible Ischaemia Trial (SPIRIT) Study Group. A randomised trial of anticoagulant versus aspirin after cerebral ischemia of presumed arterial origin. *Ann Neurol* 1997;42:857–865.

42. Mohr J for the WARSS Group. Design considerations for the warfarin-antiplatelet recurrent stroke study. *Cerebrovasc Dis* 1995;5: 156–157.

43. De Schryver E for the ESPRIT Study Group. ESPRIT: mild anticoagulation, acetylsalicylic acid plus dipyridamole or acetylsalicylic acid alone after cerebral ischaemia of arterial origin [abstract]. *Cerebrovasc Dis* 1998;8(suppl 4):83.

44. Cina C, Clase C, Haynes R. Carotid endarterectomy for symptomatic stenosis. In: The Cochrane Library, Issue 1, 2001. Oxford: Update Software. Search date March 1999; primary sources Cochrane Stroke Group Specialised

Register of Trials; Medline; Embase; Healthstar; Serline; Cochrane Controlled Trials Register; DARE; Best Evidence.

45. European Carotid Surgery Trialists' Collaborative Group. Randomised trial of endarterectomy for recently symptomatic carotid stenosis: final results of the MRC European carotid surgery trial. *Lancet* 1998;351:1379–1387.

46. North American Symptomatic Carotid Endarterectomy Trial Collaborators. Beneficial effect of carotid endarterectomy in symptomatic patients with high-grade carotid stenosis. *N Engl J Med* 1991;325:445–453.

47. Barnett HJ, Taylor DW, Eliasziw M, et al. Benefit of carotid endarterectomy in patients with symptomatic moderate or severe stenosis. North American symptomatic carotid endarterectomy trial collaborators. *N Engl J Med* 1998;339:1415–1425.

48. Benavente O, Moher D, Pham B. Carotid endarterectomy for asymptomatic carotid stenosis: a meta–analysis. *BMJ* 1998;317:1477–1480. Search date 1998; primary sources Medline; CCTR Ottawa Stroke Trials Register; Current Contents; and hand searching.

49. Chambers BR, You RX, Donnan GA. Carotid endarterectomy for asymptomatic carotid stenosis. In: The Cochrane Library, Issue 1, 2001. Oxford: Update Software. Search date 1998; primary sources Cochrane Stroke Group Trials Register; Medline; Current Contents; hand searches of reference lists; and contact with researchers in the field.

50. Rothwell P, Slattery J, Warlow C. Clinical and angiographic predictors of stroke and death from carotid endarterectomy: systematic review. *BMJ* 1997;315:1571–1577. Search date 1996; primary sources Medline; Cochrane Collaboration Stroke database; and hand searching of reference lists.

51. Whitty C, Sudlow C, Warlow C. Investigating individual subjects and screening populations for asymptomatic carotid stenosis can be harmful. *J Neurol Neurosurg Psychiatry* 1998;64:619–623.

52. Halliday A, Thomas D, Manssfield A. The asymptomatic carotid surgery trial (ACST). Rationale and design. *Eur J Vascular Surg* 1994; 8:703–710.

53. Brown MM, for the CAVATAS Investigators. Results of the carotid and vertebral artery transluminal angioplasty study (CAVATAS) [abstract]. *Cerebrovasc Dis* 1998;8(suppl 4):21.

54. Brown M, Pereira A, McCabe D. Carotid and vertebral transluminal angioplasty study (CAVATAS): 3 year outcome data [abstract]. *Cerebrovasc Dis* 1999;9(suppl 1):66.

55. Brown M. The International Carotid Stenting Study [abstract]. *Stroke* 2000;31:2812.

56. Al-Mubarek N, Roubin G, Hobson R, Ferguson R, Brott T, Moore W. Credentialing of Stent Operators for the Carotid Revascularization Endarterectomy vs Stenting Trial (CREST) [abstract]. *Stroke* 2000; 31:292.

57. Atrial Fibrillation Investigators. Risk factors for stroke and efficacy of antithrombotic therapy in atrial fibrillation. *Arch Intern Med* 1994;154: 1449–1457.

58. Stroke Prevention in Atrial Fibrillation Investigators. Adjusted-dose warfarin versus low-intensity, fixed-dose warfarin plus aspirin for high-risk patients with atrial fibrillation: stroke prevention in atrial fibrillation III randomised clinical trial. *Lancet* 1996;348:633–638.

59. Koudstaal P. Anticoagulants for preventing stroke in patients with non-rheumatic atrial fibrillation and a history of stroke or transient ischemic attacks. In: The Cochrane Library, Issue 1, 2001. Oxford: Update Software. Search date not stated; primary source Cochrane Stroke Group Trials

Register, and contact with trialists.

60. Hart R, Benavente O, McBride R, Pearce L. Antithrombotic therapy to prevent stroke in patients with atrial fibrillation: a meta-analysis. *Ann Intern Med* 1999;131:492–501. Search date 1999; primary sources Medline; Cochrane Database and Antithrombotic Trialists Collaboration.

61. European Atrial Fibrillation Trial Study Group. Secondary prevention in non-rheumatic atrial fibrillation after transient ischaemic attack or minor stroke. *Lancet* 1993;342:1255.

62. The European Atrial Fibrillation Trial Study Group. Optimal oral anticoagulant therapy in patients with non-rheumatic atrial fibrillation and recent cerebral ischemia. *N Engl J Med* 1995;333:5–10.

63. Pengo V, Zasso Z, Barbero F, et al. Effectiveness of fixed minidose warfarin in the prevention of thromboembolism and vascular death in nonrheumatic atrial fibrillation. *Am J Cardiol* 1998; 82:433–437.

64. Gullov A, Koefoed B, Petersen P, et al. Fixed minidose warfarin and aspirin alone and in combination vs adjusted-dose warfarin for stroke prevention in atrial fibrillation. Second Copenhagen Atrial Fibrillation, Aspirin, and Anticoagulation Study. *Arch Intern Med* 1998; 158:1513–1521.

65. Hellemons B, Langenberg M, Lodder J, et al. Primary prevention of arterial thrombo-embolism in non-rheumatic atrial fibrillation in primary care: randomised controlled trial comparing two intensities of coumarin with aspirin. *BMJ* 1999; 319:958–964

66. Hylek EM, Skates SJ, Sheehan MA, Singer DE. An analysis of the lowest effective intensity of prophylactic anticoagulation for patients with non-rheumatic atrial fibrillation. *N Engl J Med* 1996; 335:540–546.

67. Koudstaal P. Anticoagulants versus antiplatelet therapy for preventing stroke in patients with non-rheumatic atrial fibrillation and a history of stroke or transient ischemic attacks. In: The Cochrane Library, Issue 1, 2001. Oxford: Update Software. Search date not stated; primary source Cochrane Stroke Group Trials Register, and contact with trialists.

68. Morocutti C, Amabile G, Fattapposta F, et al for the SIFA Investigators. Indobufen versus warfarin in the secondary prevention of major vascular events in non-rheumatic atrial fibrillation. *Stroke* 1997;28:1015–1021.

69. Atrial Fibrillation Investigators. The efficacy of aspirin in patients with atrial fibrillation: analysis of pooled data from 3 randomized trials. *Arch Intern Med* 1997;157:1237–1240.

70. Benavente O, Hart R, Koudstaal P, Laupacis A, McBride R. Oral anticoagulants for preventing stroke in patients with non-valvular atrial fibrillation and no previous history of stroke or transient ischemic attacks. In: The Cochrane Library, Issue 1, 2001. Oxford: Update Software. Search date 1999; primary sources Cochrane Stroke Group Specialised Register of Trials; Medline; Antithrombotic Trialists Collaboration database; and hand searches of reference lists of relevant articles.

71. Benavente O, Hart R, Koudstaal P, Laupacis A, McBride R. Antiplatelet therapy for preventing stroke in patients with non-valvular atrial fibrillation and no previous history of stroke or transient ischemic attacks. In: The Cochrane Library, Issue 1, 2001. Oxford: Update Software. Search date June 1999; primary sources Medline; Cochrane Register of Trials; and hand searches of reference lists of relevant articles.

72. Lip G. Thromboprophylaxis for atrial fibrillation. *Lancet* 1999;353:4–6.

73. Ezekowitz M, Levine J. Preventing stroke in patients with atrial fibrillation. *JAMA* 1999;281: 1830–1835.

74. Hart R, Sherman D, Easton D, Cairns J. Prevention of stroke in patients with non-valvular atrial fibrillation. *Neurology* 1998;51:674–681.

75. Feinberg W. Anticoagulation for prevention of stroke. *Neurology* 1998;51(suppl 3):20–22.

76. Albers G. Choice of antithrombotic therapy for stroke prevention in atrial fibrillation. Warfarin, aspirin, or both? *Arch Intern Med* 1998;158: 1487–1491.

77. Nademanee K, Kosar E. Long-term antithrombotic treatment for atrial fibrillation. *Am J Cardiol* 1998; 82:37N–42N.

78. Green CJ, Hadorn DC, Bassett K, Kazanjian A. Anticoagulation in chronic non-valvular atrial fibrillation: a critical appraisal and meta-analysis. *Can J Cardiol* 1997;13:811–815.

79. Blakely J. Anticoagulation in chronic non-valvular atrial fibrillation: appraisal of two meta-analyses. *Can J Cardiol* 1998;14:945–948.

Cathie Sudlow
Specialist Registrar in Neurology
Department of Neurology
Derriford Hospital
Plymouth
UK

Peter Sandercock
Professor in Neurology
Neurosciences Trials Unit
University of Edinburgh
Edinburgh
UK

Gord Gubitz
Assistant Professor
Division of Neurology
Dalhousie University
Halifax
Canada

Gregory Lip
Consultant Cardiologist
and Reader in Medicine
City Hospital
Birmingham
UK

Competing interests: GL is UK principal investigator for the ERAFT Trial (Knoll) and has been reimbursed by various pharmaceutical companies for attending several conferences, running educational programmes and research projects. PS has given lectures and symposia, and received lecture fees and travel expenses from Boehringer Ingelheim, Sanofi, BMJ Publishing Group, and a variety of other companies, and he has received support from Boehringer Ingelheim and GlaxoWellcome for trials and research. GG and CS, none declared.

Cardiovascular disorders

TABLE 1 Effects of cholesterol lowering on risk of stroke: results of two systematic reviews of RCTs of non-statin and statin interventions in the primary and secondary prevention of coronary heart disease* (see text, p 143).

Overview	Number of		Mean reduction in cholesterol (%)	Summary OR (95% CI) for active treatment v control	
	Participants	Strokes		Fatal or non-fatal stroke	Fatal stroke
Non-statin interventions					
1995 overview (11 trials)[14]	36 000	435	11%	0.99 (0.82 to 1.21)	1.10 (0.79 to 1.54)
Statin interventions					
1997 overview (14 trials)[15] + LIPID trial[16]	38 000	827	21%	0.76 (0.66 to 0.87)	0.99 (0.67 to 1.45)
Subtotal, primary prevention trials	8 000	108	20%	0.80 (0.54 to 1.16)	–
Subtotal, secondary prevention trials	30 000	719	22%	0.75 (0.65 to 0.87)	–

* The findings of other published overviews are consistent with the results shown here.

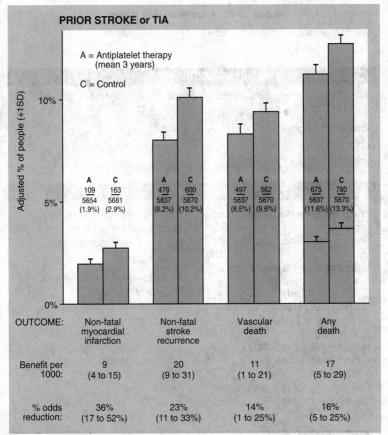

FIGURE 1	Absolute effects of antiplatelet treatment on various outcomes in people with a prior stroke or TIA: results of a systematic review.[5] The columns show the absolute risks over 3 years for each outcome; the error bars represent standard deviations. In the "any death" column, non-vascular deaths are represented by lower horizontal lines (see text, p 144). Adapted with permission.[5]

Thromboembolism

Cardiovascular disorders

Search date September 2000: expanded this issue

David Fitzmaurice, FD Richard Hobbs and Richard McManus

QUESTIONS

INTERVENTIONS

Trade off between benefits and harms

Unknown effectiveness

To be covered in future issues of *Clinical Evidence*

Thrombolysis for pulmonary
embolism

Compression stockings for DVT

Oral antithrombotic agents (such as
glycoprotein IIb/IIIa antagonists)

Inferior vena cava filters

Aspirin

Thromboembolism in pregnancy

Key Messages

Proximal DVT

- One RCT has found that combined intravenous unfractionated heparin and oral anticoagulant reduce recurrent thromboembolic events in people with proximal deep vein thrombosis (DVT) compared with oral anticoagulants alone.

- Two systematic reviews have found good evidence that longer duration of anticoagulation is associated with significantly fewer recurrent DVTs. One systematic review has found limited evidence that longer duration of anticoagulation is associated with significantly increased risk of major haemorrhage, but the other systematic review has found no significantly increased risk of major haemorrhage.

- Systematic reviews have found that low molecular weight heparin (LMWH) (see glossary, p 167) is at least as effective as unfractionated heparin in reducing the incidence of recurrent thromboembolic disease.

- Systematic reviews have found that LMWH is at least as safe as unfractionated heparin for the treatment of DVT.

Isolated calf vein thrombosis

- One RCT has found that warfarin plus unfractionated heparin reduce the risk of recurrence in isolated calf vein thrombosis compared with unfractionated heparin alone.

■ We found insufficient evidence on optimal duration or intensity of anticoagulation.

Pulmonary embolism

■ One RCT has found that combined treatment with oral anticoagulant plus intravenous unfractionated heparin reduces mortality compared with unfractionated heparin alone. One RCT found no evidence of a difference in the benefits and harms of LMWH versus unfractionated heparin in people with pulmonary embolism.

Duration of warfarin treatment

■ Evidence for intensity and duration of treatment has been extrapolated from studies in people with proximal DVT and any venous thromboembolism.

■ Two systematic reviews have found good evidence of a significant reduction in recurrent venous thromboembolism with longer duration of anticoagulation. One systematic review found limited evidence of increased risk of major haemorrhage with longer periods of anticoagulation. The other systematic review found no significantly increased risk of major haemorrhage with longer versus shorter durations of anticoagulation.

■ The absolute risk of recurrent venous thromboembolism decreases with time whereas the relative risk reduction with therapy remains constant. Harms of therapy, including major haemorrhage, continue during prolonged treatment. People with thromboembolism have different risk profiles, and it is likely that the optimal duration of anticoagulation will vary between people.

Intensity of warfarin treatment

■ One RCT in people with a first episode of idiopathic venous thromboembolism treated for 3 months with warfarin found no significant difference in recurrence between treatment targeted at an international normalised ratio (INR) (see glossary, p 167) of 2.0–3.0 versus an INR of 3.0–4.5. Treatment targeted at the higher INR was associated with a greater risk of bleeding.

Computerised decision support of oral anticoagulation

■ We found no RCTs of computerised decision support versus usual management of oral anticoagulation that used clinically important outcomes (major haemorrhage or death). Systematic reviews and RCTs have found limited evidence that computerised decision support of oral anticoagulation improves time spent in the target INR range.

DEFINITION **Venous thromboembolism** is any thromboembolic event occurring within the venous system, including DVT and pulmonary embolism. **Deep vein thrombosis (DVT)** is a radiologically confirmed partial or total thrombotic occlusion of the deep venous system of the legs sufficient to produce symptoms of pain or swelling. **Proximal DVT** affects the veins above the knee (popliteal, superficial femoral, common femoral, and iliac veins). **Isolated calf vein thrombosis** is confined to the deep veins of the calf and does not affect the veins above the knee. **Pulmonary embolism** is radiologically confirmed partial or total thromboembolic occlusion of pulmonary arteries, sufficient to cause symptoms of breathlessness, chest pain, or both. **Post-thrombotic syndrome** is oedema, ulceration, and impaired viability of the subcutaneous tissues of

Thromboembolism

the leg occurring after DVT. **Recurrence** refers to symptomatic deterioration due to a further (radiologically confirmed) thrombosis, after a previously confirmed thromboembolic event, where there had been an initial partial or total symptomatic improvement. **Extension** refers to a radiologically confirmed new, constant, symptomatic intraluminal filling defect extending from an existing thrombosis.

INCIDENCE/ PREVALENCE We found no reliable study of the incidence/prevalence of DVT or pulmonary embolism in the UK. A prospective Scandinavian study found an annual incidence of 1.6–1.8 per 1000 people in the general population.[1,2] One post mortem study extrapolated that 600 000 people develop pulmonary embolism each year in the USA, of whom 60 000 die as a result.[3]

AETIOLOGY/ RISK FACTORS Risk factors for DVT include immobility, surgery (particularly orthopaedic), malignancy, smoking, pregnancy, older age, and inherited or acquired prothrombotic clotting disorders.[4] Evidence for these factors is mainly observational. The oral contraceptive pill is associated with death due to venous thromboembolism (ARI with any combined oral contraception 1 to 3 per million women per year).[5] The principal cause of pulmonary embolism is a DVT.[4]

PROGNOSIS The annual recurrence rate of symptomatic calf vein thrombosis in people not having surgery is over 25%.[6,7] Between 40–50% of people with symptomatic calf vein thrombosis develop proximal extension.[8] Proximal DVT may cause fatal or non-fatal pulmonary embolism, recurrent venous thrombosis, and the post-thrombotic syndrome. One observational study published in 1946 found a 20% mortality from pulmonary emboli in people in hospital with untreated DVT.[9] One non-systematic review of observational studies found that, in people after surgery who have an asymptomatic calf vein DVT, the rate of fatal pulmonary embolism was 13–15%.[10] The incidence of other complications without treatment is not known. The risk of recurrent venous thrombosis and complications is related to the presence of thrombotic risk factors.[11]

AIMS To reduce acute symptoms of DVT and to prevent morbidity and mortality associated with thrombus extension, the post-thrombotic syndrome and pulmonary embolisation; to reduce recurrence; and to minimise any adverse effects of treatment.

OUTCOMES Rates of symptomatic recurrence, post-thrombotic syndrome, symptomatic pulmonary embolism, and death. Proxy outcomes include radiological evidence of clot extension or pulmonary embolism.

METHODS *Clinical Evidence* update search and appraisal September 2000. Observational studies were used for estimating incidence, prevalence, and adverse event rates. RCTs were included only if cases and outcomes were objectively defined, and if the trial provided dose ranges (with adjusted dosing schedules for oral anticoagulation and unfractionated heparin) and independent, blinded outcome assessment.

OPTION ANTICOAGULATION

We found no RCTs comparing warfarin with placebo. One RCT found that combined warfarin and intravenous unfractionated heparin for initial treatment reduced recurrence of proximal DVT compared with warfarin alone. Two systematic reviews have found that longer duration of anticoagulation is associated with significantly fewer DVT recurrences. Systematic reviews have found that LMWH (see glossary, p 167) is at least as effective as unfractionated heparin in reducing the incidence of recurrent thromboembolic disease. We found evidence from systematic reviews that LMWH is at least as safe as unfractionated heparin for the treatment of DVT.

Benefits: **Warfarin versus placebo:** We found no RCTs. **Warfarin plus heparin versus warfarin alone:** One RCT (120 people with proximal DVT) found that combined intravenous unfractionated heparin plus warfarin reduced recurrence compared with warfarin alone at interim analysis at 6 months, and as a result the trial was stopped (rate of recurrence 12/60 [20%] with warfarin alone v 4/60 [6.7%] with combined treatment, P = 0.058; NNT 8, 95% CI 4 to 71).[12] **Duration of anticoagulation:** We found two systematic reviews. The first systematic review (search date 2000, 4 RCTs, 1500 people)[13] included two RCTs of people with a first episode of venous thromboembolism, one RCT in people with a second episode of venous thromboembolism, and a fourth RCT in people with acute proximal DVT. The periods of treatment compared were different in all four RCTs: 4 weeks versus 3 months, 6 weeks versus 6 months, 3 months versus 27 months, and 6 months versus 4 years. In all RCTs, anticoagulant doses were adjusted to achieve an INR (see glossary, p 167) between 2.0 and 3.0. Individual RCTs found significant protection from thromboembolic complications with prolonged versus shorter treatment (on pooling, 7/758 [0.9%] in the long arm v 91/742 [12%] in the short arm; OR 0.15, 95% CI 0.10 to 0.23). None of the individual RCTs found a significant reduction in mortality. Analysis of pooled results also found no significant reduction in mortality with prolonged versus shorter treatment (OR 0.70, 95% CI 0.45 to 1.09). The second systematic review (search date not stated, 7 RCTs, 2304 people) included three of the same RCTs as the first systematic review plus four RCTs that had been excluded on methodological grounds from the first systematic review (either because of problems with blinding of outcomes or lack of an objective test to confirm thromboembolism).[14] There was wide variation in the duration of short term (3–12 weeks) and longer term (12 weeks–2 years) RCTs. This review also found that longer versus short duration of anticoagulation reduced the risk of recurrent thromboembolism (ARs 74/1156 events per person with longer anticoagulation v 127/1148 with shorter duration; RR 0.60, 95% CI 0.45 to 0.79). **Intensity of anticoagulation:** We found one RCT comparing INR targets of 2.0–3.0 versus 3.0–4.5 for 12 weeks treatment with warfarin following an initial course of intravenous heparin in people with a first episode of idiopathic venous thromboembolism. It found similar recurrence rates at 10 months for both

INR target ranges (recurrence rate 1/47 [2.1%] with lower range v 1/49 [2%] with higher range; P = NS), but found significantly more haemorrhagic events with the higher target range (2/47 [4.3%] v 11/49 [22.4%]; P = 0.015).[15] **Abrupt versus gradual discontinuation of warfarin:** We found one RCT (41 people with DVT), which compared abrupt withdrawal of warfarin versus an additional month of warfarin at a fixed low dose of 1.25 mg/day. It found no significant difference in recurrence rates between the two groups (recurrence in 3 people who stopped warfarin abruptly v 1 person who reduced warfarin gradually).[16] **LMWH versus unfractionated heparin:** We found two systematic reviews confined to symptomatic proximal DVT.[17,18] One (search date 1993, 16 RCTs, 2045 people) found that LMWH reduced thrombus extension compared with unfractionated heparin (ARs not given; OR for thrombus extension 0.45, 95% CI 0.25 to 0.81).[17] The other review (search date 1994, 10 RCTs, 1424 people) found that, compared with unfractionated heparin, low molecular weight heparin reduced symptomatic thromboembolic complications (ARs not given; RR 0.47, 95% CI 0.27 to 0.82) and mortality (RR 0.53, 95% CI 0.31 to 0.90).[18] We also found four systematic reviews comparing LMWH with unfractionated heparin in people with radiologically confirmed symptomatic venous thromboembolism,[19–22] and one subsequent RCT.[23] The first systematic review (search date 1999, 14 RCTs, 4754 people) included five studies (blinded and unblinded, 1636 people) examining proximal thrombosis.[19] Analysis of these trials showed statistically significant reductions in thrombotic complications (LMWH v unfractionated heparin: ARs 39/814 [4.8%] v 64/822 [7.8%]; OR 0.60, 95% CI 0.40 to 0.89). Overall mortality was also reduced (LMWH v unfractionated heparin: ARs 44/814 [5.4%] v 68/822 [8.3%]; OR 0.64, 95% CI 0.43 to 0.93). Eight of the 14 RCTs in the systematic review included people with symptomatic DVT of the leg without symptoms of pulmonary embolism, and these accounted for about 75% of all participants. Analysis of the seven RCTs that concealed treatment allocation found no significant difference between treatments for rates of recurrent venous thromboembolism during treatment (ARs 34/1569 [2.2%] v 43/1595 [2.7%]; OR 0.80, 95% CI 0.51 to 1.26), or at the end of follow up (ARs 75/1671 [4.5%] v 92/1693 [5.4%]; OR 0.82, 95% CI 0.60 to 1.12), or overall mortality (ARs 123/1671 [7.4%] v 150/1694 [8.9%]; OR 0.82, 95% CI 0.64 to 1.05), or major haemorrhage. Wider analysis that included unblinded trials, and so is likely to be more biased, found that LMWH reduced overall mortality and major haemorrhage compared with unfractionated heparin (see harms below). The other three systematic reviews included many of the same trials as the first. Results were similar with no differences between unfractionated heparin and LMWH for recurrent venous thromboembolism or pulmonary embolism, and an unexplained, significant difference in favour of LMWH for total mortality when data were pooled.[20–22] We also found one open RCT not included in the systematic reviews (294 people with acute proximal DVT), which found no significant difference in recurrent DVT rates with intravenous unfractionated heparin in hospital versus LMWH administered subcutaneously twice daily mainly at home (outpatients) or alternatively in hospital versus subcutaneous heparin calcium administered at home (6/98 [6%] with unfractionated heparin v 6/97 [6%] with LMWH v 7/99 [7%] with subcutaneous heparin calcium).[23] See systematic anticoagulation under stroke management, p 127.

Harms: **Warfarin:** Two non-systematic reviews of RCTs and cohort studies found annual bleeding rates of 0–4.8% (fatal bleeding) and 2.4–8.1% (major bleeds).[24,25] Rates depended on how bleeding was defined and the intensity of anticoagulation. No individual study in either review comparing length of anticoagulation found a significant increase in bleeding complications during prolonged versus shorter treatment for venous thromboembolism.[13–14] Both reviews included studies with different periods of treatment and the populations studied had different types of venous thromboembolism (see benefits above). Pooling the results for the first review found that prolonged versus shorter anticoagulation increased the risk of major haemorrhage (19/758 [2.5%] with prolonged anticoagulation v 4/742 [0.5%] with shorter anticoagulation; OR 3.75, 95% CI 1.63 to 8.62). Pooling the results of the second review found a greater risk of major haemorrhage with prolonged versus shorter anticoagulation, but the difference was not significant (10/917 [1.1%] with prolonged treatment v 6/906 [0.7%] with shorter treatment; RR 1.43, 95% CI 0.51 to 4.01). In the RCT of warfarin plus heparin, one person in the combined treatment group committed suicide at 6 months. There were two cancer related deaths, confirmed by post mortem examination, in the group treated with warfarin alone, one in week 11, and the other in week 12.[12] **Heparin:** One systematic review (3306 people treated for at least 5 days) found no significant difference in the risk of thrombocytopenia with LMWH versus unfractionated heparin (RR 0.85, 95% CI 0.45 to 1.62).[20] Another systematic review of blinded RCTs found no significant difference in the risk of major haemorrhage with LMWH versus unfractionated heparin in people with venous thromboembolism (ARs 27/1791 [1.5%] v 39/1827 [2.1%]; OR 0.71, 95% CI 0.43 to 1.15).[19] In this systematic review, pooling of blinded and unblinded RCTs found that the risk of major haemorrhage was 1–2% for up to 10 days treatment with either LMWH or unfractionated heparin.[19] Analysis of the five RCTs of people with proximal thrombosis (blinded and unblinded, 1636 people) found a significant reduction in major haemorrhage with LMWH versus unfractionated heparin (ARs 8/814 [1.0%] v 19/822 [2.3%]; OR 0.44, 95% CI 0.21 to 0.95). The other three systematic reviews, covering many of the same trials, found similar significant reductions in major haemorrhage.[20–22] One of the systematic reviews in people with DVT found that, compared with LMWH, unfractionated heparin was associated with higher rates of clinically important bleeding (ARs not given; RR unfractionated v LMWH 2.48, 95% CI 1.27 to 6.67) and death (see benefits above).[11]

Comment: **Studies evaluating harm:** These varied in regard to diagnostic criteria, definitions of adverse events, and intensity of anticoagulation, making interpretation difficult. **Duration of warfarin therapy:** The absolute risk of recurrent venous thromboembolism decreases with time, whereas the relative risk reduction with therapy remains constant. Harms of therapy, including major haemorrhage, continue during prolonged treatment. Individual people have different risk profiles and it is likely that the optimal duration of anticoagulation will vary between people. **Differences between LMWH:** We found no trials comparing different LMWH.

QUESTION **What are the effects of treatment for isolated calf vein thrombosis?**

OPTION ANTICOAGULATION

One RCT found that, in isolated calf vein thrombosis, warfarin plus intravenous unfractionated heparin (INR 2.5–4.2) reduced rates of proximal extension compared with heparin alone. We found insufficient evidence on optimal duration or intensity of anticoagulation.

Benefits: **Anticoagulation:** We found no systematic review and no good placebo controlled RCTs. We found one RCT that compared intravenous unfractionated heparin for at least 5 days with or without 3 months of warfarin. It found that heparin plus warfarin reduced proximal extension of clot at 1 year compared with heparin alone (proximal extension occurred in 1/23 people with heparin plus warfarin v 9/28 people with heparin alone; ARR 28%, 95% CI 8.6% to 47%).[6] **Duration and intensity of anticoagulation:** We found insufficient evidence in people with isolated calf vein thrombosis.

Harms: See harms of anticoagulation, p 163.

Comment: Many reported cases of isolated calf vein thrombosis are asymptomatic but detected radiologically for research purposes. We found very limited evidence on the clinical significance of asymptomatic calf vein thrombosis. Similarly, studies into the incidence of pulmonary embolism associated with isolated calf vein thrombosis detected asymptomatic embolism by ventilation–perfusion scanning, and it is not clear what the clinical significance of these findings are.

QUESTION **What are the effects of treatments for pulmonary embolism?**

OPTION ANTICOAGULATION

One small RCT has found that heparin plus warfarin significantly reduces mortality in people with pulmonary embolism, compared with no anticoagulant treatment. Two RCTs found that LMWH was at least as effective as unfractionated heparin in people with pulmonary embolism.

Benefits: **Anticoagulation:** We found no systematic review. We found one RCT (published 1960; 35 people with pulmonary embolism) comparing heparin plus warfarin with no anticoagulation.[26] It found that anticoagulation reduced mortality (0/16 deaths [0%] with anticoagulation v 5/19 deaths [26%] with no anticoagulation; NNT 4, 95% CI 2 to 16). We found no RCTs of heparin versus placebo, warfarin versus placebo, or heparin plus warfarin versus heparin alone or warfarin alone. **Duration and intensity of anticoagulation:** We found no direct evidence in people with pulmonary embolism alone.

Evidence for intensity and duration of treatment has been extrapolated from studies in people with proximal DVT and any venous thromboembolism. These trials found that bleeding rates were increased by higher INR target ranges (INR 3.0–4.5), but recurrence rates were not significantly different compared with a lower range (INR 2.0–3.0), and that longer courses of anticoagulation reduced recurrence compared with shorter courses (see benefits of anticoagulation under treatments for isolated calf vein thrombosis, p 164). **LMWH versus unfractionated heparin:** We found no systematic review. We found two RCTs. The first (612 people with symptomatic pulmonary embolism who did not receive thrombolysis or embolectomy) found no significant difference in the death rate with subcutaneous LMWH (tinzaparin) versus intravenous heparin (AR 12/304 [3.9%] with tinzaparin v 14/308 [4.5%] with heparin; P = 0.7) or recurrent thromboembolism (5/304 [1.6%] with tinzaparin v 6/308 [1.9%] with heparin; P = 0.8).[27] The second RCT (200 people at study entry with proximal DVT without clinical signs or symptoms of pulmonary embolism but with high probability lung scan findings) found that fixed dose subcutaneous heparin given once daily versus dose adjusted intravenous heparin reduced the number of new episodes of venous thromboembolism (ARs 0/97 [0%] with LMWH v 7/103 [6.8%] with intravenous heparin; P = 0.01).[28]

Harms: The first RCT comparing LMWH versus unfractionated heparin found no significant difference in the rate of major haemorrhage (3/304 [1.0%] with LMWH v 5/308 [1.6%] with unfractionated heparin; P = 0.5).[27] The second RCT also found no significant difference in the risk of major bleeding with LMWH and intravenous heparin (1/97 [1%] with LMWH v 2/103 [2%] with intravenous heparin; P = 0.6).[28] (See harms of anticoagulants under treatments for proximal DVT, p 163).

Comment: In the two RCTs,[27–28] the incidence of major haemorrhage was low and the number of people in these RCTs was too small to detect a clinically important difference.

QUESTION **What are the effects of computerised decision support on oral anticoagulation management?** New

We found no RCTs of computerised decision support versus usual management of oral anticoagulation that used clinically important outcomes (major haemorrhage or death). Three systematic reviews and three subsequent RCTs have found that computerised decision support in oral anticoagulation improves time spent in the target INR range. Most RCTs were small and brief.

Benefits: **Clinical outcomes:** We found no systematic review and no RCTs. **Laboratory outcomes:** We found three systematic reviews[29–31] and three subsequent RCTs.[32–34] One systematic review specifically addressed computerised decision support (see glossary, p 166) in oral anticoagulation management and two included oral anticoagulation management in addition to other forms of computerised decision support. The first (search date 1997, 9 RCTs, 1336 people) included eight RCTs using warfarin and one using heparin.[29] The computer systems advised the doses for initiation of anticoagulation (2 RCTs) and for maintenance of anticoagulation (6 RCTs).

Follow up was short (15 days–12 months). Indication for treatment included cardiac diseases and venous thrombosis. The outcome reported by seven of the nine RCTs (1327 people) in the systematic review was the proportion of days within the target range of anticoagulation. The review found that computerised decision support versus usual care increased the time that the INR was in the target range (OR 1.29, 95% CI 1.17 to 1.49). One included trial (small and with the largest effect) introduced significant heterogeneity between the trials and was therefore excluded (OR for remaining RCTs 1.25, 95% CI 1.1 to 1.5). The other two systematic reviews included a wider range of computer support for determining drug dose and included seven[30] and four[31] RCTs of the nine found by the first systematic review.[29] The first subsequent RCT assessed warfarin management after hip replacement (71 people with usual care and 51 people managed with computerised decision support).[32] Only initiation of warfarin was studied. It found no significant difference in the time taken to reach therapeutic levels of anticoagulation (4.7 v 2.8 days). The second RCT compared a specific computerised decision support with physician adjusted dosing in five hospitals.[33] People who were taking warfarin for at least 6 days were selected (285 people) and followed for at least 3 months (results from 254 [89%] were analysed). People managed by computerised decision support spent more time with their INR in the target range than people managed conventionally (63% v 53%; P < 0.05). The third study compared a package of care that included computerised decision support with traditional hospital outpatient management. The intervention was based in primary care: a practice nurse clinic included near patient INR testing and computerised decision support. After 12 months, analysis of 224 people (122 intervention, 102 controls) found more time spent in the target range (69% v 57%; P < 0.001) but no difference in the proportion of tests in range (61% with intervention v 51% with control) or in the point prevalence of tests in range (71% v 62%).[34]

Harms: **Major haemorrhage:** See glossary, p 167. One systematic review (7 RCTs, 1336 people) reported the incidence of major haemorrhage.[29] There were 14 major haemorrhages among 700 (2%) people with computerised decision support and 25 among 636 (3.9%) in the control group. Most of the events occurred in one study making meta-analysis inappropriate. One RCT found no significant difference in overall death rates or serious adverse events with computerised decision support versus usual care.[34]

Comment: We found only limited evidence (from small trials with short follow up of proxy outcomes) on the use of computerised decision support in oral anticoagulation management. Computerised decision support for oral anticoagulation appears at least as effective as human performance in terms of time spent in the target INR range. It is not clear if this will translate to improved clinical outcomes. Larger and longer trials that measure clinical outcomes (particularly harms) are needed.

GLOSSARY

Computerised decision support system A computer program that provides advice on the significance and implications of clinical findings or laboratory results.

International normalised ratio (INR) A value derived from a standardised laboratory test that measures the effect of an anticoagulant. The laboratory materials used in the test are calibrated against internationally accepted standard reference preparations, so that variability between laboratories and different reagents is minimised. Normal blood has an INR of 1. Therapeutic anticoagulation often aims to achieve an INR value of 2–3.5.

Low molecular weight heparins (LMWH) are manufactured from heparin, by using chemical or enzymatic methods. The various formulations of LMWH differ in mean molecular weight, composition, and anticoagulant activity. As a group, LMWHs have distinct properties and it is not yet clear that one LMWH will behave exactly like another. Some subcutaneously administered LMWHs do not require monitoring.

Major haemorrhage Exact definitions vary between studies but usually a major haemorrhage is one involving intracranial, retroperitoneal, joint or muscle bleeding leading directly to death or requiring admission to hospital to stop the bleeding or provide a blood transfusion. All other haemorrhages are classified as minor.

Substantive changes since last issue

Proximal DVT anticoagulation A second systematic review[14] that included four RCTs excluded on methodological grounds from the first systematic review.[13] The new review found that longer versus short duration of anticoagulation reduced the risk of recurrent thromboembolism but had no significant effect on major haemorrhage; overall conclusions unaltered.

Proximal DVT anticoagulation A new systematic review[22] including many of the same trials as earlier reviews. It found similar results as the earlier reviews.[19-21]

Intervention table Reinterpretation of available evidence has led to recategorisation of most options to the "Trade off between benefits and harms" category. People with thromboembolism have different risk profiles. The balance of benefit and harms will vary between people.

REFERENCES

1. Nordstrom M, Linblad B, Bergqvist D, Kjellstrom. A prospective study of the incidence of deep-vein thrombosis within a defined urban population. *Arch Intern Med* 1992;326:155–160.
2. Hansson PO, Werlin L, Tibblin G, Eriksson H. Deep vein thrombosis and pulmonary embolism in the general population. *Arch Intern Med* 1997;157: 1665–1670.
3. Rubinstein I, Murray D, Hoffstein V. Fatal pulmonary emboli in hospitalised patients: an autopsy study. *Arch Intern Med* 1988;148:1425–1426.
4. Hirsh J, Hoak J. Management of deep vein thrombosis and pulmonary embolism. *Circulation* 1996;93:2212–2245.
5. Farley TMM, Meirik O, Chang CL, Marmot MG, Poulter NR. Effects of different progestogens in low oestrogen oral contraceptives on venous thromboembolic disease. *Lancet* 1995;346: 1582–1588.
6. Lagerstedt C, Olsson C, Fagher B, Oqvist B, Albrechtsson U. Need for long term anticoagulant treatment in symptomatic calf vein thrombosis. *Lancet* 1985;334:515–518.
7. Lohr J, Kerr T, Lutter K, Cranley R, Spirtoff K, Cranley J. Lower extremity calf thrombosis: to treat or not to treat? *J Vasc Surg* 1991;14:618–623.
8. Kakkar VV, Howe CT, Flanc C, Clarke MB. Natural history of postoperative deep vein thrombosis. *Lancet* 1969;2:230–232.
9. Zilliacus H. On the specific treatment of thrombosis and pulmonary embolism with anticoagulants, with a particular reference to the post thrombotic sequelae. *Acta Med Scand* 1946; 170:1–221.
10. Giannoukas AD, Labropoulos N, Burke P, Katsamouris A, Nicolaides AN. Calf deep vein thrombosis: a review of the literature. *Eur J Vasc Endovasc Surg* 1995;10:398–404.
11. Lensing AWA, Prandoni P, Prins MH, Buller HR. Deep-vein thrombosis. *Lancet* 1999;353:479–485.
12. Brandjes DPM, Heijboer H, Buller HR, Rijk M, Jagt H, ten Cate JW. Acenocoumarol and heparin compared with acenocoumarol alone in the initial treatment of proximal thrombosis. *N Engl J Med* 1992;327:1485–1489.
13. Hutten BA, Prins MH. Duration of treatment with vitamin K antagonists in symptomatic venous thromboembolism. In: The Cochrane Library. Issue 4, 2000. Oxford: Update Software. Search date January 2000; primary sources Medline; Embase; hand searching relevant journals, and personal contacts.
14. Pinede L, Duhaut P, Cucherat M, Ninet J, Pasquier J, Boissel JP. Comparison of long versus short duration of anticoagulant therapy after a first episode of venous thromboembolism: a meta-analysis of randomized, controlled trials. *J Intern Med* 2000;247:553–562. Search date not specified; primary sources Medline, Embase, Cochrane Controlled Trials Register, and hand searched reference lists.
15. Hull R, Hirsh J, Jay RM, et al. Different intensities of oral anticoagulant therapy in the treatment of

proximal vein thrombosis. *N Engl J Med* 1982; 307:1676–1681.

16. Ascani A, Iorio A, Agnelli G. Withdrawal of warfarin after deep vein thrombosis: effects of a low fixed dose on rebound thrombin generation. *Blood Coagul Fibrinolysis* 1999;10:291–295.

17. Leisorovicz A, Simonneau G, Decousous H, Boissel JP. Comparison of efficacy and safety of low molecular weight heparins and unfractionated heparin in initial treatment of deep venous thrombosis: a meta-analysis. *BMJ* 1994;309: 299–304. Search date December 1993; primary sources Medline and hand searched references.

18. Lensing AWA, Prins MH, Davidson BL, Hirsh J. Treatment of deep venous thrombosis with low-molecular weight heparins. *Arch Intern Med* 1995; 155:601–607. Search date 1994; primary sources Medline 1984 to 1994; manual search and hand searched references.

19. Van den Belt AGM, Prins MH, Lensing AWA, et al. Fixed dose subcutaneous low molecular weight heparins versus adjusted dose unfractionated heparin for venous thromboembolism. In: The Cochrane Library, Issue 4. Oxford: Update Software. Search date July 1999; primary sources Medline, Embase, and LILACS; contact with researchers and pharmaceutical companies; and hand searched references.

20. Dolovich LR, Ginsberg JS, Douketis JD, Holbrook AM, Cheah G. A meta-analysis comparing low-molecular-weight heparins with unfractionated heparin in the treatment of venous thromboembolism. *Arch Intern Med* 2000;160: 181–188. Search date 1996; primary sources Medline; HEALTH; and The Cochrane Library; and hand searched references.

21. Bijsterveld NR, Hettiarachchi R, Peters R, Prins MH, Levi M, Buller HR. Low-molecular weight heparins in venous and arterial thrombotic disease. *Thromb Haemost* 1999;82(suppl 1):139–147. Search date 1999; primary sources Medline 1996 to 1999; Embase 1996 to 1999; principal study investigators; and hand searched references.

22. Rohan JK, Hettiarachchi RJ, Prins MH, Lensing AW, Buller HR. Low molecular weight heparin versus unfractionated heparin in the initial treatment of venous thromboembolism. *Curr Opin Pulmon Med* 1998;4:220–225. Search date not stated; primary sources Medline, Current Contents, Embase.

23. Belcaro G, Nicolaides AN, Cesarone MR, et al. Comparison of low-molecular-weight heparin, administered primarily at home, with unfractionated heparin, administered in hospital, and subcutaneous heparin, administered at home for deep-vein thrombosis. *Angiology* 1999;50:781–787.

24. Landefeld CS, Beyth RJ. Anticoagulant related bleeding: clinical epidemiology, prediction, and prevention. *Am J Med* 1993;95:315–328.

25. Levine MN, Hirsh J, Landefeld CS, Raskob G. Haemorrhagic complications of anticoagulant treatment. *Chest* 1992;102(suppl):352–363.

26. Barrit DW, Jordan SC. Anticoagulant drugs in the treatment of pulmonary embolism: a controlled trial. *Lancet* 1960;i:1309–1312.

27. Simonneau G, Sors H, Charbonnier B, et al. A comparison of low-molecular weight heparin with unfractionated heparin for acute pulmonary embolism. *N Engl J Med* 1997;337:663–669.

28. Hull RD, Raskob GE, Brant RF, et al. Low-molecular-weight heparin vs heparin in the treatment of patients with pulmonary embolism. American-Canadian Thrombosis Study Group. *Arch Intern Med* 2000;160:229–236.

29. Chatellier G, Colombet I, Degoulet P. An overview of the effect of computer-assisted management of anticoagulant therapy on the quality of anticoagulation. *Int J Med Informatics* 1998;49: 311–320. Search date 1997; primary source Medline.

30. Hunt DL, Haynes RB, Hanna SE, Smith, K. Effects of computer-based clinical decision support systems on physician performance and patient outcomes: a systematic review. *JAMA* 1998;280: 1339–1346. Search date not specified; primary sources Medline, Embase, Inspec, SciSearch, Cochrane Library, and hand searching of reference lists and personal contact with authors.

31. Walton R, Dovey S, Harvey E, Freemantle N. Computer support for determining drug dose: systematic review and meta-analysis. *BMJ* 1999; 318:984–990. Search date 1996, primary sources Specialised Register of Studies from Cochrane Collaboration on Effective Professional Practice, Medline, Embase, hand search of *Therapeutic Drug Monitoring* 1993–1996; contact with experts and pharmaceutical companies.

32. Motykie GD, Mokhtee D, Zebala LP, Caprinin JA, Kudma JC, Mungall DR. The use of a Bayseian Forecasting Model in the management of warfarin therapy after total hip arthroplasty. *J Arthroplasty* 1999;14:988–993.

33. Poller L, Shiach CR, MacCallum PK, et al. Multicentre randomised study of computerised anticoagulant dosage. European Concerted Action on Anticoagulation *Lancet* 1998;352:1505–1509.

34. Fitzmaurice DA, Hobbs FDR, Murray ET, Holder RL, Allan TF, Rose PE. Oral anticoagulation management in primary care with the use of computerized decision support and near-patient testing. Randomized Controlled Trial. *Arch Intern Med* 2000;160:2343–2348.

David Fitzmaurice
Senior Lecturer

FD Richard Hobbs
Professor

Richard McManus

Clinical Research Fellow, Department of Primary Care and General Practice, The Medical School, University of Birmingham, Birmingham, UK

Competing interests: RM none declared. FDRH is a member of the European Society of Cardiology (ESC) Working Party on Heart Failure, Treasurer of the British Society for Heart Failure, and Chair of the British Primary Care Cardiovascular Society (PCCS). He has received travel sponsorship and honoraria from a number of multinational biotechnology and pharmaceutical companies with cardiovascular products for plenary talks and attendance at major cardiology scientific congresses and conferences. DF has received reimbursement for attendance at scientific meetings from Leo Laboratories who make tinzaparin, a low molecular weight heparin. The Department of Primary Care and General Practice at the University of Birmingham, where the authors work, has a computerised decision support programme that is commercially available.

Search date November 2000: expanded this issue

Madhu Natarajan

INTERVENTIONS

Beneficial
Aspirin 171
Low molecular weight heparins
    added to aspirin. 174

Likely to be beneficial
Intravenous glycoprotein IIb/IIIa
    inhibitors. 172
Unfractionated heparin added
    to aspirin. 174

**Trade off between benefits and
    harms**
Ticlopidine 171
Hirudin. 175

Unknown effectiveness
Nitrates 176
β Blockers 176
Routine early invasive treatment
    for all people with unstable
    angina 177

Unlikely to be beneficial
Calcium channel blockers 176

Likely to be ineffective or harmful
Oral glycoprotein IIb/IIIa
    inhibitors New 173

**To be covered in future issues of
    *Clinical Evidence***
Clopidogrel

Key Messages

- One systematic review of RCTs has found that aspirin reduces the risk of death or myocardial infarction (MI) in people with unstable angina.
- One RCT found that ticlopidine was significantly more effective than conventional treatment (without aspirin) in unstable angina, but was associated with a significant risk of neutropenia.
- RCTs have found that intravenous glycoprotein IIb/IIIa inhibitors may improve outcome in people who undergo early percutaneous interventions when added to aspirin plus heparin, or heparin alone.
- Two RCTs have no significant difference in outcome between oral glycoprotein IIb/IIIa inhibitors versus, or in addition to, aspirin. One RCT has found that orbofiban versus placebo significantly increased mortality at 30 days.
- Two systematic reviews have found that the benefit of adding unfractionated heparin to aspirin is small. One systematic review has found that adding low molecular weight heparins (LMWH) to aspirin significantly reduces the short term rates of death and MI in people with unstable angina. One systematic review found no significant difference in benefits between LMWH and unfractionated heparin. One systematic review comparing short term treatment with LMWH versus unfractionated heparin found no significant difference in the frequency of major bleeding, and found that long term LMWH is associated with a significant increase in the risk of major bleeding compared with placebo.

Unstable angina

- RCTs have found that hirudin versus unfractionated heparin in people also taking aspirin reduces short term but not medium term rates of death or MI.
- One systematic review found no evidence that calcium channel blockers prevent death or MI in people with unstable angina.
- We found that the effects of nitrates or β blockers in people with unstable angina have not yet been adequately evaluated.
- Three RCTs found little evidence that routine early invasive treatment reduces mortality compared with initial medical treatment plus, later, more selective intervention.

DEFINITION Unstable angina is distinguished from stable angina, acute MI, and non-cardiac pain, by the pattern (characteristic pain present at rest or on lower levels of activity) or severity (recently increasing intensity, frequency, or duration) of symptoms, and the absence of persistent ST elevation on a resting electrocardiogram (ECG). Unstable angina includes a variety of different clinical patterns: angina at rest of up to 1 week's duration; angina increasing in severity to moderate or severe pain; non-Q wave MI; and post-MI angina continuing for more than 24 hours.

INCIDENCE/ PREVALENCE In industrialised countries the annual incidence of unstable angina is about six of 10 000 people in the general population.

AETIOLOGY/ RISK FACTORS Risk factors are the same as for other manifestations of ischaemic heart disease: older age, previous atheromatous cardiovascular disease, diabetes mellitus, smoking cigarettes, hypertension, hypercholesterolaemia, male sex, and a family history of ischaemic heart disease. Unstable angina can also occur in association with other disorders of the circulation, including heart valve disease, arrhythmia, and cardiomyopathy.

PROGNOSIS In people taking aspirin, the incidence of serious adverse outcomes (such as death, acute MI, or refractory angina requiring emergency revascularisation) is 5–10% within the first 7 days and about 15% at 30 days. Between 5% and 14% of people with unstable angina die in the year after diagnosis, with about half of these deaths occurring within 4 weeks of diagnosis. No single factor identifies people at higher risk of an adverse event. Risk factors include severity of presentation (e.g. duration of pain, rapidity of progression, evidence of heart failure), medical history (e.g. previous unstable angina, acute MI, left ventricular dysfunction), other clinical parameters (e.g. age, diabetes), ECG changes (e.g. severity of ST segment depression, deep T wave inversion, transient ST elevation), biochemical parameters (e.g. troponin concentration), and change in clinical status (e.g. recurrent chest pain, silent ischaemia, haemodynamic instability).

AIMS To relieve pain and ischaemia; to prevent death and MI; to identify people at high risk requiring revascularisation; to facilitate early hospital discharge in people at low and medium risk; to modify risk factors; to prevent death, MI, and recurrent ischaemia after discharge from hospital, with minimum adverse effects.

OUTCOMES	Rate of death or MI (often measured at 2, 7, and 30 days, and 6 months after randomisation); adverse effects of treatment. Some RCTs include rates of refractory ischaemia or re-admission for unstable angina.
METHODS	*Clinical Evidence* update search and appraisal November 2000.

QUESTION What are the effects of antiplatelet treatments?

OPTION ASPIRIN

One systematic review has found that aspirin alone reduces the risk of death and MI in people with unstable angina. The evidence suggests no added cardiovascular benefit, and possible added harm, from doses of aspirin over 325 mg daily.

Benefits:	One systematic review (search date 1990, 145 RCTs, 100 000 people) compared antiplatelet treatment versus placebo.[1] Seven of these trials included a total of 4000 people with unstable angina. The review found that antiplatelet treatment (mostly medium dose aspirin, 75–325 mg daily) reduced the combined outcome of vascular death, MI, or stroke at 6 months (AR 14% on placebo v 9% on antiplatelet treatment; RR 0.65, 95% CI 0.51 to 0.79). This means that 20 people would need to be treated with aspirin rather than placebo to prevent one additional event in 6 months (NNT 20, 95% CI 15 to 34). Individual trials within the systematic review showed consistent benefit from daily aspirin in terms of reduced deaths and MI.
Harms:	The review found that people taking doses of aspirin ranging from 75 to 1200 mg daily had no significant adverse events, including gastrointestinal intolerance or bleeding.[1] However, the sum of the evidence suggests no added cardiovascular benefit, and greater incidence of gastrointestinal effects, for aspirin doses greater than 325 mg daily. Some people are allergic to aspirin.
Comment:	The systematic review covered a wide range of people with different morbidities and levels of risk. Its results should be generalisable to routine practice.[1] People with unstable angina who are allergic or who do not respond to aspirin will need alternative antiplatelet treatment.

OPTION TICLOPIDINE

One RCT found that ticlopidine was more effective than conventional treatment (without aspirin) in people with unstable angina, but it was associated with a significant risk of reversible neutropenia. Ticlopidine may therefore be an alternative in people who are intolerant of, or allergic to, aspirin.

Benefits:	We found no systematic review of ticlopidine in unstable angina. One RCT compared ticlopidine versus conventional treatment without aspirin in 652 people (72% male) with unstable angina treated within 48 hours of admission.[2] At 6 months, there were significantly fewer vascular deaths or non-fatal MI in people taking ticlopidine (RR compared with control 0.54, 95% CI 0.19 to 0.88; NNT for 6

Cardiovascular disorders

months 16, 95% CI 9 to 62). We found no trial of ticlopidine versus aspirin in the treatment of unstable angina.

Harms: Reversible neutropenia was reported in 1–2% of people taking ticlopidine. Other adverse effects include diarrhoea and rash.

Comment: Ticlopidine is an alternative for people with unstable angina who are intolerant of, or allergic to, aspirin. A large study is currently comparing clopidogrel plus aspirin versus aspirin alone in this group of people.

OPTION **INTRAVENOUS GLYCOPROTEIN IIB/IIIA PLATELET RECEPTOR INHIBITORS**

RCTs have found that adding parenteral glycoprotein IIb/IIIa inhibitors to unfractionated heparin alone or unfractionated heparin plus aspirin reduces deaths and MI. However, this was in the context of high rates of early percutaneous interventions.

Benefits: We found no systematic review, but found three RCTs that assessed adding intravenous glycoprotein IIb/IIIa inhibitors to standard treatment,[3–5] and three RCTs that compared a glycoprotein IIb/IIIa inhibitor versus heparin.[3,5,6] The primary end points varied, but all trials included data on death rates and MI at 30 days (see table 1, p 180). **Added to heparin or aspirin or both:** The first RCT (1915 people with unstable angina or non-Q wave MI) with three treatment arms compared tirofiban, heparin, or both, as an infusion for a mean of 72 hours.[3] The tirofiban alone group was stopped early because of excess mortality at 7 days (AR of death at 7 days, 4.6% with tirofiban alone v 1.1% with heparin alone). The RCT found that compared with heparin alone, tirofiban plus heparin reduced rates of death, MI, or refractory ischaemia (at 7 days, AR 12.9% with tirofiban plus heparin v 17.9% with heparin, RR 0.68, 95% CI 0.53 to 0.88, P = 0.004; at 30 days, AR 18.5% with tirofiban plus heparin v 22.3% with heparin, P = 0.03; at 6 months, AR 27.7% with tirofiban plus heparin v 32.1% with heparin, P = 0.02). Early angiography and intervention were encouraged in this trial. The second RCT (9461 people with unstable angina) compared eptifibatide plus heparin plus aspirin versus heparin plus aspirin. The trial found modest benefit when eptifibatide was added to aspirin and unfractionated heparin (deaths and non-fatal MI at 30 days, eptifibatide 11.6% v placebo 16.7%, P = 0.01). No benefit was seen in people with low rates of intervention with percutaneous transluminal coronary angioplasty (PTCA).[4] The third RCT (2282 people), which included five treatment arms, compared high dose lamifiban with and without heparin versus low dose lamifiban with and without heparin versus heparin plus placebo.[5] The trial found that rates of ischaemic events were similar with high dose lamifiban plus heparin versus heparin plus placebo, but that the combination of low dose lamifiban and heparin reduced ischaemic events (AR of ischaemic event at 6 months, 12.6% with low dose lamifiban plus heparin v 17.9% with heparin plus placebo, P = 0.025). **Versus heparin:** One RCT (3232 people who were already taking aspirin) compared intravenous tirofiban versus heparin for 48 hours.[6] The primary composite end point of death, MI, or refractory ischaemia at 48 hours was significantly lower on tirofiban (AR 3.8% v 5.6%; RR

0.67, 95% CI 0.48 to 0.92), but at 30 days there was no significant difference in the end point of death or MI (see table 1, p 180). The RCT that included five treatment arms (high and low dose lamifiban ± heparin versus heparin plus placebo) was able to compare low and high dose lamifiban alone versus heparin. It found no significant difference in combined outcome of death or non-fatal MI at 30 days between heparin alone, low dose lamifiban alone, or high dose lamifiban alone (AR of death or MI, 11.7% with heparin v 10.6% with low dose lamifiban v 12.0% with high dose lamifiban, P = 0.67).[5] However, at 6 months there were significantly fewer deaths or MI in people on low dose lamifiban alone, compared with high dose lamifiban alone or heparin alone (AR of death or MI, 13.7% with low dose lamifiban v 16.4% with high dose lamifiban v 17.9% with heparin). One further RCT, which included three arms (tirofiban v heparin v both) found that tirofiban alone increased mortality at 7 days compared with other treatments.[3] This arm of the trial was therefore stopped early (see benefits section above).[3]

Harms: No significant difference was reported in rates of major bleeding between tirofiban and heparin (AR 0.4% in both groups).[6] When high dose lamifiban was added to heparin, there were significantly more intermediate or major bleeds versus heparin alone (AR 12.1% v 5.5%, P = 0.002), although bleeding rates were similar with low dose lamifiban plus heparin compared with heparin plus placebo.[5] Reversible thrombocytopenia occurred more frequently with tirofiban than with heparin (AR 1.1% v 0.4%, P = 0.04).[6]

Comment: The smaller trial of adding a glycoprotein IIb/IIIa inhibitor to standard treatment[5] suggests that a "dose ceiling" may exist beyond which escalation of dose results in higher bleeding complications with no increase in efficacy.

OPTION	ORAL GLYCOPROTEIN IIB/IIIA PLATELET RECEPTOR INHIBITORS

New

Two RCTs have found no significant difference in outcome between oral glycoprotein IIb/IIIa inhibitors versus, or in addition to, aspirin. One RCT found that orbofiban versus placebo significantly increased mortality at 30 days.

Benefits: We found no systematic review. **Versus aspirin:** One RCT (9233 people, 75% with non-Q wave MI) compared aspirin versus low dose sibrafiban (designed to achieve ≥25% inhibition of platelet aggregation) or high dose sibrafiban (designed to achieve ≥50% inhibition of platelet aggregation).[7] The dose of sibrafiban ranged from 3–6 mg. The RCT found no significant difference between aspirin versus sibrafiban in the primary composite end point of death, MI, or severe recurrent ischaemia after 90 days of treatment (aspirin v low dose sibrafiban [9.8%] v [10.1%]; OR 1.03, 95% CI 0.87 to 1.21: aspirin v high dose sibrafiban [9.8%] v [10.1%]; OR 1.03, 95% CI 0.87 to 1.21). **Versus placebo:** One RCT (10 288 people, 60% with non-Q wave MI) compared orbofiban (50 mg twice daily) or orbofiban (50 mg twice daily for 30 days, then 30 mg twice daily thereafter) versus placebo.[8] All people received aspirin prior to randomisation. It found no significant difference between orbofiban versus placebo in the primary composite end point of death, MI, recurrent ischaemia, urgent revascularisation, or stroke after 30 days (orbofiban groups combined v placebo, 9.9% v 10.8%, P = 0.12), or after 10 months (orbofiban fixed dose v placebo, 22.8% v 22.9%, P = 0.59; variable dose v placebo, 23.1% v 22.9%, P = 0.41), but found a significant increase in mortality at 30 days (orbofiban groups combined v placebo, 2.0% v 1.4%, P = 0.02), which did not quite reach significance at 10 months (orbofiban variable dose v placebo, 5.1% v 3.7%, P = 0.09). The unexpected increased mortality resulted in premature termination of the trial.[8]

Harms: The first RCT found that major bleeding was increased in people taking sibrafiban versus placebo, but was only significant for high dose sibrafiban.[7] The second RCT found that major or severe bleeding (excluding intracranial haemorrhage) was significantly increased in both orbofiban groups (fixed dose v placebo, 4.5% v 2.0%, P < 0.0001; variable dose 3.7% v 2.0%, P = 0.0004).[8]

Comment: None.

QUESTION   What are the effects of antithrombin treatments?

OPTION   UNFRACTIONATED HEPARIN

Two systematic reviews of six small RCTs have found benefit from adding unfractionated heparin to aspirin in people with unstable angina, but this may have occurred by chance.

Benefits: **Added to aspirin:** We found two systematic reviews that met our quality criteria.[9,10] Both included the same six RCTs in 1353 people with unstable angina who were treated with either heparin and aspirin or aspirin alone for 2–7 days. The first review (search date not stated) found that the risk of death or MI during treatment with heparin plus aspirin was less than that for aspirin alone (AR 55/698 [8%] v 68/655 [10%]); but was not significantly different (OR 0.67, 95% CI 0.44 to 1.02).[9] The second review (search date not stated) used a different statistical method for meta-analysis and found a result that just reached statistical significance (OR 0.67, 95% CI 0.45 to 0.99).[10] The first systematic review also found no significant difference between the two groups (from 4 RCTs with data available) in the rate of death or MI at 12 weeks (AR 12% on heparin plus aspirin v 14% on aspirin alone; RR 0.82, 95% CI 0.56 to 1.20).[9] **Versus LMWH:** See benefits of LMWH, p 175.

Harms: Major bleeding occurred in 0.4% of people on aspirin and 1.5% of those on aspirin plus heparin (RR 1.89, 95% CI 0.66 to 5.38).[9]

Comment: In this situation it is not clear which statistical method is preferred.

OPTION   LOW MOLECULAR WEIGHT HEPARINS

One systematic review has found that aspirin plus LMWH is more effective than aspirin alone in the first 30 days after an episode of unstable angina. One systematic review found no significant difference in benefits between LMWH and unfractionated heparin. One systematic review comparing short term treatment with LMWH versus unfractionated

heparin found no significant difference in the frequency of major bleeding, and found that long term LMWH is associated with a significant increase in the risk of major bleeding compared with placebo.

Benefits: **Adding LMWH to aspirin:** We found one systematic review (search date not stated, 2 RCTs, 1639 people),[10] which compared LMWH for up to 7 days versus placebo or untreated control. The review found a reduction in death or MI with LMWH (OR 0.34, 95% CI 0.20 to 0.58). The same systematic review found five RCTs (12 099 people) comparing long term LMWH versus placebo. The review found no benefit of long term LMWH given for up to 90 days (OR for death or MI, LMWH v placebo 0.98, 95% CI 0.81 to 1.17). **Versus unfractionated heparin:** We found one systematic review of five RCTs (12 171 people),[10] which compared an equal duration (maximum 8 days) of LMWH versus unfractionated heparin. The review found no significant difference between treatments (OR for death or MI, LMWH v unfractionated heparin 0.88, 95% CI 0.69 to 1.12).

Harms: One systematic review comparing LMWH versus unfractionated heparin found no significant difference in the frequency of major bleeds between treatments (OR 1.00, 95% CI 0.64 to 1.57)[10] (see harms of unfractionated heparin, p 174). Long term LMWH versus placebo significantly increases the risk of major bleeding (OR 2.26, 95% CI 1.63 to 3.14), equivalent to an excess of 12 bleeds for every 1000 people treated.[10]

Comment: LMWH may be more attractive than unfractionated heparin for routine short term use because coagulation monitoring is not required and it can be self administered after discharge.

OPTION   **HIRUDIN**

RCTs have found that in people with unstable angina taking aspirin, rates of death and MI are significantly lower during infusion of hirudin than during infusion of unfractionated heparin. However, no added benefit is found once the infusion stops. Longer durations of hirudin infusion (> 72 hours) are currently being evaluated. Compared with heparin, hirudin causes significantly more major bleeds requiring transfusion but no more life threatening bleeds or haemorrhagic strokes.

Benefits: We found no systematic review. **Versus unfractionated heparin:** Three large RCTs (>19 000 people with unstable angina taking aspirin, compared R-hirudin versus unfractionated heparin given for 2–3 days.[11–13] A pooled analysis of these trials found reduced risk of cardiovascular death or MI at the end of the 72 hour treatment period (AR 233/9615 [2.4%] for hirudin, 315/9446 [3.3%] for heparin; ARR 0.9%, 95% CI 0.5% to 1.3%; RR 0.77, 95% CI 0.61 to 0.86), with some loss of this early benefit at 7 days (RR 0.83, 95% CI 0.73 to 0.94) and 35 days (RR 0.91, 95% CI 0.83 to 1.0).

Harms: In the largest RCT, hirudin versus unfractionated heparin was associated with a significant increase in the need for transfusion (AR 10.2% v 8.4%, P = 0.01), and a trend for increased extracranial haemorrhage (AR 10.2% v 8.6%, P = 0.06) and intracranial haemorrhage (AR 0.2% v 0.02%, P = 0.06).[11] In the second largest RCT, hirudin was associated with an excess of major bleeding

(AR 1.2% v 0.7%; RR 1.71, 95% CI 1.13 to 2.58) but no increase in life threatening bleeds or strokes at day 7.[13] The smallest RCT reported no haemorrhagic strokes and no difference in the rate of major bleeds (about 1% in all groups).[12] Hirudin was associated with a higher rate of minor bleeding (AR 16.2% low dose hirudin [LDHir] v 21.3% medium dose hirudin [MDHir] v 10.5% heparin; RR LDHir v heparin 1.54, 95% CI 1.03 to 2.31; RR MDHir v heparin 2.03, 95% CI 1.39 to 2.96).[12]

Comment: Whether longer duration of treatment has greater benefits is the target of future trials (S Yusuf, personal communication). Two of the RCTs gave doses of hirudin in proportion to the body weight, but gave heparin as a fixed dose.[11,12]

QUESTION What are the effects of anti-ischaemic treatments?

OPTION NITRATES, β BLOCKERS, AND CALCIUM CHANNEL BLOCKERS

We found insufficient evidence on the effects of nitrates, β blockers, and calcium channel blockers on rates of death or MI. Short acting dihydropyridine calcium channel blockers may increase mortality.

Benefits: **Nitrates:** We found no systematic reviews or RCTs of nitrates versus placebo in unstable angina. We found one RCT (162 people with unstable angina) of intravenous glyceryl trinitrate versus placebo for 48 hours. Those receiving glyceryl trinitrate had fewer episodes of chest pain, less severe episodes (pain lasting ≥20 minutes), and less need for additional sublingual glyceryl trinitrate.[14] We found one RCT (200 people with unstable angina within 6 months of PTCA) comparing intravenous glyceryl trinitrate, heparin, and glyceryl trinitrate plus heparin versus placebo. The trial found that recurrent angina occurred significantly less frequently in people treated with glyceryl trinitrate alone and glyceryl trinitrate plus heparin compared with placebo, but there was no benefit from heparin alone or additional benefit from combination treatment (P < 0.003 for glyceryl trinitrate alone and for glyceryl trinitrate plus heparin v placebo)[15] **β Blockers:** We found no systematic review of β blockers versus placebo in unstable angina. We found two RCTs. The first RCT (338 people with rest angina not receiving β blocker) compared nifedipine, metoprolol, both, or neither versus placebo.[16] The main outcome was recurrent angina or MI within 48 hours. Metoprolol was significantly more effective than nifedipine. The second RCT (81 people with unstable angina on "optimal doses" of nitrates and nifedipine) compared placebo versus at least 160 mg a day of propranolol.[17] The incidence of cardiac death, MI, and requirement for coronary artery bypass grafting or percutaneous coronary interventions at 30 days did not differ significantly between the two groups (propranolol 16/42 v placebo 18/39, P = NS). People taking propranolol had a lower cumulative probability of experiencing recurrent rest angina over the first 4 days of the trial. The mean number of clinical episodes of angina, duration of angina, glyceryl trinitrate requirement, and ischaemic ST changes by continuous ECG monitoring was also lower. **Calcium channel blockers:** We found one systematic review (search date not stated). It found that calcium channel blockers reduced symptoms and ischaemia but had no effect on rates of MI or death.[18]

Harms: Hypotension is a potential adverse effect of nitrates. However, both older and more recent large RCTs in people with other ischaemic conditions showed that nitrates were safe and well tolerated when used judiciously in clinically appropriate doses. Potential adverse effects of β blockers include bradycardia, exacerbation of reactive airways disease, and hypoglycaemia in diabetics. Observational studies have reported increased mortality with short acting dihydropyridine calcium channel blockers (such as nifedipine) in people with coronary heart disease.[19,20]

Comment: We found no good evidence that anti-ischaemic drugs (nitrates, β blockers, calcium channel blockers) prevent death or MI. By consensus, until further data are available, intravenous nitrates remain a first line treatment together with heparin and aspirin in unstable angina.

QUESTION What are the effects of invasive treatments?

OPTION EARLY ROUTINE CARDIAC CATHETERISATION AND REVASCULARISATION

RCTs have found that early invasive treatment reduces symptoms and promotes early discharge compared with early conservative treatment in people with unstable angina. However, they found that early invasive treatment did not reduce rates of death and MI. We found insufficient evidence to ascertain whether certain people (e.g. those who are refractory to medical treatment) are more likely than others to benefit from early invasive treatment.

Benefits: We found no systematic review. We found three RCTs comparing early routine angiography/revascularisation versus medical treatment alone.[21–24] The largest, most recent RCT (2457 people with unstable angina) compared early invasive treatment (within the first 7 days) versus non-invasive treatment plus planned coronary angiography, followed by placebo controlled long term dalteparin for 3 months, using a factorial randomisation protocol.[24] All people were initially treated with open label dalteparin or standard heparin for up to 72 hours after admission. In people randomised to invasive treatment, 96% underwent cardiac catheterisation, and 71% underwent revascularisation within the first 10 days. The trial found that compared with early non-invasive treatment, early invasive treatment reduced the risk of the primary end point of combined death and MI at 6 months (113/1207 [9.4%] v 148/1226 [12.1%]; RR 0.78, 95% CI 0.62 to 0.98), but did not significantly reduce mortality at 6 months (23/1207 [1.9%] with early invasive treatment v 36/1226 [2.9%] with non-invasive treatment; RR 0.65, 95% CI 0.39 to 1.09). The trial also found that invasive treatment significantly reduced angina and re-admission rates (presence of angina at 6 months, 256/1174 [22%] with invasive treatment v 455/1177 [39%] with non-invasive treatment; RR 0.56, 95% CI 0.50 to 0.64, P < 0.001; re-admission during 6 month period, 357/1167 [31%] with invasive treatment v 594/1204 [49%] with non-invasive treatment, RR 0.62, 95% CI 0.60 to 0.69,

Cardiovascular disorders

$P < 0.001$). The second RCT (1473 people with unstable angina presenting within 24 hours of ischaemic chest discomfort) used a factorial design to compare tissue plasminogen activator versus placebo, and early invasive treatment (cardiac catheterisation at 18–48 hours) versus early conservative treatment.[21,22] All people received aspirin and unfractionated heparin. Within 6 weeks, 64% of people randomised to conservative treatment underwent cardiac catheterisation, 26% underwent percutaneous transluminal coronary angioplasty, and 24% underwent coronary artery bypass grafting. At 6 weeks, there was no significant difference in the composite end point of death, MI, or a symptom limited exercise stress test (invasive 18.1% v conservative 16.2%, $P = 0.78$). However, invasive treatment significantly reduced re-admission (7.8% v 14.1%, $P < 0.001$), total duration of all re-admissions (total 365 days v 930 days, $P < 0.001$), and need for antianginal medications ($P < 0.02$). At 1 year, there was no significant difference in rates of death or MI (invasive 10.8% v conservative 12.2%, $P = 0.42$), but the lower numbers of repeat hospital admissions and hospital days with invasive treatment persisted. The third and smallest RCT (920 people) compared invasive versus conservative treatment.[23] Over 23 months of follow up (range 12–44 months) there was no significant difference in the combined primary end point of death or MI (RR 0.87, 95% CI 0.68 to 1.10).

Harms: The largest, most recent RCT found that early invasive treatment increased major bleeding compared with early non-invasive treatment, but found no significant difference between treatments for ischaemic or haemorrhagic stroke (major bleeds, AR 1.6% with invasive treatment v 0.7% with non-invasive treatment, P value not given).[24] The second RCT reported no differences in complication rates (death, MI, emergency coronary artery bypass grafting, abrupt vessel closure, haemorrhage, serious hypotension) between invasive and conservative treatment (14% v 13%, $P = 0.38$).[21,22] In the smallest RCT, people who underwent early invasive treatment were significantly more at risk of death or MI at hospital discharge (36 v 15 people, $P = 0.004$), 30 days after randomisation (48 v 26 people, $P = 0.012$), and at 1 year (111 v 85 people, $P = 0.05$).[23]

Comment: All trials have reported only short term and medium term follow up, so we cannot exclude a long term difference in effect between early invasive and early non-invasive strategies. It is not clear yet whether there are subgroups of people that benefit particularly from either invasive or conservative treatment. Advances in catheterisation and revascularisation technology and periprocedural management may reduce the early risks of invasive treatment in the future.

REFERENCES

1. Antiplatelet Trialists' Collaboration. Collaborative overview of randomised trials of antiplatelet therapy. I: Prevention of death, myocardial infarction, and stroke by prolonged antiplatelet therapy in various categories of patients. *BMJ* 1994;308:81–106. Search date 1990; primary sources Medline, Current Contents.
2. Balsano F, Rizzon P, Violi F, et al, and the Studio della Ticlopidina nell'Angina Instabile Group. Antiplatelet treatment with ticlopidine in unstable angina: a controlled multicentre clinical trial.

Circulation 1990;82:17–26.
3. PRISM-PLUS Study Investigators. Inhibition of the platelet glycoprotein IIb/IIIa receptor with tirofiban in unstable angina and non-Q-wave myocardial infarction. *N Engl J Med* 1998;338:1488–1497.
4. Pursuit Trial Investigators. Inhibition of platelet glycoprotein IIb/IIIa with eptifibatide in patients with acute coronary syndromes. *N Engl J Med* 1998;339:436–443.
5. PARAGON Investigators. International, randomized, controlled trial of lamifiban (a platelet glycoprotein

IIb/IIIa inhibitor), heparin, or both in unstable angina. *Circulation* 1998;97:2386–2395.

6. PRISM Study Investigators. A comparison of aspirin plus tirofiban with aspirin plus heparin for unstable angina. *N Engl J Med* 1998;338:1498–1505.

7. The SYMPHONY Investigators. Sibrafiban versus Aspirin to Yield Maximum Protection from Ischemic Heart Events Post-acute Coronary Syndromes. *Lancet* 2000;355:337–345. Comparison of sibrafiban with aspirin for prevention of cardiovascular events after acute coronary syndromes: a randomised trial.

8. Cannon CP, McCabe CH, Wilcox RG, et al. Oral glycoprotein IIb/IIIa inhibition with orbofiban in patients with unstable coronary syndromes (OPUS-TIMI 16) trial. *Circulation* 2000;102:149–156.

9. Oler A, Whooley MA, Oler J, Grady D. Adding heparin to aspirin reduces the incidence of myocardial infarction and death in patients with unstable angina: a meta-analysis. *JAMA* 1996; 276:811–815. Search date 1995; primary sources Medline 1966 to September 1995, hand search of reference lists, consultation with experts.

10. Eikelboom JW, Anand SS, Malmberg K, et al. Unfractionated heparin and low molecular weight heparin in acute coronary syndrome without ST elevation: a meta-analysis. *Lancet* 2000;355: 1936–1942. Search date not stated; primary sources Medline and Embase, reference lists of published papers were scanned, experts canvassed for unpublished trials, personal data.

11. GUSTO IIb Investigators. A comparison of recombinant hirudin for the treatment of acute coronary syndromes. *N Engl J Med* 1996; 335:775–782.

12. OASIS Investigators. Comparison of the effects of two doses of recombinant hirudin compared with heparin in patients with acute coronary ischemia without ST elevation: a pilot study. *Circulation* 1997;96:769–777.

13. OASIS-2 Investigators. Effects of recombinant hirudin (lepirudin) compared with heparin on death, myocardial infarction, refractory angina, and revascularisation procedures in patients with acute myocardial ischaemia without ST elevation: a randomised trial. *Lancet* 1999;353:429–38.

14. Karlberg KE, Saldeen T, Wallin R, et al. Intravenous nitroglycerine reduces ischaemia in unstable angina pectoris: a double-blind placebo-controlled study. *J Intern Med* 1998;243:25–31.

15. Douchet S, Malekianpour M, Theroux P, et al. Randomized trial comparing intravenous nitroglycerin and heparin for treatment of unstable angina

secondary or restenosis after coronary artery angioplasty. *Circulation* 2000;101:955–961.

16. HINT Research Group. Early treatment of unstable angina in the coronary care unit: a randomized, double blind, placebo controlled comparison of recurrent ischaemia in patients treated with nifedipine or metoprolol or both. *Br Heart J* 1986; 56:400–413.

17. Gottlieb SO, Weisfeldt ML, Ouyang P, et al. Effect of the addition of propranolol to therapy with nifedipine for unstable angina pectoris: a randomized, double-blind, placebo-controlled trial. *Circulation* 1986;73:331–337.

18. Held PH, Yusuf S, Furberg CD. Calcium channel blockers in acute myocardial infarction and unstable angina: an overview. *BMJ* 1989;299: 1187–1192. Search date not stated; primary sources not specified in detail.

19. Furberg CD, Psaty BM, Meyer JV. Nifedipine: dose-related increase in mortality in patients with coronary heart disease. *Circulation* 1995;92: 1326–1331. Search date and primary sources not specified.

20. WHO-ISH Study. Ad hoc subcommittee of the liaison committee of the World Health Organisation and the International Society of Hypertension: effects of calcium antagonists on the risks of coronary heart disease, cancer and bleeding. *J Hypertens* 1997:15:105–115.

21. The TIMI IIIB Investigators. Effects of tissue plasminogen activator and a comparison of early invasive and conservative strategies in unstable angina and non-Q-wave myocardial infarction. Results of the TIMI IIIB trial. *Circulation* 1994;89: 1545–1556.

22. Anderson V, Cannon CP, Stone PH, et al, for the TIMI IIIB Investigators. One-year results of the thrombolysis in myocardial infarction (TIMI) IIIB clinical trial: a randomized comparison of tissue-type plasminogen activator versus placebo and early invasive versus early conservative strategies in unstable angina and non-Q wave myocardial infarction. *J Am Coll Cardiol* 1995;26:1643–1650.

23. Boden WE, O'Rourke RA, Crawford MH, et al, for the VANQWISH Trial Investigators. Outcomes in patients with acute non-Q-wave myocardial infarction randomly assigned to an invasive as compared with a conservative management strategy. *N Engl J Med* 1998;338:1785–1792.

24. Yusuf S, Zucker D, Peduzzi P, et al. Effect of coronary artery bypass graft surgery on survival: overview of 10-year results from randomized trials by the coronary artery bypass graft surgery trialists collaboration. *Lancet* 1994;344:563–570.

Madhu Natarajan
Division of Cardiology
McMaster University
Hamilton
Canada

Competing interests: None declared.

Cardiovascular disorders

TABLE 1 Effects of intravenous glycoprotein IIb/IIIa inhibitors in unstable angina and non-Q wave myocardial infarction: results of main RCTs (see text, p 172).

Trial	Total participants	Comparison	Odds reduction for death or MI at 30 days* (95% CI)	NNT to avoid one additional death or MI at 30 days
PRISM-PLUS[3]	1570	Tirofiban + heparin v heparin alone	30% (4% to 49%)	31
PURSUIT[4]	10 948	Eptifibatide + heparin v heparin alone	11% (1.3% to 20%)	67
PARAGON[5]	2282	Lamifiban + heparin v heparin alone	4% (−32% to +30%)	NA
PRISM[6]	3232	Aspirin + tirofiban v aspirin + heparin	20% (−5% to +39%)	NA

* = 1-OR, equivalent to RRR; NA, not applicable; MI, myocardial infarction.

Search date October 2000

Paddy O'Neill

QUESTIONS

INTERVENTIONS

TREATMENT

Likely to be beneficial
Non-steroidal anti-inflammatory
   drugs (NSAIDs) 183
Paracetamol. 183

Trade off between benefits and harms
Antibiotics 183

Unlikely to be beneficial
Antibiotics in children under
   2 years old with uncomplicated
   acute otitis media (AOM) . . .183

PREVENTION

Trade off between benefits and harms
Long term antibiotic
   prophylaxis 186
Xylitol syrup or gum 187

To be covered in future issues of *Clinical Evidence*
Myringotomy
Surgery

Covered elsewhere in this issue
Otitis media with effusion, p 359

Key Messages

Treatment

- We found limited evidence from one RCT that non-steroidal anti-inflammatory drugs (NSAIDs) and paracetamol may be more effective than placebo in relieving pain.
- We found conflicting evidence from two systematic reviews on the effects of antibiotics in uncomplicated acute otitis media (AOM). Rates of adverse effects are higher in children taking antibiotics compared with placebo. We found no clear evidence favouring a particular antibiotic.
- One systematic review and one subsequent RCT found no evidence that antibiotics improved outcome in children aged less than 2 years with uncomplicated AOM.
- One systematic review found greater immediate benefit but no difference in long term outcome with 10 day courses of antibiotics compared with shorter (5 day) courses.

Prevention

- One systematic review has found that long term antibiotic prophylaxis has an effect in preventing recurrence of AOM. One subsequent RCT found no significant difference between antibiotic prophylaxis and placebo.
- We found insufficient evidence on which antibiotic to use, for how long, and how many episodes of AOM justify treatment.
- We found limited evidence from one RCT that xylitol syrup or gum is effective in preventing AOM, but has significant adverse effects.

DEFINITION Otitis media is inflammation in the middle ear. Subcategories include AOM (see otitis media with effusion — also known as "glue ear", p 359), recurrent AOM, and chronic suppurative otitis media. AOM presents with systemic and local signs, and has a rapid onset. The persistence of an effusion beyond 3 months without signs of infection defines otitis media with effusion, whereas chronic suppurative otitis media is characterised by continuing inflammation in the middle ear causing otorrhoea and a perforated tympanic membrane.

INCIDENCE/ PREVALENCE AOM is common, with a high morbidity and low mortality. In the UK about 30% of children under 3 years old visit their general practitioner with AOM each year, and 97% receive antimicrobial treatment.[1] By 3 months of age, 10% of children have had an episode of AOM. It is the most common reason for outpatient antimicrobial treatment in the USA.[2] The World Health Organization estimates that each year 51 000 children under the age of 5 years die from otitis media in developing countries.[3]

AETIOLOGY/ RISK FACTORS The most common bacterial causes for AOM in the USA and UK are *Streptococcus pneumoniae*, *Haemophilus influenzae*, and *Moraxella catarrhalis*. A review that included a study conducted in Colombia showed similar pathogens in that setting.[4] The incidence of penicillin resistant *S pneumoniae* has risen, but rates differ between countries. The most important risk factors for AOM are young age and attendance at day care centres such as nursery schools. Others include white race, male sex, and a history of enlarged adenoids, tonsillitis, or asthma. Other aetiological factors include multiple previous episodes, bottle feeding, a history of ear infections in parents or siblings, and use of a soother or pacifier. The evidence for an effect of environmental tobacco smoke is controversial.[1]

PROGNOSIS In about 80% of children the condition resolves in about 3 days without antibiotic treatment. Complications are rare but include hearing loss, mastoiditis, meningitis, and recurrent attacks.[1]

AIMS To reduce the severity and duration of pain and other symptoms; to prevent complications; and to minimise adverse effects of treatment.

OUTCOMES Pain control (in infants this can be assessed by proxy measures such as parental observation of distress/crying and analgesic use); incidence of complications such as deafness (usually divided into short and long term hearing loss), recurrent attacks of AOM, mastoiditis, and meningitis; resolution of otoscopic appearances; incidence of adverse effects of treatment.

METHODS *Clinical Evidence* update search and appraisal October 2000.

QUESTION What are the effects of treatments?

OPTION ANALGESIA

One RCT found that NSAIDs and paracetamol were more effective than placebo in relieving pain. The dosing regimen for paracetamol may not have been optimal.

Benefits: We found no systematic review. We found one double blind multi-centre RCT (219 children aged 1–6 years with otoscopically diagnosed AOM) comparing three times daily treatment with ibuprofen, paracetamol, or placebo for 48 hours.[5] All children received antibiotic treatment with cefaclor. Ibuprofen was more effective than placebo in controlling pain after 2 days (AR 5/71 [7%] had otalgia after 2 days with ibuprofen v 19/75 [25%] with placebo; RR 0.28, 95% CI 0.11 to 0.71; NNT 5, 95% CI 3 to 15). In a similar way, paracetamol was more effective than placebo in controlling otalgia after 2 days (AR 7/73 [10%] with paracetamol v 19/75 [25%] with placebo; RR 0.38, 95% CI 0.17 to 0.85; NNT 6, 95% CI 3 to 28). There was no significant difference between paracetamol and ibuprofen in pain relief. There was no significant difference between placebo and active treatments for other outcomes (appearance of the tympanic membrane, rectal temperature, and parental assessment).

Harms: All treatments were well and equally tolerated.

Comment: The evidence from this trial may be limited because the assessment of the child's pain relief was based on parental observation, using a scale of 0 or 1. A reader informed us that, contrary to our conclusions, recalculation from the raw data did in fact find a significant difference between paracetamol and placebo at the 95% significance level (J Mrukowicz, personal communication, 2000). This contradicts the conclusions presented in the original article[5] and previous issues of *Clinical Evidence*. Our statisticians confirmed these figures and the text has been amended accordingly.

OPTION ANTIBIOTICS

We found conflicting evidence from systematic reviews. The more recent review found that antibiotics reduce the proportion of children still in pain at 2–7 days and reduce the risk of developing contralateral AOM. The review found that antibiotics have no effect on pain within 24 hours, and no effect on incidence of AOM or deafness at 1 month. Rates of adverse effects were higher in children on antibiotics compared with placebo. We found no clear evidence favouring a particular antibiotic. One systematic review and one subsequent RCT have found no evidence that antibiotics improve outcomes in children aged under 2 years with uncomplicated AOM.

Benefits: **Versus placebo or no treatment:** We found two systematic reviews.[6,7] The first (search date June 1992) identified four RCTs comparing antibiotics versus placebo or no treatment in 535 children aged 4 months to 18 years with AOM.[6] Co-intervention with analgesics and other symptomatic relief was allowed in most trials.

Rate of treatment success (absence of all presenting symptoms and signs about 7–14 days after treatment started) was significantly greater on active treatment (4 studies, 535 participants: ARR 13.7%, 95% CI 8.2% to 19.2%). The second systematic review (search date March 1999) identified nine RCTs comparing early use of antibiotics versus placebo in children aged 7 months to 15 years with AOM.[7] Most trials did not state the time interval between onset of symptoms and starting treatment: the two that did stated 1–24 hours and about 30 hours. Four studies reported pain outcomes 24 hours after presentation (717 children). All four found that antibiotic treatment was no more effective than placebo during that time frame (RR 1.02, 95% CI 0.85 to 1.22). Nine trials found that, 2–7 days after presentation, fewer children were still in pain after treatment with antibiotics compared with placebo (106/1043 children in pain after antibiotics v 145/1005 after placebo, ARR 4.8%, 95% CI 2.1% to 7.5%; RR 0.67, 95% CI 0.53 to 0.85), and fewer children experienced contralateral AOM (35/329 with antibiotic v 56/337 with placebo, ARR 5.9%, 95% CI 1.0% to 10.8%; RR 0.65, 95% CI 0.45 to 0.94). The trial found no significant difference in the rate of subsequent attacks of AOM (187/864 with antibiotics v 175/804 with placebo; RR 1.00, 95% CI 0.83 to 1.19), abnormal tympanometry at 1 month (85/234 with antibiotic v 91/238 with placebo; RR 0.94, 95% CI 0.74 to 1.19), or abnormal tympanometry at 3 months (38/182 with antibiotic v 49/188 with placebo; RR 0.80, 95% CI 0.55 to 1.16). Only 1 of 1962 children developed mastoiditis (in a penicillin treated group).[6] **Choice of antibiotic regimen:** The first systematic review (search date June 1992) identified 33 RCTs of antibiotics in 5400 children aged 4 months to 18 years with AOM.[6] Compared with placebo or no treatment, the rate of treatment success (absence of all presenting signs and symptoms of AOM about 7–14 days after treatment was started) was significantly higher with penicillin (2 trials, 242 participants: OR 2.13, 95% CI 1.16 to 3.96; ARI 15.7%, 95% CI 4.7% to 26.7%), ampicillin/amoxicillin (3 trials, 386 participants: OR 3.02, 95% CI 1.62 to 5.81; ARI 12.9%, 95% CI 6.8% to 19.0%), and for any antibiotic (4 trials, 535 participants: OR 2.9, 95% CI 1.76 to 4.88; ARI 13.7%, 95% CI 8.2% to 19.2%). The review found no significant differences between antimicrobial agents in rate of treatment success at 7–14 days or of middle ear effusion at 30 days. **Antibiotics in children aged under 2 years:** We found one systematic review and one subsequent RCT. The review (search date 1997) found four RCTs in 741 children with AOM under the age of 2 years, which compared antibiotics versus placebo alone or versus placebo with myringotomy.[8] The outcome measured was symptomatic clinical improvement. The review found no significant difference between the two groups (OR 1.31, 95% CI 0.83 to 2.08). The subsequent RCT compared amoxicillin (40 mg/kg per day in three doses) versus placebo in 240 children aged 6 months to 2 years. The trial found that amoxicillin reduced persistence of symptoms after 4 days (AR 69/117 [59%] children had persistent symptoms with amoxicillin v 89/123 [72%] with placebo; RR 0.82, 95% CI 0.6.8 to 0.98; NNT 7, 95% CI 4 to 72) and slightly reduced duration of fever (mean duration with amoxicillin 2 days v 3 days with placebo, mean reduction 1 day, no CI given, P = 0.004).

However, the trial found that amoxicillin did not alter duration of pain, otoscopic appearances at 4 days, or clinically judged treatment failure rate after 11 days (mean duration of pain or crying: 8 days with amoxicillin v 9 days with placebo (P = 0.43); otoscopic appearance (AR 88/114 [77%] not improved with amoxicillin v 99/120 [83%] with placebo; RR 0.94, 95% CI 0.82 to 1.07); treatment failure defined as persistent symptoms or eardrum signs (AR 72/112 [64%] with amoxicillin v 84/120 [70%] with placebo; RR 0.92, 95% CI 0.77 to 1.10).[9]

Harms: The first review gave no information on adverse events.[6] In the second review, antibiotics were associated with an increased risk of vomiting, diarrhoea, or rashes (AR 57/345 [17%] with antibiotics v 38/353 [11%] in control groups; RR 1.55, 95% CI 1.11 to 2.16; NNH 17, 95% CI 9 to 152).[7] The recent RCT in children under 2 years found no significant difference in rates of diarrhoea developing after either 4 days (AR 20/117 [17%] with amoxicillin v 12/123 [10%] with placebo, RR 1.75, 95% CI 0.9 to 3.4) or 10 days of treatment (AR 14/117 [12%] with amoxicillin v 10/123 [8%] with placebo, RR 1.47, 95% CI 0.68 to 3.18). Three children withdrew from the placebo group because of skin rashes and two from the antibiotic group because of diarrhoea.[9]

Comment: The first review[6] excluded two placebo controlled trials that were included in the second,[7] on the basis that they included myringotomy as part of treatment. This may have biased results in favour of antibiotic treatment and may explain the higher absolute risk reduction quoted in the first review. We found inadequate evidence for the effectiveness of antibiotics in areas where the incidence of complicating mastoiditis is high. Children with AOM aged under 2 years are at greater risk of a poorer outcome than older children. An update of the second review has been recently published and will be appraised for the next issue.

OPTION   **SHORT VERSUS LONGER COURSES OF ANTIBIOTICS**

One systematic review found greater immediate benefit but no difference in long term outcome with 10 day courses of antibiotics compared with shorter (5 day) courses.

Benefits: We found one systematic review[10] and two subsequent RCTs.[11,12] The systematic review (search date March 1998) identified 30 RCTs of antibiotic treatment in children aged 4 weeks to 18 years with AOM. Treatment failure, relapse, or reinfection at an early evaluation (8–19 days) were significantly more likely to occur with shorter courses of antibiotics (5 days) than with longer courses (8–10 days) (OR compared with longer courses 1.52, 95% CI 1.17 to 1.98). However, by 20–30 days, there were no significant differences between treatment groups (OR 1.22, 95% CI 0.98 to 1.54). The first trial was a double blind RCT that included 385 younger children (mean age 13.3 months, range 4–30 months) with newly diagnosed AOM.[11] They were given either amoxicillin/clavulanate in three divided doses for 10 days or for 5 days, followed by 5 days of placebo. Clinical success or failure was assessed at 12–14 days, then again at 28–42 days after starting treatment. Intention to treat analysis found that the 10 day regimen increased clinical success on days 12–14 compared with the 5 day regimen (AR 158/186 [85%] for the 10 day active treatment v 141/192 [73%] for the 5 day active treatment group; RR 1.16, 95% CI 1.04 to 1.28; NNT 8, 95% CI 5 to 30). However, by days 28–42, there was no significant difference in clinical success between the two groups (AR 108/185 [58%] for the 10 day active treatment v 102/190 [54%] for the 5 day active treatment group; RR 1.09, 95% CI 0.91 to 1.30). Similar results were obtained in a subsequent trial comparing cefpodoxime-proxetil twice daily at 8 mg/dg per day for 10 days v for 5 days followed by placebo for 5 additional days. It found significant differences showing success rates were higher in the 10 day active treatment group after 12–14 days, than in the 5 day treatment group (AR 199/222 [90%] for 10 days v 180/226 [80%] for 5 day treatment; RR 1.13, 95% CI 1.04 to 1.22; NNT 10, 95% CI 6 to 30), but no significance was found after 28–42 days (AR 149/222 [67%] for 10 days v 141/226 [62%] for 5 day treatment; RR: 1.08, 95% CI 0.94 to 1.23).[12]

Harms: One RCT of amoxicillin plus clavulanate in 868 children between 2 months and 12 years reported higher incidence of diarrhoea in children receiving a three times daily treatment compared with children on twice daily treatment for 10 days (AR 74/277 [27%] for the three times daily group v 27/280 [10%] for two times daily treatment during 10 days; RR 2.77, 95% CI 1.84 to 4.17; NNH 5, 95% CI 4 to 9).[13] No clear difference was found for the comparison between 10 and 5 day twice daily treatments (AR 27/280 [10%] for 10 day treatment twice daily v 25/286 [9%] for the 5 day treatment twice daily; RR 1.10, 95% CI 0.66 to 1.85). The trial made no mention of other adverse effects.

Comment: In the trial addressing harms, the 5 day treatment group did not receive a placebo from days 6–10, which may have biased the results.[13]

QUESTION   What are the effects of preventive interventions?

OPTION   LONG TERM ANTIBIOTIC TREATMENT

One systematic review found that long term antibiotic prophylaxis has an effect in preventing recurrences of AOM. However, one subsequent RCT found no significant difference between antibiotic prophylaxis and placebo. We found insufficient evidence on which antibiotic to use, for how long, and how many episodes of AOM justify treatment.

Benefits: **Versus placebo:** We found one systematic review and one subsequent RCT. The systematic review (search date April 1993) identified 33 RCTs comparing antibiotics versus placebo to prevent recurrent AOM and otitis media with effusion.[14] Nine of the trials (945 participants) looked at recurrent AOM only. It was not clear from the review which of the studies referred only to children; four either included the word "children" in the title or appeared in paediatric journals. Most studies defined recurrent AOM as at least three episodes of AOM in 6 months. The most commonly used antibiotics were amoxicillin, cotrimoxazole, and sulphamethoxazole, given for 3 months to 2 years. All nine studies showed a lower rate of recurrence with antibiotic treatment although, in seven, the difference was not significant. Overall, the review found that antibiotics slightly reduced recurrence of AOM (AR of recurrence per person per month 0.08 with antibiotics v 0.19 with placebo; ARR 11%, 95% CI 3% to 19%; NNT per month to prevent one acute episode 9, 95% CI 5 to 33). The later RCT included 194 children aged 3 months to 6 years with three documented episodes of AOM within the preceding 6 months who were randomised to amoxicillin 20 mg/kg per day either once or twice daily, or placebo.[15] The children were followed up monthly if asymptomatic, or within 3–5 days if they had symptoms of upper respiratory tract infection, for up to 90 days. The trial found that antibiotics were no more effective than placebo in preventing recurrent AOM (RR of remaining AOM free, diagnosed by otoscopy and tympanometry 1.00, 95% CI 0.66 to 1.52 using complete analysis, 36 lost to follow up). Including those lost to follow up yielded similar results, whether these children's outcomes were assumed in favour of placebo or in favour of antibiotics. **Choice and duration of antibiotic:** The systematic review found no significant difference in rate of recurrence between antibiotics. Greater treatment effect was seen with treatment lasting less than 6 months, but the confidence intervals overlapped (ARR for recurrence with courses < 6 months 21%, 95% CI 7% to 49%; ARR with courses > 6 months 4%, 95% CI 1% to 9%).[14]

Harms: The studies gave no information on harms.

Comment: None.

OPTION   **XYLITOL SYRUP AND XYLITOL CHEWING GUM**

We found limited evidence that xylitol syrup or gum reduces the incidence of AOM. Adverse effects included abdominal discomfort.

Benefits: We found no systematic review. We found one RCT (857 children, 54% boys), which compared xylitol sugar given five times daily for 3 months in the form of syrup, chewing gum, or lozenges, versus placebo.[16] Children deemed too young to chew gum (mean age 2.2 years) were allocated to xylitol syrup (10 g xylitol per day, 159 children) or a control syrup (0.5 g xylitol per day, 165 children). Children deemed old enough to chew gum (mean age 4.6 years) were given xylitol chewing gum (8.4 g xylitol per day, 179 children), control chewing gum (0.5 g of xylitol per day, 178 children) or xylitol lozenges (10 g xylitol per day, 176 children). Each time the child showed any signs of acute respiratory infection, AOM was excluded using tympanometry and otoscopy. Follow up was for 3 months. The trial found that children who received xylitol syrup were less likely than those receiving control syrup to have one or more episodes of AOM (AR 46/159 [029%] with xylitol syrup v 68/165 [41%] with control syrup; RR 0.70, 95% CI 0.52 to 0.95; NNT 8, 95% CI 4 to 53). Chewing xylitol gum reduced the incidence of AOM compared with control gum (AR 29/179 [16%] with xylitol gum v 49/178 [28%] with control gum; RR 0.59, 95% CI 0.39 to 0.89; NNT 8, 95% CI 5 to 36) but xylitol lozenges were not significantly more effective than control gum (AR 39/176 [22%] with xylitol lozenges v 49/178 [28%]; RR 0.81, 95% CI 0.56 to 1.16).

Child health

Harms: Abdominal discomfort was reported as a reason for withdrawals in children taking syrup, although no significant differences were found with respect to control syrup (AR 8/189 with xylitol syrup v 5/182 with control syrup; RR 1.54, 95% CI 0.51 to 4.62). Few children receiving xylitol lozenges retired from the study because of abdominal discomfort (AR 7/202 [3.5%]). A single child retired from the trial because of abdominal discomfort in the xylitol chewing gum group. The overall withdrawal rate in the xylitol group was twice as high as for those receiving placebo (AR 68/582 [12%] receiving xylitol v 25/368 [7%] in control groups; RR 1.72, 95% CI 1.11 to 2.67; NNH 20, 95% CI 11 to 96). We found no evidence about the long term effects of xylitol.

Comment: The children in this study received xylitol or the control intervention five times daily, a regimen that might be difficult to maintain long term. We found no evidence about optimum duration of treatment.

Substantive changes since last issue

Paracetamol versus placebo Conclusions changed following recalculation from raw data;[5] paracetamol recategorised as "likely to be beneficial".

Short versus longer courses of antibiotics An updated systematic review and a new trial have been added;[10,12] conclusions unchanged.

REFERENCES

1. Froom J, Culpepper L, Jacobs M, et al. Antimicrobials for acute otitis media? A review from the International Primary Care Network. BMJ 1997;315:98–102.
2. Del Mar C, Glasziou P, Hayem M. Are antibiotics indicated as initial treatment for children with acute otitis media? A meta-analysis. BMJ 1997; 314:1526–1529. Search date 1966 to August 1994; primary sources Medline, Current Contents.
3. World Health Organization. World Development Report 1993: Investing in health. Oxford: Oxford University Press, 1993:215–222.
4. Berman S. Otitis media in developing countries. Pediatrics 1995;96:126–131.
5. Bertin L, Pons G, d'Athis P, et al. A randomized double blind multicentre controlled trial of ibuprofen versus acetaminophen and placebo for symptoms of acute otitis media in children. Fundam Clin Pharmacol 1996;10:387–392.
6. Rosenfeld RM, Vertrees JE, Carr J, et al. Clinical efficacy of antimicrobial drugs for acute otitis media: meta-analysis of 5400 children from thirty-three randomised trials. J Pediatr 1994;124:355–367. Search date 1966 to June 1992; primary sources Medline, Current Contents.
7. Glasziou PP, Hayem M, Del Mar CB. Antibiotics for acute otitis media in children. In: The Cochrane Library, Issue 3, 2000. Oxford: Update Software. Search date 1999; primary sources Cochrane Controlled Trials Register, Medline, Index Medicus, Current Contents, and reference lists of articles.
8. Damoiseaux RA, van Balen FAM, Hoes AW, de Melker RA. Antibiotic treatment of acute otitis media in children under two years of age: evidence based? Br J Gen Pract 1998;48:1861–1864. Search date January 1997; primary sources Medline, Embase, and hand searched references.
9. Damoiseaux RA, van Balen FA, Hoes AW, Verheij TJ, de Melker RA. Primary care based randomised,

double blind trial of amoxicillin versus placebo for acute otitis media in children aged under 2 years. BMJ 2000;320:350–354.
10. Kozyrskj AL, Hildes-Ripstein GE, Longstaffe SEA, et al. Short course antibiotics for acute otitis media. In: the Cochrane Library, Issue 3, 2000. Oxford: Update Software. Search date 1998; primary sources Medline, Embase, Science Citation Index, Current Contents, and hand searches of reference lists, and personal contacts.
11. Cohen R, Levy C, Boucherat M, Langue J, de la Rocque F. A multicenter randomized, double blind trial of 5 versus 10 days of antibiotic therapy for acute otitis media in young children. J Pediatr 1998;133:634–639.
12. Cohen R, Levy C, Boucherat M, et al. Five vs. ten days of antibiotic therapy for acute otitis media in young children. Pediatr Infect Dis J 2000;19:458–463.
13. Hoberman A, Paradise JL, Burch DJ, et al. Equivalent efficiency and reduced occurrence of diarrhoea from a new formulation of amoxycillin/clavulanate potassium (Augmentin) for treatment of acute otitis media in children. Pediatr Infect Dis J 1997;16:463–470.
14. Williams RL, Chalmers TC, Stange KC, Chalmers FT, Bowin SJ. Use of antibiotics in preventing recurrent acute otitis media and in treating otitis media with effusion: a meta-analytic attempt to resolve the brouhaha. JAMA 1993;270:1344–1351. [Published erratum appears in JAMA 1994; 27:430.] Search date 1966 to April 1993; primary sources Medline, Current Contents.
15. Roark R, Berman S. Continuous twice daily or once daily amoxycillin prophylaxis compared with placebo for children with recurrent acute otitis media. Pediatr Infect Dis J 1997;16:376–378.
16. Uhari M, Kontiokari T, Niemela MA. Novel use of xylitol sugar in preventing acute otitis media. Pediatrics 1998;102:879–884.

Paddy O'Neill
General Practitioner, Norton Medical Centre, Stockton on Tees, UK
Competing interests: None declared.

Search date October 2000: expanded this issue

Duncan Keeley

INTERVENTIONS

TREATING ACUTE CHILDHOOD ASTHMA

Beneficial

Oxygen* 191

Ipratropium bromide added to
β_2 agonists 192

Spacer devices for delivery of
β_2 agonists (as effective as
nebulisers) 192

Systemic corticosteroids 193

High dose inhaled
corticosteroids New 193

Likely to be beneficial

Intravenous theophylline 194

SINGLE AGENT PROPHYLAXIS IN CHILDREN WITH ASTHMA

Beneficial

Inhaled corticosteroids. 195

Oral theophylline 195

Inhaled sodium cromoglycate. .195

Inhaled nedocromil New 195

Inhaled long acting
β_2 agonists 195

Oral leukotriene receptor
antagonists New 196

ADDITIONAL TREATMENTS IN ASTHMA INADEQUATELY CONTROLLED BY REGULAR LOW DOSE INHALED STEROIDS

Unknown effectiveness

Increased dose of inhaled
corticosteroid New 198

Long acting β_2 agonists New .198

Oral theophylline New 199

Oral leukotriene receptor
antagonists New 199

TREATING ACUTE WHEEZE IN INFANCY

Unknown effectiveness

β_2 agonists 200

Inhaled anticholinergic drugs . .200

Oral corticosteroids 201

PROPHYLAXIS IN WHEEZING INFANTS (see bronchiolitis, p 214)

Unknown effectiveness

Inhaled corticosteroids. 200

Oral theophylline 200

Inhaled sodium cromoglycate. .200

*No RCT, but strong consensus
belief that oxygen is beneficial.

Key Messages

Treating acute childhood asthma

- Strong consensus supports the use of oxygen for acute asthma. We found one prospective cohort study suggesting that it is effective.

- One systematic review has found that adding ipratropium bromide to β_2 agonists in acute asthma leads to marginal improvement.

- One systematic review found no difference between nebuliser and metered dose inhaler plus spacer for delivering β_2 agonists in acute asthma, in children old enough to use a spacer.

- Systematic reviews of RCTs have found that systemic corticosteroids in acute asthma reduce the likelihood of hospital admission and length of hospital stay.

- RCTs have found that high dose inhaled steroids may be as effective as systemic steroids in moderately severe episodes of acute asthma.

- We found conflicting evidence from one systematic review and one large RCT on the effects of intravenous theophylline in acute asthma.

Prophylaxis in childhood asthma

- One systematic review has found that prophylactic inhaled corticosteroids improve symptoms compared with placebo.

- RCTs have found that prophylactic inhaled steroids are more effective than oral theophylline, sodium cromoglycate, or inhaled long acting β_2 agonists. We found no good evidence on the comparative efficacy of inhaled steroids and oral leukotriene receptor antagonists in children.

- One systematic review of long term follow up studies and a subsequent long term RCT found no evidence of growth retardation in asthmatic children treated with inhaled steroids, although another systematic review of short term studies and a subsequent short term RCT found reduced growth velocity in some children.

- One RCT found no significant long term benefit from the addition of an increased dose of inhaled corticosteroid or a β_2 agonist for asthma inadequately controlled on low dose inhaled steroids.

- One small brief RCT found that the addition of theophylline to previous treatment significantly improved the number of symptom free days and significantly reduced the use of additional β_2 agonist and additional corticosteroid medication, but it was too brief to rule out possible long term harms.

- We found no good evidence on the effects of adding leukotriene antagonists to previous treatment.

Treatment and prophylaxis in infants with wheeze

- We found only weak and conflicting evidence on the effects of treatment and prophylaxis in wheezy infants. The main problem is probably the difficulty of distinguishing asthmatic from non-asthmatic wheezing in infancy (see bronchiolitis, p 214).

DEFINITION **Childhood asthma** is characterised by chronic or recurrent cough and wheeze. The diagnosis is confirmed by demonstrating reversible airway obstruction in children old enough to perform peak flow measurements or spirometry. Diagnosing asthma in children requires exclusion of other causes of recurrent respiratory symptoms. **Wheezing in infancy** may be caused by acute viral infection (see bronchiolitis, p 214), episodic viral associated wheeze, or asthma. These are not easy to distinguish clinically.

INCIDENCE/ PREVALENCE	Surveys have found increasing prevalence of wheeze and shortness of breath, and diagnosed asthma in children. The increase is more than can be explained by an increased readiness to diagnose asthma. One questionnaire study from Aberdeen, Scotland, surveyed 2510 children aged 8–13 years in 1964 and 3403 children in 1989. Over the 25 years, prevalence of wheeze rose from 10.4% to 19.8%; episodes of shortness of breath from 5.4% to 10.0%; and diagnosis of asthma from 4.1% to 10.2%.[1] One prospective cohort study (826 neonates reviewed at 3 and 6 years of age) found that 34% had experienced at least one wheezing illness before age 3, 14% wheezed before age 3 and were still wheezing at age 6, and 15% had a wheezing illness in the past year at age 6 but had not wheezed before age 3.[2]
AETIOLOGY/ RISK FACTORS	Asthma is more common in children with a personal or family history of atopy. Precipitating factors include infection, house dust mites, allergens from pet animals, exposure to tobacco smoke, and anxiety.
PROGNOSIS	A retrospective cohort study of wheezing in the first year of life found that 14% of children with one attack and 23% of children with four or more attacks (recalled at age 5) had experienced at least one wheezing illness in the past year at age 10.[3]
AIMS	To reduce or abolish cough and wheeze; to attain best possible lung function; to reduce the risk of severe attacks; to minimise sleep disturbance and absence from school; to minimise adverse effects of treatment; and to allow normal growth.
OUTCOMES	Wheeze; cough; nights disturbed by asthma; days lost from school or normal activities; hospital admission; duration of stay in hospital; lung function tests (peak expiratory flow rate [PEFR]) and forced expiratory volume in one second (FEV_1); blood oxygen saturation in acute attacks; airway hyper-responsiveness, measured using methacholine challenge tests.
METHODS	*Clinical Evidence* update search and appraisal October 2000.

QUESTION   How effective are treatments for acute asthma in children?

OPTION   OXYGEN

One prospective cohort study and clinical experience support the need for oxygen in acute asthma.

Benefits:	We found no systematic review or RCTs. One double blind, prospective cohort study (280 children) found that decreased oxygen saturation upon entry to an emergency department was correlated with increased treatment with intravenous aminophylline (see glossary, p 202) and steroids, and increased rates of hospital admission or subsequent re-admission (arterial oxygen saturation ≤ 91% v arterial oxygen saturation ≥ 96%: OR 35, 95% CI 11 to 150; for arterial oxygen saturation 92–95% v ≥ 96%: OR 4.2, 95% CI 2.2 to 8.8).[4]
Harms:	We found no evidence of harm.
Comment:	An RCT of oxygen in acute severe asthma would be considered unethical. The cohort study does not directly address whether

oxygen should be given therapeutically but it does suggest, along with clinical experience, that oxygen should continue to be given promptly to children with acute asthma.[4]

IPRATROPIUM BROMIDE ADDED TO β_2 AGONISTS

We found good evidence from one systematic review and one subsequent RCT that combination treatment with an anticholinergic agent plus a β_2 agonist improves lung function and may reduce admission rates compared with a β_2 agonist alone or placebo.

Benefits:
We found one systematic review (search date 1997, 10 RCTs, 836 children aged 18 months to 17 years)[5] and one subsequent RCT.[6] The systematic review compared combined inhaled anticholinergics plus β_2 agonists versus β_2 agonists alone. Two RCTs in the systematic review found that combination treatment compared with β_2 agonists alone improved FEV_1 in children with milder asthma at 1 hour (WMD 16%, 99% CI 2% to 30%) and 2 hours (WMD 17.5%, 99% CI 0.4% to 35%), but found no reduction in hospital admission. With multiple dose protocols for severe exacerbations (5 RCTs), combination treatment reduced hospital admissions (OR 0.6, 99% CI 0.3 to 0.98; NNT 11) and improved FEV_1 (mean increase 9.8% of predicted, 99% CI 5% to 14%). The subsequent RCT (90 children aged 6–18 years) compared nebulised salbutamol plus ipratropium versus nebulised salbutamol plus saline and found greater improvement in lung function with salbutamol plus ipratropium (between 30 and 120 minutes: mean increase in PEFR 23% v 15%; mean increase in FEV_1 19% v 14%; P = 0.0001 for all results), but found no reduction in rates of admission.[6]

Harms:
No difference in the rate of adverse effects was noted in the systematic review or in the subsequent RCT.

Comment:
None.

SPACER WITH METERED DOSE INHALER β_2 AGONISTS

One systematic review of RCTs found no significant difference between a metered dose inhaler plus spacer and nebulisation for delivering β_2 agonists in children with acute asthma who are old enough to use a spacer.

Benefits:
Spacer versus placebo: We found no systematic review and no RCTs. **Spacer versus nebuliser:** We found one systematic review (search date 1998, 12 RCTs) comparing metered dose inhaler with spacer versus nebuliser for the administration of β_2 agonists to children with acute asthma.[7] Six RCTs studied children aged over 2 years, excluding life threatening episodes, and three RCTs studied children under 5 years. The review found no significant difference in hospital admission rates (OR 0.71, 95% CI 0.2 to 2.2). One large RCT in the systematic review (152 children, aged 2 years and older) found that time spent in the emergency department was lower in children treated with spacers (WMD –32 minutes, 95% CI –50 to –24 minutes).[8] The increase in pulse rate was higher with nebulisers (WMD 10% from baseline, 95% CI 6% to 14%). Two RCTs

reported blood gas results showing less deterioration with spacer than with nebuliser. No outcomes were worse with spacer.

Harms: There were no reports of serious adverse effects with either mode of delivery.[7]

Comment: These findings suggest that, in children old enough to use a spacer, metered dose inhalers plus spacers could be substituted for nebulisation in the treatment of acute asthma in emergency departments and hospital wards.

| OPTION | SYSTEMIC CORTICOSTEROIDS |

Two systematic reviews of RCTs have found that systemic corticosteroids reduce hospital admission and improve lung function.

Benefits: We found two systematic reviews.[9,10] One review (search date 1991, 2 placebo controlled RCTs in children) evaluated hospital stay after acute asthma.[9] The first RCT in the review (30 children) found reduced admission rates with methylprednisolone (OR 0.42, 95% CI 0.0 to 1.0). The second RCT found briefer hospital stays for children on prednisolone (median length of stay 24 hours v 39 hours; P = 0.001). The second review (search date 1997) identified two different RCTs (61 children). It found that pulmonary function test scores improved with steroids (WMD 14, 95% CI 5.4 to 23).[10]

Harms: We found few reports of adverse effects with short courses of systemic corticosteroids. Several case reports have associated systemic corticosteroid treatment with severe varicella infection. One case control study (167 cases, 134 controls) in otherwise immunocompetent children with complicated and uncomplicated varicella infection did not find significant risk attributable to corticosteroid exposure (OR 1.6, 95% CI 0.2 to 17) but was too small to exclude a clinically important risk.[11]

Comment: None.

| OPTION | HIGH DOSE INHALED CORTICOSTEROIDS   New |

One systematic review and two subsequent RCTs found no consistent differences between initial treatment with high dose inhaled steroids versus oral steroids in acute moderately severe asthma on hospital admission rates or increased FEV_1. These RCTs excluded children with the most severe attacks. One RCT in 100 children with severe attacks found oral steroids to be more effective.

Benefits: **High dose inhaled steroids versus oral steroids:** We found one systematic review[12] and two subsequent RCTs.[13,14] The systematic review (search date not stated, 3 RCTs with 213 children) compared initial treatment with high dose inhaled steroids versus oral steroids in hospital emergency departments.[12] One RCT used nebulised dexamethasone 1.5 mg/kg,[15] one used budesonide 1600 µg by turbohaler,[16] and one used three doses of 800 µg of nebulised budesonide at 0, 30, and 60 minutes.[17] Children with the most severe asthma were excluded from these RCTs. There was no significant difference between the groups in admission rates (OR for inhaled steroids v oral steroids 0.49, 95% CI 0.22 to 1.07). In the largest RCT (111 children aged 1–17 years),[15] there were fewer relapses within 48 hours in the inhaled steroid group (0/44 [0%] v 6/38 [16%]; ARR −16%, 95% CI −27% to −4.5%), but all children in the RCT received a 5 day course of prednisolone on discharge. The first subsequent RCT (100 children with acute asthma ≥5 years, mean initial FEV_1 45%) compared 2 mg fluticasone by MDI/spacer with 2 mg/kg prednisolone. It found that prednisolone reduced hospital admission (31% fluticasone v 10% prednisolone) and increased mean FEV_1 at 4 hours (9% fluticasone v 19% prednisolone).[13] The second subsequent RCT (46 children, aged 15–16 years, admitted to hospital with severe exacerbations of asthma) compared nebulised budesonide 2 mg hourly with oral prednisolone 2 mg/kg at admission and after 24 hours.[14] It found no significant difference between groups at 24 hours or at 3 and 24 days after admission. All children in this trial were treated with 800 µg budesonide daily following discharge from hospital.

Harms: No significant harms from short term high dose inhaled steroids were reported in these trials.

Comment: These RCTs suggest that high dose inhaled corticosteroids may be substituted for oral corticosteroids in the initial phase of treatment of moderately severe acute episodes. This may be useful for children who vomit oral steroids or for children with frequent exacerbations where there is concern about the cumulative dose of oral steroids.

OPTION   **INTRAVENOUS THEOPHYLLINE**

We found conflicting evidence of benefit from one systematic review of small RCTs and from one subsequent large RCT. Treatment was frequently stopped because of adverse effects.

Benefits: We found one systematic review (search date 1994, 6 small RCTs, 164 children aged 1.5–18 years), which found no significant benefit from intravenous theophylline added to routine treatment (mean difference in FEV_1 +39% of predicted; P = 0.25).[18] One subsequent RCT (163 children aged 1–19 years with acute asthma, 43% admitted to intensive care) found greater improvement in FEV_1 at 6 hours (mean increase in FEV_1 10%, 95% CI 4% to 17%), less additional oxygen needed in the first 30 hours (median 6 hours with additional intravenous aminophylline v 18 hours with placebo; P = 0.015), and reduced likelihood of intubation (AR 0% with aminophylline v 6% with placebo; P = 0.03).[19]

Harms: Theophylline has serious adverse effects (cardiac arrhythmia, convulsion) if therapeutic blood concentrations are exceeded. In one RCT, 32% of children receiving aminophylline had their infusion stopped because of adverse effects (mainly nausea and vomiting).[19]

Comment: The trials in the review were too small to exclude a clinically important effect.

QUESTION	What are the effects of single agent prophylaxis in childhood asthma?

RCTs have found that prophylactic inhaled steroids, oral theophylline, inhaled sodium cromoglycate, nedocromil, long acting β_2 agonists, and oral leukotriene receptor antagonists compared with placebo improve symptoms and lung function in children with asthma (see comment p 197). RCTs have found that inhaled steroids are more effective than theophylline, sodium cromoglycate, or inhaled long acting β_2 agonists for improving symptoms and lung function in children with asthma. Two systematic reviews of studies with long term follow up and a subsequent long term RCT have found no evidence of growth retardation in asthmatic children treated with inhaled steroids. Some shorter term studies found reduced growth velocity.

Benefits: **Inhaled corticosteroids versus placebo:** We found one systematic review (search date 1996, 24 RCTs, 1087 children, 10/24 RCTs in pre-school children, duration 4–88 weeks), which compared regular inhaled steroids versus placebo.[20] It found that steroids improved symptom score (overall weighted relative improvement in symptom score 50%, 95% CI 49% to 51%), reduced β_2 agonist use (RR 0.37, 95% CI 0.36 to 0.38), reduced oral steroid use (RR 0.68, 95% CI 0.66 to 0.70), and improved peak flow rate (weighted mean improvement in PEFR 11% predicted, 95% CI 9.5% to 12.5%). **Inhaled corticosteroids versus theophylline:** We found no systematic review. One double blind RCT (195 children aged 6–16 years, followed for 12 months) compared oral theophylline versus inhaled beclomethasone (360 µg daily).[21] It found that beclomethasone gave similar symptom control with less use of bronchodilators and oral steroids. **Inhaled corticosteroids versus sodium cromoglycate:** We found no systematic review. Several small comparative RCTs have found sodium cromoglycate to be less effective than inhaled steroids in improving symptoms and lung function. **Inhaled corticosteroids versus nedocromil:** We found one RCT (1041 children aged 5–12 years, FEV_1 94% predicted), which compared inhaled budesonide (200 µg twice daily), inhaled nedocromil (8 mg twice daily) versus placebo for 4–6 years.[22] It found that budesonide was superior to nedocromil, and that nedocromil was superior to placebo in several measures of asthma symptoms and morbidity (see table 1, p 204). The mean change in postbronchodilator FEV_1 over the study period was no different in the three groups. **Inhaled corticosteroids versus inhaled long acting β_2 agonists:** We found no systematic review but found two RCTs of beclomethasone 200 µg twice daily versus salmeterol 50 µg twice daily for 1 year. The first RCT (67 children aged 6–16 years) found that beclomethasone was more effective than salmeterol in improving FEV_1 (mean change of FEV_1 –4.5% of predicted with salmeterol, 95% CI –9.0% to +0.1% v 10% with beclomethasone, 95% CI not given; mean difference beclomethasone v salmeterol 14.2%, 95% CI 8.3% to 20%), reducing use of rescue salbutamol (0.44 uses per day with salmeterol v 0.07 uses per day with beclomethasone; $P \le 0.001$).[23] Both treatments improved symptom scores (3% of children asymptomatic before the trial with salmeterol v 6% with beclomethasone; 36% at 1 year with salmeterol v 55% with beclomethasone) and PEFR (improvement in morning PEFR 49 l/minute with salmeterol v 61 l/minute with beclomethasone), but there was no significant difference between treatments at 1 year. There were two exacerbations in the beclomethasone group compared with 17 in the salmeterol group. The second RCT (241 children aged 6–14 years) compared beclomethasone (81 children) versus salmeterol (80 children) versus placebo (80 children).[24] It found that beclomethasone reduced airway hyper-responsiveness more than salmeterol (P = 0.003). Beclomethasone versus placebo reduced rescue bronchodilator use (P ≤ 0.001) and treatment withdrawals because of exacerbations (P = 0.03). Salmeterol versus placebo did not significantly reduce the use of a rescue bronchodilator (P = 0.09) or treatment withdrawals because of exacerbations (P = 0.55). Both salmeterol and beclomethasone improved FEV_1 compared with placebo, but the difference between beclomethasone and salmeterol was not significant. **Inhaled corticosteroids versus oral leukotriene receptor antagonists:** We found one systematic review (search date 1999, 10 RCTs).[25] All studies were brief (6–12 weeks), although some had longer unblinded extensions. Only two studies included children. One of these (involving montelukast) remains unpublished. The other study (451 people aged 12 years and older) compared zafirlukast and low dose fluticasone. It found that fluticasone caused greater improvement in lung function (increase in mean morning PEFR 50 l/minute v 12 l/minute) and symptoms (change in percentage of symptom free days 28% v 16%).[26] The systematic review, mainly of results for adults, found similar exacerbation rates but inhaled steroids resulted in better improvements in lung function and symptoms when compared with leukotriene antagonists.

Harms: **Inhaled steroids:** One systematic review (search date December 1996) found no significant adverse effects, including no documented effects on growth (monitored in 8 studies) or adrenal function (monitored in 12 studies).[20] Observational studies found little or no biochemical evidence of change in bone metabolism with inhaled steroids. Two cross sectional studies used a slit lamp to screen for lenticular changes in 198 children taking long term inhaled steroids.[27,28] The only posterior subcapsular cataract was in a child who had also received several prolonged courses of oral steroids. **Effects of inhaled steroids on growth:** Another systematic review (search date 1993) identified 21 studies that reported height for age in asthmatic children treated with steroids. No evidence of growth impairment was found in the 12 studies involving beclomethasone (331 children).[29] A more recent systematic review (search date 1999) found three RCTs comparing the effects of beclomethasone and non-steroidal medication on linear growth in children with asthma (200 µg twice daily, duration up to maximum 54 weeks) suggesting a short term decrease in linear growth of –1.54 cm a year.[30] One RCT of inhaled beclomethasone (360 µg daily) compared with oral theophylline for 1 year[21] found a significantly higher rate of growth (more notable in boys) with the theophylline group (mean rate of growth in prepubescent boys 4.3 cm/year v 6.2 cm/year). This effect was not sufficient to be noticed by the children or by their parents, and no child was withdrawn from the study on this account. The two RCTs comparing beclomethasone with salmeterol found a similar slowing in linear growth with beclomethasone (growth over year of treatment 5.4 cm[23] and 6.1 cm in the salmeterol groups, 4.0 cm[23] and 4.7 cm[24] in beclomethasone groups, P = 0.004,[23] P = 0.007).[24] One controlled, prospective parallel group study compared 216 children treated with 400–600 µg budesonide daily with 62 children treated with theophylline or sodium cromoglycate, with 3–5 years' follow up.[31] No significant changes in growth velocity were found (budenoside 5.5 cm/year v controls 5.6 cm/year) at doses up to 400 µg. The adult height of 142 of these budesonide treated children (mean treatment period 9.2 years, mean daily dosage 412 µg) was compared with 18 controls never treated with inhaled steroids and 51 healthy siblings. There were no significant differences. Children in all groups attained their target adult height (mean difference between measured and target adult height: +0.3 cm, 95% CI –0.6 to +1.2 for budesonide treated children; –0.2 cm, 95% CI –2.4 to +2.1 for control children with asthma; +0.9 cm, 95% CI –0.4 to +2.2 for healthy siblings).[32] A large RCT (1041 children with mild to moderate asthma) compared budesonide (400 µg daily) versus nedocromil versus placebo with follow up for 4–6 years.[22] The mean increase in height in the budesonide group was 1.1 cm less than in the placebo group (22.7 cm v 23.8 cm; P = 0.005) the difference occurring largely within the first year of treatment. **Theophylline:** One RCT found that continuous oral theophylline was associated with a higher frequency of headache, gastric irritation, and tremor than beclomethasone (360 µg daily).[21] One systematic review (12 studies, 340 children) of the behavioural and cognitive effects of theophylline found no evidence of significant adverse effects.[33] **Sodium cromoglycate:** Sodium cromoglycate may cause cough, throat irritation, and bronchoconstriction, but no long term adverse effects have been reported. **Inhaled long acting β_2 agonists:** These agents occasionally cause tremor or tachycardia. Three large RCTs found no evidence of important adverse effects from salmeterol over 1 year.[23,24,34] **Oral leukotriene receptor antagonists:** Placebo controlled RCTs found similar incidence of adverse effects with leukotriene receptor antagonists and placebo, but the systematic review found that anti-leukotrienes compared with corticosteroids were associated with increased risk of withdrawal because of adverse effects (3 RCTs, RR 1.9, 95% CI 1.1 to 3.3).[25] Gastrointestinal symptoms and headaches have been reported with both montelukast and zafirlukast. Churg Strauss syndrome has been reported in people taking either drug, possibly because of reduction in steroid therapy unmasking a pre-existing condition.

Comment: In school age children with asthma, benefit compared with placebo has been found in RCTs for theophylline,[35] sodium cromoglycate,[36] nedocromil,[22] long acting β_2 agonists,[34] and oral leukotriene receptor antagonists.[37]

OPTION INCREASED DOSE OF INHALED CORTICOSTEROID

One RCT, of the addition to previous treatment of a second dose of inhaled corticosteroids, has found no significant differences in lung function, symptom scores, exacerbation rates, or bronchial reactivity, and has found an adverse effect on growth velocity at 1 year.

Benefits: We found no systematic review but found one RCT (177 children, age 6–16 years, 1 year follow up, mean pre-bronchodilator FEV_1 86% predicted) comparing beclomethasone (200 µg twice daily), salmeterol (50 µg twice daily), and placebo in children already taking beclomethasone (200 µg twice daily).[38] No significant differences were found at 1 year in lung function (mean change in FEV_1: 5.8% of predicted, 95% CI 2.9% to 8.7% with double dose beclomethasone v 4.3%, 95% CI 2.1 to 6.5 with placebo), symptom scores, exacerbation rates, bronchial reactivity or changes in airway responsiveness (1.30 units of methacholine, 95% CI 0.73 to 1.87 with salmeterol v 0.80, 95% CI 0.33 to 1.27 with placebo). No benefit of either adding salmeterol or a second dose of beclomethasone was demonstrated in this group of children whose compliance with pre-existing medication was good.

Harms: Growth was significantly slower in the group receiving higher dose inhaled steroids (3.6 cm, 95% CI 3.0 to 4.2 with double dose beclomethasone v 5.1 cm, 95% CI 4.5 to 5.7 with salmeterol v 4.5 cm, 95% CI 3.8 to 5.2 with placebo).

Comment: Higher dose inhaled steroids are frequently used despite lack of evidence of benefit. In some children, higher prescribed doses may compensate for poor compliance or incorrect inhaler technique.

OPTION ADDITION OF REGULAR LONG ACTING β_2 AGONIST

One RCT found that additional salmeterol increased PEFRs in the first few months of treatment but found no increase after 1 year. A second short term RCT also found increased morning PEFRs and more symptom free days at 3 months.

Benefits: We found no systematic review but found two RCTs.[38,39] One RCT (177 children) found that at 1 year the addition of salmeterol did not improve lung function, airway responsiveness, symptom scores, exacerbation rates, or bronchial reactivity.[38] Salmeterol versus placebo increased mean morning PEFRs slightly after 3 months (difference: +12 l/minute). There were no significant differences in symptom scores at any time. The second RCT (210 children, 4–16 years, 12 week follow up, mean morning PFER 79% predicted) compared salmeterol (50 µg twice daily) versus placebo in children inadequately controlled on inhaled steroids (average dose 750 µg daily).[39] At 12 weeks, mean morning PEFR (as percent predicted) was 4% higher in the salmeterol group. Mean evening PEFR was not significantly different. The median proportion of symptom free days improved more with salmeterol than with placebo (60% v 30% for the third month of treatment).

Harms: The RCTs found no significant adverse effects associated with salmeterol.[38,39]

Comment: The second RCT was organised and funded by the manufacturer of salmeterol. Studies of adults with poor control on low dose inhaled steroids have found greater benefit with additional long acting β_2 agonists than with higher doses of inhaled steroid (see salmeterol v high dose inhaled steroids under adult asthma, p 1011).

OPTION   ADDITION OF ORAL THEOPHYLLINE

One small brief RCT found that addition of theophylline versus placebo to previous treatment significantly increased the number of symptom free days and significantly reduced the use of additional β agonist and additional corticosteroid medication. We found insufficient evidence to weigh these short term benefits and possible long term harms.

Benefits: We found no systematic review but found one RCT (double blind crossover trial, 33 children, age 6–19 years, recruited from a hospital asthma clinic, 22 children used inhaled beclomethasone [mean 533 µg/day], 11 used oral prednisolone [mean 30 mg alternate days]).[40] It found that the addition for 4 weeks of oral theophylline (serum concentration 10–20 µg/ml) versus placebo increased the mean number of symptom free days (63% with theophylline v 42% with placebo; $P \leq 0.01$). Inhaled beta agonist was needed twice as often with placebo (0.5 doses per day with theophylline v 1.0 with placebo; $P \leq 0.01$). Additional daily prednisolone was needed by fewer children while on theophylline than while on placebo (3/32 with theophylline v 10/32 with placebo; $P = 0.02$).

Harms: In the RCT, short term adverse effects included mild transient headache and nausea in six children after the crossover from placebo to the theophylline dose that they had previously tolerated.

Comment: One child was excluded from the analysis because of poor compliance. The RCT was too brief to exclude long term harms.

OPTION   ADDITION OF ORAL LEUKOTRIENE RECEPTOR ANTAGONISTS

We found no good evidence of the effects of adding oral leukotriene receptor antagonists to low dose inhaled steroids in children.

Benefits: We found no systematic review and no RCTs in children.

Harms: None.

Comment: One large RCT of the use of montelukast added to beclomethasone in adults with inadequately controlled asthma (funded by the manufacturer of montelukast) found benefit over a 16 week period.[41]

OPTION   β₂ AGONISTS DELIVERED BY NEBULISER OR METERED DOSE INHALER/SPACER

We found conflicting evidence from RCTs. Transient hypoxia may be caused by nebulised bronchodilators, particularly with air driven nebulisers, and seems less likely when using metered dose inhalers/spacers (see bronchiolitis, p 214).

Benefits: We found no systematic review. We found many hospital based RCTs of nebulised β_2 agonists compared with normal saline in infants and young children with acute wheezing. Some, but not all, have found short term improvements in clinical respiratory distress scores with β_2 agonists.[42] We found no large RCTs with clinical outcomes. Small RCTs with physiological rather than clinical end points found that giving β_2 agonists by metered dose inhaler with spacer to wheezy infants was effective, with less likelihood than nebulisation to show transient adverse effects on lung function.[43,44] A large single blind RCT (123 children, aged 1–24 months [mean age 8 months], based in an inner city hospital emergency department in Santiago, Chile) compared nebulised salbutamol 0.25 mg/kg three times in 1 hour with salbutamol by MDI/spacer two puffs five times in 1 hour for the treatment of moderate to severe wheezing. Treatment was repeated for a second hour together with intramuscular betamethasone in children assessed as non-responders after the first hour. Withholding of β_2 agonist treatment from a control group was considered unethical. Success of treatment as measured by reduction in clinical severity score after 1 hour was 71% (nebuliser group) and 90% (spacer group) and at 2 hours 94% (nebuliser group) and 100% (spacer group). Only one child (in the nebuliser group) was hospitalised owing to treatment failure.[45]

Harms: Some infants have transiently decreased oxygen saturation after nebulisation, especially with air driven nebulisers.[42] Nebulised β_2 agonists are known to cause tachycardia, tremor, and hypokalaemia, but serious adverse effects are rare.

Comment: None.

OPTION   INHALED ANTICHOLINERGIC DRUGS

We found limited and conflicting evidence from one systematic review of small RCTs on the effects of inhaled anticholinergic drugs for clinical outcomes.

Benefits: We found one systematic review (search date 1998, 321 children, 6 RCTs) of ipratropium bromide for wheeze in children under 2 years.[46] One included RCT found that adding ipratropium bromide to β_2 agonists resulted in fewer children receiving further treatment 45 minutes after initial treatment in the emergency room (OR 0.22, 95% CI 0.08 to 0.61), but a second similar study found no additional benefit. A third included RCT (31 hospitalised children) comparing ipratropium bromide versus placebo found no significant difference in the duration of hospitalisation (WMD −0.4 days, 95% CI −1.4 to +0.61). Adding ipratropium bromide to β_2 agonist had no effect on duration of hospitalisation compared with β_2 agonist alone (WMD −0.4 days, 95% CI −1.41 to +0.61). In one home based, 2 month crossover trial, parents preferred regular nebulised ipratropium bromide to nebulised water, but there was no significant reduction in the frequency of reported symptoms during treatment.[46]

Harms: No evidence of harm specific to the use of ipratropium bromide was found in these studies.

Comment: The studies were too small to exclude a clinically important effect of ipratropium bromide.

OPTION	ORAL CORTICOSTEROIDS

We found no evidence that oral steroids improve outcomes in acute wheezing infants.

Benefits: We found no systematic review. One outpatient study compared oral prednisolone with placebo (38 acutely wheezing children aged 3–17 months, including 30 children previously admitted with wheeze). It found no significant differences in outcome between the two groups in the 56 episodes studied.[47]

Harms: No important adverse effects were identified.

Comment: Acute infantile wheezing may be because of bronchiolitis. This is often difficult to separate from other acute wheezing, and is dealt with elsewhere (see bronchiolitis, p 214).

QUESTION	What are the effects of prophylaxis in wheezing infants?

We found weak and conflicting evidence on the effects of prophylaxis in wheezing infants.

Benefits: We found no systematic review. We found inconsistent results of placebo controlled trials on inhaled steroids in recurrent or persistent infant wheezing. Some found improvements in symptom scores and reduced administration of additional treatments. Other studies did not find beneficial effect. We found a greater tendency for positive findings in studies of older children and in studies involving administration by metered dose inhaler and spacer rather than nebuliser. We found no RCTs of continuous oral theophylline in infants, and the small numbers of trials with inhaled sodium cromoglycate were mainly negative.

Harms: We found no good evidence on the long term safety of treatment with continuous inhaled steroids in infancy. Known effects of using nebuliser and facemasks include oral candidiasis and thinning of facial skin.

Comment: Administering inhaled treatments to infants is difficult. RCTs of treatment for infant wheezing used a variety of drugs, dosages, and devices, and were sometimes conducted in populations with differing proportions of children with asthma rather than other types of infant wheeze. These factors may explain the inconsistent results.

GLOSSARY

Aminophylline A stable combination of theophylline and ethylenediamine: the ethylenediamine is added to increase the solubility of theophylline in water.

REFERENCES

1. Russell G, Ninan TK. Respiratory symptoms and atopy in Aberdeen school children: evidence from two surveys 25 years apart. BMJ 1992;304:873–875.
2. Martinez FD, Wright AL, Taussig L, et al. Asthma and wheezing in the first six years of life. N Engl J Med 1995;333:132–138.
3. Park ES, Golding J, Carswell F, et al. Pre-school wheezing and prognosis at 10. Arch Dis Child 1986;61:642–646.
4. Geelhoed GC, Landau LI, Le Souef PN. Evaluation of SaO₂ as a predictor of outcome in 280 children presenting with acute asthma. Ann Emerg Med 1994;23:1236–1241.
5. Plotnick LH, Ducharme FM. Combined inhaled anticholinergics and β₂ agonists in the initial management of acute paediatric asthma. In: The Cochrane Library, Issue 3, 2000. Oxford: Update Software. Search dates 1997; primary sources Medline; Embase; Cinahl; hand searches of bibliographies of references; and contact with pharmaceutical companies for details of unpublished trials and personal contacts.
6. Qureshi F, Zaritsky A, Lakkis H. Efficacy of nebulised ipratropium in severely asthmatic children. Ann Emerg Med 1997;29:205–211.
7. Cates CJ. Holding chambers versus nebulisers for β-agonist treatment of acute asthma. In: The Cochrane Library, Issue 3, 2000. Oxford: Update Software. Search date February 1998; primary sources Medline and Cochrane Airways Review Group Register.
8. Chou KJ, Cunningham SJ, Crain EF. Metered-dose inhalers with spacers vs nebulizers for pediatric asthma. Arch Pediatr Adolesc Med 1995;149:201–205.
9. Rowe BH, Kelleher JL, Oxman AD. Effectiveness of steroid therapy in acute exacerbations of asthma: a meta-analysis. Am J Emerg Med 1992;10:301–310. Search date February 1991; primary sources Medline 1966 to February 1991; Science Citation Search 1980 to 1990; and content experts, review papers, textbooks.
10. Rowe BH, Spooner CH, Ducharme FM, Bretzlaff JA, Bota GW. Corticosteroids for preventing relapse following acute exacerbations of asthma In: The Cochrane Library, Issue 3, 2000. Oxford: Update Software. Search date May 1997; primary source Cochrane Airways Group Register.
11. Patel H, Macarthur C, Johnson D. Recent corticosteroids use and the risk of complicated varicella in otherwise immunocompetent children. Arch Pediatr Adolesc Med 1996;150:409–414.
12. Edmonds ML, Camargo CA Jr, Pollack CV Jr, Rowe BH. Early use of inhaled corticosteroids in the emergency department treatment of acute asthma. In: The Cochrane Library, Issue 3, 2000. Oxford: Update Software. Search date not stated; primary sources Cochrane Airways Group Register, and hand searches of bibliographies.
13. Schuh S, Resiman J, Alshehri M, et al. A comparison of inhaled fluticasone and oral prednisone for children with severe acute asthma. N Engl J Med 2000;343:689–694.
14. Matthews EE, Curtis PD, McLain B, Morris L, Turbitt M. Nebulized budesonide versus oral steroid in severe exacerbations of childhood asthma. Acta Paediatr 1999;88:841–843.
15. Scarfone RJ, Loiselle JM, Wiley JF II, et al. Nebulized dexamethasone versus oral prednisone in the emergency treatment of asthmatic children. Ann Emerg Med 1995;26:480–486.
16. Volowitz B, Bentur L, Finkelstein Y, et al. Effectiveness and safety of inhaled corticosteroids in controlling acute asthma attacks in children who were treated in the emergency department: a controlled comparative study with oral prednisolone. J Allergy Clin Immunol 1998;102:1605–1609.
17. Devidayal S, Singhi S, Kumar L, Jayshree M. Efficacy of nebulized budesonide compared to oral prednisolone in acute bronchial asthma. Acta Paediatr 1999;88:835–840.
18. Goodman DC, Littenberg B, O'Connor GT, et al. Theophylline in acute childhood asthma: a meta-analysis of its efficacy. Pediatr Pulmonol 1996;21:211–218. Search date May 1994; primary sources Medline 1966 to May 1994.
19. Yung M, South M. Randomised controlled trial of aminophylline for severe acute asthma. Arch Dis Child 1998;79:405–410.
20. Calpin C, Macarthur C, Stephens D, et al. Effectiveness of prophylactic inhaled steroids in childhood asthma: a systematic review of the literature. J Allergy Clin Immunol 1997;100:452–457. Search date December 1996; primary source Medline.
21. Tinkelman DG, Reed C, Nelson H, et al. Aerosol beclomethasone diproprionate compared with theophylline as primary treatment of chronic, mild to moderately severe asthma in children. Pediatrics 1993;92:64–77.
22. The Childhood Asthma Management Program Research Group. Long term effects of budesonide or nedocromil in children with asthma. N Engl J Med 2000;343:1054–1063.
23. Verberne A, Frost C, Roorda R, et al. One year treatment with salmeterol compared with beclomethasone in children with asthma. Am J Respir Crit Care Med 1997;156:688–695.
24. Simons FER and the Canadian Beclomethasone Diproprionate – Salmeterol Xinafoate Study Group. A comparison of beclomethasone, salmeterol and placebo in children with asthma. N Engl J Med 1997;337:1659–1665.

25. Ducharme FM, Hicks GC. Anti-leukotriene agents compared to inhaled corticosteroids in the management of recurrent and/or acute asthma. In: The Cochrane Library, Issue 3, 2000. Search date 1999; primary sources Medline; Embase; Cinahl; hand searches of reference lists; and personal contact with colleagues and internal headquarters of leukotriene producers.

26. Bleecker ER, Welch MJ, Weinstein SF, et al. Low dose inhaled fluticasone proprionate versus oral zafirlukast in the treatment of persistent asthma. *J Allergy Clin Immunol* 2000;105(6 Pt 1):1123–1129.

27. Simons FE, Persaud MP, Gillespie CA, et al. Absence of posterior subcapsular cataracts in young patients treated with inhaled corticosteroids. *Lancet* 1993;342:776–778.

28. Abuektish F, Kirkpatrick JN, Russell G. Posterior subcapsular cataract and inhaled steroid therapy. *Thorax* 1995;50:674–676.

29. Allen DB, Mullen M, Mullen B. A meta-analysis of the effect of oral and inhaled steroids on growth. *J Allergy Clin Immunol* 1994;93:967–976. Search date January 1993; primary sources literature search of leading medical journals 1956 to 1993.

30. Sharek PJ, Bergman DA. Beclomethasone for asthma in children: effects on linear growth. In: The Cochrane Library, Issue 3, 2000. Oxford: Update Software. Search date March 1999; primary source Cochrane Airways Group Asthma Trials Register.

31. Agertoft L, Pedersen S. Effects of long-term treatment with an inhaled corticosteroid on growth and pulmonary function in asthmatic children. *Respir Med* 1994;88:373–381.

32. Agertoft L, Pedersen S. Effect of long term treatment with inhaled budesonide on adult height in children with asthma. *N Engl J Med* 2000;343:1064–1069.

33. Stein MA, Krasowski M, Leventhal BL, et al. Behavioural and cognitive effects of theophylline and caffeine. *Arch Pediatr Adolesc Med* 1996:50:284–288. Search date not given; primary sources Medline; Psychlit; Dissertation Abstracts; and hand searched references.

34. Lenney W, Pedersen S, Boner AL, Ebbutt A, Jenkins M, on behalf of an international study group. Efficacy and safety of salmeterol in childhood asthma. *Eur J Pediatr* 1995;154:983–990.

35. Dusdieker L, Green M, Smith GD, Ekwo EE, Weinberger M. Comparison of orally administered metaproterenol and theophylline in the control of chronic asthma. *J Pediatr* 1982;101:281–287.

36. Eigen H, Reid JJ, Dahl R, et al. Evaluation of the addition of cromolyn sodium to bronchodilator maintenance therapy in the long term management of asthma. *J Allergy Clin Immunol* 1987;80:612–621.

37. Knorr B, Matz J, Bernstein JA, et al. Montelukast for chronic asthma in 6–14 year old children. *JAMA* 1998;279:1181–1186.

38. Verberne A, Frost C, Duiverman E, Grol M, Kerrebijn K. Addition of salmeterol versus doubling the dose of beclomethasone in children with asthma. *Am J Respir Crit Care Med* 1998;158:213–219.

39. Russell G, Williams DAJ, Weller P, Price J. Salmeterol xinafoate in children on high dose inhaled steroids. *Ann Allergy Asthma Immunol* 1995;75:423–428.

40. Nassif EG, Weinberger M, Thompson R, Huntley W. The value of maintenance theophylline in steroid dependent asthma. *N Engl J Med* 1981;304:71–75.

41. Laviolette M, Malmstrom K, Lu S, et al. Montelukast added to inhaled beclomethasone in treatment of asthma. *Am J Respir Crit Care Med* 1999;160:1862–1868.

42. Alario AJ, Lewander W, Dennehy P, et al. The efficacy of nebulised metaproterenol in wheezing infants and young children. *Am J Dis Child* 1992;146:412–418.

43. Kraemer R, Frey U, Sommer CW, et al. Short term effect of albuterol, delivered via a new auxiliary device, in wheezy infants. *Am Rev Respir Dis* 1991;144:347–351.

44. Yuksel B, Greenough A. Comparison of the effects on lung function of different methods of bronchodilator administration. *Respir Med* 1994;88:22.

45. Rubilar L, Castro-Rodrguez JA, Girardi G. Randomized controlled trial of salbutamol via metered-dose inhaler with spacer verus nebuliser for acute wheezing in children less than 2 years of age. *Pediatr Pulmonol* 2000;29:264–269.

46. Everard M, Kurian M. Anticholinergic drugs for wheeze in children under the age of two years. In: The Cochrane Library, Issue 3, 2000. Oxford: Update Software. Search date 1998; primary sources Cochrane Airways Group Register 1966 to May 1998; hand search of respiratory care and paediatric journals.

47. Webb M, Henry R, Milner AD. Oral corticosteroids for wheezing attacks under 18 months. *Arch Dis Child* 1986;61:15–19.

Duncan Keeley
General Practitioner
Thame
Oxfordshire
UK

Competing interests: The author has received occasional consultancy fees or assistance with organisation of, or travel to, meetings from companies including Allen and Hanburys, Astra, MSD, Zeneca, 3M, and Boots.

| TABLE 1 | Comparison of inhaled budesonide, nedocromil, and placebo over 4–6 years on several measures of asthma symptoms and morbidity (see text, p 195).[22] |

Intervention	Budesonide (311 children)	Nedocromil (312 children)	Placebo (418 children)
Prednisone courses per 100 person years	70	102	122
Urgent care visits due to asthma per 100 person years	12	16	22
Hospitalisations due to asthma per 100 person years	2.5	4.3	4.4
Beclomethasone or other asthma medications added	6.6%	17.1%	18.7%

Attention deficit hyperactivity disorder in children

Search date August 2000: new for this issue

Carol Joughin, Morris Zwi and Paul Ramchandani

QUESTIONS

INTERVENTIONS

Key Messages

- One systematic review has found that methylphenidate compared with placebo reduces core symptoms of attention deficit hyperactivity disorder (ADHD) in the short term but may disturb sleep and appetite. Adding methylphenidate to behavioural treatment consistently improved outcomes.

- Limited evidence from one systematic review of four small RCTs comparing dexamfetamine with placebo suggests significant improvement of some outcomes.

- Benefits have usually been reported as outcomes on rating scales that are difficult to interpret in every day use. The clinical importance of these results is unclear.

- Limited evidence from one recent systematic review found that clonidine may be more effective than placebo on ADHD symptoms, but the clinical importance of these findings is unclear.

- Systematic reviews and a subsequent RCT have found inconclusive results for psychological/behavioural treatments used alone or when added to drug treatment of ADHD.

Attention deficit hyperactivity disorder in children

DEFINITION
ADHD is "a persistent pattern of inattention and/or hyperactivity–impulsivity that is more frequent and severe than is typically observed in individuals at a comparable level of development" (DSM-IV).[1] Inattention, hyperactivity, and impulsivity are commonly known as the core symptoms of ADHD. Symptoms must be present for at least 6 months, observed before the age of 7 years, and "clinically significant impairment in social, academic, or occupational functioning" must be evident in more than one setting. The symptoms must not be better explained by another disorder such as an anxiety disorder, mood disorder, psychosis or autistic disorder.[1] The World Health Organization's International Statistical Classification of Diseases and Related Health Problems (ICD-10)[2] uses the term "hyperkinetic disorder" for a more restricted diagnosis. It differs from the DSM-IV classification[3] as all three problems of attention, hyperactivity, and impulsiveness must be present, more stringent criteria for "pervasiveness" across situations must be met, and the presence of another disorder is an exclusion criterion.

INCIDENCE/ PREVALENCE
Prevalence estimates of ADHD vary according to the diagnostic criteria used and the population sampled. DSM-IV prevalence estimates among school children range from 3% to 5%,[1] but other estimates vary from 1.7% to 16%.[4,5] No objective test exists to confirm the diagnosis of ADHD, which remains a clinical diagnosis. Other conditions frequently coexist with ADHD. Oppositional defiant disorder is present in 35% (CI 27% to 44%) of children with ADHD, conduct disorder in 26% (CI 13% to 41%), anxiety disorder in 26% (CI 18% to 35%), and depressive disorder (see glossary, p 212) in 18% (CI 11% to 27%).[6]

AETIOLOGY/ RISK FACTORS
The underlying causes are not known.[6] There is limited evidence that it has a genetic component.[7–9] Risk factors also include psychosocial factors.[10] There is increased risk in boys compared to girls, with ratios varying from $3:1$[6] to $4:1$.[3]

PROGNOSIS
More than 70% of hyperactive children may continue to meet criteria for ADHD in adolescence, and up to 65% of adolescents may continue to meet criteria for ADHD in adulthood.[5] Changes in diagnostic criteria cause difficulty with interpretation of the few outcome studies. One cohort of boys followed up for an average of 16 years found a ninefold increase in antisocial personality disorder and a fourfold increase in substance misuse disorder.[7]

AIMS
To reduce inattention, hyperactivity and impulsivity, and to improve psychosocial and educational functioning in affected children and adolescents, with minimal adverse effects of treatment.

OUTCOMES
Children's behaviour (e.g. Conners Rating Scales); school performance; adverse effects.

METHODS
Clinical Evidence search and appraisal August 2000.

| OPTION | METHYLPHENIDATE |

One recent systematic review has found that methylphenidate compared with placebo reduces core symptoms of ADHD (see glossary, p 212) in the short term but may disturb sleep and appetite. Few trials have compared methylphenidate with dexamfetamine, and results are inconsistent and inconclusive. Two small brief RCTs compared methylphenidate with imipramine, but found inconclusive results. Methylphenidate was consistently better than non-drug interventions, but the clinical importance of the results is unclear. Adding methylphenidate to behavioural treatment (see glossary, p 211) consistently improved outcomes.

Benefits: We found one recent systematic review (search date 2000).[11] Most studies were conducted in the USA, used a diagnosis of attention deficit disorder (DSM-III) or ADHD (DSM-IIIR or DSM-IV), and included children aged between 5–18 years, mostly recruited from psychiatric and other hospital outpatient clinics. **Versus placebo:** The systematic review[11] included, but did not pool results from, 13 rigorously selected short term RCTs (1177 children, aged 5–18 years). Three RCTs (99 children) did not find significant benefits in favour of methylphenidate. The other 10 RCTs found significant benefit in favour of methylphenidate (dose range 0.56–0.72 mg/kg per day or 5–35 mg/day for trials reporting in those units) on the Conners Teacher's Rating Scale hyperactivity index (see comment below). The same systematic review found similar results in 17 other RCTs (643 children), which were less stringent in terms of homogeneity of participants, outcome measures, and methodological quality. **Versus dexamfetamine:** The systematic review[11] identified four poorly reported crossover RCTs (224 children, aged 5–18 years) comparing methylphenidate (dose range 0.6 mg–4.5 mg/kg per day or 20 mg/day for trials reporting in those units) with dexamfetamine (dose 0.39–2.6 mg/kg per day or 10 mg/day for trials reporting in those units) but, because of heterogeneity, could not pool their results. Three RCTs (99 children aged 5–12 years) did not report any significant differences in the outcomes of interest. The other RCT found better outcomes with methylphenidate than with dexamfetamine for some, but not all measures. No firm conclusions can be drawn. **Versus tricyclic antidepressants:** The systematic review[11] identified, but could not pool, the results of two poorly reported crossover RCTs (105 children) comparing methylphenidate (dose 0.4 mg/kg or mean 20 mg/day for trials reporting in those units) with imipramine (dose 1–2 mg/kg/day or mean 65 mg per day for trials reporting in those units). One RCT (75 children) found no significant differences in clinical outcomes after 1 year, and the other (30 children) found imipramine versus methylphenidate improved some but not all outcomes in the short term. No firm conclusions can be drawn. **Versus non-drug treatments:** The systematic review identified four RCTs comparing methylphenidate and non-drug treatments.[11] Three of the RCTs were poorly reported (192 children aged 5–12 years) and compared methylphenidate (5–60 mg/day) with a variety of non-drug treatments (individual cognitive training over 12 weeks; parent and teacher training; behaviour therapy for 8 weeks). Overall these three RCTs found limited evidence that, in the medium term, methylphenidate versus non-drug treatment improves symptoms. The fourth RCT (579 children aged 7–10 years) compared medication treatment (144 children, double blind titration of methylphenidate dose, switched to alternative medication after 28 days if response unsatisfactory, mean initial dose 30.5 mg/day) versus intensive behavioural management (144 children) versus combined medication and intensive behavioural management (145 children) versus standard community care (146 children). A total of 74% of the children in the medication group were taking methylphenidate at the end of the study. Results were not presented as the number of children who improved, but only as P values. Methylphenidate versus non-drug treatments improved some but not all of the symptoms of ADHD. **As an adjunct to non-drug interventions:** See option, p 211.

Harms:
We found one recent systematic review (search date 2000),[11] which did not combine results because of heterogeneity and incomplete data reporting. It presented the number of RCTs that had found significant results (see comment below). **Versus placebo:** The following symptoms were found by at least one RCT to be significantly more common in children receiving methylphenidate: sleep disorders; anorexia or appetite disturbance; headache; motor tics; irritability; and abdominal pain (see table 1, p 213). We found no good evidence of effects of methylphenidate on growth rates in children. **Versus dexamfetamine:** The systematic review found that two of five RCTs recorded no significant differences for anorexia or appetite disturbance between methylphenidate and dexamfetamine. Motor tics, abdominal pain, and irritability were not significantly different in the single RCT that reported these. **Versus non-drug interventions:** The one large study comparing medication with intensive behavioural treatment[12] found that, of the children receiving either medication management or combined medication and intensive behavioural treatment, 50% reported mild adverse effects, 11% had moderate adverse effects, and 3% experienced severe adverse effects.

Comment:
The RCT comparing medication treatment versus intensive behavioural treatment versus combined medication plus intensive behavioural treatment versus standard community care is the largest and most rigorous currently available RCT of ADHD treatments.[12] However, there are concerns about the methods used in the RCT, which raise doubts about the firmness of its conclusions.[13] The principal outcome measures were rating scales based on impressions of parents and teachers. It did not include the child's view or direct measures of their response to treatment. Other outcomes such as school achievement were not measured. Long term effects on psychosocial adjustment, educational success, or behavioural improvement are unclear. We found no evidence about methylphenidate for pre-school children.[14] A systematic review is being prepared on the efficacy and safety of methylphenidate in attention deficit disorder (H Schachter, personal communication, 2000).

OPTION   DEXAMFETAMINE SULPHATE

One systematic review combined four small RCTs comparing dexamfetamine with placebo, but the clinical importance of the significant findings is unclear. Few trials compare methylphenidate with dexamfetamine, and the results are inconsistent and inconclusive.

Benefits: **Versus placebo:** We found one systematic review (search date 1997, 4 relevant RCTs, 61 children aged 6–12 years, dexamfetamine 0.46–0.75 mg/kg per day).[14] It found that dexamfetamine improved the change in the abbreviated Conners Teacher Rating Scale more than placebo (WMD −4.8, 95% CI −6.4 to −2.9). **Versus methylphenidate:** See option, p 207.

Harms: We found one recent high quality systematic review (search date 1997),[5] which did not combine results because of heterogeneity of studies and incomplete data reporting, but presented the number of RCTs with significant results. **Versus placebo:** The systematic review found that anorexia and appetite disturbance were significantly increased in the group receiving dexamfetamine in three RCTs.[5] **Versus methylphenidate:** See option, p 207.

Comment: The abbreviated Conners Teacher Rating Scale has been used widely in treatment studies and has been researched, validated, and standardised to measure treatment effects in ADHD.[15] However, the clinical importance of the effect of methylphenidate versus placebo on the abbreviated Conners Teacher Rating Scale remains unclear (see comment under methylphenidate for the principal outcome measures, p 208).

OPTION   CLONIDINE

Limited evidence from one recent systematic review found that clonidine was more effective than placebo in reducing ADHD symptoms, but the clinical importance of these findings is unclear.

Benefits: **Versus placebo:** We found one relevant systematic review (search date 1999, 6 RCTs, 143 children, mean age 11 years, dose of clonidine 0.1–0.24 mg/day for 4–12 weeks).[16] One of the six RCTs was a comparison of clonidine versus methylphenidate, rather than versus placebo,[17] but the other five RCTs were not analysed separately. Rating scales of the clinical features of ADHD completed by parents, teachers, and clinicians were combined. A meta-analysis of the six RCTs found that clonidine improved this combined rating scale more than placebo (effect size 0.58, 95% CI 0.27 to 0.89). The clinical importance of this result is not clear (see comment below), and the results should be treated with caution. **Versus other drugs:** We found no systematic review but found one small RCT (3 groups of 8 boys aged 6–16 years with ADHD and either co-morbid oppositional defiant disorder [see glossary, p 212] or conduct disorder [see glossary, p 212]), which compared clonidine (mean dose 0.17 mg/day) versus methylphenidate (mean dose 35 mg/day) versus both drugs.[17] Most outcomes were not significantly different between the three groups. The teacher reported School Situations Questionnaire improved more with methylphenidate than with clonidine (P < 0.009). The clinical importance of this isolated result from a single small RCT is unclear.

Harms: **Versus placebo:** The systematic review[16] included information from 10 studies of harms. Not all were high quality RCTs, and their results are difficult to interpret. Nine of 10 studies found sedation in children taking clonidine. Six studies found increased irritability. Electrocardiographs were recorded in two placebo controlled RCTs, which found no abnormalities. **Versus other drugs:** One small RCT (24 boys)[17] found that two of eight children on clonidine developed new onset bradycardia. Four of eight children on a combination of clonidine and methylphenidate developed bradycardia.

Comment: The systematic review[16] noted larger effect sizes in smaller and lower quality studies. Inclusion of the RCT of clonidine versus methylphenidate[17] in the systematic review creates difficulties in using that review to indicate the effects of clonidine versus placebo. The RCT[17] had a larger effect size than most other included studies, and it is likely to have inflated the final result of the meta-analysis. The results used by the systematic review for that RCT were not described in the original RCT report, and may have been a less reliable comparison of baseline and end of the study measures, rather than a rigorous comparison of randomly allocated groups. The results of the systematic review may not provide a good estimate of the effects of clonidine versus placebo. Harms were reported as the number of studies that recorded a specific adverse effect or not, rather then the number of children experiencing adverse effects.

OPTION	PSYCHOLOGICAL/BEHAVIOURAL TREATMENT

One systematic review found insufficient evidence about psychological/behavioural treatment used alone. Psychological/ behavioural therapy appears inferior to methylphenidate in the short term, but the clinical importance of the results is unclear.

Benefits: **Versus standard care:** We found one systematic review (search date 1997, 2 RCTs, 50 children aged 6–13 years),[14] which found that psychological/behavioural treatment (see glossary, p 212) versus standard care did not significantly improve teacher rating scales (SMD –0.40, 95% CI –1.28 to +0.48), or parent ratings (1 RCT, 26 children, WMD –3.8, CI –9.6 to +2.0). The RCTs were small and the clinical importance of these results is unclear. One RCT (290 children)[12] compared intensive behavioural treatments versus standard community care. Substantial improvement occurred in both groups. Intensive behavioural treatment was not significantly different from standard community care. For children with comorbid anxiety disorders (see glossary, p 211), intensive behavioural treatment was found to give better outcomes. **Versus methylphenidate:** See option, p 207. **Versus combined medication management and psychological/behavioural treatments:** See option, p 207.

Harms: Harms were not reported.

Comment: Children in the trials had differing diagnoses, presentations, and clinical needs.[18] Complex clinical outcomes, such as social adjustment or improved educational functioning, are difficult to measure. High quality psychological/behavioural trials are difficult to design and conduct. Caution is needed in the interpretation of findings regarding psychological/behavioural therapies alone or in combination with drug treatments because of methodological difficulties.[14]

OPTION	DRUGS PLUS PSYCHOLOGICAL/BEHAVIOURAL TREATMENT

One systematic review found inconsistent results for combination treatments in ADHD. A subsequent RCT found combined treatments were more effective than standard community treatment and behavioural/psychological treatments. The results were less clear comparing combined treatments to medication alone, with both treatments broadly equally effective for ADHD symptoms.

Benefits: We found one systematic review (search date 1997, 3 RCTs, 35 children, aged 5–13 years),[14] which found inconsistent results. **Versus control/placebo:** Combinations of medication with psychological/behavioural therapies were more effective than various control/placebo conditions for parent ratings of ADHD (Conners Parent Rating Scale WMD −7.3, 95% CI −12.3 to −2.4), but not teacher ratings of ADHD (Conners Teacher Rating Scale WMD 1.3, 95% CI −0.7 to +3.2). The clinical importance of these results is unclear. **Versus stimulant drugs alone:** See option, p 207. **Versus psychological/behavioural treatments alone:** We found one systematic review[11] and one subsequent RCT.[12] The systematic review (search date 2000, 11 RCTs, 428 children aged 5–18 years)[11] found that methylphenidate plus behavioural treatments versus behavioural treatments alone significantly improved ADHD behaviours, symptoms, and measures of academic achievement. The subsequent RCT[12] found that combined drug and intensive behavioural treatment versus intensive behavioural treatment alone significantly improved three of five measures of ADHD core symptoms, one of three measures of aggression/oppositional behaviour, one of three measure of anxiety depression, and one of three measures of academic achievement. No significant difference was found in social skills or in measures of the relationship between parents and children.[11]

Harms: We found no evidence of adverse effects other than those for the drug alone.

Comment: The recent RCT[12] is the largest and most methodologically rigorous study of ADHD treatments with high standards for reporting and follow up of nearly all children (see comment under methylphenidate, p 208).[13]

GLOSSARY

Anxiety disorder A range of conditions with features, including apprehension, motor tension, and autonomic overactivity.

Behavioural treatment Treatment using insights from learning theory to achieve specific changes in behaviour. It is usually highly structured. It can be used with either children with ADHD or their parents/carers.

Cognitive training Brief structured treatment aimed at changing dysfunctional beliefs.

Conduct disorder Conduct disorders include a repetitive pattern of antisocial, aggressive, or defiant conduct, which violate age appropriate social expectations.[2]

Core symptoms of ADHD Inattention, hyperactivity, and impulsivity are commonly known as the core symptoms of ADHD.[5]

Depressive disorder Characterised by persistent low mood, loss of interest and enjoyment, and reduced energy.

Oppositional defiant disorder Presence of markedly defiant, disobedient, provocative behaviour, but without the severely dissocial or aggressive acts seen in conduct disorder.[2]

Psychological/behavioural treatments Include any of the following methods: contingency management methods (e.g. behaviour modification); cognitive–behavioural therapy; individual psychotherapy; parent training or education; teacher training and education; parent and family counselling/therapy; social skills training; and electroencephalogram, biofeedback, or relaxation therapy.

REFERENCES

1. American Psychiatric Association. *Diagnostic and Statistical Manual of Mental Disorders, 4th Edition (DSM-IV)*. American Psychiatric Association, Washington, DC, 1994.
2. The International Statistical Classification of Diseases and Related Health Problems, 10th Revision. 10th Edition. World Health Organisation, 1994.
3. Taylor E, Sergeant J, Doepfner M, et al. Clinical guidelines for hyperkinetic disorder. European Society for Child and Adolescent Psychiatry. *Eur Child Adolesc Psychiatry* 1998;7:184–200.
4. Goldman LS, Genel M, Bezman RJ, Slanetz PJ. Diagnosis and treatment of attention-deficit/hyperactivity disorder in children and adolescents. Council on Scientific Affairs, American Medical Association. *JAMA* 1998;279:1100–1107.
5. Jadad AR, Boyle M, Cunningham C, Kim M, Schachar R. Treatment of attention-deficit/hyperactivity disorder. Evidence report/technology assessment: No 11 (Prepared by McMaster University under Contract No. 290–97–0017). 1999. Agency for Health Care Policy and Research and Quality. Search date November 1997; primary sources Medline; Cinahl; HealthStar; Psycinfo; Embase; Cochrane Library; hand searched reference lists; organisations funding research on ADHD and researchers contacted.
6. Green M, Wong M, Atkins D, et al. *Diagnosis and treatment of attention-deficit/hyperactivity disorder in children and adolescents*. Council on Scientific Affairs, American Medical Association. Technical Review No.3 (Prepared by Technical Resources International, Inc. under Contract No. 290–94–2024.). Agency for Health Care Policy and Research, AHCPR Publication No. 99–0050. Rockville, MD, 1999.
7. Finkel MF. The diagnosis and treatment of the adult attention deficit hyperactivity disorders. *Neurologist* 1997;3:31–44.
8. Hertzig MEE, Farber EAE. *Annual progress in child psychiatry and child development, 1996*. New York: Brunner/Mazel Inc, 1997:602.
9. Kaminester DD. Attention deficit hyperactivity disorder and methylphenidate: When society misunderstands medicine. *McGill J Med* 1997;3:105–114.
10. Taylor E, Sandberg S, Thorley G, Giles S. *The epidemiology of childhood hyperactivity*. London, Institute of Psychiatry. Maudsley Monographs 1991;33.
11. Lord J, Paisley S. The clinical effectiveness and cost-effectiveness of methylphenidate for hyperactivity in childhood. London: National Institute for Clinical Excellence, Version 2, August 2000. Search date 2000; primary sources Jadad, et al, reference 5 above; Medline; Cinahl; Healthstar; Psychinfo; and Embase.
12. A 14-month randomized clinical trial of treatment strategies for attention-deficit/hyperactivity disorder. The MTA Cooperative Group. Multimodal Treatment Study of Children with ADHD. *Arch Gen Psychiatry* 1999;56:1073–1086.
13. Boyle MH, Jadad AR. Lessons from large trials: the MTA study as a model for evaluating the treatment of childhood psychiatric disorder. *Can J Psychiatry* 1999;44:991–998.
14. Miller A, Lee SK, Raina P, Klassen A, Zupanic J, Olsen L. A review of therapies for attention-deficit/hyperactivity disorder. 1998. Canadian Coordinating Office for Health Technology Assessment. Search date not given; primary sources Medline; Current Contents; hand search of review articles and textbooks and British Columbia Methylphenidate Survey and Intercontinental Medical Statistics for information on drug prescription and utilization in Canada.
15. Goyette CH, Conners CK, Ulrich RF. Normative data on revised Conners parent and teacher rating scales. *J Abnorm Child Psychol* 1978;6:221–236.
16. Connor DF, Fletcher KE, Swanson JM. A meta-analysis of clonidine for symptoms of attention-deficit hyperactivity disorder. *J Am Acad Child Adolesc Psychiatry* 1999;38:1551–1559. Search date 1999; primary sources Medline; PsychInfo; Current Contents; Social and Behavioral Sciences; and Current Contents Clinical Medicine and hand searches of non peer reviewed research reports; book chapters; chapter bibliographies; and individual report references.
17. Connor DF, Barkley RA, Davis HT. A pilot study of methylphenidate, clonidine, or the combination in ADHD comorbid with aggressive oppositional defiant or conduct disorder. *Clin Pediatr (Phila)* 2000;39:15–25.
18. Klassen A, Miller A, Raina P, et al. Attention-deficit hyperactivity disorder in children and youth: A quantitative systematic review of the efficacy of different management strategies. *Can J Psychiatry* 1999;44:1007–1016. Search date 1997; primary sources Current Index to Journals in Education, Healthstar, Medline, Psycinfo, Embase, Current Contents, Cochrane Library, and hand searches of reference lists, and contact with manufacturers.

Carol Joughin
Project Manager
FOCUS
Royal College of Psychiatrists
Research Unit
London
UK

Morris Zwi
Consultant Child and Adolescent
Psychiatrist
Child and Family Consultation Centre
Richmond
Surrey
UK

Paul Ramchandani
Specialist Registrar
Park Hospital for Children
Oxford
UK

Competing interests: None declared. The opinions expressed are those of the authors and do not necessarily reflect those of the Royal College of Psychiatrists.

TABLE 1 The number of RCTs reporting significant adverse effects with methylphenidate versus placebo (see text, p 208).[11]

Adverse effect	Number of trials (%)
Anorexia or appetite disturbance	7/12 (58%)
Motor tics	1/2 (50%)
Irritability	2/9 (22%)
Sleep disorder	4/20 (20%)
Abdominal pain	2/10 (20%)
Headache	2/10 (20%)

Bronchiolitis

Search date May 2000

Nancy Tang and Elaine Wang

Child health

INTERVENTIONS

Key Messages

Treatment

- Two small, good quality systematic reviews of RCTs have found that inhaled bronchodilators improve overall clinical scores in children in the short term, although they found no evidence that bronchodilators reduce admission rates or improve oxygen saturation.

- One systematic review and seven RCTs found limited and conflicting evidence on the effects of corticosteroids in children with bronchiolitis.

- One RCT found no evidence that routine use of antibiotics improved clinical scores in children with bronchiolitis.

- One systematic review of small RCTs found no evidence that ribavirin reduces mortality or the risk of respiratory deterioration in children admitted to hospital with respiratory syncytial virus (RSV) bronchiolitis. One additional RCT found no evidence that ribavirin reduces duration of ventilation or hospital stay in children intubated for bronchiolitis.

- We found insufficient evidence to determine the effect of immunoglobulin treatment on clinical outcomes for children with bronchiolitis.

Preventing transmission in hospital

- We found no evidence from RCTs that cohort segregation, handwashing, or the wearing of gowns, masks or eye-nose goggles by carers reduced transmission rates between children in hospital.

Prevention in high risk children

- One systematic review of RCTs has found that, in children born prematurely, in children with bronchopulmonary dysplasia, and in children with a combination of risk factors, prophylactic immunoglobulin (RSVIg) or monoclonal antibody reduces admission rates to hospital and intensive care.

DEFINITION Bronchiolitis is a virally induced acute bronchiolar inflammation that is associated with signs and symptoms of airway obstruction. Diagnosis is based on clinical findings. Clinical manifestations include fever, rhinitis (inflammation of the nasal mucosa), tachypnoea, expiratory wheezing, cough, rales, use of accessory muscles, apnoea (absence of breathing), dyspnoea (difficulty in breathing), alar flaring (flaring of the nostrils), and retractions (in-drawing of the intercostal soft tissues on inspiration). Clinically, disease severity (see glossary, p 221) of bronchiolitis may be classified as mild, moderate, or severe.

INCIDENCE/ PREVALENCE Bronchiolitis is the most common lower respiratory tract infection in infants, occurring in a seasonal pattern with highest incidence in the winter in temperate climates[1] and in the rainy season in warmer countries. Each year in North America, about 21% of infants have lower respiratory tract disease and 6–10 per 1000 infants require admission to hospital for bronchiolitis (1%–2% of children under 12 months of age[2]). The peak rate of admission occurs in infants aged between 2–6 months.[3]

AETIOLOGY/ RISK FACTORS Respiratory syncytial virus (RSV) is responsible for bronchiolitis in 70% of cases. This figure reaches 80–100% in the winter months. However, in early spring, parainfluenza virus type 3 is often responsible.[1]

PROGNOSIS **Morbidity and mortality:** Disease severity is directly related to the size of the infant, and proximity and frequency of contact with infective infants. Children at increased risk of morbidity and mortality are those with congenital heart disease, chronic lung disease, history of premature birth, hypoxia, and age less than 6 weeks.[4] Other factors associated with a prolonged or complicated hospital stay include a history of apnoea or respiratory arrest, pulmonary consolidation as shown on a chest radiograph, and (in North America) native American or Inuit race.[5] The risk of death within 2 weeks is high for children with congenital heart disease (3.4%) or chronic lung disease (3.5%) compared with other groups combined (0.1%).[4] Rates of admission to the intensive care unit (ICU) (range 31% to 36%) and need for mechanical ventilation (range 11% to 19%) is similar among all high risk groups.[4] The percentage of these children needing oxygen supplementation is also high (range 63% to 80%).[4] In contrast, mortality in children with bronchiolitis, but without these risk factors, is less than 1%, and rates of ICU admission and ventilation in such children are markedly lower (15% and 8%).[6] **Long term prognosis:** Information on long term prognosis varies depending on inception cohort. One small prospective study of two matched cohorts (one with bronchiolitis, 25 children;

one without, 25 children) found no evidence that bronchiolitis requiring outpatient treatment was associated with an increased risk of asthma in the long term.[7] Possible confounding factors include differences in illness severity, smoke exposure, and crowding.[8] We found one prospective study in 50 randomly selected infants admitted with bronchiolitis, followed up by questionnaire for 5 years, and a visit in the fifth year. It found a doubling of asthma incidence compared with the general population, although there was large (30%) loss to follow up, and no matched control group.[9]

AIMS	To decrease morbidity and mortality, shorten hospital stay, and prevent transmission of infection, with minimum adverse effects.
OUTCOMES	Death rate; rate of intubation or admission to ICU; clinical score (clinical score is a subjective, unvalidated measure that is based on judgements made by the clinician); rates of clinical and serological infection.
METHODS	*Clinical Evidence* search and appraisal May 2000. Studies were appraised independently by the two authors and then reviewed again together to resolve differences by consensus. Titles were scanned and, if the article seemed relevant, the abstract was obtained and appraised to determine if the complete article was to be reviewed.

QUESTION What are the effects of treatment for children with bronchiolitis?

OPTION BRONCHODILATORS (INHALED SALBUTAMOL, INHALED EPINEPHRINE/ADRENALINE)

Two small, good quality systematic reviews of RCTs have found that inhaled bronchodilators achieve short term improvement in overall clinical scores in children treated in hospitals, emergency departments, and outpatient clinics, although they found no evidence that bronchodilators reduced admission rates or improved oxygen saturation.

Benefits: We found two systematic reviews. The first (updated in 1998) found eight RCTs in a total of 485 children treated in outpatient clinics or the emergency department and after admission to hospital.[10] The second review (search date 1995) found five RCTs in 251 children treated in outpatient clinics.[11] Four RCTs were common to both reviews. The first review found that, in the short term, bronchodilators improved clinical scores in children with mild and moderately severe bronchiolitis (RR for lack of improvement in clinical score, bronchodilator v placebo, 0.76, 95% CI 0.60 to 0.95).[10] Both reviews found no evidence that bronchodilators improved oxygen saturation by a clinically important amount (effect size for oxygen saturation 0.14, 95% CI −0.04 to +0.33;[10] mean difference in oxygen saturation 1.2%, 95% CI 0.8% to 1.6%[11]). Both reviews found no evidence that bronchodilators versus placebo reduced admission rates in children treated in outpatient clinics or the emergency department (RR 0.85, 95% CI 0.47 to 1.53;[10] 23 children treated with bronchodilator admitted v 21 with placebo, P = NS[11]).

Harms: One systematic review reported tachycardia, increased blood pressure, decreased oxygen saturation, flushing, hyperactivity, prolonged cough, and tremor following use of bronchodilators. The review did not report frequency of adverse events.[10] The second review did not report on harms.[11]

Comment: None of the trials used respiratory failure as an outcome. Discrepancies in primary studies included differences in study populations, such as inclusion of sedated children, short duration of follow up, and validity of clinical scores. Results of individual trials were contradictory. Bronchodilators may improve the clinical appearance of a child through a general stimulatory effect rather than by improving respiratory function.[12]

OPTION   CORTICOSTEROIDS

One systematic review and seven RCTs found limited and conflicting evidence on the effects of corticosteroids in children with bronchiolitis.

Benefits: We found one systematic review[13] (6 RCTs, search date 1999; 347 children in hospital) and seven additional RCTs of corticosteroids versus placebo in children with bronchiolitis.[14–20] Three of the additional RCTs had been mentioned in the systematic review but excluded because of data inconsistency,[18] treatment outside hospital,[19] or failure to report the outcome markers sought by the systematic review.[20] The systematic review found no significant difference in the mean length of stay in all the RCTs that reported length of stay (5 RCTs; mean –0.43 days, 95% CI –1.05 to +0.18 days), in the four RCTs with clearly identified randomisation methods (mean –0.35 days, 95% CI –0.84 to +0.14 days) and after exclusion of RCTs that included children with previous wheezing (4 RCTs; mean –0.29 days, 95% CI –0.71 to +0.13 days).[13] Interpretation of the effect of corticosteroids versus placebo on clinical symptoms found by the systematic review is difficult (see comment below). The RCTs in the systematic review reported different clinical scales at varying times after starting treatment. The scales usually included measurements of oxygen saturation, wheezing, accessory muscle use, and respiratory rate. Results 72 hours after starting treatment were too heterogeneous for analysis. Only three RCTs (197 children) provided results for 24 hours after starting treatment. The systematic review pooled the standardised effect size for clinical scores from these three RCTs and found that corticosteroids versus placebo produced a significant improvement (1.60, 95% CI 1.28 to 1.92). Six of the seven additional RCTs comparing corticosteroids (360 children) versus placebo reported a clinical score: all found no significant difference for corticosteroids (355 children) versus placebo.[14–17,19,20]

Harms: The acute adverse effects of oral steroids are well documented, and include hyperglycaemia and immunosuppression. The trials did not give information on these.

Comment: The evidence presented in the published systematic review[13] is difficult to interpret because some of the RCTs did not exclude children with a history of wheezing who may have asthma, a condition likely to respond to steroids. The clinical scales used in the RCTs included oxygen saturation, but the clinical relevance of changes in this item are unclear. Even if the results are accepted at face value, the clinical significance of an effect size of 1.6 is unclear.

Another systematic review is under way (E Wang, personal communication, 2000). We found inadequate evidence to evaluate the effects of systemic versus inhaled corticosteroids.

| OPTION | ROUTINE ANTIBIOTICS |

One unblinded RCT found no evidence that routine antibiotics are of clinical benefit in children admitted to hospital with bronchiolitis and uncomplicated RSV pneumonia, although the study was not powerful enough to rule out an effect.

Benefits: We found no systematic review. We found one unblinded RCT comparing the routine use of antibiotics versus no antibiotics (no placebo) in 138 children admitted to hospital with clinically apparent pneumonia, 45% of whom were diagnosed with RSV infection. It found no significant difference between treatment groups in the proportion infected with RSV. It found no evidence that antibiotics reduced duration of hospital stay or respiratory rate, or improved clinical symptoms, clinical signs or radiographic assessment scores for pulmonary disease.[21]

Harms: The trial did not report on harms, although potential risks include superinfection with resistant bacteria and drug reactions.

Comment: The trial was unblinded and used block randomisation (children randomised in groups of 20). This reduces confidence in the results. Two children initially treated without antibiotics were switched to antibiotics owing to complicating purulent infections.

| OPTION | RIBAVIRIN |

One systematic review of small RCTs found no evidence that ribavirin reduced mortality or the risk of respiratory deterioration in children admitted to hospital with RSV bronchiolitis. One additional RCT found no evidence that ribavirin reduced duration of ventilation or hospital stay in children intubated for bronchiolitis.

Benefits: We found one systematic review (search date 1995, update 1997, 8 small RCTs, 250 children) and one subsequent RCT. The review found that, in children and infants hospitalised with RSV bronchiolitis, ribavirin did not significantly reduce mortality or the risk of respiratory deterioration compared with placebo (rate of respiratory depression with ribavirin v placebo 4/56 [7.1%] v 11/60 [18.3%], RR 0.42, 95% CI 0.16 to 1.34; mortality with ribavirin v placebo 3/56 [5.4%] v 6/43 [13.9%], RR 0.42, 95% CI 0.13 to 1.44).[22] The high mortality in both groups may have been due to severe disease at baseline. The RCT published after the review compared ribavirin aerosol versus placebo in 41 children within 24 hours of intubation for severe bronchiolitis. It found no difference in duration of ventilation (102 hours, 95% CI 37 to 167 hours with ribavirin v 126 hours, 95% CI 47 to 205 hours with placebo, P = 0.29) or hospital stay (256 hours, 95% CI 131 to 381 hours with ribavirin v 295 hours, 95% CI 171 to 419 hours; P = 0.32).[23]

Harms: We found no prospective data. The review and RCTs did not report on harms. We found case reports of headaches and contact lens dysfunction in carers. Ribavirin has been reported to be associated with acute bronchospasm in treated children. The standard aerosol is sticky, and clogging of ventilatory equipment has been reported.[24]

Comment: We found one small prospective study, which compared pulmonary function tests in 54 children who had previously been randomised to inpatient treatment with ribavirin or placebo. It found no evidence of long term differences in outcome, although the study was not powerful enough to rule out a difference.[25]

OPTION	IMMUNOGLOBULINS (POOLED IMMUNOGLOBULINS, RSV IG)

We found no evidence from small, low powered RCTs that immunoglobulins improve clinical outcomes in children admitted to hospital with bronchiolitis.

Benefits: We found no systematic review. We found five RCTs (4 using albumin solution as control, 1 using saline, 335 children in total).[26–30] Two trials used pooled immunoglobulin, two trials used RSV Ig, and one trial used a synthetic monoclonal antibody. Neither trial using RSV Ig found evidence that RSV Ig shortened hospital stay compared with albumin (in high risk children—see glossary, p 221, mean duration hospital stay RSV Ig v albumin 8.41 days v 8.89 days, P = NS; in non-high risk children, mean stay RSV Ig v albumin 4.58 days v 5.52 days, P = NS).[26,27] The third RCT found no evidence in 35 children that monoclonal antibody reduced hospital stay, duration of ventilation, or duration of treatment with supplemental oxygen (hospital stay, placebo v antibody 11.5 days, 95% CI 10.0 to 13.0 days v 14.5 days, 95% CI 12.4 to 16.6 days, P = 0.25; duration of oxygen treatment, placebo v antibody 9.5 days, 95% CI 7.9 to 11.1 days v 12.3 days, 95% CI 10.0 to 14.6 days, P = 0.47; duration of ventilation, placebo v antibody 6.2 days, 95% CI 4.7 to 7.7 days v 8.8 days, 95% CI 6.5 to 11.1 days, P = 0.45).[30] Neither of the remaining trials found any evidence that pooled immunoglobulin improved outcome in children with bronchiolitis.

Harms: The RCTs found that RSV Ig was associated with elevation of liver enzymes and anoxic spells (no frequency data given).[26] One open label RCT of prophylactic RSV Ig in 249 children found that adverse effects occurred in about 3% of treated children.[31] This trial and a subsequent analysis of the data found that effects included increased respiratory rate, mild fluid overload during the first infusion, urticarial reaction at the infusion site, mild decreases in oxygen saturation, and fever (no frequency data given).[31,32]

Comment: Four trials used albumin as control rather than placebo. The effects of albumin itself in bronchiolitis are not known.

QUESTION	What are the effects of measures to prevent transmission in hospital?

OPTION	NURSING INTERVENTIONS (COHORT SEGREGATION, HANDWASHING, GOWNS, MASKS, GLOVES, AND GOGGLES)

We found no direct evidence from RCTs that cohort segregation (see glossary, p 221), handwashing, use of gowns, masks, gloves, or goggles

reduce nosocomial transmission of RSV to other children. Handwashing is a well established technique for reducing cross infection in other contexts, so RCTs may not be ethically feasible.

Benefits: We found no systematic review and no good quality RCTs examining effects of cohort segregation, handwashing, gowns, masks, gloves, or goggles, used either singly or in combination, on nosocomial transmission of bronchiolitis in children.

Harms: **Cohort segregation:** Potential risks of cohort segregation include misdiagnosing RSV infection and putting non-infected patients at risk by subsequent placement into the wrong cohort. **Handwashing:** Dermatitis is a well recognised adverse effect of repeated handwashing. **Other interventions:** No harms reported.

Comment: **Single nursing interventions:** We found four observational studies comparing nosocomial infection rates in separate series of children before and after introduction of cohort segregation, handwashing, gowns and masks, and goggles. No study adjusted results for variations in baseline incidence. Three found a lower incidence of transmission after introduction of cohort segregation alone, handwashing alone, and eye-nose goggles alone.[33–35] The fourth found no significant difference in transmission after introducing gowns and masks.[36] **Combinations of nursing interventions:** We found one RCT in 58 medical personnel caring for children admitted with bronchiolitis, which found no significant difference in nosocomial infection rate in staff when they used gowns and masks, in addition to handwashing (5/28 [18%] of those using gowns, masks, and handwashing v 4/30 [13%] in the control group; RR 1.3, 95% CI 0.4 to 3.6).[37] The trial did not report on transmission rates in the children. One non-randomised prospective trial in 233 children at risk of severe nosocomial infection compared transmission rates in wards adopting different nursing policies. It found that a combination of cohort segregation, gowns, and gloves reduced nosocomial transmission rates, compared with all other policies (cohort segregation alone, gown and gloves alone, no special precautions) taken together. However, the control interventions did not remain constant throughout the trial, the results were based on an interim analysis, and the definition of "at risk" children was not clearly stated.[38]

QUESTION What are the effects of prophylactic measures in high risk children?

OPTION IMMUNOGLOBULIN

One systematic review of RCTs has found that, in children born prematurely, or children with bronchopulmonary dysplasia, prophylactic RSV Ig or monoclonal antibody given monthly reduces hospital admission. and admission to intensive care.

Benefits: We found one systematic review (updated March 1999, 4 RCTs, 2598 children) comparing monthly RSV Ig or monoclonal antibody versus placebo or no prophylaxis. Three of the trials used intravenous RSV Ig, and one used intramuscular monoclonal antibody. Two of the trials using RSV Ig were unblinded, and both of these used no prophylaxis as the control intervention. The review found that Ig reduced admission to hospital and intensive care but did not reduce the incidence of mechanical ventilation (OR prophylaxis v placebo for hospital admission 0.48, 95% CI 0.37 to 0.64; for ICU admission 0.47, 95% CI 0.29 to 0.77; for ventilation 0.99, 95% CI 0.48 to 2.07).[31]

Harms: See harms of immunoglobulins, p 219.

Comment: Premature infants included in the trials were children under 6 months old, with gestational age at birth less than either 32 or 35 weeks. Children with bronchopulmonary dysplasia were under 2 years old and still undergoing treatment for this anomaly. Planned subgroup analysis in the review found that prophylaxis reduced hospital admission in children whose only risk factor was prematurity (OR 0.27, 95% CI 0.15 to 0.49), and in children with bronchopulmonary dysplasia alone (OR 0.54, 95% CI 0.37 to 0.80), but not in children with cardiac comorbidity alone (OR 0.64, 95% CI 0.37 to 1.10).

GLOSSARY

Cohort segregation Children infected with different viral strains are segregated from each other and treated separately, with the aim of preventing cross infection.
Disease severity Mild: not requiring hospitalisation. Moderate: requiring hospitalisation but not intubation. Severe: requiring intubation or artificial ventilation.
High risk children Premature infants with or without bronchopulmonary dysplasia, or infants and children with congenital heart disease.

Substantive changes since last issue
Corticosteroids New systematic review;[13] conclusions unchanged.

REFERENCES

1. Phelan P, Olinsky A, Robertson C. *Respiratory illness in children.* 4th ed. London: Blackwell Scientific Publications, 1994.
2. Gruber W. Bronchiolitis. In: Long S, Pickering L, Prober C, eds. *Principles and practice of pediatric infectious diseases.* 1st ed. New York: Churchill Livingstone, 1997:1821.
3. Glezen WP, Taber LH, Frank AL, Kessel JA. Risk of primary infection and reinfection with respiratory syncytial virus. *Am J Dis Child* 1986;140:543–546.
4. Navas L, Wang E, de Carvalho V, Robinson J, PICNIC. Improved outcome of respiratory syncytial virus infections in a high-risk hospitalized population of Canadian children. *J Pediatr* 1992; 121:348–354.
5. Wang EEL, Law BJ, Stephens D, PICNIC. Pediatric Investigators Collaborative Network on Infections in Canada (PICNIC) study of morbidity and risk factors with RSV disease. *J Pediatr* 1995;126: 212–219.
6. Wang EEL, Law BJ, Boucher F, et al. Pediatric Investigators Collaborative Network on Infections in Canada (PICNIC) study of admission and management variation in patients hospitalized with respiratory syncytial viral lower respiratory infection. *J Pediatr* 1996;129:390–395.
7. McConnochie KM, Mark JD, McBride JT, et al. Normal pulmonary function measurements and airway reactivity in childhood after mild bronchiolitis. *J Pediatr* 1985;107:54–58.
8. McConnochie KM, Roghmann KJ. Parental smoking, presence of older siblings and family history of asthma increase risk of bronchiolitis. *Am J Dis Child* 1986;140:806–812.
9. Sly PD, Hibbert ME. Childhood asthma following hospitalization with acute viral bronchiolitis in infancy. *Pediatr Pulmonol* 1989;7:153–158.
10. Kellner JD, Ohlsson A, Gadomski AM, Wang EEL. Bronchodilators for bronchiolitis. In: The Cochrane Library, Issue 1, 2000. Oxford: Update Software. Search date June 1998; primary sources Medline from 1966; Embase from 1974; Reference Update, reference lists of articles, and files of two of the authors.
11. Flores G, Horwitz RI. Efficacy of beta 2-agonists in bronchiolitis: A reappraisal and meta-analysis. *Pediatrics* 1997;100:233–239. Search date 1995; primary sources Medline 1966 to January 1995, and hand searched references and selected journals.
12. Gadomski AM, Lichenstein R, Horton L, King J, Keane V, Permutt T. Efficacy of albuterol in the management of bronchiolitis. *Pediatrics* 1994;93: 907–912.
13. Garrison MM, Christakis DA, Harvey E, Cummings P, Davis RL. Systemic corticosteroids in infant bronchiolitis: A meta-analysis. *Pediatrics* 2000; 105:849. Search date 1999; primary sources Medline, Embase, Cochrane Clinical Trials Registry.
14. Richter H, Seddon P. Early nebulized budesonide in the treatment of bronchiolitis and the prevention

of postbronchiolitic wheezing. *J Pediatr* 1998;132: 849–853.

15. Bulow SM, Nir M, Levin E. Prednisolone treatment for respiratory syncytial virus infection: a randomized controlled trial of 147 infants. *Pediatrics* 1999;104:77.

16. Tal A, Bavilski C, Yohai D, Bearman JE, Gorodischer R, Moses SW. Dexamethasone and salbutamol in the treatment of acute wheezing in infants. *Pediatrics* 1983;71:13–18.

17. Cade A, Brownlee KG, Conway, SP. Randomised placebo-controlled trial of nebulised corticosteroids in acute respiratory syncytial viral bronchiolitis. *Arch Dis Child* 2000;82:126–130.

18. Connolly JH, Field CM, Glasgow JF, Slattery CM, MacLynn DM. A double blind trial of prednisolone in epidemic bronchiolitis due to respiratory syncytial virus. *Acta Paediatr Scand* 1969;58: 116–120.

19. Berger I, Argaman Z, Schwartz SB. Efficacy of corticosteroids in acute bronchiolitis: short-term and long- term follow-up. *Pediatr Pulmonol* 1998; 26:162–166.

20. Leer JA, Green JL, Heimlich EM, et al. Corticosteroid treatment in bronchiolitis. A controlled collaborative study in 297 infants and children. *Am J Dis Child* 1969;117:495–503.

21. Fris B, Andersen P, Brenoe E, et al. Antibiotic treatment of pneumonia and bronchiolitis: a prospective randomised study. *Arch Dis Child* 1984;59:1038–1045.

22. Randolph AG, Wang EEL. Ribavirin for respiratory syncytial virus lower respiratory tract infection. In: The Cochrane Library, Issue 1, 2000. Oxford: Update Software. Search date 1997; primary sources Medline from 1975; hand searched references and noted experts contacted.

23. Guerguerian AM, Gauthier M, Lebel MH, Farrell CA, Lacroix J. Ribavirin in ventilated respiratory syncytial virus bronchiolitis. *Am J Respir Crit Care Med* 1999;160:829–834.

24. Johnson EM. Developmental toxicity and safety evaluations of ribavirin. *Pediatr Infect Dis J* 1997; 9(suppl):85–87.

25. Long CE, Voter KZ, Barker WH, Hall CB. Long term follow-up of children hospitalized with respiratory syncytial virus lower respiratory tract infection and randomly treated with ribavirin or placebo. *Pediatr Infect Dis J* 1997;16:1023–1028.

26. Rodriguez WJ, Gruber WC, Welliver RC, et al. Respiratory syncytial virus (RSV) immune globulin intravenous therapy for RSV lower respiratory tract infection in infants and young children at high risk for severe RSV infections. *Pediatrics* 1997;99: 454–461.

27. Rodriguez WJ, Gruber WC, Groothuis JR, et al. Respiratory syncytial virus immune globulin

treatment of RSV lower respiratory tract infection in previously healthy children. *Pediatrics* 1997; 100:937–942.

28. Hemming VG, Rodriguez W, Kim HW, et al. Intravenous immunoglobulin treatment of respiratory syncytial virus infections in infants and young children. *Antimicrob Agents Chemother* 1987;31:1882–1886.

29. Rimensberger PC, Burek-Kozlowska A, Morell A, et al. Aerosolized immunoglobulin treatment of respiratory syncytial virus infection in infants. *Pediatr Infect Dis J* 1996;15:209–216.

30. Malley R, DeVincenzo J, Ramilo O, et al. Reduction of respiratory syncytial virus (RSV) in tracheal aspirates in intubated infants by use of humanized monoclonal antibody to RSV F protein. *J Infect Dis* 1998;178:1555–1561.

31. Wang EEL, Tang NK. Immunoglobulin for preventing respiratory syncytial virus infection. In: The Cochrane Library. Issue 4, 1999. Oxford: Update Software. Search date March 1999; primary sources Cochrane Acute Respiratory Infections Trials Register, Medline, abstracts from the Pediatric Academy Meetings and the Intersciences Conference on Antimicrobial Agents and Chemotherapy from 1994 to 1997.

32. Groothuis JR, Levin MJ, Rodriguez W, et al. Use of intravenous gamma globulin to passively immunize high-risk children against respiratory syncytial virus: safety and pharmacokinetics. *Antimicrob Agents Chemother* 1991;35:1469–1473.

33. Krasinski K, LaCouture R, Holzman R, Waithe E, Bonk S, Hanna B. Screening for respiratory syncytial virus and assignment to a cohort at admission to reduce nosocomial transmission. *J Pediatr* 1990;116:894–898.

34. Isaacs D, Dickson H, O'Callaghan C, Sheaves R, Winter A, Moxon ER. Handwashing and cohorting in prevention of hospital acquired infections with respiratory syncytial virus. *Arch Dis Child* 1991;66: 227–231.

35. Gala CL, Hall CB, Schnabel KC, et al. The use of eye-nose goggles to control nosocomial respiratory syncytial virus infection. *JAMA* 1986;256:2706–2708.

36. Hall CB, Douglas RG. Nosocomial respiratory syncytial virus infections: should gowns and masks be used? *Am J Dis Child* 1981;135:512–515.

37. Murphy D, Todd JK, Chao RK, Orr I, McIntosh K. The use of gowns and masks to control respiratory illness in pediatric hospital personnel. *J Pediatr* 1981;99:746–750.

38. Madge P, Paton JY, McColl JH, Mackie PLK. Prospective controlled study of four infection-control procedures to prevent nosocomial infection with respiratory syncytial virus. *Lancet* 1992;340: 1079–1083.

Nancy Tang

Elaine Wang
Associate Professor

Hospital for Sick Children
University of Toronto and Aventis Pasteur
Toronto
Canada

Competing interests: None declared.

Search date October 2000

David Creery and Kate Ackerman

Child health

INTERVENTIONS

Key Messages

- Outcome following out-of-hospital cardiorespiratory arrest in children is poor, and it is unclear at what stage intervention becomes futile.

- Prospective and retrospective observational studies have consistently found that out-of-hospital arrest in children where the cause is uncertain (fatal and near miss sudden infant death syndrome) has a far worse prognosis than arrest from any other cause.

- It is widely accepted that cardiopulmonary resuscitation and ventilation should be undertaken in children who have arrested. Placebo controlled trials would be considered unethical. We found no prospective evidence on the effects of training parents to perform cardiopulmonary resuscitation.

- One RCT found no evidence that endotracheal intubation improves survival or neurological outcome compared with bag-mask ventilation in children who have arrested in the community.

- We found no prospective evidence on the effects of bicarbonate, calcium, different doses of adrenaline (epinephrine), or direct current cardiac shock to improve the outcome of non-submersion out-of-hospital cardiorespiratory arrest in children.

© *Clinical Evidence* 2001;5:223–230.

Cardiorespiratory arrest

DEFINITION	Non-submersion out-of-hospital cardiorespiratory arrest in children is a state of pulselessness and apnoea occurring outside of a medical facility and not apparently caused by submersion in water. The term "sudden infant death syndrome" refers to the sudden unexpected death of a child, usually between the ages of 1 month and 1 year, for which a thorough postmortem examination does not define an adequate cause of death.[1] Near miss sudden infant death syndrome refers to survival of a child after an unexpected arrest of unknown cause.
INCIDENCE/ PREVALENCE	We found 11 studies (3 prospective, 8 retrospective) reporting the incidence of non-submersion out-of-hospital cardiorespiratory arrest in children (see table 1, p 230).[2–12] Ten studies reported the incidence in both adults and children,[2–8,10–12] and seven reported the incidence in children.[2,3,6–10] Incidence of arrests in the general population ranged from 2.2 to 5.7 per 100 000 people a year (mean 3.1, 95% CI 2.0 to 4.2).[7] Incidence in children ranged from 6.9 to 18.0 arrests per 100 000 children a year (mean 11.0, 95% CI 7.0 to 15.1).[10] One prospective study in 300 children found that about 50% of out-of-hospital cardiorespiratory arrests occurred in children under 12 months, and about two thirds occurred in children under 18 months.[10]
AETIOLOGY/ RISK FACTORS	We found 26 studies reporting the causes of non-submersion pulseless arrests in a total of 1574 children. The commonest causes of arrest were sudden infant death syndrome (39.1%), trauma (17.6%), chronic disease (7.1%), and pneumonia (4.2%) (see table 2, p 230).[2–29]
PROGNOSIS	We found no systematic review that investigated non-submersion arrests alone. We found one systematic review (search date 1997; primary sources Medline and bibliographic search), which reported outcomes after cardiopulmonary resuscitation for both in-hospital and out-of-hospital arrests of any cause, including submersion in children.[29] Studies were excluded if they did not report on survival. The review found evidence from prospective and retrospective observational studies that out-of-hospital arrest of any cause in children carries a poorer prognosis than arrest within hospital (132/1568 children [8.4%] survived to hospital discharge after out-of-hospital arrest v 129/544 children [24%] after in-hospital arrests). About half of the survivors were involved in studies that reported on neurological outcome. Of these, survival with "good neurological outcome" (i.e. normal or mild neurological deficit) was higher in children who arrested in hospital, compared with those who arrested elsewhere (60/77 surviving children [78%] v 28/68 [41%]).[29] We found 26 studies (5 prospective, 21 retrospective) in a total of 1734 children that reported only on out-of-hospital arrest (22 studies were included in the review; the remainder were published subsequent to the review search date).[2–11,13–28] The overall survival rate following out-of-hospital arrest was 5% (87 children). Nineteen of these studies (1140 people) found that, of the 48 surviving children, 12 (25%) had no or mild neurological disability, and 36 (75%) had moderate or severe neurological disability. Survival rates are listed according to cause of arrest (see table 2, p 230).

AIMS	To improve survival and minimise neurological sequelae in children suffering out-of-hospital cardiorespiratory arrest.
OUTCOMES	Out-of-hospital death rate; rate of death in hospital without return of spontaneous circulation; return of spontaneous circulation with subsequent death in hospital; and return of spontaneous circulation with successful hospital discharge with mild, moderate, severe, or no neurological sequelae; adverse effects of treatment.
METHODS	*Clinical Evidence* update search and appraisal October 2000. In addition, we searched citation lists of retrieved articles and relevant review articles. Studies reporting out-of-hospital arrest in adults that listed "adolescent" as a MeSH heading were also reviewed. Both authors reviewed the retrieved studies independently, and differences were resolved by discussion. We selected studies reporting out-of-hospital cardiorespiratory arrests in children. Studies were excluded if data relating to submersion could not be differentiated from non-submersion data (except where we found no data relating exclusively to non-submersion arrest; in such cases we have included studies that did not differentiate these types of arrest, and have made it clear that such evidence is limited by this fact). Likewise, as the pathogenesis of arrest in adults appears to be different from arrest in children, studies were excluded if data relating to adults could not be differentiated from data relating to children.

QUESTION What are the effects of treatments?

OPTION AIRWAY MANAGEMENT AND VENTILATION

It is widely accepted that good airway management and rapid ventilation should be undertaken in a child who has arrested, and it would be considered unethical to test its role in a placebo controlled trial.

Benefits: We found no studies comparing airway management and ventilation versus no intervention.

Harms: We found insufficient information.

Comment: It would be considered unethical to test the role of airway management and ventilation in a placebo controlled trial.

OPTION INTUBATION VERSUS BAG-MASK VENTILATION

One controlled trial found no evidence of a difference in survival or neurological outcome between bag-mask ventilation and endotracheal intubation in children requiring airway management in the community.

Benefits: We found no systematic review. We found one high quality controlled trial (830 children requiring airway management in the community, including 98 children who had arrested after submersion) of bag-mask ventilation versus endotracheal intubation (given by paramedic staff trained in these techniques).[30] Treatments were not randomised; each was allocated on alternate days. Analysis was by intention to treat (see comment below). The trial found no significant difference in rates of survival or good neurological outcome (normal, mild deficit, or no change from baseline function) between the two treatment groups (123/404 [30%] survived after bag-mask ventilation v 110/416 [26%] after intubation, OR 0.82, 95% CI 0.61 to 1.11; good neurological outcome achieved in 92/404 [23%] of children after bag-mask ventilation v 85/416 [20%] after intubation, OR 0.87, 95% CI 0.62 to 1.22).

Harms: The trial found that the time at the scene of the arrest was longer when intubation was intended, and this was the only significant determinant of a longer total time from dispatch of paramedic team to arrival at hospital (mean time at scene 9 minutes with bag-mask v 11 minutes with intubation, P < 0.001; mean total time 20 minutes with bag-mask v 23 minutes with intubation, P < 0.001).[30] However, the trial found no significant difference between bag-mask ventilation and intubation for complications common to both treatments (complications in 727 children for whom data were available, bag-mask v intubation: gastric distension 31% v 7%, P = 0.20; vomiting 14% v 14%, P = 0.82; aspiration 14% v 15%, P = 0.84; oral or airway trauma 1% v 2%, P = 0.24). A total of 186 children across both treatment groups were thought by paramedical staff to be successfully intubated. Of these, oesophageal intubation occurred in three children (2%); the tube became dislodged in 27 children (14%; unrecognised in 12 children, recognised in 15); right main bronchus intubation occurred in 33 children (18%); and an incorrect size of tube was used in 44 children (24%). Death occurred in all but one of the children with oesophageal intubation or unrecognised dislodging of the tube.[30]

Comment: **Population characteristics:** The baseline characteristics of children did not differ significantly between groups in age, sex, ethnicity, or cause of arrest. The trial did not report the frequency of pulseless arrest versus respiratory arrest. **Intention to treat:** Intubation and bag-mask ventilation are not mutually exclusive. The study protocol allowed bag-mask ventilation before intubation and after unsuccessful intubation. Of 420 children allocated to intubation, 115 received bag-mask ventilation before intubation, 128 received bag-mask ventilation after attempted intubation, four were lost to follow up, and the remainder received intubation that was believed to be successful. Of 410 children allocated to bag-mask ventilation, 10 children were intubated successfully (although in violation of study protocol), nine received bag-mask ventilation after attempted intubation, six were lost to follow up, and the remainder received bag-mask ventilation in accordance with study protocol.[30]

| OPTION | INTRAVENOUS ADRENALINE (EPINEPHRINE) |

Intravenous adrenaline (epinephrine) at "standard dose" (0.01 mg/kg) is a widely accepted treatment for establishing return of spontaneous circulation. We found no prospective evidence comparing adrenaline versus placebo, or comparing standard or single doses versus high or multiple doses of adrenaline, in children who have arrested in the community.

Benefits: We found no systematic review, no RCTs, and no prospective observational studies.

Harms: We found no prospective data in this context.

Comment: **Versus placebo:** Standard dose adrenaline is a widely accepted treatment for arrests in children. Placebo controlled trials would be considered unethical. **High versus low dose:** Two small retrospective studies (128 people) found no evidence of a difference in survival to hospital discharge between low or single dose epinephrine and high or multiple dose adrenaline, although the studies were too small to rule out an effect.[7,9]

OPTION	INTRAVENOUS BICARBONATE

We found insufficient evidence on the effects of intravenous bicarbonate in cardiorespiratory arrest in children.

Benefits: We found no RCTs.

Harms: We found insufficient evidence.

Comment: Bicarbonate is widely believed to be effective in arrest associated with hyperkalaemic ventricular tachycardia or fibrillation, but we found no prospective evidence supporting this.

OPTION	INTRAVENOUS CALCIUM

We found insufficient evidence on the effects of intravenous calcium in cardiorespiratory arrest in children.

Benefits: We found no RCTs.

Harms: We found insufficient evidence.

Comment: Calcium is widely believed to be effective in arrest associated with hyperkalaemic ventricular tachycardia or fibrillation, but we found no prospective evidence supporting this.

OPTION	BYSTANDER CARDIOPULMONARY RESUSCITATION

It is widely accepted that cardiopulmonary resuscitation and ventilation should be undertaken in children who have arrested. Placebo controlled trials would be considered unethical. We found no prospective evidence on the effects of training parents to perform cardiopulmonary resuscitation. One systematic review of observational studies found that children who were witnessed having an arrest and who received bystander cardiopulmonary resuscitation were more likely to survive to hospital discharge.

Benefits: We found no RCTs. We found one systematic review of prospective and retrospective studies. This concluded that survival was improved in children who were witnessed to arrest and received cardiopulmonary resuscitation from a bystander. Of 150 witnessed arrests outside hospital, 28 of 150 (19%) survived to hospital discharge Of those children who received bystander cardiopulmonary resuscitation, 20 of 76 (26%) survived to discharge.[29] The review did not report survival rates in children whose arrests were not witnessed, but the overall survival rate for out-of-hospital cardiac arrest was 8.4%. **Training parents to perform cardiopulmonary resuscitation:** We found no systematic review and no RCTs examining the effects of training parents to perform cardiopulmonary resuscitation in children who have arrested outside hospital.

Harms: Potential harms include those resulting from unnecessary chest compression after respiratory arrest with intact circulation.

Comment: The review of observational studies found that children who received bystander cardiopulmonary resuscitation had a hospital discharge rate of 26% (20/76) versus 11% (8/74) for children who also had their arrests witnessed but had not received cardiopulmonary resuscitation. Cardiopulmonary resuscitation was not randomly allocated and children resuscitated may be systematically different from those who did not receive resuscitation. The apparent survival rates for witnessed arrests and arrests with bystander initiated cardiopulmonary resuscitation may be artificially high because of inappropriate evaluation of true arrest. However, assuming confounding variables were evenly distributed between groups, then the best estimate of the benefit of cardiopulmonary resuscitation is a 15% absolute increase in the probability that children will be discharged alive from hospital (7 children).

OPTION	DIRECT CURRENT CARDIAC SHOCK

It is widely accepted that children who arrest outside hospital and are found to have ventricular fibrillation or pulseless ventricular tachycardia should receive direct current cardiac shock treatment. Placebo controlled trials would be considered unethical. We found insufficient evidence on the effects of direct current cardiac shock in children who have arrested in the community, regardless of the heart rhythm.

Benefits: We found no systematic review and no RCTs.

Harms: We found insufficient evidence.

Comment: **In children with ventricular fibrillation:** One retrospective study (29 children with ventricular fibrillation who had arrested out-of-hospital from a variety of causes, including submersion) found that of 27 children who were defibrillated, 11 survived (5 with no sequelae, 6 with severe disability). The five children with good outcome all received defibrillation within 10 minutes of arrest (time to defibrillation not given for those who died). Data on the two children who were not defibrillated were not presented.[31] **In children with asystole:** One retrospective study in 90 children with asystole (including those who had arrested after submersion) found that 49 (54%) had received direct current cardiac shock treatment. None of the children survived to hospital discharge, regardless of whether or not direct current cardiac shock was given.[32] We found one systematic review of observational studies (1420 children who had arrested outside hospital) that recorded electrocardiogram rhythm. Bradyasystole or pulseless electrical activity was found in 73%, whereas ventricular fibrillation or pulseless ventricular tachycardia were found in 10%.[29] The review found that survival after ventricular fibrillation or ventricular tachycardia arrest was higher than after asystolic arrest in children. Survival to discharge reported in the systematic review was 5% (39/802) for children with initial rhythm asystole and 30% (29/97) with initial rhythm ventricular fibrillation or ventricular tachycardia.[29]

REFERENCES

1. Gausche M, Barkin RM, eds. Sudden infant death syndrome (SIDS). In: *Pediatric Emergency Medicine*. Toronto: Mosby, 1997;1115–1116.
2. Eisenberg M, Bergner L, Hallstrom A. Epidemiology of cardiac arrest and resuscitation in children. *Ann Emerg Med* 1983;12:672–674.
3. Applebaum D, Slater PE. Should the Mobile Intensive Care Unit respond to pediatric emergencies? *Clin Pediatr (Phila)* 1986;25: 620–623.
4. Tsai A, Kallsen G. Epidemiology of pediatric prehospital care. *Ann Emerg Med* 1987;16: 284–292.
5. Thompson JE, Bonner B, Lower GM. Pediatric cardiopulmonary arrests in rural populations. *Pediatrics* 1990;86:302–306.
6. Safranek DJ, Eisenberg MS, Larsen MP. The epidemiology of cardiac arrest in young adults. *Ann Emerg Med* 1992;21:1102–1106.
7. Dieckmann RA, Vardis R. High-dose epinephrine in pediatric out-of-hospital cardiopulmonary arrest. *Pediatrics* 1995;95:901–913.
8. Kuisma M, Suominen P, Korpela R. Paediatric out-of-hospital cardiac arrests: epidemiology and outcome. *Resuscitation* 1995;30:141–150.
9. Ronco R, King W, Donley DK, Tilden SJ. Outcome and cost at a children's hospital following resuscitation for out-of-hospital cardiopulmonary arrest. *Arch Pediatr Adolesc Med* 1995;149: 210–214.
10. Sirbaugh PE, Pepe PE, Shook JE, et al. A prospective, population-based study of the demographics, epidemiology, management, and outcome of out-of-hospital pediatric cardiopulmonary arrest. *Ann Emerg Med* 1999; 33:174–184.
11. Friesen RM, Duncan P, Tweed WA, Bristow G. Appraisal of pediatric cardiopulmonary resuscitation. *Can Med Assoc J* 1982;126:1055–1058.
12. Hu SC. Out-of-hospital cardiac arrest in an oriental metropolitan city. *Am J Emerg Med* 1994;12: 491–494.
13. Barzilay Z, Somekh E, Sagy M, Boichis H. Pediatric cardiopulmonary resuscitation outcome. *J Med* 1988;19:229–241.
14. Bhende MS, Thompson AE. Evaluation of an end-tidal CO_2 detector during pediatric cardiopulmonary resuscitation. *Pediatrics* 1995; 95:395–399.
15. Brunette DD, Fischer R. Intravascular access in pediatric cardiac arrest. *Am J Emerg Med* 1988;6: 577–579.
16. Clinton JE, McGill J, Irwin G, Peterson G, Lilja GP, Ruiz E. Cardiac arrest under age 40: etiology and prognosis. *Ann Emerg Med* 1984;13:1011–1015.
17. Hazinski MF, Chahine AA, Holcomb GW III, Morris JA Jr. Outcome of cardiovascular collapse in pediatric blunt trauma. *Ann Emerg Med* 1994;23: 1229–1235.
18. Losek JD, Hennes H, Glaeser P, Hendley G, Nelson DB. Prehospital care of the pulseless, nonbreathing pediatric patient. *Am J Emerg Med* 1987;5:370–374.
19. Ludwig S, Kettrick RG, Parker M. Pediatric cardiopulmonary resuscitation. A review of 130 cases. *Clin Pediatr (Phila)* 1984;23:71–75.
20. Nichols DG, Kettrick RG, Swedlow DB, Lee S, Passman R, Ludwig S. Factors influencing outcome of cardiopulmonary resuscitation in children. *Pediatr Emerg Care* 1986;2:1–5.
21. O'Rourke PP. Outcome of children who are apneic and pulseless in the emergency room. *Crit Care Med* 1986;14:466–468.
22. Rosenberg NM. Pediatric cardiopulmonary arrest in the emergency department. *Am J Emerg Med* 1984;2:497–499.
23. Schindler MB, Bohn D, Cox PN, et al. Outcome of out-of-hospital cardiac or respiratory arrest in children. *N Engl J Med* 1996;335:1473–1479.
24. Sheikh A, Brogan T. Outcome and cost of open- and closed-chest cardiopulmonary resuscitation in pediatric cardiac arrests. *Pediatrics* 1994;93: 392–398.
25. Suominen P, Rasanen J, Kivioja A. Efficacy of cardiopulmonary resuscitation in pulseless paediatric trauma patients. *Resuscitation* 1998; 36:9–13.
26. Suominen P, Korpela R, Kuisma M, Silfvast T, Olkkola KT. Paediatric cardiac arrest and resuscitation provided by physician-staffed emergency care units. *Acta Anesthesiol Scand* 1997;41:260–265.
27. Torphy DE, Minter MG, Thompson BM. Cardiorespiratory arrest and resuscitation of children. *Am J Dis Child* 1984;138:1099–1102.
28. Walsh R. Outcome of pre-hospital CPR in the pediatric trauma patient. *Crit Care Med* 1994;22: A162.
29. Young KD, Seidel JS. Pediatric cardiopulmonary resuscitation: a collective review. *Ann Emerg Med* 1999;33:195–205. Search date 1966–1997; primary sources Medline and bibliographic search.
30. Gausche M, Lewis RJ, Stratton SJ, et al. Effect of out-of-hospital pediatric endotracheal intubation on survival and neurological outcome. *JAMA* 2000;283:783–790.
31. Mogayzel C, Quan L, Graves JR, Tiedeman D, Fahrenbruch C, Herndon P. Out-of-hospital ventricular fibrillation in children and adolescents: causes and outcomes. *Ann Emerg Med* 1995;25: 484–491.
32. Losek JD, Hennes H, Glaeser PW, Smith DS, Hendley G. Prehospital countershock treatment of pediatric asystole. *Am J Emerg Med* 1989;7: 571–575.

David Creery
Children's Hospital of Eastern Ontario
Ottawa
Canada

Kate Ackerman
The Children's Hospital
Boston
USA

Competing interests: None declared.

Cardiorespiratory arrest

TABLE 1 Incidence of non-submersion pre-hospital cardiorespiratory arrest in children* (see text, p 224).

Reference	Location	Year	Incidence per 100 000 people in total population	Incidence per 100 000 children
11	Manitoba, Canada	1982	2.9	–
2	King County, USA	1983	2.4	9.9
3	Jerusalem, Israel	1986	2.5	6.9
4	Fresno, USA	1987	5.7	–
5	Midwestern USA	1990	4.7	–
6	King County, USA	1992	2.4	10.1
12	Taipei, Taiwan	1994	1.3	–
7	San Francisco, USA	1995	2.2	16.1
8	Helsinki, Finland	1995	1.4	9.1
9	Birmingham, USA	1995	–	6.9
10	Houston, USA	1999	4.9	18.0

* Incidence represents arrests per 100 000 population per year.

TABLE 2 Causes of non-submersion pre-hospital cardiorespiratory arrest in children* (see text, p 224).

Cause	Number of arrests (%)	Number of survivors (%)
SIDS	691 (39.1)	1 (0.1)
Trauma	311 (17.6)	10 (3.2)
Chronic disease	126 (7.1)	9 (7.1)
Pneumonia	75 (4.2)	6 (8.0)
Non-accidental injury	23 (1.3)	2 (8.7)
Aspiration	20 (1.1)	0 (0)
Overdose	19 (1.1)	3 (15.8)
Other	309 (17.6)	28 (9.1)
Total	**1574 (88.1)**	**87 (3.7)**

*Figures represent the numbers of arrests/survivors in children with each diagnosis. SIDS, sudden infant death syndrome.

Search date December 2000

Gregory Rubin

QUESTIONS

INTERVENTIONS

Likely to be beneficial

Unknown effectiveness

Trade off between benefits and harms

*Not widely licensed for use in
    children. Clinical use in adults
    recently restricted because of
    heart rhythm abnormalities.

Key Messages

- We found no direct evidence that increased fibre intake is effective in childhood constipation.

- Two small RCTs have found that cisapride increases stool frequency and reduces gut transit time in children with constipation. Cisapride is not widely licensed for use in children; clinical use in adults is restricted because of heart arrhythmias.

- We found no placebo controlled trials of osmotic or stimulant laxatives. Small RCTs, comparing osmotic versus stimulant laxatives, have found limited evidence that both are effective. One small RCT found benefit from the addition of toilet training or biofeedback.

- Limited evidence from RCTs suggests short term but no long term benefit from adding biofeedback training to conventional treatment.

Constipation

DEFINITION Constipation is characterised by infrequent bowel evacuations, hard, small faeces, or difficult or painful defecation. The frequency of bowel evacuation varies from person to person.[1] Encopresis is defined as involuntary bowel movements in inappropriate places at least once a month for 3 months or more, in children aged 4 years and older.[2]

INCIDENCE/ PREVALENCE Constipation with or without encopresis is common in children. It accounts for 3% of consultations to paediatric outpatient clinics and 25% of paediatric gastroenterology consultations in the USA.[3] Encopresis has been reported in 1.5% of children at school entry. The peak incidence is at 2–4 years of age.

AETIOLOGY/ RISK FACTORS No cause is discovered in 90–95% of children with constipation. Low fibre intake and a family history of constipation may be associated factors.[4] Psychosocial factors are often suspected, although most children with constipation are developmentally normal.[3] Chronic constipation can lead to progressive faecal retention, distension of the rectum, and loss of sensory and motor function. Organic causes for constipation are uncommon, but include Hirschsprung's disease (1/5000 births; male : female 4 : 1; constipation invariably present from birth), cystic fibrosis, anorectal physiological abnormalities, anal fissures, constipating drugs, dehydrating metabolic conditions, and other forms of malabsorption.[3]

PROGNOSIS Childhood constipation can be difficult to treat, and often requires prolonged support, explanation, and medical treatment. In one long term follow up study of children presenting under the age of 5 years, 50% recovered within 1 year and 65–70% recovered within 2 years; the remainder required laxatives for daily bowel movements or continued to soil for years.[3] It is not known what proportion continue to have problems into adult life, although adults presenting with megarectum or megacolon often have a history of bowel problems from childhood.

AIMS To remove faecal impaction and to restore a bowel habit in which stools are soft and passed without discomfort.

OUTCOMES Number of defecations per week; number of episodes of soiling per month; gut transit time; use of laxatives.

METHODS *Clinical Evidence* update search and appraisal December 2000 using the following key words: constipation, diet therapy, diagnosis, therapy, psychology, stimulant laxatives, dietary fibre, lactulose. The search was limited to infants and children. No systematic reviews were identified. Trials were selected for inclusion if they focused on the management of constipation or encopresis, or both; if they were relevant to primary health care; and if they included children without an organic cause for constipation.

QUESTION **What are the effects of dietary and medical treatments?**

OPTION **INCREASED DIETARY FIBRE**

We found no direct evidence of benefit from increasing dietary fibre intake on colonic transit time or cure of constipation in children.

Benefits: We found no systematic review or good RCTs of the effect of increasing dietary fibre on constipation in children. We found one RCT of the effect of laxatives plus advice about dietary fibre on chronic constipation and colonic transit time in 73 children with the same mean fibre intake as healthy controls but increased colonic transit time.[5] The study found that, although advice significantly increased fibre intake, it did not significantly reduce colonic transit time or increase the cure of constipation at 6 months.

Harms: Adults who increase dietary fibre intake have reported abdominal pain and distension.

Comment: None.

OPTION **CISAPRIDE**

Two RCTs have found improvement in stool frequency and symptoms of constipation with cisapride after 8–12 weeks of treatment in an outpatient setting. We found no evidence from primary care settings. Cisapride has been suspended from the market in several countries because of adverse cardiac effects.

Benefits: We found no systematic review but found two RCTs. One RCT (69 children, aged 4–18 years, with idiopathic constipation) compared cisapride (0.3 mg/kg/day as a syrup) with placebo following clearance of accumulated stool. It found that cisapride significantly increased stool frequency and decreased gut transit time after 8 weeks (mean stool frequency per week 6.75 v 1.31).[6] The second RCT (40 children, aged 2–16 years), analysed by intention to treat, showed significant benefit for cisapride over placebo at 12 weeks, as measured by a composite of improved stool frequency, absence of faecal soiling, and no use of other laxatives (improvement in composite index AR 14/20 [70%] with cisapride v 7/20 [35%] with placebo; RR 2.0, CI 1.03 to 3.88; NNT 3, 95% CI 1 to 24).[7]

Harms: The RCTs did not report harms; see comment below.

Comment: Cisapride is licensed for use in children in the Republic of Ireland. Its license has been suspended in the UK and Germany, and its marketing stopped in the USA, because of its association with heart rhythm abnormalities in adults.

OPTION **OSMOTIC LAXATIVES**

We found limited evidence that osmotic laxatives may increase stool frequency, and in infants result in normal stools. One small RCT found short term benefit from the addition of toilet training or biofeedback.

Benefits: We found no systematic review and no placebo controlled trials of osmotic laxatives in children. We found two small RCTs comparing the effects of lactitol versus lactulose on stool frequency and consistency in 51 and 39 children with constipation.[8,9] Both preparations resulted in a significant increase in stool frequency at 4 weeks and normal consistency of stools at 2 weeks compared with baseline.[8,9] A third RCT (220 non-breastfed, constipated infants aged 0–6 months) compared 2% versus 4% lactulose mixed with an artificial milk preparation.[10] At 14 days, over 90% of parents in both groups reported easy passage of normal or thin consistency stools (P < 0.05 compared with baseline). **With toilet training or biofeedback:** One RCT (87 children with encopresis) compared medical treatment (enemas and laxatives) with and without toilet training.[11] A third arm of the trial evaluated biofeedback. Children receiving toilet training used significantly fewer laxatives and required fewer treatment sessions than those in the other two groups. Toilet training and biofeedback produced similar reductions in rates of soiling, which were greater than those achieved by medical treatment alone (P < 0.04).

Harms: One study found that children taking lactulose experienced significantly more abdominal pain and flatus than those taking lactitol (English abstract only, detailed results will be reported following translation).[8]

Comment: The benefits shown in these studies are comparisons of outcomes before and after treatment, and were not necessarily due to the treatments.[8,9] Toilet training consisted of reinforcement and scheduling to promote response to the urge to defecate, and instruction and modelling to promote appropriate straining.[11]

OPTION   STIMULANT LAXATIVES

We found no placebo controlled RCTs of the effects of stimulant laxatives in children.

Benefits: We found no systematic review or placebo controlled RCT. Studies were all comparative and used multiple interventions, had small sample sizes, or both. One quasi-randomised study (see comment below) compared senna versus mineral oil concentrate in 37 children aged 3–12 years with chronic constipation.[12] The study found that senna versus mineral oil after 6 months was less effective in reducing involuntary faecal soiling (involuntary faecal soiling AR 8/18 [44%] with senna v 1/19 [5%] with mineral oil; RR 8.44, 95% CI 1.52 to 16.72). No significant differences were found in the number of children with relapses of constipation symptoms during the treatment period (relapses of constipation AR 12/19 [63%] with senna v 16/18 [89%] with mineral oil; RR 0.71, 95% CI 0.48 to 1.04).[12] **With toilet training or biofeedback:** See osmotic laxatives, p 233.[11]

Harms: None identified.

Comment: The study used last hospital number digit to randomise patients.[12]

OPTION   BIOFEEDBACK TRAINING

RCTs found short term benefit from adding biofeedback training to conventional treatment in childhood constipation. Two RCTs found no significant benefit after 1 year.

Benefits: We found no systematic review. Four RCTs compared conventional treatment with or without biofeedback in 87,[11] 192,[13] 129,[14] and 41[15] children with constipation, encopresis, or both. The biofeedback compared 2–6 weeks of training[15] or seminars.[13] Two studies found short term benefit in defecation dynamics,[13,15] and rates of soiling,[11] but none found significant improvement in soiling, stool frequency, or laxative use at 1 year or more.

Harms: None identified.

Comment: None.

REFERENCES

1. Nelson R, Wagget J, Lennard-Jones JE, Barnes PRH. Constipation and megacolon in children and adults. In: Misiewicz JJ, Pounder RE, Venables CW, eds. *Diseases of the gut and pancreas*. 2nd ed. Oxford: Blackwell Science, 1994.

2. American Psychiatric Association. *Diagnostic and statistical manual of mental disorders*. 4th ed. Washington, DC: American Psychiatric Association, 1994.

3. Loening-Baucke V. Chronic constipation in children. *Gastroenterology* 1993;105:557–1563.

4. Roma E, Adamidis D, Nikolara R, Constantopoulos A, Messaritakis J. Diet and chronic constipation in children: the role of fiber. *J Pediatr Gastroenterol Nutr* 1999;28:169–174.

5. Mooren GCAH, Van der Plas RN, Bossuyt PMM, Taminiau JAJM, Buller HA. The connection between dietary fibre intake and chronic constipation in children. *Ned Tijdschr Geneeskd* 1996;140:2036–2039.

6. Halibi IM. Cisapride in the management of chronic pediatric constipation. *J Pediatr Gastroenterol Nutr* 1999;28:199–202.

7. Nurko MD, Garcia-Aranda JA, Worona LB, Zlochisty O. Cisapride for the treatment of constipation in children: a double blind study. *J Pediatr* 2000;136:35–40.

8. Pitzalis G, Mariani P, Chiarini-Testa MR, et al. Lactitol in chronic idiopathic constipation of childhood. *Pediatr Med Chir* 1995;17:223–226.

9. Martino AM, Pesce F, Rosati U. The effects of lactitol in the treatment of intestinal stasis in childhood. *Minerva Pediatr* 1992;44:319–323.

10. Hejlp M, Kamper J, Ebbesen F, Hansted C. Infantile constipation and allomin-lactulose. Treatment of infantile constipation in infants fed with breast milk substitutes: a controlled trial of 2% and 4% allomin-lactulose. *Ugeskr Laeger* 1990;152:1819–1822.

11. Cox DJ, Sutphen J, Borowitz S, et al. Contribution of behaviour therapy and biofeedback to laxative therapy in the treatment of pediatric encopresis. *Ann Behav Med* 1998;20:70–76.

12. Sondheimer JM, Gervaise EP. Lubricant versus laxative in the treatment of chronic functional constipation of children: a comparative study. *J Pediatr Gastroenterol Nutr* 1982;1:223–226.

13. Van der Plas RN, Benninga MA, Büller HA, et al. Biofeedback training in treatment of childhood constipation: a randomised controlled study. *Lancet* 1996;348:776–780.

14. Loening-Baucke V. Biofeedback treatment for chronic constipation and encopresis in childhood: long term outcome. *Pediatrics* 1995;96:105–111.

15. Loening BV. Modulation of abnormal defecation dynamics by biofeedback treatment in chronically constipated children with encopresis. *J Pediatr* 1990;116:214–222.

Gregory Rubin
Professor of Primary Care
University of Sunderland
Sunderland
UK

Competing interests: None declared.

Croup

Search date September 2000

Martin Osmond and David Evans

QUESTIONS

INTERVENTIONS

Key Messages

- We found that treatment of croup in primary care has not yet been evaluated adequately in RCTs.

- RCTs in primary paediatric assessment units (PAUs) (see glossary, p 244) have found that systemic steroids, nebulised steroids, and nebulised adrenaline (epinephrine) all improve symptoms. Systemic and nebulised steroids have also been found to reduce hospital admissions.

- RCTs have found no evidence of a difference between systemic and nebulised steroids, but the trials were too limited to rule out a clinically important difference.

- In children admitted to hospital, RCTs have found that systemic steroids, nebulised steroids in PAUs, and nebulised adrenaline all improve symptoms. Systemic and nebulised steroids have also been found to reduce hospital stay and reattendance.

- We found no good evidence to compare the effectiveness of systemic and nebulised steroids in hospitals.

- We found no good evidence to compare the effectiveness of nebulised adrenaline and steroids in hospitals.

- None of the RCTs we reviewed described any deaths in over 1000 infants with childhood croup, related either to croup itself or to any associated treatment.

© Clinical Evidence 2001;5:236–245.

DEFINITION Croup is an acute clinical syndrome characterised by a harsh, barking cough, inspiratory stridor, and hoarse voice, caused by laryngeal or tracheal obstruction. Mild fever and rhinorrhoea may also be present. The most important differential diagnoses are acute epiglottitis, inhalation of a foreign body, and bacterial tracheitis.

INCIDENCE/ Croup occurs in about 3% of children aged under 6 years per year,[1]
PREVALENCE and causes 2–3% of hospital admissions in young children in the UK.[2] One retrospective Belgian study of 5–8 year olds found that 15.5% of children had suffered from croup, and 5% had experienced recurrent croup (3 or more episodes).[3]

AETIOLOGY/ Croup is believed to be mainly viral in origin, but atopy plays a part
RISK FACTORS in some children. The most common virus isolated is parainfluenza types 1, 2, or 3. Others include influenza, adenovirus, respiratory syncytial virus, and rhinovirus.

PROGNOSIS Fewer than 2% of children with croup are admitted to hospital in the UK.[1] Of those admitted, only 0.5–1.5% require intubation. Mortality is low: of 208 children who were given artificial airways over a 10 year period, two died.[4] Symptoms of upper airway obstruction can be extremely distressing to the child and the family.

AIMS To reduce suffering and distress, need for hospital admission, duration of hospital stay, rates of intubation, and mortality, without undue adverse effects.

OUTCOMES Severity of symptoms and signs of upper airway obstruction, rates of hospital admission, visits to a medical practitioner or reattendance to an accident and emergency department, intubation rates, mortality, and adverse effects of treatment. A commonly used definition of a clinically significant improvement is 2 points or more of the validated Westley croup score (maximum score, or most severe, 17)[5] within a predefined timescale. The Westley score comprises the sum of five clinical parameters: conscious level, cyanosis, stridor, air entry, and chest wall retractions. Intubation and death are rare in children with croup, so trials recruiting large numbers of children would be needed to exclude a difference in rates between interventions.

METHODS *Clinical Evidence* update search and appraisal September 2000, covering croup, laryngotracheitis, and laryngotracheobronchitis. Data were extracted from trials that used randomisation (not quasi-randomisation) and intention to treat analysis. Common exclusion criteria were previous upper airway abnormalities, previous prolonged intubation, severe croup (cyanosis with impaired consciousness), and recent treatment with steroids. The conclusions presented below should not be applied to children with these clinical features. Most children in the studies were cared for in institutions with excellent staffing and monitoring facilities. RCTs performed in hospital settings studied children with more severe croup than those based in assessment units.

QUESTION   **What are the effects of treatment in primary care settings?**

We found insufficient evidence about the treatment of croup in primary care settings.

Benefits: We found no systematic review or RCTs evaluating interventions in acute childhood croup in primary care settings.

Harms: Insufficient data.

Comment: It is surprising that there is no evidence relating to children with croup in the primary care setting as this is where the great majority of children with croup are treated.

QUESTION   **What are the effects of treatment in primary paediatric assessment units?**

OPTION   SYSTEMIC STEROIDS VERSUS PLACEBO IN PAEDIATRIC ASSESSMENT UNITS

Three RCTs found that a single dose of oral or intramuscular steroids significantly improved symptoms within 5 hours, reduced the likelihood of admission to hospital by 75%, and reduced the need for further treatment after discharge by 70%.

Benefits: We found two systematic reviews (search dates 1997), which included relevant trials of systemic steroids versus placebo for children with croup in paediatric assessment units (PAUs).[6,7] However, they did not analyse these three trials[8–10] separately from other included studies. The three RCTs included 230 children seen at primary PAUs in Australia, Canada, and the USA. One compared a single intramuscular dose of 0.6 mg/kg dexamethasone, given shortly after arrival in the assessment unit, versus placebo.[8] The others compared 0.15 mg/kg oral dexamethasone[9] and 0.6 mg/kg intramuscular dexamethasone[10] versus placebo in children ready for discharge from the assessment unit. **Symptom improvement:** Intramuscular dexamethasone (0.6 mg/kg) significantly improved the croup score within 5 hours (96 children; change in croup score: dexamethasone v placebo, -2.9 v -1.3).[8] **Admission to hospital:** Intramuscular dexamethasone given shortly after arrival in the assessment unit reduced admissions to hospital (RR of admission compared with placebo 0.25, 95% CI 0.13 to 0.49; NNT to prevent one additional admission 2, 95% CI 1 to 3).[8] **Reattendance:** For the week after discharge, all three RCTs reported lower rates of reattendance to any medical practitioner or institution in children given steroids (RR for reattendance compared with placebo 0.33, 95% CI 0.19 to 0.56; NNT to prevent one additional child reattending 12, 95% CI 6 to 60).[8–10]

Harms: None reported.

Comment: The children were observed for up to 5 hours in a PAU before discharge was decided. Some children were treated with nebulised adrenaline.[10]

NEBULISED STEROIDS VERSUS PLACEBO IN PAEDIATRIC ASSESSMENT UNITS

RCTs have found that nebulised steroids versus placebo reduce the likelihood of a poor response within 2–5 hours by more than half, and halve the risk of hospital admission.

Benefits: We found three systematic reviews,[6,7,11] which included four RCTs comparing nebulised steroids versus placebo for children with croup in PAUs.[8,12–14] However, the reviews combined the results with RCTs of hospital based treatment. **Symptom improvement:** The four relevant RCTs (250 children) evaluated treatment in assessment units. They compared a single dose of inhaled steroids versus placebo, given after humidified oxygen.[8,12–14] Combined data from the three RCTs that dichotomised outcomes into either good (improvement in croup score of 2 or more) or poor response showed a significantly reduced likelihood of a poor response within 2–5 hours after treatment (RR 0.44, 95% CI 0.29 to 0.67).[12–14] **Admission to hospital:** Rate of admission was halved (RR 0.55, 95% CI 0.38 to 0.81; NNT to prevent one additional admission 4, 95% CI 3 to 8).[8,12–14] **Reattendance:** The four RCTs found no evidence of a significant difference in rates of further admission (RR 0.74, 95% CI 0.26 to 2.08)[8,12–14] or consultations with other health practitioners (RR 0.86, 95% CI 0.34 to 2.19) in the week after discharge from the assessment unit.[8,12–14]

Harms: Nebulised steroids seem to be well tolerated. In one of these four RCTs, two neutropenic children suffered bacterial tracheitis after treatment with nebulised dexamethasone.[14]

Comment: We found insufficient evidence to compare regimens of nebulised steroids. In the RCTs, children were observed for up to 5 hours in the assessment unit, and all received humidified air or oxygen; in one RCT, both groups also received oral dexamethasone 0.6 mg/kg.[13] One pilot RCT (in 17 hospitalised children) compared inhaled steroid (fluticasone propionate 1000 µg, 2 doses) versus placebo delivered by a metered dose inhaler and spacing device, as a potential treatment that could be given at home. It found no evidence of benefit, but was too small to rule out a clinically significant effect.[15] We found another systematic review that did not analyse separately data from trials of nebulised steroids versus placebo.[6]

SYSTEMIC VERSUS NEBULISED STEROIDS IN PAEDIATRIC ASSESSMENT UNITS

RCTs have found that systemic dexamethasone and nebulised budesonide are equally effective in reducing symptoms. In one RCT, oral dexamethasone reduced the rate of admission compared with nebulised budesonide.

Benefits: We found one systematic review,[7] which included a single RCT,[16] and we found two additional RCTs.[8,17] The RCTs compared oral dexamethasone 0.6 mg/kg versus nebulised budesonide 2 mg,[16,17] and intramuscular dexamethasone 0.6 mg/kg versus nebulised budesonide 4 mg[8] for 280 children with acute croup attending an assessment unit. The RCTs found no significant difference between nebulised budesonide and systemic dexamethasone in rates of symptom resolution or reattendance after discharge, although fewer children on oral dexamethasone were admitted (RR oral v nebulised steroids 0.53, 95% CI 0.34 to 0.81).[8]

Harms: None reported.

Comment: None.

OPTION NEBULISED ADRENALINE (EPINEPHRINE) IN PAEDIATRIC ASSESSMENT UNITS

One small RCT found that nebulised adrenaline versus placebo given in the assessment unit to children suffering from croup significantly improved symptoms within 30 minutes. Symptoms returned to preintervention severity in a third of children within 2 hours.

Benefits: We found no systematic review. **Adrenaline versus placebo:** We found one RCT (54 children with stridor at rest seen in an assessment unit) comparing nebulised racemic adrenaline (0.5 mg/kg diluted to 2 ml with 0.9% sodium chloride) versus saline placebo.[18] It found a significant improvement in croup scores 30 minutes after treatment with epinephrine (mean scores 2.0 v 3.6 on placebo; P < 0.01).[18] The trial found no significant reduction in duration of stay in the assessment unit (mean stay [range]: 11.5 hours [5–21] v 13.3 hours [6–24]). **Adrenaline combined with steroids:** We found no RCTs. Two prospective cohort studies assessed 115 children treated with nebulised adrenaline and dexamethasone 0.6 mg/kg in an assessment unit. Of the 55–66% who responded satisfactorily, all were discharged after 3–4 hours' observation, and none reattended for further medical care within 24–48 hours.[19,20]

Harms: We found no evidence of a significant difference in adverse effects after treatment with adrenaline or placebo. Of the children who had improved by 30 minutes, a considerable proportion relapsed, although there was no significant difference in the rate of relapse (return of croup scores to the pretreatment value) between the two groups (35% with adrenaline v 25% with placebo; RR adrenaline v placebo 1.41, 95% CI 0.36 to 5.51). This raises the question of whether children given nebulised adrenaline and then discharged may come to harm when symptoms recur. No children discharged in the RCT reattended for further treatment.[18] Children were observed for a minimum of 5 hours (up to 24 hours). During this time, 40% of treated children and 48% of controls were given a further dose of adrenaline, whereas 52% of treated children and 58% of controls received oral betamethasone (6 mg) before final discharge. These differences were not significant.

Comment: None.

What are the effects of treatment in hospital?

OPTION **INHALATION OF HUMIDIFIED AIR/OXYGEN IN HOSPITAL**

The effectiveness of inhaling humidified air/oxygen has not been evaluated adequately.

Benefits: We found no systematic review. We found one RCT (16 children), which compared up to 12 hours' care in a humidified atmosphere (air with relative humidity 87–95%) versus normal care.[21] It found no significant difference in recovery rates (mean croup scores at 6 hours were 3.1 v 3.8).

Harms: None reported.

Comment: The study was not blinded, and selection, performance, and detection biases remain possible.

OPTION **SYSTEMIC STEROIDS IN HOSPITAL**

RCTs have found that giving systemic corticosteroids to children admitted with croup significantly improves symptoms by 12 hours, and reduces hospital stay. Limited evidence suggests that a single dose of oral dexamethasone 0.3 mg/kg is as effective as 0.6 mg/kg in children admitted with croup.

Benefits: We found two systematic reviews (search dates 1999, and not specified),[22,11] which combined data from 11 relevant RCTs (904 children), and we found one additional RCT not included in either review (41 children).[23] The most common regimen was intramuscular or oral dexamethasone 0.3–0.6 mg/kg as a single dose on admission or repeated over 24–48 hours. **Symptom improvement:** RCTs that evaluated symptomatic improvement at 12–24 hours found that significantly more children responded to steroids than to placebo (response defined as ≥2 points improvement of croup score; RR of response 1.23, 95% CI 1.13 to 1.33; NNT to achieve response in one additional child 7, 95% CI 5 to 10). **Hospital stay:** Four RCTs evaluated duration of hospital stay. Three found a significant reduction in hospital stay on dexamethasone compared with placebo (median stay 20 v 13 hours,[17] mean stay 91 v 49 hours,[24] and 9 v 3 days[23]). The fourth RCT found no significant difference.[25] **Intubation rates:** Seven RCTs in the systematic review and two subsequent RCTs gave data on intubation rates.[17,22,23] Children given systemic steroids were less at risk of intubation than infants taking placebo (RR 0.21, 95% CI 0.06 to 0.69). This combined estimate is dominated by one small study with a much higher than average rate of intubation (5/32 children).[23]

Harms: Systemic steroids seem to be well tolerated. We found three RCTs (130 children) reporting rates of secondary bacterial infection.[23,25,26] These reported nine cases of pneumonia, one of septicaemia, one of bacterial tracheitis, one of otitis media, and one of sinusitis. Six cases were in treated children and seven in controls (RR for infection compared with placebo 0.94, 95% CI 0.33 to 2.69).

Comment: A significant reduction in time to symptom resolution may not reduce hospital stay, which is influenced by hospital policies and referral patterns, availability of treatment in the community, parental access to transportation and communications, and the tendency to discharge children at a certain time each day.[27]

OPTION **HIGH VERSUS LOW DOSE SYSTEMIC STEROID REGIMENS IN HOSPITAL**

Limited evidence suggests that a single dose of oral dexamethasone 0.3 mg/kg is as effective as 0.6 mg/kg in children admitted with croup.

Benefits: We found one systematic review,[7] which included one RCT (120 children admitted with croup) comparing different single doses of oral dexamethasone (0.6 v 0.3 mg/kg and 0.3 v 0.15 mg/kg).[24] It found no significant differences in rate of improvement in croup score, duration of hospital stay, or intubation rates. However, children given the lower dose of dexamethasone were more likely to be given nebulised adrenaline than those given the higher dose (RR 2.32, 95% CI 1.02 to 5.28). We found no studies comparing other systemic regimens.

Harms: None reported.

Comment: None.

OPTION **NEBULISED STEROIDS IN HOSPITAL**

RCTs have found that children admitted with croup given corticosteroids versus placebo improve more rapidly, leave hospital sooner, and are less likely to reattend. We found insufficient evidence on the effect of nebulised steroids on intubation rates.

Benefits: We found one systematic review (4 RCTs, 252 children admitted to hospital with croup),[11] comparing nebulised steroids with placebo.[17,28–30] However, this review combined the results with RCTs conducted in PAUs. **Symptom improvement:** One RCT evaluated budesonide 1 mg, two doses 30 minutes apart.[28] The risk of an inadequate response by 2 hours was significantly reduced (RR 0.40, 95% CI 0.19 to 0.83; NNT to prevent one additional inadequate response 2, 95% CI 1 to 8). **Hospital stay:** Another RCT compared nebulised budesonide 2 mg initially, followed by 1 mg every 12 hours, versus placebo and found a significant reduction in hospital stay (mean stay 36 v 55 hours).[29] The third RCT compared budesonide 2 mg single dose versus placebo and reported a significant reduction in the number of children staying in hospital for more than 24 hours (RR 0.37, 95% CI 0.16 to 0.88; NNT 3, 95% CI 2 to 14).[17] **Intubation rates:** Using data from the three RCTs, there was no significant effect on intubation rates (RR of intubation 0.18, 95% CI 0.01 to 3.67).[17,28,29] **Relapse rate:** The fourth RCT compared nebulised budesonide 2 mg versus placebo given every 12 hours while in hospital.[30] It found that budesonide accelerated clinical improvement (decrease in croup score by 2 points or more) compared with placebo (P = 0.013), and reduced the rate of further medical attendance in the 3 days after discharge (reattendance rate 1/34 with budesonide v 7/32 with placebo; P = 0.02).

Harms: Nebulised steroids seem to be well tolerated. Two RCTs have reported adverse effects. One reported one episode of nausea and one episode of distress caused by firm application of the face mask for 10 minutes.[29] The other reported emotional distress in six of 42 children treated with budesonide nebulisers and nine of 40 children treated with placebo.[30] In four children with severe croup (1 treated with budesonide and 3 with placebo), this led to interventional treatment outside of the protocol (nebulised adrenaline).

Comment: The optimal regimen of nebulised steroids has not yet been established.

OPTION   SYSTEMIC VERSUS NEBULISED STEROIDS IN HOSPITAL

We found no RCTs undertaken outside of PAUs of oral versus nebulised steroids for croup.

Benefits: We found no systematic review and no RCTs investigating the effects of oral versus nebulised steroids in hospital.

Harms: We found no evidence.

Comment: None.

OPTION   NEBULISED ADRENALINE (EPINEPHRINE) IN HOSPITAL

One small RCT found that nebulised adrenaline versus placebo given in the assessment unit to children suffering from croup significantly improved symptoms within 30 minutes. Symptoms returned to preintervention severity in a third of children within 2 hours.

Benefits: We found no systematic review. **Versus placebo:** We found three RCTs (53 children admitted to hospital with croup) comparing nebulised adrenaline versus placebo. Two RCTs did not show improvement with adrenaline, but were too small to exclude a clinically significant difference.[31,32] The other small RCT compared aerosolised racemic adrenaline versus 0.9% sodium chloride placebo, both delivered by intermittent positive pressure breathing.[5] Children given adrenaline experienced greater reductions in croup score. The reduction was greatest within 30 minutes of treatment and was not apparent at 2 hours (mean croup scores at 30 minutes 1.7 v 3.1). **Nebuliser versus intermittent positive pressure breathing:** We found one RCT (14 children) comparing nebulised adrenaline delivered by intermittent positive pressure breathing versus nebulised adrenaline alone.[33] It found no significant difference in resolution of symptoms (mean croup scores at 30 minutes 3.1 v 2.4). **L-adrenaline versus racemic adrenaline:** We found one RCT (31 children) comparing racemic adrenaline versus L-adrenaline.[34] It found no significant difference in croup scores (mean scores at 30 minutes, 3.8 v 4.8).

Harms: There was no significant difference in the risk of cardiovascular adverse effects with L-adrenaline or racemic adrenaline. Three children receiving racemic adrenaline were intubated (RR of intubation with racemic v L-adrenaline 6.59, 95% CI 0.37 to 118).[34] Children given nebulised adrenaline need medical observation because symptoms may return to pretreatment severity (see harms of nebulised adrenaline in paediatric assessment units, p 240).

Comment: Racemic adrenaline comprises equal amounts of D- and L-isomers and was historically chosen in favour of the more readily available L-form in the belief that it caused fewer adverse cardiovascular effects.

OPTION | **NEBULISED ADRENALINE VERSUS STEROIDS IN HOSPITAL**

We found no good evidence to compare the effectiveness of nebulised adrenaline and steroids.

Benefits: We found one systematic review,[7] which identified one RCT (66 children admitted to hospital with croup) comparing nebulised adrenaline 4 mg versus nebulised budesonide 2 mg (66 children admitted to hospital with croup).[35] This trial found no significant difference in duration of hospital stay (mean difference in hospital stay adrenaline v budesonide -5.8 hours, 95% CI -22.8 to $+11.2$) or in croup scores (mean change -2.9 v -1.7; P = 0.08). We found no RCTs comparing nebulised adrenaline versus oral steroids.

Harms: None reported.

Comment: Nebulised adrenaline and steroids may have an additive effect through different modes of action, although whether this leads to improved outcomes is unknown.

GLOSSARY

Primary paediatric assessment unit An emergency room or accident and emergency department with the facilities to monitor closely the clinical condition of a child with acute onset of inspiratory stridor.

REFERENCES

1. Denny FW, Murphy TF, Clyde WA Jr, Collier AM, Henderson FW. Croup: an 11-year study in a pediatric practice. *Pediatrics* 1983;71:871–876.

2. Phelan PD, Landau LI, Olinsily A. *Respiratory illness in children.* 2nd ed. Oxford: Blackwell Science, 1982:32–33.

3. Van Bever HP, Wieringa MH, Weyler JJ, et al. Croup and recurrent croup: their association with asthma and allergy. *Eur J Pediatr* 1999;158:253–257.

4. McEniery J, Gillis J, Kilham H, Benjamin B. Review of intubation in severe laryngotracheobronchitis. *Pediatrics* 1991;87:847–853.

5. Westley CR, Cotton EK, Brooks JG. Nebulized racemic epinephrine by IPPB for the treatment of croup: a double-blind study. *Am J Dis Child* 1978; 132:484–487.

6. Ausejo M, Saenz A, Pham B, et al. The effectiveness of glucocorticoids in treating croup: meta-analysis. *BMJ* 1999;319:595–600. Search date 1997; primary sources Cochrane Controlled Trials Register, Embase 1974 to August 1997, Medline 1966 to August 1997; letters to authors.

7. Ausejo M, Saenz A, Pham B, et al. Glucocorticoids for Croup. In: The Cochrane Library, Issue 3, 2000. Oxford: Update software. Search date 1997; primary sources Cochrane Controlled Trials Register, Embase 1974 to August 1997, Medline 1966 to August 1997, letters to authors. Substantially amended June 1999.

8. Johnson DW, Jacobson S, Edney PC, et al. A comparison of nebulised budesonide, intramuscular dexamethasone, and placebo for moderately severe croup. *N Engl J Med* 1998; 339:498–503.

9. Geelhoed GC, Turner J, Macdonald WBG. Efficacy of a small single dose of oral dexamethasone for outpatient croup: a double blind placebo controlled clinical trial. *BMJ* 1996;313:140–142.

10. Cruz MN, Stewart G, Rosenberg N. Use of dexamethasone in the outpatient management of acute laryngotracheitis. *Pediatrics* 1995;96:220–223.

11. Griffin S, Ellis S, Fitzgerald-Barron A, Rose J, Egger M. Nebulised steroid in the treatment of croup: a systematic review of randomised controlled trials. *Br J Gen Pract* 2000;50:135–141. Search date not specified; primary sources Cinahl, Cochrane Controlled Trials Register, Embase, Medline; hand searching of article bibliographies, pharmaceutical industry database.

12. Klassen TP, Feldman ME, Watters LK, Sutcliffe T, Rowe PC. Nebulized budesonide for children with mild-to-moderate croup. *N Engl J Med* 1994;331: 285–289.

13. Klassen TP, Watters LK, Feldman ME, Sutcliffe T, Rowe PC. The efficacy of nebulized budesonide in dexamethasone-treated outpatients with croup. *Pediatrics* 1996;97:463–466.

14. Johnson DW, Schuh S, Koren G, Jaffe DM. Outpatient treatment of croup with nebulized dexamethasone. *Arch Pediatr Adolesc Med* 1996; 150:349–355.

15. Jan Roorda R, Walhof CM. Effects of inhaled fluticasone propionate administered with metered dose inhaler and spacer in mild to moderate croup: A negative preliminary report. *Pediatr Pulmonol* 1998;25:114–117.

16. Klassen TP, Craig WR, Moher D, et al. Nebulized budesonide and oral dexamethasone for the treatment of croup: a randomized controlled trial. *JAMA* 1998;279:1629–1632.

17. Geelhoed GC, Macdonald WB. Oral and inhaled steroids in croup: a randomized, placebo-controlled trial. *Pediatr Pulmonol* 1995;20:355–361.

18. Kristjansson S, Berg-Kelly K, Winso E. Inhalation of racemic adrenaline in the treatment of mild and moderately severe croup. Clinical symptom score and oxygen saturation measurements for evaluation of treatment effects. *Acta Paediatr* 1994;83:1156–1160.

19. Ledwith CA, Shea LM, Mauro RD. Safety and efficacy of nebulized racemic epinephrine in conjunction with oral dexamethasone and mist in the outpatient treatment of croup. *Ann Emerg Med* 1995;25:331–337.

20. Kunkel NC, Baker MD. Use of racemic epinephrine, dexamethasone, and mist in the outpatient management of croup. *Pediatr Emerg Care* 1996;12:156–159.

21. Bourchier D, Dawson KP, Fergusson DM. Humidification in viral croup: a controlled trial. *Aust Paediatr J* 1984;20:289–291.

22. Kairys SW, Olmstead EM, O'Connor GT. Steroid treatment of laryngotracheitis: a meta-analysis of the evidence from randomized trials. *Pediatrics* 1989;83:683–693. Search date June 1999; primary sources Medline, Embase, and Cochrane Library.

23. Sumboonnanonda A, Suwanjutha S, Sirinavin S. Randomized controlled trial of dexamethasone in infectious croup. *J Med Assoc Thai* 1997;80:262–265.

24. Geelhoed GC, Macdonald WBG. Oral dexamethasone in the treatment of croup: 0.15 mg/kg versus 0.3 mg/kg versus 0.6 mg/kg. *Pediatr Pulmonol* 1995;20:362–368.

25. Super DM, Cartelli NA, Broosks LJ, Lembo RM, Kumar ML. A prospective randomized double-blind study to evaluate the effect of dexamethasone in acute laryngotracheitis. *J Pediatr* 1989;115:323–329.

26. Kuusela AL, Vesikari T. A randomized double-blind, placebo-controlled trial of dexamethasone and racemic epinephrine in the treatment of croup. *Acta Paediatr Scand* 1988;77:99–104.

27. Kemper KJ. Medically inappropriate hospital use in a pediatric population. *N Engl J Med* 1988;318: 1033–1037.

28. Husby S, Agertoft L, Mortensen S, Pedersen S. Treatment of croup with nebulised steroid (budesonide): a double blind, placebo controlled study. *Arch Dis Child* 1993;68:352–355.

29. Godden CW, Campbell MJ, Hussey M, Cogswell JJ. Double blind placebo controlled trial of nebulised budesonide for croup. *Arch Dis Child* 1997;76: 155–158.

30. Roberts GW, Master VV, Staugas RE, et al. Repeated dose inhaled budesonide versus placebo in the treatment of croup. *J Paediatr Child Health* 1999;35:170–174.

31. Gardner HG, Powell KR, Roden VJ, Cherry JD. The evaluation of racemic epinephrine in the treatment of infectious croup. *Pediatrics* 1973;52:52–55.

32. Taussig LM, Castro O, Beaudry PH, Fox WW, Bureau M. Treatment of laryngotracheobronchitis (croup). *Am J Dis Child* 1975;129:790–793.

33. Fogel JM, Berg IJ, Gerber MA, Sherter CB. Racemic epinephrine in the treatment of croup: nebulization alone versus nebulization with intermittent positive pressure breathing. *J Pediatr* 1982;101:1028–1031.

34. Waisman Y, Klein BL, Boenning DA, et al. Prospective randomized double-blind study comparing L-epinephrine and racemic epinephrine aerosols in the treatment of laryngotracheitis (croup). *Pediatrics* 1992;89:302–306.

35. Fitzgerald D, Mellis C, Johnson M, et al. Nebulized budesonide is as effective as nebulized adrenaline in moderately severe croup. *Pediatrics* 1996;97: 722–725.

Martin Osmond
Associate Professor of Pediatrics
University of Ottawa
Ottawa
Canada

David Evans
Lecturer in Paediatrics
and Child Health
University of Leeds
Leeds
UK

Competing interests: None declared.

Child health

Search date September 2000

Philip Hazell

INTERVENTIONS

Key Messages

- One systematic review found evidence of no benefit from tricyclic antidepressants in prepubertal children, and no clear benefit in adolescents. Fluoxetine may be of some benefit in child and adolescent depression, but more research is needed. We found no evidence to support the use of other serotonin reuptake inhibitor drugs. We found equivocal evidence to support the use of the reversible monoamine oxidase inhibitor moclobemide. We found no evidence supporting the use of non-reversible monoamine oxidase inhibitors. Preliminary data do not support the use of the selective noradrenergic reuptake inhibitor venlafaxine, nor the mood stabiliser lithium.

- We found insufficient evidence on the effects of St John's Wort (*Hypericum perforatum*) and electroconvulsive therapy in children and adolescents with depression.

- One systematic review of RCTs has found cognitive behavioural therapy to be superior to non-specific supportive therapies for mild to moderate depression in children and adolescents. Two RCTs of interpersonal therapy also suggested benefit compared with no treatment. We found insufficient evidence to conclude that family therapy, or group treatments other than cognitive behavioural therapy, are effective treatments for depression in children and adolescents.

- We found no systematic reviews or RCTs looking at long term outcomes for psychological or pharmacological treatments.

DEFINITION See depressive disorders, p 652. Compared with adult depression, depression in children and adolescents may have a more insidious onset, may be characterised more by irritability than sadness, and occurs more often in association with other conditions such as anxiety, conduct disorder, hyperkinesis, and learning problems.[1]

INCIDENCE/ PREVALENCE Estimates of prevalence of depression among children and adolescents in the community range from 1.7% to 5.9%.[2,3] Prevalence tends to increase with age, with a sharp rise around onset of puberty. Preadolescent boys and girls are equally affected by the condition, but depression is seen more frequently among adolescent girls than boys.[4]

AETIOLOGY/ RISK FACTORS Uncertain, but may include childhood events and current psychosocial adversity.

PROGNOSIS See prognosis under depressive disorders, p 652. In children and adolescents, the recurrence rate of depressive episodes first occurring in childhood or adolescence is 70% by 5 years, which is similar to the recurrence rate in adults.[5] Young people experiencing a moderate to severe depressive episode may be more likely than adults to have a manic episode within the next few years.[4] Trials of treatment for child and adolescent depression have found high rates of spontaneous remission (as much as two thirds of people in some inpatient studies).

AIMS To improve mood, social and occupational functioning, and quality of life; to reduce morbidity and mortality; to prevent recurrence of depressive disorder; and to minimise adverse effects of treatment.

OUTCOMES See depressive disorders, p 652. In children and adolescents, there are developmentally specific continuous measures such as the Children's Depression Rating Scale and the Children's Depression Inventory. Categorical outcomes are sometimes expressed as people no longer meeting DSM criteria for depression on a structured psychiatric interview such as the Kiddie-SADS.

METHODS *Clinical Evidence* update search and appraisal September 2000.

QUESTION What are the effects of treatments?

OPTION PRESCRIPTION ANTIDEPRESSANT DRUGS

One systematic review found no evidence of benefit from tricyclic antidepressants in prepubertal children, and no clear benefit in adolescents. We found limited evidence that fluoxetine may be of some benefit for child and adolescent depression. We found no evidence about other serotonin reuptake inhibitor drugs. We found little high quality evidence regarding moclobemide. We found no evidence on the effectiveness of non-reversible monoamine oxidase inhibitors. We have found no evidence that venlafaxine or lithium are beneficial, although the power of the trials was too low to rule out a clinically important difference.

Benefits: **Tricyclic antidepressants:** We found one systematic review (search date 1997, 14 RCTs)[6] and one subsequent RCT.[7] The systematic review found no significant reduction in non-response

Child health

with the active drug versus placebo (273 children and adolescents; OR 0.83, 95% CI 0.48 to 1.42). Analyses for children (2 trials) and adolescents (5 trials) also found no significant benefit of treatment, (children RR of failure to recover 0.9, 95% CI 0.7 to 1.2; adolescents RR of failure to recover 0.9, 95% CI 0.7 to 1.3). However, using the weighted mean difference, trials found a modest but significant difference in adolescents (WMD in depression checklist scores −2.3, 95% CI −3.3 to −1.4) but not in children. Inclusion of the subsequent RCT (meta-analysis personal communication from the author) produced little changes in the estimate of effectiveness but narrowed the 95% confidence intervals.[7] **Pulsed intravenous clomipramine:** We found no systematic review. One small RCT (including 16 non-suicidal adolescent outpatients with major depression) found that significantly more people (7/8) responded to intravenous clomipramine 200 mg than to saline (3/8).[8] **Monoamine oxidase inhibitors:** We found no systematic review. In one small RCT, 20 adolescents treated with moclobemide showed greater improvement on one clinician rated scale than those treated with placebo, but not on other clinician rated and self reported measures.[9] We found no trials of non-reversible monoamine oxidase inhibitors. **Selective serotonin reuptake inhibitors:** We found one systematic review addressing both adults and children (search date 1998, 2 RCTs, 126 children).[10] The first RCT in the systematic review (30 children) found no global benefit. The second RCT (96 children) found significant benefit on clinician reported global rating and on self reported depressive symptoms, but not on other measures. The systematic review did not pool data from the two RCTs. However, combination of the results for clinician global rating, using a random effects model, found an insignificant pooled odds ratio for non-improvement (0.5, 95% CI 0.22 to 1.12). **Selective noradrenergic reuptake inhibitors:** We found one systematic review (search date 1998, 1 RCT, 33 children).[10] The one small RCT compared a combination of venlafaxine and psychotherapy with a combination of placebo and psychotherapy. It found no significant difference with regard to improvement. **Lithium:** We found no systematic review. One small placebo controlled RCT compared lithium versus placebo in 30 depressed prepubertal children with a family history of bipolar affective disorder.[11] It found no significant difference of global assessment or of depression scores at follow up.

Harms: See harms of antidepressants under depressive disorders, p 652. We found one unpublished systematic review, see comment. We found single case reports and case series of toxicity and death from tricyclic antidepressants in overdose and therapeutic doses (see harms of antidepressants under depressive disorders, p 652). Of the 17 children randomised to lithium treatment, four were withdrawn because of adverse effects (3 had confusion, 1 had nausea and vomiting).[11]

Comment: One systematic review awaiting publication found that tricyclic antidepressants were more commonly associated with vertigo (OR 8.47, 95% CI 1.40 to 51.0), orthostatic hypotension (OR 4.77, 95% CI 1.11 to 20.5), and dry mouth (OR 5.19, 95% CI 1.15 to 23.5) than placebo (P Hazell, et al, personal communication,

2000). It found no significant differences for other adverse effects (tiredness, sleep problems, headache, palpitations, tremor, perspiration, constipation, or problems with micturition). Further research is needed to determine long term effects of intravenous clomipramine.

OPTION   **ST JOHN'S WORT (*HYPERICUM PERFORATUM*)**

We found no evidence on the effects of St John's Wort (*Hypericum perforatum*) in children and adolescents with depression.

Benefits: We found no systematic review and no RCTs in children or adolescents.

Harms: See harms of St John's Wort under depressive disorders, p 652. We found no evidence on adverse effects in children and adolescents.

Comment: None.

OPTION   **ELECTROCONVULSIVE THERAPY**

We found insufficient evidence about the routine use of electroconvulsive therapy in children and adolescents with depression.

Benefits: We found no systematic reviews or RCTs.

Harms: Despite widespread concern about potentially harmful effects of electroconvulsive therapy, especially on memory loss, we found no evidence on harms in children or adolescents.

Comment: None.

OPTION   **SPECIFIC PSYCHOLOGICAL TREATMENTS**

One systematic review of RCTs has found cognitive behavioural therapy increases the rate of resolution of the symptoms of depression compared with non-specific supportive therapies for children and adolescents with mild to moderate depression. One RCT of interpersonal therapy found slightly more people recovered than with clinical monitoring alone. A further RCT did not find a significant difference in the recovery rate with interpersonal therapy compared with waiting list control. We found insufficient evidence to conclude that family therapy, or group treatments other than cognitive behavioural therapy, are effective treatments for depression in children and adolescents.

Benefits: **Cognitive behavioural therapy:** See glossary, p 251. We found one systematic review (search date 1997, 6 RCTs, 376 people) of cognitive behavioural therapy compared with "inactive" treatment that ranged from waiting list control to supportive psychotherapy.[12] Cognitive behavioural therapy was associated with increased rate of resolution of symptoms of depression (OR 3.2, 95% CI 1.9 to 5.2; NNT 4, 95% CI 3 to 5), a finding consistent with two non-systematic meta-analytic studies.[13,14] **Interpersonal therapy:** See glossary, p 251. We found no systematic review. We found two RCTs, which compared 12 weekly sessions of interpersonal therapy versus clinical monitoring or waiting list control in adolescents with depression. In the first RCT, sessions were augmented by telephone contact. In the first RCT, 18 of 24 adolescents receiving interpersonal therapy recovered versus 11 of 24 adolescents receiving clinical monitoring alone (RR 1.64, 95% CI 1.00 to 2.68; ARR 0.29, 95% CI 0.03 to 0.56).[15] In the second RCT, 17 of 19 adolescents receiving interpersonal therapy recovered versus 12 of 18 adolescents on the waiting list (RR 1.33, 95% CI 0.94 to 1.93; ARR 0.22, 95% CI −0.03 to +0.49).[16] **Systemic behaviour family therapy:** See glossary, p 251. We found no systematic review. One RCT of family therapy versus non-specific supportive therapy did not find a significant difference in remission rates (29% v 34%).[17] **Group administered cognitive behavioural therapy:** We found no systematic review. One RCT group, administered cognitive behavioural therapy for adolescents with depression, produced a significantly higher remission rate among those receiving treatment (67%) compared with those on a waiting list (48%).[18] **Group therapeutic support versus group social skills training:** We found no systematic review. One RCT in 47 adolescents comparing group therapeutic support versus group social skills training found no significant difference in remission rates (50% v 40%).[19]

Harms: See harms of specific psychological treatments under depressive disorders, p 652. We found no report of harms specifically for children and adolescents.

Comment: See comment of specific psychological treatments under depressive disorders, p 652.

> **QUESTION   Which treatments are most effective at improving long term outcome?**

We found no systematic reviews and no RCTs looking at long term outcomes.

Benefits: We found no systematic reviews and no RCTs. We found no trials comparing structured psychotherapy with pharmacotherapy in children and adolescents. We found no trials comparing combined pharmacotherapy and psychotherapy with either treatment alone. We found no trials comparing different psychotherapies.

Harms: See harms of prescription antidepressant drugs, p 248, and under depressive disorders, p 652. See also harms of cognitive behavioural therapy, in table 2 under depressive disorders, p 652.

Comment: See depressive disorders, p 652. We found one prospective cohort study in which adolescents with depression, randomised to cognitive behavioural therapy, systemic behavioural family therapy, or non-directive supportive therapy (see glossary, p 251), were assessed at 3 monthly intervals for the first 12 months and then once again at 24 months. The study found no significant difference between the groups. Of 106 adolescents, 38% experienced sustained recovery, 21% experienced persistent depression, and 41% had a relapsing course.[20]

GLOSSARY

Cognitive behavioural therapy A brief (20 sessions over 12–16 weeks) structured treatment aimed at changing the dysfunctional beliefs and negative automatic thoughts that characterise depressive disorders.[21] Cognitive behavioural therapy requires a high level of training in the therapist, and has been adapted for children and adolescents suffering depression. A course of treatment is characterised by 8–12 weekly sessions, in which the therapist and the child collaborate to solve current difficulties. The treatment is structured, and often directed by a manual. Treatment generally includes cognitive elements, such as the challenging of negativistic thoughts, and behavioural elements such as structuring time to engage in pleasurable activity.

Interpersonal therapy A standardised form of brief psychotherapy (usually 12–16 weekly sessions) primarily intended for outpatients with unipolar non-psychotic depressive disorders. It focuses on improving the individual's interpersonal functioning and identifying the problems associated with the onset of the depressive episode.[22] In children and adolescents, interpersonal therapy has been adapted for adolescents to address common adolescent developmental issues, for example separation from parents, exploration of authority in relationship to parents, development of dyadic interpersonal relationships, initial experience with the death of relative or friend, and peer pressure.

Non-directive supportive treatment See brief, non-directive counselling under depressive disorders, p 652.

Systemic behaviour family therapy A combination of two treatment approaches that have been used effectively for dysfunctional families. In the first phase of treatment the therapist clarifies the concerns that brought the family into treatment, and provides a series of reframing statements designed to optimise engagement in therapy and identification of dysfunctional behaviour patterns (systemic therapy). In the second phase the family members focus on communication and problem-solving skills and the alteration of family interactional patterns (family behaviour therapy).

REFERENCES

1. Costello EJ, Angold A, Burns BJ, et al. The Great Smoky Mountains Study of Youth. Goals, design, methods, and the prevalence of DSM-III-R disorders. *Arch Gen Psychiatry* 1996;53:1129–1136.

2. Costello EJ. Developments in child psychiatric epidemiology. *J Am Acad Child Adolesc Psychiatry* 1989;28:836–841.

3. Lewinsohn PM, Rohde P, Seely JR. Major depressive disorder in older adolescents: Prevalence, risk factors, and clinical implications. *Clin Psychol Rev* 1998;18:765–794.

4. Birmaher B, Ryan ND, Williamson DE, Brent DA. Childhood and adolescent depression: A review of the past 10 years, Part I. *J Am Acad Child Adolesc Psychiatry* 1996;35:1427–1439.

5. Geller B, Fox LW, Fletcher M. Effect of tricyclic antidepressants on switching to mania and on the onset of bipolaria in depressed 6- to 12-year-olds. *J Am Acad Child Adolesc Psychiatry* 1993;32:43–50.

6. Hazell P, O'Connell D, Heathcote D, Henry D. Tricyclic drugs for depression in children and adolescents. In: The Cochrane Library, Issue 3, 2000. Oxford: Update software. Search date 1997; primary sources Medline, Excerpta Medica, Cochrane trials database.

7. Bernstein, GA, Borchardt, CM, Perwien, AR, et al. Imipramine plus cognitive-behavioral therapy in the treatment of school refusal. *J Am Acad Child Adolesc Psychiatry* 2000;39:276–283.

8. Sallee FR, Vrindavanam NS, Deas-Nesmith D, Carson SW, Sethuraman G. Pulse intravenous clomipramine for depressed adolescents: Double-blind, controlled trial. *Am J Psychiatry* 1997;154:668–673.

9. Avci A, Diler RS, Kibar M, Sezgin F. Comparison of moclobemide and placebo in young adolescents with major depressive disorder. *Ann Med Sci* 1999;8:31–40.

10. Williams JW, Mulrow CD, Chiquette E, Noel PH, Aguilar C, Cornell J. A systematic review of newer pharmacotherapies for depression in adults: Evidence report summary. *Ann Intern Med* 2000;132:743–756. Search date 1998; primary sources Medline, Embase, Psychlit, Lilacs, Psyindex, Sigle, Cinahl, Biological Abstracts, Cochrane Controlled Trials, hand searches, and personal contacts.

11. Geller B, Cooper TB, Zimerman B, et al. Lithium for prepubertal depressed children with family history predictors of future bipolarity: A double-blind, placebo-controlled study. *J Affect Disord* 1998;51:165–175.

12. Harrington R, Whittaker J, Shoebridge P, Campbell F. Systematic review of efficacy of cognitive behavioural therapies in childhood and adolescent depressive disorder. *BMJ* 1998;316:1559–1563. Search date 1997; primary sources Medline, Psychlit, Cochrane, and hand searches of reference lists, book chapters, conference proceedings, and relevant journals in the field.

13. Lewinsohn PM, Clarke GN. Psychosocial treatments for adolescent depression. *Clin Psychol Rev* 1999;19:329–342.

14. Reinecke MA, Ryan NE, DuBois DL. Cognitive-behavioral therapy of depression and depressive symptoms during adolescence: A review and meta-analysis. *J Am Acad Child Adolesc Psychiatry* 1998;37:26–34.

15. Mufson L, Weissman MM, Moreau D, Garfinkel R. Efficacy of interpersonal psychotherapy for depressed adolescents. *Arch Gen Psychiatry* 1999;56:573–579.

16. Rossello J, Bernal G. The efficacy of cognitive-behavioral and interpersonal treatments for depression in Puerto Rican adolescents. *J Consult Clin Psychol* 1999;67:734–745.

17. Brent DA, Holder D, Kolko D, et al. A clinical psychotherapy trial for adolescent depression comparing cognitive, family, and supportive therapy. *Arch Gen Psychiatry* 1997;54:877–885.

18. Clarke GN, Rohde P, Lewinsohn PM, Hops H, Seeley JR. Cognitive-behavioral treatment of adolescent depression: Efficacy of acute group treatment and booster sessions. *J Am Acad Child Adolesc Psychiatry* 1999;38:272–279.

19. Fine S, Forth A, Gilbert M, Haley G. Group therapy for adolescent depressive disorder: a comparison of social skills and therapeutic support. *J Am Acad Child Adolesc Psychiatry* 1991;30:79–85.

20. Birmaher B, Brent DA, Kolko D, et al. Clinical outcome after short-term psychotherapy for adolescents with major depressive disorder. *Arch Gen Psychiatry* 2000;57:29–36.

21. Haaga DAF, Beck AT. Cognitive therapy. In: Paykel ES, ed. *Handbook of affective disorders*. Edinburgh: Churchill Livingstone, 1992;511–523.

22. Klerman GL, Weissman H. Interpersonal psychotherapy. In: Paykel ES, ed. *Handbook of affective disorders*. Edinburgh: Churchill Livingstone, 1992;501–510.

Philip Hazell
Conjoint Professor of
Child and Adolescent Psychiatry/Director
Child and Youth Mental Health Service
University of Newcastle
New South Wales
Australia

Competing interests: The author has been paid a fee for speaking to general practitioners about the evidence for the treatment of depression in young people by Pfizer, the manufacturer of sertraline.

Search date January 2001

Yadlapalli Kumar and Rajini Sarvananthan

QUESTIONS

INTERVENTIONS

**To be covered in future issues of
    *Clinical Evidence***
Bethanecol
Domperidone
Metoclopramide

Key Messages

- Small RCTs have found that prone and left lateral positioning reduce reflux, but both are known risk factors for sudden infant death syndrome (SIDS).

- One small RCT has found that carob flour is superior to rice flour in reducing symptoms and vomiting.

- One small RCT has found that sodium alginate improves parent reported symptoms of gastro-oesophageal reflux disease (GORD).

- One systematic review of cisapride versus placebo found no clinical improvement in symptoms in childhood GORD. Cisapride is not widely licensed for use in children, and clinical use in adults is restricted because of heart arrhythmias. Cisapride has been withdrawn from several markets.

- One small RCT has found that cimetidine versus placebo is effective for GORD complicated by oesophagitis.

- We found insufficient evidence on the use of proton pump inhibitors for GORD.

- We found insufficient evidence on the effect of surgical fundoplication. Although most children improve after surgical fundoplications, surgery is associated with significant mortality and morbidity.

Gastro-oesophageal reflux in children

DEFINITION GORD is the passive transfer of gastric contents into the oesophagus due to transient or chronic relaxation of the lower oesophageal sphincter.[1] A survey of 69 children with GORD attending a tertiary referral centre (median age 16 months) found that presenting symptoms were recurrent vomiting (72%), epigastric and abdominal pain (36%), feeding difficulties (29%), failure to thrive (28%), and irritability (19%).[2] Over 90% of children with GORD have vomiting before 6 weeks of age.[1] Rare complications of the condition include oesophagitis with haematemesis and anaemia, respiratory problems such as cough, apnoea and recurrent wheeze, and failure to thrive.[1] A small comparative study (40 children) suggested that, when compared with healthy children, infants with GORD display slower development of feeding skills and problems affecting behaviour, swallowing, food intake, and mother–child interaction.[3]

INCIDENCE/ Gastro-oesophageal regurgitation is considered a problem if it is
PREVALENCE frequent and persistent.[1] Eighteen per cent of the general infant population has regurgitation.[4] In a study comparing the prevalence of GORD in children with respiratory dysfunction (62 children) to a control group (387 children), the prevalence of excessive gastro-oesophageal reflux, diagnosed by pH-metric criteria, was 42% and 8%, respectively.[5]

AETIOLOGY/ Factors favouring GORD are immaturity of the lower oesophageal
RISK FACTORS sphincter, chronic relaxation of the sphincter, increased abdominal pressure, gastric distension, hiatus hernia, and oesophageal dysmotility.[1] Premature infants and children with severe neurodevelopmental problems or congenital oesophageal anomalies are particularly at risk.

PROGNOSIS Regurgitation is considered benign, and most cases resolve spontaneously by 12–18 months of age.[6] However, with GORD caused by hiatus hernia, 30% of cases persist until the age of 4 years.[7]

AIMS To relieve symptoms, maintain normal growth, prevent complications such as oesophagitis, and minimise adverse effects of treatment.

OUTCOMES Clinical condition (in terms of symptoms and growth); parental distress; incidence of complications (e.g. oesophagitis). Reflux Index, a measure of the percentage of time with a low oesophageal pH (frequently < 4), is an intermediate outcome often used in RCTs. Clinical interpretation of the resulting data is problematic.

METHODS *Clinical Evidence* update search and appraisal January 2001. We searched Best Evidence, Cinahl, The Cochrane Library, Embase, and Medline for systematic reviews and RCTs relevant to GORD in children.

OPTION DIFFERENT POSTURES

We found two small RCTs that did not measure clinical outcomes. Both found that prone positioning significantly improved pH, compared with supine positioning. A third small RCT in preterm infants found that prone positioning decreased the number of episodes of reflux. Prone positioning is associated with SIDS.

Benefits: We found no systematic review. We found no RCTs investigating the effects of posture on clinical symptoms. Three small RCTs all reported effects of posture on oesophageal pH variables, such as Reflux Index. One RCT (crossover, 24 children, age < 5 months) found that the severity of GORD, expressed as Reflux Index, was significantly less in the prone and left lateral positions compared with the supine and right lateral positions (P < 0.001).[8] In this RCT, head elevation did not affect Reflux Index significantly. A second RCT (crossover, 15 children, age < 6 months) also found significantly less reflux in the prone position (head elevated in a harness) compared with supine positioning in an infant seat where the head and trunk were elevated to 60° (P < 0.001). Again, results were expressed in terms that are difficult to interpret clinically (Reflux Index).[9] The third RCT (crossover, 18 children, < 37 weeks gestation but > 7 days old) compared prone versus left and right lateral positions over 24 hours.[10] The findings favoured the prone and left lateral positions (P < 0.001). This trial found the number of episodes of reflux to be less with prone positioning (mean prone 15.4, 95% CI 9.9 to 20.9 v mean left lateral 24.6, 95% CI 17.7 to 31.5 v mean right 41.6, 95% CI 32.6 to 50.1, P < 0.001).

Harms: None reported.

Comment: Both prone and left lateral positions are known risk factors for SIDS. In a large, prospective cohort study prone sleeping position compared with supine position was associated with an increased risk of SIDS (OR 4.47, 95% CI 1.30 to 15.43).[11] The side sleeping position was found to increase the risk of SIDS compared with the supine position (at 2 months, adjusted OR 6.57, 95% CI 1.71 to 25.2).[12]

OPTION FEED THICKENERS

One small RCT found no significant difference between carob flour thickened feeds and a placebo thickener. A second small RCT found that carob flour was more effective than a traditional formula with rice flour in reducing symptoms and vomiting.

Benefits: We found no systematic review. **Versus placebo:** We found two RCTs. The first (double blind, 20 children, age 1–16 weeks) compared feeds thickened with carob flour (locus bean gum preparation) versus Saint John's bread, which is free of fibre and polysaccharides.[13] Regurgitation, as documented by parents after 1 week of treatment, decreased, but the difference was not significant (mean regurgitation score 2.2 *v* 3.3). It is unclear how to interpret regurgitation scores. This RCT also found no significant decrease in the Reflux Index after 1 week. The second RCT compared dry rice cereal with isocaloric unthickened feeds but did not seek to report benefits (see harms below).[14] **Versus each other:** We found one RCT (24 children, age 5–11 months) that compared feeds thickened with carob flour versus a traditional formula thickened with rice flour.[15] At the end of the 2 week treatment period, babies receiving the carob flour formula had a significant decrease in both symptomatic score (mean percentage reduction 70.4% *v* 48.7%, P < 0.01) and number of episodes of vomiting (58.1% *v* 34.1%, P < 0.05), recorded by parents.

Harms: The second RCT (24 children, age 0–6 months) of thickened versus unthickened feeds found that coughing occurred more frequently after feedings thickened with dry rice cereal than after isocaloric unthickened feedings (cough salvos per hour, thickened feeds mean 3.1, 95% CI 1.5 to 4.7 *v* unthickened feeds mean 2.0, 95% CI 1.2 to 2.8, P = 0.034).[15]

Comment: None.

OPTION SODIUM ALGINATE

One small RCT found that parents of children taking sodium alginate reported fewer episodes of regurgitation than those of infants given placebo.

Benefits: We found no systematic review. We found one RCT (20 children, mean age 28 months, treatment duration 8 days).[16] Sodium alginate reduced episodes of regurgitation to 25–33% of the former level whereas no clinical improvement was noted with placebo (lactose powder). Sodium alginate significantly reduced all pH variables compared to placebo (P< 0.05, CI not available).

Harms: None reported.

Comment: The high sodium load of sodium alginate may be inappropriate in preterm babies.[17]

OPTION CISAPRIDE

One systematic review found no significant improvement in clinical symptoms when comparing cisapride with placebo. Cisapride has been suspended from the market in several countries because of adverse cardiac effects.

Benefits: We found one good quality systematic review (8 RCTs, search date not stated).[18] Seven RCTs compared cisapride with placebo (236 children). There was no statistically significant difference in clinical improvement (being "same or worse" versus "improved symptoms" at the end of treatment, 7 RCTs, 236 children, OR 0.34, 95% CI 0.10 to 1.19). In these studies the "same or worse" categories included slight improvement, and significant heterogeneity was found when pooling data for this outcome, therefore the central effect estimate should be regarded with caution. Evidence suggesting publication bias favouring trials with a positive outcome was found. Use of cisapride was associated with a reduction in Reflux Index (5 RCTs, 176 children, weighted mean difference −6.49, 95% CI −10.13 to −2.85), but as Reflux Index and clinical symptoms are poorly correlated, the clinical importance of this finding is uncertain.

Harms: In the systematic review, adverse events were reported in four trials (190 people). There were more adverse events in the cisapride group, but the difference was not statistically significant (4 RCTs, 190 children, OR 1.8, 95% CI 0.87 to 3.70). Information on specific adverse effects was not provided by the systematic review.[18]

Comment: Cisapride is licensed for use in children in the Republic of Ireland. In the UK and Germany its license has been suspended and in the USA its marketing stopped because of an association with heart rhythm abnormalities in adults. Cisapride has been withdrawn from various markets because of its adverse effects. A recent case control study (201 children, age 1–12 months) found cisapride significantly prolonged the QTc interval on electrocardiogram in a subgroup of infants younger than 3 months, whereas in older infants the difference was not significant.[19] These changes are associated with sudden death. Gastrointestinal adverse effects (borborygmi, cramps, and diarrhoea) occur in 2% of infants.[19] Rash, pruritus, urticaria, bronchospasm, extrapyramidal effects, headache, dose-related increases in urinary frequency, hyperprolactinaemia, and reversible liver function abnormalities are extremely rare.[19] Most macrolide antibiotics and cimetidine elevate plasma cisapride levels, which may be clinically significant.[19]

OPTION	H₂ ANTAGONISTS

One small RCT has found that cimetidine is an effective treatment for GORD complicated by oesophagitis in children.

Benefits: We found no systematic review. We found one RCT (double blind, 37 children with GORD complicated by oesophagitis, age range 1 month to 14 years) comparing cimetidine 30–40 mg/kg a day versus placebo over 12 weeks.[20] More children improved on cimetidine (ARR 51%, 95% CI 21% to 81%; NNT 2, 95% CI 2 to 5). Improvement was defined in terms of either clinical or endoscopic findings. A second crossover RCT (27 children with GORD) compared different doses of cimetidine but reported only physiological outcomes (gastric pH, gastric acid suppression).[21] We found no RCTs of ranitidine in children.

Harms: None reported.

Comment: Cimetidine has been reported to cause bradycardia in a small subgroup of people and may increase cisapride plasma levels.[19] Bronchospasm, acute dystonic reactions, sinus node dysfunction, bradycardia, and increases in parasympathetic tone reactions have been reported with ranitidine, although this information was not obtained from controlled studies.[19]

Gastro-oesophageal reflux in children

OPTION   PROTON PUMP INHIBITORS (OMEPRAZOLE)

We found insufficient evidence on the effects of proton pump inhibitors on GORD.

Benefits: We found no systematic review or RCT. One small case series did not report clinical outcomes.[22]

Harms: None reported.

Comment: Proton pump inhibitors have been reported to cause hepatitis, and omeprazole chronically elevates serum gastrin.[22]

OPTION   SURGERY

We found insufficient evidence on the effects of surgery on GORD. Although most children improve after fundoplication, surgery is associated with significant mortality and morbidity.

Benefits: We found no systematic review or RCT comparing surgery with medical interventions, or one surgical procedure with another. We found a cohort study of 22 children who had undergone anterior gastric fundoplication.[23] Twenty children (91%) remained asymptomatic by 2 years.

Harms: A retrospective review (106 children) of modified Nissen's fundoplication showed a failure rate of 7.5% and, when neurologically impaired children were included, a long-term mortality of 7.8%.[24] If only neurologically normal children were considered, the mortality was 1.6% in the immediate postoperative period and 3.2% on long term follow up (3 deaths out of 62; all with associated congenital abnormalities).

Comment: Complications of surgical treatment include dumping, retching, intestinal obstruction, "gas bloat", and recurrence of GORD.[17]

Substantive changes since last issue

Cisapride versus placebo New systematic review;[18] conclusion unchanged.

REFERENCES

1. Herbst JJ. *Textbook of Gastroenterology and Nutrition in Infancy.* 2nd ed. New York: Raven Press, 1989:803–813.

2. Lee WS, Beattie RM, Meadows N, et al. Gastro-oesophageal reflux: Clinical profiles and outcome. *J Paediatr Child Health* 1999;35:568–571.

3. Mathisen B, Worrall L, Masel J, et al. Feeding problems in infants with gastro-oesophageal reflux disease: a controlled study. *J Paediatr Child Health* 1999;35:163–169.

4. Boulton TJ, Rowley MP. Nutritional studies during early childhood. III. Incidental observations of temperament, habits, and experiences of ill-health. *Aust Paediatr J* 1979;15:87–90.

5. Sacré L, Vandenplas Y. Gastroesophageal reflux associated with respiratory abnormalities during sleep. *J Pediatr Gastroenterol Nutr* 1989;9: 28–33.

6. Vandenplas Y, Belli D, Benhamou P, et al. A critical appraisal of current management practices for infant regurgitation – recommendations of a working party. *Eur J Pediatr* 1997;156:343–357.

7. Carre IJ. Natural history of partial thoracic stomach ("hiatus hernia") in children. *Arch Dis Child* 1959;34:344–353.

8. Tobin JM, McCloud P, Cameron DJS. Posture and gastro-oesophageal reflux: a case for left lateral positioning. *Arch Dis Child* 1997;76:254–258.

9. Orenstein SR, Whitington PF. Positioning for prevention of infant gastroesophageal reflux. *J Pediatr* 1983;103:534–537.

10. Ewer AK, James ME, Tobin JM. Prone and left lateral positioning reduce gastro-oesophageal reflux in preterm infants. *Arch Dis Child Fetal Neonatal Ed* 1999;81:F201–205.

11. Dwyer T, Ponsonby AB, Newman NM, et al. Prospective cohort study of prone sleeping position and sudden infant death syndrome. *Lancet* 1991;337:1244–1247.

12. Mitchell EA, Tuohy PG, Brunt JM, et al. Risk factors for sudden infant death following the prevention campaign in New Zealand. *Pediatrics* 1997;100:835–840.

13. Vandenplas Y, Hachimi-Idrissi S, Casteels A, et al. A clinical trial with an "anti-regurgitation" formula. *Eur J Pediatr* 1994;153:419–423.

14. Orenstein SR, Shalaby TM, Putnam PE. Thickening feedings as a cause of increased coughing when used as therapy for gastroesophageal reflux in infants. *J Pediatr* 1992;121:913–915.

15. Borrelli O, Salvia G, Campanozzi A, et al. Use of a new thickened formula for treatment of symptomatic gastroesophageal reflux in infants. *Ital J Gastroenterol Hepatol* 1997;29:237–242.

16. Buts JP, Barudi C, Otte JB. Double-blind controlled study on the efficacy of sodium alginate (Gaviscon) in reducing gastroesophageal reflux assessed by 24 hour continuous pH monitoring in infants and children. *Eur J Pediatr* 1987;146: 156–158.

17. Davies AEM, Sandhu BK. Diagnosis and treatment of gastro-oesophageal reflux. *Arch Dis Child* 1995; 73:82–86.

18. Augood C, MacLennan S, Gilbert R, Logan S. Cisapride treatment for gastro-oesophageal reflux in children (Cochrane Review). In: The Cochrane Library, Issue 4, 2000. Oxford: Update Software. Search date not stated; primary sources Cochrane Central Trials Register, Cochrane Specialised Trials register of the Cochrane Upper Gastrointestinal and Pancreatic Diseases Group, Medline, Embase, Science Citation Index, and hand searched reference lists.

19. Vandenplas Y, Belli DC, Benatar A, et al. The role of cisapride in the treatment of pediatric gastroesophageal reflux. *J Pediatr Gastroenterol Nutr* 1999;28:518–528.

20. Cucchiara S, Gobio-Casali L, Balli F, et al. Cimetidine treatment of reflux esophagitis in children: An Italian multicentre study. *J Pediatr Gastroenterol Nutr* 1989;8:150–156.

21. Lambert J, Mobassaleh M, Grand RJ. Efficacy of cimetidine for gastric acid suppression in pediatric patients. *J Pediatr* 1992;120:474–478.

22. Gunasekaran TS, Hassall EG. Efficacy and safety of omeprazole for severe gastroesophageal reflux in children. *J Pediatr* 1993;123:148–154.

23. Bliss D, Hirschl R, Oldham K, et al. Efficacy of anterior gastric fundoplication in the treatment of gastroesophageal reflux in infants and children. *J Paediatr Surg* 1994;29:1071–1075.

24. Spillane AJ, Currie B, Shi E. Fundoplication in children: Experience with 106 cases. *Aust NZ J Surg* 1996;66:753–756.

Yadlapalli Kumar
Specialist Registrar in Paediatrics
Alder Hey Children's Hospital
Liverpool
UK

Rajini Sarvananthan
Specialist Registrar in Paediatrics
St Luke's Hospital
Bradford
UK

Competing interests: None declared.

Infantile colic

Search date January 2001: expanded this issue

Sally Wade and Teresa Kilgour

QUESTIONS

INTERVENTIONS

Key Messages

- Two systematic reviews have found that dicyclomine reduces infantile colic, but may be associated with adverse events.

- Two systematic reviews found no evidence that simethicone reduces infantile colic.

- We found limited evidence from one small RCT that soya milk may reduce duration of crying compared with standard formula milk.

- We found insufficient evidence from small RCTs on the effects of low lactose milk.

- We found limited evidence from small RCTs that herbal tea or sucrose solution were effective.

- Four small RCTs of modification of parental responses to the infant found inconsistent effects on infantile colic. We found no clear evidence that any form of behaviour modification reduces infantile colic.

- One small RCT has found that replacing the standard formula milk with whey hydrolysate reduces infant colic.

- Two systematic reviews found limited evidence that casein hydrolysate milk reduces infant colic.

DEFINITION	Infantile colic is defined as excessive crying in an otherwise healthy baby. The crying typically starts in the first few weeks of life and ends by 4–5 months. Excessive crying is defined as crying that lasts at least 3 hours a day, for 3 days a week, for at least 3 weeks.[1]
INCIDENCE/ PREVALENCE	Infantile colic causes one in six families to consult a health professional. One population based study (409 breast or formula fed infants) found the incidence of infantile colic to be 3.3–17%, depending on the definition used and whether the symptoms were reported prospectively or retrospectively. The incidence was 9% using the definition given above.[2] One RCT (89 breast and formula fed infants) found that, at 2 weeks of age, the incidence of crying more than 3 hours a day was 43% (formula fed) and 16% (breast fed) infants. The incidence at 6 weeks was 12% (formula fed) and 31% (breast fed).[3]
AETIOLOGY/ RISK FACTORS	The cause of infantile colic is unclear. It may be part of the normal distribution of crying. Other possible explanations are painful gut contractions, lactose intolerance, gas, or parental misinterpretation of normal crying.[1] One large survey found that older primigravid women, mothers in non-manual occupations, or those who stayed in full time education, had the greatest risk of reporting infantile colic.[4]
PROGNOSIS	Infantile colic improves with time. One study found that 29% of infants aged 1–3 months cried for more than 3 hours a day, but by 4–6 months of age the prevalence had fallen to 7–11%.[5]
AIMS	To reduce infant crying and distress, and the anxiety of the family, with minimal side effects of treatment.
OUTCOMES	Duration of crying or colic, as measured on dichotomous, ordinal, or continuous scales. Parents' perceptions of severity (recorded in a diary).
METHODS	*Clinical Evidence* update search and appraisal January 2001. We searched Cinahl, the Cochrane Library, Embase, and Medline for publications using reduction in crying or colic as the main outcome. Trials were excluded for the following reasons: infants studied had normal crying patterns, infants were older than 6 months, interventions lasted less than 3 days, trials had no control groups or had low Jadad quality scores (see glossary, p 266).[6] Sometimes we pooled results from RCTs with different but comparable outcomes; effect sizes were calculated using a random effects model.

QUESTION What are the effects of treatments for infantile colic?

OPTION ANTICHOLINERGIC DRUGS

Two systematic reviews have found that anticholinergic drugs (dicyclomine or dicycloverine) significantly reduce infantile colic, but may be associated with more frequent minor adverse effects.

Benefits: We found two systematic reviews.[1,7] The first systematic review (search date 1996, 5 RCTs, 177 infants)[1] found that anticholinergic drugs (most frequently dicyclomine 5 mg four times daily) were more effective than placebo (effect size SMD 0.46, 95% CI 0.33 to

0.60) (see comment below). The clinical importance of this result is unclear. A second systematic review (search date 1999, 4 of the same RCTs) found similar results (3 of 4 RCTs found that dicyclomine was more effective than placebo).[7]

Harms: Two of five RCTs[8,9] in the systematic reviews[1,7] compared harms of dicyclomine versus placebo. The first RCT (crossover design, 30 infants) found more drowsiness with dicyclomine versus placebo (4/30 v 1/30; P = 0.16).[8] The second RCT (crossover design, 25 infants) found more loose stools or constipation in infants on dicyclomine versus placebo (3/25 v 1/25; P = 0.3).[9] Case reports of harms have included breathing difficulties, seizures, syncope, asphyxia, muscular hypotonia, and coma.[10]

Comment: Most RCTs used dicyclomine; dicycloverine was used in only one of the RCTs. Only one RCT stated measures to make the control syrup taste the same as the drug syrup.[8] The first review is limited because it pooled different outcome measures from RCTs and included crossover studies.[1] The crossover design is unlikely to provide valid evidence because infantile colic is an unstable condition, and the effects of dicyclomine may continue even after a washout period.[11]

OPTION   SIMETHICONE

Two systematic reviews of the same three RCTs found no evidence that simethicone reduced infantile colic.

Benefits: We found two systematic reviews (search dates 1996 and 1999, same 3 RCTs, 136 infants with infantile colic),[1,7] which found no evidence that simethicone was more effective than placebo. One RCT was of unsatisfactory quality. The second RCT (double blind, crossover, 83 infants) compared 0.3 ml of simethicone versus placebo before feeds.[12] It found no significant difference for colic when rated by carers (28% improved with simethicone, 37% with placebo, 20% with both; effect size for simethicone versus placebo: −0.10, 95% CI −0.27 to +0.08). The third RCT (double blind, crossover trial, 27 infants) compared simethicone with placebo and found no improvement as rated by parental interview, 24 hour diary, or behavioural observation (effect size +0.06, 95% CI −0.17 to +0.28).[13]

Harms: None reported.

Comment: The crossover design limits the validity and clinical utility of the RCTs.

OPTION   REPLACEMENT OF COW'S MILK WITH SOYA

One small RCT has found that soya replacement of standard formula milk reduced crying time.

Benefits: We found two systematic reviews (search dates 1996 and 1999, 1 RCT).[1,7] The RCT (19 infants) found that soya milk versus standard milk formula reduced the duration of crying (4.3–12.7 hours with soya milk v 17.3–20.1 hours with formula milk; mean difference 10.3 hours, 95% CI −16 to −4 hours).[14]

Harms: None reported.

Comment: Mothers were not told which milk the babies received, but differences between the milks could be detected by smell and texture.

OPTION **REPLACEMENT OF COW'S MILK WITH CASEIN HYDROLYSATE**

Two RCTs of cow's milk formula versus casein hydrolysate found insufficient evidence.

Benefits: We found two systematic reviews (search dates 1996 and 1999, identified the same 2 RCTs).[1,7] The first RCT (double blind, cross-over, 17 infants) studied the effect of each of three changes of infant diet for 4 days.[15] Colicky, bottle fed infants received casein hydrolysate and cow's milk alternatively. By the third change there was no notable difference in the incidence of colic between groups, but 47% of infants left the study before completion. The second RCT (122 infants) compared bottle fed infants given casein hydrolysate versus cow's milk formula. It also compared breast fed infants with mothers on a hypoallergenic diet (see glossary, p 266) versus controls on an unmodified diet.[16] Thirty eight infants were bottle fed, but the RCT did not report how many of these babies received the active diet. This RCT pooled the results of breast and bottle fed babies and found that the active diet reduced infant distress as measured by parents on a validated chart. The number of bottle fed infants was too small to establish any important effect in the bottle fed subgroup.

Harms: None reported.

Comment: None.

OPTION **REPLACEMENT OF COW'S MILK FORMULA BY WHEY HYDROLYSATE** New

One RCT found limited evidence that replacing cow's milk formula by whey hydrolysate reduces infant colic.

Benefits: We found two systematic reviews (search dates 1996 and 1999)[1,7] and one subsequent RCT.[17] The systematic reviews found no RCTs of adequate quality. The subsequent, double blind RCT (43 infants) found that whey hydrolysate formula (23 infants) versus standard cow's milk formula reduced the time that babies cried each day, measured by a validated parental diary (crying reduced by 63 minutes/day, 95% CI 1 to 127).[17]

Harms: None identified in the RCT.

Comment: Parents may not have been blind to the intervention. When asked, six indicated that they were aware, but two of these falsely identified the formula. When these infants' results were removed from the analysis, the calculated reduction in crying time with whey hydrolysate formula versus standard cow's milk formula was 58 minutes a day (P = 0.03).[17]

| OPTION | LOW LACTOSE MILK |

We found insufficient evidence from RCTs on the effects of low lactose milk.

Benefits: We found two systematic reviews (search dates 1996 and 1999, 2 RCTs),[1,7] and one additional small RCT.[18] The first RCT in the systematic reviews (double blind, crossover, 10 weaned infants) compared bottle feeding using pooled breast milk versus lactase treated breast milk versus formula milk versus lactase treated formula milk.[19] It found no evidence that low lactose milk reduced the time, severity, or duration of colic, as recorded by parents. The second RCT (12 breast fed infants) compared lactase versus placebo drops given within 5 minutes of feeding, and found no differences in the duration of time spent feeding, sleeping, or crying. The additional small crossover RCT (13 infants) compared lactase treated milk versus milk with placebo drops added.[18] It found that the lactase treated milk reduced crying time (1.1 hours/day, 95% CI 0.2 to 2.1).

Harms: None reported.

Comment: The RCTs are too small to allow confident conclusions to be drawn. The babies were not selected on the basis of any prior history of confirmed lactose intolerance.

| OPTION | SUCROSE SOLUTION |

We found limited evidence from one small RCT that sucrose solution may benefit infantile colic.

Benefits: We found one systematic review (search date 1999, 1 RCT).[7] The small crossover RCT (19 infants), compared 2 ml of 12% sucrose solution versus placebo given to babies when they continued to cry despite comforting.[20] Parents, blind to the intervention, scored the effect of the treatment on a scale of 1–5. Treatments were crossed over after 3–4 days and again after 6–8 days. The RCT found that parent rated improvement was more likely with sucrose than with placebo (12/19 [63%] with sucrose v 1/19 [5%] with placebo; ARI 58%, 95% CI 10% to 89%; NNT 2, 95% CI 1 to 10; RR 12, 95% CI 3.0 to 19).

Harms: None reported.

Comment: Publication bias has not been excluded.

| OPTION | HERBAL TEA |

One small RCT found limited evidence that herbal tea is effective for infantile colic.

Benefits: We found two systematic reviews (search dates 1996 and 1999, 1 RCT[21]).[1,7] The RCT compared herbal tea containing extracts of chamomile, vervain, licorice, fennel, and balm-mint in a sucrose solution (33 infants) versus sucrose control (35 infants) given by parents up to three times daily in response to episodes of colic.

Coding was only known to the pharmacist and the taste and smell of the tea and placebo were similar. Parents rated response using a symptom diary. The RCT found that, at 7 days, herbal tea eliminated colic in more infants than sucrose controls (number of infants colic free: 19/33 [58%] with herbal tea v 9/5 [26%] with sucrose; ARI 32%, 95% CI 7% to 53%; RR 2.2, 95% CI 1.3 to 3.1; NNT 3, 95% CI 2 to 14).

Harms: None reported.

Comment: One additional RCT, evaluating herbal drops, was not considered suitable for inclusion. The possibility of publication bias has not been excluded.

| OPTION | BEHAVIOURAL MODIFICATION |

Two systematic reviews found conflicting evidence from four small RCTs of the effects of behavioural modification (see glossary, p 266) of parents in response to their baby's crying.

Benefits: We found two systematic reviews (search dates 1996 and 1999, 4 RCTs).[1,7] **Focused counselling versus non-specific reassurance:** One RCT (22 infants) assessed maternal anxiety and the hours of crying each day by questionnaire. It found no evidence that counselling mothers about specific management techniques (responding to crying with gentle soothing motion, avoidance of over stimulation, using a pacifier, and prophylactic carrying) was any better than reassurance (see glossary, p 266) and support.[22] **Focused counselling versus car ride simulation:** The same RCT also allocated 16 infants (mean age 6.8 weeks) to car ride simulation for up to 1 hour. There were no important differences between this group and the control group (11 infants) for crying times or maternal anxiety.[22] **Focused counselling versus elimination of cow's milk protein:** One RCT (20 infants) found that counselling parents to respond to their baby's cries by feeding, holding, offering a pacifier, stimulating, or putting the baby down to sleep, decreased duration and extent of crying more quickly than substitution of soya or cow's milk with hydrolysed casein formula. Mean decrease in crying (hours/day) as recorded by parent diary was 2.1 hours with counselling versus 1.2 hours with dietary change.[23] **Increased carrying versus general advice:** The third RCT (66 infants) randomised mothers of babies with colic to carry their infant, even when not crying, for at least an additional 3 hours a day or to a general advice group (to carry, check baby's nappy, feed, offer pacifier, place baby near mother, or use background stimulation such as music). The first group carried their babies for 4.5 hours a day compared with 2.6 hours a day in the general advice group. There was no effect on daily crying time (mean difference 3 minutes less, 95% CI 37 minutes less to 32 minutes more).[24] **Reducing stimulation versus non-specific interview:** The fourth RCT (42 infants, median age 10 weeks) allocated mothers of infants to a low stimulation group (mothers were advised to reduce stimulation by not patting, lifting, winding or jiggling the baby, or reducing auditory stimulation) or a group that was given an empathetic interview. For infants under 12 weeks, advice to reduce stimulation versus no advice improved a change rating scale for more infants (after 7 days: 14/15 [95%] improved with advice v 6/12 [50%] with control; ARI 43%, 95% CI 8% to 49%; RR 1.9, 95% CI 1.2 to 2.0; NNT 2, 95% CI 2 to 13).[25] Improvement in the change rating scale was defined as a score of +2 or better on a scale from –5 to +5 that was meant to indicate perceived change in crying since the start of the trial. It is unclear if this scale has been validated (see comment).

Harms: None reported.

Comment: Mothers given advice to reduce stimulation were also given permission to leave their infants if they felt they could no longer tolerate the crying. It is unclear whether the improved change score represents a true change in the hours that the baby cried, or altered maternal perception.

GLOSSARY

Behavioural modification Changing the way in which parents respond to their babies crying from colic.

Hypoallergenic diet In bottle fed infants, a hypoallergenic diet uses a casein hydrolysate formula. In breast fed infants, a hypoallergenic diet involves a maternal diet, free of artificial colourings, preservatives, and additives, and low in common allergens (e.g. milk, egg, wheat, nuts).

Jadad Scale This measures factors that impact on trial quality. Poor description of the factors, rated by low figures, are associated with greater estimates of effect. The scale includes three items: was the study described as randomized? (0–2); was the study described as double blind? (0–2); was there a description of withdrawals and drop-outs? (0–1).[6]

Reassurance Informing the parent that infantile colic is a self limiting condition resolving by 3–4 months of age, and is not caused by disease or any fault in parental care.

Substantive changes since last issue

All options New systematic review;[7] conclusions unchanged.

REFERENCES

1. Lucassen PLB, Assendelf WJJ, Gubbels JW, Van Eijk JTM, Van Geldrop WJ, Knuistingh Neven A. Effectiveness of treatments for infantile colic: a systematic review. *BMJ* 1998;316:1563–1569. Search date 1996: primary sources Cochrane Controlled Trials Register, Embase, Medline, and reference searching.
2. Canivet C, Hagander B, Jakobsson I, Lanke J. Infantile colic – less common than previously estimated? *Acta Paediatr* 1996;85:454–458.
3. Lucas A, St James-Roberts I. Crying, fussing and colic behaviour in breast and bottle-fed infants. *Early Human Development* 1998;53:9–19.
4. Crowcroft NS, Strachan DP. The social origins of infantile colic; questionnaire study covering 76 747 infants. *BMJ* 1997;314:1325–1328.
5. St James Roberts I, Halil A. Infant crying patterns in the first year: Normal community and clinical findings. *J Child Psychol Psychiatry* 1991;32:951–968.
6. Jadad AR, Moore RA, Carroll D, et al. Assessing the quality of reports of randomized clinical trials: is blinding necessary? *Control Clin Trials* 1996;17:1–12.
7. Garrison MM, Christakis DA. A systematic review of treatments for infant colic. *Pediatrics* 2000; 106:184–190. Search date May 1999; primary sources English language sources in Medline,

Cochrane Clinical Trials Registry, hand searches of reference lists, authors.
8. Hwang CP, Danielsson B. Dicyclomine hydrochloride in infantile colic. *BMJ* 1985;291:1014.
9. Gruinseit F. Evaluation of the efficacy of dicyclomine hydrochloride ("Merbentyl") syrup in the treatment of infantile colic. *Curr Med Res Opin* 1977;5:258–261.
10. Williams J, Watkin Jones R. Dicyclomine: worrying symptoms associated with its use in some small babies. *BMJ* 1984;288:901.
11. Fleiss JL. The crossover study. In: Fleiss JL, ed. *The design and analysis of clinical experiments.* New York: John Wiley and Sons, 1986.
12. Metcalf TJ, Irons TG, Sher LD, Young PC. Simethicone in the treatment of infantile colic: a randomized, placebo-controlled, multicenter trial. *Pediatrics* 1994;94:29–34.
13. Danielsson B, Hwang CP. Treatment of infantile colic with surface active substance (simethicone). *Acta Paediatr Scand* 1985;74:446–450.
14. Campbell JPM. Dietary treatment of infantile colic: a double-blind study. *J R Coll Gen Pract* 1989;39:11–14.
15. Forsythe BWC. Colic and the effect of changing formulas: a double blind, multiple-crossover study. *J Pediatr* 1989;115:521–526.

16. Hill DJ, Hudson IL, Sheffield LJ, Shelton MJ, Menahem S, Hosking CS. A low allergen diet is a significant intervention in infantile colic: Results of a community based study. *J Allergy Clin Immunol* 1995;96:886–892.

17. Lucassen LB, Assendelft WJ, Gubbels LW, Van Eijk, Douwes AC. Infantile colic: crying time reduction with a whey hydrolysate; a double blind, randomized placebo-controlled trial. *Pediatrics* 2000;106:1349–1354.

18. Kearney PJ, Malone AJ, Hayes T, Cole M, Hyland M. A trial of lactase in the management of infant colic. *J Hum Nutrition Dietetics* 1998;11:281–285.

19. Stahlberg MR, Savilahti E. Infantile colic and feeding. *Arch Dis Child* 1986;61:1232–1233

20. Markestad T. Use of sucrose as a treatment for infant colic. *Arch Dis Child* 1997;77:356–357

21. Weizman Z, Alkrinawi S, Goldfarb D, Bitran C. Herbal teas for infantile colic. *J Pediatr* 1993;123: 670–671.

22. Parkin PC, Schwartz CJ, Manuel BA. Randomised controlled trial of three interventions in the management of persistent crying of infancy. *Pediatrics* 1993;92;197–201.

23. Taubman B. Parental counselling compared with elimination of cow's milk or soy milk protein for the treatment of infant colic syndrome: a randomized trial. *Pediatrics* 1988;81:756–761.

24. Barr RG, McMullen SJ, Spiess H, Leduc DG, Yaremko J, Barfield R, et al. Carrying as a colic "therapy": a randomized controlled trial. *Pediatrics* 1991;87:623–630.

25. McKenzie S. Troublesome crying in infants: effect of advice to reduce stimulation. *Arch Dis Child* 1991;66:1461–1420.

Sally Wade
Staff Grade Community Paediatrician
Archer Street Clinic
Darlington
UK

Teresa Kilgour
Staff Grade Community Paediatrician
City Hospitals Sunderland
Sunderland
UK

Competing interests: None declared.

Search date February 2001

Sara Bosson and Natalie Lyth

INTERVENTIONS

Key Messages

- Systematic reviews have found that desmopressin and tricyclic drugs are more effective than placebo for short term symptom relief. The reviews found that desmopressin was associated with fewer adverse effects than tricyclic drugs.

- One good quality RCT has found that indomethacin versus placebo significantly increases the number of dry nights.

- We found limited evidence from one small RCT that carbamazepine versus placebo increases the number of dry nights in nocturnal enuresis caused by detrusor instability.

- One systematic review has found that enuresis alarms are associated with good initial success, low relapse rates, and few adverse effects, with drugs and behavioural treatments providing some additional benefit. One RCT found that an alarm clock used at a critical time of night increased the number of dry nights.

- We found insufficient evidence indicating the youngest age at which treatment becomes effective.

DEFINITION Nocturnal enuresis is the involuntary discharge of urine at night in the absence of congenital or acquired defects of the central nervous system or urinary tract in a child aged 5 years or older.[1] Disorders that have bed wetting as a symptom (termed "nocturnal incontinence") can be excluded by a thorough history, examination, and urinalysis. "Monosymptomatic" nocturnal enuresis is characterised by night time symptoms only and accounts for 85% of cases. Nocturnal enuresis is defined as primary if the child has never been dry for a period of more than 6 months, and secondary if such a period of dryness preceded the onset of wetting.

INCIDENCE/ PREVALENCE Between 15% and 20% of 5 year olds, 7% of 7 year olds, 5% of 10 year olds, 2–3% of 12–14 year olds, and 1–2% of people aged 15 years and over wet the bed twice a week on average.[2]

AETIOLOGY/ RISK FACTORS Nocturnal enuresis is associated with several factors, including small functional bladder capacity, nocturnal polyuria, and arousal dysfunction. Linkage studies have identified associated genetic loci on chromosomes 8q, 12q, 13q, and 22q11.[3–6]

PROGNOSIS Nocturnal enuresis has widely differing outcomes, from spontaneous resolution to complete resistance to all current treatments. About 1% of adults remain enuretic. Without treatment, about 15% of children with enuresis become dry each year.[7]

AIMS To stay dry on particular occasions (e.g. when visiting friends); to reduce the number of wet nights; to reduce the impact of the enuresis on the child's lifestyle; to initiate successful continence; to avoid relapse, with minimal adverse effects.

OUTCOMES Rate of initial success (defined as 14 consecutive dry nights); average number of wet nights per week; number of relapses after initial success; average number of wet nights after treatment has ceased.

METHODS *Clinical Evidence* update search and appraisal February 2001. Three large systemic reviews were identified as the best available evidence.[8–10]

QUESTION **What are the effects of treatments for short term relief of symptoms?**

OPTION **DESMOPRESSIN**

Systematic reviews have found that desmopressin is more effective than placebo for rapid symptom relief.

Benefits: We found two systematic reviews.[8,9] The more recent review (search date 1997, 21 RCTs, 948 children)[9] found that desmopressin versus placebo significantly reduced the number of wet nights (1.56, 95% CI 1.19 to 1.94 fewer wet nights per week), and increased the chance of attaining 14 consecutive dry nights (RR with desmopressin v placebo 4.6, 95% CI 1.4 to 15.0).

Harms: Adverse effects were reported in a small number of children: anorexia, headache, rash, sight disturbance, upset stomach, an unpleasant taste in the mouth, epistaxis, and nasal discomfort.[8,9] Rarely, water intoxication has been reported.

Comment: The systematic reviews included only studies of interventions used to remedy either primary or secondary nocturnal enuresis (incontinence was excluded by medical examination or explicitly mentioned in the inclusion/exclusion criteria of included RCTs), and included a systematic measurement of baseline wetting and outcomes. Many of the included RCTs were of poor quality.

OPTION   TRICYCLIC DRUGS

Systematic reviews have found that tricyclic drugs significantly increase the chance of attaining 14 consecutive dry nights compared with placebo.

Benefits: **Versus placebo:** We found two systematic reviews.[8,10] The more recent review (search date 1997, 22 RCTs, 1100 children) evaluated imipramine, amitriptyline, viloxazine, clomipramine, and desipramine.[10] Many of the trials were of poor quality. It found that tricyclic drugs significantly increased the chance of attaining 14 consecutive dry nights (RR for 14 consecutive dry nights with tricyclic drugs v placebo 5.0, 95% CI 2.4 to 10.4) and reduced the number of wet nights (tricyclic drugs v placebo, WMD 0.99 fewer wet nights per week, 95% CI 0.71 to 1.27). **Versus alarms:** Three small RCTs (103 people) compared imipramine versus an alarm, and found no significant difference in effectiveness, during the treatment period.[10] However, two of the RCTs found that when the treatment had stopped, children taking imipramine had one fewer wet night per week (WMD 1.03, 95% CI 0.19 to 1.87).[10]

Harms: In the systematic reviews, reported adverse effects included anorexia, anxiety reaction, burning sensation, constipation, depression, diarrhea, dizziness, drowsiness, dry mouth, headache, irritability, lethargy, sleep disturbance, upset stomach, and vomiting.[8,10] When reported, tricyclic drugs were associated with more adverse effects than desmopressin (tricyclic drugs 83/480 [17.3%] v desmopressin 41/579 [7.1%]). Tricyclic drugs have been reported as fatal in overdose.

Comment: We found no good studies directly comparing tricyclic drugs versus desmopressin.

OPTION   INDOMETHACIN

We found limited evidence from one small RCT that indomethacin significantly reduces the number of wet nights compared with placebo.

Benefits: We found no systematic review. One good quality RCT (85 children aged over 6 years with primary nocturnal enuresis) compared desmopressin versus indomethacin versus placebo. It found that indomethacin, given by suppository, significantly increased the number of dry nights compared with placebo over 3 weeks (mean number of dry nights 8.9 with indomethacin v 3.8 with placebo, P < 0.005).[11]

Harms: The study did not report any adverse effects (see harms of NSAIDs under osteoarthritis, p 808).

Comment: None.

| OPTION | CARBAMAZEPINE |

We found limited evidence from one small RCT that carbamazepine versus placebo increases the number of dry nights in nocturnal enuresis caused by detrusor instability.

Benefits: We found no systematic review. We found one small double blind crossover study (26 people with detrusor instability on videocystourethrography) of carbamazepine versus placebo.[12] It found that carbamazepine significantly increased the number of dry nights over 30 days (mean number of dry nights 18.8 with carbamazepine v 3.9 with placebo, $P < 0.001$).

Harms: The study did not report any adverse effects (see harms of carbamazepine under epilepsy, p 876).

Comment: The study population had proven detrusor instability. It may not be possible to generalise these results to all people with nocturnal enuresis.

| QUESTION | What are the effects of long term treatments? |

| OPTION | ENURESIS ALARMS, DRY BED TRAINING, DRUG TREATMENTS, ALARM CLOCK |

One systematic review has found that enuresis alarms are associated with good initial success, low relapse rates, and few adverse effects, with drugs and behavioural treatments providing some additional benefit. One RCT found that a simple alarm clock was effective for initial success when used for 16 weeks.

Benefits: We found one systematic review (search date 1997, 62 RCTs) of interventions in people with primary or secondary nocturnal enuresis.[8] Table 1, p 273 summarises results of studies in children that compared behavioural, pharmacological, and non-drug treatments versus placebo, enuresis alarm, or no treatment controls. Also included are the results from one additional RCT that compared a standard home alarm clock (to wake the child just before the usual time of enuresis) versus waking the child after 3 hours of sleep.[13]

Harms: **Medication:** See harms of desmopressin, p 269, and harms of tricyclic drugs, p 270. **Enuresis alarms:** Four trials reported adverse effects, most commonly alarm failure, as well as failure to wake the person, false alarms, fright, and disturbance to others. **Standard home alarm clock:** None reported.

Comment: Medication acts rapidly (see desmopressin, indomethacin, imipramine, and carbamazepine above) and may be an alternative where alarms are unacceptable.

Child health

QUESTION   What is the best age to start treatment?

We found insufficient evidence indicating the youngest age at which treatment becomes effective.

Benefits: We found no systematic review or RCTs.

Harms: We found no evidence.

Comment: Anecdotal experience suggests that reassurance is often all that is needed below the age of 7 years. Behavioural treatments, such as alarms, require motivation and commitment on the part of the child and parent. Anecdotal experience suggests that children under the age of 7 years may not exhibit the commitment needed. Minimum ages for which drugs are licensed vary according to local policy.

REFERENCES

1. Forsythe WI, Butler R. 50 years of enuretic alarms; a review of the literature. Arch Dis Child 1991;64: 879–885.
2. Blackwell C. A guide to enuresis: a guide to treatment of enuresis for professionals. Bristol: Eric, 1989.
3. Eiberg H. Total genome scan analysis in a single extended family for primary nocturnal enuresis: Evidence for a new locus (ENUR 3) for primary nocturnal enuresis on chromosome 22q11. Eur Urol 1998;33:34–36.
4. Eiberg H. Nocturnal enuresis is linked to a specific gene. Scand J Urol Nephrol 1995;173(suppl):15–17.
5. Arnell H, Hjalmas M, Jagervall G, et al. The genetics of primary nocturnal enuresis: Inheritance and suggestion of a second major gene on chromosome 12q. J Med Genet 1997;34:360–365.
6. Eiberg H, Berendt I, Mohr J. Assignment of dominant inherited nocturnal enuresis (ENUR 1) to chromosome 13q. Nat Genet 1995;10:354–356.
7. Forsythe WI, Redmond A. Enuresis and spontaneous cure rate of 1129 enuretics. Arch Dis Child 1974;49:259–263.
8. Lister-Sharp D, O'Meara S, Bradley M, Sheldon TA. University of York. NHS Centre for Reviews and Dissemination. August 1997. A systematic review of the effectiveness of interventions for managing childhood nocturnal enuresis. CRD Report 11. Search date 1996; primary sources Cochrane Library, Medline, Embase, Psychlit.
9. Glazener CMA, Evans JHC. Desmopressin for nocturnal enuresis in children. In: The Cochrane Library, Issue 3, 2000. Oxford: Update Software. Search date 1997; primary sources Medline, Embase, Amed, Assia, Bids, Cinahl, Psychlit, SIGLE, DHSS data.
10. Glazener CMA, Evans JHC. Tricyclic and related drugs for nocturnal enuresis in children. In: The Cochrane Library, Issue 3, 2000. Oxford: Update Software. Search date 1997; primary sources Medline, Embase, Amed, Assia, Bids, Cinahl, Psychlit, SIGLE, DHSS data.
11. Sener F, Hasanoglu E, Soylemezoglu O. Desmopressin versus indomethacin treatment in primary nocturnal enuresis and the role of prostaglandins. Urology 1998;52:878–881.
12. Al Waili NS. Carbamazepine to treat primary nocturnal enuresis: double-blind study. Eur J Med Res 2000;5:40–44.
13. El-Anany FG, Maghraby HA, Shaker SED, Abdel-Moneim AM. Primary nocturnal enuresis: a new approach to conditioning treatment. Urology 1999;53:405–409.

Sara Bosson
Staff Grade Community Paediatrician
Mancunian Community Health NHS Trust
Manchester
UK

Natalie Lyth
Staff Grade Community Paediatrician
Northallerton Health Service Trust
Northallerton
UK

Competing interests: SB, none declared. NL has been reimbursed for attending a symposium by Ferring Pharmaceuticals, the manufacturer of desmotabs.

TABLE 1 Effective treatments for enuresis: advantages and disadvantages (see text, p 271).[8-10]

	Initial success (14 consecutive dry nights)	Long term success	Evidence	Advantages	Disadvantages
Desmopressin	RR v placebo 4.6, 95% CI 1.4 to 15.0	No better than placebo	Meta-analysis of three RCTs	Effective within days, safe, few adverse effects with appropriate pretreatment advice	Case reports of water intoxication
Tricyclic drugs	RR v placebo 5.0, 95% CI 2.4 to 10.4	No better than placebo (RR 1.1)	Meta-analysis of 4 RCTs	Effective within days	Risk of lethal overdose, frequent significant adverse effects
Alarm	RR v no treatment 13.3, 95% CI 5.6 to 31.5	31–61% still dry at 3 months. Nine times less likely relapse than with desmopressin	Meta-analysis of 4 RCTs	Safe	Takes longer to become dry, needs good cooperation from child and family
Alarm and medication	75% v 46% with alarm alone	Not studied	1 RCT, 71 people (not in systematic review)	More rapid effect than alarm alone	Same adverse effects as medication
Dry bed training without alarm	RR v no treatment 2.5, 95% CI 0.55 to 11.4	No better than no treatment (RR 0.4, 95% CI 0.14 to 1.13)	1 good quality RCT, 45 people	Safe	Requires high degree of motivation
Dry bed training with alarm	RR v no treatment 10, 95% CI 2.69 to 37.24	No better than alarm alone (RR 1.0, 95% CI 0.7 to 1.5)	1 RCT, 45 people	Safe	Requires an even greater input from the family than either treatment alone
Standard home alarm clock	77.1% v 61.8% with waking after 3 hours' sleep (RR 1.3, P = 0.03)	No better at 3 months than waking after 3 hours' sleep (66% dry v 56%; P = 0.19)	1 RCT, 125 people	Safe, does not require bed wetting to initiate alarm	None reported

Recurrent idiopathic epistaxis (nosebleeds)

Search date February 2000

Martin Burton and Robert Walton

QUESTIONS

INTERVENTIONS

Key Messages

- One small RCT found that chlorhexidine/neomycin cream and silver nitrate cautery were of similar effectiveness. Some children found the smell and taste of the antiseptic cream unpleasant. All children found cautery painful despite the use of local anaesthesia.
- One small RCT found no advantage to adding once only silver nitrate cautery to standard treatment with a chlorhexidine/neomycin cream.

DEFINITION Recurrent idiopathic epistaxis is recurrent, self limiting nasal bleeding in children for which no specific cause has been identified. There is no consensus on how frequent or severe recurrences need to be. A cross sectional study of a sample of 1218 children aged 11–14 years found that 9% had frequent episodes of epistaxis.[1] It is likely that most nosebleeds in children are not brought to the attention of health professionals, and that only the most severe are considered for treatment.

AETIOLOGY/ In children, most epistaxis occurs from the anterior part of the
RISK FACTORS septum in the region of Little's area.[2] Common local factors are inflammation of the nasal mucosa, excessive nasal dryness and trauma, including nose-picking.[2] Epistaxis caused by other specific local (e.g. tumours) or systemic factors (e.g. clotting disorders) is not considered here.

PROGNOSIS Clinical experience suggests that recurrent epistaxis is less common in adolescents over 14 years and that many children "grow out" of this problem.

AIMS To reduce the number and severity of nosebleeds.

OUTCOMES Number and severity of nosebleeds.

METHODS *Clinical Evidence* search and appraisal February 2000. One author reviewed all RCTs and excluded those not relating to recurrent idiopathic epistaxis in children.

QUESTION	What are the effects of treatments in children with recurrent idiopathic epistaxis?

OPTION	ANTISEPTIC CREAMS

We found no placebo controlled trials. One small RCT found that chlorhexidine/neomycin cream and silver nitrate cautery were of similar effectiveness. Some children found the smell and taste of antiseptic cream unpleasant. All children found cautery painful despite the use of local anaesthesia.

Benefits: We found no systematic review. **Versus placebo:** We found no RCTs. **Versus cautery:** We found one RCT, although the method of randomisation was not explicit. It involved 48 children, age 3–14 years, who had at least one nosebleed in the previous 4 weeks and a "history of repeated epistaxis".[3] They were randomised to antiseptic cream (chlorhexidine hydrochloride 0.1%, neomycin sulphate 3250 units/g) applied to both nostrils twice daily for 4 weeks (24 children), or one episode of cautery (24 children). Cautery was undertaken in secondary care using sliver nitrate applied on a stick to prominent vessels or bleeding points. After 8 weeks, this small study found no significant difference between treatments. About half of the children in both groups had complete resolution (no bleeding in past 4 weeks, RR 0.92, 95% CI 0.54 to 1.59). Rates of other outcomes were also similar between groups at 8 weeks: partial success (50% reduction in number of bleeds in past 4 weeks, 4/24 v 3/24), failure (less than 50% reduction in number of bleeds in past 4 weeks, 7/24 v 6/24) and lost at 8 weeks (1/24 v 2/24). **Plus cautery:** See silver nitrate cautery, p 276.

Recurrent idiopathic epistaxis (nosebleeds)

Harms: No adverse reactions were observed with antiseptic cream, but some children found the smell and taste unpleasant. No percentages were reported. Chlorhexidine/neomycin cream may cause occasional skin reactions. Some commercial antiseptic creams contain arachis (peanut) oil. All children undergoing cautery experienced pain even with the use of 5% cocaine as local anaesthetic.[3]

Comment: Both trials involving silver nitrate cautery were undertaken in the context of secondary care.[3,4] Silver nitrate cautery is also used in primary care. It is unknown if complication rates differ.

OPTION   SILVER NITRATE CAUTERY

We found no placebo controlled trials of cautery. Small short term trials in secondary care found no significant differences between silver nitrate cautery and an antiseptic preparation. One small RCT found no advantage to adding once only silver nitrate cautery to standard treatment with a chlorhexidine/neomycin cream. All children found cautery painful.

Benefits: We found no systematic review. **Versus placebo:** We found no RCTs. **Versus antiseptic cream:** See antiseptic creams, p 275. **Plus antiseptic cream:** One RCT (40 adults, 24 children) compared once only silver nitrate cautery plus chlorhexidine hydrochloride 0.1% neomycin sulphate 3250 units/g cream twice daily for 2 weeks with antiseptic cream alone. The study included too few children to allow conclusions to be drawn.[4]

Harms: The RCT reported no harms.[4] Recognised complications of cautery include septal perforation, although the incidence following unilateral cautery in children is not known. Simultaneous bilateral cautery in children is not recommended because of an expected increased risk of perforation.

Comment: See comment under antiseptic creams above.

REFERENCES

1. Rodeghiero F, Castaman G, Dini E. Epidemiological investigation of the prevalence of von Willebrand's disease. *Blood* 1987;69:454–459.
2. Watkinson JC, Epistaxis. In: Kerr AG, Mackay IS, Bull TR eds. *Scott-Brown's Otolaryngology*, Volume 4 Rhinology. Oxford: Butterworth-Heinemann, 1997;18:1–19
3. Ruddy J, Proops DW, Pearman K, Ruddy H. Management of epistaxis in children. *Int J Paediatr Otorhinolaryngol* 1991;21:139–142.
4. Murthy P, Nilssen ELK, Rao S, McClymont LG. A randomised clinical trial of antiseptic nasal carrier cream and silver nitrate cautery in the treatment of recurrent anterior epistaxis. *Clin Otolaryngol* 1999;228:231.

Martin Burton
Consultant Otolaryngologist
The Radcliffe Infirmary
Oxford
UK

Robert Walton
Honorary Senior Clinical Lecturer
Department of Public Health and
Primary Care, University of Oxford
Institute of Health Sciences
Oxford
UK

Competing interests: None declared.

Search date August 2000: new for this issue

Ruth Gilbert and Linda Franck

QUESTIONS

INTERVENTIONS

Key Messages

- Three RCTs have found that venepuncture compared with heel puncture substantially reduces pain responses and the need for repeat punctures.
- Eighteen RCTs have found that oral sucrose or glucose reduces pain responses compared with water or no treatment in neonates undergoing heel puncture or venepuncture. We found no evidence about the optimal concentration or dose, or whether sucrose or glucose is most effective.
- Six RCTs have found that topical anaesthetics reduce pain responses compared to placebo for venepuncture. RCTs found that topical anaesthetics were ineffective in reducing pain responses to heel puncture.
- We found no evidence of clinically important adverse effects associated with a single application of EMLA in term or preterm infants.
- Six RCTs found small but significant reduction in pain responses in infants given a pacifier compared with no pacifier during heel puncture or venepuncture.
- We found limited evidence that physical manoeuvres (rocking, prone position, tucking in arms and legs, or skin to skin contact) reduce pain responses during blood sampling.

© *Clinical Evidence* 2001;5:277–286.

Reducing pain during blood sampling in infants

DEFINITION Methods of sampling blood in infants include heel puncture, venepuncture, and arterial puncture. Heel puncture involves lancing of the lateral aspect of the infant's heel, squeezing the heel, and collecting the pooled capillary blood. Venepuncture involves aspirating blood through a needle in a peripheral vein. Arterial blood sampling is not discussed in this review.

INCIDENCE/ PREVALENCE Almost every infant in the developed world undergoes heel puncture to screen for metabolic disorders (e.g. phenylketonuria). Many infants have repeated heel punctures or venepunctures to monitor blood glucose or haemoglobin levels. Preterm or ill neonates receiving intensive care may have one to 21 painful procedures a day.[1–3] Heel punctures comprised 61–87% and venepuncture comprised 8–13% of the invasive procedures performed on ill infants. Analgesics were rarely given specifically for blood sampling procedures but 5–19% of infants received analgesia for other indications.[2,3] In one study, comfort measures were provided during 63% of venepunctures and 75% of heel punctures.[3]

AETIOLOGY/ RISK FACTORS Blood sampling in infants can be difficult to perform, particularly in preterm or ill infants. Young infants may have increased sensitivity and more prolonged responses to pain than older age groups.[4] Factors that may affect the infant's pain responses include postconceptual age, previous pain experience, and procedural technique.

PROGNOSIS Pain caused by blood sampling is associated with acute behavioural and physiological deterioration.[4] Other adverse effects of blood sampling include bleeding, bruising, haematoma, and infection. Extremely rarely, heel puncture can result in cellulitis, osteomyelitis, calcaneal spurs, and necrotising chondritis.[5–7]

AIMS To obtain an adequate blood sample with minimal pain for the infant and minimal adverse effects of treatments.

OUTCOMES We found no easily administered, widely accepted assessment of pain in infants. Where available, we have analysed the proportion of infants crying at all, or the duration of crying. Other behavioural outcomes include facial expressions (the number of specific expressions or the duration of those expressions). We have not pooled differences in pain responses reported in different studies.

METHODS *Clinical Evidence* search and appraisal August 2000, and additional hand searches to November 2000.

QUESTION What are the effects of interventions to reduce pain responses during blood sampling in infants?

OPTION VENEPUNCTURE VERSUS HEEL PUNCTURE

Three RCTs have found that venepuncture versus heel puncture significantly reduces pain responses, particularly crying, during blood sampling and also reduces the need for repeat samples.

Benefits: We found one systematic review (search date 1999, 2 RCTs)[8] and one subsequent RCT.[9] All three RCTs (264 full term healthy neonates) found that venepuncture versus heel puncture significantly reduced pain responses and the number of repeat punctures (264 infants; RR 0.34, 95% CI 0.34 to 0.51; NNT 3, 95% CI 2 to 4). Each study used different measures of pain responses. Two of the RCTs found that fewer infants cried during venepuncture compared with heel puncture (237 infants; RR 0.61, 95% CI 0.50 to 0.74; NNT 3, 95% CI 2 to 4).[9,10]

Harms: One of the RCTs reported bruising in a single infant following heel puncture and higher maternal anxiety during venepuncture than during heel puncture.[11] Too few infants were studied to detect infection or rare complications.

Comment: Of the three RCTs, only one reported adequate concealment of randomisation and blinded assessment of pain responses.[10] All three RCTs compared blood sampling procedures performed by a single individual in each study. Larger, well conducted trials with many people who routinely perform blood sampling in infants are needed to provide generalisable evidence about optimal sampling methods. Pain responses should be assessed blind to the puncture technique.

OPTION   ORAL SWEET SOLUTIONS

Eighteen RCTs have found that oral sucrose and glucose versus water or no treatment in infants undergoing heel puncture or venepuncture significantly reduce pain responses, particularly the duration of crying. We found no clear evidence about the optimal concentration of sucrose or glucose for pain relief with heel puncture or venepuncture. One RCT did not find a beneficial effect of multiple compared with a single dose of sucrose for heel puncture. One RCT found no evidence that sucrose and glucose differ in their effects on pain in term infants.

Benefits: **Sucrose for heel puncture:** We found three systematic reviews (search dates 1995,[12] 1997,[13] 1998,[14] 9 RCTs[15-23]) and four additional RCTs[24-27] of oral sucrose (0.05–2 ml of 12–70%) versus water or no treatment in newborns undergoing heel puncture. The 13 RCTs included 184 preterm neonates[16,19,21,26,27] and 542 healthy term neonates.[15,18,21-25,27] Five RCTs in preterm neonates found that sucrose (24–70%)[16,19,20,26,27] versus water significantly reduced pain responses and pain scores. The time spent crying during the procedure was significantly reduced (by 30 seconds) and the total duration of crying was significantly reduced (by 39 seconds).[16,20] Four RCTs[21,24,25,27] (213 term neonates) found that sucrose (12–70%)[25,27] versus water significantly reduced pain responses. Eight RCTs (525 term neonates) compared sucrose versus water.[15,17,18,21-25] Seven of the RCTs found significantly reduced crying time (mean differences 16–90 seconds).[15,18,23] In one RCT, a significant difference was found only for neonates given 50% sucrose, and not for those given lower concentrations.[18] Another RCT found significantly shorter crying with infants given sucrose and carried compared with infants given sucrose and not carried or compared with infants carried but not given sucrose.[17] One RCT used a low concentration of sucrose (2 ml of 7.5%) and found no significant difference in duration of crying.[22] **Glucose for heel puncture:** We found three systematic reviews (search dates 1995,[12] 1997,[13] and 1998;[14] 3 RCTs[15,21,28]) and two additional

RCTs.[9,29] The five RCTs included term infants. One RCT included an unknown number of preterm infants over 30 weeks' gestation with a mean gestation of 35.5 weeks.[28] A total of 330 neonates were given 1–2 ml of glucose or hydrogenated glucose[21] versus water prior to heel puncture. Two RCTs found significant reduction of pain responses with glucose versus water.[9,21,29] Three RCTs found significantly briefer crying in infants given 30–35% glucose versus water (mean differences 28 seconds,[28] 50 seconds,[21] and 107 seconds[9]). Three RCTs found significantly reduced pain responses after 30–35% glucose versus water.[9,21] One RCT (85 infants) found no significant change in crying time for infants given 12% glucose versus water (mean crying time 60 seconds with water v 56 seconds with glucose).[15] **Sucrose for venepuncture:** We found two systematic reviews (search dates 1995,[12] 1997,[13] 1 RCT,[30] 28 preterm neonates) and one additional RCT (term neonates),[31] which compared sucrose with water in neonates having venepuncture. Mean crying time was reduced in eight preterm neonates given 2 ml of 24% sucrose (mean duration of crying 19 seconds) compared with 12 neonates given water (73 seconds), but was not reduced in eight neonates given 12% sucrose (63 seconds).[30] The other RCT (75 term infants) found significantly reduced pain responses with sucrose versus water or no treatment.[31] **Glucose for venepuncture:** We found two RCTs, which compared 2 ml of 30% glucose with water in term infants undergoing venepuncture.[9,31] One RCT (60 infants) found significantly reduced pain scores but no difference in the proportion of infants crying (46% with glucose v 39% with water).[9] The other RCT (75 infants) found significantly reduced median pain scores with glucose versus water or no treatment.[31] **Concentration of glucose or sucrose:** We found one systematic review (search date 1998,[14] 1 RCT) and four additional RCTs[15,18,21,31] of the effects of glucose or sucrose concentration in heel puncture. We found no studies of the effects of glucose or sucrose concentration in venepuncture. Three RCTs in term neonates compared different concentrations of sucrose during heel puncture.[15,18,21] One RCT (75 neonates) found that increasing concentrations of sucrose (2 ml of 12.5%, 25%, and 50%) produced significantly greater reductions in the duration of crying.[18] The other two trials found no difference in crying duration with different sucrose concentrations (56 infants in all, given 2 ml of 25–50% or 12–25% sucrose).[15,21] Two RCTs compared different concentrations of glucose during heel puncture.[28,31] One RCT (60 term and preterm infants) compared 1 ml of 10% versus 1 ml of 30% glucose; it found no significant difference in the duration of crying or the proportion of babies who cried at all (no crying in 40% with dilute glucose v 53% with more concentrated glucose, $P > 0.05$).[28] **Multiple doses:** We found one RCT (32 preterm neonates, mean gestation 31 weeks), which compared a single dose (0.05 ml) of 24% sucrose 2 minutes before heel puncture with three doses given 2 minutes prior, immediately before the procedure, and during the procedure.[26] Pain scores measured at five points during the procedure were significantly different only at the latest time. **Sucrose versus glucose:** We found one RCT (50 term infants undergoing venepuncture) comparing 30% sucrose with 30% glucose.[29] Median pain scores in the two groups were not significantly different. **Repeated doses for repeated blood sampling:** We found no RCTs.

Harms: No adverse effects from oral sucrose or glucose administered to full term or preterm infants have been reported in any of the RCTs. The safety of repeated oral administration of sucrose or glucose has not been adequately investigated. Theoretical adverse effects include hyperglycaemia and necrotising enterocolitis.

Comment: Some studies were crossover RCTs, which might produce biased estimates of the effect of sucrose if neonates become habituated to pain or if the washout period between interventions is too short.[16,20,27] Only some RCTs reported adequate allocation concealment.[9,16,17,19,24,26,29,31] Most had blinded measurement of at least some of the pain responses, particularly crying, on the basis of independent audio or video tape recordings. One RCT had no blinded outcome assessment.[20] We found inadequate evidence about the benefits or harms of repeated administration of sucrose or glucose for repeated blood sampling.

OPTION BREAST MILK

Two RCTs found no evidence that breast milk reduced pain or crying compared with water in neonates undergoing heel puncture.

Benefits: We found one systematic review (search date 1998,[14] 2 RCTs,[23,28] 126 preterm and term neonates undergoing heel puncture) comparing breast milk (1–2 ml) versus water. Neither RCT found a significant effect of breast milk on duration of crying[23,28] or proportion of infants not crying.[28]

Harms: None reported.

Comment: Concealment of allocation and whether pain responses were assessed blind to the intervention were not clearly stated in either study. We found no RCTs on the effects of breast milk during venepuncture.

OPTION TOPICAL ANAESTHETICS

Systematic reviews and additional RCTs found no evidence of reduced pain responses, particularly crying, in infants who received either lidocaine or lidocaine–prilocaine emulsion (EMLA) versus placebo prior to heel puncture or venepuncture. One small RCT found substantial benefit for amethocaine compared with placebo in preterm and term neonates during venepuncture.

Benefits: **Lidocaine or EMLA for heel puncture:** We found three systematic reviews (search dates 1996,[32] 1998,[14] 1998,[33] 5 RCTs)[34–38] and one additional RCT,[1] which compared lidocaine or EMLA with placebo in neonates undergoing heel puncture. Three RCTs included 186 preterm neonates[1,34,35] and three RCTs included 192 infants who were mainly term neonates.[36–38] The RCTs compared lidocaine analgesic ointment or EMLA versus placebo. Treatments were usually given 30–60 minutes before heel puncture, with the exception of one RCT that randomised infants to eight application times (10–120 minutes before heel puncture).[37] The five studies used different assessments of pain responses. No RCT found a significant difference in the pain score between lidocaine or EMLA versus placebo. One RCT found no significant difference with EMLA versus placebo in the proportion of infants who cried during the procedure (54/56 [96%] v 52/54 [96%]).[37] **EMLA for venepuncture:** We found two systematic reviews (search dates 1996,[32] 1998,[14] 2 RCTs)[39,40] and three additional RCTs,[41–43] which compared EMLA versus placebo in infants having venepuncture. One RCT[43] included 19 preterm neonates, and the other three RCTs[39–41] included 240 term neonates. Pain responses were reported in three RCTs[39,42,43] but they could not be pooled. In one RCT, pain scores for preterm neonates were not reduced by EMLA versus placebo (median difference 0, 95% CI –2.0 to +1.75).[43] One RCT (120 term infants) found a significant difference in pain score 15 seconds after puncture (P = 0.016) but not at 60 seconds.[39] Two RCTs (169 babies) reported the proportion of babies who cried at all during the procedure.[39,41] The difference between EMLA and placebo was not significant (pooled ARR –10%; 95% CI –24% to +4%). One RCT of term neonates reported that the duration of crying was greater with EMLA, but did not present any results.[40] **Amethocaine:** We found one RCT (40 neonates, median gestation 33 weeks) comparing amethocaine gel with placebo applied 1 hour before venepuncture.[44] Amethocaine significantly increased the proportion of infants with a low pain score (defined as less than 10 out of 25 points), which was assessed blind based on videotape recordings (16/19 [84%] with amethocaine v 6/20 [30%] with placebo; ARR 54%; NNT 2, 95% CI 1 to 4). The difference in the proportion of infants who cried at all was similar. **Topical anaesthetic versus sweet solutions:** We found no relevant RCTs. **Topical anaesthetic versus pacifiers:** We found no RCTs.

Harms: We found six RCTs (250 infants) that reported the absence of adverse reactions to EMLA, or to placebo, or no difference in minor, transient local reactions.[1,36–38,42,43] One cohort study (500 neonates) found unusual cutaneous effects in four neonates under 32 weeks gestation.[45] Methaemoglobinaemia can occur with the prilocaine constituent of EMLA. Levels of methaemoglobin over 25–30% can cause clinical symptoms.[46] We found one systematic review (search date not stated, 12 RCTs or cohort studies, > 355 neonates)[32] and two subsequent RCTs (167 neonates)[1,46] of EMLA for heel puncture, venepuncture, circumcision, or lumbar puncture. All but one of these studies found mean methaemoglobin levels less than 1.5% in groups given EMLA. The other RCT (47 preterm and term infants given EMLA) found that the highest mean methaemoglobin levels (2.3%, range 0.6–6.2%) occurred after 15 days of repeated doses of EMLA.[45] A systematic review found two case reports of neonates who were treated with oxygen at methaemoglobin levels of 12% and 16%.[32]

Comment: Some of the studies reported adequate allocation concealment.[36,37,39,43] Three RCTs used video taped recordings of pain responses to blind assessors to the intervention.[39,42,43] In the other RCTs, although placebo ointment was used, pain responses were assessed by observers at the time of the procedure, rather than by scoring of video film. Deduction of treatment allocation may not have been possible in all studies because of the smell and skin blanching caused by EMLA. One study excluded 25% of children who had high behaviour scores before puncture, and presented results only for selected subgroups.[42] Its findings may be difficult to generalise.

OPTION   PACIFIERS

Six RCTs found reduced pain responses in term and preterm infants given pacifiers (see glossary, p 285) compared with no treatment prior to heel puncture. One RCT found significant reduction in pain responses in term infants given a pacifier compared with water or no treatment during venepuncture. Two RCTs found that pacifier plus sucrose versus pacifier alone had no significant effect on pain responses.

Benefits:
: **Heel puncture:** We found two systematic reviews (search dates 1997,[13] 1998,[14] 1 RCT)[47] and five additional RCTs (409 infants of which 254 are preterm)[25,48–51] comparing pacifiers versus no treatment. Pacifiers were given 2–5 minutes before heel puncture. Three RCTs were crossover trials.[40,47,49] Four studies in preterm infants[47–50] reported some measure of behavioural response to pain but only one used a validated pain score.[47] All four RCTs found that pacifier versus no pacifier significantly reduced pain responses[47,49] or the percentage of time spent in a distressed, fussy, or awake state.[48,50] In the three RCTs in term infants, those given a pacifier cried for significantly less time[25,51] or spent less time in fussy or awake states.[50,51] However, reductions were not significant for all measures of pain: in one study, grimacing was not significantly reduced by the pacifier[25] and in another, the pain score was similar during the procedure but fell more quickly in babies given pacifiers.[49] **Venepuncture:** We found one RCT (75 term infants undergoing venepuncture) that compared pacifier versus no treatment or 2 ml of water orally.[30] It found a significant reduction in the pain score during the procedure (median difference in 10 point pain score was 5, P < 0.0001). **Pacifier plus sucrose versus pacifier plus water:** We found two RCTs.[30,47] One RCT (50 term neonates having venepuncture) compared 2 ml of 30% sucrose versus 2 ml of water from a pacifier.[30] The second RCT (crossover, 122 preterm neonates having heel puncture) compared a pacifier dipped in 24% sucrose versus dipped in water.[47] Neither RCT found significant differences in pain responses between the interventions.

Harms:
: No adverse effects were reported in any of these studies.

Comment:
: None of the studies explicitly defined the method of allocation to pacifier or no treatment. Two RCTs blinded assessors to the intervention by analysing audio tapes of crying during the procedure.[47,51] Measurement of pain responses on the basis of facial expressions could not be blinded to the pacifier intervention.

OPTION   SKIN TO SKIN CONTACT

One RCT found a significant reduction in crying in babies held skin to skin during heel puncture.

Benefits:
: We found no systematic review but found one RCT (30 term babies undergoing heel puncture) comparing holding the baby with skin to skin

Reducing pain during blood sampling in infants

contact versus being swaddled in a crib.[52] Crying and grimacing were significantly reduced in the babies held skin to skin (proportion crying during procedure 8% v 45%; ARR 37%; NNT 3, 95% CI 2 to 13).

Harms: None reported.

Comment: Assessment of crying was based on analysis of audiotape recordings and was blind to the intervention. Assessments based on facial expressions were not blind to the intervention.

OPTION   ROCKING

Two RCTs comparing rocking with no intervention in neonates undergoing heel puncture found limited evidence that rocking reduced pain.

Benefits: We found no systematic review but found two RCTs comparing rocking with no intervention.[19,51] One RCT (44 preterm infants, 25 to 34 weeks gestation)[19] compared 0.05 ml water given before heel puncture versus simulated rocking using a respirator attached to an air mattress. No significant differences were reported in facial expressions of pain. The other RCT (40 term neonates)[51] compared no intervention with being held vertically and rocked by the examiner; it found that rocking reduced the duration of crying during the procedure and the risk of persistent crying (crying persistently: 2/20 [10%] with rocking v 9/20 [45%] with no intervention; ARR 35%; NNT 3, 95% CI 2 to 10).

Harms: None reported.

Comment: The method of allocation to rocking or standard care was adequate in one study[19] and unclear in the other.[51] Both studies used blinded assessment of pain responses based on video[19] and audio-tape[51] recordings.

OPTION   POSITION, SWADDLING, AND PRIOR HANDLING

Four RCTs found limited evidence that pain responses were reduced by tucking the arms and legs into a midline flexed position during heel puncture, or by avoiding handling before heel puncture. RCTs found no evidence of benefit from positioning or swaddling.

Benefits: We found four RCTs comparing positioning, swaddling, or handling with no intervention.[47,53–55] One crossover RCT (122 preterm infants, 25–34 weeks gestation having heel puncture) compared prone position versus side or supine position. It found no difference in the mean pain score.[47] One RCT (crossover, 15 preterm neonates)[53] compared swaddling immediately after heel puncture versus standard care (no swaddling). No difference in facial expressions of pain or arousal state were detected. Another RCT (crossover, 30 preterm neonates, 25–35 weeks gestation)[54] compared facilitative tucking during and after heel puncture (defined as the gentle containment of arms and legs in a flexed, midline position) with no intervention. It found a significant reduction in the total crying time and time to quietening (mean cry duration 2.2 v 0.3 minutes, P < 0.001). The fourth RCT (48 mainly preterm infants, mean gestation 35 weeks) compared handling (as if being prepared for a lumbar puncture) with avoidance of handling for 10 minutes prior to heel puncture.[55] It found that prior handling increased facial expressions of pain, the proportion of time crying, and crying at all during the 2 minutes after heel puncture (21/21 [100%] handled babies cried v 21/27 [78%] non-handled babies; ARR 22%; NNT 5, 95% CI 3 to 17).

Harms: No adverse events were reported for any of these interventions.

Comment: None of the studies explicitly reported the method of allocation to the interventions and only the study comparing handling versus no handling[55] assessed pain responses blind to the intervention.

GLOSSARY

Pacifier A device with a teat that a baby sucks on for comfort. Some pacifiers can deliver a liquid to the baby. Also known as a "dummy", "soother", or "plug" in some countries.

REFERENCES

1. Stevens B, Johnston C, Taddio A, Jack A, Narciso J, Stremler R, et al. Management of pain from heel lance with lidocaine-prilocaine (EMLA) cream: is it safe and efficacious in preterm infants? *J Dev Behav Pediatr* 1999;20:216–221.
2. Johnston CC, Collinge JM, Henderson SJ, Anand KJ. A cross-sectional survey of pain and pharmacological analgesia in Canadian neonatal intensive care units. *Clin J Pain* 1997;13:308–312.
3. Porter FL, Anand KJS. Epidemiology of pain in neonates. *Res Clin Forum* 1998;20:9–18.
4. Anand K, Stevens BJ, McGrath PJ. *Pain in neonates*. Amsterdam: Elsevier Science BV, 2000.
5. Meehan RM. Heel sticks in neonates for capillary blood sampling. *Neonatal Netw* 1998;17:17–24.
6. Lilien LD, Harris VJ, Ramamurthy RS, Pildes RS. Neonatal osteomyelitis of the calcaneus: complications of heel puncture. *J Pediatr* 1976; 88:478–480.
7. Blumenfeld TA, Turi GK, Blanc WA. Recommended site and depth of newborn heel skin punctures based on anatomical measurements and histopathology. *Lancet* 1979;1:230–233.
8. Shah V, Ohlsson A. Venepuncture versus heel lance for blood sampling in term neonates. In: The Cochrane Library, Issue 3, 2000. Oxford: Update Software 2000. Search date 1999; primary sources Cochrane Library; Medline; Embase; and Cinahl.
9. Eriksson M, Gradin M, Schollin J. Oral glucose and venepuncture reduce blood sampling pain in newborns. *Early Hum Dev* 1999;55:211–218.
10. Larsson BA, Tannfeldt G, Lagercrantz H, Olsson GL. Venepuncture is more effective and less painful than heel lancing for blood tests in neonates. *Pediatrics* 1998;101:882–886.
11. Shah VS, Taddio A, Bennett S, Speidel BD. Neonatal pain response to heel stick vs venepuncture for routine blood sampling. *Arch Dis Child Fetal Neonatal Ed* 1997;77:F143–F144.
12. Stevens B, Taddio A, Ohlsson A, Einarson T. The efficacy of sucrose for relieving procedural pain in neonates: a systematic review and meta-analysis. *Acta Paediatr* 1997;86:837–842. Search date 1995; primary sources Medline; Embase; Reference Update; and hand searches of personal files, bibliographies, most recent neonatal and pain journals, and conference proceedings.
13. Stevens B, Ohlsson A. Sucrose for analgesia in newborn infants undergoing painful procedures. In: The Cochrane Library, Issue 3, 2000. Oxford: Update Software. Search date 1997; primary sources Medline; Embase; Reference Update; Cochrane Library; and hand searches of personal files, bibliographies, recent neonatal and pain journals, and conference proceedings.
14. Ohlsson A, Taddio A, Jadad AR, Stevens B. Evidence-based decision making, systematic reviews and the Cochrane collaboration: implications for neonatal analgesia. In: Anand K, Stevens B, McGrath PJ, eds. *Pain in Neonates*. Amsterdam: Elsevier Science BV, 2000:251–268. Search date August 1998; primary sources Medline; Cochrane Library; and hand searches of personal files and reference lists.
15. Abad Massanet F, Diaz Gomez NM, Domenech Martinez E, Robayna Curbelo M, Rico Sevillano J. Analgesic effect of oral sweet solution in newborns. *An Esp Pediatr* 1995;43:351–354.
16. Bucher HU, Moser T, von Siebenthal K, Keel M, Wolf M, Duc G. Sucrose reduces pain reaction to heel lancing in preterm infants: a placebo-controlled, randomized and masked study. *Pediatr Res* 1995;38:332–335.
17. Gormally SM, Barr RG, Young SN, Alhawaf R, Wersheim L. Combined sucrose and carrying reduces newborn pain response more than sucrose or carrying alone [abstract]. *Arch Pediatr Adolesc Med* 1996;150:47.
18. Haouari N, Wood C, Griffiths G, Levene M. The analgesic effect of sucrose in full term infants: a randomised controlled trial. *BMJ* 1995;310: 1498–1500.
19. Johnston CC, Stremler RL, Stevens BJ, Horton LJ. Effectiveness of oral sucrose and simulated rocking on pain response in preterm neonates. *Pain* 1997;72:193–199.
20. Ramenghi LA, Wood CM, Griffith GC, Levene MI. Reduction of pain response in premature infants using intraoral sucrose. *Arch Dis Child Fetal Neonatal Ed* 1996;74:F126–F128.
21. Ramenghi LA, Griffith GC, Wood CM, Levene MI. Effect of non-sucrose sweet tasting solution on neonatal heel prick responses. *Arch Dis Child Fetal Neonatal Ed* 1996;74:F129–F131.
22. Rushforth JA, Levene MI. Effect of sucrose on crying in response to heel stab. *Arch Dis Child* 1993;69:388–389.
23. Ors R, Ozek E, Baysoy G, et al. Comparison of sucrose and human milk on pain response in newborns. *Eur J Pediatr* 1999;158:63–66.
24. Overgaard C, Knudsen A. Pain-relieving effect of sucrose in newborns during heel prick. *Biol Neonate* 1999;75:279–284.

25. Blass EM, Watt LB. Suckling- and sucrose-induced analgesia in human newborns. Pain 1999;83: 611–623.

26. Johnston CC, Stremler R, Horton L, Friedman A. Effect of repeated doses of sucrose during heel stick procedure in preterm neonates. Biol Neonate 1999;75:160–166.

27. Mellah D, Gourrier E, Merbouche S, Mouchnino G, Crumiere C, Leraillez J. Analgesia with saccharose during heel capillary prick. A randomized study in 37 newborns of over 33 weeks of amenorrhea. Arch Pediatr 1999;6:610–616.

28. Skogsdal Y, Eriksson M, Schollin J. Analgesia in newborns given oral glucose. Acta Paediatr 1997; 86:217–220.

29. Guala A, Giroletti G. Glucose as an analgesic in neonatology [in Italian]. A blind randomized controlled study. (Italian). Pediatr Med Chir 1998; 20:201–203.

30. Abad F, Diaz NM, Domenech E, Robayna M, Rico J. Oral sweet solution reduces pain-related behaviour in preterm infants. Acta Paediatr 1996; 85:854–858.

31. Carbajal R, Chauvet X, Couderc S, Olivier-Martin M. Randomised trial of analgesic effects of sucrose, glucose, and pacifiers in term neonates. BMJ 1999;319:1393–1397.

32. Taddio A, Ohlsson A, Einarson TR, Stevens B, Koren G. A systematic review of lidocaine-prilocaine cream (EMLA) in the treatment of acute pain in neonates. Pediatrics 1998;101:E1. Search date not stated; primary sources Medline; Embase; Reference Update; and hand searches of personal files and meeting proceedings.

33. Essink-Tjebbes CM, Hekster YA, Liem KD, Van Dongen RTM. Topical use of local anesthetics in neonates. Pharm World Sci 1999;21:173–176. Search date 1998; primary source Medline.

34. Ramaioli F, Amice De D, Guzinska K, Ceriana P, Gasparoni A. EMLA cream and the premature infant. Int Monitor Reg Anaesthesia 1993;59.

35. Stevens B, Johnston C, Taddio A, Koren G, Aranda J. The safety and efficacy of EMLA for heel lance in premature neonates. International Association for the Study of Pain, 8th World Congress on Pain, Vancouver, Canada 1996;239:181–182.

36. Rushforth JA, Griffiths G, Thorpe H, Levene MI. Can topical lignocaine reduce behavioural response to heel prick? Arch Dis Child Fetal Neonatal Ed 1995;72:F49–F51.

37. Larsson BA, Jylli L, Lagercrantz H, Olsson GL. Does a local anaesthetic cream (EMLA) alleviate pain from heel-lancing in neonates? Acta Anaesthesiol Scand 1995;39:1028–1031.

38. Wester U. Analgesic effect of lidocaine ointment on intact skin in neonates. Acta Paediatr 1993; 82:791.

39. Larsson BA, Tannfeldt G, Lagercrantz H, Olsson GL. Alleviation of the pain of venepuncture in neonates. Acta Paediatr 1998;87:774–779.

40. Lindh, V, Wiklund, U, Hakansson S. Does EMLA alleviate pain from venepuncture in neonates?

41. Lindh V, Wiklund U, Hakansson S. Assessment of the effect of EMLA during venipuncture in the newborn by analysis of heart rate variability. Pain 2000;86:247–254.

42. Robieux I, Kumar R, Radhakrishnan S, Koren G. Assessing pain and analgesia with a lidocaine-prilocaine emulsion in infants and toddlers during venipuncture. J Pediatr 1991;118:971–973.

43. Acharya AB, Bustani PC, Phillips JD, Taub NA, Beattie RM. Randomised controlled trial of eutectic mixture of local anaesthetics cream for venepuncture in healthy preterm infants. Arch Dis Child Fetal Neonatal Ed 1998;78:F138–F142.

44. Jain A, Rutter N. Does topical amethocaine gel reduce the pain of venepuncture in newborn infants? A randomised double blind controlled trial. Arch Dis Child Fetal Neonatal Ed 2000;83: F207–F210.

45. Gourrier E, Karoubi P, el Hanache A, Merbouche S, Mouchnino G, Leraillez J. Use of EMLA cream in a department of neonatology. Pain 1996;68:431–434.

46. Brisman M, Ljung BM, Otterbom I, Larsson LE, Andreasson SE. Methaemoglobin formation after the use of EMLA cream in term neonates. Acta Paediatr 1998;87:1191–1194.

47. Stevens B, Johnston C, Franck L, Petryshen P, Jack A, Foster G. The efficacy of developmentally sensitive interventions and sucrose for relieving procedural pain in very low birth weight neonates. Nurs Res 1999;48:35–43.

48. Corbo MG, Mansi G, Stagni A, et al. Nonnutritive sucking during heelstick procedures decreases behavioral distress in the newborn infant. Biol Neonate 2000;77:162–167.

49. Bo LK, Callaghan P. Soothing pain-elicited stress in Chinese newborns. Pediatrics 2000;105:E 49.

50. Field T, Goldson E. Pacifying effects of nonnutritive sucking on term and preterm neonates during heelstick procedures. Pediatrics 1984;74:1012–1015.

51. Campos RG. Rocking and pacifiers: two comforting interventions for heelstick pain. Res Nurs Health 1994;17:321–331.

52. Gray L, Watt L, Blass EM. Skin-to-skin contact is analgesic in healthy newborns. Pediatrics 2000; 105:e14.

53. Fearon I, Kisilevsky BS, Hains SMJ, Muir DW, Tranmer J. Swaddling after heel lance: age-specific effects on behavioural recovery in preterm infants. J Dev Behav Pediatr 1997;18:222–232.

54. Corff KE, Seideman R, Venkataraman PS, Lutes L, Yates B. Facilitated tucking: a nonpharmacologic comfort measure for pain in preterm neonates. J Obstet Gynecol Neonatal Nurs 1995;24:143–147.

55. Porter FL, Wolf CM, Miller JP. The effect of handling and immobilization on the response to acute pain in newborn infants. Pediatrics 1998; 102:1383–1389.

Ruth Gilbert
Senior Lecturer in Clinical Epidemiology/Honorary Consultant Paediatrician
Centre for Evidence-based Child Health, Institute of Child Health
London
UK

Linda Franck
Professor of Children's Nursing Research
King's College School of Nursing and Midwifery and Great Ormond Street Hospital for Children NHS Trust
London
UK

Competing interests: None declared.

Search date September 2000: expanded this issue

James Larcombe

QUESTIONS

INTERVENTIONS

PREVENTION

Likely to be beneficial

Unlikely to be beneficial

INVESTIGATION

Unlikely to be beneficial

TREATMENT

Beneficial

Likely to be beneficial

Unknown effectiveness

Key Messages

- Antibiotic treatment is accepted clinical practice in children with acute urinary tract infection (UTI), and placebo controlled trials are considered unethical.

- We found little evidence on the effects of delaying treatment while results of microscopy or culture are awaited. Five retrospective studies found that medium to long term delays (4 days to 7 years) in treatment may be associated with an increased risk of renal scarring, but we found inconclusive evidence that shorter delays cause harm.

- One systematic review of RCTs has found that antibiotic treatment for 7 days or longer is more effective than shorter courses.

- One RCT found no evidence of a difference between oral and intravenous antibiotics for acute treatment in children under the age of 2 years with an uncomplicated first UTI.

- We found no evidence of benefit from routine diagnostic imaging of all children with a first UTI. We found indirect evidence suggesting that children at increased risk of morbidity may benefit from investigation.

Urinary tract infection

- Two small RCTs found that prophylactic antibiotics prevented recurrent UTI in children, particularly during the period of prophylaxis. We found inadequate evaluation of the long term benefits of prophylaxis, even in children with vesicoureteric reflux. We found insufficient evidence to comment on the optimum duration of prophylaxis.

- One systematic review has found that, in premature and in low birthweight neonates, intravenous immunoglobulins reduce the occurrence of serious infections, including UTIs.

- One RCT has found that an immunotherapeutic agent, pidotomid, reduces UTI recurrence in children. Limited evidence suggests that other immunotherapeutic agents may be of benefit.

- One systematic review and a later RCT found no evidence of differences between surgical and medical management of vesicoureteric reflux in the prevention of recurrence of UTI or complications from UTI.

DEFINITION   UTI is defined by the presence of a pure growth of more than 10^5 colony forming units of bacteria per ml. Lower counts of bacteria may be clinically important, especially in boys and in specimens obtained by urinary catheter. Any growth of typical urinary pathogens is considered clinically important if obtained by suprapubic aspiration. In practice, three age ranges are usually considered on the basis of differential risk and different approaches to management: children under 1 year; young children (1–4, 5, or 7 years, depending on the information source); and older children (up to 12–16 years). Recurrent UTI is defined as a further infection by a new organism. Relapsing UTI is defined as a further infection with the same organism.

INCIDENCE/ PREVALENCE   Boys are more susceptible before the age of 3 months; thereafter the incidence is substantially higher in girls. Estimates of the true incidence of UTI depend on rates of diagnosis and investigation. At least 8% of girls and 2% of boys will have a UTI in childhood.[1]

AETIOLOGY/ RISK FACTORS   The normal urinary tract is sterile. Contamination by bowel flora may result in urinary infection if a virulent organism is involved or if the child is immunosuppressed. In neonates, infection may originate from other sources. *Escherichia coli* accounts for about three quarters of all pathogens. *Proteus* is more common in boys (about 30% of infections). Obstructive anomalies are found in 0–4% and vesicoureteric reflux in 8–40% of children being investigated for their first UTI.[2] Although vesicoureteric reflux is a major risk factor for adverse outcome, other as yet unidentified triggers may also need to be present.

PROGNOSIS   After first infection, about half of girls have a further infection in the first year and three quarters within 2 years.[3] We found no figures for boys, but a review suggests that recurrences are common under 1 year of age but rare subsequently.[4] Renal scarring occurs in 5–15% of children within 1–2 years of their first UTI, although 32–70% of these scars are noted at the time of initial assessment.[2] The incidence of renal scarring rises with each episode of infection in childhood.[5] An RCT comparing oral versus intravenous antibiotics found retrospectively that new renal scarring after a first UTI was more common in children with vesicoureteric reflux than in children without reflux (logistic regression model: AR of scarring 16/107

[15.0%] with reflux *v* 10/165 [6.1%] without reflux; RR 2.47, 95% CI 1.17 to 5.24).[6] An RCT of medical versus surgical management of severe vesicoureteric reflux found that younger children (under 2 years) were at greater risk of renal scarring than older children, measured by dimercaptosuccinic acid (DMSA) scintigraphy, regardless of treatment allocation (AR for deterioration in DMSA scan over 5 years 21/86 for younger children *v* 27/201 for older children; RR 1.82, 95% CI 1.09 to 3.03).[7] Renal scarring is associated with future complications: poor renal growth; recurrent adult pyelonephritis; impaired glomerular function; early hypertension; and end stage renal failure.[8–11] A combination of recurrent urinary infection, severe vesicoureteric reflux, and the presence of renal scarring at first presentation is associated with the worst prognosis.

AIMS	To relieve acute symptoms; to eliminate infection; and to prevent recurrence, renal damage, and long term complications.

OUTCOMES	**Short term:** clinical symptoms and signs (dysuria, frequency, fever); urine culture; incidence of new renal scars. **Long term:** incidence of recurrent infection; prevalence of renal scarring; renal size and growth; renal function; prevalence of hypertension and renal failure.

METHODS	*Clinical Evidence* update search and appraisal September 2000.

QUESTION   What are the effects of treatment of acute urinary tract infection in children?

Placebo controlled trials of antibiotics for symptomatic acute UTI in children are considered unethical. We found little evidence on the effects of giving early empirical treatment versus awaiting the results of microscopy or culture. Five retrospective studies found that delayed treatment may be associated with increased rates of renal scarring, but we found inconclusive evidence on the effects of shorter delays. One systematic review has found that antibiotic treatment for 7 days or longer is more effective than short courses.

Benefits: **Versus placebo:** We found no RCTs. **Immediate empirical versus delayed treatment:** We found no RCTs comparing immediate empirical treatment versus treatment delayed while microscopy or culture results are awaited. Five retrospective observational studies found increased rates of scarring in children in whom diagnosis was delayed between 4 days (in acute UTI) to 7 years (when a child presented with chronic non-specific symptoms).[2] We found one RCT that compared oral versus intravenous antibiotic treatment for UTI in children under 2 years (see below). It found no evidence that children treated 24 hours after the onset of fever were at greater risk of renal scarring than children presenting within 24 hours (9/99 [9%] children presenting before 24 hours developed scarring *v* 19/159 [12%] children presenting later; RR 1.3, 95% CI 0.6 to 2.7; P = 0.29). However, this incidental analysis was done retrospectively.[6] **Long versus short courses:** We found one systematic review (search date not stated, 14 RCTs) comparing short course (single dose to 4 days) versus longer courses (7–10 days).[12] It found two RCTs that were adequately powered to find an effect; both found that short courses were less effective than conventional

Urinary tract infection

treatment (results from the higher quality RCT: AR of failure to cure 14/38 [37%] with short course v 2/27 [8%] with long course; ARI short v long course 29%; RR 4.6, no 95% CI given; P < 0.01). The remaining 12 RCTs found no significant difference between long versus short courses but were too small to rule out a clinically important difference (see comment below). We found no RCTs comparing 5 day courses of antibiotics with other regimens. **Oral versus intravenous antibiotics:** We found one RCT (309 children, age ≤2 years, fever > 38.2 °C, first UTI confirmed from catheter specimen), which compared oral cefixime for 14 days versus intravenous cefotaxime for 3 days plus 11 days of oral cefixime.[6] It found no significant difference between treatments in mean duration of fever (24.7 hours with oral treatment v 23.9 hours with intravenous; P = 0.76), reinfection rate (132/153 [86.3%] with oral treatment v 134/153 [87.6%] with intravenous treatment; P = 0.28), incidence of renal scarring (intention to treat analysis: 15/153 [9.8%] with oral treatment [21 children not scanned and counted as having no scarring] v 11/153 [7.2%] with intravenous treatment [13 children not scanned]; P = 0.21), and mean extent of scarring (7.9% of renal parenchyma with oral treatment v 8.6% with intravenous treatment).

Harms:

Long versus short courses: The studies did not report comparative harms for long versus short courses of antibiotics nor for immediate versus delayed treatment. **Oral versus intravenous antibiotics:** We found weak evidence from a post-hoc subgroup analysis in children with grade III to IV reflux (see glossary, p 294) that renal scarring at 6 months may be more common with oral versus intravenous treatment (new renal scarring within 6 months: 8/24 [33%] after oral antibiotics v 1/22 [4.5%] after intravenous antibiotics; ARI 29%, 95% CI 8% to 49%; NNH 3, 95% CI 2 to 13).[6]

Comment:

Versus placebo: Placebo controlled trials would be considered unethical because there is a strong consensus that antibiotics are likely to be beneficial. The improved response seen with longer versus shorter courses of antibiotics is indirect evidence that antibiotics are likely to be more effective than no treatment. **Long versus short courses:** The systematic review comparing long versus short courses of antibiotics rigorously evaluated the methods of the included studies. It found that few studies accounted for confounding factors such as age, sex, and previous UTI. Those that considered these did so by selecting one subgroup only and not by stratifying children according to these factors. This limits the generalisability of the results. The 12 trials that found no evidence of a difference between long and short courses were too small to exclude a clinically important effect. **Oral versus intravenous antibiotics:** The trial comparing oral versus intravenous antibiotics excluded three of 309 children because investigators considered that the severity of symptoms in these children warranted intravenous treatment.[6]

QUESTION Which children benefit from diagnostic imaging?

We found no evidence of benefit from routine diagnostic imaging of all children with a first UTI. We found indirect evidence suggesting that subgroups at increased risk of morbidity may benefit from investigation.

Benefits: We found no RCTs. One systematic review (search date 1994, 63 descriptive studies) found no direct evidence that routine diagnostic imaging in children with UTI was effective.[2] The quality of studies was generally poor, and none included clinically important long term outcome measures.

Harms: The studies reported no evidence on harms. Potential harms include those relating to radiation, invasive procedures, and allergic reactions to contrast media.

Comment: Subgroups of children at high risk of morbidity, including those with vesicoureteric reflux, may benefit from early investigation.[2] However, it may be difficult to identify such children clinically.[13] One prospective study found that the highest rates of renal scarring after pyelonephritis occurred between 1 and 5 years of age.[14] A further study found that presentation with pyelonephritic symptoms in children of all ages is associated with high rates of renal abnormalities (abnormal initial scans in 34/65 [52%] children).[15]

QUESTION What are the effects of preventive interventions?

OPTION PROPHYLACTIC ANTIBIOTICS

We found limited evidence from two small RCTs that prophylactic antibiotics reduce UTI recurrence in children, particularly during the period of prophylaxis. We found inadequate evaluation of the long term benefits of prophylaxis, even in children with vesicoureteric reflux. We found insufficient evidence to comment on the optimum duration of prophylaxis.

Benefits: **Versus no prophylaxis:** We found one systematic review,[16] which compared antibiotics versus no antibiotics to prevent UTIs (search date 1999, 2 RCTs[17,3] of 40 children without a neurogenic bladder — see glossary, p 294). The first RCT (double blind, crossover trial, 18 girls [1 with vesicoureteric reflux] age 3–13 years) found fewer episodes of infection while taking antibiotics than while not taking antibiotics (2 episodes in 1 year with antibiotics v 35 without antibiotics; $P < 0.01$).[17] The second RCT (40 girls and 5 boys, first or subsequent acute UTI, radiologically normal urinary tracts, no vesicoureteric reflux) compared 10 months' treatment with prophylactic antibiotics versus no treatment.[3] During the prophylaxis period, recurrent UTIs were less frequent in the intervention group (AR 0/25 [0%] with antibiotics v 11/22 [50%] with control; ARR 50%, 95% CI 26% to 74%). Twelve months after stopping prophylactic antibiotics, fewer children from the intervention group had experienced a UTI compared with those in the control group (AR 32% v 64%; ARR +27%, 95% CI −1.8% to +47%). **Duration of prophylaxis:** We found no RCTs evaluating the optimum length of prophylaxis even in children with vesicoureteric reflux (although two studies of prolonged acute treatment were identified).[18]

Harms: Potential harms include those of using long term antibiotics. In one study, although gut flora were affected by treatment, E coli cultured from rectal swabs from 70% of children remained sensitive to the prophylactic antibiotic (co-trimoxazole).[19]

Comment: The systematic review[16] was thorough, but both RCTs that it identified had weak methods. One was a crossover study that did not include a washout period, and did not report separately the results for the period before the crossover.[17] The other RCT was not blinded, the control group received no treatment, and no criteria were given for the diagnosis of a UTI.[3] It may not be possible clinically to identify children who are at high risk of recurrent UTIs and long term damage.[20] Routine prophylaxis until the results of investigations are known may therefore be warranted, but we found no good evidence about the benefits or harms of antibiotic prophylaxis. The systematic review also found three other RCTs of antibiotic prophlaxis in children with a neurogenic bladder.[16]

| OPTION | IMMUNOTHERAPY | New |

One systematic review has found that, in premature and in low birthweight neonates, intravenous immunoglobulins reduce the occurrence of serious infections, including UTIs. One RCT has found that an immunotherapeutic agent, pidotomid, reduces UTI recurrence in children. Limited evidence suggests that other immunotherapeutic agents may be of benefit.

Benefits: **Intravenous immunoglobulin:** We found one systematic review (search date 1997, 15 RCTs), which compared intravenous immunoglobulin prophylaxis with placebo or no treatment. It found that immunoglobulin prophylaxis significantly reduced serious infections, including UTIs, in preterm and in low birth weight neonates (RR 0.80, 95% CI 0.68 to 0.94; NNT 24, 95% CI 15 to 83).[21] The dose varied from 120 mg/kg to 1 g/kg. The number of treatments varied from one to seven. The specific effect on UTIs was not reported. **Other immunotherapeutic agents:** We found one RCT (60 children with recurrent UTIs) comparing pidotomid versus placebo.[22] It found that pidotomid reduced recovery time (recovery time 9.6 days with pidotomid v 12.3 days with placebo) and recurrence rate for UTIs (RR recurrence 0.31). An open pilot study (40 children) compared nitrofurantoin with an antigenic extract of E coli.[23] No significant difference was found between the two treatments during active treatment or during the subsequent 6 months.

Harms: Parenteral treatment can cause pain, and there is an unquantified risk from the administration of blood products.[21] **Intravenous immunoglobulin:** Prophylactic use of intravenous immunoglobulin was not associated with any short term serious adverse effects.[21] **Other immunotherapeutic agents:** In the trial of pidotomid, the only adverse effects recorded were thought to be attributable to concomitant antibiotic therapy.[22] The open pilot study found no significant difference in withdrawal rates between the antigenic extract of E coli (1/22) and nitrofurantoin (1/18).[23]

Comment: **Intravenous immunoglobulin:** We found no evidence for or against the suggestion that preparations with specific antibodies against common pathogens are more beneficial.[24] The greatest benefits were noted in units with higher nosocomial infection rates (see glossary, p 294). It remains unclear whether intravenous immunoglobulin is only justified where infection control policies have failed to reduce the infection rate.[21] Preterm and low birth weight neonates might have greater immune deficiency than other neonates and might be expected to gain more from treatment with immunoglobulin. **Other immunotherapeutic agents:** The pidotomid study is being translated and more detail may be available in future issues of Clinical Evidence.[22] We also found one non-randomised age matched study in 10 otherwise healthy girls with recurrent UTI who were given intramuscular extracts of five uropathogenic bacteria. The girls who were injected had significantly reduced frequency of subsequent UTI who compared with 10 other age matched girls with UTI.[25] This study is limited by its non-randomised design and low sample size.

OPTION **SURGICAL CORRECTION FOR ANOMALIES OBSTRUCTING MICTURITION**

We found no good studies evaluating surgical correction.

Benefits: We found no systematic review or RCTs.

Harms: Potential harms include the usual risks of surgery.

Comment: One small prospective study (271 children) suggested that children with minor anomalies do not develop renal scarring and may therefore not benefit from surgery.[26] Renal scars were present in more children with moderate degrees of vesicoureteric reflux than in children with minor anomalies (8/20 [40%] v 0/6 [0%]). In the presence of major anomalies, the prevention of UTIs is not the prime motive of surgical intervention.

OPTION **SURGICAL CORRECTION FOR VESICOURETERIC REFLUX**

One systematic review and a later multicentre RCT found that, although surgery abolished reflux, there was no evidence of a difference between surgery and medical management in the prevention of recurrence or complications from UTIs. We found no evidence on the long term effects of surgical versus medical treatment for clinical outcomes.

Benefits: We found one systematic review[27] and one subsequent RCT.[28] The systematic review (search date 1988, 4 RCTs, 830 children with moderate/severe grade III–V vesicoureteric reflux) compared surgical correction versus medical management (continuous prophylactic antibiotics).[27] It found that surgery abolished reflux, but found no significant differences in rates of subsequent UTIs, renal function, incidence of new renal scars, hypertension, or end stage renal failure among groups over a period of 6 months to 5 years. The subsequent RCT (132 children) found that surgery reduced the incidence of pyelonephritis (pyelonephritis in 5/64 [8%] with surgery v 15/68 [22%] treated medically; ARR 14%, 95% CI 2% to 19%; RRR 65%, 95% CI 10% to 87%), although it found no significant difference in overall clinical outcome.[28] **Long term outcome:** We found no systematic review or RCTs.

Harms: The review gave no information on surgical complications, and none of the individual studies were designed to compare rates of adverse effects.[27] In one arm of the subsequent RCT, seven of nine children who had postoperative obstruction developed evidence of renal scarring on DMSA scintigraphy. This may have negated an otherwise beneficial effect of surgery over medical management.[7]

Comment: Best results were obtained by centres handling the greatest number of children.[29] Surgery is usually considered only in children with more severe vesicoureteric reflux (grade III–V), who are less likely to experience spontaneous resolution.[4,30] **Long term outcome:** We found one prospective cohort study in 226 children aged 5 days to 12 years who presented with UTI and were found to have grade III–IV vesicoureteric reflux.[8] It found that surgery was associated with a higher rate of resolution of reflux compared with medical treatment (AR of resolution from age 8–14 years on micturating cystoure-throgrophy: 29/33 [88%] with surgery v 134/193 [69%] treated medically; ARI 19%, 95% CI 6% to 31%) but did not compare clinical outcomes.

GLOSSARY

Neurogenic bladder Loss of normal bladder function from damage to the nervous system (causing dysfunction of the nerves to and from the bladder or sphincters).

Nosocomial infection Definitions vary but typically an infection arising at least 48–72 hours after admission to hospital. The infection may have been acquired from other patients, hospital staff, the hospital environment, or from within the person themselves.

Severity of vesicoureteric reflux:

Grade I Reflux into ureter only.

Grade II Reflux into ureter, pelvis, and calyces.

Grade III Mild/moderate dilatation or tortuosity of ureter, and mild/moderate dilatation of pelvis, but little or no forniceal blunting.

Grade IV As grade III, but with complete obliteration of forniceal angles, yet maintenance of papillary impressions in calyces.

Grade V Gross dilatation of ureters, pelvis, and calyces, and papillary impressions in calyces obliterated.

Substantive changes since last issue

Prophylactic antibiotics New systematic review;[16] conclusions unaltered.

REFERENCES

1. Stark H. Urinary tract infections in girls: the cost-effectiveness of currently recommended investigative routines. *Pediatr Nephrol* 1997;11: 174–177.
2. Dick PT, Feldman W. Routine diagnostic imaging for childhood urinary tract infections: a systematic overview. *J Pediatr* 1996;128:15–22. Search date 1994; primary sources Medline, hand searches of article bibliographies, and Current Contents.
3. Smellie JM, Katz G, Gruneberg RN. Controlled trial of prophylactic treatment in childhood urinary tract infection. *Lancet* 1978;ii:175–178.
4. Jodal U, Hansson S, Hjalmas K. Medical or surgical management for children with vesico-

ureteric reflux? *Acta Paediatr Suppl* 1999;431: 53–61.
5. Jodal U. The natural history of bacteriuria in childhood. *Infect Dis Clin North Am* 1987;1:713–729.
6. Hoberman A, Wald ER, Hickey RW, et al. Oral versus initial intravenous therapy for urinary tract infections in young febrile children. *Pediatrics* 1999;104:79–86.
7. Piepsz A, Tamminen-Mobius T, Reiners C, et al. Five-year study of medical and surgical treatment in children with severe vesico-ureteric reflux dimercaptosuccinic acid findings. International

Reflux Study Group in Europe. *Eur J Pediatr* 1998; 157:753–758.

8. Smellie JM, Prescod NP, Shaw PJ, Risdon RA, Bryant TN. Childhood reflux and urinary infection: a follow-up of 10–41 years in 226 adults. *Pediatr Nephrol* 1998;12:727–736.

9. Berg UB. Long-term follow-up of renal morphology and function in children with recurrent pyelonephritis. *J Urol* 1992;148:1715–1720.

10. Martinell J, Claeson I, Lidin-Janson G, Jodal U. Urinary infection, reflux and renal scarring in females continuously followed for 13–38 years. *Pediatr Nephrol* 1995;9:131–136.

11. Jacobson S, Eklof O, Erikkson CG, Lins LE, Tidgren B. Development of hypertension and uraemia after pyelonephritis in childhood: 27 year follow up. *BMJ* 1989;299:703–706.

12. Moffatt M, Embree J, Grimm P, Law B. Short-course antibiotic therapy for urinary tract infections in children: a methodological review of the literature. *Am J Dis Child* 1988;142:57–61. No search date or primary sources given.

13. Smellie JM, Normand ICS, Katz G. Children with urinary infection: a comparison of those with and those without vesicoureteral reflux. *Kidney Int* 1981;20:717–722.

14. Benador D, Benador N, Slozman D, Mermillod B, Girardin E. Are younger patients at higher risk of renal sequelae after pyelonephritis? *Lancet* 1997; 349:17–19.

15. Rosenberg AR, Rossleigh MA, Brydon MP, Bass SJ, Leighton DM, Farnsworth RH. Evaluation of acute urinary tract infection in children by dimercaptosuccinic acid scintography: a prospective study. *J Urol* 1992;148:1746–1749.

16. Le Saux N, Pham B, Moher D. Evaluating the benefits of antimicrobial prophylaxis to prevent urinary tract infections in children: a systematic review. *Can Med Assoc J* 2000;163:523–529 Search date 1999; primary sources Medline, Embase, Cochrane Library, textbooks, conference proceedings, experts; http://www.cma.ca/cmaj/vol-163/issue-5/0523.htm (last accessed 31 March 2001).

17. Lohr JA, Nunley DH, Howards SS, Ford RF. Prevention of recurrent urinary tract infections in girls. *Pediatrics* 1977;59:562–565.

18. Garin EH, Campos A, Homsy Y. Primary vesico-ureteral reflux: a review of current concepts. *Pediatr Nephrol* 1998;12:249–256.

19. Smellie JM, Gruneberg RN, Leakey A, Atkin WS. Long term low dose co-trimoxazole in prophylaxis of childhood urinary tract infection: clinical aspects/bacteriological aspects. *BMJ* 1976;2: 203–208.

20. Greenfield SP, Ng M, Gran J. Experience with vesicoureteric reflux in children: clinical characteristics. *J Urol* 1997;158:574–577.

21. Ohlsson A, Lacy JB. Intravenous immunoglobulin for preventing infection in pre-term and/or low-birth-weight infants. In: The Cochrane Library, Issue 3, 2000. Oxford: Update Software. Search date 1997; primary sources Medline, Embase, Cochrane Library, Reference Update, Science Citation Index, and hand searches of reference lists of identified RCTs and personal files.

22. Clemente E, Solli R, Mei V, et al. Therapeutic efficacy and safety of pidotomid in the treatment of urinary tract infections in children. *Arzneim Forsh* 1994;44:1490–1494.

23. Lettgen B. Prevention of urinary tract infections in female children. *Curr Ther Res* 1996;57:464–475.

24. Weisman LE, Cruess DF, Fischer GW. Opsonic activity of commercially available standard intravenous immunoglobulin preparations. *Paediatr Inf Dis J* 1994;13:1122–1125.

25. Nayir A, Emre S, Sirin A, Bulut A, Alpay H, Tanman F. The effects of vaccination with inactivated uropathogenic bacteria in recurrent urinary tract infections of children. *Vaccine* 1995;13:987–990.

26. Pylkannen J, Vilska J, Koskimies O. The value of childhood urinary tract infection in predicting renal injury. *Acta Paediatr Scand* 1981;70:879–883.

27. Shanon A, Feldman W. Methodological limitations in the literature on vesicoureteric reflux: a critical review. *J Pediatr* 1990;117:171–178. Search date 1988; primary source Medline.

28. Weiss R, Duckett J, Spitzer A. Results of a randomized clinical trial of medical versus surgical management of infants and children with grades III and IV primary vesico-ureteral reflux (United States): the international reflux study in children. *J Urol* 1992;148:1667–1673.

29. Smellie JM. Commentary: management of children with severe vesicoureteral reflux. *J Urol* 1992;148:1676–1678.

30. Sciagra R, Materassi M, Rossi V, et al. Alternative approaches to the prognostic stratification of mild to moderate primary vesicoureteral reflux in children. *J Urol* 1996;155:2052–2056.

James Larcombe
General Practitioner
Sedgefield
UK

Competing interests: None declared.

Colonic diverticular disease

Search date July 2000: new for this issue

John Simpson and Robin Spiller

INTERVENTIONS

Likely to be beneficial

Unknown effectiveness

**To be covered in future issues of
*Clinical Evidence***

Elective surgery for diverticular
disease
Antispasmodics in the treatment of
diverticular disease
Mesalazine in the treatment of
diverticular disease

Key Messages

- Two RCTs found no consistent effect of dietary fibre supplements in uncomplicated diverticular disease.
- One small RCT found limited evidence that rifaximin (an antibiotic) is effective in uncomplicated diverticular disease.
- We found no evidence that lactulose or methylcellulose is effective in uncomplicated diverticular disease.
- We found no RCT comparing medical or surgical management of acute diverticulitis versus placebo.
- We found no RCT comparing medical versus surgical management of acute diverticulitis.
- One comparative RCT and observational studies of medical treatment for acute uncomplicated diverticulitis have found high clinical cure rates, with low mortality, but a 7–28% risk of recurrent acute attacks. The RCT found no significant difference between two antibiotic regimens.
- One RCT of acute resection versus no acute resection for acute diverticulitis with diffuse peritonitis found no significant difference in mortality or adverse effects of surgery.

DEFINITION Diverticula of the colon are mucosal herniations through the large bowel wall. They are often accompanied by structural changes (elastosis of the taenia coli, muscular thickening, and mucosal folding). They are usually multiple and occur most frequently in the sigmoid colon. We found some variation among information sources in the terminology used to describe different forms and severities of illness caused by diverticula. In this review the term **diverticulosis** is used to describe diverticula that are asymptomatic. Most people with colonic diverticula have no symptoms. **Diverticular disease** is used to describe diverticula associated with any symptoms.[1] The symptoms commonly include abdominal pain and alteration in bowel habit. Diverticular disease may be complicated by abscess formation, fistulae, perforation, obstruction, or haemorrhage. **Acute diverticulitis** is presumed to occur when a diverticulum becomes acutely inflamed: there may be general symptoms and signs of infection (including fever and rapid heart rate) with local symptoms and signs (pain and localised tenderness, usually in the lower left abdomen, sometimes with a mass that can be felt through the abdomen on rectal examination).

INCIDENCE/ PREVALENCE In the UK, the incidence of diverticulosis increases with age: about 5% of people are affected in the fifth decade of life and about 50% in the ninth decade.[2]

AETIOLOGY/ RISK FACTORS Diverticulosis is common in western developed countries but is almost unknown in rural Africa and Asia. There is an association between diets low in fibre and diverticulosis of the colon.[3] There is a lower prevalence of diverticulosis in western vegetarians consuming a high roughage diet.[4] Prospective observational studies have found that physical activity[5] and a high fibre diet[6] are associated with lower risk of diverticular disease. One case control study found an association between the ingestion of non-steroidal anti-inflammatory drugs and the development of severe complications, including pericolic abscess, generalised peritonitis, bleeding, and fistula formation.[7] People in Japan, Singapore, and Thailand develop diverticula that affect predominantly the right side of the colon.[8]

PROGNOSIS Most people with diverticula remain asymptomatic. It is unclear why some people develop symptoms and some do not. Symptoms will develop at some point during their life in 10–25% of people with diverticula.[2] Even after successful medical treatment of diverticulitis, almost two thirds of people suffer recurrent pain in the lower abdomen.[9] Recurrent diverticulitis is observed in 7–35% of people and once recovered from the initial attack, the calculated yearly risk of suffering a further bout is 3%.[10] About half the recurrences occur within the first year and 90% within 5 years.[11] Complications of diverticular disease (perforation, obstruction, haemorrhage, and fistula formation) are each seen in 5% of people with diverticula when followed up for between 10 and 30 years.[12] Intra-abdominal abscess formation can occur.

AIMS To reduce mortality, symptoms and complications, with minimal adverse effects.

OUTCOMES   Subjective gastrointestinal symptoms by use of validated question-naires. Stool weight and transit time are surrogate outcomes. Admission and re-admission rates as a result of diverticular disease and its complications. Incidence of diverticulitis, haemorrhage, perforation, abscess and fistula formation, and mortality.

METHODS   *Clinical Evidence* search and appraisal July 2000.

QUESTION   **What are the effects of treatments for uncomplicated diverticular disease?**

OPTION   **BRAN AND ISPAGHULA**

Two RCTs found no consistent effect of bran or ispaghula versus placebo on symptom relief in uncomplicated diverticular disease.

Benefits: **Versus placebo:** We found no systematic review but found two RCTs of fibre supplements compared with placebo for uncompli-cated diverticular disease.[13,14] The first RCT (58 people with no other gastrointestinal disorders, no abdominal operations, and no complicated diverticular disease) was a crossover double blind RCT that compared bran crispbread (6.99 g/day fibre) versus ispaghula drink (9.04 g/day fibre) versus placebo (2.34 g/day fibre) over three periods, each of 4 months.[13] It found no significant differences between the three groups in pain score, lower bowel symptom score (combination of the pain score and sensation of incomplete emp-tying, straining, stool consistency, flatus, and aperients taken), and total symptom score (including nausea, vomiting, dyspepsia, belch-ing, and abdominal distension). Both active treatments significantly improved straining of stool (versus placebo: bran $P < 0.01$; ispa-ghula $P < 0.001$), increased wet stool weight ($P < 0.001$ for both treatments), and stool frequency ($P < 0.001$), and significantly softened the stools ($P < 0.001$). The second RCT (18 people with radiologically confirmed diverticula and no other colonic disorder) compared bran crispbread (6.7 g/day fibre) versus placebo crisp-bread (0.6 g/day fibre) over 3 months.[14] It found that fibre versus placebo significantly improved the total symptom score ($P < 0.002$) and the pain score ($P < 0.02$), but found no significant difference in the scores for bowel dysfunction (passage of excessive wind per rectum, need to strain, frequency of evacuation, consistency of motion, presence of anal pain on defaecation, feeling of incomplete evacuation, presence of blood or mucus, use of laxatives) or dyspeptic symptoms (nausea, vomiting, heartburn, belching, and abdominal distension).

Harms: No significant adverse effects were reported in the RCTs.[13,14]

Comment: Participants in the RCTs had been investigated to exclude co-existing abdominal pathology, but the extent of the investigations was not stated. Both studies were brief, small, and the difference in fibre content between control and treatment interventions was small. Both treatment and control groups improved during the RCTs.

One brief and small RCT found that methylcellulose versus placebo produced no significant clinical improvement in people with uncomplicated diverticular disease.

Benefits: We found no systematic review but found one RCT. The double blind, crossover RCT (30 people with symptomatic diverticular disease and no other gastrointestinal disease) compared methylcellulose (500 mg twice daily) versus placebo over 3 months.[15] It found that methylcellulose versus placebo had no significant effect on a symptom score.

Harms: None reported.

Comment: Both the methylcellulose and placebo groups improved during the RCT.[15] The RCT was brief and small. Diverticular disease was confirmed by barium enema, but the extent of any other investigations to exclude comorbidity was not stated. The score used to assess symptoms and signs was not clearly described, but included barium enema results.

We found no adequate evidence about the effects of lactulose versus placebo in uncomplicated diverticular disease.

Benefits: We found no systematic review. **Versus placebo:** We found no RCTs. **Versus high fibre diet:** We found one RCT (43 people with diverticular disease and no other abdominal pathology) comparing lactulose (15 ml twice daily) versus a high fibre diet (30–40 g/day) over 12 weeks.[16] Both groups improved during the RCT but statistical comparison of the groups was not performed.

Harms: More people taking high fibre versus lactulose developed symptoms during the trial period (12 v 9).[16] These were described as minor, but no further details were given. Two people taking lactulose withdrew from the trial because of symptoms, one with abdominal pain and one with nausea.

Comment: Participants were investigated to exclude coexisting abdominal pathology, but the extent of the investigations was not stated.

One RCT found limited evidence that oral antibiotic treatment improved symptoms of uncomplicated diverticular disease.

Benefits: We found no systematic review but found one RCT.[17] The multicentre, double blind RCT (168 people with uncomplicated diverticular disease) compared fibre supplementation (glucomannan 2 g/day) plus either placebo or oral rifaximin (400 mg twice daily) for 7 days a month for 1 year.[17] It found that rifaximin versus placebo increased the number of people with no symptoms or only mild symptoms after 12 months (69% with rifaximin v 39% with placebo; $P = 0.001$), improved bloating ($P < 0.001$), lower abdominal pain

(P < 0.001), and abdominal tenderness (P < 0.05), but had no significant effect on diarrhoea, tenesmus, or upper abdominal pain.

Harms: None reported. Two people in each arm developed acute diverticulitis during the RCT.

Comment: None.

QUESTION   What are the effects of treatments for acute diverticulitis?

OPTION   MEDICAL TREATMENT

We found no RCTs of medical treatment versus placebo for acute uncomplicated diverticulitis. One comparative RCT and observational studies of acute uncomplicated diverticulitis have found low mortality and high rates of clinical cure with medical treatment, but a 7–28% risk of recurrent acute attacks.

Benefits: We found no systematic review. **Versus placebo:** We found no RCTs. **Versus other medical treatment:** We found one RCT (51 people with a clinical diagnosis of acute diverticulitis that did not need immediate surgery), which found no significant difference in the clinical cure rate with cefoxitin versus gentamicin plus clindamycin (27/30 [90%] with cefoxitin v 18/21 [86%] with gentamicin plus clindamycin; ARI +4.3%, 95% CI –14% to +22%).[18]

Harms: In the RCT,[18] toxicity, possibly antibiotic related, occurred in both groups (2/30 with cefoxitinin v 3/21 with gentamicin plus clindamycin, P = 0.37).

Comment: We found many observational studies[10,19–21] with variable follow up (1–12 years) of medical treatment for acute diverticulitis. They consistently report low mortality after medical treatment of acute diverticulitis (0–5%), but 7–28% suffer recurrent acute diverticulitis.

OPTION   SURGERY

One RCT found that, for people with acute diverticulitis of the left colon complicated by diffuse peritonitis, acute resection versus no acute resection (involving a transverse colostomy) had no significant effect on mortality. We found weak evidence from a subgroup analysis that, for people with purulent rather than faecal peritonitis, acute colonic resection might increase mortality.

Benefits: We found no systematic review. **Surgery versus placebo or medical treatment:** We found no RCTs. **Open surgery versus other types of open surgery:** We found one RCT (62 people with diffuse peritonitis from perforated acute diverticulitis of the left colon, median age 72 years), which compared acute resection (with end colostomy of the proximal bowel and, for the distal bowel, formation of a mucus fistula or oversewing of the rectal stump) versus no acute resection (acute transverse colostomy, suture, and omental covering of a visible perforation).[22] The RCT found that acute resection versus no resection had no significant effect on mortality within 30 days (8/31 [26%] with resection v 6/31 [19%]

with no acute resection; ARI with resection +6.5%, 95% CI −14% to +27%; P = 0.54). However, for people with purulent peritonitis, postoperative mortality was significantly higher with acute resection versus no acute resection (6/25 [24%] with acute resection v 0/21 [0%] without acute resection; ARI 24%, 95% CI 4.5% to 44%). For people with faecal peritonitis, acute resection versus no acute resection had no significant effect on mortality (2/6 [33%] with acute resection v 6/10 [60%] without acute resection; ARI −27%, 95% CI −77% to +24%). **Open surgery versus laparoscopic surgery:** We found no RCTs.

Harms: The RCT of acute resection versus no acute resection for acute diverticulitis complicated by diffuse peritonitis found that both forms of emergency surgery in elderly people had significant risks. It found similar rates of cardiopulmonary complications (13/31 with acute resection v 14/31 without acute resection), thromboembolism (3/31 v 5/31), mental confusion (4/31 v 4/31), wound dehiscence (3/31 v 3/31), wound infection but no dehiscence (2/31 v 4/31), intraperitoneal abscess (4/31 v 5/31), ileus (2/31 v 0/31), colo-cutaneous fistula (1/31 v 2/31), and revision of colostomy (1/31 v 2/31).

Comment: The RCT was conducted in a single centre and took 14 years to recruit 62 people. The high complication rates are not unexpected in predominantly elderly people following a perforation of the large bowel. The wide spectrum of presentation and operative treatment options for acute complicated diverticulitis makes RCTs difficult to perform.

QUESTION **What are the effects of a high fibre diet to prevent complications of diverticular disease?**

We found no systematic review and no RCTs.

Benefits: We found no systematic review and no RCTs of high fibre versus placebo to prevent complications in people with diverticular disease.

Harms: We found no evidence.

Comment: None.

REFERENCES

1. Kohler L, Sauerland S, Neugebauer E. Diagnosis and treatment of diverticular disease: results of a consensus development conference. The Scientific Committee of the European Association for Endoscopic Surgery. Surg Endosc 1999;13:430–436.

2. Parks TG. Natural history of diverticular disease of the colon. Clin Gastroenterol 1975;4:53–69.

3. Painter NS, Burkitt DP. Diverticular disease of the colon, a 20th century problem. Clin Gastroenterol 1975;4:3–21.

4. Gear JS, Ware A, Fursdon P, et al. Symptomless diverticular disease and intake of dietary fibre. Lancet 1979;1:511–514.

5. Aldoori WH, Giovannucci EL, Rimm EB, et al. Prospective study of physical activity and the risk of symptomatic diverticular disease in men. Gut 1995;36:276–282.

6. Aldoori WH, Giovannucci EL, Rimm EB, Wing AL, Trichopoulos DV, Willett WC. A prospective study of diet and the risk of symptomatic diverticular disease in men. Am J Clin Nutr 1994;60:757–764.

7. Campbell K, Steele RJ. Non-steroidal anti-inflammatory drugs and complicated diverticular disease: a case-control study. Br J Surg 1991;78:190–191.

8. Sugihara K, Muto T, Morioka Y, Asano A, Yamamoto T. Diverticular disease of the colon in Japan. A review of 615 cases. Dis Colon Rectum 1984;27:531–537.

9. Munson KD, Hensien MA, Jacob LN, Robinson AM, Liston WA. Diverticulitis. A comprehensive follow-up. Dis Colon Rectum 1996;39:318–322.

10. Haglund U, Hellberg R, Johnsen C, Hulten L. Complicated diverticular disease of the sigmoid

colon. An analysis of short and long term outcome in 392 patients. *Ann Chir Gynaecol* 1979;68:41–46.

11. Parks TG, Connell AM. The outcome in 455 patients admitted for treatment of diverticular disease of the colon. *Br J Surg* 1970;57:775–778.

12. Boles RS, Jordon SM. The clinical significance of diverticulosis. *Gastroenterology* 1958;35:579–581.

13. Ornstein MH, Littlewood ER, Baird IM, Fowler J, North WR, Cox AG. Are fibre supplements really necessary in diverticular disease of the colon? A controlled clinical trial. *BMJ* 1981;282:1353–1356.

14. Brodribb AJ. Treatment of symptomatic diverticular disease with a high-fibre diet. *Lancet* 1977;1:664–666.

15. Hodgson WJ. The placebo effect. Is it important in diverticular disease? *Am J Gastroenterol* 1977;67:157–162.

16. Smits BJ, Whitehead AM, Prescott P. Lactulose in the treatment of symptomatic diverticular disease: a comparative study with high-fibre diet. *Br J Clin Pract* 1990;44:314–318.

17. Papi C, Ciaco A, Koch M, Capurso L. Efficacy of rifaximin in the treatment of symptomatic diverticular disease of the colon. A multicentre double-blind placebo-controlled trial. *Aliment Pharmacol Ther* 1995;9:33–39.

18. Kellum JM, Sugerman HJ, Coppa GF, et al. Randomized, prospective comparison of cefoxitin and gentamicin–clindamycin in the treatment of acute colonic diverticulitis. *Clin Ther* 14:376–384.

19. Larson DM, Masters SS, Spiro HM. Medical and surgical therapy in diverticular disease: a comparative study. *Gastroenterology* 1976;71:734–737.

20. Sarin S, Boulos PB. Long-term outcome of patients presenting with acute complications of diverticular disease. *Ann R Coll Surg Engl* 1994;76:117–120.

21. Farthmann EH, Ruckauer KD, Haring RU. Evidence-based surgery: diverticulitis – a surgical disease? *Langenbecks Arch Surg* 2000;385:143–151.

22. Kronborg O. Treatment of perforated sigmoid diverticulitis: a prospective randomised trial. *Br J Surg* 1993;80:505–507.

John Simpson

Robin Spiller

Division of Gastroenterology
University Hospital
Nottingham
UK

Competing interests: None declared.

INTERVENTIONS

Beneficial
Adjuvant chemotherapy in
    Dukes' C colorectal cancer . .304

Likely to be beneficial
Adjuvant chemotherapy in
    Dukes' B colorectal cancer . .304
Portal vein infusion with
    5-fluorouracil in Dukes' A, B
    and C colon cancer 304
Colonoscopy to detect
    metachronous cancers and
    polyps. 306
3–5 yearly follow up 306

**Trade off between benefits and
    harms**
Preoperative radiotherapy 305

Unknown effectiveness
Preoperative versus postoperative
    radiotherapy 306
Total mesorectal excision 307

Unlikely to be beneficial
Levamisole for adjuvant therapy
    (colorectal cancer, no residual
    disease) 304
Annual or biannual follow up
    (no better than less
    frequent). 306

**To be covered in future issues of
    *Clinical Evidence***
Surgery
Colonoscopic polypectomy
Immunotherapy
Specialist versus generalist surgical
    care
Liver resection for metastases

Key Messages

■ RCTs have found that adjuvant chemotherapy improves 5 year survival by at least 5% in people with Dukes' B and C tumours. The evidence of benefit in people with Dukes' B tumours is less clear. We found no good evidence about harmful effects.

■ RCTs have found that, compared with surgery alone, preoperative radiotherapy significantly reduces the risk of local recurrence and can improve survival in some people with rectal cancer. About a third of people develop associated impairment of bowel function. One RCT found no significant survival benefit from short course preoperative radiotherapy compared with a longer course of postoperative radiotherapy.

■ We found limited evidence that annual or biannual follow up is not significantly different from 3–5 yearly follow up in terms of detection of recurrence or survival. The harms of follow up are poorly described.

■ We found no RCTs that evaluated mesorectal excision for rectal cancer. Non-randomised studies suggest that it may reduce the rate of recurrence.

DEFINITION   Colorectal cancer is a malignant neoplasm arising from the lining (mucosa) of the large intestine (colon and rectum). Nearly two thirds of colorectal cancers occur in the rectum or sigmoid colon. It is categorised as Dukes' A, B, or C (see glossary, p 308).

INCIDENCE/ PREVALENCE   Colorectal cancer is the third most common malignancy in the developed world. It accounts for about 20 000 deaths a year in the UK and 60 000 deaths a year in the USA. Although the incidence of and mortality from colorectal cancer has changed little over the past 40 years, the incidence of the disease has fallen recently in both the UK and the USA.[1,2] In the UK, about a quarter of people with colorectal cancer present as emergencies with either intestinal obstruction or perforation.[3,4]

AETIOLOGY/ RISK FACTORS   Colon cancer affects almost equal proportions of men and women, most commonly between the ages of 60 and 80 years. Rectal cancer is more common in men.[1] The pathogenesis of colorectal cancer involves genetic and environmental factors. The most important environmental factor is probably diet.[5]

PROGNOSIS   Overall 5 year survival is about 50% and has not changed over the past 40 years. Disease specific mortality in both USA and UK cancer registries is decreasing but reasons are unclear.[1,2] Surgery is undertaken with curative intent in over 80% of people, but about half suffer recurrence.

AIMS   To reduce mortality and morbidity (e.g. bowel obstruction or perforation) associated with the tumour; to minimise adverse effects of treatment (e.g. avoiding permanent stoma by restoring intestinal continuity); to maximise quality of life.

OUTCOMES   Survival, proportion of people with permanent stoma, incidence of local recurrence, rates of metastasis, adverse effects of treatment, quality of life.

METHODS   *Clinical Evidence* update search and appraisal December 2000, using the following key words: colorectal cancer, neoplasia, adjuvant chemotherapy, surgery, follow up, recurrence.

QUESTION   What are the effects of adjuvant chemotherapy?

RCTs have found that adjuvant systemic chemotherapy improves survival by at least 5% in people with Dukes' B and C tumours. The evidence of benefit in people with Dukes' B tumours is less clear. One systematic review found evidence of a modest improvement in 5 year survival after 7 days of portal vein infusion with 5-fluorouracil versus no infusion, mainly in people within colon cancer. One RCT found no significant improvement with levamisole versus placebo, or high dose folinic acid versus low dose folinic acid. We found no good evidence about harmful effects.

Benefits: **Versus placebo or no treatment:** We found two systematic reviews[6,7] and one subsequent RCT.[8] The first systematic review (search date 1993, 29 RCTs, 1673 people with Dukes' C colon cancer and 695 with Dukes' B or C rectal cancer) found a small but significant improvement in overall survival with adjuvant treatment versus no adjuvant treatment (OR for death 0.91, 95% CI 0.83 to 0.99).[6] There was a 5% overall improvement in 5 year survival for people with colon cancer, and 9% for people with rectal cancer. Publication of 24 of the 29 RCTs was before 1990. The results were less clear for Dukes' B than for Dukes' C tumours, partly because of the smaller numbers of Dukes' B tumours. Pooled analysis of three RCTs of adjuvant fluouracil and folinic acid in colon cancer found an absolute increase in survival of 5–10% for Dukes' C tumours at 3 years but no significant survival advantage for Dukes' B tumours.[9] The second systematic review (search date 1994–1995, 10 RCTs, 3499 people with Dukes' A, B, or C colorectal cancer) compared 1 week of continuing portal vein infusion of 5-fluorouracil within 5–7 days of surgery versus no further treatment after surgery.[7] It found significant improvement in survival at 6 years with portal vein infusion versus no infusion (RRR of death 10%, 95% CI 3% to 16%; ARR of death 4.7%; NNT 22, 95% CI 13 to 67). The benefit was restricted to those with colon cancer. The subsequent RCT (4927 people with colorectal cancer and no evident residual disease) compared levamisole versus placebo.[8] It found no significant reduction of recurrence at 3 years (37% with levamisole v 35% with placebo, P = 0.16), and no significant effect on survival (69% with levamisole v 72% with placebo). **Versus higher dose:** The subsequent RCT (4927 people with colorectal cancer and no evident residual disease) also compared high dose folinic acid versus low dose folinic acid.[8] It found no significant difference in recurrence at 3 years (36% high dose v 36% low dose, P = 0.94) or in survival (70% high dose v 71% low dose, P = 0.43).

Harms: We found little good evidence on the harms of chemotherapy, partly because many different regimens were used.[6] In the RCTs included in one systematic review, the incidence of severe adverse effects (stomatitis, diarrhoea, nausea, and leukopenia) with 5-fluorouracil and levamisole ranged from 10–30%, with life threatening toxicity occurring in about 5% of people.[6] For every 10 people treated, about three will experience an additional, severe adverse effect. Three studies reported deaths related to chemotherapy in about 2% of people with advanced disease.

Comment: A much larger RCT of the effects of adjuvant chemotherapy in people with Dukes' B tumours is underway in the UK (D Kerr, personal communication, 1999). Further RCTs are required to assess the benefits of portal vein infusion.

| QUESTION | What is the effect of preoperative radiotherapy for rectal cancer? |

One systematic review and a number of RCTs have found that, compared with surgery alone, preoperative radiotherapy significantly reduces the risk of local recurrence and can improve survival in some people with rectal cancer. About a third of the people have associated impairment of bowel function. One RCT found no significant survival benefit from short course preoperative radiotherapy compared with a longer course of postoperative radiotherapy.

Benefits: **Versus surgery alone:** We found one systematic review (search date December 1999, 14 RCTs, 5974 people with rectal adeno-carcinoma), which found that surgery plus radiotherapy versus surgery alone significantly reduced overall mortality after 5 years

(OR 0.84, 95% CI 0.72 to 0.98; P = 0.03; NNT 25), local recurrence (11 RCTs, 4494 people; OR 0.49, 95% CI 0.38 to 0.62; NNT 10), but did not significantly reduce the risk of distant metastases.[10] **Versus postoperative radiotherapy:** We found no systematic review. One RCT compared a short course of preoperative radiotherapy (25.5 Gy in 1 week) versus postoperative radiotherapy (60 Gy over 7–8 weeks) in people with Dukes' B or C rectal carcinoma. After 5 years, there was no significant difference in overall survival (P = 0.5), but preoperative radiotherapy significantly reduced local recurrence (27/209 [13%] with preoperative v 45/204 [22%] with postoperative treatment; ARR 9%, 95% CI 4% to 14%; RR 0.59, 95% CI 0.37 to 0.91; NNT 11, 95% CI 7 to 49).[11]

Harms: We found one systematic review (search date 1998) of harms associated with adjuvant radiotherapy.[12] **Versus surgery alone:** The review identified 19 RCTs of preoperative radiotherapy versus surgery alone (5110 people). Preoperative radiotherapy compared with surgery alone increased early postoperative morbidity and mortality. Early harms included diarrhoea, wound infections (20% with preoperative radiotherapy v 10% with surgery alone), bowel obstruction, cardiovascular problems, and pain. Two RCTs (1027 people) found that preoperative radiotherapy significantly increased the risk of venous thromboembolism, fracture of the hip, intestinal obstruction, postoperative fistulae, cardiovascular, and thrombotic events compared with surgery alone.[13] Increased bowel frequency and urgency impaired social life in about 30% of people after preoperative radiotherapy.[14] In people with low rectal tumours, who underwent abdominoperineal excision, preoperative radiotherapy was associated with twice the rate of perineal wound breakdown compared with surgery alone (20% v 10%).[12] **Versus postoperative radiotherapy:** The systematic review[12] identified nine RCTs of postoperative radiotherapy. It found a greater risk of anastomotic complications (breakdown and stricture formation) after postoperative compared with preoperative radiotherapy.

Comment: There are reductions in local recurrence and modest improvements in survival following preoperative radiotherapy compared with surgery alone for rectal cancer; but the risk of local recurrence for T1 and T2 tumours is so low that preoperative radiotherapy is unlikely to provide much absolute benefit. There are unresolved issues about preoperative staging of rectal cancers and case selection for preoperative radiotherapy.

QUESTION What are the effects of routine follow up for colorectal cancer?

We found limited evidence that surveillance (colonoscopy and computerised tomography scan every 3–5 years) may be beneficial, but that more intensive, annual or biannual follow up confers no additional benefit. Whether the interval between follow up visits should be 3 or 5 years is uncertain. The harms of follow up are poorly described. Limited evidence suggests that follow up is reassuring to most people.

Benefits: We found one systematic review[15] and two additional RCTs.[16,17] The systematic review (search date not specified, 10 RCTs, 37 000 people) found no significant benefit from follow up on either survival, liver metastasis, lung metastasis, or local recurrence.[15] The first additional RCT (1418 people who had undergone removal of adenomatous polyps) compared follow up colonoscopy at 1 and 3 years versus 3 years only.[16] More frequent follow up detected new polyps in a greater proportion of people (42% v 32%; RR of detection 1.3, 95% CI 1.1 to 1.6), but there was no significant difference in the proportion of detected polyps with advanced pathology (about 3% in both groups; RR 1.0, 95% CI 0.5 to 2.2). The second additional RCT (325 people who had undergone curative resection for newly diagnosed Dukes' A, B, or C colorectal cancer) compared standard versus intensive follow up.[17] Standard follow up comprised clinical review (history, examination, liver function tests, carcinoembryonic antigen, and faecal occult blood testing) three monthly for 2 years, and thereafter six monthly for 5 years or until a major end point was reached. Intensive follow up comprised standard clinical review (as above) plus annual chest radiograph, computerised tomography scan of the liver, and colonoscopy. After 5 years there was no significant difference in survival between the two groups. Annual colonoscopy did not detect any asymptomatic local recurrences.

Harms: Presymptomatic diagnosis of incurable recurrent disease may increase anxiety and reduce quality of life. Invasive tests such as colonoscopy also carry risks. These outcomes were not reported in the trials.

Comment: One RCT (212 people being followed up after treatment for colorectal cancer) found that 78% were "rather reassured" or "very reassured" by follow up. However, follow up had no effect on quality of life. Most people in the trial said that they would still prefer follow up even if it did not lead to earlier detection of recurrence.[18] Current follow up regimens are variable in frequency and intensity. We found no evidence on whether follow up should be stopped in elderly people (aged > 75 years), although many people with colorectal cancer are in this age group. In the UK, people over 75 years are not routinely considered for chemotherapy because of its potential toxicity. We found no evidence for or against this policy. The role of carcino-embryonic antigen monitoring is also uncertain, as 30% of colorectal cancers do not express this antigen.

QUESTION What are the effects of total mesorectal excision for rectal cancer?

We found no RCTs evaluating total mesorectal excision for rectal cancer. Non-randomised studies suggest that it may reduce the rate of local recurrence.

Benefits: We found no systematic review or RCTs. We found several non-randomised studies[19–23] (see table 1, p 310).

Harms: Increased stool frequency is found after total mesorectal excision compared with techniques leaving a rectal stump (median 4–5/day v 1–2/day). Observational studies have found that total mesorectal excision also carries a higher incidence of anastomotic leakage (11–15% v 8–10%).[23]

Colorectal cancer

Comment: Rectal cancer surgery is more technically demanding than colon cancer resection. With conventional anterior resection, some of the rectum is retained. The removal of the rectum in total mesorectal excision necessitates coloanal anastomosis. Some observational studies (but no RCTs) suggest that surgical technique is especially important in resecting rectal cancer. Many surgeons routinely use a temporary defunctioning stoma after total mesorectal excision in an attempt to reduce the incidence of anastomotic leakage.[19]

GLOSSARY

Dukes' classification Dukes' classification of the pathologic stages of carcinoma of the colon or rectum includes four stages: A, limited to mucosa and submucosa; B, penetration of the entire bowel wall and serosa or pericolic fat; C, stages A and B, and invasion into the regional draining lymph node system; D, advanced and widespread regional involvement (metastasis).

Substantive changes since last issue

Portal vein infusion with 5-fluorouracil versus no other treatment New systematic review;[7] likely to be beneficial.

Levamisole versus placebo and high dose folinic acid versus low dose folinic acid New RCT;[8] no significant benefit.

Preoperative radiotherapy plus surgery versus surgery alone New systematic review;[10] conclusion unchanged.

Effect of routine follow up New systematic review;[15] conclusion unchanged.

REFERENCES

1. *Mortality statistics, cause, England and Wales 1993*. OPCS dh22. London: HMSO, 1995.
2. Miller BA, Ries LA, Hankey BF, et al. *Cancer statistics review 1973–1989*. Rockville (MD): National Institutes of Health, National Cancer Institute. Report No: NIH-NCI 92–2789.
3. Mella J, Biffen A, Radcliffe AG, Stamatakis JD, Steele RJ. A population based on audit of colorectal cancer management in two United Kingdom health districts. *Br J Surg* 1997;84: 1731–1736.
4. Scholefield JH, Robinson MHE, Mangham C, Hardcastle JD. Screening for colorectal cancer reduces emergency admissions. *Eur J Surg Oncol* 1998;24:47–50.
5. Kune G, ed. *Causes and control of colorectal cancer: a model for cancer prevention*. Boston: Kluwer Academic Publishers, 1996.
6. Dube S, Heyen, F Jenicek M. Adjuvant chemotherapy in colorectal carcinoma. Results of a meta analysis. *Dis Colon Rectum* 1997;40:35–41. Search date June 1993; primary source Medline, January 1959 to June 1993.
7. Liver Infusion Meta-analysis Group. Portal vein chemotherapy for colorectal cancer: A meta-analysis of 4000 patients in 10 studies. *J Natl Cancer Inst* 1997;89:497–505. Search date not given; primary sources Medline, Cancerlit, Excerpta Medica; hand searched books, journals, registers of trials.
8. QUASAR Collaborative Group. Comparison of fluouracil with additional levamisole, higher dose folinic acid or both as adjuvant chemotherapy for colorectal cancer: a randomised trial. *Lancet* 2000;355:1588–1596.
9. International Multicenter Pooled Analysis of Colon Cancer Trials (IMPACT) Investigators. Efficacy of adjuvant fluouracil and folinic acid in colon cancer. *Lancet* 1995;348:939–944.
10. Camma C, Giunta M, Pagliaro L. Preoperative radiotherapy for resectable rectal cancer. A meta analysis. *JAMA* 2000:284:1008–1015. Search date December 1999; primary sources, Medline and Cancerlit 1970–1999; handsearches of reference lists. No company sponsorship stated.
11. Jansson-Frykholm G, Glimelius B, Pahlman L. Preoperative or postoperative irradiation in adenocarcinoma of the rectum. Final treatment results of a randomised trial and an evaluation of late secondary effects. *Dis Colon Rectum* 1993; 36:564–572.
12. Ooi B, Tjandra J, Green M. Morbidities of adjuvant chemotherapy and radiotherapy for resectable rectal cancer: an overview. *Dis Colon Rectum* 1999;42:403–418. Search date 1998; primary source Medline.
13. Holm T, Singnomklao T, Rutqvist LE, Cedermark B. Adjuvant preoperative radiotherapy in patients with rectal carcinoma. Adverse effects during long term follow-up of two trials. *Cancer* 1996;78:968–976.
14. Dahlberg M, Glimelius B, Graf W, Pahlman L. Preoperative irradiation affects functional results after surgery for rectal cancer: results from a randomised study. *Dis Colon Rectum* 1998;41:543–549.
15. Kievit J. Colorectal cancer follow up: a reassessment of empirical evidence on effectiveness. *Eur J Surg Oncol* 2000;26:322–328. Search date not given; primary sources Medline. No company sponsorship stated.
16. Winawer SJ, Zauber AG, O'Brien MJ, et al. Randomised comparison of surveillance intervals after colonoscopic removal of newly diagnosed adenomatous polyps: the national polyp study workgroup. *N Engl J Med* 1993;328:901–906.

17. Shoemaker D, Black R, Giles L, Toouli J. Yearly colonoscopy, liver CT and chest radiography do not influence 5 year survival of colorectal cancer patients. *Gastroenterology* 1998;114:7–14.

18. Stiggelbout AM, de Haes JCJM, Vree R, et al. Follow up of colorectal cancer patients: quality of life and attitudes towards follow up. *Br J Cancer* 1997;75:914–920.

19. McFarlane JK, Ryall RDH, Heald RJ. Mesorectal excision for rectal cancer. *Lancet* 1993;341:457–460.

20. Enker WE, Thaler HT, Cranor ML, Polyak T. Total mesorectal excision in the operative treatment of carcinoma of the rectum. *J Am Coll Surg* 1995;181:335–346.

21. Singh S, Morgan MBF, Broughton M, Caffarey S, Topham C, Marks CG. A ten-year prospective audit of outcome of surgical treatment for colorectal carcinoma. *Br J Surg* 1995;82:1486–1490.

22. Arbman G, Nilsson E, Hallbook O, Sjodahl R. Local recurrence following total mesorectal excision for rectal cancer. *Br J Surg* 1996;83:375–379.

23. Karanja ND, Corder AP, Bearn P, Heald RJ. Leakage from stapled low anastomosis after total mesorectal excision for carcinoma of the rectum. *Br J Surg* 1994;81:1224–1226.

John Scholefield
Professor of Surgery
University Hospital
Nottingham
UK

Competing interests: None declared.

Digestive system disorders

TABLE 1 Effects of total mesorectal excision: results of non-randomised studies (see text, p 307).

Reference	Duke's stage (number of patients)	Intervention	Recurrence at 5 years (95% CI)		RRR of death by 5 years (95% CI)	Incidence of anastomic leak (95% CI)
			Local	Overall		
19	B (88) C (73)	TME	5% (0% to 7.5%)	18% (10% to 25%)	78% (68% to 88%)	11% clinical 6.4% radiological
20	B (99) C (147)	TME	7.3%	23%	74%	NA
21	A, B, and C (158 in total)	TME	8%	24%	60%	10%
22	A (67) B (89) C (100)	TME Non-TME	6% at 1 year 14% at 1 year	NA	NA	8% (57% stoma rate) 9% (15% stoma rate)

TME, total mesorectal excision; NA, not applicable.

Search date June 2000

Paul Moayyedi, Brendan Delaney, David Katzka and David Forman

QUESTIONS

INTERVENTIONS

Beneficial

Proton pump inhibitors
(PPIs) 313

H_2 antagonists (less so than
PPIs) 313,314

Fundoplication for erosive
oesophagitis. 318,319

Unknown effectiveness

Different surgical techniques for
non-erosive oesophagitis . . .314

Surgical treatment for non-erosive
oesophagitis 314

Long term effects of medical and
surgical treatments for erosive
and non-erosive
oesophagitis. 314,318

Different surgical techniques for
erosive oesophagitis. 319

Medical and surgical treatment of
gastro-oesophageal reflux in
people with Barrett's
oesophagus. 320

Medical and surgical treatment of
gastro-oesophageal reflux in
selected people with
extraoesophageal
manifestations. 321

To be covered in future issues of
Clinical Evidence

Diet and lifestyle changes

Key Messages

In people with non-erosive reflux disease

- One systematic review of RCTs that directly compared H_2 antagonists and proton pump inhibitors (PPIs) versus placebo has found both are more effective than placebo for symptom relief.
- One systematic review of RCTs that directly compared daily H_2 antagonists with PPIs has found PPIs are more effective for symptom relief.
- One RCT found PPIs are better than H_2 antagonists for maintaining remission.
- We found no evidence about surgical treatment for non-erosive disease.

In people with erosive oesophagitis

- One systematic review of indirect comparisons found that PPIs were more effective than H_2 antagonists at healing erosive oesophagitis, and that both were more effective than placebo. RCTs found no significant difference in rates of short term adverse events. We found no good data on long term risks of treatment or on possible long term benefits. One RCT found no evidence of a difference in relapse rates between PPIs and H_2 antagonists when used intermittently, although relief of symptoms was more rapid with PPIs.

© *Clinical Evidence* 2001;5:311–323.

Gastro-oesophageal reflux disease

- One RCT found no significant difference in effectiveness among different PPIs for people with erosive disease.

- We found no good evidence adequately comparing medical and surgical treatments in RCTs. One RCT found fundoplication to be significantly more effective than medical treatment, but it did not use PPIs, which might have increased the effectiveness of the medical treatment. We found no good comparative data on preventing relapse or complications.

- One RCT found that fundic mobilisation had no effect on postoperative symptoms or rates of cure, but increased rates of sliding hiatus hernia. One RCT found no difference in outcomes between total or partial fundoplication, other than increased flatulence with total fundoplication.

In people with gastro-oesophageal reflux complicated by erosive gastritis or Barrett's oesophagus

- We found no good evidence on the effects of treatment for gastro-oesophageal reflux in people with Barrett's oesophagus.

In people with extraoesophageal symptoms

- One systematic review did not find any evidence of an improvement in lung function in people with asthma treated for gastro-oesophageal reflux disease.

DEFINITION	Gastro-oesophageal reflux occurs when gastric contents enter the oesophagus because of transient or chronic relaxation of the lower oesophageal sphincter. Excessive reflux causes symptoms of gastro-oesophageal reflux disease (heartburn, acid taste in the mouth). It can be divided into non-erosive oesophagitis (predominant heartburn with a normal endoscopy, also termed "endoscopy negative reflux disease") and erosive oesophagitis (endoscopy shows inflammation and erosions).
INCIDENCE/ PREVALENCE	Gastro-oesophageal reflux disease is common. Weekly heartburn occurs in up to 20% of people questioned in population surveys. Up to 10% of these will have erosive disease.
AETIOLOGY/ RISK FACTORS	We found no evidence of clear predictive factors for gastro-oesophageal reflux disease.
PROGNOSIS	Gastro-oesophageal reflux disease is generally benign with little mortality. However, persistent symptoms can interfere with normal activities and cause considerable morbidity. Long term retrospective data (up to 22 years) suggest that in people with an initially normal endoscopy, endoscopy tends to remain normal.[1] A small subset of people develop strictures, Barrett's oesophagus, adenocarcinoma, or extraoesophageal manifestations (see table 1, p 323).[2]
AIMS	To relieve symptoms; to prevent complications in those with severe oesophagitis; to control extraoesophageal manifestations; to minimise adverse effects of treatment; to improve quality of life.
OUTCOMES	Frequency and severity of symptoms, degree of oesophagitis, prevalence and severity of extraoesophageal manifestations, incidence of stricture, adenocarcinoma. Symptoms do not correlate closely with the extent of oesophagitis. People with Barrett's oesophagus may have minimal symptoms, whereas people with severe symptoms may have no evidence of oesophagitis on

endoscopy. Proxy outcomes include atrophic gastritis and Barrett's oesophagus, which some studies have found to be associated with adenocarcinoma.[3,4]

METHODS *Clinical Evidence* search and appraisal June 2000.

QUESTION What are the effects of treatment in non-erosive oesophagitis?

OPTION PROTON PUMP INHIBITORS VERSUS PLACEBO

One systematic review of RCTs has found PPIs to be more effective than placebo at relieving symptoms. We found no good evidence on recurrence.

Benefits: **Symptom relief:** We found one systematic review (search date 1999), which identified five RCTs evaluating the effect of PPIs in endoscopy negative reflux disease.[5] Meta-analysis of four trials with heartburn as an outcome found PPIs were significantly better than placebo (n = 1017; AR of still having heartburn 40% v 67%; RR 0.68, 95% CI 0.53 to 0.88). One subsequent RCT (241 people) also found that PPI treatment was superior to placebo (complete resolution of heartburn during week 2: 41% v 5%, P < 0.001).[6] **Recurrence:** We found no placebo controlled trials with recurrence as an outcome.

Harms: See harms under erosive oesophagitis, p 315.

Comment: None.

OPTION PROTON PUMP INHIBITORS VERSUS H_2 ANTAGONISTS

One systematic review found limited evidence that PPIs are more effective at relieving symptoms than H_2 antagonists. One RCT found limited evidence that PPIs are better at preventing recurrence than H_2 antagonists.

Benefits: **Symptom relief:** We found one systematic review (search date 1999) comparing PPIs versus H2 antagonists.[5] This review identified two RCTs (776 people) in endoscopy negative reflux disease. Meta-analysis found more people improved with PPIs but the difference was not significant for heartburn remission (AR of still having heartburn: 47% v 58%; RR 0.81, 95% CI 0.70 to 0.94). We found one subsequent RCT (901 people), which compared lansoprazole 30 mg once daily versus lansoprazole 15 mg once daily versus ranitidine 150 mg twice daily for 8 weeks.[7] This trial found that people treated with PPIs had significantly lower heartburn scores (symptom free for at least 80% of treatment days: 37% with lansoprazole 15 mg, 35% with lansoprazole 30 mg, 23% with ranitidine, P < 0.05 for each lansoprazole group v ranitidine). The trials also found omeprazole was more likely than ranitidine to improve symptom and psychological wellbeing scores. **Recurrence:** We found one RCT in people in remission comparing omeprazole (134 people) versus ranitidine (129 people).[8] At 12 months, significantly more people were still in remission with omeprazole (68% v 39%, P < 0.0001).

Harms: See harms of erosive oesophagitis, p 315.

Comment: None.

OPTION **H_2 ANTAGONISTS VERSUS PLACEBO**

One systematic review of RCTs has found H_2 antagonists are more effective than placebo at relieving heartburn.

Benefits: **Symptom relief:** We found one systematic review comparing H_2 antagonists versus placebo (search date 1999, 2 RCTs, 514 people).[5] The review found H_2 antagonists were more likely than placebo to relieve heartburn (AR of still having heartburn 65% v 78%; RR 0.84, 95% CI 0.74 to 0.95). **Recurrence:** We found no systematic reviews or RCTs.

Harms: See harms of erosive oesophagitis, p 315.

Comment: None.

OPTION **SURGICAL TREATMENT**

We found insufficient evidence on the effects of surgical treatment for non-erosive oesophagitis.

Benefits: We found no systematic review or RCTs comparing medical versus surgical treatment in people with non-erosive oesophagitis, nor any comparing different surgical techniques.

Harms: We found no good evidence.

Comment: Good long term trials are needed to compare laparoscopic fundoplication with PPIs, taking into account symptom relief, adherence, prevention of complications, and adverse effects of treatment.

QUESTION **What are the effects of treatments for erosive oesophagitis?**

OPTION **PROTON PUMP INHIBITORS VERSUS PLACEBO**

One systematic review of pooled results across treatment arms found PPIs had faster healing rates than placebo. RCTs found PPIs were better than placebo at preventing recurrence.

Benefits: **Healing:** One systematic review (published in 1997) identified 43 single and double blind RCTs in 7635 people which compared different drug treatments versus each other, versus placebo, or both (total of 95 study arms, treatment given for 2–12 weeks).[9] By pooling results across treatment arms, PPIs provided the fastest overall healing rate (12% healed per week, 95% CI 10.7% to 12.6%), four times faster than placebo (3% healed per week, 95% CI 2.4% to 3.4%). Doses of PPIs varied, not routinely exceeding 40 mg omeprazole or 30 mg lansoprazole. **Preventing recurrence:** One RCT found omeprazole was more effective than placebo at preventing relapse (193 people). At 12 months, remission rates with omeprazole 20 mg daily were 74% (95% CI 62% to 86%), with omeprazole 10 mg daily 50%, (95% CI 34% to 66%), and with placebo 14% (95% CI 2% to 26%).[10] One RCT in people who had already responded symptomatically to lansoprazole found that it was more effective than placebo at preventing relapse (173 people; 12 months' remission rates 67% with lansoprazole 30 mg, 72% with lansoprazole 15 mg, 35% with placebo, CIs not reported).[11] **Preventing complications:** We found no good evidence.

Harms: **Short term adverse effects:** Rare adverse events of PPIs in people with gastro-oesophageal reflux disease include liver function test abnormalities, increased bowel bacterial counts, cytopenias, hypersensitivity reactions, and decreased (but not clinically important) vitamin B12 levels. **Long term adverse effects:** In two studies of chronic use of PPIs in the presence of *Helicobacter pylori,* infection has been linked to atrophic gastritis after 3–5 years.[12,13] Among people treated with omeprazole, none of whom had atrophic gastritis at baseline, atrophic gastritis developed in 18 of the 59 people infected with *H pylori* and two of the 46 people who were not infected.[12] A further study reported that out of 14 people with persistent *H pylori* infection, six developed mild to severe atrophy in 5 years.[13] Subgroup analysis from one RCT comparing long term omeprazole treatment with fundoplication found more people infected with *H pylori* who were treated with omeprazole developed gastric atrophy at 3 years' follow up but, the difference was not significant (8/31 [26%] v 3/31 [10%]; RR 2.6, 95% CI 0.8 to 6.1).[14]

Comment: The meta-analysis[9] did not compare groups as they were randomised, but compared one group from one trial with another group from another trial. This loses the benefits of randomisation since the groups being compared may not have had the same characteristics. The next issue of *Clinical Evidence* will consider the results from the individual trials. The clinical significance of atrophic gastritis is as a risk factor for gastric cancer, but there is debate about whether a clear definition of atrophic gastritis exists.[3–4]

| OPTION | PROTON PUMP INHIBITORS VERSUS H₂ ANTAGONISTS |

One systematic review of indirect comparative data found that PPIs were more likely than H₂ antagonists to heal erosive oesophagitis and prevent recurrence. RCTs found no significant difference in short term rates of adverse events. We found no good data on long term risks of treatment or on possible long term benefits. One RCT found no evidence of a difference in relapse rates between a PPI and H₂ antagonist when used intermittently, although relief of symptoms was more rapid with PPIs.

Benefits: One systematic review (published in 1997) indirectly compared PPIs versus H₂ antagonists. It identified 43 single and double blind RCTs in 7635 people that compared different drug treatments versus each other, versus placebo, or both (total of 95 study arms, treatment given for 2–12 weeks).[9] **Healing:** By pooling results across treatment arms (omeprazole 20–80 mg daily, lansoprazole 30–60 mg daily, pantoprazole 40 mg daily, cimetidine 800–1600 mg daily, ranitidine 300–1200 mg daily, famotidine 40–80 mg daily, nizatidine 300–600 mg daily), the review found a higher healing rate by 12 weeks of erosive oesophagitis on endoscopic examination with PPIs (84% with PPIs, 95% CI 79% to 88%, v 52% with H_2 antagonists, 95% CI 47% to 57%). PPIs provided the fastest overall healing rate with 12% healed per week (95% CI 10.7% to 12.6%), twice as fast as H_2 antagonists (6% healed per week, 95% CI 5.5% to 6.3%). Two of the RCTs added a prokinetic agent to the H_2 antagonist, but results still strongly favoured the PPI.[15,16] One subsequent RCT (133 people) also found that PPIs were more effective for healing (confirmed endoscopically after 4 weeks 79% v 42%, P < 0.001).[17] Doses of PPIs varied, not routinely exceeding 40 mg omeprazole or 30 mg lansoprazole. **Preventing recurrence:** We found no systematic review. We found three RCTs looking at recurrence rates. Two RCTs (one double blind and one single blind) compared omeprazole versus ranitidine (with or without cisapride) in people with endoscopically confirmed oesophagitis who had already received omeprazole for 4 weeks.[18,19] At 1 year, people treated with daily omeprazole were significantly less likely to relapse than those on ranitidine. In the first RCT, 159 people were randomised to either omeprazole 20 mg daily, omeprazole 20 mg on 3 consecutive days per week ("weekend omeprazole"), or ranitidine 150 mg twice daily. At 12 months, a significantly greater proportion of people treated with daily omeprazole remained in remission compared with daily ranitidine (ARR daily omeprazole v ranitidine 64%, 95% CI 50% to 78%). The trial found no significant difference between weekend omeprazole and daily ranitidine treatments (ARR weekend omeprazole v daily ranitidine 7%, 95% CI –11% to +25%).[18] In the second RCT, 175 people were randomised to omeprazole, ranitidine, or cisapride, alone and in various combinations. At 12 months, people on omeprazole were significantly more likely to be in remission than those on either ranitidine or cisapride alone (80% still in remission with omeprazole v 50% with ranitidine or cisapride, CIs not reported).[19] **Preventing complications:** We found no RCTs that examined possible longer term benefits of medical treatment. **Intermittent treatment:** We found one recent, multicentre, double blind RCT trial of intermittent, symptomatic treatment with omeprazole (10 mg or 20 mg) versus ranitidine (150 mg) over a 12 month period (677 people).[20] The trial found that intermittent treatment with any of these regimens was moderately effective at controlling symptoms (40% had no relapse within 12 months; 93% had three or fewer relapses in the intermittent treatment phase), and that there was no significant difference between the three groups in terms of long term relapse rates. However, symptoms were controlled more rapidly by omeprazole than ranitidine (by the second week of symptom onset, proportion of people with symptom relief was 55% with 20 mg omeprazole, 40% with 10 mg omeprazole, and 26% with ranitidine). The trial did not compare intermittent treatment with maintenance treatment.

Harms: **Short term:** The placebo controlled RCTs found similar rates of adverse effects with PPIs and H_2 antagonists. Most data on significant adverse effects come from case reports or uncontrolled trials. H_2 antagonists have been associated rarely with cytopenias, gynaecomastia, liver function test abnormalities, and hypersensitivity reactions. Rare adverse effects of PPIs in people with gastro-oesophageal reflux disease include liver function test abnormalities, increased small bowel bacterial counts, cytopenias, hypersensitivity reactions, and decreased (but not clinically important) vitamin B_{12} levels. **Long term:** We found no RCTs with long term follow up on the safety of chronic use of H_2 antagonists. Chronic use of PPIs in the presence of *H pylori* infection has been linked in two studies to atrophic gastritis after 3–5 years.[12,13] Among people treated with omeprazole, none of whom had atrophic gastritis at baseline, atrophic gastritis developed in 18 out of 59 people infected with *H pylori* and two out of 46 people who were not infected, compared with no new cases of atrophic gastritis among 72 people treated with fundoplication (31 with *H Pylori* and 41 without).[12] One further study reported that out of 14 people with persistent *H pylori* infection, six developed mild to severe atrophy in 5 years.[13]

Comment: The meta-analysis did not compare groups as they were randomised, but compared one group from one trial with another group from another. This loses the benefits of randomisation since the groups being compared may have different characteristics. The next issue of *Clinical Evidence* will consider the results from the individual trials. The clinical significance of atrophic gastritis is as a risk factor for gastric cancer but there is debate whether a clear definition of atrophic gastritis exists.[3,4] Cisapride has recently been withdrawn in the UK and other countries because of associated mortality.

OPTION	DIFFERENT PROTON PUMP INHIBITORS

One RCT found no evidence of a difference between PPIs in healing erosive oesophagitis.

Benefits: **Healing:** We found no systematic review, but found one good multicentre, double blind RCT (225 people).[21] The trial found no significant difference in the proportion healed at 8 weeks by lansoprazole 30 mg versus 20 mg omeprazole in people with erosive oesophagitis (AR healing at 8 weeks 85% with lansoprazole, 87% with omeprazole; ARR 2%, 95% CI −6% to +14%; RRR 2%, 95% −7% to +16%). Relapse rates were not evaluated. Another double blind RCT (n = 202) compared 20 mg rabeprazole with 20 mg omeprazole and found no significant difference in healing of erosive and ulcerative oesophagitis at 4 weeks (81% v 81%) and at 8 weeks (92% rabeprazole v 94% omeprazole; ARR 2%, 95% CI −3% to +15%).[22] **Preventing recurrence:** We found no systematic review or RCTs that compared different maintenance treatments. **Preventing complications:** We found one small double blind RCT with three-arms (30 participants) in people who responded to omeprazole treatment.[23] All participants were treated with dilatation of the stenosis weekly and at the clinician's discretion. The trial compared omeprazole 20 mg twice daily versus lansoprazole 30 mg twice daily versus pantoprazole 40 mg twice daily. The trial found omeprazole was superior at maintaining remission (relapse rates 10%, 80%, 70%, omeprazole v other groups combined, P = 0.001).

Harms: See PPIs versus placebo, p 315.

Comment: None.

Digestive system disorders

One systematic review found indirect evidence that H$_2$ antagonists are more effective than placebo.

Benefits: **Healing:** One systematic review (published in 1997) indirectly compared H$_2$ antagonists versus placebo.[9] The review identified 43 single blind and double blind RCTs in 7635 people that compared different drug treatments versus each other, versus placebo, or both (total of 95 study arms, treatment given for 2–12 weeks). By pooling results across treatment arms, the review found that people in trials on H$_2$ antagonists had faster healing rates (6% healed per week, 95% CI 5.5% to 6.3%) than people in trials on placebo (3% healed per week, 95% CI 2.4% to 3.4%). **Preventing recurrence:** We found no systematic review. **Preventing complications:** We found no systematic review.

Harms: We found no RCTs examining the course of incompletely treated gastro-oesophageal reflux disease, nor any good data on the natural history of inflammatory oesophageal disease.[1] We also found no data on the level of gastric acid suppression needed to ensure adequate oesophageal healing. **Short term:** The RCTs with people on placebo found similar rates of adverse effects to the RCTs with people on H$_2$ antagonists. Most evidence about adverse effects is from case reports or uncontrolled trials. H$_2$ antagonists have been associated rarely with cytopenias, gynaecomastia, liver function test abnormalities, and hypersensitivity reactions. **Long term:** We found no controlled trials with long term follow up on the safety of chronic use of H$_2$ antagonists.

Comment: The meta-analysis did not compare groups as they were randomised, but compared one group from one trial with another group from another. This loses the benefits of randomisation since the groups being compared may have different characteristics. The results from the individual trials will be considered in a future issue of *Clinical Evidence*.

We found no RCTs that adequately compared medical and surgical treatments. One RCT found fundoplication to be significantly more effective than medical treatment, but it did not use PPIs, which would probably have increased the effectiveness of the medical treatment. We found preliminary data suggesting that PPIs and fundoplication are almost equally effective at healing. We found no good comparative data on preventing relapse or complications.

Benefits: We found no systematic review. **Healing:** We found one RCT (243 men and 4 women) comparing medical versus surgical treatment in people with complicated gastro-oesophageal reflux disease (defined as erosive oesophagitis, Barrett's oesophagus, stricture, or oesophageal ulcer).[24] The trial compared continuous medical treatment (antacids, ranitidine, metoclopramide, or sucralfate), medical treatment for symptoms only, and open fundoplication. Evaluation was performed at 6 weeks (201 people), 1 year (176 people), and 2 years (106 people), using symptom score (range 74 [least severe] to 172 [most severe]) and grade of oesophagitis (range 1 [least severe] to 4 [most severe]). People receiving fundoplication had significantly better symptom scores (mean symptom score 78 with fundoplication v 88 with symptomatic medical treatment v 90 with continuous medical treatment; P value for improvement, surgery v either medical treatment < 0.003) and grade of oesophagitis (mean decrease in grade of oesophagitis 1.5 with fundoplication v 1.9 with symptomatic medical treatment v 2.2 with continuous medical treatment; P < 0.03). **Preventing relapse:** The trial did not evaluate relapse rates. Uncontrolled trials on the long term results of open fundoplication found that up to 90% of people continued to benefit 6–20 years after surgery in terms of relief of symptoms, reduced acid exposure on pH monitoring, and absence of inflammation on endoscopy.[25–27] **Preventing complications:** We found no good data.

Harms: **Medical treatment:** See harms under PPIs versus placebo, p 315. **Surgery:** The RCT found no operative deaths, but operative complications occurred in 15% and postoperative complications occurred in 18% of people.[24] Uncontrolled studies found that intraoperative complications included splenic trauma (0–4%), viscus perforation (1–2%), and, less commonly, abscess or inadvertent vagotomy. Immediate postoperative complications included pleural effusion, pulmonary embolism, or late abscess formation. Mortality related to surgery was usually less than 1%. Late adverse effects related to fundoplication included bloating, dysphagia, gastric herniation, or breakdown of the fundoplication. Up to 15% of people underwent reoperation.

Comment: Given the evidence that PPIs are more effective than H_2 antagonists for healing and maintenance of remission (see harms of proton pump inhibitors versus H_2 antagonists, p 314),[11,18,19,28] the use of only an H_2 antagonist in the RCT[24] may have biased the results in favour of fundoplication. Preliminary data from one RCT suggest similar efficacy when comparing fundoplication with omeprazole for people with erosive oesophagitis at 3 years' follow up.[29] Individual patient characteristics may direct the clinician towards medical or surgical treatment. Some people are refractory to PPIs[30] or have severe "mechanical" reflux requiring surgery. Some people may be high risk surgical candidates or have relative contraindications to reflux surgery (e.g. scleroderma, multiple previous laparotomies, or previous gastric surgery). Younger people may prefer surgery to lifelong drug treatment. We found no studies addressing these issues.

OPTION **DIFFERENT SURGICAL TECHNIQUES**

One RCT found no difference in outcomes between total or partial fundoplication other than increased flatulence with total fundoplication. We found no RCTs comparing major kinds of surgical techniques. One RCT found no evidence that fundic mobilisation improved postoperative symptoms or rates of cure, but found that it increased rates of sliding hiatus hernia. One RCT found laparoscopic fundoplication was associated with more dysphagia than open surgery.

Benefits: **Total versus partial fundoplication:** We found one RCT comparing a total Nissen versus Toupet partial posterior fundoplication in

106 people with endoscopically proven gastro-oesophageal reflux.[31] The trial found no significant difference over a 3 year period in recurrent reflux symptoms or dysphagia between groups. **Fundic mobilisation:** We found one RCT of fundic mobilisation versus no mobilisation of Nissen fundoplication in 40 people undergoing surgery for confirmed gastro-oesophageal reflux.[32] It found no significant difference in recurrent reflux symptoms or oesophagitis between the two groups over a 3 year follow up period. We found no RCTs comparing techniques with Dor fundoplication or Hill gastro-plasty. **Laparoscopic versus open surgery:** We found one RCT, which compared laparoscopic with open Nissen fundoplication in people with gastro-oesophageal reflux disease.[33] The trial found laparoscopic Nissen fundoplication was as effective as open surgery in controlling reflux symptoms but was associated with more dysphagia (7/46 with laparoscopic treatment v 0/57 with open treatment; $P = 0.02$), and the trial was discontinued at the interim analysis stage.

Harms:　Individuals undergoing total fundoplication reported significantly more flatulence ($P < 0.01$).[31] Sliding hiatus hernia was significantly more common in those with fundic mobilisation (9/21 v 1/19; $P = 0.02$).[32]

Comment:　None.

QUESTION　**Does treatment for gastro-oesophageal reflux disease reduce the risk of progression of Barrett's oesophagus?**

We found no good evidence on the effects of treatment for gastro-oesophageal reflux in people with Barrett's oesophagus. One RCT found no significant difference in symptom control with omeprazole compared with ranitidine but it provided no clinical relevant outcomes on progression of Barrett's oesophagus.

Benefits:　One double blind RCT randomised 68 people with Barrett's oesophagus to omeprazole 40 mg twice daily or ranitidine 150 mg twice daily.[34] Symptomatic control was better in the omeprazole arm, although this did not reach statistical significance. This was reflected in a significantly lower percentage of acid reflux after 3 months' treatment (0.1% v 9.4%, $P < 0.001$). The trial found a significant reduction in the area of Barrett's oesophagus in people allocated to omeprazole but the clinical significance of this finding is uncertain. Uncontrolled studies looking at the long term effect of cimetidine,[35] ranitidine,[35] or fundoplication[36] in people with Barrett's oesophagus found no significant effect. One uncontrolled study of PPIs found evidence of regression of Barrett's oesophagus,[37] but other uncontrolled studies found no evidence of regression.[38,39] None of these studies followed more than 27 people. Small, long term studies of the effects of fundoplication on Barrett's oesophagus found that effective fundoplication (defined by ambulatory pH monitoring, symptoms, and endoscopy) may lead to regression.[40,41]

Harms:　We found no good evidence on harms of treatments for gastro-oesophageal reflux in people with Barrett's oesophagus. Small, long term studies of fundoplication suggest that after failed procedures there may be progression to dysplasia and carcinoma.[40,41]

Comment: Few centres see enough people with Barrett's oesophagus to perform long term RCTs. In addition, our poor understanding of the pathophysiology of Barrett's oesophagus means that we do not know what end point of treatment for gastro-oesophageal reflux (symptom relief, healing, elimination of acid reflux) may change the course of Barrett's metaplasia. It is also not clear whether progression can be measured endoscopically.[42,43] Only a long term, multicentre trial will be able to answer these questions.

QUESTION Does treatment for gastro-oesophageal reflux alter outcome in people with extraoesophageal manifestations of gastro-oesophageal reflux disease?

We found one systematic review which found no improvement in lung function in asthmatics treated for gastro-oesophageal reflux. We found no RCTs that looked at effects of treatment on other extraoesophageal manifestations (see table 1, p 323).

Benefits: **Asthma:** We found one systematic review of the effects of treatments in gastro-oesophageal reflux on asthma severity.[44] The review identified nine RCTs (3 of PPIs, 5 of H_2 antagonists, and one of long term conservative management). It found anti-reflux treatment did not consistently improve asthma symptoms, lung function, or the use of asthma medications compared with placebo. The reviewers concluded that there is no evidence that treating gastro-oesophageal reflux improves asthma symptoms, although they could not exclude the possibility that specific subgroups may benefit from this approach. **Other extraoesophageal manifestations:** We found no RCTs. One prospective open label cohort study of omeprazole in 182 people with chronic laryngitis and reflux found an improvement in symptoms.[45]

Harms: We found no good data on harms of treatment for gastro-oesophageal reflux specifically in people with extraoesophageal symptoms.

Comment: The link between extraoesophageal symptoms and gastro-oesophageal reflux is by association and it is often difficult to prove that gastro-oesophageal reflux is the primary cause. There was little standardisation in these trials with regard to treatments used or patient characteristics. Before good RCTs can be performed, further research must first identify clear criteria for reflux as the cause of these syndromes.

REFERENCES

1. Isolauri J, Luostarinen M, Isolauri E, et al. The natural course of gastroesophageal reflux disease: 17–22 year follow-up of 60 patients. *Am J Gastroenterol* 1997;92:37–41.

2. Richter JE. Extraesophageal manifestations of gastroesophageal reflux disease. *Clin Perspectives* 1998;1:28–39.

3. Genta RM. Review article: gastric atrophy and atrophic gastritis – nebulous concepts in search of a definition. *Aliment Pharmacol Ther* 1998; 12(suppl 1):17–23.

4. Kokkola A, Haapianinen R, Laxen F, et al. Risk of gastric carcinoma in patients with mucosal dysplasia associated with atrophic gastritis: a follow up study. *J Clin Pathol* 1996;49:979–984.

5. Van Pinxteren B, Numans ME, Bonis PA, Lau J. Short-term treatment with proton pump inhibitors, H2-receptor antagonists and prokinetics in gastro-oesophageal reflux disease-like symptoms and endoscopy negative reflux disease. In: The Cochrane Library, Issue 2, 2000. Oxford: Update Software. Search date 1999.

Gastro-oesophageal reflux disease

6. Richter JE, Peura D, Benjamin SB, Joelsson B, Whipple J. Efficacy of omeprazole for the treatment of symptomatic acid reflux disease without esophagitis. *Arch Intern Med* 2000;160: 1810–1816.

7. Richter JE, Campbell DR, Kahrilas PJ, Huang B, Fludas C. Lansoprazole compared with ranitidine for the treatment of nonerosive gastroesophageal reflux disease. *Arch Intern Med* 2000;160:1803–1809.

8. Festen HPM, Shenk E, Tan G, et al. Omeprazole versus high-dose ranitidine in mild gastroesophageal reflux disease: short- and long-term treatment. *Am J Gastroenterol* 1999;94:931–936.

9. Chiba N, DeGara CJ, Wilkinson JM, Hunt RH. Speed of healing and symptom relief in grade II to IV gastroesophageal reflux disease: a metaanalysis. *Gastroenterology* 1997;112:1798–1810. Search date July 1996; primary sources Medline plus manual search of earlier issues of *Eur J Gastroenterol Hepatol*. Reference lists of retrieved articles searched.

10. Bate CM, Booth SN, Crowe JP, et al. Omeprazole 10 mg or 20 mg once daily in the prevention of recurrence of reflux oesophagitis. *Gut* 1995;36:492–498.

11. Robinson M, Lanza F, Avner D, Haber M. Effective maintenance treatment of reflux esophagitis with low-dose lansoprazole: a randomized double blind placebo-controlled trial. *Ann Intern Med* 1996;124:859–867.

12. Kuipers EJ, Lundell L, Klinkenberg-Knol EC, et al. Atrophic gastritis and *Helicobacter pylori* infection in patients with reflux esophagitis treated with omeprazole or fundoplication. *N Engl J Med* 1996;334:1018–1022.

13. Eissele R, Brunner G, Simon B, Solcia E, Arnold R. Gastric mucosa during treatment with lansoprazole: *Helicobacter pylori* is a risk factor for argyrophil cell hyperplasia. *Gastroenterology* 1997;112:707–717.

14. Lundell L, Miettinen P, Myrvold HE, et al. Lack of effect of acid suppression therapy on gastric atrophy. *Gastroenterology* 1999;117:319–326.

15. Richter JE, Sabesin SM, Kogut DG, et al. Omeprazole versus ranitidine or ranitidine/ metoclopramide in poorly responsive symptomatic gastroesophageal reflux disease. *Am J Gastroenterol* 1996;91:1766–1772.

16. Robinson M, Decktor DL, Maton PN, et al. Omeprazole is superior to ranitidine plus metoclopramide in the short-term treatment of erosive esophagitis. *Aliment Pharmacol Ther* 1993;7:67–73.

17. Jansen JB, Van Oene JC. Standard-dose lansoprazole is more effective than high-dose ranitidine in achieving endoscopic healing and symptom relief in patients with moderately severe reflux oesophagitis. *Aliment Pharmacol Ther* 1999;13:1611–1620.

18. Dent J, Yeomans ND, Mackinnon M, et al. Omeprazole v ranitidine for prevention of relapse in reflux esophagitis: a controlled double blind trial of their efficacy and safety. *Gut* 1994;35:590–598.

19. Vigneri S, Termini R, Leandro G, et al. A comparison of five maintenance therapies for reflux esophagitis. *N Engl J Med* 1995;333:1106–1110.

20. Bardhan KD, M ller-Lissner S, et al. Symptomatic gastro-oesophageal reflux disease: double blind controlled study of intermittent treatment with omeprazole or ranitidine. *BMJ* 1999;318:502–507.

21. Hatlebakk JG, Berstad A, Carling L, et al. Lansoprazole versus omeprazole in short-term treatment of reflux oesophagitis. Results of a Scandinavian multicentre trial. *Scand J Gastroenterol* 1993;28:224–228.

22. Dekkers CP, Beker JA, Thjodleifsson B, et al. Double-blind, placebo-controlled comparison of rabeprazole 20 mg vs omeprazole 20 mg in the treatment of erosive or ulcerative gastro-oesophageal reflux disease. The European Rabeprazole Study Group. *Aliment Pharmacol Ther* 1999;13:49–50.

23. Jaspersen D, Diehl KL, Schoeppner H, Geyer P, Martens E. A comparison of omeprazole, lansoprazole and pantoprazole in the maintenance treatment of sever reflux oesophagitis. *Aliment Pharmacol Ther* 1998;12:49–52.

24. Spechler SJ. Comparison of medical and surgical therapy for complicated gastroesophageal reflux disease in veterans. *N Engl J Med* 1992;326:786–792.

25. Martinez de Haro LF, Ortiz A, Parrilla P, et al. Long-term results of Nissen fundoplication in reflux esophagitis without strictures: clinical, endoscopic, and pH–metric evaluation. *Dig Dis Sci* 1992;37:523–527.

26. Bjerkeset T, Edna T-H, Fjosne U. Long-term results after 'floppy' Nissen/Rosetti fundoplication for gastroesophageal reflux disease. *Scand J Gastroenterol* 1992;27:707–710.

27. Luostarinen M, Isolauri J, Laitinen J, et al. Fate of Nissen fundoplication after 20 years: a clinical, endoscopical, and functional analysis. *Gut* 1993;34:1015–1020.

28. Klinkenberg-Knol EC, Festen HPM, Jansen JBMJ, et al. Long-term treatment with omeprazole for refractory reflux oesophagitis: efficacy and safety. *Ann Intern Med* 1994;121:161–167.

29. Lundell L, Dalenback J, Hattlebakk J, et al. Omeprazole or antireflux surgery in the long term management of gastroesophageal reflux disease: results of a multicenter, randomized clinical trial. *Gastroenterology* 1998;114:A207.

30. Leite L, Johnston B, Just R, Castell DO. Persistent acid secretion during omeprazole therapy: a study of gastric acid profiles in patients demonstrating failure of omeprazole therapy. *Am J Gastroenterol* 1996;91:1527–1531.

31. Rydberg L, Ruth M, Abrahamsson H, Lundel L. Tailoring antireflux surgery: a randomized clinical trial. *World J Surg* 1999;23:612–618.

32. Luostarinen MES, Isolauri JO. Randomized trial to study the effect of fundic mobilization on long-term results of Nissen fundoplication. *Br J Surg* 1999;86:614–618.

33. Bais JE, Bartelsman JF, Bonjer HJ, et al. Laparoscopic or conventional Nissen fundoplication for gastro-oesophageal reflux disease: randomised clinical trial. *Lancet* 2000;355:170–174.

34. Peters FTM, Ganesh S, Kuipers EJ, et al. Endoscopic regression of Barrett's oesophagus during omeprazole treatment: a randomised double blind study. *Gut* 1999;45:489–494.

35. Sampliner RE, Garewal HS, Fennerty MB, Aickin M. Lack of impact of therapy on extent of Barrett's esophagus in 67 patients. *Dig Dis Sci* 1990;35:93–96.

36. Williamson WA, Ellis FH Jr, Gibb SP, Shahian DM, Aretz T. Effect of antireflux operation on Barrett's mucosa. *Ann Thorac Surg* 1990;49:537–542.

37. Gore S, Healey CJ, Sutton R, et al. Regression of columnar lined (Barrett's) esophagus with continuous omeprazole therapy. *Aliment Pharmacol Ther* 1993;7:623–628.

38. Sampliner RE. Effect of up to 3 years of high-dose lansoprazole on Barrett's esophagus. *Am J Gastroenterol* 1994;89:1844–1848.

39. Sharma P, Sampliner RE, Camargo E.

Normalization of esophageal pH with high-dose proton pump inhibitor therapy does not result in regression of Barrett's esophagus. *Am J Gastroenterol* 1997;92:582–585.

40. Sagar PM, Ackroyd R, Hosie KB, et al. Regression and progression of Barrett's esophagus after antireflux surgery. *Br J Surg* 1995;82:806–810.

41. Csendes A, Braghetto I, Burdiles P, et al. Long-term results of classic antireflux surgery in 152 patients with Barrett's esophagus: clinical, radiologic, endoscopic, manometric and acid reflux test analysis before and late after operation. *Surgery* 1998;123:645–657.

42. Kim R, Baggott BB, Rose S, et al. Quantitative endoscopy: precise computerized measurement of metaplastic epithelial surface area in Barrett's esophagus. *Gastroenterology* 1995;108:360–366.

43. Sharma P, Morales TG, Bhattacharyya A, Garewal HS, Sampliner RE. Squamous islands in Barrett's esophagus: what lies underneath? *Am J Gastroenterol* 1998;93:332–335.

44. Gibson PG, Henry RL, Coughlan JL. Gastro-oesophageal reflux treatment for asthma in adults and children. In: The Cochrane Library, Issue 2, 2000. Oxford: Update Software. Search date not given; primary sources Cochrane Airways Group trials register; hand searched references.

45. Hanson DG, Kamel PL, Kahrilas PJ. Outcomes of anti-reflux therapy in the treatment of chronic laryngitis. *Ann Otol Rhinol Laryngol* 1995;104:550–555.

Paul Moayyedi
Senior Lecturer
Centre for Digestive Diseases
The General Infirmary
Leeds
UK

Brendan Delaney
Senior Lecturer
University of Birmingham
Birmingham
UK

David Katzka
Cochrane Upper Gastrointestinal and
Pancreatic Diseases Group
University of Leeds
Leeds
UK

David Forman
Professor
University of Leeds
Leeds
UK

Competing interests: PM has received lecture fees from AstraZeneca, and TAP-Abbott. DF has received lecture fees from AstraZeneca, Glaxo-Wellcome, Wyeth, and Takeda.

TABLE 1 **Extraoesophageal manifestations of gastro-oesophageal reflux disease (see text, p 312, p 321).[2]**

Pulmonary	Ear, nose, and throat	Other
Asthma, chronic bronchitis, aspiration pneumonia, sleep apnoea, atelectasis, interstitial pulmonary fibrosis	Chronic cough, hoarseness, enamel erosion, halitosis, pharyngitis, subglottic stenosis, vocal cord inflammation, granuloma, possible cancer	Non-cardiac chest pain, chronic hiccups, nausea

Digestive system disorders

Search date October 2000: new for this issue

Brendan Delaney, Paul Moayyedi and David Forman

INTERVENTIONS

Key Messages

- Three systematic reviews have found that *Helicobacter pylori* eradication treatment in people with duodenal ulcers increases the proportion of ulcers healed 6 weeks after treatment was started (to 96%), and reduces 1 year recurrence rates from 58% to 12%. Three RCTs have found that, in people with a bleeding duodenal ulcer, eradication treatment versus no eradication treatment reduces the risk of re-bleeding during the subsequent year.

- One systematic review has found that *H pylori* eradication treatment heals 83% of gastric ulcers within 6 weeks of starting treatment and reduces the risk of recurrence by 1 year from 49% to 9%. We found no evidence about the effect of *H pylori* eradication treatment on the complication rates of gastric ulcers.

- One RCT found that *H pylori* eradication treatment has neither a beneficial nor a harmful effect in people with gastro-oesophageal reflux disease (GORD). About 25% of people with successful eradication treatment have persisting reflux symptoms.

- Observational studies found limited evidence that 60–93% of people with localised, low grade B cell lymphoma respond to *H pylori* eradication treatment and avoid the need for radical surgery, radiotherapy, or chemotherapy. We found no evidence from RCTs.

- We found consistent evidence from observational studies of an association between *H pylori* infection and increased risk of distal gastric adenocarcinoma of the stomach. We found no evidence of a reduced incidence of gastric cancer with eradication therapy. One RCT has found that *H pylori* eradication treatment versus no eradication treatment increases the regression of high risk lesions.

- One systematic review of *H pylori* eradication versus placebo in people with non-ulcer dyspepsia has found a reduction in dyspeptic symptoms.

- In people with uninvestigated dyspepsia, two RCTs have found that initial *H pylori* testing and eradication treatment is at least as effective in relieving dyspeptic symptoms as endoscopy-guided management. We found no evidence of benefit from initial *H pylori* eradication versus empirical acid suppression treatment.

Choice of *H pylori* eradication treatment:

- Three systematic reviews have found that dual eradication regimens versus triple eradication regimens eradicate *H pylori* from fewer people.

- We found no evidence about the effects of different eradication regimens on clinical outcomes. Systematic reviews are limited by a lack of head-to-head comparisons. Three systematic reviews found limited evidence from indirect comparisons of RCTs that triple regimens containing omeprazole and two antibiotics give consistently high eradication rates. One systematic review found limited evidence that metronidazole resistance established by laboratory testing is associated with reduced eradication of *H pylori* by regimens containing metronidazole.

- One systematic review found limited evidence, from indirect comparisons of *H pylori* eradication treatments, that 2 week regimens are no more effective than 1 week regimens at increasing the eradication risk.

- One systematic review has found that minor adverse effects are common (20–40% of people), but less than 4% of people taking any regimen have to discontinue treatment.

Helicobacter pylori infection

DEFINITION	*H pylori* is a Gram negative flagellated spiral organism found in the stomach, which is predominantly acquired in childhood. The organism is associated with a lifelong chronic gastritis and may cause other gastroduodenal disorders and their complications.
INCIDENCE/ PREVALENCE	Prevalence rates vary with birth cohort and social class in the developed world. Prevalence rates of infection in most developed countries tend to be much higher (50–80%) in those born prior to 1950, in comparison to rates (less than 20%) in those born more recently. In many developing countries the infection has a very high prevalence (80–95%) irrespective of the period of birth.[1] Adult prevalence is believed to represent the persistence of a historically higher rate of infection acquired in childhood, rather than increasing acquisition of infection during life.
AETIOLOGY/ RISK FACTORS	Overcrowded conditions associated with childhood poverty lead to increased transmission and higher prevalence rates. Adult reinfection rates are low, less than 1% per annum.[1]
PROGNOSIS	*H pylori* infection is believed to be causally related to the development of duodenal and gastric ulceration, gastric B cell lymphoma, and distal gastric cancer. About 15% of people infected with *H pylori* will develop a peptic ulcer, and 1% of people will develop gastric cancer during their lifetime.[2] *H pylori* infection is not associated with a specific type of dyspeptic symptom.
AIMS	Improvement in dyspeptic symptoms; reduction in peptic ulcer complications; reduced mortality from peptic ulcer complications of gastric cancer; improved quality of life.
OUTCOMES	Dyspeptic symptom scores and proportion of subjects with symptoms; quality of life; mortality.
METHODS	*Clinical Evidence* search and appraisal October 2000. The authors searched Medline, Embase, and the Cochrane Library for systematic reviews of *H pylori* eradication treatment from 1986 to October 2000. Further searches for additional RCTs were conducted from January 1998 to October 2000.

QUESTION What are the effects of *H pylori* eradication treatment in people with a proven duodenal ulcer?

Three systematic reviews have found that *H pylori* eradication treatment in people with duodenal ulcers increases the proportion of ulcers healed 6 weeks after treatment started (to 96%), and reduces 1 year recurrence rates from 58% to 12%. Three RCTs have found that, in people with a bleeding duodenal ulcer, eradication treatment versus no eradication treatment reduces the risk of re-bleeding during the subsequent year.

Benefits: We found three systematic reviews of *H pylori* eradication treatment in people with proven duodenal ulcers.[3–5] **Endoscopic healing:** The first systematic review (search date 1994, 7 RCTs)[3] found in indirect comparisons that triple therapy (see glossary, p 334) versus acid suppressing drugs alone healed more duodenal ulcers at 6 weeks (299/310 [96%] with triple therapy v 191/251 [76%] with omeprazole alone). The second systematic review (search date 1995, 15 RCTs that directly compared treatments)[4] found that triple therapy versus 4 weeks of antisecretory treatment increased healing rates (91–97% with eradication v 20–90% with antisecretory drugs; no statistical comparison performed).[4] The third systematic review (search date 1996, 7 RCTs conducted in the USA, 989 *H pylori* positive people with duodenal ulcer given eradication treatment)[5] found that most duodenal ulcers were endoscopically healed 6 weeks after the start of eradication treatment (68%, 95% CI 65% to 71% with eradication treatment). This review did not make any comparison with the ulcer healing rate in people given control treatment. **Prevention of recurrence:** We found two systematic reviews[3,4] that compared the effects of eradication treatment versus antisecretory drugs alone on ulcer recurrence 1 year after treatment (see table 1, p 336). The first systematic review (search date 1994) made indirect comparisons by analysing single arms from different RCTs, and as a result the comparison loses some of the benefits of randomisation. The second systematic review (search date 1995, included 20 RCTs) directly compared eradication treatment versus antisecretory treatment alone. Both systematic reviews found that eradication treatment versus antisecretory treatment produced a large reduction in ulcer recurrence rates within 1 year (NNT about 3; see table 1, p 336). **Prevention of bleeding:** We found no systematic review but found three RCTs that compared re-bleeding rates with *H pylori* eradication treatment versus no eradication treatment in people with a history of bleeding duodenal ulcer and a positive test for *H pylori* (see table 2, p 336).[6–8] The three RCTs found consistent results (overall risk of re-bleeding 6/105 [6%] with eradication treatment v 23/97 [24%] with control treatment; ARR 18%, 95% CI 8% to 28%; RR 0.28, 95% CI 0.13 to 0.61; NNT 6, 95% CI 4 to 13). **Prevention of perforation or obstruction:** We found no systematic reviews and no RCTs.

Harms: The harms of *H pylori* eradication treatment are mainly the short term effects of the antibiotics, particularly nausea from metronidazole or clarithromycin, and diarrhoea. Bismuth (see glossary, p 334) compounds may turn the stools black. One review found that side effects reported in RCTs[9] are common with bismuth (40% of people), metronidazole (39%), clarithromycin (22%), and tinidazole (7%). Discontinuation of treatment because of severe adverse effects is rare (bismuth 4%, metronidazole 2%, clarithromycin 1%, and tinidazole < 1%). Poor adherence and the use of less effective regimens might lead to increased antibiotic resistance in *H pylori*, but we found no direct evidence.

Comment: We excluded analyses that grouped people by *H pylori* status at the end of the trial. Observational evidence from RCTs suggests that duodenal ulcer recurrence rates 1 year after treatment are lower in people with successful *H pylori* eradication treatment (in the review of US RCTs: 20%, 95% CI 14% to 26% in people cured of *H pylori* v 56%, 95% CI 50% to 61% for people remaining infected).[5] The recurrence rate in non-US trials was lower than the recurrence rate found in the US trials (6% for people cured of *H pylori*). The difference in recurrence rates between US and non-US studies may be explained partially by the marked loss to follow up in the US trials (9–41%). However, countries with low prevalence of *H pylori* infection also have a low prevalence of duodenal ulcer, but a greater proportion of those ulcers arise from causes other than *H pylori*. Eradication may, therefore, be less effective where *H pylori* prevalence is low.

QUESTION What are the effects of *H pylori* eradication treatment for people with a proven gastric ulcer?

One systematic review has found that *H pylori* eradication treatment heals 83% of gastric ulcers within 6 weeks of starting treatment and reduces the risk of recurrence by 1 year from 49% to 9%. We found no evidence about the effect of *H pylori* eradication treatment on the complication rates of gastric ulcers.

Benefits: **Endoscopic healing:** We found one systematic review (search date 1995, 14 studies of people with uncomplicated gastric ulcer),[4] which analysed single arms from 14 studies. It found that, 6 weeks after the start of *H pylori* eradication treatment, 83% of gastric ulcers (95% CI 78% to 88%) were healed.[4] This systematic review found, but did not analyse, the results of six RCTs that directly compared eradication treatment versus no eradication treatment on the healing of gastric ulcers. **Prevention of recurrence:** We found one systematic review (search date 1995, 6 RCTs)[4] comparing the effects of *H pylori* eradication treatment versus 4–6 weeks antisecretory treatment on ulcer recurrence at 1 year after treatment. It found that *H pylori* eradication compared with antisecretory treatment alone significantly reduced the risk of recurrent ulcers (9% with eradication treatment v 49% with no eradication treatment; ARR 40%, 95% CI 29 to 50%; RR 0.18, 95% CI 0.1 to 0.3; NNT 3, 95% CI 2 to 4). **Prevention of complications:** We found no systematic reviews or RCTs reporting complication rates specifically for gastric ulcers.

Harms: See harms under effects of eradication treatment for *H pylori* in people with a proven duodenal ulcer, p 327.

Comment: None.

QUESTION What are the effects of *H pylori* eradication treatment in people with proven gastro-oesophageal reflux disease?

One RCT found that *H pylori* eradication treatment has neither a beneficial nor a harmful effect in people with GORD. About 25% of people with successful eradication treatment have persisting reflux symptoms.

Benefits: We found no systematic review but found one RCT (190 *H pylori* positive people with GORD but no duodenal ulcer). It found that *H pylori* eradication treatment versus placebo had no significant effect on symptomatic relapse rates (83% in both groups; difference 0%, 95% CI –11% to +11%).[10]

Harms: We found insufficient evidence about the harms of *H pylori* eradication treatment in people with GORD. Case control studies have found increased risk of reflux symptoms after *H pylori* eradication.[11] However, discontinuation of acid suppression treatment after *H pylori* eradication might have unmasked symptoms of co-existing GORD. Two RCTs (in people with duodenal ulcer) compared the effect of *H pylori* eradication treatment versus placebo on heartburn symptoms, but no analysis by intention to treat was reported.[12,13] One RCT (2324 people from the general population) found no significant increase in reflux symptoms 2 years after *H pylori* eradication versus placebo treatment.[14]

Comment: None.

QUESTION **What are the effects of *H pylori* eradication treatment in people with B cell lymphoma of the stomach?**

Observational studies found limited evidence that 60–93% of people with localised, low grade B cell lymphoma respond to *H pylori* eradication treatment, avoiding the need for radical surgery, radiotherapy, or chemotherapy. We found no evidence from RCTs.

Benefits: We found no systematic review and no RCTs of *H pylori* eradication treatment for B cell gastric lymphoma (see glossary, p 334).

Harms: We found insufficient evidence about the harms of *H pylori* eradication treatment in people with B cell gastric lymphoma.

Comment: Treatment options for primary gastric lymphoma include surgery, radiotherapy, chemotherapy, and *H pylori* eradication. We found no direct comparative studies. We found six prospective cohort studies of *H pylori* eradication therapy in people with localised, low grade lymphomas.[15] Tumour regression occurred in 60–93% of people, but responses were sometimes delayed and some people relapsed within 1 year of treatment.

QUESTION **What are the effects of *H pylori* eradication treatment in people at increased risk of gastric cancer?**

We found consistent evidence from observational studies of an association between *H pylori* infection and increased risk of distal gastric adenocarcinoma of the stomach. We found no evidence of a reduced incidence of gastric cancer with eradication therapy. One RCT has found that *H pylori* eradication treatment versus no eradication treatment increases the regression of high risk lesions.

Benefits: **General population:** We found no systematic review and no RCTs of *H pylori* eradication treatment to prevent gastric cancer (adenocarcinoma) in the general population. **In people at high risk of gastric cancer:** We found no systematic review and no RCTs that reported the rate of development of gastric cancer. One RCT (852 people with gastric atrophy or intestinal metaplasia found at screening endoscopy) compared *H pylori* eradication treatment, β carotene, ascorbic acid, and placebo in a factorial design.[16] It found that *H pylori* eradication treatment versus no eradication treatment increased the relative risk of lesion regression (calculated by multivariate modelling) for both atrophy (4.8, 95% CI 1.6 to 14.2) and intestinal metaplasia (3.1, 95% CI 1.0 to 9.3).

Harms: We found insufficient evidence in people at high risk of gastric cancer.

Comment: We found four systematic reviews of observational studies of the association between *H pylori* infection and gastric cancer.[17–20] One review (search date 1999, 42 case control studies)[17] found an increased risk of gastric adenocarcinoma in people with *H pylori* (OR 2.04, 95% CI 1.69 to 2.45). The second review (search date 1998, 10 nested case control studies within prospective cohort studies, 818 cases of adenocarcinoma)[18] performed a meta-analysis, which also found increased risk in people with *H pylori* (RR 2.5, 95% CI 1.1 to 3.2). Observational studies with short follow up periods may underestimate the risk of gastric cancer from *H pylori* infection (because gastric cancer is associated with gastric atrophy and serological tests for *H pylori* infection may give false negative results in people with gastric cancer and atrophy). A meta-analysis of prospective case control studies found that the odds ratio increased to 8.7 (95% CI 2.7 to 45) when the interval between serological sampling and diagnosis of cancer was over 14 years.[19] A further systematic review (search date 1996, 19 studies, 2491 subjects, 3959 controls)[20] found that the apparent risk of adenocarcinoma from *H pylori* infection decreased significantly with increasing age (OR 9.29, 95% CI 3.4 to 34 at age 20–29 years; OR 1.05, 95% CI 0.73 to 1.52 at age > 70 years).

QUESTION **What are the effects of *H pylori* eradication treatment in people with proven non-ulcer dyspepsia?**

One systematic review of *H pylori* eradication versus placebo in people with non-ulcer dyspepsia has found a reduction in dyspeptic symptoms.

Benefits: We found one systematic review (search date 2000, 9 RCTs, 2541 people),[21] which found that *H pylori* eradication versus placebo produced a small but significant improvement in dyspeptic symptoms 3–12 months after the treatment started (AR of recurrent symptoms: 72% with placebo v 64% with eradication treatment; ARR 7%, 95% CI 3% to 10%; RR 0.91, 95% CI 0.86 to 0.96; NNT 15, 95% CI 10 to 31).[21] Three of the RCTs also measured the effect of *H pylori* eradication treatment on quality of life; no significant effect was found.

Harms: See harms under effects of eradication treatment for *H pylori* in people with a proven duodenal ulcer, p 327. We found two RCTs[22,23] that assessed whether *H pylori* eradication treatment increases the prevalence of oesophagitis in people with non-ulcer dyspepsia. They found that *H pylori* eradication treatment versus placebo increased endoscopically assessed oesophagitis (5.7% with eradication treatment v 2.9% with placebo; ARI +2.8%, 95% CI −0.5% to +6%; RR 2.1, 95% CI 0.94 to 4.6). No trial evaluated individual dyspeptic symptoms, so the effect on reflux symptoms cannot be estimated separately from epigastric pain.

Comment: None.

QUESTION **What are the effects of *H pylori* eradication treatment in people with uninvestigated dyspepsia?**

Two RCTs have found that initial *H pylori* testing and eradication treatment is at least as effective in relieving dyspeptic symptoms as endoscopy-guided management. We found no evidence about initial *H pylori* eradication versus empirical acid suppression treatment.

Benefits: **Initial *H pylori* testing versus initial endoscopy:** We found one systematic review of initial management strategies for dyspepsia, which did not find any RCTs of *H pylori* testing plus eradication.[24] We found two subsequent RCTs comparing *H pylori* testing plus eradication versus prompt endoscopy. The first RCT (500 people with >2 weeks' epigastric pain) found that ^{13}C-urea breath testing plus (if positive) *H pylori* eradication treatment versus prompt endoscopy produced no significant difference in symptom free days, but reduced the endoscopy rate (to 40% of the rate with prompt endoscopy).[25] The second RCT (104 *H pylori* positive people, aged < 45 years) compared *H pylori* testing and (where positive) eradication treatment versus endoscopy plus tailored treatment (*H pylori* eradication treatment for people with peptic ulcer; treatment with a proton pump inhibitor [see glossary, p 334] for oesophagitis; step up acid suppression treatment for non-ulcer dyspepsia).[26] The RCT found that the "test and eradicate" strategy compared with endoscopy reduced the number of people who were symptomatic after 1 year (57% with initial *H pylori* testing v 70% with initial endoscopy; ARR +13%, 95% CI –6% to +31%; RR 0.82, 95% CI 0.59 to 1.1). **Initial *H pylori* testing versus initial empirical acid suppression:** We found no RCTs of *H pylori* eradication treatment versus empirical acid suppression treatment.

Harms: A few people given *H pylori* eradication treatment discontinued treatment because of short term side effects (14/104 [13%] people in the first RCT[25] and 4/80 [5%] in the second RCT[26]).

Comment: The results of the two RCTs will not be applicable to all people with dyspepsia. People with "alarm" symptoms (dysphagia, weight loss, jaundice, epigastric mass, or anaemia), or over the age of 55 years, with either continuous epigastric pain or first onset of symptoms in the previous year, may have a significant risk of upper gastrointestinal malignancy. For these people prompt endoscopy should be considered. Both RCTs[25,26] were conducted in a hospital setting. The first RCT stipulated that all eligible people with dyspepsia consulting with a general medical practitioner should be included.[25] The second RCT entered only routine referrals.[26] The results might not apply directly to primary care, where people with less severe dyspepsia might be treated and *H pylori* eradication rates might be lower, and the reassuring or anxiety provoking effect of specialist consultation might not be replicated. At least four primary care RCTs are in progress: a comparison of "test and treat" versus prompt endoscopy in Nottingham, UK (RFA Logan, personal communication, 2001); a multicentre comparison of *H pylori* "test and treat" versus treatment with a proton pump inhibitor in the UK (BC Delaney, personal communication, 2001); a comparison of *H pylori* eradication treatment versus placebo in *H pylori* positive people with dyspepsia in Guelph, Canada (N Chiba, personal communication, 2001); a comparison of *H pylori* eradication treatment versus omeprazole in *H pylori* positive people with dyspepsia in Helsinki, Finland (P Sipponen, personal communication, 2001).

OPTION   DUAL VERSUS TRIPLE REGIMENS

Three systematic reviews have found that dual versus triple eradication regimens eradicate *H pylori* from fewer people.

Benefits: **Duodenal ulcer complication rates:** We found no systematic review and no RCTs. **Eradication rates:** We found one systematic review (search date 1995, 19 RCTs of omeprazole plus amoxicillin versus triple regimens containing bismuth, 17 RCTs of dual regimens containing a proton pump inhibitor versus triple regimens [see glossary, p 334]).[9] No formal meta-analysis was performed, but dual regimens versus triple regimens (two antibiotics plus either a proton pump inhibitor or bismuth) reduced the number of people with successful *H pylori* eradication. For omeprazole 20 mg twice daily plus amoxicillin 1 g twice daily in 4137 people, the overall eradication rate was 59% (95% CI 58% to 61%). For omeprazole 20 mg twice daily plus clarithromycin 250 mg twice daily in 1265 people, the eradication rate was 68% (95% CI 65% to 70%). The review found 31 studies of amoxicillin or clarithromycin in combination with other proton pump inhibitors in dual regimens: the pooled eradication rates by intention to treat analysis (see glossary, p 334) were less than 55%.

Harms: See harms under effects of eradication treatment for *H pylori* in people with a proven duodenal ulcer, p 327.

Comment: Systematic reviews of *H pylori* eradication treatments are difficult to interpret because they rarely pool RCTs in an analysis that maintains the randomised comparison. Instead, all treatment arms for one combination from any one trial are pooled together. This greatly weakens the strength of the evidence to that of a non-randomised study. Many RCTs have additional design problems, such as lack of a gold standard for defining cure and publication only as an abstract. A systematic review of this topic is in progress.[27] Despite the limitations, the evidence suggests that the highest *H pylori* eradication rates occur with combinations of two antibiotics plus a proton pump inhibitor or bismuth. Factors that might influence the choice of eradication treatment for an individual also include ease of adherence, potential harms, allergy or sensitivity, drug resistance, and cost.

OPTION   WHAT ARE THE EFFECTS OF DIFFERENT TRIPLE REGIMENS?

We found no evidence about the effects of different eradication regimens on clinical outcomes. Three systematic reviews found limited evidence from indirect comparisons of RCTs that triple regimens containing omeprazole and two antibiotics give consistently high eradication rates. One systematic review found limited evidence that metronidazole resistance established by laboratory testing is associated with reduced eradication of *H pylori* by regimens containing metronidazole.

Benefits: **Complication rates:** We found no systematic review and no direct comparison of the effect of different eradication treatments on complication rates. **Eradication rates:** We found three systematic reviews, most of which included indirect comparisons between RCTs (see table 3, p 337).[9,28,29] An intention to treat analysis of direct (head-to-head) comparisons in 4 RCTs[29] found that more people had successful *H pylori* eradication with clarithromycin 500 mg twice daily versus 250 mg twice daily in combination with a proton pump inhibitor and amoxicillin (AR 90% v 80%; ARR 10%, 95% CI 3% to 17%; RR 0.89, 95% CI 0.81 to 0.97; NNT 11, 95% CI 6 to 38). There was no significant difference in eradication rates between clarithromycin 500 mg twice daily and clarithromycin 250 mg twice daily in combination with a proton pump inhibitor and metronidazole (AR 89% with clarithromycin 500 mg twice daily v 87% with clarithromycin 250 mg twice daily; ARR +1.5%, 95% CI −3.6% to +6.6%; RR 0.98, 95% CI 0.93 to 1.04). We found no clear evidence of clinically important differences between the eradication rates for the different triple regimens. The limited evidence from the indirect comparisons found the highest eradication rates (85–90%) with omeprazole (20 mg daily, or equivalent) plus a combination of two of the following: amoxicillin (1–1.5 g daily), metronidazole (1.2 g daily), or clarithromycin (500 mg daily with metronidazole or 1 g daily with amoxicillin). **Antibiotic resistance:** We found one systematic review (search date 1995, 19 RCTs, 10 006 people with metronidazole sensitive *H pylori*, 452 with metronidazole resistant *H pylori*), and one RCT that assessed the efficacy of metronidazole (or other nitroimidazole) based triple and quadruple regimens with strains of *H pylori* that were resistant in the laboratory.[30] They found that nitroimidazole based regimens achieved *H pylori* eradication in significantly fewer people with strains showing nitroimidazole resistance in the laboratory than in people with sensitive strains (99%, 95% CI 95% to 100% eradication in people with sensitive strains v 69%, 95% CI 60% to 67% in people with resistant strains).

Harms: See harms under effects of eradication treatment for *H pylori* in people with a proven duodenal ulcer, p 327.

Comment: The systematic review of nitroimidazole resistance concluded that clinically important reduction of eradication rates is unlikely with a proportion of resistant strains below 15–25%.[30]

OPTION   **ONE WEEK VERSUS 2 WEEK *H PYLORI* ERADICATION TREATMENT**

One systematic review found limited evidence, from indirect comparisons of *H pylori* eradication treatments, that a 2 week triple regimen versus a 1 week regimen does not increase the eradication rate.

Benefits: **Complication rates:** We found no systematic review and no RCTs. **Eradication rates:** We found one systematic review (search date 1996, 74 RCTs, 1169 people with 1 week regimens, 3203 people with 2 week regimens), comparing the effect of duration of eradication treatment on the number of people from whom *H pylori* was eradicated.[31] The systematic review did not make any direct comparisons, but compared the results of different RCTs that had used different lengths of treatment. It found that 2 week versus 1 week regimens did not increase the eradication rate (84%, 95% CI 81%

to 86% with 1 week omeprazole based triple regimens v 71%, 95% CI 69% to 73% with 2 week regimens).[31]

Harms: See harms under effects of eradication treatment for *H pylori* in people with a proven duodenal ulcer, p 327.

Comment: The indirect comparison is a weak form of evidence, equivalent to an observational study. The characteristics of the people, settings, and procedures in the different RCTs may not be comparable.

GLOSSARY

Bismuth A compound containing bismuth, such as bismuth subsalicilate or ranitidine bismuth citrate.

Dual regimen *H pylori* eradication regimen consisting of two components.

Intention to treat analysis All subjects analysed according to the group to which they were randomised, rather than some other grouping, such as post-treatment *H pylori* status, or an analysis based merely on those who completed the study.

MALT "Mucosa-associated lymphoid tissue" is constitutionally found in the intestine but not in the stomach. MALT lymphoma is also known as B cell gastric lymphoma.

Proton pump inhibitor A drug that directly inhibits the mechanism within the stomach that secretes acid, such as esomeprazole, lansoprazole, omeprazole, or rabeprazole.

Triple regimen *H pylori* eradication regimen consisting of three components. The original "triple therapy" was bismuth subsalicilate, metronidazole, and either amoxicillin or tetracycline. Now the term usually applies to a proton pump inhibitor plus two antibiotics.

REFERENCES

1. Axon AT. *Helicobacter pylori* infection. *J Antimicrob Chemother* 1993;32(suppl A):61–68.

2. Graham DY. Can therapy ever be denied for *Helicobacter pylori* infection? *Gastroenterology* 1997;113:S113–S117.

3. Moore RA. Helicobacter pylori and peptic ulcer. Cortecs Diagnostics and the Health Technology Association. Oxford, 1995. Search date 1994; primary sources Medline, survey of pharmaceutical companies. http://195.172.98.196/bandopubs/hpyl/hp0.html (last accessed 27 March 2001).

4. Penston JG. Review article: Clinical aspects of *Helicobacter pylori* eradication therapy in peptic ulcer disease. *Aliment Pharmacol Ther* 1996;10:469–486. Search date October 1995; primary sources Medline, conference abstracts 1990–1994.

5. Laine L, Hopkins RJ, Girardi LS. Has the impact of *Helicobacter pylori* therapy on ulcer recurrence in the United States been overstated? A meta-analysis of rigorously designed trials. *Am J Gastroenterol* 1998;93:1409–1415. Search date 1996; primary sources Medline, conference abstracts, pharmaceutical companies (US trials only).

6. Lai K-C, Hui W-M, Wong B C-Y, Hu WHC, Ching C-K, Lam S-K. Treatment of *Helicobacter pylori* in patients with duodenal ulcer haemorrhage–a long term randomised controlled study. *Am J Gastroenterol* 2000;95:2225–2232.

7. Rokkas T, Karameris A, Mavrogeorgis A, Rallis E, Giannikos N. Eradication of *Helicobacter pylori* reduces the possibility of rebleeding in peptic ulcer disease. *Gastrointest Endosc* 1995;41:1–4.

8. Jaspersen D, Koerner T, Schorr W, Brennenstuhl M, Raschka C, Hammar CH. *Helicobacter pylori* eradication reduces the rate of rebleeding in ulcer hemorrhage. *Gastrointest Endosc* 1995;41:5–7.

9. Penston JG, McColl KEL. Eradication of *Helicobacter pylori*: An objective assessment of current therapies. *Br J Clin Pharmacol* 1997;43:223–243. Search date October 1995; primary sources Medline, conference abstracts.

10. Moayyedi P, Bardhan KD, Wrangstadh M, Dixon MF, Brown L, Axon ATR. Does eradication of *Helicobacter pylori* influence the recurrence of symptoms in patients with symptomatic gastro-oesophageal reflux disease? A randomised double blind study. *Gut* 1999;44(suppl 1):A112.

11. Labenz J, Blum AL, Bayerdorffer E, Meining A, Stolte M, Borsch G. Curing *Helicobacter pylori* infection in patients with duodenal ulcer may provoke reflux esophagitis. *Gastroenterology* 1997;112:1442–1447.

12. Vakil N, Hahn B, McSorley D. Recurrent symptoms and gastro-oesophageal reflux disease in patients with duodenal ulcer treated for *Helicobacter pylori* infection. *Aliment Pharmacol Ther* 2000;14:45–51.

13. Fallone CA, Barkun AN, Friedman G, et al. Is *Helicobacter pylori* eradication associated with gastroesophageal reflux disease? *Am J Gastroenterol* 2000;95:914–920.

14. Moayyedi P, Feltbower R, Brown J, et al. Effect of population screening and treatment for *Helicobacter pylori* on dyspepsia and quality of life in the community: a randomised controlled trial. *Lancet* 2000;355:1665–1669.

15. Roher HD, Vereet PR, Wormer O, Muller FP, Ohmann C, Fisbach W. *Helicobacter pylori* in the upper gastrointestinal tract: medical or surgical treatment of gastric lymphoma? *Langenbeck's Arch Surg* 2000;385:97–105. Search date

unavailable; primary sources Medline and hand searches.

16. Correa P, Fontham ETH, Bravo JC, et al. Chemoprevention of gastric dysplasia: Randomized trial of antioxidant supplements and anti-*Helicobacter pylori* therapy. *J Natl Cancer Inst* 2000;92:1881–1888.

17. Eslick GD, Lim LLY, Byles JE, Xia HHX, Talley NJ. Association of *Helicobacter pylori* infection with gastric carcinoma: A meta-analysis. *Am J Gastroenterol* 1999;94:2373–2379. Search date March 1999; primary sources Medline, Cinahl, Cancer CD, Biological Abstracts, Current Contents, survey of experts.

18. Danesh J. *Helicobacter pylori* infection and gastric cancer: systemic review of the epidemiological studies. *Aliment Pharmacol Ther* 1999;13:851–856. Search date 1998; primary sources Medline, hand searches.

19. Forman D, Webb P, Parsonnet J. *Helicobacter pylori* and gastric cancer. *Lancet* 1994;343:243–244. Search date 1994; primary source expert group.

20. Huang JQ, Sridhar S, Chen Y, Hunt RH. Meta-analysis of the relationship between *Helicobacter pylori* seropositivity and gastric cancer. *Gastroenterology* 1998;114:1169–79. Search date April 1996; primary source Medline.

21. Soo S, Moayyedi P, Deeks J, et al. Eradication *Helicobacter pylori* for non-ulcer dyspepsia. In: The Cochrane Library, Issue 3, 2000. Oxford: Update Software. Search date May 2000; primary sources Medline, Embase, Science Citation Index, conference abstracts, survey of experts.

22. Blum AL, Talley NJ, O'Morain C, et al. Lack of effect of treating *Helicobacter pylori* infection in patients with nonulcer dyspepsia. *N Engl J Med* 1998;339:1875–1881.

23. Koelz HR, Arnold R, Stolte M, Blum AL. Treatment of *Helicobacter pylori* (HP) does not improve symptoms of functional dyspepsia. *Gastroenterology* 1998;114:G0747.

24. Delaney BC, Innes MA, Deeks J, et al. Initial management strategies for dyspepsia. In: The Cochrane Library, Issue 3, 2000. Oxford: Update Software. Search date January 1999; primary sources Medline, Embase, Science Citation Index, conference abstracts, survey of experts.

25. Lassen AT, Pedersen FM, Bytzer P, Scaffalitzky de Muckadell OB. *Helicobacter pylori* "test and eradicate" or prompt endoscopy for management of dyspeptic patients. A randomised controlled trial with one year follow-up. *Lancet* 2000;356:455–460.

26. Heaney A, Collins JSA, Watson RGP, McFarland RJ, Bamford KB, Tham TCK. A prospective randomised trial of a "test and treat" policy versus endoscopy based management in young *Helicobacter pylori* positive patients with ulcer-like dyspepsia, referred to a hospital clinic. *Gut* 1999;45:186–190.

27. Forman D, Bazzoli F, Bennett C, et al. Therapies for the eradication of *Helicobacter pylori* (protocol for a Cochrane Review). In: The Cochrane Library, Issue 4, 2001. Oxford: Update Software.

28. Pipkin GA, Dixon JS, Williamson R, Wood JR. Clarithromycin dual therapy regimens for eradication of *Helicobacter pylori*: A review. *Helicobacter* 1997;2:159–171. Search date May 1997; primary sources Medline, conference abstracts.

29. Huang JQ, Hunt RH. The importance of clarithromycin dose in the management of *Helicobacter pylori* infection: a meta-analysis of triple therapies with a proton pump inhibitor, clarithromycin and amoxicillin or metronidazole. *Aliment Pharmacol Ther* 1999;13:719–729. Search date March 1998; primary sources Medline, conference abstracts.

30. Lind T, Peal MFU. The Mach 2 study: Role of omeprazole in eradication of *Helicobacter pylori* with 1 week triple therapies. *Gastroenterology* 1999;116:248–253.

31. Schmid CH, Whiting G, Cory D, Ross SD, Chalmers TC. Omeprazole plus antibiotics in the eradication of *Helicobacter pylori* infection: a meta-regression analysis of randomised controlled trials. *Am J Therapeutics* 1999;6:25–36. Search date April 1996; primary sources Medline, conference abstracts.

Brendan Delaney
Department of Primary Care and
General Practice
University of Birmingham
Birmingham
UK

Paul Moayyedi
Centre for Digestive Disease
University of Leeds
Leeds
UK

David Forman
Cochrane Upper Gastrointestinal and
Pancreatic Disease Collaborative
Review Group
University of Leeds
Leeds
UK

Competing interests: PM has acted as an independent medical advisor for AstraZeneca. DF has received lecture fees from AstraZeneca, GlaxoSmithKline, Wyeth, and Takeda. BD, none declared.

Helicobacter pylori infection

TABLE 1 Results of systematic reviews that compared the effects of eradication treatment versus non-eradication treatment on the rate of ulcer recurrence 1 year after treatment (see text, p 327).[3,4]

Reference	Treatment		Ulcer recurrence by 1 year	
	Eradication	Control	Eradication	Control
3	Bismuth, tetracycline, metronidazole, and ranitidine or omeprazole	Histamine receptor antagonist alone 4–6 weeks	13/148 (8.8%) 7 RCTs	100/121 (83%) 5 RCTs
4 (20 RCTs)	Any type of eradication treatment	Antisecretory treatment	128/1059 (12%)	575/988 (58%)

TABLE 2 Effect of *H pylori* eradication therapy versus no eradication treatment on re-bleeding in people with a history of bleeding duodenal ulcer and positive test for *H pylori* (see text, p 327).[6–8]

Reference	Treatment		Re-bleeding (%)	
	Eradication	Control	Eradication	Control
6	Bismuth, amoxicillin, metronidazole	Bismuth	6/60 (10%)	12/60 (20%)
7	Omeprazole, amoxicillin (2 weeks)	Omeprazole	0/16 (0%)	5/15 (33%)
8	Omeprazole, amoxicillin (2 weeks)	Omeprazole	0/29 (0%)	6/22 (27%)

TABLE 3 *H pylori* eradication rates for triple regimens containing bismuth versus triple regimens containing proton pump inhibitors (see text, p 337).[9,28,29]

Regimen	Source	Eradication rate (95% CI)
Bismuth triple regimens		
Bismuth, metronidazole, amoxicillin/tetracycline	7979 people[9]	78%* (77% to 79%)
Ranitidine, bismuth citrate, clarithromycin	11 RCTs[28]	85%* (83% to 87%)
Proton pump inhibitor triple regimens		
Triple therapy (PPI, two antibiotics)	79 RCTs 3389 people[9]	86%* (95% CI 85% to 87%)
Clarithromycin 250 mg bd, PPI, amoxicillin	4 RCTs[29]	80%†
Clarithromycin 500 mg bd, PPI, amoxicillin		89%†
Clarithromycin 250 mg bd, PPI, metronidazole		90%†
Clarithromycin 500 mg bd, PPI, metronidazole		87%†
Bismuth and proton pump inhibitor triple regimens		
Bismuth, tetracycline, amoxicillin, PPI	No evidence found	–

*Rates are indirect comparisons based on pooled results from many different RCTs. †Rates represent direct comparisons. bd, twice daily; PPI, proton pump inhibitor.

Digestive system disorders

Search date January 2001

Peter McCulloch

INTERVENTIONS

Likely to be beneficial

Complete surgical resection (cancer confined to stomach and perigastric lymph nodes). . . .340

Palliative partial gastrectomy (symptomatic cancer that cannot be curatively resected) 340

Subtotal gastrectomy for operable distal tumours 340

Trade off between benefits and harms

Palliative total gastrectomy (symptomatic cancer, spread preventing curative resection) 340

Unknown effectiveness

Removal of adjacent organs. . .341

Radical versus conservative lymphadenectomy 342

Adjuvant chemotherapy 343

Unlikely to be beneficial

Palliative gastrectomy (asymptomatic or mildly symptomatic cancer, spread preventing curative resection) 340

Total gastrectomy "de principe" for cancer of the distal stomach (no evidence of greater benefit than subtotal gastrectomy, and evidence of greater harm). . .340

To be covered in future issues of *Clinical Evidence*

Adjuvant radiotherapy

Adjuvant chemoradiotherapy

Endoscopic mucosal resection for early gastric cancer

Addition of bacterial and fungal extracts to adjuvant chemotherapy

Regional chemotherapy

Key Messages

- Prospective and retrospective cohort studies have found a strong association between survival and complete excision of all tumour, with microscopic confirmation of clear resection margins.

- Retrospective cohort studies found short survival and high perioperative mortality but improved quality of life in symptomatic people undergoing palliative gastrectomy.

- Two RCTs found similar survival after total gastrectomy (see glossary, p 345) and subtotal gastrectomy in people with primary tumours in the distal stomach.

- Retrospective subgroup analysis of RCTs and prospective cohort studies have found increased morbidity and mortality from resection of additional organs (spleen and distal pancreas) versus no resection.

- Four RCTs found no clear evidence of benefit or harm from extended lymph node dissection.

- Three systematic reviews of RCTs found weak evidence of improved survival from adjuvant pre or postoperative chemotherapy for stomach cancer.

DEFINITION Stomach cancer is an adenocarcinoma arising in the stomach, including tumours arising at or just below the gastro-oesophageal junction (type 2 and 3 junctional tumours). Tumours are staged according to degree of invasion and spread (see table 1, p 347).

INCIDENCE/ PREVALENCE The incidence of stomach cancer varies among countries and by sex (incidence per 100 000 population per year in Japanese men is about 80, Japanese women 30, British men 18, British women 10, white American men 11, white American women 7).[1] Incidence has declined dramatically in North America, Australia, and New Zealand since 1930, but decline in Europe has been slower.[2] In the USA, stomach cancer remains relatively common among particular ethnic groups, especially Japanese Americans and some Hispanic groups. The incidence of cancer of the proximal stomach and gastro-oesophageal junction is rising rapidly in most Western countries; the reasons for this are poorly understood.[3,4]

AETIOLOGY/ RISK FACTORS Distal stomach cancer is strongly associated with lifelong infection with *Helicobacter pylori* and poor dietary intake of antioxidant vitamins (A, C, E).[5,6] In Western Europe and North America, distal stomach cancer is associated with relative socioeconomic deprivation. Proximal cancer is strongly associated with smoking (OR about 4)[7] and is probably associated with gastro-oesophageal reflux, obesity, high fat intake, and medium to high socioeconomic status.

PROGNOSIS Invasive cancer (stages T_2–T_4) is fatal without surgery. Mean survival without treatment is less than 6 months from diagnosis.[8,9] Intramucosal or submucosal cancer (stage T_1) may progress slowly to invasive cancer over several years.[10] The prognosis after macroscopically and microscopically complete resection (R0) is related strongly to disease stage (see glossary, p 345), particularly penetration of the serosa (stage T_3) and lymph node involvement. Five year survival rates range from over 90% in intramucosal cancer to about 20% in people with stage T_3N_2 disease (see table 1, p 347). In the USA, over 50% of people recently diagnosed with stomach cancer have regional lymph node metastasis or involvement of adjacent organs. In Japan, the 5 year survival rate for advanced disease is reported to be about 50%, but the explanation of the difference remains unclear. Comparisons between Japanese and Western practice are confounded by factors such as age, fitness, and disease stage, as well as by tumour location, because many Western series include gastro-oesophageal junction adenocarcinoma with a much lower survival after surgery.

AIMS To prevent progression; extend survival; and relieve symptoms, with minimal adverse effects.

OUTCOMES Survival; quality of life; adverse effects of treatment.

METHODS *Clinical Evidence* update search and appraisal January 2001. Hand searches of conference proceedings and consultations with experts were also used to identify relevant studies.

OPTION COMPLETE VERSUS INCOMPLETE TUMOUR RESECTION

Prospective and retrospective cohort studies have found a strong association between survival and complete excision of the primary tumour.

Benefits:
Surgery versus no surgery: We found no systematic reviews or RCTs. We found two observational studies of surgery versus no surgery. People who did not undergo resection (generally those with the most advanced disease and highest comorbidity) had a near zero 5 year survival in all case series.[8,9] In people with similar stage weight loss and performance status, macroscopically incomplete tumour resection (palliative gastrectomy) was associated with twice the survival time of non-resection and with better quality of life owing to relief of tumour symptoms.[11] **Positive versus clear microscopic resection margins:** We found no systematic reviews or RCTs comparing these options directly. Multivariate risk factor analysis of RCTs and retrospective cohort studies have found that failure to achieve microscopically clear resection margins was associated with a poor outcome independently of other indicators of tumour spread and behaviour.[12–14]

Harms:
We found no systematic reviews or RCTs.

Comment:
Current consensus is that improving long term survival is best achieved by complete resection of the primary tumour with microscopic confirmation of clear resection margins ("curative" gastrectomy).

OPTION TOTAL VERSUS SUBTOTAL GASTRECTOMY FOR RESECTABLE DISTAL TUMOURS

Two RCTs have found similar survival after total and distal subtotal gastrectomy in people with primary tumours in the distal stomach.

Benefits:
We found no systematic reviews, but we found two RCTs (787 people) comparing total versus subtotal gastrectomy.[15–18] Neither RCT used blinded allocation. **Five year survival:** The larger RCT involved 648 people aged under 76 years with a resectable tumour and a macroscopic proximal margin of more than 6 cm.[17,18] All had regional lymphadenectomy (D2). There was no significant difference between the groups in the incidence of microscopic resection margin involvement (found in 15/315 [4.8%] with subtotal gastrectomy v 6/303 [2.0%] with total gastrectomy; ARI +2.8%, 95% CI –0.1% to +9.6%) or in 5 year survival (Kaplan–Meier 5 year survival estimates 65% for subtotal v 62% for total gastrectomy; HR 0.89, 95% CI 0.68 to 1.17). Multivariate analysis found that after adjustment for covariates, the type of stomach surgery had no influence on survival (5 year HR 1.01, 95% CI 0.76 to 1.33). The other RCT included 169 people with potentially curable distal stomach cancer. No difference was found in 5 year survival (48% in each group, CI not available). **Nutritional function and quality of life:** These outcomes were better after distal subtotal gastrectomy than after total gastrectomy.[19–22]

Harms: **Postoperative morbidity:** Included intra-abdominal sepsis, chest infections, wound sepsis, and fistulae. The larger RCT found that subtotal gastrectomy reduced postoperative morbidity (29/320 [9%] for subtotal gastrectomy v 40/304 [13%] after total gastrectomy), and mean duration of hospital stay (13.8 days for subtotal v 15.4 days for total gastrectomy).[17,18] The other RCT found no significant differences in postoperative morbidity (25/76 [32%] for total gastrectomy v 32/93 [34%] for subtotal gastrectomy).[15,16] **Postoperative mortality:** In the larger RCT, postoperative mortality was lower in the subtotal gastrectomy group, but not significantly so (4/320 [1%] for subtotal v 7/304 [2%] for total). The other RCT found no significant differences in postoperative mortality (1/76 [1.3%] for total v 3/93 [3.2%] for subtotal gastrectomy). Nearly all non-randomised studies that we identified reported higher mortality after total gastrectomy compared with subtotal gastrectomy, but total gastrectomy tended to be performed on people with more extensive disease.

Comment: Infiltration of the proximal resection margin by microscopic tumour deposits is perceived as a problem in people with poorly differentiated "diffuse" cancer of the distal stomach undergoing distal subtotal gastrectomy. Some surgeons have therefore recommended total gastrectomy "de principe" (see glossary, p 345) for these tumours. The two RCTs have found similar survival after total and distal subtotal gastrectomy in people with primary tumours in the distal stomach.[15–18] Both RCTs recruited otherwise fit people, which may explain the low postoperative mortality rates. The lack of any evidence of survival benefit, and the poorer nutritional and quality of life outcome, argue against total gastrectomy where subtotal distal gastrectomy (see glossary, p 345) is technically possible with an adequate margin.

OPTION **REMOVAL OF ADJACENT ORGANS**

Retrospective analyses of removal of additional organs (spleen and distal pancreas) versus no removal have found increased morbidity and mortality.

Benefits: We found no systematic reviews and no RCTs that randomised people with stomach cancer to removal or no removal of adjacent organs.

Harms: Retrospective analyses of RCTs and cohort studies in which removal of the spleen and distal pancreas had been performed routinely during radical total gastrectomy (D2) (see table 2, p 347), and at the surgeon's discretion during non-radical total gastrectomy (D1), found that removal of the spleen or distal pancreas was associated with increased perioperative mortality (OR about 2) and no evidence of improved long term survival.[23,24]

Comment: Some advocates of radical surgery have suggested routine removal of the spleen and distal pancreas to ensure complete regional lymph node dissection during total gastrectomy. Current consensus is that removal of adjacent organs is justified only when necessary to ensure complete tumour removal, or when required because of trauma during surgery.

OPTION **RADICAL VERSUS CONSERVATIVE LYMPHADENECTOMY**

Four RCTs have found no clear benefit from extended lymph node removal. The results may be affected by lack of experience with the extended dissection technique.

Benefits:

Regional (D2, D3) versus local lymphadenectomy (D1): We found no systematic review. Four RCTs (711, 400, 55, and 43 people) compared radical removal of regional and local perigastric lymph nodes (see glossary, p 345) versus conservative removal of just the local lymph nodes.[25–28] There were no significant differences in overall 5 year survival. The largest RCT reported 5 year survival rates of 45% after D1 resection and 47% after D2 resection (ARR +2%, 95% CI −5.6% to +9.6%).[28] The second largest RCT reported non-significantly lower survival with radical removal (survival at 5 years 35% v 33%; HR 1.1, 95% CI 0.87 to 1.39).[27] Subgroup analysis suggests a possible advantage for D2 resection in people with stage II and IIIA disease (corresponding to $T_1N_2M_0$, $T_2N_1M_0$, $T_3N_0M_0$, $T_2N_2M_0$, $T_3N_1M_0$, and $T_4N_0M_0$), particularly in people who did not have additional organ removal. **Para-aortic (D4) versus regional and local (D3, D2) lymphadenectomy:** We found one small RCT (70 people with stomach cancer that had spread to the serosa or adjacent organs, T_3 or T_4) performed in Japan, which compared removal of local, regional, and para-aortic lymph nodes versus removal of only local and regional lymph nodes (see glossary, p 345).[29] This pilot study was too small to detect clinically important differences in survival.

Harms:

The four RCTs of regional and local versus local lymphadenectomy found increased perioperative mortality with the more extensive operation.[23–26] In the second largest RCT, mortality was 13% with D2 resection versus 6% with D1 (P < 0.04).[24] In the largest RCT, the difference in mortality nearly achieved significance (10% with D2 v 6% with D1, P = 0.06).[23] In both of these large trials, the excess mortality was associated closely with greater frequency of pancreatic and splenic removal with D2 resection.[23,24]

Comment:

One large prospective cohort study (1654 people with gastric cancer) found no benefit from D2 resection (defined within this study as over 25 lymph nodes removed; 300 people) versus D1 resection (25 or fewer nodes removed; 1096 people) in the entire cohort of people with gastric cancer after 10 years' follow up. A subgroup analysis found that there may be a beneficial effect of D2 versus D1 resection in the subgroup of people with stage II tumours (230 people; RR of long term survival 1.8, 95% CI 1.3 to 2.7).[30] Cohort studies comparing radical and conservative lymphadenectomy are affected by numerous biases, including selection bias owing to a recent tendency towards more radical treatment, patient differences (age, cancer stage, comorbidity), definition differences (in the meaning of "limited" and "extended"), and stage migration bias (see glossary, p 345). These biases make the interpretation of observational data difficult. The randomised trials were conducted by surgeons with limited prior experience and training in D2 resection, and may have been affected by both learning curve effects[31] and failure to apply the assigned treatment (contamination and non-compliance).[32] Differences in age, cancer stage, and comorbidity may explain why mortality for gastrectomy in Western countries remains high at 5–10%, compared with about 1% in many Japanese reports.[33]

| QUESTION | What are the effects of adjuvant chemotherapy? |

Three systematic reviews of RCTs found weak evidence of a beneficial effect of adjuvant chemotherapy (see glossary, p 345). The size of any benefit remains uncertain, but the treatment is frequently associated with morbidity and can be associated with mortality. Modern regimens have not been evaluated fully in RCTs.

Benefits: **Adjuvant chemotherapy versus surgery alone:** We found three systematic reviews,[34–36] which compared adjuvant chemotherapy versus surgery alone. The first systematic review (search date 1991, 11 RCTs, 2096 people)[34] found that adjuvant chemotherapy compared with surgery alone reduced the risk of death by the end of follow up, but the result was not significant (OR 0.88, 95% CI 0.78 to 1.08). This review was criticised for involving trials that included people with known residual tumour after surgery, and trials that also included immunotherapy and intraperitoneal delivery of the adjuvant therapy. A subsequent update by the authors revised the meta-analysis (OR 0.82, 95% CI 0.68 to 0.97).[37] The second systematic review (search date 1999, 13 RCTs, 1990 people in non-Asian countries) excluded trials of people with known residual tumour after surgery or that also included immunotherapy and intraperitoneal therapy.[35] The review found that adjuvant chemotherapy versus surgery alone reduced the risk of death slightly (AR 595/979 [61%] with chemotherapy v 660/1011 [65%] for controls; OR 0.80, 95% CI 0.66 to 0.97; RRR 6%, 95% CI 0% to 11%). The third systematic review (search date 2000, 20 RCTs, 3658 people) included most of the RCTs from the first two systematic reviews, but included two RCTs published after the earlier reviews. It found that adjuvant chemotherapy compared with surgery alone significantly reduced the risk of death (HR 0.82, 95% CI 0.75 to 0.89). However, there are difficulties interpreting the result of the meta-analysis. **Japanese RCTs:** We found eight Japanese trials that compared adjuvant chemotherapy versus surgery alone. Most were not included in the systematic reviews. One recent and large Japanese RCT (579 people after curative gastrectomy for early cancer, stage T1 or T2) was included in the third systematic review. This review compared adjuvant chemotherapy (mitomycin, fluorouracil, uracil, tegafur) versus no further treatment.[38] After a median follow up of 72 months, it found no significant difference in the death rate (47/288 [16%] with chemotherapy v 59/291 [20%] with no further treatment; OR 0.77, 95% CI 0.50 to 1.17). Of seven older Japanese studies published before 1985, only one found a significant benefit for chemotherapy.[39] This study included 120 people in three arms, and found a significant benefit for adjuvant mitomycin, cytarabine, and fluorouracil over both adjuvant mitomycin and surgery alone. However, a multi-institutional study of the same regimens with over 1200 patients failed to confirm this.[40] One recent small RCT (248 people thought to have stage II or stage III gastric cancer before surgery) found that surgery plus postoperative intraperitoneal chemotherapy versus surgery alone had no significant effect on 5 year survival (39% with surgery and chemotherapy v 29% with surgery only, $P = 0.22$).[41] Subgroup analysis found that in people with stage III gastric cancer, adjuvant intraperitoneal chemotherapy may increase 5 year survival (49% v 18%). **Adjuvant chemotherapy in palliative care:** We found no systematic review, but found one RCT that compared no preoperative adjuvant treatment versus intravenous chemotherapy versus superselective intra-arterial chemotherapy in 386 consecutive people diagnosed with gastric cancer in a Ukrainian cancer centre who preoperatively were thought to have no liver or peritoneal metastases, no enlarged lymph nodes, and no locally advanced disease. All had surgery and 74 were then discovered to be inoperable. Subgroup analysis of these people found that, compared with no adjuvant treatment, 1 year survival was significantly increased by selective intra-arterial chemotherapy but not by intravenous chemotherapy (11/20 survivors at 1 year with intra-arterial chemotherapy v 0/43 in the other groups; ARR 54%, 95% CI 5% to 95%; RR 47, 95% CI 5.3 to 82; NNT 2, 95% CI 1 to 20). The median survival was 91 days with no adjuvant treatment, 96 days with intravenous treatment, and 401 days with intra-arterial treatment.[42]

Harms: Two RCTs reported toxicity (mainly nausea and vomiting) in 53% of people.[43,44] Serious toxicity was usually because of cardiac or cumulative haematological problems; treatment related mortality was 1–2%. We found no definitive evidence from completed studies to justify the concern that preoperative chemotherapy increases postoperative morbidity or mortality. Two RCTs found significant increases in some types of postoperative complications after intraperitoneal chemotherapy.[45,46]

Comment: The three systematic reviews included seven RCTs in common. Only published trials were included. All included trials were reported in English. There was no evidence of publication bias. No statistical heterogeneity of effects was found by the first two systematic reviews, but random effects meta-analysis was used, which may give a conservative estimate of the treatment effect. The third systematic review is difficult to interpret. Some of the results, included in the meta-analysis as if they are independent trials, appear to be duplicate versions of the same RCT.[47,48] This systematic review found significant heterogeneity of the results ($P = 0.028$) but a fixed effects model was used. These factors reduce confidence in the published estimate of effect. The significant effect observed by all three systematic reviews might indicate a true effect or the impact of undetected biases. It is not known whether certain subgroups respond more than others. A subgroup analysis in the second systematic review suggested an effect only in RCTs in which at least two thirds had node positive disease, but the power was insufficient to draw definite conclusions and the result was not confirmed in the third systematic review. Japanese adjuvant chemotherapy regimens often contain bacterial or fungal extracts. We found some evidence from one well designed RCT that addition of these substances to combined surgery and chemotherapy was associated with improved 5 year survival; this will be reviewed in a future issue.[49] The RCT of adjuvant chemotherapy in palliative care identified people before surgery who appeared to have no tumour spread, but who during surgery were found to have tumour spread. The analysis applies to only 19% of those randomised and may not generalise to all people with inoperable gastric cancer.

GLOSSARY

Adjuvant chemotherapy Treatment with cytotoxic drugs given in addition to surgery in an attempt to achieve cure.

Disease stage Surgical and microscopic assessment of the primary tumour. Microscopic spread to distant sites can be detected only by radical surgery, creating a potential bias.

Perigastric lymph nodes Lymph nodes that lie adjacent to the stomach.

Regional lymph nodes Lymph nodes that lie along the blood vessels that supply the stomach.

Stage migration bias Apparent increase in stage specific survival without influencing overall survival caused by recategorisation of the stage following removal of diseased lymph nodes.

Subtotal distal gastrectomy Removal of lower part (usually two thirds or four fifths) of the stomach.

Total gastrectomy Removal of the whole stomach.

Total gastrectomy "de principe" Total gastrectomy where it is not technically necessary to resect a distal tumour; this technique is used minimise the risk of resection line involvement or later second cancer of the gastric stump.

Substantive changes since last issue

Adjuvant chemotherapy New systematic review;[36] conclusion unchanged.

REFERENCES

1. Whelan SL, Parkin DM, Masuyer E, eds. *Trends in cancer incidence and mortality* (IARC scientific publication no. 102). Lyon: IARC Scientific Publications, 1993.
2. Cancer Research Campaign. *Factsheet 18.* London: Cancer Research Campaign, 1993.
3. Powell J, McConkey CC. Increasing incidence of adenocarcinoma of the gastric cardia and adjacent sites. *Br J Cancer* 1990;62:440–443.
4. Devesa SS, Blot WJ, Fraumeni JF Jr. Changing patterns in the incidence of esophageal and gastric carcinoma in the United States. *Cancer* 1998;83:2049–2053.
5. EUROGAST study group. An international association between *Helicobacter pylori* infection and gastric cancer. *Lancet* 1993;341:1359–1362.
6. Buiatti E, Palli D, Decarli A, et al. A case-control study of gastric cancer and diet in Italy. II Association with nutrients. *Int J Cancer* 1990;45:896–901.
7. Rios-Castellanos E, Sitas F, Shepherd NA, et al. Changing pattern of gastric cancer in Oxfordshire. *Gut* 1992;33:1312–1317.
8. Boddie AW Jr, McMurtrey MJ, Giacco GG, et al. Palliative total gastrectomy and oesophagogastrectomy: an evaluation. *Cancer* 1983;51:1195–2000.
9. McCulloch P. Should general surgeons treat gastric carcinoma? An audit of practice and results. *Br J Surg* 1994;81:417–420.
10. Kohli Y, Kawai K, Fujita S. Analytical studies of the growth of human gastric cancer. *J Clin Gastroenterol* 1981;3:129–133.
11. Haugstvedt T. Benefits of resection in palliative surgery. *Dig Surgery* 1994;11:121–125.
12. Maruyama K, Okabayashi K, Kinoshita T. Progress in gastric cancer surgery in Japan and its limits of radicality. *World J Surg* 1987;11:418–425.
13. Jakl RJ, Miholic J, Koller R, et al. Prognostic factors in adenocarcinoma of the cardia. *Am J Surg* 1995;169:316–319.
14. Allum WH, Hallissey MT, Kelly KA. Adjuvant chemotherapy in operable gastric cancer: 5 year follow-up of the first British Stomach Cancer Group trial. *Lancet* 1989;1:571–574.
15. Gouzi JL, Huguier M, Fagniez PL, et al. Gastrectomie totale contre gastrectomie partielle pour adeno-cancer de l'antre. Une etude francaise prospective controlee. *Ann Chir* 1989;43:356–360.
16. Gouzi JL, Huguier M, Fagniez PL, et al. Total versus subtotal gastrectomy for adenocarcinoma of the gastric antrum. A French prospective controlled study. *Ann Surg* 1989;209:162–166.
17. Bozzetti F, Marubini E, Bonfanti G, et al, for the Italian Gastrointestinal Tumor Study Group. Total versus subtotal gastrectomy: surgical morbidity and mortality rates in a multicenter Italian randomized trial. *Ann Surg* 1997;226:613–620.
18. Bozzetti F, Marubini E, Bonfanti G, et al, for the Italian Gastrointestinal Tumor Study Group. Subtotal versus total gastrectomy for gastric cancer: five-year survival rates in a multicenter randomized Italian Trial. *Ann Surg* 1999;230:170–178.
19. Davies J, Johnston D, Sue-Ling H, et al. Total or subtotal gastrectomy for gastric carcinoma? A study of quality of life. *World J Surg* 1998;22:1048–1055.
20. Wu CW, Hsieh MC, Lo SS, et al. Quality of life of patients with gastric adenocarcinoma after curative gastrectomy. *World J Surg* 1997;21:777–782.

Digestive system disorders

21. Svedlund J, Sullivan M, Liedman B, et al. Quality of life after gastrectomy for gastric carcinoma: controlled study of reconstructive procedures. *World J Surg* 1997;21:422–433.

22. Roder JD, Stein HJ, Eckel F, et al. Quality of life after total and subtotal gastrectomy for gastric carcinoma. *Dtsch Med Wochenschr* 1996;121:543–549.

23. Bonenkamp JJ, Songun I, Hermans J, et al. Randomised comparison of morbidity after D1 and D2 dissection for gastric cancer in 996 Dutch patients. *Lancet* 1995;345:745–748.

24. Cuschieri A, Fayers P, Fielding J, et al. Postoperative morbidity and mortality after D1 and D2 resections for gastric cancer: preliminary results of the MRC randomised controlled surgical trial. *Lancet* 1996;347:995–999.

25. Dent DM, Madden MV, Price SK. Randomised comparison of R1 and R2 gastrectomy for gastric carcinoma. *Br J Surg* 1988;75:110–112.

26. Robertson CS, Chung SCS, Woods SDS, et al. A prospective randomised trial comparing R1 subtotal gastrectomy with R3 total gastrectomy for antral cancer. *Ann Surg* 1994;220:176–182.

27. Cuschieri A, Weedon S, Fielding J, et al. Patient survival after D1 and D2 resections for gastric cancer: long-term results of the MRC randomised surgical trial. *Br J Cancer* 1999;79:1522–1530.

28. Bonenkamp JJ, Hermans J, Sasako M, et al. Extended lymph-node dissection for gastric cancer. Dutch Gastric Cancer Group. *N Engl J Med* 1999;340:908–914.

29. Maeta M, Yamashiro H, Saito H, et al. A prospective pilot study of extended (D3) and superextended para-aortic lymphadenectomy (D4) in patients with T3 or T4 gastric cancer managed by total gastrectomy. *Surgery* 1999;125:325–331.

30. Siewert JR, Bottcher K, Stein HJ, et al. Relevant prognostic factors in gastric cancer: ten-year results of the German Gastric Cancer Study. *Ann Surg* 1998;228:449–461.

31. Parikh D, Chagla L, Johnson M, et al. D2 gastrectomy: lessons from a prospective audit of the learning curve. *Br J Surg* 1996;83:1595–1599.

32. Bunt AMG, Hermans J, Boon MC, et al. Evaluation of the extent of lymphadenectomy in a randomised trial of Western versus Japanese style surgery in gastric cancer. *J Clin Oncol* 1994;12:417–422.

33. Bonenkamp JJ, van de Velde CJH, Kampschoer GHM, et al. A comparison of factors influencing the prognosis of Japanese, German and Dutch gastric cancer patients. *World J Surg* 1993;17:410–415.

34. Hermans J, Bonenkamp JJ, Ban MC, et al. Adjuvant therapy after curative resection for gastric cancer: a meta-analysis of randomised trials. *J Clin Oncol* 1993;11:1441–1447. Search date June 1991; primary sources Medline from 1980, and hand searched references.

35. Earle CC, Maroun JA. Adjuvant chemotherapy after curative resection for gastric cancer in non-Asian patients: revisiting a meta-analysis of randomised trials. *Eur J Cancer* 1999;35:1059–1064. Search date to January 1999; primary sources Medline, CancerLit.

36. Mari E, Floriani I, Tinazzi A, et al. Efficacy of adjuvant chemotherapy after curative resection for gastric cancer: a meta-analysis of published randomised trials. A study of the GISCAD (Gruppo Italiano per lo Studio dei Carcinomi dell'Apparato Digerente). *Ann Oncol* 2000;11:837–843. Search date December 1999, primary sources Medline, Embase, Cancerlit, and handsearched references.

37. Hermans J, Bonenkamp H. In reply [letter]. *J Clin Oncol* 1994;12:879–880.

38. Nakajima T, Nashimoto A, Kitamura M, et al. Adjuvant mitomycin and fluorouracil followed by oral uracil plus tegafur in serosa-negative gastric cancer: a randomised trial. Gastric Cancer Surgical Study Group. *Lancet* 1999;354:273–277.

39. Nakajima T, Fukami A, Takagi K, et al. Adjuvant chemotherapy with mitomycin C and with a multi drug combination of mitomycin, fluoro-uracil and cytosine arabinoside, after curative resection of gastric cancer. *Jpn J Clin Oncol* 1990;10:187–194.

40. Imanaga H, Nakazato H. Results of surgery for gastric cancer, and effect of adjuvant mitomycin C on cancer recurrence. *World J Surg* 1977;1:213–221.

41. Yu W, Whang I, Suh I, et al. Prospective randomized trial of early postoperative intraperitoneal chemotherapy as an adjuvant to resectable gastric cancer. *Ann Surg* 1998;228:347–354.

42. Shchepotin IB, Chorny V, Hanfelt J, et al. Palliative superselective intra-arterial chemotherapy for advanced nonresectable gastric cancer. *J Gastrointest Surg* 1999;3:426–431.

43. Coombes RC, Schein PS, Chilvers CE, et al. A randomised trial comparing adjuvant 5-fluoro-uracil, doxorubicin and mitomycin C with no treatment in operable gastric cancer. International Collaborative Cancer Group. *J Clin Oncol* 1990;8:1362–1369.

44. Hallissey MT, Dunn JA, Ward LC, et al. The second British Stomach Cancer Group trial of adjuvant radiotherapy or chemotherapy in advanced gastric cancer: 5 year follow-up. *Lancet* 1994;343:1309–1312.

45. Rosen HR, Jatzko G, Repse S, et al. Adjuvant intraperitoneal chemotherapy with carbon-adsorbed mitomycin in patients with gastric cancer: results of a randomized multicenter trial of the Austrian Working Group for Surgical Oncology. *J Clin Oncol* 1998;16:2733–2738.

46. Yu W, Whang I, Averbach A, Chang D, Sugarbaker PH. Morbidity and mortality of early postoperative intraperitoneal chemotherapy as adjuvant therapy for gastric cancer. *Am Surg* 1998;64:1104–1108.

47. Alcobendas F, Milla A, Estape J, Curto J, Pera C. Mitomycin C as an adjuvant in resected gastric cancer. *Ann Surg* 1983;198:13–17.

48. Grau JJ, Estape J, Alcobendas F. Positive results of adjuvant mitomycin C in resected gastric cancer: a randomised trial on 134 patients. *Eur J Cancer* 1993;29A:340–342.

49. Nakazato H, Koike A, Saji S, et al. Efficacy of immunochemotherapy as adjuvant treatment after curative resection of gastric cancer. Study Group of Immunochemotherapy with PSK for Gastric Cancer. *Lancet* 1994;343:1122–1126.

Peter McCulloch

Consultant Surgeon, University Hospital Aintree and Senior Lecturer, University of Liverpool, Liverpool, UK

Competing interests: The author has received research funding and assistance with travel to meetings from British Biotech Ltd and the Aphton Corporation, two companies involved in research on non-cytotoxic medical treatments for gastric cancer.

TABLE 1	Staging of stomach cancer (see text, p 339).

Stage	Description
T1	Involvement of mucosa +/– submucosa
T2	Involvement of muscularis propria
T3	Involvement of serosa but no spread to adjacent organs
T4	Involvement of adjacent organs
N0	No lymph node involvement
N1	Local (perigastric) nodes involved
N2	Regional nodes involved
N3	More distant intra-abdominal nodes involved
M0	No metastases
M1	Metastases

TABLE 2	Different types of surgical resection for stomach cancer (see text, p 341).

Resection	Description
R0	Removal of all detectable tumour, with a margin of healthy tissue confirmed microscopically: synonymous with "curative" resection.
R1	Incomplete removal, with histological evidence of cancer at the resection margin.
R2	Incomplete removal, with macroscopically obvious remnants of the main tumour: synonymous with "palliative" resection.
D1	Removal of all or part of the stomach, together with local (perigastric) nodes.
D2	Removal of all or part of the stomach, together with local and regional nodes, which lie along the branches of the coeliac axis.
D3/D4	More radical lymph node resection, including removal of para-aortic nodes and nodes within the small bowel mesentery.

Ear, nose, and throat

Search date June 2000: new for this issue

Adrian James and Marc Thorp

INTERVENTIONS

Key Messages

Treatment of acute attacks

- We found no systematic reviews or RCTs of treatments in acute attacks of Meniere's disease.

Prophylactic treatment

- We found insufficient evidence on the effect of diuretics on Meniere's disease.
- We found conflicting evidence from four RCTs on the effect of betahistine on the frequency and severity of attacks of vertigo, tinnitus, and aural fullness.
- We found conflicting evidence of the effect of trimetazidine on vertigo in Meniere's disease. No significant effect on tinnitus has been found.
- Two RCTs have found no significant effect of lithium on Meniere's disease.
- RCTs have found no significant effect of medication on hearing.

© *Clinical Evidence* 2001;5:348–355.

DEFINITION Meniere's disease is characterised by recurrent episodes of spontaneous rotational vertigo and sensorineural hearing loss with tinnitus and a feeling of fullness or pressure in the ear. It may be unilateral or bilateral. Acute episodes may occur in clusters of about 6–11 a year, although remission may last several months.[1] The diagnosis is made clinically.[2] It is important to distinguish Meniere's disease from other types of vertigo that might occur independently with hearing loss and tinnitus, and respond differently to treatment (e.g. benign positional vertigo, acute labyrinthitis). Strict diagnostic criteria help. In this review we applied the classification of the American Academy of Otolaryngology–Head and Neck Surgery (AAO–HNS) to RCTs to indicate the diagnostic rigour used in RCTs (see table 1, p 355).

INCIDENCE/ PREVALENCE Meniere's disease is most common between 40–60 years of age, although younger people can be affected.[6,7] In Europe, the incidence is about 50–200 per 100 000 a year. A survey of general practitioner records of 27 365 people in the UK found an incidence of 43 affected people in a 1 year period (157 per 100 000).[8] Diagnostic criteria were not defined in this survey. A survey of over 8 million people in Sweden found an incidence of 46 per 100 000 a year with diagnosis strictly based on the triad of vertigo, hearing loss, and tinnitus.[9] From smaller studies, the incidence appears lower in Uganda[10] and higher in Japan (350 per 100 000 based on a national survey of hospital attendances during a single week).[7]

AETIOLOGY/ RISK FACTORS Meniere's disease is associated with endolymphatic hydrops (raised endolymph pressure in the membranous labyrinth of the inner ear),[11] but a causal relationship between Meniere's disease and endolymphatic hydrops remains unproven.[12] Specific disorders associated with hydrops (such as temporal bone fracture, syphilis, hypothyroidism, Cogan's syndrome, and Mondini dysplasia (see glossary, p 354) can produce similar symptoms to Meniere's disease.

PROGNOSIS Meniere's disease is progressive, but fluctuates unpredictably. It is difficult to distinguish natural resolution from the effects of treatment. Significant improvement of vertigo is usually seen in the placebo arm of RCTs.[13,14] Acute attacks of vertigo often increase in frequency during the first few years after presentation then decrease in frequency in association with sustained deterioration in hearing.[6] In most people, vertiginous episodes eventually cease completely.[15] In one 20 year cohort study in 34 people, 28 (82%) people had at least moderate hearing loss (mean pure tone hearing loss > 50 dB),[1] and 16 (47%) developed bilateral disease. Symptoms other than hearing loss improve in 60–80% of people, irrespective of treatment.[16]

AIMS To prevent attacks of Meniere's disease; to reduce the severity of vertigo in acute attacks; to relieve chronic symptoms of hearing loss and tinnitus; to improve quality of life, with minimum adverse effects of treatment.

OUTCOMES Frequency and severity of acute attacks of vertigo; hearing acuity; severity of tinnitus; sensation of aural fullness; functional impairment and quality of life; adverse effects of treatment.

METHODS   *Clinical Evidence* search and appraisal June 2000. We excluded studies with loss to follow up over 20%. The authors categorised each RCT according to the classification of the AAO–HNS to indicate the diagnostic rigour used in each RCT (see table 1, p 355). Agreement was obtained by discussion. We excluded RCTs that did not use diagnostic criteria similar to those of AAO–HNS. Several non-English language studies were identified; they are being translated for future issues.

QUESTION   What are the effects of treatment for acute attacks?

OPTION   ANTICHOLINERGIC DRUGS

We found no systematic review or RCTs of anticholinergics for acute attacks of Meniere's disease.

Benefits: We found no systematic review and no randomised trials.

Harms: No adverse effects were reported in this trial.

Comment: We found one non-randomised trial (37 people with definite Meniere's disease) comparing an anticholinergic (glycopyrolate 2 mg twice daily as required) versus placebo for 4 weeks.[17] Glycopyrolate significantly reduced a symptom score based on a validated scale,[18] including questions about the severity of vertigo and its impact on quality of life (Dizziness Handicap Inventory, 76 to 37 v 73 to 75; P < 0.001). An RCT of diphenidol (an antimuscarinic) is being translated.[19]

OPTION   BENZODIAZEPINES

We found no RCTs of benzodiazepines for acute attacks of Meniere's disease.

Benefits: We found no systematic reviews or RCTs.

Harms: We found no evidence about harms from benzodiazepines in people with Meniere's disease.

Comment: An RCT of clonazepam is being translated.[20]

OPTION   BETAHISTINE

We found no RCTs of betahistine versus placebo in which the intervention was taken when required for relief of acute attacks of Meniere's disease.

Benefits: We found no systematic review or RCTs.

Harms: We found no evidence.

Comment: Intravenous histamine was found in an observational study in 1940 to be associated with a reduced severity of acute attacks of Meniere's disease.[21]

OPTION DIURETICS

We found insufficient evidence to comment on the effect of diuretics on vertigo and tinnitus in Meniere's disease. No effect on hearing was found in one RCT.

Benefits: We found no systematic review but found one RCT of a diuretic (triamterene 50 mg plus hydrochlorothiazide 25 mg) versus placebo in 33 people with possible Meniere's disease.[22] It found no significant audiological change in hearing over 17 weeks (P > 0.2).

Harms: No significant adverse effects were reported in this trial.

Comment: In the RCT, frequency of vertigo attacks was reduced and tinnitus was unchanged, but valid statistical analyses cannot be performed because only the mean of categorical data was presented. A trial of hydrochlorothiazide and betahistine is being translated.[23]

OPTION TRIMETAZIDINE

We found conflicting evidence of the effect of trimetazidine on vertigo in Meniere's disease. No significant effect on hearing or tinnitus has been found.

Benefits: We found no systematic review. **Versus placebo:** We found no RCTs. **Versus betahistine:** We found two RCTs.[24,25] One RCT (20 people with definite or probable Meniere's disease) compared trimetazidine (20 mg three times daily) with betahistine (8 mg three times daily) over 3 months. It found no difference in hearing, tinnitus, aural fullness, or quality of life (RR improved quality of life 1.0, 95% CI 0.34 to 2.93). Trimetazidine versus betahistine increased the number of people reporting that the duration of vertigo was substantially better or cured (RR 1.8, 95% CI 1.0 to 3.2), or reporting the intensity of vertigo was substantially better or cured (RR 1.7, 95% CI 1.0 to 2.8). Trimetazidine also improved the global impression of vertigo scale more than betahistine, but it is not clear if this scale has been validated (RR 2.5, 95% CI 1.17 to 5.34).[24] The second RCT (45 people with possible Meniere's disease) of trimetazidine (20 mg three times daily) versus betahistine (12 mg three times daily) over 2 months found no difference in hearing or tinnitus. A beneficial effect of trimetazidine on vertigo intensity was reported but is not confirmed by analysis of the available data (P = 0.23, 2-sided Fisher's exact test).[25]

Harms: No significant adverse effects were reported in these trials.

Comment: None.

| OPTION | BETAHISTINE |

We found no systematic review. Only one of four RCTs of betahistine versus placebo found a reduction in vertigo and tinnitus. None found any change in hearing.

Benefits: We found no systematic review. **Versus placebo:** We found four RCTs of betahistine versus placebo in Meniere's disease.[13,26–28] A 6 week RCT (30 people with possible Meniere's disease) of betahistine (8 mg three times daily) versus placebo did not report the number of people with stated outcomes, but merely reported significant reduction in vertigo (P = 0.0001), tinnitus (P = 0.001), and aural fullness (P = 0.02) with betahistine.[26] A second crossover RCT (35 people with possible Meniere's disease) of two 16 week periods of betahistine (24 mg three times daily in a slow release formulation) versus placebo found no significant difference in tinnitus (P = 0.68) or aural fullness (P = 0.63). Vertigo was not adequately assessed.[13] In the third RCT (betahistine 18 mg twice daily versus placebo for 2 weeks) 16 of the 36 people included had symptoms of possible Meniere's disease. It found no significant improvement in vertigo (RR 1.17, 95% CI 0.86 to 1.58) or tinnitus (RR 2.4, 95% CI 0.11 to 51.3).[27] The fourth RCT (10 people with possible Meniere's disease) of betahistine (8 mg three times daily) versus placebo found no significant difference in the number of people with improved vertigo (RR 5.0, 95% CI 0.3 to 84), tinnitus, or aural fullness over 6–12 months.[28] None of the four RCTs found any change in pure tone audiograms. **Versus trimetazidine:** See trimetazidine option, p 351.

Harms: None of the trials reported any significant adverse effects. Because of its histaminergic action, betahistine is usually avoided in asthma and peptic ulcer disease.

Comment: Crossover studies are more useful if the condition is stable and the interventions have no carry over effects.[29] Meniere's disease is not a stable condition and it is feasible that the effects of treatments extend beyond their presence in the blood stream. A systematic review of the effects of betahistine is in press.[30] RCTs of hydrochlorothiazide and betahistine[23] and a crossover trial of betahistine[31] are being translated.

| OPTION | LITHIUM |

Two RCTs found no significant effect of lithium on Meniere's disease.

Benefits: We found no systematic review but found two crossover RCTs of lithium versus placebo (47 people with possible Meniere's disease). They found no difference in vertigo, tinnitus, aural fullness, or hearing, but no analysable results were presented.[32–34]

Harms: Serum lithium concentration was checked every 2 weeks to reduce the risk of adverse effects. Two people withdrew from one study because of adverse effects from lithium (tremor, thirst, polyuria).

Comment: The crossover RCT design may be inappropriate because Meniere's disease is not stable and it is not clear that the lithium is free of any other effects. Dosage was adjusted to maintain serum lithium concentration between 0.7–1.1 mmol/l.

OPTION   DIETARY MODIFICATION

We found no evidence about dietary modification in Meniere's disease.

Benefits: We found no systematic reviews or RCTs.

Harms: None reported.

Comment: It has been suggested that a low salt diet reduces endolymphatic pressure in endolymphatic hydrops,[35] but we found no RCTs of dietary modification.

OPTION   SYSTEMIC AMINOGLYCOSIDES

We found no systematic review or RCTs of systemic aminoglycosides in Meniere's disease.

Benefits: We found no systematic review or RCTs of systemic aminoglycosides in Meniere's disease.

Harms: There is a risk of severe disruption of balance (including oscillopsia) and sensorineural hearing loss.

Comment: This treatment has been used in severe bilateral disease,[36–38] but we found no evidence from RCTs to support or to refute this.

OPTION   PSYCHOLOGICAL SUPPORT

We found no evidence about psychological suppport in Meniere's disease.

Benefits: We found no evidence about psychological support in Meniere's disease.

Harms: None reported.

Comment: We found no good evidence that Meniere's disease responds to psychological support.[32] However, symptomatic improvement is seen with all treatments, including placebo,[16] or being put on a waiting list for surgery.[39] The improvements, which occur after psychological support, have not been distinguished from the improvement attributable to the natural history of Meniere's disease.

OPTION   VESTIBULAR REHABILITATION

We found no evidence about the effects of vestibular rehabilitation exercises (see glossary, p 354) on Meniere's disease.

Benefits: We found no systematic review or RCTs.

Harms: None reported.

Comment: Improvements noted after vestibular rehabilitation have not been distinguished from spontaneous improvement of Meniere's disease.

Ear, nose, and throat

GLOSSARY

Cogan's syndrome Episodic vertigo of the Meniere's type, hearing loss and interstitial keratitis, without syphilis.[5]

Mondini dysplasia A congenital deformity of the cochlea in which only the basal turns are present.

Vestibular rehabilitation Involves a series of exercises intended to improve the sense of balance through controlled movements of the head and body.[40] They are usually recommended for stable vestibular disorders.[41]

REFERENCES

1. Friberg U, Stahle J, Svedberg A. The natural course of Menière's disease. *Acta Otolaryngol Suppl* 1984;406:72–77.
2. Kitahara M. Concepts and diagnostic criteria of Menière's disease. In: Kitahara M, ed. *Menière's disease*. Tokyo: Springer–Verlag; 1990:3–12.
3. Alford BR. Menière's disease: criteria for diagnosis and evaluation of therapy for reporting. Report of subcommittee on equilibrium and its measurement. *Trans Am Acad Opthalmol Otolaryngol* 1972;76:1462–1464.
4. Pearson BW, Brackmann DE. Committee on hearing and equilibrium guidelines for reporting treatment results in Menière's disease. *Otolaryngol Head Neck Surg* 1985;93:578–581.
5. Committee on hearing and equilibrium. Guidelines for the diagnosis and evaluation of therapy in Menière's disease. *Otolaryngol Head Neck Surg* 1995;113:181–185.
6. Moffat DA, Ballagh RH. Menière's Disease. In: Kerr AG, Booth JB, eds. *Scott-Brown's Otolaryngology*. 6th ed. Oxford, Butterworth-Heinemann, 1997:3/19/1–50.
7. Watanabe I. Incidence of Menière's disease, including some other epidemiological data. In: Oosterveld WJ, ed. *Menière's disease: A comprehensive appraisal*. Chichester: John Wiley & Sons Ltd, 1983:9–23.
8. Cawthorne T, Hewlett AB. Menière's disease. *Proc Royal Soc Med* 1954;47:663–670.
9. Stahle J, Stahle C, Arenberg IK. Incidence of Menière's disease. *Arch Otolaryngol* 1978;104:99–102.
10. Nsamba C. A comparative study of the aetiology of vertigo in the African. *J Laryngol Otol* 1972;86:917–925.
11. Hallpike C, Cairns H. Observations on the pathology of Menière's syndrome. *J Laryngol Otol* 1938;53:625–655.
12. Ruckenstein MJ, Harrison RV. Cochlear pathology in Menière's disease. In: Harris JP, ed. Menière's disease. The Hague: Kugler Publications, 1999:195–202.
13. Schmidt JT, Huizing EH. The clinical drug trial in Menière's disease with emphasis on the effect of betahistine SR. *Acta Otolaryngol* 1992;497(suppl):1–189.
14. Moser M, Ranacher G, Wilmot TJ, Golden GJ. A double-blind clinical trial of hydroxyethylrutosides in Menière's disease. *J Laryngol Otol* 1984;98:265–272.
15. Silverstein H, Smouha E, Jones R. Natural history versus surgery for Menière's disease. *Otolaryngol Head Neck Surg* 1989;100:6–16.
16. Torok N. Old and new in Menière's disease. *Laryngoscope* 1977;87:1870–1877.
17. Storper IS, Spitzer JB, Scanlan M. Use of glycopyrrolate in the treatment of Menière's disease. *Laryngoscope* 1998;108:1442–1445.
18. Jacobson GP, Newman CW. The development of the Dizziness Handicap Inventory. *Arch Otolaryngol Head Neck Surg* 1990;116:424–427.
19. Vasil'eva VP, Romanenko DA. Cephadol in the treatment of patients with Menière's disease and labyrinthopathies. [in Russian] *Vestnik Otorinolaringologii* 1985:28–31.
20. Mangabuira Albernaz PL, Ganança MM, Da Fonseca MC. Clonazepam in the treatment of vestibular disorders. *Folha Medica* 1984;88.
21. Sheldon CH, Horton BT. Treatment of Menière's disease with histamine administered intravenously. *Proceedings of the Staff Meetings of the Mayo Clinic*. 1940;15:17–21.
22. van Deelen GW, Huizing EH. Use of a diuretic (Dyazide) in the treatment of Menière's disease. A double-blind cross-over placebo-controlled study. *ORL J Otorhinolaryngol Relat Spec* 1986;48:287–292.
23. Petermann W, Mulch G. Long-term therapy of Menière's disease. Comparison of the effects of betahistine dihydrochloride and hydrochlorothiazide [in German]. *Fortschr Medizin* 1982;100:431–435.
24. Kluyskens P, Lambert P, D'Hooge D. Trimetazidine contre betahistine dans le vertiges vestibulaires. *Ann Otolaryngol Chir Cervicofac* 1990;107(suppl 1):11–19.
25. Martini A, De Domenico F. Trimetazidine versus betahistine in Menière's disease. A double blind method [in French]. *Ann Otolaryngol Chir Cervicofac* 1990;107(suppl 1):20–27.
26. Salami A, Dellepiane M, Tinelle E, Jankowska B. Studio a doppia cecita' tra cloridrato di betaistina e placebo nel trattamento delle sindromi Menieriformi. *Valsalva* 1984;60:302–312.
27. Okamato K, Hazeyama F, Taira T, Yoshida A. Therapeutic results of betahistine in Menière's disease with statistical analysis. *Iryo* 1968;22:650–666.
28. Ricci V, Sittoni V, Nicora M. Valutazione terapeutica e tollerabilita del chloridrato di betaistina (Microser) in confronto a placebo nella malattia di Meniere. *Riv Ital Ornitolog Audiolog Foniat* 1987;7:347–350.
29. Fleiss JL. The crossover study. In: *The design and analysis of clinical experiments*. Chichester: John Wiley & Sons, 1984.
30. James AL, Burton MJ. Betahistine for Menière's disease or syndrome [protocol]. In: The Cochrane Library, Issue 3, 2000. Oxford: Update Software; 1999.
31. Watanabe K, Fukami J, Yoshimoto H, Ueda M, Suzuki J. Evaluation of the effect of betahistine in Menière's disease by double-blind test and multivariate analysis. *Jibiinkoka* 1967;39: 1237–1250.
32. Thomsen J, Bech P, Prytz S, Vendsbourg P, Zilstorff K. Menière's disease: lithium treatment (demonstration of placebo effect in a double blind cross-over trial). *Clin Otolaryngol* 1979;4:119–123.
33. Thomsen J, Bech P, Geisler A, et al. Lithium treatment of Menière's disease: results of a double-blind cross-over trial. *Acta Otolaryngol* 1976;82:294–296.

34. Thomsen J, Bech P, Geisler A, et al. Menière's Disease. Preliminary report of lithium treatment. *Acta Otolaryngol* 1974;78:59–64.
35. Furstenburg AC, Richardson G, Lathrop FD. Menière's disease. Addenda to medical therapy. *Arch Otolaryngol* 1941;34:1083–1092.
36. Wilson WR, Schuknecht HF. Update on the use of streptomycin therapy for Menière's disease. *Am J Otol* 1980;2:108–111.
37. Graham MD. Bilateral Menière's disease. Treatment with intramuscular titration streptomycin sulfate. *Otolaryngol Clin North Am* 1997;30:1097–1100.
38. Shea JJ, Ge X, Orchik DJ. Long-term results of low dose intramuscular streptomycin for Menière's disease. *Am J Otol* 1994;15:540–544.
39. Kerr AG, Toner JG. A new approach to surgery for Menière's disease: talking about surgery. *Clin Otolaryngol* 1998;23:263–264.
40. Dix MR. The rationale and technique of head exercises in the treatment of vertigo. *Acta Otorhinolaryngol Belg* 1979;33:370–384.
41. Clendaniel RA, Tucci DL. Vestibular rehabilitation strategies in Menière's disease. *Otolaryngol Clin North Am* 1997;30:1145–1158.

Adrian James
Department of Otolaryngology
Radcliffe Infirmary
Oxford
UK

Marc Thorp
Department of Otolaryngology
University of Toronto
Toronto
Canada

Competing interests: None declared.

TABLE 1	American Academy of Otolaryngology–Head and Neck Surgery (AAO–HNS) definition of the certainty of diagnosis of Meniere's disease (see text, p 349).[3–5]
Certain	Definite Meniere's + postmortem confirmation
Definite	Two or more episodes of vertigo* + audiometrically confirmed sensorineural hearing loss + tinnitus or aural fullness + other causes excluded
Probable	One episode of vertigo* + audiometrically confirmed sensorineural hearing loss + tinnitus or aural fullness + other causes excluded
Possible	Episodes of vertigo* with no hearing loss, or sensorineural hearing loss with dysequilibrium; other causes excluded

*Defined as spontaneous, rotational vertigo lasting more than 20 minutes.

Middle ear pain and trauma during air travel

Search date November 2000

Simon Janvrin

QUESTIONS

INTERVENTIONS

Likely to be beneficial

Unknown effectiveness

Key Messages

- We found only limited evidence that oral decongestants are effective in reducing ear pain and hearing loss during air travel in adults. One small RCT found no evidence of benefit in children.

- We found insufficient evidence on the effects of topical decongestants in this setting.

DEFINITION	The effects of air travel on the middle ear can include tympanic membrane pain, vertigo, hearing loss, and perforation.
INCIDENCE/ PREVALENCE	The prevalence of symptoms depends on the altitude, type of aircraft, and characteristics of the passengers. One point prevalence study found that 20% of adult and 40% of child passengers had negative pressure in the middle ear after flight, and that 10% of adults and 22% of children had auroscopic evidence of damage to the tympanic membrane.[1] We found no data on the incidence of perforation, which seems to be extremely rare in commercial passengers.
AETIOLOGY/ RISK FACTORS	During aircraft descent, the pressure in the middle ear drops relative to that in the ear canal. A narrow, inflamed, or poorly functioning Eustachian tube impedes the necessary influx of air. As the pressure difference between the middle and outer ear increases, the tympanic membrane is pulled inward.
PROGNOSIS	In most people, symptoms resolve spontaneously. Experience in military aviation shows that most ear drum perforations will heal spontaneously.[2]
AIMS	To prevent ear pain and trauma during air travel.
OUTCOMES	Incidence and severity of pain and hearing loss; incidence of perforation of tympanic membrane.
METHODS	*Clinical Evidence* update search and appraisal November 2000.

QUESTION What are the effects of preventive interventions?

OPTION ORAL DECONGESTANTS

We found limited evidence from two RCTs suggesting that oral pseudoephedrine may reduce the incidence of pain and hearing loss during flight in adult passengers prone to symptoms. One small RCT found no evidence of benefit in children.

Benefits:	We found no systematic review. We found three RCTs. Two RCTs (350 adult passengers) compared oral pseudoephedrine (120 mg given 30 minutes before flight) versus placebo.[3,4] All people had a history of ear pain during air travel. Those with acute or chronic ear problems were excluded. A total of 272 passengers completed the post flight questionnaires. The RCTs found that pseudoephedrine versus placebo significantly reduced pain and hearing loss (incidence of symptoms in combined treatment groups: 33% v 64%; RR 0.51, 95% CI 0.31 to 0.84). The third RCT (50 children up to the age of 6 years) compared oral pseudoephedrine versus placebo.[5] It found no significant difference in ear pain between children taking treatment versus placebo, at either take off or landing.
Harms:	"Dry mouth or drowsiness" was reported by 7–15% of adult participants taking pseudoephedrine versus 2% on placebo.[3,4] More children taking pseudoephedrine were drowsy on take off compared with placebo (60% v 13%).[5]
Comment:	None.

| OPTION | TOPICAL NASAL DECONGESTANTS |

We found insufficient evidence on the effects of topical decongestants in this setting.

Benefits: We found no systematic review. We found one RCT comparing oxymetazoline nasal spray versus placebo nasal spray in 83 participants during air travel.[3] It found no significant difference in reported ear pain between the two groups.

Harms: Nasal irritation was reported by 14% of people taking oxymetazoline. The rate in people taking placebo was not reported.

Comment: The RCT was too small to rule out an effect of topical decongestants.

REFERENCES

1. Stangerup S-E, Tjernstrom O, Klokke M, Harcourt J, Stokholm J. Point prevalence of barotitis in children and adults after flight, and the effect of autoinflation. *Aviat Space Environ Med* 1998;69: 45–49.
2. O'Reilly BJ. Otorhinolaryngology. In: Ernsting J, Nicholson AN, Rainford DJ, eds. *Aviation Medicine*. 3rd edition. Oxford: Butterworth-Heinemann, 1999:319–336.
3. Jones JS, Sheffield W, White LJ, Bloom MA. A double-blind comparison between oral pseudoephedrine and topical oxymetazoline in the prevention of barotrauma during air travel. *Am J Emerg Med* 1998;16:262–264.
4. Csortan E, Jones J, Haan M, Brown M. Efficacy of pseudoephedrine for the prevention of barotrauma during air travel. *Ann Emerg Med* 1994;23:1324–1327.
5. Buchanan BJ, Hoagland J, Fischer PR. Pseudoephedrine and air travel-associated ear pain in children. *Arch Pediatr Adolesc Med* 1999; 153:466–468.

Simon Janvrin
Former Senior Medical Officer
Civil Aviation Authority
West Sussex
UK

Competing interests: None declared.

QUESTIONS

INTERVENTIONS

Key Messages

- We found insufficient evidence on the effects of strategies for preventing otitis media with effusion (OME).
- One systematic review of RCTs found that antimicrobial drugs speed the resolution of OME, but are not effective in the long term. Adverse effects were reported frequently.
- We found little evidence of clinically significant benefit with oral steroids, but some evidence of adverse effects.
- RCTs found short term benefit from autoinflation with a nasal balloon.
- We found insufficient evidence about sustained benefits from mechanical and surgical treatment.

Otitis media with effusion

DEFINITION	OME, or "glue ear", is serous or mucoid but not mucopurulent fluid in the middle ear. Children usually present with hearing loss and speech problems. In contrast to those with acute otitis media (see topic, p 181), children with OME do not suffer from acute ear pain, fever, or malaise. Hearing loss is usually mild and often identified when parents express concern about their child's behaviour, school performance, or language development.
INCIDENCE/ PREVALENCE	At any time 5% of children aged 2–4 years have persistent (at least 3 months) bilateral hearing loss associated with OME. The prevalence declines considerably over age 6.[1] About 80% of children aged 10 years have been affected by OME at some time in the past. OME is the most common reason for referral for surgery in children in the UK. Middle ear effusions also occur infrequently in adults after upper respiratory tract infection or after air travel.
AETIOLOGY/ RISK FACTORS	Contributory factors include upper respiratory tract infection and narrow upper respiratory airways. Prospective case control studies have found established risk factors, including age 6 years or younger at first onset, day care centre attendance, high number of siblings, low socioeconomic group, frequent upper respiratory tract infection, bottle feeding, and household smoking.[2,3] Most factors are associated with about double the risk of developing OME.[4]
PROGNOSIS	In 5% of preschool children, OME (identified by tympanometric screening) persists for at least 1 year.[5,6] One large cohort study (534 children) found that middle ear disease increased reported hearing difficulty at age 5 years (OR 1.44, 95% CI 1.18 to 1.76) and was associated with delayed language development in children up to age 10 years.[7]
AIMS	To improve hearing and wellbeing; to avoid poor behavioural, speech and educational development; and to prevent recurrent earache and otitis media.
OUTCOMES	Resolution of effusion (both speed and completeness) assessed by otoscopy, tympanometry, or global clinical assessment; hearing impairment, assessed by audiometry or tympanometry (although the positive predictive value of these tests has been reported as low as 49%);[8] developmental and behavioural tests; language and speech development; adverse effects of treatment. Hearing losses as small as 15 dB above the normal hearing threshold can be disabling in children. Patient centred outcomes in children with OME (e.g. disability or quality of life) need further development and evaluation.
METHODS	*Clinical Evidence* update search and appraisal November 2000.

QUESTION   What are the effects of preventive interventions?

OPTION   AVOIDANCE OF MODIFIABLE RISK FACTORS

We found no RCTs that evaluated interventions to modify risk factors for OME, such as passive smoking and bottle feeding.

Benefits:	We found no systematic review or RCTs of interventions aimed at modifying risk factors for OME.

Harms: We found insufficient data.

Comment: There is good epidemiological evidence that the risk of OME is increased by passive smoking,[2] bottle feeding,[3] low socioeconomic group, and exposure to a large number of other children.[8] Feasible preventive interventions may include strategies to reduce household smoking and encourage breast feeding.

QUESTION   What are the effects of treatments?

OPTION   ANTIMICROBIAL DRUGS

Two systematic reviews of RCTs and one subsequent non-systematic review have found that resolution of OME occurred faster with antibiotics versus placebo or no treatment. They found no significant effect on longer term outcomes. Adverse effects with antibiotics were frequent.

Benefits: We found two systematic reviews (search dates 1992 and 1993) and one subsequent non-systematic review.[8–10] Both systematic reviews found that OME resolves faster with antimicrobial drugs. **Short term outcomes:** The first review (search date 1992, 10 blinded RCTs in 1041 children with OME), compared antimicrobial drugs (amoxicillin with or without clavulanic acid, cefaclor, erythromycin, sulphisoxazole, sulfamethoxazole, or trimethoprim) versus placebo or versus no treatment.[8] Treatment duration varied from 2–5 weeks. Follow up was from 10–60 days. At 1 month, resolution of effusion (assessed by pneumatic otoscopy, tympanometry, and audiometry) was significantly more likely with antimicrobial treatment (pooled ARR for non-resolution compared with placebo or no treatment 14%, 95% CI 4% to 24%; NNT 7). **Longer term outcomes:** The second systematic review (8 RCTs) found no significant difference in presence of effusions between 6 weeks and 11 months after treatment (pooled ARR for presence of effusion compared with placebo 6%, 95% CI –3% to +14%).[9] This review also found no significant differences in effectiveness between antibiotics. A more recent meta-analysis based on eight RCTs (7 of 18 previously included RCTs and 1 newer RCT) compared antibiotics versus placebo in OME (1292 children) and found no significant effect (cure rate 179/813 [22%] for antibiotics v 85/479 [18%] for placebo; ARI of cure 4.3%, RR 1.24, 95% CI 0.99 to 1.54).[10]

Harms: The systematic reviews did not report rates of adverse events in children on placebo or no treatment. Adverse events on antibiotics were frequent. For amoxicillin, diarrhoea was reported in 20–30% and rashes in 3–5% of children. For co-amoxiclav, diarrhoea was reported in 9%, nausea and vomiting in 4%, and skin rashes and urticaria in 3% of children.[8,11] For antibiotics overall, nausea and vomiting, diarrhoea, or both were reported in 2–32% of children, and cutaneous reactions in less than 5%.[11] Adherence to long courses of antibiotics is poor. Prescribing antibiotics for minor illness encourages further consultations[12] and antibiotic resistance.[13]

Comment: In the third meta-analysis the timing to outcomes was not clear.[10]

| OPTION | STEROIDS |

A systematic review of RCTs found no evidence of long term benefit from oral steroids in children with OME. We found no RCTs that adequately evaluated topical steroids.

Benefits: We found one systematic review (search date 2000).[14] **Oral steroids versus placebo:** The review identified three placebo controlled RCTs of oral steroids in 108 children with OME. Presence of effusion was assessed clinically by pneumatic otoscopy, tympanometry, and audiometry after 7–14 days of treatment. There was no significant difference in mean improvement at 2 weeks after treatment (AR of clearance compared with placebo 0.18, 95% CI −0.03 to +0.39). There were no available summary data beyond 6 weeks. **Added to antibiotic:** The systematic review identified four RCTs (292 children) comparing antibiotic plus oral steroids versus antibiotic alone. Time to measurement of results varied from 1 week to 2 months. There was a significant difference in clearance rates with combined treatment versus antibiotic alone (ARR for non-clearance versus antibiotic alone at 2 weeks 0.32, 95% CI 0.2 to 0.5), but there was significant heterogeneity between studies ($P < 0.01$). **Topical steroids:** We found one RCT (61 children with chronic middle ear infection), which compared intranasal beclomethasone with placebo as an adjunct to prophylactic antibiotics.[15] It found significant improvement in middle ear pressure at 12 weeks ($P < 0.05$) and fewer effusions at 4 and 8 weeks ($P < 0.05$) in those treated with intranasal steroids and antibiotics, compared with either antibiotics alone or placebo spray.

Harms: Short courses of steroids can cause behavioural changes, increased appetite, and weight gain. Idiosyncratic reactions have been reported such as avascular necrosis of the femoral head and fatal varicella infections.

Comment: The trials were small. Use of secondary care populations weakens the applicability of results to primary care.

| OPTION | ANTIHISTAMINES AND DECONGESTANTS |

One systematic review of RCTs found no benefit from antihistamines and decongestants versus placebo in children with OME.

Benefits: We found one systematic review (search date 1992, 4 placebo controlled RCTs, 1202 infants and older children).[8] Treatment lasted for 4 weeks. Meta-analysis found that combined antihistamine/decongestants versus placebo had no significant effect on effusion clearance rate, as assessed by history, otoscopy, and tympanometry (difference in clearance rate −0.009, 95% CI −0.036 to +0.054).

Harms: Adverse effects of antihistamines include hyperactivity, insomnia, drowsiness, behavioural change, blood pressure variability, and seizures. Decongestant nose drops given for 3 weeks or more can lead to iatrogenic rhinitis.

Comment: The RCTs included clinically heterogeneous groups (e.g. infants and older children) and selected individuals from ambulatory care or waiting lists. There were too few children with allergies for subgroup analysis.

| OPTION | MUCOLYTICS |

One systematic review of RCTs found that 1–3 month courses of mucolytics compared with placebo or no treatment had no significant effect on effusion resolution.

Benefits: We found one systematic review (search date 1993, 6 RCTs, 430 children) comparing S-carboxymethylcysteine, its lysine salt, or both, versus placebo or no treatment.[16] Treatment lasted for 15–90 days. Increased frequency of complete resolution with mucolytics did not quite reach significance (178 children; OR 2.25, 95% CI 0.97 to 5.22). Three small RCTs comparing another mucolytic, bromhexine, versus placebo in 155 children and 195 ears found conflicting results.

Harms: The review gave no information on adverse effects.[16] Reported adverse effects of S-carboxymethylcysteine include gastric irritation, nausea, and rashes.

Comment: The RCTs were heterogeneous in their clinical outcomes and treatment duration.

| OPTION | AUTOINFLATION |

One systematic review of RCTs found benefit from autoinflation using a nasal balloon, although some children may find autoinflation difficult. The value of all methods of autoinflation has not yet been adequately evaluated.

Benefits: We found one systematic review (search date not given, 6 RCTs) comparing autoinflation versus no treatment.[17] Improvement was variously defined as being effusion free, improved tympanogram, or improvement in hearing. The RCTs assessing different treatment effects had different results. However, trials evaluating nasal balloons in children found a homogeneous effect size (3 RCTs, 386 children). Children in the treatment group were more likely than controls to improve within 1 week to 3 months, using tympanometric and audiometric criteria (RR 1.12, 95% CI 1.03 to 1.22).[17]

Harms: No serious adverse effects have been reported.

Comment: The Eustachian tubes can be inflated by several methods, including blowing up a balloon through a plastic tube inserted into the nostril. In one RCT, 12% of children aged 3–10 years were unable to use the balloon.[18] Most trials appeared not to use intention to treat analysis, and beneficial effects were noted only when adherence was 70% or greater. The evidence is suboptimal because different methods were used, outcome assessments were not blinded, and follow up was short. Other methods of autoinflation (such as inflating a carnival blower through the nostril, or forcible exhalation through the nostrils, with closed mouth, into an anaesthetic mask with a flowmeter attachment) have not been adequately evaluated.

OPTION	SURGERY

One systematic review of heterogeneous RCTs has found that surgery (insertion of grommets, adenoidectomy, or both) results in short term hearing gain. Grommets and adenoidectomy alone were of similar effectiveness. A subsequent RCT has found that grommets and adenoidectomy combined were more effective than adenotonsillectomy or grommets, either alone or combined. Two subsequent RCTs found no benefit in language development with grommets. We found no good evidence of the effects of tonsillectomy.

Benefits: We found one systematic review of surgery in children with OME (search date 1992, 19 RCTs). Nine reported the data per child (1508 children) and 10 reported data per ear (1452 children). None were placebo controlled, although some used children as their own controls.[19] Outcomes were mean change in audiometry, tympanometry, and clinical and otoscopic evidence of OME. The review concluded that evidence for the effectiveness of surgical interventions was still confused. **Grommets:** The review reported a mean 12 dB improvement in hearing after insertion of grommets (CI not available). However, the authors concluded that this was difficult to interpret clinically. Two subsequent RCTs (369 children) found that grommets do not improve language development in infants.[20,21] However, one RCT (182 children) found early insertion of bilateral grommets significantly reduced behavioural problems at 9 months compared with watchful waiting (24 withdrawals from watchful waiting, 8 from early surgery, no intention to treat analysis: Richman behaviour check list 25/84 [30%] v 31/66 [47%], RR 0.63, 95% CI 0.30 to 0.96).[21] **Grommets plus adenoidectomy:** The review found that adenoidectomy gave little additional benefit over grommets alone in terms of mean hearing gain, which varied from 1.1 to 2.6 dB. A subsequent RCT (228 children) compared adenotonsillectomy or adenoidectomy (analysed together) versus neither procedure.[22] All children had a grommet inserted into one ear. Outcomes were mean audiometric change and tympanometric and otoscopic clearance assessed over 6 months to 10 years after treatment. The trial found benefit in combining adenoidectomy with grommets. Median duration of glue ear assessed tympanometrically was reduced from 7.8 years without treatment to 4.9 years with grommets, 4 years with adenoidectomy, and 2.8 years with adenoidectomy and grommets combined. The difference between duration for adenoidectomy alone and grommets alone was not significant ($P = 0.2$), but all other comparisons were significant. **Tonsillectomy:** The review found no good RCTs of tonsillectomy alone in OME.

Harms: Otorrhoea occurred postoperatively in 13% of children after grommet insertion (AR 0.13, 95% CI 0.05 to 0.21) and persisted in 5% at 1 year.[23] The true incidence of persistent perforation beyond 1 year is not known. A systematic review of observational and experimental studies (search date 1998)[24] of the complications following grommet insertion found a reported prevalence of tympanosclerosis in 39–65% of ventilated ears as opposed to 0–10% of untreated ears. Partial atrophy was noted in 16–73% of ears treated, and in 5–31% of those untreated. Atelectasis ranged from 10–37% of

ears treated as opposed to 1–20% untreated, and attic retraction between 10–52% and 29–40%, respectively. The average hearing loss associated with these abnormalities was less than 5 dB.
Adenoidectomy: Deaths have been reported in 1 of 16 700–25 000 children when combined with tonsillectomy (no figures available for adenoidectomy alone), and postoperative haemorrhage in 0.5%.[25]

Comment: About half of children who have grommets inserted will undergo reinsertion within 5 years.[26] Resolution after surgery takes longer in younger children and in those whose parents smoke, irrespective of treatment.[22] The RCT of early insertion of grommets versus watchful waiting claims to use intention to treat analysis because people randomised to watchful waiting who actually received early surgery were excluded from analysis rather than counted in the early surgery group.[21]

Substantive changes since last issue

Steroids New systematic review of steroids versus placebo;[14] conclusion unchanged.
Grommets Two RCTs of grommets found no significant effect on language outcomes.[20,21] One RCT found a significant improvement in behaviour.[21]

REFERENCES

1. Williamson IG, Dunleavey J, Bain J, Robinson D. The natural history of otitis media with effusion: a three year study of the incidence and prevalence of abnormal tympanograms in four SW Hampshire infant and first schools. *J Laryngol Otol* 1994;108: 930–934.
2. Strachan DP, Cook DG. Health effects of passive smoking. 4. Passive smoking, middle ear disease and adenotonsillectomy in children. *Thorax* 1998; 53:50–56. Search date 1997; primary sources Medline, Embase.
3. Paradise JL, Rockette HE, Colborn DK, et al. Otitis media in 2253 Pittsburgh area infants: prevalence and risk factors during the first two years of life. *Pediatrics* 1997;99:318–333.
4. Haggard M, Hughes E. *Objectives, values and methods of screening children's hearing – a review of the literature*. London: HMSO, 1991.
5. Zeilhuis GA, Rach GH, Broek PV. Screening for otitis media with effusion in pre-school children. *Lancet* 1989;1:311–314.
6. Fiellau-Nikolajsen M. Tympanometry in three year old children: prevalence and spontaneous course of MEE. *Ann Otol Rhinol Laryngol* 1980;89(suppl 68):233–237.
7. Bennett KE, Haggard MP. Behaviour and cognitive outcomes in middle ear disease. *Arch Dis Child* 1999;80:28–35.
8. Stool SE, Berg SO, Berman S, et al. *Otitis media with effusion in young children: clinical practice guideline number 12*. AHCPR Publication 94–0622. Rockville, Maryland: Agency for Health Care Policy and Research, Public Health Service, United States Department of Health and Human Services, July, 1994. Search date 1992; primary sources online database of National Library of Medicine, 10 specialised bibliographic databases.
9. Williams RL, Chalmers TC, Strange KC, Chalmers FT, Bowlin SJ. Use of antibiotics in preventing recurrent acute otitis media and in treating otitis media with effusion: a meta-analytic attempt to resolve the brouhaha. *JAMA* 1993;270:1344–1351. Search date 1966 to 1993; primary source Medline, Current Contents.
10. Cantekin EI, McGuire TW. Antibiotics are not effective for otitis media with effusion: reanalysis of meta-analysis. *Otorhinolaryngol Nova* 1998;8: 214–222.
11. Computerised clinical information system. Denver, Colorado: Micromedex Inc, June 1993.
12. Little P, Gould C, Williamson I, Warner G, Gantley M, Kinmonth AL. Reattendance and complications in a randomised trial of prescribing strategies for sore throat: the medicalising effect of prescribing antibiotics. *BMJ* 1997;315:350–352.
13. Anonymous. Antimicrobial resistance is a major threat to public health [Editorial]. *BMJ* 1998;317: 609–610.
14. Butler CC, van der Voort JH. Oral or nasal steroids for hearing loss associated with otitis media with effusion in children. In: The Cochrane Library, Issue 4, 2000. Oxford: Update Software. Search date February 2000; primary sources Cochrane Controlled Trials Register, Embase, Medline.
15. Tracy TM, Demain JG, Hoffman KM, Goetz DW. Intranasal beclomethasone as an adjunct to treatment of chronic middle ear effusion. *Ann Allergy Asthma Immunol* 1998;80:198–206.
16. Pignataro O, Pignataro LD, Gallus G, Calori G, Cordaro CI. Otitis media with effusion and S-carboxymethylcysteine and/or its lysine salt: a critical overview. *Int J Pediatr Otorhinolaryngol* 1996;35:231–241. Search date 1993; primary sources Medline, Embase, Biosis.
17. Reidpath DD, Glasziou PP, Del Mar C. Systematic review of autoinflation for treatment of glue ear in children. *BMJ* 1999;318:1177–1178. Search date not stated; primary sources Medline, Cochrane Library, and pharmaceutical company database.
18. Blanshard JD, Maw AR, Bawden R. Conservative treatment of otitis media with effusion by autoinflation of the middle ear. *Clin Otolaryngol* 1993;18:188–192.
19. University of York. Centre for Reviews and Dissemination. 1992. The treatment of persistent glue ear in children. *Effective Health Care* 1(4).

Search date 1992; primary sources BIDS, Medline, Embase.

20. Rovers MM, Stratman H, Ingels K, van der Wilt GJ, van den Broek P, Zielhuis GA. The effect of ventilation tubes on language development in infants with otitis media with effusion: A randomised trial. Pediatrics 2000;106:3–42.

21. Wilks J, Maw R, Peters TJ, Harvey I, Golding J. Randomised controlled trial of early surgery versus watchful waiting for glue ear: The effect on behavioural problems in pre-school children. Clin Otol Allied Sci 2000;25:209–214.

22. Maw R, Bawden R. Spontaneous resolution of severe chronic glue ear in children and the effect of adenoidectomy, tonsillectomy, and insertion of ventilation tubes. BMJ 1993;306:756–760.

23. Mclelland CA. Incidence of complications from tympanostomy tubes. Arch Otolaryngol 1980;106: 97–99.

24. Schilder AG. Assessment of complications of the conditions and of the treatment of otitis media with effusion. Int J Pediatr Otolaryngol 1999;49: 247–251. Search date 1998; primary sources not stated.

25. Yardley MP. Tonsillectomy, adenoidectomy and adenotonsillectomy; are they safe day case procedures. J Laryngol Otol 1992;106:299–300.

26. Maw AR. Development of tympanosclerosis in children with otitis media with effusion and ventilation tubes. J Laryngol Otol 1991;105:614–617.

Ian Williamson
Senior Lecturer in Primary Medical Care
Southampton University
Southampton
UK

Competing interests: None declared.

Search date May 2000

Martin Burton

Key Messages

- We found no RCTs evaluating tonsillectomy in adults, and we found inconclusive evidence from RCTs in children.

DEFINITION	Tonsillitis is infection of the parenchyma of the palatine tonsils. It is only one cause of "sore throat," which may be caused by infection of other pharyngeal tissues. Severe tonsillitis has been defined as seven episodes in the preceding year, five episodes per year in the preceding 2 years, or three per year in the preceding 3 years.[1]
INCIDENCE/ PREVALENCE	Recurrent sore throat has an incidence in general practice in the UK of 100 per 1000 population per year.[2] Acute tonsillitis is more common in childhood.
AETIOLOGY/ RISK FACTORS	Common bacterial pathogens include β haemolytic and other streptococci. The part played by viruses is uncertain.
PROGNOSIS	We found no good data on the natural history of tonsillitis or recurrent sore throat in children or adults. Participants in RCTs who were randomised to medical treatment (courses of antibiotics as required) have shown a tendency towards improvement over time.[1,3]
AIMS	To abolish tonsillitis; to reduce the frequency and severity of throat infections; to improve general wellbeing, behaviour, and educational achievement, with minimal adverse effects.
OUTCOMES	Number and severity of episodes of tonsillitis or sore throat; requirement for antibiotics and analgesics; time off work or school; behaviour, school performance, general wellbeing; morbidity and mortality of surgery, and adverse effects of drugs.
METHODS	We searched Medline and Embase up to 1997 for RCTs and controlled clinical trials using the key words tonsillitis, tonsillectomy, and tonsil. *Clinical Evidence* search and appraisal May 2000.

QUESTION Is tonsillectomy effective in severe tonsillitis in children and adults?

OPTION TONSILLECTOMY VERSUS ANTIBIOTICS

Limited evidence from one RCT suggests that tonsillectomy may benefit some children with severe tonsillitis. We found no good evidence on tonsillectomy in adults. We found that many important outcome measures have not been considered.

Benefits: We found two systematic reviews (search dates 1997 and 1998).[4,5] **Children:** Both reviews identified the same two RCTs as being the only ones that met quality inclusion criteria.[1,3] The smaller RCT involved 91 children who fulfilled stringent diagnostic criteria for "severe tonsillitis" (see definition above).[1] The children were randomised to tonsillectomy alone (n = 27), adenotonsillectomy (n = 16), or intermittent courses of antibiotics as needed (n = 48). Some children (n = 16) were withdrawn from the non-surgical group by their parents and had surgery, and children who developed infections after surgery received antibiotics as necessary for each episode of infection. Secondary outcome measures such as time off school were also considered. The authors concluded that children undergoing tonsillectomy experienced significantly fewer throat infections than those on antibiotics, amounting to an average of three fewer throat infections in the first 2 years, but by the third year the difference was no longer significant. The larger RCT, in 246 "less severely affected children" is published only in abstract form.[3] Some children in this study also underwent adenoidectomy. The limited data available provide no evidence of a difference between surgical and medical treatment. The second review concluded that it was not possible to determine the effectiveness of tonsillectomy from these RCTs.[5] **Adults:** The reviews found no RCTs that evaluated tonsillectomy in adults with recurrent tonsillitis or sore throats.

Harms: The risks of tonsillectomy include those associated with general anaesthesia and those specific to the procedure. The overall complication rate in the smaller RCT was 14%[1] (all were "readily managed or self limiting") compared with 2.3–7.8% in one Scottish tonsillectomy audit.[6] Haemorrhage, either primary (in the immediate postoperative period) or secondary, occurred in 4% of children studied in the larger RCT[3] and fewer than 1% of children in the Scottish tonsillectomy audit.[6] Potentially harmful effects of non-surgical treatment are principally those associated with antibiotic usage. In the smaller RCT,[1] erythematous rashes occurred in 4% of children in the non-surgical group while taking penicillin.

Comment: In the smaller RCT,[1] there were significant baseline differences between groups before treatment, and the authors pooled the results of tonsillectomy and adenotonsillectomy, making it impossible to assess the effectiveness of tonsillectomy alone. Tonsillectomy is one of the most frequently performed surgical procedures in the UK, particularly in children, and accounts for about 20% of all operations performed by otolaryngologists.[6] We found no RCT that found improved general wellbeing, development, or behaviour—despite suggestions that these are influenced by tonsillectomy.[6] Adenoidectomy is now only performed with tonsillectomy when there is a specific indication to remove the adenoids as well as the tonsils.

REFERENCES

1. Paradise JL, Bluestone CD, Bachman RZ, et al. Efficacy of tonsillectomy for recurrent throat infection in severely affected children. *N Engl J Med* 1984;310:674–683.
2. Shvartzman P. Careful prescribing is beneficial. *BMJ* 1994;309:1101–1102.
3. Paradise JL, Bluestone CD, Rogers KD, et al. Comparative efficacy of tonsillectomy for recurrent throat infection in more versus less severely affected children [abstract]. *Pediatric Res* 1992; 31:126A.
4. Marshall T. A review of tonsillectomy for recurrent throat infection. *Br J Gen Pract* 1998;48:1331–

1335. Search date 1997; primary sources Cochrane Library; Medline.
5. Burton MJ, Towler B, Glasziou P. Tonsillectomy versus non-surgical treatment for chronic/recurrent acute tonsillitis. In: The Cochrane Library, Issue 4, 1999. Oxford: Update Software. Search date 1998; primary sources Medline; Embase; Cochrane Controlled Trials Register, and hand searched references..
6. Blair RL, McKerrow WS, Carter NW, Fenton A. The Scottish tonsillectomy audit. *J Laryngol Otol* 1996; 110(suppl 20):1–25.

Martin Burton
Consultant Otolaryngologist
Department of Otolaryngology
Radcliffe Infirmary NHS Trust
Oxford
UK

Competing interests: None declared.

Wax in ear

Search date March 2000

Martin Burton and Elizabeth Mogg

Ear, nose, and throat disorders

QUESTIONS

Effects of methods to remove symptomatic ear wax 371

INTERVENTIONS

Trade off between benefits and harms
Ear syringing* 372

Unknown effectiveness
Wax softeners 371
Manual removal* 372

*Although many practitioners consider these to be standard treatments, we found no RCTs regarding the benefits or harms of these interventions.
See glossary, p 373

Key Messages

- We found no good evidence about mechanical methods of removing ear wax.
- One small RCT found that wax softeners were better than no treatment at completely removing ear wax without syringing.

DEFINITION	Ear wax is normal and becomes a problem only if it produces deafness, pain, or other aural symptoms. Ear wax may also need to be removed if it prevents inspection of the ear drum. The term "impacted" is used in different ways, and may merely imply the coexistence of wax obscuring the ear drum with symptoms in that ear.[1,2]
INCIDENCE/ PREVALENCE	A survey found that 289 Scottish general practitioners each saw an average of nine people a month requesting removal of ear wax.[1]
AETIOLOGY/ RISK FACTORS	Factors that prevent the normal extrusion of wax from the ear canal (e.g. wearing a hearing aid, using cotton buds) increase the chance of ear wax accumulating.
PROGNOSIS	Most ear wax emerges from the external canal spontaneously. Without impaction or adherence to the drum, there is likely to be minimal, if any, hearing loss. One survey of 21 unselected outpatients with completely obstructing wax found that the average improvement in hearing following syringing was 5.5 dB (95% CI 0.6 to 10.5 dB).[1]
AIMS	To relieve symptoms or to allow examination by completely removing impacted wax or obstructing wax; to soften impacted wax to ease mechanical removal.
OUTCOMES	Proportion of people (or ears) with relief of hearing loss or discomfort; total removal of wax, proportion of people requiring further intervention to improve symptoms, ease of mechanical removal measured, for example, by the volume of water used to accomplish successful syringing.
METHODS	*Clinical Evidence* search and appraisal March 2000.

QUESTION   What are the effects of methods to remove ear wax?

OPTION   WAX SOFTENERS

One RCT found limited evidence that using a wax softener for 5 days increases the chance of an ear being cleared of wax compared with no treatment. One third of untreated ears cleared in the same period. Nine RCTs found no consistent evidence that any one type of wax softener was superior to the others.

Benefits: We found no systematic review. **Versus placebo:** We found one RCT in 113 people with impacted wax (see glossary, p 373) in one or both ears.[2] The ears were randomly allocated to treatment by the nursing staff with sterile water, sodium bicarbonate, a proprietary softening agent (arachis oil/chlorobutanol/p-dichlorobenzene), or no treatment. Active treatment allocation was double blind. The participants were recruited in a hospital for the elderly. People already using ear drops, and people with known pathology of the ear canal or ear drum, were excluded. Of those recruited, 13 left hospital and three died before completing the trial. Analysis of the remaining 97 people (155 ears) found that the risk of persisting impaction at the end of the trial was reduced by any active form of treatment compared with no treatment (AR of persistent impaction: 26/38 [68%] ears with no treatment; 55/117 [47%] with any active treatment; ARR 21%, 95% CI 3% to 35%; RRR 31%, 95% CI 6% to 75%; NNT 5, 95% CI 3 to 34). **Versus other wax softeners:** We found nine RCTs reported in seven publications comparing wax softeners (see table 1, p 374).[1-8] Three of these, rather than using randomisation used alternate allocation, and an additional four did not state their methods of randomisation. The trials were conducted in a variety of settings. They varied in size from 35 people to 286 ears. The commonest outcomes were a subjective assessment of the amount of wax remaining, the need for syringing, or the perceived ease, the result of syringing, or both. The RCTs found no consistent evidence that any one type of wax softener was clinically superior to any other.

Harms: Six RCTs did not report complications or adverse effects. Two found single cases of irritation, itch, or buzzing.[3,4] One study found that 16% (17/106) using either arachis oil/chlorobutanol/p-dichlorobenzene or a proprietary agent whose composition was not stated (Otocerol®) reported adverse effects, including pain or irritation, giddiness, and dislike of the smell of the wax softener.[6]

Comment: We found no good evidence about the optimal duration of treatment. Most trials did not use rigorous methods of randomisation. Many trials were sponsored by companies that manufactured only one of the products being tested, but the possibility of publication bias has not been assessed. The inclusion criteria for the RCTs were not always clear: many stated that the participants had impacted wax without defining how this was assessed. The RCT that included a no-treatment group found that 32% of ears with impacted wax showed spontaneous resolution after 5 days.[2]

| OPTION | MECHANICAL METHODS |

We found no good evidence concerning the benefits or harms of mechanical removal of wax.

Benefits: We found no systematic review and no RCTs comparing mechanical methods intended to remove ear wax with no treatment or alternative treatment.

Harms: A survey found that 38% of 274 general practitioners performing ear syringing reported complications, including otitis externa, perforation of the tympanic membrane, damage to the skin of the external canal, tinnitus, pain, and vertigo.[1] We found no study of the incidence of these complications. People may experience dizziness when wax is removed by suction.

Comment: There is consensus that syringing is effective, and that training can reduce complications, but we found no evidence establishing these points. Other mechanical techniques include manual removal under direct vision, with or without a microscope, using suction, probes, or forceps. These methods require specific training and access to appropriate equipment.

GLOSSARY

Impacted wax Wax that has accumulated in the ear canal, completely obstructing the lumen. In practice, many RCTs define impaction as the presence of symptoms associated with obstructing wax.

Obstructing wax Wax that obscures direct vision of the ear drum.

REFERENCES

1. Sharp JF, Wilson JA, Ross L, Barr-Hamilton RM. Ear wax removal: a survey of current practice. *BMJ* 1990;301:1251–1252.

2. Keane EM, Wilson H, McGrane D, Coakley D, Walsh JB. Use of solvents to disperse ear wax. *Br J Clin Pract* 1995;49:7–12.

3. Dummer DS, Sutherland IA, Murray JA. A single-blind, randomized study to compare the efficacy of two ear drop preparations ('Andax' and 'Cerumol') in the softening of ear wax. *Curr med Res Opin* 1992;13:26–30.

4. Lyndon S, Roy P, Grillage MG, Miller AJ. A comparison of the efficacy of two ear drop preparations ('Aurax' and 'Earex') in the softening and removal of impacted ear wax. *Curr Med Res Opin* 1992;13:21–25.

5. Fahmy S, Whitefield M. Multicentre clinical trial of Exterol as a cerumenolytic. *Br J Clin Pract* 1982; 36:197–204.

6. Jaffe G, Grimshaw J. A multicentric clinical trial comparing Otocerol with Cerumol as cerumenolytics. *J Int Med Res* 1978;6:241–244.

7. Amjad AH, Scheer AA. Clinical evaluation of cerumenolytic agents. *Eye Ear Nose Throat Mon* 1975;54:76–77.

8. Chaput de Saintonge DM, Johnstone CI. A clinical comparison of triethanolamine polypeptide oleate-condensate ear drops with olive oil for the removal of impacted wax. *Br J Clin Pract* 1973;27:454–455.

Martin Burton
Consultant Otolaryngologist

Elizabeth Mogg
Senior House Officer

The Radcliffe Infirmary
Oxford
UK

Competing interests: None declared.

Ear, nose, and throat disorders

TABLE 1 Effects of wax softeners: results of comparative RCTs (see text, p 372).

Reference	Wax softener	Administration	Selection characteristic; setting	Number of people (ears)	Randomisation; blind	Outcome	Results	Adverse effects
2	(a) Arachis oil Chlorobutanol P-dichlorobenzene (b) Sodium bicarbonate (in glycerol) (c) Sterile water (d) Nothing	4 drops twice a day for 5 days	Impacted ear(s); hospital	113 recruited; 97 completed (155)	Double blind (active treatments)	Residual wax; 3 tiered clinical rating scale	Treatment better than no treatment; no difference between agents	None
3	(a) Ethyleneoxide-polyoxypropylene glycol Choline salicylate (b) Arachis oil Chlorobutanol P-dichlorobenzene	Drops to fill ear twice a day for 4 days	Impacted or hardened wax; general practice	50 (100)	Not stated; single blind	Wax amount, colour and consistency; objective hearing; global impression of efficiency	No difference	Two irritation with (a); one itch, one buzzing with (b)
4	(a) Ethyleneoxide-polyoxypropylene glycol Choline salicylate (b) Arachis oil Almond oil Rectified camphor oil	Drops to fill ear twice a day for 4 days	Symptoms requiring wax softener; general practice	36 (72)	Not stated; not blind	Need for syringing; ease of syringing; global impression of efficiency	(a) better than (b); easy removal: 37/38 v 19/30	One irritation with (b); one disliked smell

TABLE 1 continued

	Intervention	Dosage	Population; setting	Number (n)	Method	Outcome measure	Results	Adverse effects
5	(a) 5% urea hydrogen peroxide in glycerol (b) Glycerol	5–10 drops twice a day for a week	Ear wax problems; ENT dept	40 (80)	Alternation; double blind	Need for syringing; ease of syringing	(a) better than glycerol; success: 35/40 v 20/40	None
5	(a) 5% urea hydrogen peroxide in glycerol (b) Arachis oil Chlorobutanol P-dichlorobenzene	5–10 drops twice a day for a week	Ear wax problems; ENT dept	50 (100)	Alternation; double blind	Need for syringing; ease of syringing	(a) better than (b); success: 47/50 v 24/50	None
5	(a) 5% urea hydrogen peroxide in glycerol (b) Arachis oil Chlorobutanol P-dichlorobenzene	5–10 drops twice a day for a week	Ear wax problems; general practice	160 (286)	Alternation; double blind	Need for syringing; ease of syringing	(a) better than (b); success: 146/157 v 93/129	None
6	(a) Otocerol® (b) Arachis oil Chlorobutanol P-dichlorobenzene	Three consecutive nights	For whom a wax softener would normally be prescribed; general practice	106 (not stated)	Random allocation; double blind	3 tiered clinical rating scale	No difference overall; (38/53 v 33/53)	Pain; irritation; giddiness; smell (Otocero; 7/53) (Cerumol; 10/53)
7	(a) Triethanolamine polypeptide oleate condensate (b) Carbamide peroxide	One dose 30 minutes before syringing	Hard or impacted wax; setting unclear	80 (not stated)	Random allocation; double blind	Result of syringing; 4 tiered clinical rating scale	(a) better than (b), but (b) normally used as multiple installations	None
8	(a) Triethanolamine polypeptide oleate condensate (b) Olive oil	One dose 20 minutes before syringing	Impacted wax suitable for syringing; hospital outpatient dept	67 (number of patients not stated)	Random order; double blind	3 tiered clinical rating scale	No difference overall (20/32 v 21/35); (a) needed less water	None

ENT, ear, nose, and throat.

Endocrine disorders

Cardiovascular disease in diabetes

Search date December 2000: expanded this issue

Ronald Sigal and Janine Malcolm

INTERVENTIONS

Key Messages

- Diabetes mellitus increases the risk of cardiovascular disease. Cardiovascular risk factors in people with diabetes include conventional risk factors (age, prior cardiovascular disease, cigarette smoking, hypertension, dyslipidaemia, sedentary lifestyle, family history of premature cardiovascular disease), and more diabetes specific risk factors (elevated urinary protein excretion, poor glycaemic control).

- We found no good evidence on the effects of screening people with diabetes for high cardiovascular risk.
- We found no direct evidence on the effects of promoting smoking cessation in people with diabetes. Observational evidence and extrapolation from people without diabetes suggest that promotion of smoking cessation is likely to reduce cardiovascular events.

RCTs have found:

- Antihypertensive treatment in people with diabetes reduces cardiovascular events.
- Aggressive blood pressure control with target diastolic blood pressures of ≤ 80 mmHg compared with less tight control reduces cardiovascular morbidity and mortality.
- Weak and conflicting evidence comparing the effects of angiotensin enzyme (ACE) inhibitors with other antihypertensive treatments.
- Statins and fibrates are effective in primary and secondary prevention of cardiovascular disease in people with diabetes and dyslipidaemia.
- Aspirin is effective in primary and secondary prevention of cardiovascular disease in people with diabetes.
- Aggressive control of blood glucose with insulin and oral agents, or both, does not increase the risk of cardiovascular disease, and may decrease this risk.
- Coronary artery bypass grafting (CABG) reduces the death rate more than percutaneous transluminal coronary angioplasty (PTCA) in people with diabetes and multivessel coronary artery disease.
- In people with diabetes and acute myocardial infarction (AMI), one RCT found that PTCA significantly reduced the risk of death or cardiovascular events within 30 days of treatment.
- The combination of stent and glycoprotein IIb/IIIa inhibition in people with diabetes undergoing percutaneous coronary revascularisation reduces restenosis rates and serious morbidity.

DEFINITION	**Diabetes mellitus:** See definition under glycaemic control in diabetes, p 403. **Cardiovascular disease:** Atherosclerotic disease the heart and/or the coronary, cerebral, or peripheral vessels leading to clinical events such as AMI, congestive heart failure, sudden cardiac death, stroke, gangrene, and/or need for revascularisation procedures.
INCIDENCE/ PREVALENCE	Diabetes mellitus is a major risk factor for cardiovascular disease. In the USA, 60–75% of people with diabetes die from cardiovascular causes.[1] The annual incidence of cardiovascular disease is increased in diabetic men (RR 2–3) and in diabetic women (RR 3–4) after adjusting for age and other cardiac risk factors.[2] About 45% of middle aged and older white people with diabetes have evidence of coronary artery disease, compared with about 25% of people without diabetes in the same populations.[2] In a population based cohort study of 1059 diabetic and 1373 non-diabetic Finnish adults aged 45–64 years, the 7 year risk of AMI was as high in adults with diabetes without previous cardiac disease as it was in people without diabetes with previous cardiac disease.[3]
AETIOLOGY/ RISK FACTORS	Conventional risk factors for cardiovascular disease contribute to increasing its relative risk in people with diabetes to about the same extent as in those without diabetes (see aetiology under primary

prevention, p 63). The absolute risk of cardiovascular disease is almost the same in diabetic women as in diabetic men. Cardiovascular risk factors relatively specific to people with diabetes include longer duration of diabetes during adulthood (the years of exposure to diabetes before age 20 add little to risk of cardiovascular disease);[4] raised blood glucose concentrations (reflected in fasting blood glucose or HbA1c); and microalbuminuria (albuminuria 30–299 mg/24 hours). People with diabetes and microalbuminuria have a higher risk of coronary morbidity and mortality than people with normal levels of urinary albumin and a similar duration of diabetes (RR 2–3).[5,6] Clinical proteinuria increases the risk of major cardiac events in type 2 diabetes (RR 3)[7] and in type 1 diabetes (RR 9),[4,8,9] compared with individuals with the same type of diabetes having normal albumin excretion. Physical inactivity is a significant risk factor for cardiovascular events in both men and women. A cohort study of diabetic women found that participation in little or no physical activity (< 1 hour per week) compared with participation in physical activity for at least 7 hours a week was associated with doubling of the risk of a cardiovascular event.[10] A cohort study of 1263 diabetic men (mean follow up 12 years) found that low baseline cardiorespiratory fitness compared with moderate or high fitness increased overall mortality (RR 2.9); and overall mortality was higher in those reporting no recreational exercise in the previous 3 months compared with those reporting any recreational physical activity in the same period (RR 1.7).[11]

PROGNOSIS Diabetes mellitus increases the risk of mortality or serious morbidity after a coronary event (RR 1.5–3).[2,3,12,13] This excess risk is partly accounted for by increased prevalence of other cardiac risk factors in people with diabetes. A systematic review found that "stress hyperglycaemia" in diabetic people on admission to hospital for AMI compared with diabetic people with lower glucose levels was associated with increased mortality in hospital (RR 1.7, 95% CI 1.2 to 2.4).[14]

AIMS To reduce mortality and morbidity from cardiovascular disease, with minimum adverse effects.

OUTCOMES Incidence of fatal or non-fatal AMI; congestive heart failure; sudden cardiac death; coronary revascularisation; stroke; gangrene; angiographic evidence of coronary, cerebral vascular, or peripheral arterial stenosis.

METHODS *Clinical Evidence* update search and appraisal December 2000. We searched for systematic reviews and RCTs with at least 10 confirmed clinical cardiovascular events among people with diabetes. Studies reporting only intermediate end points (e.g. regression of plaque on angiography, lipid changes) were not considered.

QUESTION **What are the effects of screening for high cardiovascular risk in people with diabetes?**

We found no good evidence about screening people with diabetes for cardiovascular risk.

Benefits: We found no systematic review and no large RCTs.

Harms: We found inadequate evidence.

Comment: Screening for conventional risk factors as well as regular determination of HbA1c (see glossary, p 389), lipid profile, and urinary albumin excretion will identify people at high risk.[15,16] Consensus opinion in the USA recommends screening for cardiovascular disease with exercise stress testing in previously sedentary adults with diabetes who are planning to undertake vigorous exercise programmes.[15,17] We found no evidence that such testing prevents cardiac events.

QUESTION   What are the effects of promoting smoking cessation in people with diabetes?

Observational studies have found that cigarette smoking is associated with increased cardiovascular death in people with diabetes. In non-diabetic people, smoking cessation has been found to be associated with reduced risk.

Benefits: We found no systematic review or RCTs of the promotion of smoking cessation specifically in people with diabetes.

Harms: We found no evidence of harms.

Comment: People with diabetes are likely to benefit from smoking cessation at least as much as people who do not have diabetes but have other risk factors for cardiovascular events (see smoking cessation under secondary prevention of ischaemic cardiac events, p 95).

QUESTION   What are the effects of antihypertensive drugs in people with diabetes?

OPTION   ANTIHYPERTENSIVE TREATMENT VERSUS NO ANTIHYPERTENSIVE TREATMENT

Systematic reviews of RCTs have found that diuretics, ACE inhibitors, and β blockers reduce cardiovascular events in people with diabetes and no previous cardiovascular events. One large RCT found that an ACE inhibitor reduced subsequent cardiovascular events and overall mortality in people with diabetes aged over 55 with additional cardiac risk factors, previously diagnosed coronary vascular disease (CVD), or both. No class of medication had significant adverse effects on metabolism or quality of life at the doses used in the trials reviewed.

Benefits: **Primary prevention:** See table 1, p 392. We found one systematic review (published 1997, 2 RCTs included a subgroup of 1355 people with diabetes who had no previous cardiovascular events)[18] and one subsequent RCT.[19] The systematic review found that active treatment (stepped care beginning with a diuretic) versus less active treatment (either placebo[20] or referral to usual care in the community[21]) significantly reduced cardiovascular morbidity and mortality (OR for morbidity and mortality 0.64, 95% CI 0.50 to 0.82; for overall mortality 0.85, 95% CI 0.62 to 1.17) and major cardiovascular events (AR 27% with control v 19% with active treatment over 5 years; NNT 13 middle aged and older adults with diabetes for 5 years). The subsequent RCT (4695 people, 495 with diabetes, aged ≥60 years with blood pressure 165–220/ <95 mmHg) found that active treatment (beginning with nitrendipine) versus placebo reduced all cardiovascular events over a median of 2 years (AR 13/252 [5.2%] for active treatment v 31/240 [12.9%] for controls; ARR 8%, 95% CI 3% to 10%; RR 0.4, 95% CI 0.21 to 0.75; NNT 13, 95% CI 10 to 31) but had no significant effect on overall mortality (AR 16/252 for active treatment v 26/240 for controls; ARR +4.5%, 95% CI −0.7% to +7.4%; RR 0.96, 95% CI 0.32 to 1.06).[19] **Primary and secondary prevention:** See table 3, p 396. We found one systematic review (search date not stated, 4 RCTs, 1100 people with diabetes out of 15 843 people aged > 55 years)[22] and one subsequent RCT.[23] The systematic review found that diuretics (1008 people) versus placebo reduced the risk of major CVD events (fatal or non-fatal coronary events or stroke, sudden death, or death from embolism; RR 0.8). No conclusion was reached regarding initial treatment with β blockers because so few people with diabetes (92 people) received them.[22] The subsequent RCT (3577 diabetic people out of 9541 people aged ≥55 years with at least 1 of the following risk factors: diagnosed CVD, current smoker, hypercholesterolaemia, hypertension, or microalbuminuria) compared ramipril (10 mg) versus placebo and vitamin E versus placebo over 4.5 years in a 2 x 2 factorial design (see table 3, p 396).[23] Compared with placebo, ramipril reduced major cardiovascular events (CVD death, AMI, or stroke 277/1808 with ramipril v 351/1769 with placebo; RR 0.75, 95% CI 0.64 to 0.88; ARR 4.5%; NNT 22 older people with diabetes and additional risk factors treated for 4.5 years to prevent 1 major cardiovascular event, 95% CI 14 to 43), and death from any cause (196/1808 v 248/1769; RR 0.76, 95% CI 0.67 to 0.92; ARR 3.2%; NNT 32, 95% CI 19 to 98). The relative effect of ramipril was present in all subgroups regardless of hypertensive status, microalbuminuria, type of diabetes, and nature of diabetes treatment (diet, oral agents, or insulin). Vitamin E treatment had no effect on morbidity or mortality.[23] **Secondary prevention:** See table 2, p 394. We found one systematic review (7 RCTs with follow up ≥ 1 year; 2564 people with diabetes and previous cardiovascular events).[18] It found that both ACE inhibitors and β blockers reduced the risk of subsequent cardiac events in people with diabetes and previous myocardial infarction, with or without hypertension. Active treatment versus placebo significantly reduced overall mortality (6 RCTs, 2402 people; OR 0.82, 95% CI 0.69 to 0.99). Cardiovascular morbidity plus mortality was reduced by a similar amount, but was reported by only two RCTs in the systematic review and the reduction was not significant (2 RCTs, 654 people; OR 0.82, 95% CI 0.60 to 1.13).

Harms: No class of medication had significant adverse effects on metabolism or quality of life at the doses used in the trials reviewed. More people allocated to ramipril than to placebo withdrew because of cough (7% v 2%). This was the only adverse effect occurring more frequently in the ACE inhibitor recipients than in controls.[22]

Comment: None.

One systematic review of large RCTs has found that ACE inhibitors versus calcium channel blockers as initial therapy for hypertension significantly reduce cardiovascular events in people with type 2 diabetes aged 50–65 years. We found no clear evidence directly comparing ACE inhibitors and diuretics. One large RCT found that an ACE inhibitor versus a β blocker had similar effect on cardiovascular events. One large RCT has found that doxazosin (an α blocker) versus chlorthalidone (a diuretic) increases the risk of congestive heart failure.

Benefits: We found one systematic review (search date 2000, 4 RCTs, 2180 people with diabetes)[24] and two subsequent RCTs.[25,26] The systematic review compared ACE inhibitors (1133 people) versus other antihypertensive drugs (diuretics, β blockers, or calcium channel blockers; 1047 people).[24] **ACE inhibitors versus calcium channel blockers:** We found one systematic review,[24] which found two RCTs[27,28] comparing ACE inhibitors versus calcium channel blockers in people with diabetes, and one subsequent RCT[25] comparing ACE inhibitors versus calcium channel antagonists versus conventional treatment (β blockers or hydrochlorothiazide plus amiloride). The two RCTs in the systematic review found that ACE inhibitors versus calcium channel blockers significantly reduced cardiovascular events (34/424 [8%] with ACE inhibitor v 151/526 [16%] with calcium channel blocker; ARR 8%, 95% CI 4% to 13%; RR 0.49, 95% CI 0.33 to 0.72; NNT 13, 95% CI 7 to 25). ACE inhibitors versus calcium channel blockers also reduced the three outcomes of death, AMI, and stroke, but the reductions were not significant. The subsequent RCT (6614 people, 719 with diabetes, mean age 76 years, mean blood pressure 190/99 mmHg) found (among the subgroup of people with diabetes) no significant difference in the incidence of major cardiovascular events over 4 years (64.2 events/1000 person years with ACE inhibitors v 67.7 with calcium antagonists v 75.0 with conventional agents).[25] **ACE inhibitors versus diuretics:** We found one systematic review,[24] which found no RCTs specifically comparing ACE inhibitors versus diuretics in people with diabetes, but found one RCT (572 people, 6.1 years) comparing ACE inhibitors versus alternative treatment that included β blockers, combination β blockers and diuretics, and diuretics in people with and without diabetes. Fewer people allocated to captopril experieinced AMI, stroke or death compared to diuretics or β blockers (43/263 [18%] with diuretics/β blockers v 30/309 [10%] with captopril; ARR 6.6%, 95 CI 1.1% to 12.2%; NNT 15).[24] **ACE inhibitors versus β blockers:** We found one systematic review, which included one RCT (758 people, 456 cardiovascular events) comparing an ACE inhibitor (captopril) versus a β blocker (atenolol) over 8.4 years.[29] The RCT found that captopril versus atenolol did not significantly reduce the number of cardiovascular events (102/400 [25.5%] with captopril v 75/358 [20.9%] with atenolol; ARI +5%, 95% CI −1% to +11%; RR 1.22, 95% CI 0.94 to 1.58). **Other comparisons:** We found no systematic review but found one RCT[26] (age ≥ 55 years, with hypertension and either previous CVD or at least 1 additional CVD risk factor) comparing chlorthalidone, doxazosin, amlodipine, and lisinopril. After 3.3 years of follow up there was no difference between doxazosin (3183 people with diabetes) and chlorthalidone (5481 people) in the primary outcome (fatal coronary heart disease [CHD] or non-fatal AMI), but the doxazosin arm was terminated because of an excess risk of combined CVD events (coronary heart disease death, non-fatal AMI, stroke, revascularisation procedures, angina, congestive heart failure, and peripheral vascular disease) compared with chlorthalidone (OR 1.24, 95% CI 1.12 to 1.38). The RCT is still in progress.[26]

Harms: In one RCT, people taking atenolol gained more weight than those taking captopril (3.4 kg with atenolol v 1.6 kg with captopril, P = 0.02).[29] Over the first 4 years of the trial, people allocated to atenolol had higher mean HbA1c (7.5% v 7.0%, P = 0.004), but there was no difference between groups over the subsequent 4 years. There was no difference between atenolol and captopril in rates of hypoglycaemia, lipid concentrations, tolerability, blood pressure lowering, or prevention of disease events.

Comment: We found evidence that ACE inhibitors are superior to calcium channel blockers as initial therapy. We found no clear evidence directly comparing ACE inhibitors and diuretics. It is unclear whether ACE inhibitors or β-blockers are superior to each other. In most trials, combination therapy with more than one agent was required to achieve target blood pressures.

| OPTION | DIFFERENT TARGET BLOOD PRESSURE |

RCTs have found that setting lower target blood pressures reduces cardiovascular events.

Benefits: We found several recent trials with large numbers of participants with diabetes (see table 1, p 392, and table 3, p 396). In two large RCTs, tighter control of blood pressure reduced the risk of major cardiovascular events.[29–31] In one, people with diabetes who were randomised to target diastolic blood pressure ≤ 80 mmHg had half the risk of major cardiovascular events compared with their counterparts randomised to target blood pressure ≤ 90 mmHg.[31] In the other large RCT, people with hypertension and type 2 diabetes randomised to tight blood pressure control (< 150/ < 85 mmHg) with atenolol (358 people) or captopril (400 people) had reduced incidence of "any diabetes related end point" deaths (primarily cardiovascular deaths), stroke, and microvascular disease.[29,30]

Harms: We found no good evidence of a threshold below which it is harmful to lower blood pressure.

Comment: Aggressive lowering of blood pressure in people with diabetes and hypertension reduces cardiovascular morbidity and mortality. In most trials, combination therapy with more than one agent was required to achieve target blood pressures.

Subgroup analyses of results for people with diabetes enrolled into large RCTs of statins or fibrates versus placebo have found benefit in primary and secondary prevention of AMI.

Benefits: **Primary prevention:** We found no systematic review. Three large RCTs with significant numbers of diabetic participants have compared lipid lowering agents with placebo, and found reductions in the risk of cardiovascular events (see table 1, p 392). In the first, men aged 45–73 years and women aged 55–73 years were randomised to diet plus lovastatin 20–40 mg/day or diet plus placebo, and followed for a mean of 5.2 years.[32] Only people with total cholesterol 4.65–6.82 mmol/l, low density lipoprotein cholesterol (LDL-C) 3.36–4.91 mmol/l, high density lipoprotein cholesterol (HDL-C) ≤ 1.16 mmol/l (men) or ≤ 1.22 mmol/l (women), and triglycerides ≤ 4.52 mmol/l were included in the trial. The second RCT (4081 Finnish men aged 40–55 years) compared gemfibrozil 600 mg twice daily versus placebo over 5 years. Required baseline lipid concentrations were (total minus HDL-C) ≥ 5.2 mmol/l; participants were not excluded on the basis of triglyceride level.[33] The third RCT (164 men and women with type 2 diabetes aged 35–65 years) compared bezafibrate versus placebo for 3 years.[34] Required baseline lipids included one or more of the following: total cholesterol 5.2 to 8.0 mmol/l, serum triglyceride 1.8–8.0 mmol/l, HDL-C ≤ 1.1 mmol/l, or total to HDL-C ratio ≥ 4.7. **Secondary prevention:** We found no systematic review but found four RCTs involving people with diabetes (see table 2, p 394). One RCT (4444 men and women aged 35–70 years with previous AMI or angina pectoris, total cholesterol concentrations of 5.5–8.0 mmol/l, and triglycerides ≤ 2.5 mmol/l) compared simvastatin versus placebo over a median of 5.4 years.[35] Simvastatin dosage was initially 20 mg daily, with blinded dosage titration up to 40 mg daily, according to cholesterol response during the first 6–18 weeks. The relative risk of main end points in people with diabetes treated with simvastatin were as follows: total mortality 0.57 (95% CI 0.30 to 1.08), major cardiovascular events 0.45 (95% CI 0.27 to 0.74), and any atherosclerotic event 0.63 (95% CI 0.43 to 0.92).[23] The second RCT (4159 men and women aged 21–75 years, 3–20 months after MI and with total cholesterol < 6.2 mmol/l, triglycerides < 3.92 mmol/l, and LDL-C 3.0–4.5 mmol/l) compared pravastatin 40 mg/day versus placebo over a median of 5 years.[36] Among the people with diabetes, the relative risk of major coronary events (death from coronary disease, non-fatal AMI, CABG, or PTCA) was 0.75 (95% CI 0.57 to 1.0). The third RCT (9014 men and women aged 31–75 with AMI or unstable angina, plasma total cholesterol 4.0–7.0 mmol/l, and plasma triglycerides < 5.0 mmol/l) compared pravastatin 40 mg daily versus placebo for a mean of 6.1 years.[37] Among the 782 participants with diabetes, the relative risk of CHD death or non-fatal AMI was 0.84 (95% CI 0.59 to 1.10). The fourth RCT (2531 men aged < 74 with previous CVD, AMI, angina, revascularisation, or angiographically documented coronary stenosis), (HDL-C ≤ 1.0 mmol/l, LDL-C ≤ 3.6 mmol/l and triglycerides ≤ 3.4 mmol/l) compared gemfibrozil 1200 mg daily with placebo for a median of

5.1 years (treatment was intended to raise HDL-C levels rather than reduce LDL-C).[38] Among the 627 participants with diabetes, the relative risk of CHD death or non-fatal MI was 0.76 (95% CI 0.57 to 1.0).

Harms: None reported.

Comment: Most published clinical trials with sufficient statistical power to detect effects on cardiovascular events have enrolled comparatively small numbers of diabetic people or excluded them altogether. The available evidence is therefore based almost entirely on subgroup analyses of larger trials. Several large ongoing trials are evaluating the effects of fibrates in people with diabetes.

QUESTION What are the effects of blood glucose control on cardiovascular disease in people with diabetes?

In most cohort studies, higher average concentrations of blood glucose in people with diabetes were associated with a higher incidence of cardiovascular disease. RCTs provide modest support for glucose lowering with insulin, sulphonylureas, or metformin in primary prevention of cardiovascular disease, and strong support for intensive insulin treatment after AMI.

Benefits: **Primary prevention:** See table 1, p 392. We found no systematic review. In people with diabetes, higher average levels of blood glucose are associated with a higher incidence of cardiovascular disease.[39-42] Both found that intensive hypoglycaemic treatment reduced the risks of microvascular diabetic complications in both type 1 and type 2 diabetes, although neither trial found that intensive glycaemic control significantly reduced cardiovascular risk. In the first trial, 1441 people with type 1 diabetes aged 13–39 years and free of cardiovascular disease, hypertension, hypercholesterolaemia, and obesity at baseline, were randomly assigned to conventional or intensive diabetes treatment and followed for a mean of 6.5 years.[41,42] Major macrovascular events were almost twice as frequent in the conventionally treated group (40 events) as in the intensive treatment group (23 events), although the differences were not significant (ARR 2.2%; RR 0.59, 95% CI 0.32 to 1.1). In the second trial, 3867 people aged 25–65 years (median 54 years) with type 2 diabetes that was inadequately controlled on diet alone, were randomised to conventional treatment (diet only, 1138 people, drugs added only if needed to keep fasting glucose < 15.0 mmol/l), intensive treatment with a sulphonylurea (1573 people), or insulin (1156 people).[39] People who were ≥ 120% of ideal body weight were randomised to conventional treatment (411 people), metformin (342 people), sulphonylureas (542 people), or insulin (409 people).[40] Intensive treatment beginning with a sulphonylurea or insulin improved glycaemic control (HbA1c 7.9% with conventional treatment compared with 7% with intensive treatment). Compared with conventional treatment, intensive treatment reduced diabetes related end points (RR 0.88, 95% CI 0.80 to 0.99; NNT 39 for 5 years to prevent 1 additional diabetes related end point) and the risk of AMI (ARs 14.7/1000 person years for intensive v 17.4/1000 person years for conventional; RR 0.84, 95% CI 0.71 to 1.0). Risks of stroke and amputation did not differ significantly among groups.[39] **Secondary prevention:** See table 3, p 396. We found no systematic review but found two RCTs. One small RCT (153 men with type 2 diabetes, mean age 60 years, many of whom had previous cardiovascular events) compared standard insulin (once daily) with intensive treatment with a stepped plan designed to achieve near normal blood sugar levels.[43] After 27 months, the rate of new cardiovascular events was not significantly different between the groups (24/75 [32%] with intensive therapy v 16/80 [20%] with standard insulin; RR 1.6, 95% CI 0.92 to 2.5). In the second trial, 620 people (mean age 68 years, 63% men, 84% with type 2 diabetes) with random blood glucose ≥ 11 mmol/l were randomised within 24 hours of an AMI to either standard treatment or intensive insulin treatment.[44,45] The intensive insulin group received an insulin glucose infusion for 24 hours followed by subcutaneous insulin four times daily for at least 3 months. The standard treatment group received insulin only when it was clinically indicated. HbA1c fell significantly with intensive insulin treatment (absolute fall of 1.1% with intensive treatment v 0.4% with standard treatment at 3 months and 0.9% v 0.4% at 12 months). Intensive treatment lowered mortality (ARs 19% v 26% at 1 year and 33% v 44% at a mean of 3.4 years; RR 0.72, 95% CI 0.55 to 0.92; NNT 9 treated for 3.4 years to prevent 1 additional premature death). The absolute reduction in the risk of mortality was particularly striking in people who were not previously taking insulin and had no more than one of the following risk factors before the AMI that preceded randomisation: age ≥ 70 years, history of previous AMI, history of congestive heart failure, current treatment with digitalis. In this low risk subgroup, the ARR was 15% (NNT 7 for 3.4 years).

Harms: Sulphonylureas and insulin, but not metformin, increased the risks of weight gain and hypoglycaemia. On an intention to treat basis, the proportions of people per year with severe hypoglycaemic episodes were 0.7%, 1.2%, 1%, 2%, and 0.6% for conventional, chlorpropamide, glibenclamide, insulin, and metformin groups. These frequencies of hypoglycaemia were much lower than those observed with intensive treatment in people with type 1 diabetes in the first primary prevention RCT.[41,42] One RCT found no evidence that any specific treatment (insulin, sulphonylurea, or metformin) increased overall risk of cardiovascular disease.[39,40]

Comment: The role of intensive glucose lowering in primary prevention of cardiovascular events remains unclear. However, such treatment clearly reduces the risk of microvascular disease and does not increase the risk of cardiovascular disease. The potential of the second and larger primary prevention RCT to demonstrate an effect of tighter glycaemic control was limited by the small difference achieved in median HbA1c between intensive and conventional treatment. In contrast, in the first primary prevention trial, a larger 1.9% difference in median HbA1c was achieved between groups, but the young age of the participants and consequent low incidence of cardiovascular events limited the power of the study to detect an effect of treatment on incidence of cardiovascular disease.[41,42] The study of insulin in type 2 diabetes[43] included men with a high baseline risk of cardiovascular events and achieved a 2.1%

absolute difference in HbA1c. The RCT was small and the observed difference between groups could have arisen by chance. The design of the trial of intensive versus standard glycaemic control following AMI does not distinguish whether the early insulin infusion or the later intensive subcutaneous insulin treatment was the more important determinant of improved survival in the intensively treated group. The larger primary prevention trial found no evidence that oral hypoglycaemics increase cardiovascular mortality,[39,40] but the possibility that oral hypoglycaemics may be harmful after AMI cannot be ruled out.

QUESTION What is the effect of aspirin in people with diabetes?

Very large RCTs of primary and mixed primary and secondary prevention, and a systematic review of secondary prevention, support a cardioprotective role for aspirin.

Benefits:

Primary prevention: We found no systematic review but found two RCTs. In the only large primary prevention RCT comparing aspirin versus placebo and reporting results for people with diabetes, 22 701 US male physicians aged 40–85 years were assigned to aspirin 325 mg every other day or to placebo, and followed for an average of 5 years.[46] The trial found that, after 5 years, among the 533 physicians with diabetes, aspirin versus placebo reduced the risk of AMI (11/275 [4%] with aspirin v 26/258 [10.1%] with placebo; RR 0.39, 95% CI 0.20 to 0.79; NNT 16, 95% CI 12 to 47). A second RCT comparing aspirin with placebo did not specify the number of people with diabetes, but it did report that aspirin reduced AMI to a similar degree in the subgroup of people with diabetes and in the overall trial population (RR 0.85).[31] **Primary and early secondary prevention:** We found one RCT. The largest RCT of aspirin prophylaxis in people with diabetes involved 3711 diabetic men and women (30% with type 1 diabetes, 48% with prior cardiovascular disease).[47] It compared aspirin (650 mg/day) with placebo and followed the participants for a mean of 5 years. It found a non-significant reduction in overall mortality in those treated with aspirin (RR 0.91, 95% CI 0.75 to 1.11). AMI occurred in 289 people (16%) in the aspirin group and 336 (18%) in the placebo group (ARR 2%, 95% CI 0.1% to 4.9%). Fifty people would need to be treated for 5 years with aspirin 650 mg/day to prevent one additional AMI. **Secondary prevention:** We found one systematic review (search date 1990, 145 RCTs of antiplatelet treatment, primarily aspirin).[48] Results for people with diabetes are tabulated (see table 3, p 396).

Harms:

In the large trial comparing aspirin versus placebo for primary and secondary prevention, fatal or non-fatal stroke occurred in 5% on aspirin and 4.2% on placebo (P = NS).[47] There was no significant increase with aspirin in the risks of vitreous, retinal, gastrointestinal, or cerebral haemorrhage. In the systematic review, doses of aspirin ranged from 75–1500 mg/day. Most trials used 75–325 mg/day of aspirin. Doses higher than 325 mg/day increased the risk of haemorrhagic adverse effects without improving preventive efficacy. No difference in efficacy or adverse effects was found in the dose range 75–325 mg.[48]

Comment: We found insufficient evidence to define precisely which people with diabetes should be treated with aspirin. The risk of cardiovascular disease is very low before age 30; most white diabetic adults aged over 30 are at increased risk of cardiovascular disease. Widely accepted contraindications to aspirin treatment include aspirin allergy, bleeding tendency, anticoagulant treatment, recent gastrointestinal bleeding, and clinically active liver disease.[15,49]

QUESTION What are the effects of treating proteinuria in people with diabetes?

Elevated urinary protein excretion is a risk factor for cardiovascular disease. One large RCT has found that an ACE inhibitor reduces cardiovascular risk compared with placebo in people with or without microalbuminuria.

Benefits: We found no good evidence.

Harms: We found no good evidence.

Comment: One large RCT found that the ACE inhibitor ramipril, which reduces urinary protein excretion, also reduced cardiovascular morbidity and mortality in older diabetic people with other cardiac risk factors.[23] However, the relative cardioprotective effect was present to the same extent in people with or without microalbuminuria.

QUESTION Coronary artery bypass graft versus percutaneous transluminal coronary angioplasty in people with diabetes

One RCT has found that coronary artery bypass graft (CABG) reduces the death rate more than percutaneous transluminal coronary angioplasty (PTCA) in people with diabetes and multivessel coronary artery disease.

Benefits: We found no systematic review but found one RCT (1829 people with two or three vessel coronary disease, 353 with diabetes; mean age 62 years) comparing CABG with PTCA, without stenting or glycoprotein IIb/IIIa blockade (see table 3, p 396).[50] After a mean 7.7 years, fewer diabetic people assigned to CABG than PTCA died or suffered Q-wave myocardial infarction (85/170 [50%] with PTCA v 60/173 [34.7%] with CABG; ARR 15%, 95% CI 5% to 26%; RR 0.69, 95% CI 0.54 to 0.89; NNT 7, 95% CI 4 to 20). This survival benefit was confined to those receiving at least one internal mammary graft.

Harms: In the RCT, in-hospital mortality among people with diabetes was 1.2% after CABG versus 0.6% after PTCA. Myocardial infarction during the initial hospitalisation was three times more common after CABG than after PTCA (5.8% v 1.8%). None of these differences was significant.

Comment: Adjunctive therapies (heparin or abciximab) were not used in the RCT.

What are the effects of primary coronary angioplasty versus thrombolysis for acute myocardial infarction in people with diabetes? New

One RCT has found that treatment of AMI in diabetic people with primary coronary angioplasty rather than thrombolytic therapy results in a non-significant reduction of death and cardiovascular events at 30 days.

Benefits: We found no systematic review. One RCT (1138 people with AMI presenting within 12 hours of chest pain onset, 177 with diabetes, mean age of diabetic people 65 years) compared primary angioplasty with thrombolysis (alteplase) (see table 3, p 396).[51] At 30 days, fewer diabetic people assigned to primary angioplasty experienced the composite end point of death, reinfarction or disabling stroke, but the difference was not significant (11/99 [11%] with primary angioplasty v 13/78 [17%] with alteplase; ARR +5.6%, 95% CI −4.8 to +15.9%). In the RCT, 30 day mortality among people with diabetes was eight of 99 people (81%) after angioplasty versus five of 78 people (6.4%) after alteplase. This difference was not significant.

Harms: See harms of CABG versus PTCA, p 387.

Comment: None.

Glycoprotein IIb/IIIa inhibitors and intracoronary stenting (as adjunct to percutaneous coronary revascularisation) in people with diabetes

Two RCTs have that the combination of stent and glycoprotein IIb/IIIa inhibition (abciximab) reduces restenosis rates and serious morbidity in people with diabetes undergoing percutaneous coronary angioplasty.

Benefits: We found no systematic review but found two RCTs (see table 3, p 396).[52–55] The first RCT (2792 people, 638 with diabetes, mean age 61 years, 38% female, all undergoing PTCA or directional atherectomy without stenting) compared placebo plus standard dose heparin versus abciximab plus standard dose heparin versus abciximab plus low dose heparin. Abciximab was given as a bolus plus 12 hour infusion. The primary indications for intervention were unstable angina (51%), stable ischaemia (33%), and recent AMI (16%). A total of 44% had a prior coronary intervention, 56% had multivessel disease, and 74% a history of hypertension. Compared with placebo, abciximab reduced the combined end point of death or AMI in both standard dose and low dose heparin arms (at 30 days by over 60% and at 6 months by over 50%). Abciximab reduced the rate of restenosis in people without diabetes (hazard ratio 0.78) but not in people with diabetes. The second RCT (2401 people, 491 with diabetes, mean age 60 years, 29% female, 69% hypertensive, 30% recent smokers, 48% prior AMI, 10% prior CABG) compared stent plus placebo (173 people) versus stent plus abciximab (162 people) versus balloon angioplasty plus abciximab (156 people). At 12 months, death or large AMI occurred in 13.9% of those receiving stent and placebo, 8.3% with PTCA and abciximab, and 4.9% with stent and abciximab. Subsequent revascularisation rates following stent and abciximab (13.7%) were much lower than those following stent and placebo (22.4%) or PTCA and abciximab (25.3%).[53-55] For both outcomes, the difference between the stent plus abciximab group and the other two groups was significant. We found an analysis of individual person results of these two trials and a third, earlier trial.[56] In the 1462 diabetic people, abciximab reduced overall mortality (26/540 [4.8%] v 21/844 [2.5%]; ARR 2.3%; NNT 43, 95% CI 23 to 421).

Harms: There was slightly more bleeding in people given abciximab than in those given placebo (4.3% v 3.0% for major bleeding; 6.9% v 6.3% for minor bleeding; 0% v 0.17% for intracranial haemorrhage). None of these differences were significant.[57]

Comment: For people with diabetes undergoing percutaneous procedures, the combination of stent and glycoprotein IIb/IIIa inhibition reduces restenosis rates and serious morbidity. It is unclear whether these adjunctive therapies would reduce morbidity, mortality, and restenosis associated with percutaneous revascularisation procedures to the levels seen with CABG. There was imbalance of the baseline characteristics among the study groups of the second RCT.[53] However, in a multivariate analysis, the treatment effects remained after adjusting for baseline differences.

GLOSSARY

HbA1c The haemoglobin A1c test is the commonest laboratory test of glycated haemoglobin (haemoglobin that has glucose irreversibly bound to it). HbA1c provides an indication of the "average" blood glucose over the last 3 months. The HbA1c is a weighted average over time of the blood glucose level; many different glucose profiles can produce the same level of HbA1c.

Substantive changes since last issue

Diuretics versus placebo New systematic review;[22] evidence that diuretics are more effective than placebo.

ACE inhibitors versus diuretics or calcium channel blockers New systematic review comparing ACE inhibitors versus other antihypertensive drugs;[24] no consistent results from four RCTs.

ACE inhibitors versus calcium channel blockers versus β blockers or diuretics New RCT;[25] conclusion unchanged.

REFERENCES

1. Geiss LS, Herman WH, Smith PJ. Mortality in non-insulin-dependent diabetes. In: Harris MI, ed. *Diabetes in America*. 2nd ed. Bethesda, MD: National Institutes of Health, 1995:233–255.

2. Wingard DL, Barrett-Connor E. Heart disease and diabetes. In: Harris MI, ed. *Diabetes in America*. 2nd ed. Bethesda, MD: National Institutes of Health, 1995:429–448.

3. Haffner SM, Lehto S, Ronnemaa T, et al. Mortality from coronary heart disease in subjects with type 2 diabetes and in nondiabetic subjects with and without prior myocardial infarction. *N Engl J Med* 1998;339:229–234.

4. Krolewski AS, Warram JH, Freire MB. Epidemiology of late diabetic complications. A basis for the development and evaluation of preventive programs. *Endocrinol Metab Clin North Am* 1996; 25:217–242.

5. Messent JW, Elliott TG, Hill RD, et al. Prognostic significance of microalbuminuria in insulin-dependent diabetes mellitus: a twenty-three year follow-up study. *Kidney Int* 1992;41:836–839.

6. Dinneen SF, Gerstein HC. The association of microalbuminuria and mortality in non-insulin-dependent diabetes mellitus: a systematic overview of the literature. *Arch Intern Med* 1997; 157:1413–1418. Search date 1995; primary sources Medline 1966 to 1994, Scisearch, hand-searching of bibliographies.

7. Valmadrid CT, Klein R, Moss S E, Klein BE. The risk of cardiovascular disease mortality associated with microalbuminuria and gross proteinuria in persons with older-onset diabetes mellitus. *Arch Intern Med* 2000;160:1093–1100.

8. Borch Johnsen K, Andersen PK, Deckert T. The effect of proteinuria on relative mortality in type 1 (insulin-dependent) diabetes mellitus. *Diabetologia* 1985;28:590–596.

9. Warram JH, Laffel LM, Ganda OP, et al. Coronary artery disease is the major determinant of excess mortality in patients with insulin-dependent diabetes mellitus and persistent proteinuria. *J Am Soc Nephrol* 1992;3(suppl 4):104–110.

10. Hu FB, Stampfer MJ, Solomon C, et al. Physical activity and risk for cardiovascular events in diabetic women. *Ann Intern Med* 2001;134:96–105.

11. Wei M, Gibbons LW, Kampert JB, Nichaman MZ, Blair SN. Low cardiorespiratory fitness and physical inactivity as predictors of mortality in men with type 2 diabetes. *Ann Intern Med* 2000;132:605–611.

12. Behar S, Boyko V, Reicher-Reiss H, et al. Ten-year survival after acute myocardial infarction: comparison of patients with and without diabetes. SPRINT Study Group. Secondary Prevention Reinfarction Israeli Nifedipine Trial. *Am Heart J* 1997;133:290–296.

13. Mak KH, Moliterno DJ, Granger CB, et al. Influence of diabetes mellitus on clinical outcome in the thrombolytic era of acute myocardial infarction: GUSTO-I Investigators: global utilization of streptokinase and tissue plasminogen activator for occluded coronary arteries. *J Am Coll Cardiol* 1997;30:171–179.

14. Capes SE, Hunt D, Malmberg K, Gerstein HC. Stress hyperglycaemia and increased risk of death after myocardial infarction in patients with and without diabetes: a systematic overview. *Lancet* 2000;355:773–778. Search date 1998; primary sources Medline, Science Citation Index, hand searches of bibliographies of relevant articles, and contact with experts in the field.

15. Meltzer S, Leiter L, Daneman D, et al. Clinical practice guidelines for the management of diabetes in Canada. *Can Med Assoc J* 1998; 159(suppl 8):1–29.

16. American Diabetes Association. Clinical practice recommendations 2000. *Diabetes Care* 2000; 23(suppl 1):1–116.

17. American Diabetes Association. Diabetes mellitus and exercise. *Diabetes Care* 2000;23(suppl 1):50–54.

18. Fuller J, Stevens LK, Chaturvedi N, et al. Antihypertensive therapy in preventing cardiovascular complications in people with diabetes mellitus. In: The Cochrane Library, Issue 4, 2000. Oxford, Update Software. Search date not given; primary sources Medline; Embase; and hand searches of speciality journals in cardiovascular disease, stroke, renal disease, and hypertension.

19. Tuomilehto J, Rastenyte D, Birkenhäger WH, et al. Effects of calcium-channel blockade in older patients with diabetes and systolic hypertension. *N Engl J Med* 1999;340:677–684.

20. Curb JD, Pressel SL, Cutler JA, et al. Effect of diuretic-based antihypertensive treatment on cardiovascular disease risk in older diabetic patients with isolated systolic hypertension. Systolic Hypertension in the Elderly Program Cooperative Research Group. *JAMA* 1996;276:1886–1892.

21. Davis BR, Langford HG, Blaufox MD, et al. The association of postural changes in systolic blood pressure and mortality in persons with hypertension: the Hypertension Detection and Follow-up Program experience. *Circulation* 1987; 75:340–346.

22. Lievre M, Guyffier F, Ekomb T, et al. Efficacy of diuretics and β blockers in diabetic hypertensive patients. *Diabetes Care* 2000;23:B65–B71. Search date not stated; primary source Individual Data Analysis of Antihypertensive Drug Interventions (INDANA) project database.

23. Heart Outcomes Prevention Evaluation (HOPE) Study Investigators. Effects of ramipril on cardiovascular and microvascular outcomes in people with diabetes mellitus: results of the HOPE study and the MICRO-HOPE substudy. *Lancet* 2000;355:253–259.

24. Pahor M, Psaty BM, Alderman MH, Applegate WB, Williamson JD, Furberg CD. Therapeutic benefits of ACE inhibitors and other antihypertensive drugs in patients with type 2 diabetes. *Diabetes Care* 2000;23:888–892. Search date January 2000; primary source Medline.

25. Lindholm LH, Hansson L, Ekbom T, et al. Comparison of antihypertensive treatment in preventing cardiovascular events in elderly diabetic patients: results from the Swedish trial in old patients with hypertension-2. *J Hypertens* 2000; 18:1671–1675.

26. ALLHAT Collaborative Research Group. Major cardiovascular events in hypertensive patients randomised to doxazosin vs chlorthalidone: the antihypertensive and lipid-lowering treatment to prevent heart attack trial (ALLHAT). *JAMA* 2000; 283:1967–1975.

27. Estacio RO, Jeffers BW, Hiatt WR, et al. The effect of nisoldipine as compared with enalapril on cardiovascular events in patients with non-insulin-dependent diabetes and hypertension. *N Engl J Med* 1998;338:645–652.

28. Tatti P, Pahor M, Byington RP, et al. Outcome results of the Fosinopril versus Amlodipine Cardiovascular Events randomised Trial (FACET) in patients with hypertension and NIDDM. *Diabetes Care* 1998;21:597–603.

29. UK Prospective Diabetes Study Group. Efficacy of atenolol and captopril in reducing risk of macrovascular and microvascular complications in type 2 diabetes: UKPDS 39. *BMJ* 1998;317:713–720.

30. UK Prospective Diabetes Study Group. Tight blood pressure control and risk of macrovascular and microvascular complications in type 2 diabetes: UKPDS 38. *BMJ* 1998;317:703–713.

31. Hansson L, Zanchetti A, Carruthers SG, et al. Effects of intensive blood-pressure lowering and low-dose aspirin in patients with hypertension: principal results of the Hypertension Optimal Treatment (HOT) randomised trial. *Lancet* 1998; 351:1755–1762.

32. Downs JR, Clearfield M, Weis S, et al. Primary prevention of acute coronary events with lovastatin in men and women with average cholesterol levels: results of AFCAPS/TexCAPS. Air Force/Texas Coronary Atherosclerosis Prevention Study. *JAMA* 1998;279:1615–1622.

33. Koskinen P, Manttari M, Manninen V, et al. Coronary heart disease incidence in NIDDM patients in the Helsinki Heart Study. *Diabetes Care* 1992;15:820–825.

34. Elkeles RS, Diamond JR, Poulter C, et al. Cardiovascular outcomes in type 2 diabetes. A double-blind placebo-controlled study of bezafibrate: the St Mary's, Ealing, Northwick Park Diabetes Cardiovascular Disease Prevention (SENDCAP) Study. *Diabetes Care* 1998;21:641–648.

35. Pyorala K, Pedersen TR, Kjekshus J, et al. Cholesterol lowering with simvastatin improves prognosis of diabetic patients with coronary heart disease. A subgroup analysis of the Scandinavian Simvastatin Survival Study (4S). *Diabetes Care* 1997;20:614–620.

36. Sacks FM, Pfeffer MA, Moye LA, et al. The effect of pravastatin on coronary events after myocardial infarction in patients with average cholesterol levels. Cholesterol and Recurrent Events Trial investigators. *N Engl J Med* 1996;335:1001–1009.

37. The Long-term Intervention with Pravastatin in Ischemic Disease (LIPID) Study Program. Prevention of cardiovascular events and death with pravastatin in patients with coronary heart disease and a broad range of initial cholesterol

levels. *N Engl J Med* 1998;339:1349–1357.

38. Rubins HB, Robins SJ, Collins D, et al. Gemfibrozil for the secondary prevention of coronary heart disease in men with low levels of high-density lipoprotein cholesterol. Veterans Affairs High-Density Lipoprotein Cholesterol Intervention Trial Study Group. *N Engl J Med* 1999;341:410–418.

39. UK Prospective Diabetes Study Group. Intensive blood-glucose control with sulphonylureas or insulin compared with conventional treatment and risk of complications in patients with type 2 diabetes (UKPDS 33). *Lancet* 1998;352:837–853.

40. UK Prospective Diabetes Study Group. Effect of intensive blood-glucose control with metformin on complications in overweight patients with type 2 diabetes (UKPDS 34). *Lancet* 1998;352:854–865.

41. DCCT Research Group. The effect of intensive treatment of diabetes on the development and progression of long-term complications in insulin-dependent diabetes mellitus. *N Engl J Med* 1993;329:977–986.

42. DCCT Research Group. Effect of intensive diabetes management on macrovascular events and risk factors in the Diabetes Control and Complications Trial. *Am J Cardiol* 1995;75:894–903.

43. Abraira C, Colwell J, Nuttall F, et al. Cardiovascular events and correlates in the Veterans Affairs Diabetes Feasibility Trial: Veterans Affairs Cooperative Study on glycemic control and complications in type II diabetes. *Arch Intern Med* 1997;157:181–188.

44. Malmberg K, Ryden L, Efendic S, et al. Randomised trial of insulin-glucose infusion followed by subcutaneous insulin treatment in diabetic patients with acute myocardial infarction (DIGAMI study): effects on mortality at 1 year. *J Am Coll Cardiol* 1995;26:57–65.

45. Malmberg K. Prospective randomised study of intensive insulin treatment on long term survival after acute myocardial infarction in patients with diabetes mellitus. DIGAMI (Diabetes Mellitus, Insulin Glucose Infusion in Acute Myocardial Infarction) Study Group. *BMJ* 1997;314:1512–1515.

46. Steering Committee of the Physicians' Health Study Research Group. Final report on the aspirin component of the ongoing Physicians' Health Study. *N Engl J Med* 1989;321:129–135.

47. ETDRS Investigators. Aspirin effects on mortality and morbidity in patients with diabetes mellitus. *JAMA* 1992;268:1292–1300.

48. Collaborative overview of randomised trials of antiplatelet therapy–I: Prevention of death, myocardial infarction, and stroke by prolonged antiplatelet therapy in various categories of patients. Antiplatelet Trialists' Collaboration. *BMJ* 1994;308:81–106. Search date March 1990; primary sources Medline; Current Contents; manual searches of journals; reference lists from clinical trial and review articles; inquiry among colleagues, and manufacturers of antiplatelet agents for unpublished studies.

49. American Diabetes Association. Aspirin therapy in diabetes. *Diabetes Care* 1997;20:1772–1773.

50. The BARI Investigators. Seven-year outcome in the Bypass Angioplasty Revascularization Investigation (BARI) by treatment and diabetic status. *J Am Coll Cardiol* 2000;35:1122–1129

51. Hasdai D, Granger CB, Srivatsa S, et al. Diabetes mellitus and outcome after primary coronary angioplasty for acute myocardial infarction: lessons from the GUSTO-IIb angioplasty study. *J Am Coll Cardiol* 2000;35:1502–1512.

52. Kleiman NS, Lincoff AM, Kereiakes DJ, et al. Diabetes mellitus, glycoprotein IIb/IIIa blockade, and heparin: evidence for a complex interaction in a multicenter trial. EPILOG Investigators. *Circulation* 1998;97:1912–1920.

53. Marso SP, Lincoff AM, Ellis SG, et al. Optimizing the percutaneous interventional outcomes for patients with diabetes mellitus: results of the EPISTENT (Evaluation of platelet IIb/IIIa inhibitor for stenting trial) diabetic substudy. *Circulation* 1999;100:2477–2484.

54. The EPISTENT Investigators. Randomised placebo-controlled and balloon-angioplasty-controlled trial to assess safety of coronary stenting with use of platelet glycoprotein- IIb/IIIa blockade. The EPISTENT Investigators. Evaluation of platelet IIb/IIIa inhibitor for stenting. *Lancet* 1998;352:87–92.

55. Topol EJ, Mark DB, Lincoff AM, et al. Outcomes at 1 year and economic implications of platelet glycoprotein IIb/IIIa blockade in patients undergoing coronary stenting: results from a multicentre randomised trial. EPISTENT Investigators. Evaluation of Platelet IIb/IIIa Inhibitor for Stenting (published erratum appears in Lancet 2000 Mar 25;355:1104). *Lancet* 1999;354:2019–2024.

56. The EPIC Investigation. Use of a monoclonal antibody directed against the platelet glycoprotein IIb/IIIa receptor in high-risk coronary angioplasty. *N Engl J Med* 1994;330:956–961.

57. Bhatt DL, Marso SP, Lincoff AM, Wolski KE, Ellis SG, Topol EJ. Abciximab reduces mortality in diabetics following percutaneous coronary intervention. *J Am Coll Cardiol* 2000;35:922–928.

Ronald Sigal

Assistant Professor of Medicine

University of Ottawa

Ottawa

Canada

Janine Malcolm

Fellow, Endocrinology and Metabolism

Ottawa Hospital

Ottawa

Canada

Competing interests: RS has been reimbursed by Bristol Myers Squibb, manufacturer of atorvastatin, for attending conferences. He has received speaker's fees from Eli Lilly (manufacturer of insulin and proglitazone), Novo Nordisk (manufacturer of insulin and repaglinide), GlaxoSmithkline (manufacturer of rosiglitazone), and Bayer (manufacturer of cerivastatin, aspirin, and home glucose testing devices). JM, none declared.

TABLE 1 Primary prevention of cardiovascular events in people with diabetes: evidence from systematic reviews and randomised trials (see text, p 379).

Study	Interventions	Study type	Duration (years)	Outcome	Events / Sample size (%)* Intervention	Events / Sample size (%)* Control	NNT	95% CI for NNT
Antihypertensive medication								
Cochrane meta-analysis: diabetes and hypertension[18]	Various	SR	5	CVD mortality and morbidity	121/647 (19%)	188/708 (27%)	13	9 to 28
UKPDS Hypertension Study[29,30]	"Tight" target BP (≤150/≤ 85) with captopril or atenolol v "less tight" target (≤ 180/ ≤105)	RCT	8.4	AMI (fatal or non-fatal)	107/758 (14%)	83/390 (21%)	14	9 to 35
				Stroke	38/758 (5.0%)	34/390 (8.7%)	27	18 to 116
				Peripheral vascular events	8/758 (1.1%)	8/390 (2.1%)	–	–
HOT[31]	Felodipine and ACE-inhibitor, or β blocker, with 3 distinct target BPs	RCT	3.8	AMI (fatal or non-fatal), stroke (fatal or non-fatal) or other cardiovascular death	22/499 (4.4%) Target diastolic BP 80 mmHg	45/501 (9.0%) Target diastolic BP 90 mmHg	22	16 to 57
FACET[28]	Fosinopril v amlodipine	RCT	2.9	AMI, stroke, or admission to hospital for angina	14/189 (7.4%) Fosinopril	27/191 (14%) Amlodipine	15	10 to 199
ABCD[27]	Enalapril v nisoldipine	RCT	5	AMI (fatal or non-fatal)	5/235 (2.1%) Enalapril	25/235 (11%) Nisoldipine	12	10 to 19
Syst-Eur[19]	Nitrendipine; enalapril ± hydrochlorothiazide (20 mmHg BP lowering v placebo	RCT	2	MI, CHF, or sudden cardiac death	13/252 (5%)	31/240 (13%)	13	10 to 31

TABLE 1 continued

							NNT	
Lipid-lowering								
AFCAPS/TexCAPS[32]	Lovastatin	RCT	5	MI, unstable angina, or sudden cardiac death	4/84 (4.8%)	6/71 (8.5%)	27	NS
SENDCAP[34]	Bezafibrate	RCT	3	MI or new ischaemic changes on ECG	5/64 (7.8%)	16/64 (25%)	6	5 to 20
Helsinki[33]	Gemfibrozil	RCT	5	MI or cardiac death	2/59 (3.4%)	8/76 (10.5%)	14	NS
Blood glucose control								
DCCT[41,42]	Intensive insulin therapy in Type 1 diabetes	RCT	6.5	Major macrovascular events†	23/711 (3.2%)	40/730 (5.5%)	45	28 to 728
UKPDS[39]	Intensive therapy with insulin and/or sulphyoaylurea v conventional therapy	RCT	5	MI (fatal or non-fatal)	387/2729 (14.2%)	186/1138 (16.3%)	46	NS
UKPDS[40]	Intensive therapy with metformin v conventional therapy	RCT	5	MI (fatal or non-fatal)	39/342 (11%)	73/411 (18%)	16	10 to 71
Aspirin								
Physicians' Health Study[46]	Aspirin	RCT	5	MI (fatal or non-fatal)	11/275 (4.0%)	26/258 (10%)	16	12 to 47
ETDRS (mixed primary & secondary prevention)[47]	Aspirin	RCT	5	MI (fatal or non-fatal)	289/1856 (15.6%)	336/1855 (18.1%)	39	21 to 716

*Diabetic patients only. †Combined MI (fatal or non-fatal), sudden cardiac death, revascularisation procedure, angina with coronary artery disease confirmed by angiography or by noninvasive testing, stroke, lower limb amputation, peripheral arterial events requiring revascularisation, claudication with angiographic evidence of peripheral vascular disease. AMI, acute myocardial infarction; CHF, chronic heart failure; CVD, cardiovascular disease; MI, myocardial infarction; NNT, number needed to treat; RCT, randomised controlled trials; SR, systematic review.

TABLE 2 Secondary prevention of cardiovascular events in people with diabetes: evidence from systematic reviews and randomised trials (see text, p 380)

Study	Interventions	Study Type	Duration (years)	Outcome	Events / Sample size (%)* Intervention	Events / Sample size (%)* Control	NNT	95% CI for NNT
Antihypertensive medication								
Cochrane review: long-term secondary prevention[18]	Various antihypertensive medications	SR	≥ 1	CVD mortality and morbidity	130/316 (41%)	157/338 (46%)	19	NS
Cochrane review: short-term secondary prevention[18]	Various antihypertensive medications	SR	< 1	CVD mortality and morbidity	8/245 (3.3%)	21/288 (7.3%)	25	17 to 1145
Lipid-lowering								
4S[35]	Simvastatin	RCT	5.4	CHD death or non-fatal MI	24/105 (23%)	44/97 (45%)	5	3 to 10
CARE[36]	Pravastatin	RCT	5	Coronary disease death, non-fatal MI, or revascularisation	81/282 (29%)	112/304 (37%)	12	7 to 194
LIPID[37]	Pravastatin	RCT	6.1	CHD death or non-fatal MI	76/396 (19%)	88/386 (23%)	28	NS
Veterans[38]	Gemfibrozil	RCT	5.1	CHD death or non-fatal MI	88/309 (29%)	116/318 (37%)	13	7 to 144

TABLE 2 continued

Blood glucose control								
DIGAMI[44,45]	Insulin infusion followed by intensive insulin therapy v usual care	RCT	3.4	Overall mortality	102/306 (33%)	138/314 (44%)	9	6 to 33
Aspirin								
Antiplatelet trialists[48]	Aspirin v placebo	SR	Median 2 years	CVD mortality and morbidity	415/2248 (19%)	502/2254 (22%)	26	17 to 66
Revascularization								
GUSTO IIb[51]	PTCA v alteplase	RCT	2	Death, nonfatal reirfarction or disabling stroke	PTCA 11/99 (11%)	Alteplase 13/78 (16%)	18	NS
BARI[50]	CABG v PTCA	RCT	7.7	Death or non-fatal q wave MI	CABG 60/173 (35%)	PTCA 85/170 (50%)	7	4 to 21
Glycoprotein IIb/IIIa blockers								
EPIC[56]/EPILOG[52]/ EPISTENT[53-55]	Abciximab v control	Pooled	1	Overall death rate	26/540 (4.8%)	21/844 (2.5%)	43	23 to 422
EPIC[56]/EPILOG[52]/ EPISTENT[53-55]	Abciximab v control	Pooled	1	Death or non-fatal MI	185/540 (34%)	246/844 (29%)	20	9 to 1423

*Diabetic patients only. CABG, coronary artery bypass grafting; CHD, coronary heart disease; CVD, cardiovascular disease; MI, myocardial infarction; NNT, number needed to treat; PTCA, percutaneous transluminal coronary angioplasty; RCT, randomised controlled trials; SR, systematic review.

TABLE 3 Mixed primary and secondary prevention of cardiovascular events in people with diabetes (see text, p 380, p 382, pp 385-388).

Interventions	Study type	Duration (years)	Outcome	Events/sample size (%) (diabetic people only)		NNT	95% CI for NNT
				Intervention	Control		
Antihypertensive medication							
ACE Inhibitors v diuretics or calcium channel blockers[24]	Meta-analysis	2.8 to 6.2	CVD death, MI, CHF, angina, or stroke.	ACE inhibitor 158/733	Diuretics or calcium channel blockers 266/789	6	4 to 8
Diuretics v placebo[22]	Meta-analysis	2.2 to 4.8	Any coronary event, any stroke, sudden death, or death from embolism.	Diuretics 151/1000	Placebo 189/1000	26	Unavailable
Ramipril 10 mg daily versus placebo[23]	RCT	4.5	MI, stroke, or CVD. Overall mortality	277/1808 (15%) 196/1808 (11%)	351/1769 (20%) 240/1769 (14%)	22 32	14 to 43 19 to 98

ACE; angiotensin converting enzyme; CHF, congestive heart failure; CVD, cadiovascular disease; MI, myocardial infarction.

Search date November 2000

Dereck Hunt and Hertzel Gerstein

QUESTIONS

INTERVENTIONS

Key Messages

- One RCT has found that screening and referral to a footcare clinic for people with diabetes who are at high risk of developing foot ulcers reduces the risk of foot ulcers and major amputation.
- Limited evidence from two RCTs suggests that pressure off-loading using total contact casting or non-removable fibreglass casts improves the healing of chronic, non-infected diabetic foot ulcers.
- One systematic review of RCTs has found that cultured human dermis and topical growth factors may improve the rate of healing of chronic, non-infected foot ulcers.
- Limited evidence from two small RCTs suggests that systemic hyperbaric oxygen reduces the risk of foot amputation in people with severe infected foot ulcers.
- We found limited evidence from one non-randomised trial that therapeutic footwear reduces the recurrence of foot ulceration.
- We found limited evidence from one non-randomised trial that patient education, provided after acute foot complications, decreases the risks of ulcer recurrence and major amputation.

DEFINITION Diabetic foot ulceration is full thickness penetration of the dermis of the foot in a person with diabetes. Non-traumatic lower limb amputation is the surgical removal of all or part of the lower extremity. Minor amputations involve partial removal of a foot, including toe or forefoot resections. Major amputations are above or below knee amputations.

INCIDENCE/ PREVALENCE The annual incidence of foot ulcers among people with diabetes is 2.5–10.7%, and the annual incidence of amputation is 0.25–1.8%.[1-8]

AETIOLOGY/ RISK FACTORS Risk factors for foot ulcers and amputation include duration of diabetes, poor glycaemic control, and the presence of microvascular complications (retinopathy, nephropathy, and neuropathy). However the strongest predictors are altered foot sensation and previous foot ulcer.[1-8]

PROGNOSIS People with diabetes are at risk of developing complications in the lower extremities. These include foot ulcers, infections, and vascular insufficiency. Amputation of a lower extremity is indicated if complications are severe or do not improve with appropriate treatment. As well as affecting quality of life, these complications form a large proportion of the healthcare costs of diabetes. For people with healed diabetic foot ulcers, the 5 year cumulative rate of ulcer recurrence is 66% and of amputation is 12%.[9]

AIMS To prevent diabetic foot complications, including ulcers and amputations; and to improve ulcer healing and prevent amputations where ulcers already exist, with minimum adverse effects.

OUTCOMES Rates of development or recurrence of foot ulcers or major foot lesions; rate of amputation; time ulcers take to heal, or the proportion healed in a given period; rates of hospital admission; rates of foot infection; adverse effects of treatment.

METHODS *Clinical Evidence* update search and appraisal November 2000.

QUESTION	What are the effects of preventive and therapeutic interventions?

OPTION	SCREENING AND REFERRAL TO FOOTCARE CLINIC

One RCT has found that, compared with usual care, screening for altered sensation and absent pedal pulses followed by referral to footcare clinics (for education, footwear, and podiatry) reduces the risk of foot ulcers and major amputation.

Benefits: We found one systematic review (search date 1998, 1 RCT, 2001 people attending a general diabetes clinic).[10] The RCT compared usual care versus a diabetes screening and protection programme. People in the intervention group were screened for deficits in pedal pulses, light touch, and vibration sensation. People with persistent abnormal findings were referred to the diabetic foot clinic if they had a history of foot ulcer, were found to have a low ankle-brachial index (< 0.75), or were noted to have foot deformities. The clinic provided podiatry and protective shoes as well as education regarding foot care. Follow up 2 years after enrolment found that significantly more people receiving usual care needed amputation (AR 12/1000 [1.2%] *v* 1/1000 [0.1%]; ARR 1.1%, 95% CI 0.4% to 1.9%; NNT 91, 95% CI 53 to 250).

Harms: No harms were reported.

Comment: None.

| OPTION | PRESSURE OFF-LOADING |

We found limited evidence from two small RCTs that, compared with traditional care, pressure off-loading using total contact casting or non-removable fibreglass casts increases the likelihood and speed of healing of chronic, non-infected diabetic foot ulcers. We found no direct comparison of off-loading techniques with topical growth factors.

Benefits: We found one systematic review (search date 1998, 1 RCT, 40 people with diabetes and plantar foot ulcers but free of signs of infection or gangrene)[11] and one additional RCT.[12] The review compared total contact casting versus traditional dressing changes. All participants were told to minimise weightbearing during treatment. Casts were applied by an experienced physical therapist, changed after 5–7 days, and then every 2–3 weeks until healing occurred. Control participants were provided with accommodative footwear and crutches or a walker. They were instructed to complete wet to dry dressing changes two to three times daily. Ulcer healing occurred in significantly more people treated with total contact casting (91% *v* 32%; absolute difference 59%, 95% CI 31% to 87%; NNT 2, 95% CI 1 to 3). Healing was quicker in people treated with total contact casting than controls (a mean of 42 days *v* 65 days). Five control participants were admitted to hospital because of infection, and two required amputation. No participants in the total contact casting group required hospital admission. The additional RCT (50 people with diabetes mellitus and non-infected neuropathic plantar foot ulcers) compared non-removable fibreglass casts versus specialised cloth shoes with rigid soles and off-loading insoles. All participants had dressing changes every 2 days. After 30 days, it found that non-removable casts significantly improved ulcer healing (50% of ulcers healed with cast *v* 21% with special shoe; ARR 29%, 95% CI 1.4% to 57%; NNT 4, 95% CI 2 to 72).[12]

Harms: The review found that three of 21 people treated with total contact casting developed fungal infections that required topical treatment. These events did not prevent continued casting. No adverse effects were observed in the additional RCT examining effects of non-removable fibreglass casts.[12]

Comment: Total contact casting is the application of a layer of plaster over the foot and lower leg designed to distribute pressure evenly over the entire plantar aspect of the foot to reduce exposure of plantar ulcers to pressure, even when the patient is walking. Soft tissue infections and osteomyelitis are contraindications to total contact casting. We found no RCTs evaluating other methods aimed at decreasing the pressure applied to plantar ulcers during walking, such as removable cast walkers, half shoes, healing sandals, and felted foam.

| OPTION | CULTURED HUMAN DERMIS AND TOPICAL GROWTH FACTORS |

One systematic review has found that cultured human dermis and topical growth factors may improve the rate of healing of chronic, non-infected foot ulcers. We found no comparison of these interventions with total contact casting.

Benefits: We found one systematic review (search date 1998), which identified two unblinded RCTs of cultured human dermis and six double blind RCTs of four different topical growth factors.[11] These compared topical application of cultured human dermis or a growth factor versus placebo in people attending hospital outpatient clinics with diabetic foot ulcers who were free of signs of infection or severe vascular compromise. All received wound debridement and were encouraged to avoid weight bearing on the affected limb. For cultured human dermis, one RCT (50 people) found that treatment with neonatal cultured fibroblasts (weekly for 8 weeks) significantly increased healing rates (AR non-healing 50% v 92% with placebo; RRR 46%; ARR 42%, 95% CI 5% to 80%; NNT 2, 95% CI 1 to 20). The second RCT of cultured human dermis (281 people) found a non-significant effect on healing rate (AR non-healing 61% v 68% with control; RRR 10%; ARR +7%, 95% CI –6% to +20%). For topical growth factors, one RCT (65 people) found that treatment with an arginine-glycine-aspartic (RGD) acid matrix twice weekly for up to 10 weeks significantly increased healing rates (AR non-healing 65% v 92% with placebo; RRR 29%; ARR 27%, 95% CI 6% to 48%; NNT 4, 95% CI 2 to 15). Another RCT (118 people) found that treatment with platelet derived growth factors (30 µg/g once daily for up to 20 weeks) increased healing rates (AR non-healing 52% v 75% with placebo; RRR 31%; ARR 23%, 95% CI 5% to 41%; NNT 5, 95% CI 2 to 19). A third RCT (382 people) found that treatment with platelet derived growth factors (100 µg/g once daily for up to 20 weeks) significantly increased healing rates (AR non-healing 50% v 65% with placebo; RRR 23%; ARR 15%, 95% CI 2% to 28%; NNT 7, 95% CI 4 to 42). This RCT found no benefit with platelet derived growth factors 30 µg/g once daily for up to 20 weeks versus placebo (AR non-healing 64% v 65% with placebo). Two RCTs evaluated CT-102, a growth factor derived from thrombin-induced human platelets, applied twice weekly. One small RCT (13 people) found no significant effect on healing rates (AR non-healing 29% v 83% with placebo; RRR 66%; ARR +55%, 95% CI –2% to +81%). The second, larger RCT (81 people) found a significant increase in healing rates (AR non-healing 20% v 71% with placebo; RRR 72%; ARR 51%, 95% CI 19% to 84%; NNT 2, 95% CI 1 to 5). The sixth RCT (17 people) found no benefit from recombinant platelet-derived growth factor versus control treatment.

Harms: Adverse events, when reported, occurred as frequently in the intervention arms as in the control arms.

Comment: These therapeutic agents are not widely available and may be expensive. There has been little long term follow up of people treated with these growth factors.

OPTION   **SYSTEMIC HYPERBARIC OXYGEN**

Two small RCTs have found that, compared with routine care, systemic hyperbaric oxygen reduces the risk of foot amputation in people with severe infected foot ulcers.

Benefits: We found one systematic review (search date 1998, 1 RCT)[11] and one additional RCT.[13] The RCT in the review (70 people with severe infected diabetic foot ulcers) compared usual care (aggressive debridement, broad spectrum intravenous antibiotics, revascularisation if indicated, and optimised glycaemic control) versus usual care plus daily 90 minute sessions of systemic hyperbaric oxygen at 2.2–2.5 atmospheres.[14] Participants either had full thickness gangrene or abscess, or a large infected ulcer that had not healed after 30 days. After 10 weeks, rates of major amputation were significantly lower in the intervention group (8.6% v 33% in the control group; RRR 74%, 95% CI 16% to 92%; ARR 24%, 95% CI 4% to 45%; NNT 5, 95% CI 2 to 23). The additional RCT (30 people with chronic infected foot ulcers) compared usual treatment (including debridement, intravenous antibiotics, and optimised glycaemic control) versus usual treatment plus four treatments with hyperbaric oxygen over 2 weeks. It found no significant reduction of the risk of major amputation in the intervention group (ARR +33%, 95% CI –1.6% to +68%).[13]

Harms: In the larger RCT, two people developed symptoms of barotraumatic otitis, but this did not interrupt treatment.[14]

Comment: The additional RCT may have been too small to rule out a clinically important effect.

OPTION   **APPROPRIATE FOOTWEAR**

We found limited evidence from one non-randomised trial that therapeutic footwear, made according to the Towey guidelines, decreases recurrence of ulceration.

Benefits: We found one systematic review (search date 1998, 1 non-randomised controlled trial).[10] The trial alternately allocated 69 people with a previous diabetic foot ulcer to either an intervention group, in which people received therapeutic shoes, or to a control group, in which people continued to wear their ordinary shoes. Therapeutic shoes were manufactured according to the Towey guidelines (super depth to fit customised insoles and toe deformities, and made with soft thermoformable leather along with semi-rocker soles) and fitted with custom moulded insoles. All participants received information on foot care and footwear. After 1 year, it found that wearing therapeutic shoes significantly reduced ulcer recurrence (AR 27% with intervention v 58% with control; RRR 53%; ARR 31%, 95% CI 7% to 55%; NNT 4, 95% CI 2 to 14).

Harms: The trial did not report any adverse effects associated with therapeutic shoes.

Comment: Alternate allocation leaves open the possibility of bias from non-comparability of the two treatment groups.

| OPTION | EDUCATION |

We found limited evidence from one non-randomised trial that patient education provided after the management of acute foot complications decreases ulcer recurrences and major amputations.

Benefits: We found one systematic review (search date 1998), which identified one non-randomised controlled trial.[11] The trial (227 people who presented with foot infection, ulcer, or for assistance following a previous amputation) allocated people according to their social security number and evaluated the effect of providing a single, 1 hour educational class on diabetic foot complications and important components of foot care. Surgical treatment was provided for all people when necessary. Follow up at 2 years found that allocation to the educational session significantly reduced ulcer recurrences (AR 14.7% for control group v 4.5% for education; RRR 69%; ARR 10%, 95% CI 4% to 16%; NNT 10, 95% CI 6 to 26) and major amputation (AR 10.2% v 2.8%; RRR 72%; ARR 7%, 95% CI 2% to 13%; NNT 14, 95% CI 8 to 50).

Harms: None reported.

Comment: Allocation by social security number may introduce biases and could create non-comparable groups.

Substantive changes since last issue

Pressure off-loading. One addtional RCT;[12] conclusion unchanged.

REFERENCES

1. Rith-Najarian SJ, Stolusky T, Gohdes DM. Identifying diabetic patients at high risk for lower-extremity amputation in a primary health care setting. *Diabetes Care* 1992;15:1386–1389.
2. Veves A, Murray HJ, Young MJ, et al. The risk of foot ulceration in diabetic patients with high foot pressure: a prospective study. *Diabetologia* 1992;35:660–663.
3. Young MJ, Breddy JL, Veves, et al. The prediction of diabetic neuropathic foot ulceration using vibration perception thresholds: a prospective study. *Diabetes Care* 1994;7:557–560.
4. Humphrey ARG, Dowse GK, Thoma K, et al. Diabetes and nontraumatic lower extremity amputations. Incidence, risk factors, and prevention: a 12 year follow-up study in Nauru. *Diabetes Care* 1996;19:710–714.
5. Lee JS, Lu M, Lee VS, et al. Lower-extremity amputation: incidence, risk factors, and mortality in the Oklahoma Indian diabetes study. *Diabetes* 1993;42:876–882.
6. Lehto S, Ronnemaa T, Pyorala K, et al. Risk factors predicting lower extremity amputations in patients with NIDDM. *Diabetes Care* 1996;19:607–612.
7. Moss SE, Klein R, Klein B. Long-term incidence of lower-extremity amputations in a diabetic population. *Arch Fam Med* 1996;5:391–398.
8. Nelson RG, Gohdes DM, Everhart JE, et al. Lower-extremity amputations in NIDDM: 12 year follow-up study in Pima Indians. *Diabetes Care* 1988;11:8–16.
9. Apelqvist J, Larsson J, Agardh CD. Long-term prognosis for diabetic patients with foot ulcers. *J Intern Med* 1993;233:485–491.
10. Mason J, O'Keeffe C, McIntosh A, et al. A systematic review of foot ulcer in patients with type 2 diabetes mellitus. I: prevention. *Diabet Med* 1999;16:801–812. Search date 1998; primary sources Cochrane Trials Register, Medline, Embase, Cinahl, Healthstar, Psychlit, Science Citation, Social Science Citation, Index to Scientific and Technical Conference Proceedings (ISI), HMIC database, and SIGLE.
11. Mason J, O'Keeffe C, Hutchinson A, et al. A systematic review of foot ulcer in patients with type 2 diabetes mellitus. II: treatment. *Diabet Med* 1999;16:889–909. Search date 1998, primary sources Cochrane Trials Register, Medline, Embase 1983 to 1998; Cinahl, Healthstar, Psychlit, Science Citation, Social Science Citation, Index to Scientific and Technical Conference Proceedings (ISI), HMIC database, and SIGLE 1983 to 1998.
12. Caravaggi C, Faglia E, De Giglio R, et al. Effectiveness and safety of a nonremovable fiberglass off-bearing cast versus a therapeutic shoe in the treatment of neuropathic foot ulcers: a randomized study. *Diabetes Care* 2000;23:1746–1751.
13. Doctor N, Pandya S, Supe A. Hyperbaric oxygen therapy in diabetic foot. *J Postgrad Med* 1992;38:112–114.
14. Faglia E, Favales F, Aldeghi A, et al. Adjunctive systemic hyperbaric oxygen therapy in treatment of severe prevalently ischemic diabetic foot ulcer. *Diabetes Care* 1996;19:1338–1343.

Dereck Hunt
Clinical Scholar

Hertzel Gerstein
Associate Professor of Medicine

McMaster University
Hamilton, Ontario
Canada

Competing interests: None declared.

Search date December 2000

William H Herman

QUESTIONS

INTERVENTIONS

Key Messages

- We found strong evidence from one systematic review and three large subsequent RCTs that intensive compared with conventional treatment reduces the development and progression of microvascular and neuropathic complications in both type 1 and type 2 diabetes. A second systematic review of RCTs has found that intensive treatment is associated with a small reduction in cardiovascular risk.

- We found no evidence that intensive treatment causes adverse cardiovascular outcomes. RCTs have found that intensive treatment is associated with hypoglycaemia and weight gain without adverse impact on neuropsychological function or quality of life.

- Large RCTs have found that diabetic complications increase with HbA1c concentrations above the non-diabetic range.

DEFINITION Diabetes mellitus is a group of disorders characterised by hyperglycaemia (definitions vary slightly, one current US definition is fasting plasma glucose ≥ 7.0 mmol/l or ≥ 11.1 mmol/l 2 hours after a 75 g oral glucose load, on two or more occasions). Intensive treatment is designed to achieve blood glucose values as close to the non-diabetic range as possible. The components of such treatment are education, counselling, monitoring, self management, and pharmacological treatment with insulin or oral antidiabetic agents to achieve specific glycaemic goals.

INCIDENCE/ PREVALENCE Diabetes is diagnosed in around 5% of adults aged 20 years or older in the USA.[1] A further 2.7% have undiagnosed diabetes on the basis of fasting glucose. The prevalence is similar in men and women, but diabetes is more common in some ethnic groups. The prevalence in people aged 40–74 years has increased over the past decade.

AETIOLOGY/ RISK FACTORS Diabetes results from deficient insulin secretion, decreased insulin action, or both. Many processes can be involved, from autoimmune destruction of the β cells of the pancreas to incompletely understood abnormalities that result in resistance to insulin action. Genetic factors are involved in both mechanisms. In type 1 diabetes there is an absolute deficiency of insulin. In type 2 diabetes, insulin resistance and an inability of the pancreas to compensate are involved. Hyperglycaemia without clinical symptoms but sufficient to cause tissue damage can be present for many years before diagnosis.

PROGNOSIS Severe hyperglycaemia causes numerous symptoms, including polyuria, polydipsia, weight loss, and blurred vision. Acute, life threatening consequences of diabetes are hyperglycaemia with ketoacidosis or the non-ketotic hyperosmolar syndrome. There is increased susceptibility to certain infections. Long term complications of diabetes include retinopathy (with potential loss of vision), nephropathy (leading to renal failure), peripheral neuropathy (increased risk of foot ulcers, amputation, and Charcot joints), autonomic neuropathy (cardiovascular, gastrointestinal, and genitourinary dysfunction), and greatly increased risk of atheroma affecting large vessels (macrovascular complications of stroke, myocardial infarction, or peripheral vascular disease). The physical, emotional, and social impact of diabetes and demands of intensive treatment can also create problems for people with diabetes and their families. One systematic review (search date 1998) of observational studies in people with type 2 diabetes found a positive association between increased blood glucose concentration and mortality.[2] It found no minimum threshold level.

AIMS To slow development and progression of the microvascular, neuropathic, and cardiovascular complications of diabetes, while minimising adverse effects of treatment (hypoglycaemia and weight gain) and maximising quality of life.

OUTCOMES Quality of life; short term burden of treatment; long term clinical complications; risks and benefits of treatment. Both the development of complications in people who have previously been free of them, and the progression of complications, are used as outcomes. Scales of severity are used to detect disease progression (e.g. 19

step scales of diabetic retinopathy; normoalbuminuria, microalbuminuria, and albuminuria for nephropathy; absence or presence of clinical neuropathy).

METHODS *Clinical Evidence* update search and appraisal December 2000.

| QUESTION | What are the effects of intensive versus conventional glycaemic control? |

One systematic review and three subsequent RCTs in people with type 1 and type 2 diabetes have found that intensive treatment compared with conventional treatment reduces development and progression of microvascular and neuropathic complications. A second systematic review in people with type 1 diabetes, and two additional RCTs in people with type 2 diabetes, have found no evidence that intensive treatment increases adverse cardiovascular outcomes. Intensive treatment reduced the number of macrovascular events but had no significant effect on the number of people who developed macrovascular disease. Intensive treatment is associated with hypoglycaemia and weight gain, but does not seem to affect neuropsychological function or quality of life adversely.

Benefits: **Microvascular and neuropathic complications:** We found one systematic review (search date 1991, 16 small RCTs of type 1 diabetes)[3] and three subsequent long term RCTs (see table 1, p 411),[4–6] which found the relative risks of retinopathy, nephropathy, and neuropathy were all significantly reduced by intensive treatment versus conventional treatment. In one subsequent RCT (1441 people with type 1 diabetes) about half had no retinopathy and half had mild retinopathy at baseline.[4] At 6.5 years, intensive treatment significantly reduced the progression of retinopathy and neuropathy. After a further 4 years, the benefit was maintained, regardless of whether people stayed in the groups to which they were initially randomised.[7] The difference in the median HbA1c concentration for people initially randomised to intensive or conventional care narrowed. The proportion of people with worsening retinopathy and nephropathy was also significantly lower for those who had received intensive treatment. However, another subsequent RCT[6] compared a conventional dietary treatment policy with two different intensive treatment policies based on sulfonylurea and insulin (3867 people with newly diagnosed type 2 diabetes; age 25–65 years; fasting plasma glucose 6.1–15.0 mmol/l after 3 months' dietary therapy; no symptoms of hyperglycaemia; follow up 10 years). HbA1c rose steadily in both groups. Intensive treatment was associated with a significant reduction in any diabetes related end point (40.9 v 46.0 events/1000 person years; RRR 12%, 95% CI 1% to 21%), but no significant effect on diabetes related deaths (10.4 v 11.5 deaths/1000 person years; RRR +10%, 95% CI –11% to +27%) or all cause mortality (17.9 v 18.9 deaths/1000 person years; RRR +6%, 95% CI –10% to +20%). Secondary analysis found that intensive treatment was associated with a significant reduction in microvascular end points (8.6 v 11.4/1000 person years; RRR 25%, 95% CI 7% to 40%) compared with conventional treatment (see table 1, p 411).[6] **Cardiovascular outcomes:** We found one systematic review[8] and two additional RCTs.[5,6] The systematic review (6 RCTs, 1731 people with type 1 diabetes followed for 2–8 years) found that intensive insulin treatment versus conventional treatment decreased the number of macrovascular events (OR 0.55, 95% CI 0.35 to 0.88), but had no significant effect on the number of people developing macrovascular disease (OR 0.72, 95% CI 0.44 to 1.17) or on macrovascular mortality (OR 0.91, 95% CI 0.31 to 2.65). The additional RCTs included people with type 2 diabetes.[5,6] In the first RCT the number of major cerebrovascular, cardiovascular, and peripheral vascular events in the intensive treatment group was half that of the conventional treatment group (0.6 v 1.3 events/100 person years), but the event rate in this small trial was low and the results were not significant.[5] In the second RCT, intensive treatment versus conventional treatment was associated with a non-significant reduction in the risk of myocardial infarction (AR 387/2729 [14%] with intensive treatment v 186/1138 [16%] with conventional treatment; RRR +13%, 95% CI −2% to +27%), a non-significant increase in the risk of stroke (AR 148/2729 [5.4%] v 55/1138 [4.8%]; RRI +12%, 95% CI −17% to +51%), and a non-significant reduction in the risk of amputation or death from peripheral vascular disease (AR 29/2729 [1.1%] v 18/1138 [1.6%]; RRR +33%, 95% CI −20% to +63%).[6]

Harms: **Hypoglycaemia:** We found one systematic review[9] and three additional RCTs.[5,6,10] The systematic review (search date 1996, 14 RCTs with at least 6 months' follow up and monitoring of HbA1c, 2067 people with type 1 diabetes followed for 0.5–7.5 years) found that the median incidence of severe hypoglycaemia was 7.9 episodes/100 person years among intensively treated people and 4.6 episodes/100 person years among conventionally treated people (OR 3.0, 95% CI 2.5 to 3.6). The risk of severe hypoglycaemia was associated with the degree of HbA1c lowering in the intensive treatment groups ($P = 0.005$). The three additional RCTs included people with type 2 diabetes with lower baseline rates of hypoglycaemia. In the first RCT (110 people), there was no significant difference in rates of hypoglycaemia between groups.[5] In the second RCT (3867 people), the rates of major hypoglycaemic episodes per year were 0.7% with conventional treatment, 1.0% with chlorpropamide, 1.4% with glibenclamide, and 1.8% with insulin. People in the intensive treatment group had significantly more hypoglycaemic episodes than those in the conventional group ($P < 0.0001$).[6] In the third RCT (1704 overweight people) major hypoglycaemic episodes occurred in 0.6% of overweight people in the metformin treated group.[10] **Weight gain:** Four RCTs found more weight increase with intensive treatment than with standard treatment.[4–6,11] One RCT found weight remained stable in people with type 1 diabetes in the conventional treatment group, but body mass index increased by 5.8% in the intensive treatment group (95% CI not presented, $P < 0.01$).[11] In the second RCT (1441 people with type 2 diabetes), intensive treatment was associated with increased risk of developing a body weight more than 120% above the ideal (12.7 cases per 100 person years with intensive treatment v 9.3 cases per 100 person years with conventional treatment; RR 1.33). At 5 years, people treated intensively gained 4.6 kg more than people treated conventionally (CI not presented for weight data).[4] In the third RCT, the increase in body mass index from baseline to 6 years was not significant in either group (intensive treatment group 20.5 to 21.2 kg/m², conventional treatment group 20.3 to 21.9 kg/m²).[5] In the fourth RCT, weight gain at 10 years was significantly higher in people with type 2 diabetes in the intensive treatment group compared with people in the conventional treatment group (mean 2.9 kg, P < 0.001), and people assigned insulin had a greater gain in weight (4.0 kg) than those assigned chlorpropamide (2.6 kg) or glibenclamide (1.7 kg).[6] We found one systematic review (search date 1996, 10 RCTs)[12] and one subsequent RCT[10] comparing metformin and sulfonylurea. Meta-analysis in the review found that sulfonylurea was associated with an increase in weight from baseline and metformin with a decrease (difference 2.9 kg, 95% CI 1.1 to 4.4 kg). In the subsequent RCT, overweight participants randomly assigned to intensive blood glucose control with metformin had a similar change in body weight to the conventional treatment group, and less increase in mean body weight than people receiving intensive treatment with sulfonylureas or insulin.[10] **Neuropsychological impairment:** We found no systematic review on neuropsychological impairment, but found two RCTs.[13–16] One RCT (102 people) compared intensified with standard treatment in people with type 1 diabetes. It found no cognitive impairment associated with hypoglycaemia after 3 years.[13,14] The second RCT found that intensive treatment did not affect neuropsychological performance.[15] People who had repeated episodes of hypoglycaemia did not perform differently from people who did not have repeated episodes.[16] **Quality of life:** We found three RCTs, which reported quality of life in people undergoing intensive versus conventional treatment.[17–19] Together, they suggest that quality of life is lowered by complications, but is not lowered directly by intensive versus conventional treatment. The first RCT (1441 people) found that intensive treatment did not reduce quality of life in people with type 1 diabetes.[17] Severe hypoglycaemia was not consistently associated with a subsequent increase in distress caused by symptoms or decline in the quality of life. In the primary prevention intensive treatment group, however, repeated severe hypoglycaemia (three or more events resulting in coma or seizure) tended to increase the risk of distress caused by symptoms. The second RCT (77 adolescents with type 1 diabetes) found after 1 year that behavioural intervention plus intensive diabetes management versus intensive diabetes management alone significantly improved quality of life, diabetes and medical self-efficacy, and HbA1c (7.5% v 8.5%, P = 0.001).[18] The behavioural intervention included six small group sessions and monthly follow up aimed at social problem solving, cognitive behaviour modification, and conflict resolution. The third RCT of intensive versus conventional treatment of type 2 diabetes assessed quality of life in two large cross sectional samples at 8 and 11 years after randomisation (disease specific measures in 2431 people and generic measures in 3104 people), and also in a small cohort (diabetes specific quality of life measures in 374 people 6 months after randomisation and annually thereafter for 6 years).[19] The cross sectional studies found no significant effect of intensive versus conventional treatment on scores for mood, cognitive mistakes, symptoms, work satisfaction, or general health. The longitudinal study also found no significant difference in quality of life scores other than a small increase in the number of symptoms in people allocated to conventional than to intensive treatment. In the cross sectional studies, people who had macrovascular or microvascular complications in the last year had lower quality of life than people without complications. People treated with insulin who had two or more hypoglycaemic episodes during the previous year reported more tension, more overall mood disturbance, and less work satisfaction than those with no hypoglycaemic attacks (after adjusting for age, time from randomisation, systolic blood pressure, HbA1c, and sex). It was unclear whether frequent hypoglycaemic episodes affected quality of life, or whether people with certain personality traits or symptoms simply reported increased numbers of hypoglycaemic attacks.

Comment: None.

QUESTION What is the optimum target blood glucose?

Large RCTs in people with type 1 and type 2 diabetes have found that risk of development or progression of complications increases progressively as HbA1c increases above the non-diabetic range.

Benefits: We found no systematic review but found two large RCTs.[4,6] The first RCT (1441 people with type 1 diabetes) found that lower HbA1c was associated with a lower risk of complications.[4,20] The second RCT (3867 people with type 2 diabetes) found that, as concentrations of HbA1c were reduced, the risk of complications fell but the risk of hypoglycaemia increased.[6,19] A further analysis of the second RCT (3642 people who had HbA1c measured 3 months after the diagnosis of diabetes and who had complete data whether or not they were randomised in the trial) found that each 1% reduction in mean HbA1c was associated with reduced risk of any diabetes-related microvascular or macrovascular event (RR 0.79, 95% CI 0.76 to 0.83), diabetes related death (RR 0.79, 95% CI 0.73 to 0.85), all cause mortality (RR 0.86, 95% CI 0.81 to 0.91), microvascular complications (RR 0.63, 95% CI 0.59 to 0.67), and myocardial infarction (RR 0.86, 95% CI 0.79 to 0.92).[21] These prospective observational data suggest that there is no lower glycaemic threshold for the risk of complications; the better the glycaemic control, the lower the risk of complications. They also suggest that the rate of increase of risk for microvascular disease with hyperglycaemia is greater than that for macrovascular disease.

Harms: Both RCTs found that hypoglycaemia was increased by intensive treatment.[19,20]

Comment: It is difficult to weigh the benefit of reduced complications against the harm of increased hypoglycaemia. The balance between benefits and harms of intensive treatment in type 1 diabetes may be less favourable in children under 13 years or in older adults, and in people with repeated severe hypoglycaemia or unawareness of hypoglycaemia. Similarly, the balance between benefits and harms of intensive treatment in type 2 diabetes may be less favourable in people over 65 years or in those with longstanding diabetes. The benefit of intensive treatment is limited by the complications of advanced diabetes (such as blindness, end stage renal disease or cardiovascular disease), major comorbidity, and reduced life expectancy. The risk of intensive treatment is increased by a history of severe hypoglycaemia or unawareness of hypoglycaemia, advanced autonomic neuropathy, or cardiovascular disease, and impaired ability to detect or treat hypoglycaemia (such as altered mental state, immobility, or lack of social support). For people likely to have limited benefit or increased risk with intensive treatment, it may be more appropriate to negotiate less intensive goals for glycaemic management that reflect the person's self determined goals of care and willingness to make lifestyle modifications.

Substantive changes since last issue

Intensive versus conventional control New RCT of behavioural intervention plus intensive treatment versus intensive treatment alone in adolescents;[18] conclusions unchanged.

Optimum target blood glucose New observational analysis of relationship between HbA1c and complication rates. No lower threshold of glycaemic control for reducing risk of complications;[21] conclusions unchanged.

REFERENCES

1. Harris MI, Flegal KM, Cowie CC, et al. Prevalence of diabetes, impaired fasting glucose, and impaired glucose tolerance in US adults: the third national health and nutrition examination survey, 1988–1994. *Diabetes Care* 1998;2:518–524.

2. Groeneveld Y, Petri H, Hermans J, et al. Relationship between blood glucose level and mortality in type 2 diabetes mellitus: a systematic review. *Diabet Med* 1999;16:2–13. Search date 1998; primary source Medline 1996 to 1998.

3. Wang PH, Lau J, Chalmers TC. Meta-analysis of effects of intensive blood glucose control on late complications of type I diabetes. *Lancet* 1993; 341:1306–1309. Search date 1991; primary sources Medline 1966 to December 1991.

4. The Diabetes Control and Complications Trial Research Group. The effect of intensive treatment of diabetes on the development and progression of long-term complications in insulin-dependent diabetes mellitus. *N Engl J Med* 1993;329:977–986.

5. Ohkubo Y, Kishikawa H, Arake E, et al. Intensive insulin therapy prevents the progression of diabetic microvascular complications in Japanese patients with non-insulin-dependent diabetes mellitus: a randomized prospective 6-year study. *Diabetes Res Clin Pract* 1995;28:103–117.

6. UK Prospective Diabetes Study Group. Intensive blood-glucose control with sulphonylureas or insulin compared with conventional treatment and risk of complications in patients with type 2 diabetes. *Lancet* 1998;352:837–853.

7. The DCCT/Epidemiology of Diabetes Interventions and Complications Research Group. Retinopathy and nephropathy in patients with type 1 diabetes four years after a trial of intensive therapy. *N Engl J Med* 2000;342:381–389.

8. Lawson ML, Gerstein HC, Tsui E, et al. Effect of intensive therapy on early macrovascular disease in young individuals with type 1 diabetes. *Diabetes Care* 1999;22:B35–B39. Search date 1996; primary sources Medline, Citation Index, reference lists, and personal files.

9. Egger M, Smith GD, Stettler C, et al. Risk of adverse effects of intensified treatment in insulin-dependent diabetes mellitus: a meta-analysis. *Diabet Med* 1997;14:919–928. Search date not given; primary sources Medline, reference lists, and specialist journals.

10. UK Prospective Diabetes Study Group. Effect of intensive blood-glucose control with metformin on complications in overweight patients with type 2 diabetes. *Lancet* 1998;352:854–865.

11. Reichard P, Berglund B, Britz A, et al. Intensified conventional insulin treatment retards the microvascular complications of insulin-dependent diabetes mellitus (IDDM): the Stockholm diabetes intervention study (SDIS) after 5 years. *J Intern Med* 1991;30:101–108.

12. Johansen K. Efficacy of metformin in the treatment of NIDDM. *Diabetes Care* 1999;22:33–37. Search date January 1996; primary sources current list of medical literature 1957 to 1959; Index Medicus 1959 to 1965; Medline 1966 to January 1966; Embase 1989 to January 1996, and hand searched references.

13. Reichard P, Nilsson BY, Rosenqvist U. The effect of long-term intensified insulin treatment on the development of microvascular complications of diabetes mellitus. *N Engl J Med* 1993;29:304–309.

14. Reichard P, Berglund A, Britz A, et al. Hypoglycaemic episodes during intensified insulin treatment: increased frequency but no effect on cognitive function. *J Intern Med* 1991;229:9–16.

15. The Diabetes Control and Complications Trial Research Group. Effects of intensive diabetes therapy on neuropsychological function in adults in the diabetes control and complications trial. *Ann Intern Med* 1996;124:379–388.

16. Austin EJ, Deary IJ. The effects of repeated hypoglycaemia on cognitive function. A psychometrically validated reanalysis of the diabetes control and complications trial data. *Diabetes Care* 1999;22:1273–1277.

17. The Diabetes Control and Complications Trial Research Group. Influence of intensive diabetes treatment on quality-of-life outcomes in the diabetes control and complications trial. *Diabetes Care* 1996;19:195–203.

18. Grey M, Boland EA, Davidson M, Li J, Tamborlane W. Coping skills training for youth with diabetes mellitus has long-lasting effects on metabolic control and quality of life. *J Pediatr* 2000;137:107–113.

19. UK Prospective Diabetes Study Group. Quality of life in type 2 diabetic patients is affected by complications but not by intensive policies to improve blood glucose or blood pressure control (UKPDS 37). *Diabetes Care* 1999;22:1125–1136.

20. The Diabetes Control and Complications Trial Research Group. The absence of a glycaemic threshold for the development of long-term complications: the perspective of the diabetes control and complications trial. *Diabetes* 1996; 45:1289–1298.

21. Stratton IM, Adler AI, Neil HAW, et al on behalf of the UK Prospective Diabetes Study Group. Association of glycaemia with macrovascular and microvascular complications of type 2 diabetes (UKPDS 35): prospective observational study. *BMJ* 2000;321:450–412.

William H Herman
Professor of Internal Medicine and
Epidemiology
University of Michigan Medical Center
Ann Arbor, Michigan
USA

Competing interests: None declared.

TABLE 1 Risk (odds ratio) for development or progression of microvascular, nephropathic, and neuropathic complications with intensive versus conventional treatment. Odds ratio, number needed to treat, and confidence intervals were all calculated from data in papers (see text, p 405).

	Systematic Review[3]	DCCT[4]	Kumamoto[5]	UKPDS[6]
Studies	16 RCTs	RCT	RCT	RCT
Number of participants	–	1441	110	3867
Type of diabetes	Type 1	Type 1	Type 2	Type 2*
Follow up	8 to 60 months	6.5 years	6 years	10 years
Change in HbA1c	1.4%	2.0%	2.0%	0.9%
Progression of retinopathy				
OR (95% CI)	0.49 (0.28 to 0.85)	0.39 (0.28 to 0.55)	0.25 (0.09 to 0.65)	0.66 (0.48 to 0.92)
NNT (95% CI) over duration of study	–	5 (4 to 7)	4 (3 to 11)	10 (6 to 50)
Development of retinopathy				
OR (95% CI)	–	0.22 (0.14 to 0.36)	–	–
NNT (95% CI) over duration of study	–	6 (5 to 7)	–	–
Development or progression of nephropathy				
OR (95% CI)	0.34 (0.20 to 0.58)	0.50 (0.39 to 0.63)	0.26 (0.09 to 0.76)	0.54 (0.25 to 1.18)
NNT (95% CI) over duration of study	–	7 (6 to 11)	5 (4 to 19)	–
Development or progression of neuropathy				
OR (95% CI)	–	0.36 (0.24 to 0.54)	–	0.42 (0.23 to 0.78)
NNT (95% CI) over duration of study	–	13 (11 to 18)	–	5 (3 to 16)

*All participants had fasting plasma glucose > 6.0 mmol/L on two occasions: 93% had fasting plasma glucose ≥ 7.0 mmol/L (American Diabetic Association criterion) and 86% had fasting plasma glucose ≥ 7.8 mmol/L (WHO criterion). CI, confidence interval; NNT, number needed to treat; OR, odd ratio.

Obesity

Search date January 2001

David Arterburn and Polly Hitchcock Noel

INTERVENTIONS

Key Messages

Centrally acting agents

- We found limited evidence from seven RCTs that sibutramine is more effective than placebo in promoting modest weight loss in healthy obese adults and obese adults with controlled hypertension (body mass index [BMI] 25–40 kg/m^2). Weight regain occurs after stopping treatment. We found insufficient evidence about short term safety and no evidence about long term safety.

- Small RCTs found that phentermine and mazindol versus placebo cause modest weight loss in adults more than 15% overweight. We found insufficient evidence on weight regain and long term safety.

- Small RCTs found limited and conflicting evidence on the efficacy of diethylproprion and fluoxetine for weight loss when compared with placebo.

- Dexfenfluramine and fenfluramine have been associated with valvular heart disease and pulmonary hypertension and are no longer marketed. Phenylpropanolamine has recently been linked with increased risk of haemorrhagic stroke.

Orlistat (lipase inhibitor)

- One systematic review and three subsequent RCTs have found that orlistat plus a low calorie diet has a modest effect on body weight compared with placebo plus diet in people with a BMI between 28–47 kg/m^2. We found no evidence on weight regain after stopping treatment, and no evidence on long term safety.

DEFINITION	Obesity is a chronic condition characterised by an excess of body fat. It is most often defined by the BMI (see glossary, p 418), a mathematical formula that is highly correlated with body fat. BMI is weight in kilograms divided by height in metres squared (kg/m^2). In the USA and the UK, people with BMIs between 25–30 kg/m^2 are categorised as overweight, and those with BMIs above 30 kg/m^2 are categorised as obese.[1]
INCIDENCE/ PREVALENCE	Obesity has increased steadily in many countries since 1900. In England, in 1994, it was estimated that 13% of men and 16% of women were obese.[1,2] In the past decade alone, the prevalence of obesity in the USA has increased from 12.0% in 1991 to 17.9% in 1998.[3]
AETIOLOGY/ RISK FACTORS	The aetiology of obesity includes both genetic and environmental factors. Obesity may also be induced by drugs (e.g. high dose glucocorticoids), or be secondary to a variety of neuroendocrine disorders such as Cushing's syndrome and polycystic ovary syndrome.[4]
PROGNOSIS	Obesity is a risk factor for several chronic diseases, including hypertension, dyslipidaemia, diabetes, cardiovascular disease, sleep apnoea, osteoarthritis, and some cancers.[1] The relation between increasing body weight and the mortality rate is curvilinear, with mortality rate increasing in people with low body weight. Whether this is caused by increased mortality risk at low body weights or by unintentional weight loss is not clear.[5] Results from five prospective cohort studies and 1991 national statistics suggest that the number of annual deaths attributable to obesity among US adults is approximately 280 000.[6]
AIMS	To achieve realistic gradual weight loss and prevent the morbidity and mortality associated with obesity, without undue adverse effects.
OUTCOMES	We found no studies that used the primary outcomes of functional morbidity or mortality. Proxy measures include mean weight loss (kg), number of people losing 5% or more of baseline body weight, and number of people maintaining weight loss.
METHODS	*Clinical Evidence* update search and appraisal January 2001.

QUESTION   What are the effects of drug treatments in adults?

OPTION   CENTRALLY ACTING AGENTS

We found limited evidence from six RCTs that sibutramine is more effective than placebo at promoting modest weight loss in adults with BMIs between 25–40 kg/m^2. The weight loss stabilised after 6 months of treatment and was not sustained after stopping treatment. One RCT found that sibutramine caused modest weight loss in obese adults with controlled hypertension, but we found insufficient evidence about short term safety and no evidence of long term safety. Limited evidence suggests that phentermine and mazindol, compared with placebo, result in modest weight loss over short periods in people more than 15% overweight. Weight regain was found after stopping treatment and after longer treatment periods. We found no strong evidence of serious

adverse events associated with either phentermine or mazindol. We found insufficient evidence about either diethylproprion or fluoxetine for weight loss. Dexfenfluramine, fenfluramine, and the combination of fenfluramine plus phentermine have been associated with valvular heart disease and pulmonary hypertension. Phenylpropanolamine has been associated with increased risk of haemorrhagic stroke.

Benefits: We found no systematic review or RCTs examining effects of centrally acting drugs on functional morbidity and mortality. **Sibutramine:** We found one systematic review (search date 1998, 6 RCTs, adults aged 18–65 years with BMIs 25–40 kg/m^2)[7] and one subsequent RCT[8] comparing the effect of sibutramine versus placebo on weight loss. The systematic review did not report a quantitative summary. The studies usually excluded people with other illnesses, described participants as healthy, or did not specify participants' health status. In three of the six RCTs in the systematic review, both sibutramine and placebo groups received other interventions such as diet or calorie restriction, behaviour modification, or exercise.[9-11] In a fourth RCT, participants received a diet of 220–800 kcal/day for 4 weeks before randomisation.[12] Four RCTs were 8–24 weeks and two were 12 months long. The largest RCT (1024 people) found that sibutramine (5–30 mg/day) versus placebo reduced mean weight loss at 24 weeks (5.3 kg with sibutramine 15 mg/day v 0.9 kg with placebo, 95% CI not reported, P < 0.001) and increased the percentage of people losing 5% or more of body weight at 24 weeks (53% with sibutramine 15 mg/day v 13% with placebo, 95% CI not reported; NNT 3, P < 0.001).[9] Mean weight losses for the two 12 month trials were 4.4 and 5.2 kg for people on 15 and 10 mg sibutramine versus maximal weight losses of 1.6 kg with placebo.[12,13] Weight regain of up to 25% of previously lost weight was observed within 1–6 weeks of stopping treatment in three of the RCTs.[9-11] Weight regain of up to 80% was observed within 3 months after stopping medication in one RCT.[12] The subsequent RCT (224 obese people with a diagnosis of controlled hypertension for at least 12 months, BMIs 27–40 kg/m^2) found sibutramine 20 mg/day versus placebo increased mean weight loss after treatment for 12 months (4.4 kg with sibutramine v 0.5 kg placebo, 95% CI not reported, P < 0.05).[8] In all the 12 month trials, weight loss stabilised after 6 months of sibutramine.[8,12,13] **Phentermine:** We found one RCT (108 people who were more than 20% overweight), which compared phentermine (30 mg/day) versus placebo.[14] All participants were placed on a diet of 1000 kcal/day. It found that, after 9 months, phentermine reduced weight more than placebo (–12.2 kg with phentermine v –4.8 kg with placebo; mean difference –7.4 kg, 95% CI –11.2 to –4.6 kg). **Mazindol:** We found one RCT (65 people who were more than 15% overweight), which found that mazindol (3 mg/day) reduced weight more than placebo after 3 months' treatment (–6.4 kg with mazindol v –2.6 kg with placebo; mean difference –3.8 kg, 95% CI not reported, P < 0.001). Weight loss was not sustained when treatment was discontinued.[15] **Diethylproprion:** We found two small RCTs with conflicting results. The first (20 people who were 15–20% overweight) found that diethylproprion 75 mg/day reduced weight more than placebo at 6 months (–11.6 kg with diethylproprion v –2.5 kg with placebo; mean

difference −9.1 kg, 95% CI not reported). Both groups were placed on a "strict diet".[16] The second trial (32 people with mean weight 13 kg above ideal body weight) found no significant difference in weight loss between diethylproprion (75 mg/day) and placebo after treatment for 12 months (−8.9 kg with diethylproprion v −10.5 kg with placebo; mean difference +1.6 kg, 95% CI not reported). Both groups were placed on a "low carbohydrate diet".[17] **Fluoxetine:** We found three systematic reviews (search dates 1995, 1996, 1998), which identified two RCTs of at least 1 year's duration evaluating fluoxetine, a selective serotonin reuptake inhibitor.[2,18,19] One RCT (458 people, mean BMI 35 kg/m^2) found no significant difference in weight loss between fluoxetine 60 mg/day and placebo after treatment for 1 year (−1.4 kg with fluoxetine v −1.2 kg with placebo; mean difference −0.2 kg, 95% CI not reported).[20] The second small RCT (19 people with diabetes and BMI > 30 kg/m^2) found that fluoxetine (60 mg/day) reduced weight more than placebo after treatment for 12 months (−4.3 kg with fluoxetine v +1.5 kg with placebo; mean difference −5.8 kg, 95% CI not reported).[21]
Fenfluramine: We found two RCTs (45 and 134 people who were more than 15% overweight), which found no significant difference between fenfluramine alone, fenfluramine with behavioural therapy, and behavioural therapy or diet alone (results not pooled).[22,23]
Dexfenfluramine: We found one systematic review (search date 1995, 5 RCTs), which found that dexfenfluramine (30–120 mg/day) reduced weight more than placebo after 1 year of treatment. The review pooled data from four trials in a total of 634 adults who were at least 20% overweight. The mean difference in weight at 1 year for dexfenfluramine versus placebo was −2.6 kg (95% CI −3.8 to −1.3 kg). All participants were also prescribed a calorie restricted diet.[2] **Fenfluramine plus phentermine:** We found one RCT (121 people, 30–80% overweight), which found that a combination of phentermine (15 mg/day) plus fenfluramine (60 mg/day) reduced weight more than placebo after treatment for 6 months (−14.3 kg with phentermine/fenfluramine v −4.6 kg with placebo; mean difference −9.7 kg, 95% CI −12.0 to −7.4 kg). The trial found that weight loss ceased at 18 weeks of treatment; weight regain was noted after 60 weeks of treatment.[24] **Phenylpropanolamine:** We found one non-systematic meta-analysis (7 trials, 643 obese people, BMI not stated), which found that phenylpropanolamine (dose not specified) compared with placebo reduced weight after treatment for 4 weeks (0.21 kg/week).[25] At the end of these trials (duration not specified), there was an additional weight loss of 0.14 kg/week compared with placebo.[25]

Harms: **Sibutramine:** Common adverse effects were headache, dry mouth, anorexia, constipation, insomnia, rhinitis, and pharyngitis occurring in 10–30% of people taking sibutramine versus 8–19% of people on placebo (significance of difference not reported).[7] Mean increases in systolic and diastolic blood pressure (1–3 mmHg) and heart rate (4–5 beats/minute) have been reported in people taking sibutramine at doses of 5–20 mg/day.[7] In people with controlled hypertension, the proportion who experienced a clinically significant increase in baseline systolic or diastolic blood pressure (> 10 mmHg at 3 consecutive visits) was comparable with placebo (17.6% with sibutramine v 14.5% with placebo, P value and 95% CI not reported; NNH 32). However, hypertension was the most common adverse event causing withdrawal from the study (5.3% with sibutramine v 1.4% with placebo). No serious adverse events were reported.[8] We found no evidence on long term safety. **Phentermine:** We found no evidence of serious adverse reactions. Phentermine given alone has not been associated with valvular heart disease.[26] **Mazindol and diethylproprion:** We found a single case report of pulmonary hypertension diagnosed 12 months after stopping mazindol that had been taken for 10 weeks.[27] Case reports have described pulmonary hypertension and psychosis in users of diethylproprion.[28,29] The frequency of serious adverse events with these agents is not clear. **Fluoxetine:** One RCT comparing fluoxetine versus placebo for obesity reported more frequent gastrointestinal symptoms, sleep disturbance, sweating, tremor, amnesia, and thirst in the active treatment groups (frequency of events not provided).[20] One systematic review of antidepressant treatment found that selective serotonin reuptake inhibitors were associated with a 10–15% incidence of anxiety, diarrhoea, dry mouth, headache, and nausea.[30] **Dexfenfluramine, fenfluramine, fenfluramine plus phentermine:** These agents have been associated with valvular heart disease and primary pulmonary hypertension,[31,32] and are no longer marketed.[33] One 25 centre retrospective cohort study in 1473 people found prevalence rates and relative risk of aortic regurgitation of 8.9% with dexfenfluramine (RR 2.18, 95% CI 1.32 to 3.59; NNH 20) and 13.7% with phentermine plus fenfluramine (RR 3.34, 95% CI 2.09 to 5.35; NNH 10), compared with 4.1% with no treatment.[34] One prospective study in 1072 participants found no greater risk of valvular heart disease in people taking dexfenfluramine less than 3 months than in those taking placebo (sustained release dexfenfluramine RR 1.6, 95% CI 0.8 to 3.4, regular dexfenfluramine RR 1.4, 95% CI 0.7 to 3.0, when compared with placebo).[35] One case control study in 95 people with primary pulmonary hypertension and 355 matched controls found a history of fenfluramine use was associated with increased risk of primary pulmonary hypertension (OR 6.3, 95% CI 3.0 to 13.2). The odds ratio was higher among people who had taken fenfluramine in the past year (OR 10.1, 95% CI 3.4 to 29.9), and among people treated for more than 3 months (OR 23.1, 95% CI 6.9 to 77.7).[36] **Phenylpropanolamine:** A recent case control study (men and women aged 18–49 years) found that phenylpropanolamine used as an appetite suppressant increased the risk of haemorrhagic stroke within the first 3 days of use (adjusted OR 15.9, lower confidence limit 2.04, P = 0.013). For the association between phenylpropanolamine in appetite suppressants and risk for haemorrhagic stroke among women, the adjusted odds ratio was 16.6 (lower confidence limit 2.2, P = 0.011).[37] Phenylpropanolamine is no longer marketed in the USA.[38]

Comment: **Phenylpropanolamine, phentermine, mazindol, and diethylproprion:** The few trials that we identified were small, with short duration of follow up, and high withdrawal rates. Nearly 5 million US adults used prescription weight loss pills in 1996–1998. A quarter of users were not overweight, suggesting that weight loss pills may be inappropriately used, especially among women, white people, and Hispanic people.[39]

OPTION	ORLISTAT

One systematic review and three subsequent RCTs have found that orlistat combined with a low calorie diet modestly increases weight loss in adults with obesity, compared with placebo plus diet. We found no evidence on weight gain following discontinuation, or on long term adverse effects.

Benefits: We found no systematic reviews or RCTs examining effects of orlistat on functional morbidity and mortality. We found one systematic review (search date 1999, 7 RCTs, 4188 adults with BMIs between 28–47 kg/m^2)[40] and three subsequent RCTs, comparing orlistat versus placebo.[41–43] Trials lasted 1–2 years. Meta-analysis of five of the trials found that orlistat combined with a low calorie diet (below 1500 kcal/day) reduced weight more than placebo plus diet after treatment for 1 year (mean weight loss 6.1 kg with orlistat 120 mg three times daily v 2.6 kg with placebo; P < 0.001, 95% CI not reported).[44] A greater proportion of the participants lost 10% or more of their initial weight in the orlistat groups than in the placebo groups at 12 months (20.2% v 8.3%, P < 0.001). In a 1 year trial (322 people with type 2 diabetes included in the review but not the meta-analysis), 30.2% of the orlistat plus diet group, and 13.2% of the placebo plus diet group lost 5% or more of their initial body weight.[45] We found three subsequent multicentre trials with over 30 people per trial (placebo controlled, double blind, 796,[41] 783,[42] and 376[43] people) whose results were consistent with the earlier systematic review. In the two larger trials, generally healthy obese adults (BMI 28–44 kg/m^2) were randomised to placebo or orlistat (60 or 120 mg) three times a day for 2 years after a 4 week placebo and reduced energy diet run-in, which 54 of the 796 and 161 of the 783 participants did not complete. Participants in both trials followed a reduced energy diet for the first year and a weight maintenance diet for the second year. People taking orlistat were significantly more likely to lose 10% or more of initial body weight compared with those taking placebo at the end of the first year (28.6–38.2% with orlistat 60 mg v 11.3–18.6% with placebo), and to maintain this weight loss after 2 years (28.2–33.0% with orlistat 60 mg v 6.6–18.6% with placebo). One of the trials reported significantly improved "quality of life" on orlistat compared with placebo, but this consisted of reduced obesity specific distress and reduced treatment dissatisfaction.[42] The third RCT (376 obese adults, BMI 28–38 kg/m^2 with type 2 diabetes, hypercholesterolaemia, or hypertension) compared orlistat (120 mg) versus placebo three times daily in conjunction with dietary intervention for 1 year.[43] All participants were given placebo for 2 weeks before randomisation. Orlistat versus placebo significantly increased the proportion of people who lost 5% or more of their initial body weight (54% with orlistat v 41% with placebo; P < 0.001), but did not significantly increase weight reduction of 10% or more (19.2% with orlistat v 14.6% with placebo).

Harms: Common adverse effects included oily spotting from the rectum, flatulence, and faecal urgency in 22–27% of people taking orlistat versus 1–7% of people taking placebo.[40] Four RCTs reported monitoring plasma levels of fat soluble vitamins and found a higher percentage of people treated with orlistat required vitamin supplements compared with placebo.[45–48] In the largest RCT (892 people), vitamin supplements were given to 14.1% with orlistat versus 6.5% with placebo.[47] A single case study suggests that orlistat may also reduce the intestinal absorption of contraceptive pills.[49] In the RCT of people with obesity associated coronary heart disease risk factors, more unidentified serious adverse events occurred with orlistat than with placebo (10% with orlistat v 2.6%).[43]

Comment: People in six of the seven trials in the systematic review were selected for participation after losing weight on a preliminary low calorie diet with placebo for 4–5 weeks before randomisation.[40]

GLOSSARY

Body mass index (BMI) Expressed as weight in kilograms divided by height in metres squared (kg/m^2). In the USA and UK, individuals with BMIs between $25–30\,kg/m^2$ are considered overweight; those with BMIs above $30\,kg/m^2$ are considered obese.

REFERENCES

1. National Institutes of Health. *Clinical guidelines on the identification, evaluation, and treatment of overweight and obesity in adults: the Evidence Report*. Bethesda, Maryland: US Department of Health and Human Services, 1998.

2. University of York, NHS Centre for Reviews and Dissemination. *A systematic review of the interventions for the prevention and treatment of obesity, and the maintenance of weight loss*. York, England: NHS Centre for Reviews and Dissemination, 1997. Search date 1995; primary sources Medline, Embase, Bids, Dare, Psychlit, bibliographies of review articles, and contributions from peer reviewers.

3. Mokdad AH, Serdula MK, Dietz WH, Bowman BA, Marks JS, Koplan JP. The spread of the obesity epidemic in the United States 1991–1998. *JAMA* 1999;282:1519–1522.

4. Bray GA. Obesity: etiology. *UpToDate* [serial on CD-ROM] 2000;8(1). UpToDate, Inc, Wellesley, Massachusetts, USA.

5. Bray GA. Obesity: Overview of therapy for obesity. *UpToDate* [serial on CD-ROM] 2000;8(1). UpToDate, Inc, Wellesley, Massachusetts, USA.

6. Allison DB, Fontaine KR, Manson JE, Stevens J, Vanitallie TB. Annual deaths attributable to obesity in the United States. *JAMA* 1999;282:1530–1538.

7. Luque CA, Rey JA. Sibutramine: a serotonin-norepinephrine reuptake-inhibitor for the treatment of obesity. *Ann Pharmacother* 1999;33:968–978. Search date 1998; primary sources Medline, Embase, manual search, and reference lists of relevant articles.

8. McMahon FG, Fujioka K, Singh BN, et al. Efficacy and safety of sibutramine in obese white and African American patients with hypertension: a 1-year, double-blind, placebo-controlled multicenter trial. *Arch Int Med* 2000;160:2185–2191.

9. Bray GA, Blackburn GL, Ferguson JM, et al. Sibutramine produces dose-related weight loss. *Obes Res* 1999;7:189–198.

10. Hanotin C, Thomas F, Jones SP, Leutenegger E, Drouin P. Efficacy and tolerability of sibutramine in obese patients: a dose-ranging study. *Int J Obes Relat Metab Disord* 1998;22:32–38.

11. Weintraub M, Rubio A, Golik A, Byrne L, Scheinbaum ML. Sibutramine in weight control: a dose-ranging, efficacy study. *Clin Pharmacol Ther* 1991;50:330–337.

12. Apfelbaum M, Vague P, Ziegler O, Hanotin C, Thomas F, Leutenegger E. Long-term maintenance of weight loss after a very-low calorie diet: a randomized blinded trial of the efficacy and tolerability of sibutramine. *Am J Med* 1999;106:179–184.

13. Jones SP, Smith IG, Kelly F, Gray JA. Long-term weight loss with sibutramine [abstract]. *Int J Obes Relat Metab Disord* 1995;19(suppl 2):41.

14. Munro JF, MacCuish AC, Wilson EM, et al. Comparison of continuous and intermittent anorectic therapy in obesity. *BMJ* 1968;1:352–354.

15. Vernace BJ. Controlled comparative investigation of mazindol, D-amphetamine, and placebo. *Obesity Bariatric Med* 1974;3:124–129.

16. McKay RHG. Long-term use of diethylproprion in obesity. *Curr Med Res Opin* 1973;1:489–493.

17. Silverstone JT, Solomon T. The long-term management of obesity in general practice. *Br J Clin Pract* 1965;19:395–398.

18. Douketis JD, Feightner JW, Attia J, et al. Periodic health examination, 1999 update: 1. Detection, prevention and treatment of obesity. Canadian Task Force on Preventive Health Care. *Can Med Assoc J* 1999;160:513–525. Search date 1998; primary sources Medline, bibliographies of review articles, and Current Contents listings.

19. National Task Force on the Prevention and Treatment of Obesity. Long-term pharmacotherapy in the management of obesity. *JAMA* 1996;276:1907–1915. Search date 1996; primary sources Medline and manual search of bibliographies.

20. Goldstein DJ, Rampey AH Jr, Enas GG, et al. Fluoxetine: a randomized clinical trial in the treatment of obesity. *Int J Obes* 1994;18:129–135.

21. O'Kane M, Wiles PG, Wales JK. Fluoxetine in the treatment of obese type II diabetic patients. *Diabet Med* 1994;11:105–110.

22. Ost LG, Gotestam KG. Behavioral and pharmacological treatments for obesity: an experimental comparison. *Addict Behav* 1976;1:331–338.

23. Stunkard AJ, Craighead LW, O'Brien R. Controlled trial of behavior therapy, pharmacotherapy, and their combination in the treatment of obesity. *Lancet* 1980;2:1045–1047.

24. Weintraub M. Long term weight control study: the National Heart, Lung, and Blood Institute funded multimodal intervention study. *Clin Pharmacol Ther* 1992;51:581–646.

25. Greenway FL. Clinical studies with phenylpropanolamine: a metaanalysis. *Am J Clin Nutr* 1992;55(suppl 1):203–205.

26. Gaasch WH, Aurigemma GP. Valvular heart disease induced by anorectic drugs. *UpToDate* [serial on CD-ROM][2000;8(3). UpToDate, Inc, Wellesley, Massachusetts, USA.

27. Hagiwara M, Tsuchida A, Hyakkoku M, et al. Delayed onset of pulmonary hypertension associated with an appetite suppressant, mazindol: a case report. *Jpn Circ* 2000;64:218–221.

28. Thomas SH, Butt AY, Corris PA, et al. Appetite suppressants and primary pulmonary hypertension in the United Kingdom. *Br Heart J* 1995;74:660–663.

29. Little JD, Romans SE. Psychosis following readmministration of diethylproprion: a possible role for kindling? *Int Clin Psychopharmacol* 1993;8:67–70.

30. Mulrow CD, Williams JW Jr, Trivedi M, et al. Treatment of depression – newer pharmacotherapies. *Psychopharmacol Bull* 1998;34:409–795. Search date 1998; primary sources the Cochrane and collaboration depression, anxiety and neurosis (CCDAN) Review Group's registry, and bibliographies of trial and review articles.

31. Poston WS, Foreyt JP. Scientific and legal issues in fenfluramine/dexfenfluramine litigation. *J Texas Med* 2000;96:48–56.

32. Connolly HM, Crary JL, McGoon MD, et al. Valvular heart disease associated with fenfluramine-phentermine. *N Engl J Med* 1997;337:581–588.

33. Scheen AJ, Lefebvre PJ. Pharmacological treatment of obesity: present status. *Intl J Obes Relat Metab Disord* 1999;23(suppl 1):47–53.

34. Gardin JM, Schumacher D, Constantine G, et al. Valvular abnormalities and cardiovascular status following exposure to dexfenfluramine and phentermine/fenfluramine. *JAMA* 2000;283:703–709.

35. Weissman NJ, Tighe JF, Gottdiener JS, Gwynne JT. An assessment of heart-valve abnormalities in obese patients taking dexfenfluramine, sustained-release dexfenfluramine, or placebo. Sustained release dexfenfluramine study group. *N Engl J Med* 1998;339:725–732.

36. Abenhaim L, Moride Y, Brenot F, et al. Appetite-suppressant drugs and the risk of primary pulmonary hypertension. International primary pulmonary hypertension study group. *N Engl J Med* 1996;335:609–616.

37. Horwitz RI, Brass LM, Kernan WN, Viscoli CM. Phenylpropanolamine and risk of hemorrhagic stroke: final report of the hemorrhagic stroke project. http://www.fda.gov/ohrms/dockets/ac/00/backgrd/3647b1_tab19.doc (accessed 2 Mar 2001).

38. U.S. Food and Drug Administration. Center for Drug Evaluation and Research. Phenylpropanolamine (PPA) information page. http://www.fda.gov/cder/drug/infopage/ppa/ (accessed 2 Mar 2001).

39. Khan LK, Serdula MK, Bowman BA, Williamson DF. Use of Prescription Weight Loss Pills among U.S. Adults in 1996–1998. *Ann Int Med* 2001; 134:282–286.

40. Anonymous. Orlistat: no hurry. *Can Fam Physician* 1999;45:2331–2351. Search date 1999; primary sources Medline, Embase, Reactions, Cochrane; hand searches of international journals, the Prescribe Library, and clinical pharmacology reference texts and personal contact with Produits Roche, the European Medicines Evaluation Agency, and Food and Drug Administration committees.

41. Hauptman J, Lucas C, Boldrin MN, Collins H, Segal KR. Orlistat in the long-term treatment of obesity in primary care settings. *Arch Fam Med* 2000;9:160–167.

42. Rossner S, Sjöstrom L, Noack R, Meinders AE, Noseda G. Weight loss, weight maintenance, and improved cardiovascular risk factors after 2 years treatment with orlistat for obesity. *Obes Res* 2000; 8:49–61.

43. Lindgarde F. The effect of orlistat on body weight and coronary heart disease risk profile in obese patients: the Swedish Multimorbidity Study. *J Int Med* 2000;248:245–254.

44. European Agency for the Evaluation of Medicinal Products. *Committee for proprietary medicinal products. European public assessment report (EPAR) – Xenical.* London: European Agency for the Evaluation of Medicinal Products, 1998.

45. Hollander PA, Elbein SC, Hirsch IR, et al. Role of orlistat in the treatment of obese patients with type 2 diabetes: a 1-year randomized double-blind study. *Diabetes Care* 1998;21:1288–1294.

46. Sjostrom L, Rissanen A, Anderson T, et al. Randomised placebo-controlled trial of orlistat for weight loss and prevention of weight regain in obese patients. *Lancet* 1998;352:167–173.

47. Davidson MH, Hauptman J, DiGirolamo M, et al. Weight control and risk factor reduction in obese subjects treated for 2 years with orlistat: a randomized controlled trial. *JAMA* 1999;281:235–242.

48. Finer N, James WPT, Kopelman PG, Lean MEJ, Williams G. One-year treatment of obesity: a randomized, double-blind, placebo-controlled, multicentre study of orlistat, a gastrointestinal lipase inhibitor. *Int J Obes* 2000;24:306–313.

49. Peleg R. Caution when using oral contraceptive pills with Orlistat [letter]. *Isr Med Assoc J* 2000;2:712.

David Arterburn
Chief Resident/Instructor
University of Texas, Health Science
Center at San Antonio
San Antonio
USA

Polly Hitchcock Noel
Associate Director
VERDICT, a VA HSR&D
Center of Excellence
South Texas Veterans
Health Care System
US Department of Veterans Affairs
San Antonio, Texas, USA

Competing interests: None declared. The views expressed in this article are those of the authors and do not necessarily represent the views of the US Department of Veterans Affairs.

Eye disorders

Search date October 2000

Kimble Matos, André Curi and Carlos Pavesio

QUESTIONS
Effects of topical anti-inflammatory eye drops 422

INTERVENTIONS	
Likely to be beneficial Steroid eye drops . . . . .422 **Unknown effectiveness** Non-steroidal eye drops. 423	**To be covered in future issues of** *Clinical Evidence* Mydriatics Subconjunctival steroid injection Oral steroids Slow taper of drug treatment Treatment of chronic iridocyclitis See glossary, p 423

Key Messages

- Available RCTs were too small to prove or exclude clinically important differences between steroid eye drops and placebo, or between steroid and non-steroidal eye drops. The limited evidence suggests that steroid eye drops are more effective than non-steroidal eye drops.

DEFINITION	Anterior uveitis is inflammation of the uveal tract, and includes iritis and iridocyclitis. It can be classified according to its clinical course into acute or chronic uveitis, or according to its clinical appearance into granulomatous or non-granulomatous uveitis. Acute anterior uveitis is characterised by an extremely painful red eye, often associated with photophobia and occasionally decreased visual acuity. Chronic uveitis is defined as inflammation lasting more than 6 weeks. It is usually asymptomatic, but many people have mild symptoms during exacerbations.
INCIDENCE/ PREVALENCE	Acute anterior uveitis is rare, with an annual incidence of 12 per 100 000 population.[1] It is common in Finland (annual incidence 22.6/100 000, prevalence 68.7/100 000), probably owing to genetic factors such as the high frequency of HLA-B27.[2] It occurs equally in both sexes and less than 10% of cases occur before the age of 20.[2,3]
AETIOLOGY/ RISK FACTORS	Between 60% and 80% of cases of anterior uveitis are classified as idiopathic. The range of systemic disorders associated with anterior uveitis are ankylosing spondylitis, Reiter's syndrome, juvenile chronic arthritis, Kawasaki syndrome, infectious uveitis, Behçet's syndrome, inflammatory bowel disease, interstitial nephritis, sarcoidosis, multiple sclerosis, Wegener's granulomatosis, Vogt-Koyanagi-Harada syndrome, and masquerade syndromes (see glossary, p 423). Acute anterior uveitis also occurs in association with HLA-B27 not linked to any systemic disease, and it may be the manifestation of an isolated eye disorder such as Fuchs' iridocyclitis, Posner-Schlossman syndrome, Schwartz syndrome, and it may also occur following surgery and as drug or hypersensitivity reactions.[2,3]
PROGNOSIS	Acute anterior uveitis is often self limiting, but we found no evidence about how often it resolves spontaneously, in which people, or over what time period. Complications include posterior synechiae (see glossary, p 423), cataract, glaucoma, and chronic uveitis. In a study of 154 people (232 eyes) with acute anterior uveitis (119 people HLA-B27 positive), visual acuity was better than 20/60 in 209 eyes (90%), and 20/60 or worse in 23 people and 23 eyes (10%), with 11 eyes (5%) having legal blindness (visual acuity worse than 20/200). In people with impaired visual acuity, 19 of 23 had cataract and four had secondary glaucoma and complications of surgery. HLA-B27 status made no significant difference to the rate of complications or to visual outcome.[4]
AIMS	To reduce inflammation; to relieve pain; and to prevent complications and loss of visual acuity, with minimal adverse effects.
OUTCOMES	Degree of inflammation, using scores that register cell counts and flare in the anterior chamber; keratic precipitates; ciliary flush; severity of symptoms (photophobia and pain).
METHODS	*Clinical Evidence* update search and appraisal October 2000. We found no relevant systematic reviews. Large, well designed RCTs are needed to provide adequate evidence about the effectiveness of interventions, because of the small expected differences in

outcomes with different treatments, the self limiting nature of some types of anterior uveitis, and the variation in severity of clinical manifestations.

QUESTION What are the effects of topical anti-inflammatory eye drops?

OPTION TOPICAL STEROID TREATMENTS

Available RCTs were too small to either confirm or exclude clinically important differences between steroid eye drops and placebo, or between steroid and non-steroidal eye drops. They suggest that steroid eye drops are more effective and faster acting than non-steroidal eye drops. Limited evidence suggests that new topical steroids such as rimexolone may be as effective as prednisolone but with less risk of raised intraocular pressure.

Benefits:
We found no systematic review. **Versus placebo:** We found one double blind RCT (60 people with acute unilateral, non-granulomatous anterior uveitis) comparing betamethasone phosphate 1%, clobetasone butyrate 0.1%, and placebo. Twelve participants were lost to follow up. Participants received two drops every 2 hours, atropine 1% twice daily, and acetazolamide when necessary in cases of secondary glaucoma, and were followed up for 3 weeks. There was no significant difference between the three groups, but the trial included too few people to exclude a clinically important effect.[5] **Versus each other:** We found two RCTs comparing prednisolone 1% with new topical steroids, rimexolone 1%, and loteprednol etabonate 0.5%. The rimexolone trial in people with acute uveitis, recurrent iridocyclitis, or chronic uveitis (divided into two studies with 183 people randomised and 93 people randomised) found no significant difference in cell and flare scores between groups, except at day 28 in the larger study when prednisolone 1% was associated with greater improvement in flare score.[6] Of the loteprednol trials (also divided into two studies, 245 people with acute anterior uveitis), the larger study (175 people) found that prednisolone acetate was associated with a significantly higher rate of resolution by the final visit at 28 days of treatment (72% v 87%; $P = 0.015$). The smaller study found more people achieved resolution with prednisolone acetate by 42 days of treatment but the difference was not significant.[7] **Versus topical non-steroidal treatments:** See option, p 423.

Harms:
Adverse effects of topical eye drops include local irritation, hyperaemia, oedema, and blurred vision. Rarely, topical eye drops have been associated with glaucoma, cataract, and herpes simplex keratitis. In the trials reported above,[5–7] adverse events were generally mild, resolved without treatment, and did not result in permanent harms. In one of the trials comparing loteprednol etabonate with prednisolone acetate, four people were withdrawn because of adverse effects: cystoid macular oedema and ocular symptoms in the loteprednol group, and interstitial keratitis and increase in age related macular degeneration in the prednisolone group.[7] **Raised intraocular pressure:** Clinically significant increases in intraocular pressure (defined as > 10 mmHg from

baseline) were found more frequently with prednisolone than with the new steroids (prednisolone v rimexolone[6] 11/93 v 6/88 and 8/46 v 1/46; prednisolone v loteprednol[7] 1/32 v 0/34 and 6/91 v 1/84).

Comment: Topical steroids have been standard treatment for acute anterior uveitis since the early 1950s, especially for people with acute and severe uveitis. The placebo controlled trial was too small to rule out a clinically important effect of topical steroids.[5] We are not aware of any further trials under way or planned.

OPTION **TOPICAL NON-STEROIDAL TREATMENTS**

Available RCTs were too small to either confirm or exclude clinically important differences between non-steroid eye drops and placebo, or between non-steroidal eye drops and steroid eye drops. Limited evidence suggests that non-steroidal eye drops are less effective and slower acting than steroid eye drops.

Benefits: **Versus topical steroids:** We found two RCTs. The first (71 people with acute unilateral idiopathic non-granulomatous uveitis) compared prednisolone disodium phosphate 0.5%, betamethasone disodium phosphate 0.1%, and tolmetin sodium dihydrate 5%.[8] Participants were asked to instil one drop every 2 hours during the waking period, and all received atropine 1% once daily. Clinical cure was reported in 68% on prednisolone disodium phosphate, 90% on betamethasone disodium phosphate, and 57% on tolmetin (no measure of significance reported); 11 people were excluded from statistical analysis. The second RCT (49 people with acute anterior non-granulomatous uveitis) compared dexamethasone 0.1% versus indomethacin 1% eye drops administered six times daily.[9] Most participants (equal numbers in each group) also received atropine drops three times a day. After 7 days of treatment, the inflammatory score was significantly lower in the group receiving dexamethasone. By day 14, there was no significant difference between groups. **Versus topical steroids and placebo:** We found one RCT (100 people with acute unilateral idiopathic non-granulomatous anterior uveitis) comparing prednisolone 0.5%, tolmetin 5%, and sterile saline 0.9% (placebo). Participants were asked to instil drops every 2 hours during the waking period and also atropine 1% once daily. Six people were excluded from the study. There was no significant difference between groups in cure rates (47% with tolmetin, 53% with saline, and 69% with prednisolone), but the prednisolone treated group had the highest percentage of patients cured at all stages in the trial.[10]

Harms: See harms under topical steroid treatments, p 422.

Comment: None.

GLOSSARY

Masquerade syndromes Comprise a group of disorders that occur with intraocular inflammation and are often misdiagnosed as a chronic idiopathic uveitis.

Posterior synechiae Adhesions between the iris and the lens capsule.

REFERENCES

1. Darrel RW, Wagner HP, Kurland CT. Epidemiology of uveitis: incidence and prevalence in a small urban community. *Arch Ophthalmol* 1962;68:501–514.
2. Paivonsalo-Hietanen T, Tuominen J, Vaahtoranta-Lehtonen H, Saari KM. Incidence and prevalence of different uveitis entities in Finland. *Acta Ophthalmol Scand* 1997;75:76–81.
3. Rosenbaum JT. Uveitis. An internist's view. *Arch Intern Med* 1989;149;1173–1176.
4. Linssen A, Meenken C. Outcomes of HLA-B27-positive and HLA-B27-negative acute anterior uveitis. *Am J Ophthalmol* 1995;120:351–361.
5. Dunne JA, Travers JP. Topical steroids in anterior uveitis. *Trans Ophthal Soc UK* 1979;99:481–484.
6. Foster CS, Alter G, Raymond DeBarge L, et al. Efficacy and safety of rimexolone 1% ophthalmic suspension vs prednisolone acetate in the treatment of uveitis. *Am J Ophthalmol* 1996 122: 171–182.
7. The Loteprednol Etabonate US Uveitis Study Group. Controlled evaluation of loteprednol etabonate and prednisolone acetate in the treatment of acute anterior uveitis. *Am J Ophthalmol* 1999;127:537–544.
8. Dunne JA, Jacobs N, Morrison A, Gilbert DJ. Efficacy in anterior uveitis of two known steroids and topical tolmetin. *Br J Ophthalmol* 1985;69: 120–125.
9. Sand BB, Krogh E. Topical indometacin, a prostaglandin inhibitor, in acute anterior uveitis. A controlled clinical trial of non-steroid versus steroid anti-inflammatory treatment. *Acta Ophthalmol* 1991;69:145–148.
10. Young BJ, Cunninghan WF, Akingbehin T: Double-masked controlled clinical trial of 5% tolmetin versus 0.5% prednisolone versus 0.9% saline in acute endogenous nongranulomatous anterior uveitis. *Br J Ophthalmol* 1982;66:389–391.

Kimble Matos
Research Fellow

André Curi
Clinical Research Fellow

Carlos Pavesio
Consultant Ophthalmic Surgeon

Moorfields Eye Hospital
London
UK

Competing interests: None declared.

Search date November 2000: expanded this issue

Jennifer Arnold and Shirley Sarks

INTERVENTIONS

Key Messages

Prevention

■ Two RCTs have found that laser to eyes with high risk drusen to prevent late age
related macular degeneration (AMD) causes small increases in visual acuity
but may cause a short term increase in choroidal neovascularisation, particularly in people with exudative AMD in the other eye.

Treatment

■ Four large RCTs have found that laser photocoagulation decreases the rate of
severe visual loss and preserves contrast sensitivity in selected people with
exudative age related macular degeneration (those with well demarcated
lesions on fluorescein angiography). Choroidal neovascularisation recurs within
2 years in about half of patients. Photocoagulation may reduce visual acuity
initially.

■ Three RCTs found no evidence of an effect of external beam radiation on
moderate visual loss in people with exudative AMD within 1 year. We found
insufficient evidence on long term efficacy or safety, but one RCT found no
evidence of an association with cataract formation at 1 year.

■ We found insufficient evidence on the effects of submacular surgery.

© *Clinical Evidence* 2001;5:425–435.

Age related macular degeneration

- One large multicentre RCT found no evidence of benefit from subcutaneous interferon alfa-2a, and found evidence of serious ocular and systemic adverse effects.
- One large multicentre RCT found that photodynamic treatment with verteporfin reduced the risk of moderate and severe vision loss in people with exudative AMD. Subgroup analysis suggested the benefit was only in people with predominantly classic lesions on fluorescein angiography who constitute about 10–30% of people with exudative AMD.
- Overall, we found no evidence that the main treatment options are of benefit to most people with exudative AMD.

DEFINITION   AMD is the late stage of age related maculopathy (see glossary, p 432). AMD has two forms: atrophic (or dry) AMD, characterised by geographic atrophy; and exudative (or wet) AMD, characterised by choroidal neovascularisation (see glossary, p 432), which eventually causes a disciform scar.

INCIDENCE/   AMD is the commonest cause of blind registration in industrialised
PREVALENCE   countries. Atrophic AMD is more common than the more sight threatening exudative AMD, affecting about 85% of people with AMD.[1] End stage (blinding) AMD is found in about 1.7% of all people aged over 50, and incidence rises with age (0.7–1.4% in people aged 65–75, 11.0–18.5% in people aged over 85).[2–4]

AETIOLOGY/   Age is the strongest risk factor. Ocular risk factors for the develop-
RISK FACTORS   ment of exudative AMD include the presence of soft drusen, macular pigmentary change, and choroidal neovascularisation in the other eye. Systemic risk factors are hypertension, smoking, and positive family history.[5,6] The role of diet and exposure to ultraviolet light is suspected but unproved.

PROGNOSIS   AMD impairs central vision, which is required for reading, driving, face recognition, and all fine visual tasks. **Atrophic AMD** progresses slowly over many years, and time to legal blindness (see glossary, p 433) (visual acuity < 20/200) is highly variable (usually about 5–10 years).[7,8] **Exudative AMD** is more threatening to vision; 90% of people with severe visual loss owing to AMD have the exudative type. It usually manifests with a sudden worsening and distortion of central vision. A modelling exercise derived primarily from cohort studies found the risk of developing exudative AMD in people with bilateral soft drusen has been estimated at 1–4.7% at 1 year and 13–18% at 3 years,[9] and the observed 5 year rate in a population survey was 7.1%.[10] Most people (estimates vary from 60–90%) with exudative AMD progress to legal blindness and develop a central defect (scotoma) in the visual field.[11–14] Peripheral vision is preserved, allowing the person to mobilise and be independent. The ability to read with visual aids depends on the size and density of the central scotoma and the degree to which the person retains sensitivity to contrast. Once exudative AMD has developed in one eye, the other eye is at high risk (cumulative estimated incidence: 10%, 28%, and 42% at 1, 3, and 5 years).[5]

AIMS   To minimise loss of visual acuity and central vision; to preserve the ability to read with or without visual aids; to optimise quality of life; to minimise adverse effects of treatment.

OUTCOMES   Visual acuity; rates of legal blindness; contrast sensitivity; quality of life; visual fields; rate of adverse effects of treatment. Visual acuity is measured using special eye charts, usually the Early Treatment of Diabetic Retinopathy Study (ETDRS) chart, although many studies do not specify which chart was used. Stable vision is usually defined as loss of two lines or less on the ETDRS chart. Moderate and severe visual loss is defined as a loss of greater than three and six lines, respectively, which corresponds to a doubling and quadrupling of the vision angle. Loss of vision to legal blindness (< 20/200) is also used as an outcome. A reading of 20/200 (or 6/60 in metric) on the Snellen chart means that a person can see at 20 feet (or 6 metres) what a normally sighted person can see at 200 feet (or 60 metres).

METHODS   *Clinical Evidence* update search and appraisal November 2000.

> ### QUESTION   What are the effects of interventions to prevent age related macular degeneration?   New

> ### OPTION   LASER TO DRUSEN

Two RCTs have found that laser to eyes with high risk drusen provides small improvement in visual acuity within 2 years. We found insufficient evidence that the laser induced drusen reduction results in a decreased incidence of late AMD (choroidal neovascularisation or geographic atrophy). One RCT has found that laser to drusen increases the short term incidence of choroidal neovascularisation, particularly in people with exudative AMD in the other eye.

Benefits: We found no systematic review. **Versus no treatment:** We found two large and three small unblinded RCTs using a variety of treatment protocols. The first RCT (229 eyes, 152 people) compared diode laser treatment at threshold (visible laser end point) or subthreshold (invisible laser end point) versus no laser treatment with 86% of eyes completing 24 month follow up.[15] There were 75 people with unilateral drusen and 77 people with bilateral drusen. It found a significant improvement in visual acuity associated with threshold treatment (24 month follow up, improvement in visual acuity 11.4% v 0%). The second RCT (432 eyes, 276 people) compared argon green laser versus no laser.[16,17] There were 120 people with unilateral drusen and 156 people (312 eyes) with bilateral drusen. Vision outcome at 12 months was reported for 351 eyes (81%). The analysis was not intention to treat because people with choroidal neovascularisation (see glossary, p 432) were excluded.[16] It found a significant improvement in visual acuity with active treatment and reduction in risk of vision loss (17% v 34%, P = 0.01). We found three small unblinded pilot RCTs (each < than 40 people) which reported that eyes treated with laser to drusen had better vision at follow up from 1 to 6 years.[18–20]

Harms: Macular laser may induce choroidal neovascularisation and retinal atrophy. In the first RCT, although the rate of neovascularisation was not significantly different at 24 months in treated and control groups, choroidal neovascularisation was believed to be caused in six of 105 eyes by the visible threshold diode laser.[15] In the second RCT, early analysis found an increased incidence of choroidal neovascularisation in treated eyes in the unilateral group (estimated 12 month incidence 10/59[17%] v 2/61[3%], P < 0.05).[17] The estimated 12 month incidence of choroidal neovascularisation in the bilateral group was not significantly higher (5% v 2%; RR 2.0, 95% CI 0.37 to 11.0). All RCTs sought to minimise this by using low intensity and subthreshold lasers, and by positioning laser burns at a distance (generally > 500 microns) from the fovea centre. One RCT ceased enrolment and treatment because of a higher incidence within the first 12 months of choroidal neovascularisation in treated eyes in people with unilateral (but not with bilateral) drusen,[17] and another ongoing RCT warned that preventive laser may induce choroidal neovascularisation in high risk eyes. Laser induced retinal atrophy was uncommon and seen in two of 120 and one of 105 treated eyes.

Comment: Given there is no evidence of an effective treatment for the majority of people with exudative AMD, there is considerable interest in preventive strategies to people with high risk drusen. One model estimates that a preventive measure of 10% efficacy in people with bilateral drusen would more than double the prevention of legal blindness relative to current treatment.[21] Other RCTs of laser to drusen are either ongoing[22] or planned.[15,16]

QUESTION   What are the effects of treatments for exudative AMD?

OPTION   THERMAL LASER PHOTOCOAGULATION

Four large RCTs have found that laser photocoagulation decreases the rate of severe visual loss and preserves contrast sensitivity in selected people with exudative AMD (those with well demarcated lesions). Choroidal neovascularisation recurs within 2 years in about half of those treated. Photocoagulation may reduce visual acuity initially.

Benefits: We found no systematic review. **Versus no treatment:** We found four large unblinded multicentre RCTs comparing laser photocoagulation versus no treatment (see table 1, p 435) in a selected population.[11–14,23–25] We also found four smaller RCTs that included a wider range of people.[26–29] All four of the large RCTs found that treatment conferred clinically and statistically significant benefit, in terms of reduced risk of severe visual loss (defined as loss of 6 or more lines on the special eye chart), which persisted beyond 3 years. Participants differed in terms of the position of the choroidal neovascularisation on the retina, whether far, near, or under the centre of fixation (extrafoveal,[11,13] juxtafoveal,[14,23] or subfoveal[12,24,25]). In the study of extrafoveal choroidal neovascularisation, the treatment was beneficial (by either intention to treat or on treatment analysis), despite the fact that 19% of eyes randomised to observation later received laser.[11,13] Re-analysis of people with juxtafoveal choroidal neovascularisation found that benefit was limited to those with pure classic lesions (no occult element) on fluorescein angiography (52% of randomised eyes), who were more than twice as likely to avoid developing severe visual loss at 3 years compared with people receiving no treatment (OR 2.2, 95% CI 1.4 to 3.4). The two RCTs in people with subfoveal choroidal neovascularisation found benefit from treatment despite an immediate loss of vision in the treated groups (average 3 lines on the special eye chart).[12] At 5 years after treatment, rates of recurrence of choroidal neovascularisation ranged from 39% to 76%, with most occurring within 2 years. Of the four smaller RCTs, one found that fovea sparing laser photocoagulation preserved visual acuity compared with no treatment.[26] The other three found that scatter (non-confluent) laser was no better than no treatment in occult choroidal neovascularisation.[27–29] However, the RCTs were too small to rule out a beneficial effect. **Different wavelengths:** We found three large multicentre RCTs that compared two wavelengths of laser (krypton red or argon green) for photocoagulation of choroidal neovascularisation in AMD.[30,31] All found no significant difference in outcome. **Effects in people with choroidal neovascularisation identified by indocyanine green angiography:** We found no RCTs. Uncontrolled case series have reported good outcomes in selected people.

Harms: Laser destroys new vessels and surrounding retina, and the resultant scar causes a corresponding defect in the central visual field. If the laser is applied to subfoveal lesions, or if the laser burn spreads to the fovea, visual acuity will be impaired; two of the RCTs described immediate loss of visual acuity (an average loss of 3 lines on the special eye chart).[12,25] We found no evidence of other adverse effects.

Comment: The benefits of laser photocoagulation depend on accurate, complete treatment, requiring high quality angiography and trained, experienced practitioners.[11–14,23–25] The risk of immediate loss of visual acuity with laser photocoagulation may limit its acceptability.

OPTION   **RADIOTHERAPY**

Three RCTs found no evidence of an effect of external beam radiation on the risk of moderate visual loss in people with exudative AMD within 1 year. We found insufficient evidence on long term safety, but one RCT found no evidence of an association with cataract formation at 1 year.

Benefits: We found no systematic review. **External beam radiation:** We found three RCTs. The first, large multicentre double blind RCT (205 people with new subfoveal choroidal neovascularisation) compared external beam radiation (16 Gy in 2 Gy fractions) delivered to the macula versus no treatment.[32] The control group received "sham" radiation treatment (8 fractions of 0 Gy). At 12 months, 51.1% of treated people and 52.6% of controls had moderate visual loss, defined as loss of three or more lines on a special eye chart (P = 0.88). No treatment benefit was detected for subgroups of people classified into classic and occult lesions on the basis of fluorescein angiographic appearance. The second, small, single blind RCT (74 people with new subfoveal choroidal neovascularisation) compared external beam radiation (24 Gy in 6 Gy fractions) delivered to the macula versus no treatment.[33] At 12 months, treated people had a lower risk of moderate or severe visual loss but the difference was not significant (defined as losses of 3 or 6 lines on the special eye chart; AR –20%, 95% CI –44% to +4%). The third RCT (27 people) was a small single blind pilot study comparing single fraction external beam radiation of 7.5 Gy versus no treatment.[34] It found no treatment benefit over a mean follow up of 17 months (range 7–32 months). **Other techniques:** We found conflicting and inconclusive evidence from non-randomised pilot studies using proton beam and scleral plaque (local) radiotherapy in a variety of dosing and timing schedules.

Harms: All RCTs reported no adverse effects after 12 months. Uncontrolled pilot studies suggest that the main risks using current dosing and delivery techniques are cataract (2/41 people in 1 series)[35] and transient keratoconjunctivitis with epiphora (10/75 in 1 series).[36] However, the large multicentre RCT found no significant difference in cataract formation between treated and untreated people at 12 months (10% treated v 16% control) or dry eye symptoms (40% treated v 45% control).[32] Doses of up to 25 Gy, delivered in daily fractions of 2 Gy or less, are generally claimed not to cause damage to the retina or optic nerve. However, radiotherapy is potentially toxic to the retina, optic nerve, lens, and lacrimal system, with toxic effects sometimes manifesting 2 years after treatment.[37] One case series found radiation toxicity to the retina and to the optic nerve in eight and four of 231 eyes, respectively, with 12 to 24 month follow up.[38] A two centre case series of people treated with external beam radiation reported an abnormal choroidal vascular growth pattern associated with macular bleeding and exudation, and marked loss of visual acuity.[39] This change was detected in 12 of 95 people [12%], and seven of 98 people [7.1%], 3–12 months after radiotherapy, and may explain the lack of treatment benefit.

Comment: One multicentre RCT of radiation for AMD is under way (U Chakravarthy, personal communication, 1999). RCTs with less than 2 years' follow up may miss important adverse effects.

OPTION   SUBMACULAR SURGERY

We found insufficient evidence on the effects of submacular surgery. Rates of recurrent choroidal neovascularisation are high, and there is a clinically significant risk of ocular complications resulting in visual loss and further surgical intervention.

Benefits: We found no systematic review. **Versus no treatment:** We found no RCTs. **Versus laser photocoagulation:** We found no published RCTs (see comment below). **Versus alternative surgical techniques:** We found one RCT (80 eyes with exudative AMD) comparing surgery plus subretinal injection of tissue plasminogen activator versus surgery plus subretinal injection of a control solution.[40] The RCT found no significant difference in visual or anatomic outcome.

Harms: We found one pilot RCT (70 people) comparing submacular surgery (see glossary, p 433) versus laser photocoagulation for recurrent subfoveal choroidal neovascularisation (S Bressler, Macular Society Meeting, San Francisco, personal communication, 1999). It found no significant difference between the two treatment groups. Submacular surgery can have effects that threaten vision or require further surgical intervention. However, we found no good data on the frequency of adverse events. The largest case series of people with age related and non-age related macular degeneration reported cataract formation (in up to 40%), retinal detachment (5–8%), recurrent new vessel formation (18–35% within 12 months), and macular complications (haemorrhage and pucker; no rates given).[41]

Comment: Most evidence for submacular surgery currently comes from small uncontrolled case series (< 50 people with AMD) with short follow up, often including people with other types of macular degeneration. These found that few people with AMD experienced improved vision with surgery.[37,41] Comparing results is difficult because of evolving surgical techniques, changes in outcome measures, and variations in follow up. A large non-blinded RCT is currently recruiting and will compare standardised surgical technique versus no treatment in new and haemorrhagic choroidal neovascularisation in people with AMD (S Bressler, personal communication, 1999). Other surgical techniques are being developed in volunteers, including macular translocation and retinal pigment epithelial transplantation, but these have yet to be formally evaluated.

OPTION   SUBCUTANEOUS INTERFERON ALFA-2A

One large RCT found evidence of greater loss of vision with subcutaneous interferon α-2a (an antiangiogenesis drug) compared with placebo, and evidence of serious ocular and systemic adverse effects.

Benefits: We found no systematic review. We found one multicentre, double blind RCT on 481 people with subfoveal choroidal neovascularisation owing to AMD.[41] This compared three doses of subcutaneous interferon α-2a (1.5, 3, and 6 mIU given 3 times a week for 1 year) versus placebo. At 52 weeks, treatment at all doses was associated with a higher risk of losing at least three lines of vision on the Snellen chart compared with placebo (AR 50% v 38%; ARI 12%, 95% CI 0% to 23%). No benefit was found for secondary end points or in subgroups of people.

Harms: Adverse effects of interferon α-2a were common and potentially severe in this and other poorer quality RCTs.[41] These included fatigue and influenza like symptoms, as well as gastrointestinal, and central and peripheral nervous system effects. Although at least one adverse event was reported in 86% of people taking placebo, the proportion of people on active treatment who suffered adverse effects increased with dose, as did the severity of adverse effects. Up to 5% of treated people experienced interferon α-2a induced retinopathy.[42]

Comment: There is widespread interest in safe, effective antiangiogenesis drugs for prophylaxis in exudative AMD. Several drugs are currently under preclinical and early phase clinical study. RCTs are currently investigating thalidomide, with and without concurrent laser photocoagulation, and intravitreal triamcinolone.

OPTION   PHOTODYNAMIC TREATMENT

One large multicentre RCT has found that photodynamic treatment (see glossary, p 433) with verteporfin (see glossary, p 433) reduces the risk of

moderate and severe vision loss in people with exudative AMD. Subgroup analysis suggested the benefit was only in people with predominantly classic lesions on fluorescein angiography. Subgroup analysis found no evidence that photodynamic therapy is beneficial for people with evidence of occult neovascularisation.

Benefits: We found one systematic review (search date 2000, 1 high quality multicentre, double blind placebo controlled RCT, 609 people with new and recurrent subfoveal choroidal neovascularisation due to AMD).[43] The intervention was a two stage procedure: infusion of verteporfin followed by phototherapy with activating laser light. The control group received infusion of sugar water followed by phototherapy. Twice as many participants were randomised to verteporfin. Treatments were repeated if necessary every 3 months. Outcomes were moderate and severe loss of visual acuity (defined as loss of 15 and 30 letters — about 3 and 6 lines) on a special eye chart; a change in contrast sensitivity and fluorescein angiographic appearance. At each follow up visit (up to 12 months), all outcome measures were clinically and statistically significantly better in the treatment than in the control group. At the 12 month follow up visit, significantly less treated people had lost 15 letters of vision or more (61% treated v 46% controls; RR 0.72, 95% CI 0.61 to 0.86; NNT 7, 95% CI 5 to 15). Subgroup analysis found that benefit was greater for people with predominantly classic choroidal neovascularisation lesions (67% treated v 39% control; RR 0.54, 95% CI 0.41 to 0.71), and greatest with pure classic lesions (77% treated v 27% control; RR 0.34, 95% CI 0.22 to 0.51; NNT 2, 95% CI 2 to 4). This last finding was based on only 143 eyes. No treatment benefit for visual acuity was seen in the group without predominantly classic lesions.

Harms: Verteporfin is a photosensitive dye and care must be taken to avoid tissue extravasation during infusion and exposure to bright light soon after treatment. Advice in the study was to avoid light for 48 hours but some photosensitive reactions were observed in treated people at 3 to 5 days. The treatment was well tolerated but was more likely than the control intervention to cause a transient decrease in vision (18% treated v 12% control); injection site reactions (13% treated v 3% control); photosensitivity (3% treated v 0% control); and infusion related low back pain (2% v 0% control).

Comment: The study found no common short term adverse effects of treatment. However, the possibility of rare but severe adverse events remains. The RCT is ongoing (24 months' follow up has been published subsequent to our search date) and will be included in future issues of *Clinical Evidence*.[44] A 24 month multicentre double blind RCT of photodynamic treatment versus verteporfin, in a wider range of people with exudative AMD, is underway.

GLOSSARY

Age related maculopathy Degenerative disease of the macula (centre of the retina) classified as early (marked by drusen and pigmentary change, and usually associated with normal vision) and late, when it is known as age related macular degeneration.

Choroidal neovascularisation New vessels in the choroid, classified on the basis of fluorescein angiography: in terms of its position in relation to the fovea — extrafoveal, juxtafoveal, or subfoveal; in terms of its appearance — classic (well defined) or occult (poorly defined); and in terms of its borders — well demarcated or poorly demarcated.

Drusen Small, yellow, bright objects, often near the macula, seen by ophthalmoscopy. They are usually located in or near the basement membrane of the retinal pigment layer. They are present in many older people with normal vision, but a higher number of large drusen indicate higher risk of subsequent loss of acuity from age related macular degeneration.

Legal blindness Visual acuity less than 20/200.

Photodynamic treatment A two step procedure of intravenous infusion of a photosensitive dye followed by application of a non-thermal laser that activates the dye. The treatment aims to cause selective closure of the choroidal new vessels.

Submacular surgery Removal of haemorrhage and/or choroidal neovascularisation after vitrectomy.

Verteporfin A photosensitive dye used in photodynamic treatment.

REFERENCES

1. Bressler SB, Bressler NM, Fine SL. Age-related macular degeneration. Surv Ophthalmol 1988;32: 375–413.

2. Klein R, Klein BEK, Linton KLP. Prevalence of age-related maculopathy: the Beaver Dam Eye Study. Ophthalmology 1992;99:933–943.

3. Vingerling JR, Dielemans I, Hofman A, et al. The prevalence of age-related maculopathy in the Rotterdam study. Ophthalmology 1995;102:205–210.

4. Mitchell P, Smith W, Attebo K, et al. Prevalence of age-related maculopathy in Australia. The Blue Mountains Eye Study. Ophthalmology 1995;102: 1450–1640.

5. Macular Photocoagulation Study Group. Risk factors for choroidal neovascularisation in the second eye of patients with juxtafoveal or subfoveal choroidal neovascularisation secondary to age-related macular degeneration. Arch Ophthalmol 1997;115:741–747.

6. Pieramici DJ, Bressler SB. Age-related macular degeneration and risk factors for the development of choroidal neovascularization in the fellow eye. Curr Opin Ophthalmol 1998;9:38–46.

7. Maguire P, Vine AK. Geographic atrophy of the retinal pigment epithelium. Am J Ophthalmol 1986;102:621–625.

8. Sarks JP, Sarks SH, Killingsworth M. Evolution of geographic atrophy of the retinal pigment epithelium. Eye 1988;2:552–577.

9. Holz FG, Wolfensberger TJ, Piguet B, et al. Bilateral macular drusen in age-related macular degeneration: prognosis and risk factors. Ophthalmology 1994;101:1522–1528.

10. Klein R, Klein BEK, Jensen SC, Meuer SM. The five-year incidence and progression of age-related maculopathy. The Beaver Dam Eye study. Ophthalmology 1997;104:7–21.

11. Macular Photocoagulation Study Group. Argon laser photocoagulation for neovascular maculopathy: Five-year results from randomized clinical trials. Arch Ophthalmol 1991;109:1109–1114.

12. Macular Photocoagulation Study Group. Laser photocoagulation of subfoveal neovascular lesions of age-related macular degeneration: updated findings from two clinical trials. Arch Ophthalmol 1993;111:1200–1209.

13. Macular Photocoagulation Study Group. Argon laser photocoagulation for neovascular maculopathy. Three-year results from randomized clinical trials. Arch Ophthalmol 1986;104:694–701.

14. Macular Photocoagulation Study Group. Laser photocoagulation for juxtafoveal choroidal neovascularisation. Five-year results from randomized clinical trials. Arch Ophthalmol 1994; 112:500–509.

15. Olk, RJ, Friberg TR, Stickney KL, et al. Therapeutic benefits of infrared (810 nm) diode laser macular grid photocoagulation in prophylactic treatment of nonexudative age-related macular degeneration: two-year results of a randomized pilot study. Ophthalmology 1999;106:2082–2090.

16. Ho CA, Maguire MG, Yoken J, et al. The Choroidal Neovascularization Prevention Trial research group. Laser-induced drusen reduction improves visual function at 1 year. Ophthalmology 1999;106: 1367–1373.

17. The Choroidal Neovascularization Prevention Trial research group. Laser treatment in eyes with large drusen. Short-term effects seen in a pilot randomized clinical trial. Ophthalmology 1998; 105:11–23.

18. Little HL, Showman JM, Brown BW. A pilot randomized controlled study on the effect of laser photocoagulation of confluent soft macular drusen. Ophthalmology 1997;104:623–631.

19. Frennesson C, Nilsson SEG. Prophylactic laser treatment in early age-related maculopathy reduced the incidence of exudative complications. Br J Ophthalmol 1998;82:1169–1174.

20. Figueroa MS, Regueras A, Bertrand J, Aparicio MJ, Manrique MG. Laser photocoagulation for macular soft drusen. Updated results. Retina 1997;17: 378–384.

21. Lanchoney DM, Maguire MG, Fine SL. A model of the incidence and consequences of choroidal neovascularisation secondary to age-related macular degeneration. Comparative effects of current treatment and potential prophylaxis on visual outcomes in high-risk patients. Arch Ophthalmol 1998;116:1045–1052.

22. Owens SL, Guymer RH, Gross-Jendroska M, Bird AC. Fluorescein angiographic abnormalities after prophylactic macular photocoagulation for high-risk age-related maculopathy. Am J Ophthalmol 1999;127:681–687.

23. Macular Photocoagulation Study Group. Occult choroidal neovascularization. Influence on visual outcome in patients with age-related macular degeneration. Arch Ophthalmol 1996;114:400–412.

24. Macular Photocoagulation Study Group. Persistent and recurrent neovascularization after laser photocoagulation for subfoveal choroidal

neovascularization of age-related macular degeneration. *Arch Ophthalmol* 1994;112:489–499.

25. Macular Photocoagulation Study Group. Visual outcome after laser photocoagulation for subfoveal choroidal neovascularization secondary to age-related macular degeneration. The influence of initial lesion size and initial visual acuity. *Arch Ophthalmol* 1994;112:480–488.

26. Coscas G, Soubrane G, Ramahefasolo C, et al. Perifoveal laser treatment for subfoveal choroidal new vessels in age-related macular degeneration. Results of a randomized clinical trial. *Arch Ophthalmol* 1991;109:1258–1265.

27. Bressler NM, Maguire MG, Murphy PL, et al. Macular scatter ("grid") laser treatment of poorly demarcated subfoveal choroidal neovascularisation in age-related macular degeneration. Results of a randomised pilot trial. *Arch Ophthalmol* 1996;114:1456–1464.

28. Arnold J, Algan M, Soubrane G, et al. Indirect scatter laser photocoagulation to subfoveal choroidal neovascularization in age-related macular degeneration. *Graefes Arch Clin Exp Ophthalmol* 1997;235:208–216.

29. Barondes MJ, Pagliarini S, Chisholm IH, et al. Controlled trial of laser photocoagulation of pigment epithelial detachments in the elderly: 4 year review. *Br J Ophthalmol* 1992;76:5–7.

30. Macular Photocoagulation Study Group. Evaluation of argon green vs krypton red laser for photocoagulation of subfoveal choroidal neovascularisation in the Macular Photocoagulation Study. *Arch Ophthalmol* 1994; 112:1176–1184.

31. Willan AR, Cruess AF, Ballantyne M. Argon green vs krypton red laser photocoagulation for extrafoveal choroidal neovascularization secondary to age-related macular degeneration: 3-year results of a multicentre randomized trial. *Can J Ophthalmol* 1996;31:11–17.

32. The Radiation Therapy for Age-related Macular Degeneration (RAD) study group. A prospective randomized double-masked trial on radiation therapy for neovascular age-related macular degeneration (RAD) study. *Ophthalmology* 1999; 106:2239–2247.

33. Bergink GJ, Hoyng CB, Van der Maazen RW, et al. A randomized controlled clinical trial on the efficacy of radiation therapy in the control of subfoveal choroidal neovascularization in age-related macular degeneration: radiation versus observation. *Graefes Arch Clin Exp Ophthalmol* 1998;236:321–325.

34. Char DH, Irvine AI, Posner MD, et al. Randomized trial of radiation for age-related macular

degeneration. *Am J Ophthalmol* 1999;127:574–578.

35. Hart PM, Chakravarthy U, MacKenzie G, et al. Teletherapy for subfoveal choroidal neovascularisation of age-related macular degeneration: results of follow up in a non-randomised study. *Br J Ophthalmol* 1996;80: 1046–1050.

36. Finger PT, Berson A, Sherr D, et al. Radiation therapy for subretinal neovascularization. *Ophthalmology* 1996;103:878–889.

37. Ciulla TA, Danis RP, Harris A. Age-related macular degeneration: a review of experimental treatments. *Surv Ophthalmol* 1998;43:134–146.

38. Mauget-Faysse M, Chiquet C, Milea D, et al. Long term results of radiotherapy for subfoveal choroidal neovascularisation in age-related macular degeneration. *Br J Ophthalmol* 1999;83: 923–928.

39. Spaide RF, Leys A, Herrmann-Delemazure B, et al. Radiation-associated choroidal neovasculopathy. *Ophthalmology* 1999;106:2254–2260.

40. Lewis H, Van der Brug MS. Tissue plasminogen activator-assisted surgical excision of subfoveal choroidal neovascularization in age-related macular degeneration: a randomized, double-masked trial. *Ophthalmology* 1997;104:1847–1851.

41. Thomas MA, Dickinson JD, Melberg NS, et al. Visual results after surgical removal of subfoveal choroidal neovascular membranes. *Ophthalmology* 1994;101:1384–1396.

42. Pharmacological Therapy for Macular Degeneration study group. Interferon alfa-2a is ineffective for patients with choroidal neovascularization secondary to age-related macular degeneration: results of a prospective randomized placebo-controlled clinical trial. *Arch Ophthalmol* 1997;115:865–872.

43. Wormald R, Evans J, Smeeth L. Photodynamic therapy for neovascular age-related macular degeneration. In: The Cochrane Library, Issue 4, 2000. Oxford: Update Software. Search date December 1999; primary sources Cochrane Controlled Trials Register; Cochrane Eyes and Vision Group Register; Medline; Embase; Science Citation Index; experts and hand searched references.

44. Treatment of Age-related Macular Degeneration with Photodynamic Therapy (TAP) study group. Photodynamic therapy of subfoveal choroidal neovascularization in age-related macular degeneration with verteporfin: two-year results of 2 randomized clinical trials–TAP Report 2. *Arch Ophthalmol* 2001;119:198–207.

Jennifer Arnold
Consultant Ophthalmologist, Aberdeen Royal Hospitals NHS Trust, Aberdeen, UK

Shirley Sarks
Honorary Senior Research Associate
Prince of Wales Medical Research Institute, Randwick, NSW, Australia

Competing interests: JA was a clinical investigator in the study of photodynamic treatment using verteporfin, funded by CIBA Vision/QLT and has been supported by CIBA Vision for attendance at conferences and symposia.

TABLE 1 Laser photocoagulation of choroidal neovascularisation (CNV) versus observation in exudative AMD: results of Macular Photocoagulation Study Group RCTs (see text, p 428).

Site of CNV (type of laser)	Number of eyes	Severe visual loss (6 or more lines)	Vision level treated v control	Rate of recurrence in treated eyes
Extrafoveal CNV (argon blue-green)[11,13]	236	RR 1.5 at 6 months to 5 years; P = 0.001	≥20/40 at 3 years 33% v 22%	54% at 5 years
Juxtafoveal CNV (krypton red)[14,23]	496	RR 1.2 at 6 months to 5 years; P = 0.04	≥20/40 at 3 years 13% v 7%	76% at 5 years (classic CNV only)
New subfoveal CNV (argon green or krypton)[12,24,25,27]	373	20% treated v 37% control at 2 years; P < 0.01	>20/200 at 4 years 12% v 11%	44% at 3 years
Recurrent subfoveal CNV (argon green or krypton)[12,24,27]	206	9% treated v 28% control at 2 years; P = 0.03	>20/200 at 3 years 25% v 12%	39% at 3 years

CNV, choroidal neovascularisation.

Eye disorders

Search date May 2000

Christine Chung and Elisabeth Cohen

INTERVENTIONS

Beneficial

Topical antibiotics (fluoroquinolones, polymyxin combinations, aminoglycosides, fusidic acid) 437,438

Trade off between benefits and harms

Topical chloramphenicol. 438

To be covered in future issues of *Clinical Evidence*

Propamidine isethionate ("Golden Eye")

Systemic antibiotics

Gonococcal conjunctivitis/ gonococcal ophthalmia neonatorum

Conjunctivitis in contact lens wearers

Key Messages

- Bacterial conjunctivitis is usually self limiting.

- In people with suspected bacterial conjunctivitis, one systematic review found limited evidence from one RCT that topical norfloxacin was associated with a significantly higher rate of clinical and microbiological improvement than placebo. Comparative RCTs found no significant difference between different topical antibiotics in rates of clinical or microbiological cure.

- In people with bacterial conjunctivitis proved on culture, RCTs found faster clinical and microbiological improvement with topical ciprofloxacin and ofloxacin than with placebo. Ofloxacin was associated with reduced relapse rate compared with placebo. Comparative RCTs found no significant difference between topical lomefloxacin and ciprofloxacin in clinical and microbiological cure rates. One RCT found fusidic acid to be superior to chloramphenicol.

- Chloramphenicol is the only topical antibiotic possibly associated with serious systemic adverse effects (aplastic anaemia), but we found no good evidence about the magnitude of this risk for chloramphenicol versus other topical antibiotics.

- We found no trials that examined the potential growth of resistant organisms from the use of antibiotics in bacterial conjunctivitis.

DEFINITION Conjunctivitis is any inflammation of the conjunctiva, generally characterised by irritation, itching, foreign body sensation, and tearing or discharge. Bacterial conjunctivitis may usually be distinguished from other types of conjunctivitis by the presence of a yellow–white mucopurulent discharge. There is also usually a papillary reaction (small bumps with fibrovascular cores on the palpebral conjunctiva, appearing grossly as a fine velvety surface). Bacterial conjunctivitis is usually unilateral, as opposed to viral conjunctivitis which often starts in one eye and spreads to the other. This review covers only non-gonococcal bacterial conjunctivitis.

INCIDENCE/ PREVALENCE We found no good evidence on the incidence or prevalence of bacterial conjunctivitis.

AETIOLOGY/ RISK FACTORS Conjunctivitis may be infectious (caused by bacteria or viruses) or allergic. In adults, bacterial conjunctivitis is less common than viral conjunctivitis, although estimates vary widely (viral conjunctivitis has been reported to account for 8–75% of acute conjunctivitis).[1–3] Staphylococcus species are the most common bacterial pathogens, followed by *Streptococcus pneumoniae* and *Haemophilus influenzae*.[4,5] In children, bacterial conjunctivitis is more common than viral, and is mainly caused by *H influenzae, S pneumoniae*, and *Moraxella catarrhalis*.[6,7]

PROGNOSIS Most bacterial conjunctivitis is self limiting. One systematic review of RCTs (updated in April 1999) reported clinical cure or significant improvement on placebo within 2–5 days in 64% of people (99% CI 54% to 73%).[8] Some organisms cause corneal or systemic complications, or both; otitis may develop in 25% of children with *H influenzae* conjunctivitis,[9] and systemic meningitis may complicate primary meningococcal conjunctivitis in 18% of people.[10] Conjunctivitis in children is more likely to be bacterial than viral, warranting heightened awareness of possible systemic complications.

AIMS To achieve rapid cure of inflammation, and to prevent complications, with minimum adverse effects of treatment.

OUTCOMES Time to cure or improvement. **Clinical signs/symptoms:** hyperaemia, discharge, papillae, follicles, chemosis, itching, pain, photophobia. Most studies used a numbered scale to grade signs and symptoms. Some studies also included evaluation by investigators and patients regarding success of treatment. **Culture results:** proxy outcomes usually expressed as the number of colonies, sometimes with reference to a threshold level. Results were often classified into categories such as eradication, reduction, persistence, and proliferation.

METHODS *Clinical Evidence* search and appraisal May 2000. All identified systematic reviews and subsequent RCTs were reviewed.

QUESTION **What are the effects of empirical treatment with topical antibiotics in adults and children with suspected bacterial conjunctivitis?**

One systematic review found limited evidence from one RCT that topical norfloxacin was associated with a significantly higher rate of clinical and

microbiological improvement than placebo. Comparative RCTs found no significant difference between different topical antibiotics in rates of clinical or microbiological cure.

Benefits: **Versus placebo:** We found one systematic review (updated in 1999), which identified one RCT comparing topical norfloxacin (143 adults) versus placebo (141 adults); 50% of participants were culture positive.[8] The review found significantly higher rates of clinical and microbiological cure or improvement at 5 days with norfloxacin (88%, 95% CI 81% to 93% v 72%, 95% CI 63% to 79%; P < 0.01). **Versus each other:** We found no systematic review. We found 19 comparative RCTs in adults and children. These found no significant difference between different topical antibiotics in rates of clinical or microbiological cure (see table on website; www.clinicalevidence.org). Six of the RCTs (evaluating lomefloxacin, fusidic acid, rifamycin, chloramphenicol, and tobramycin) included grading by patients of effectiveness and tolerability. No significant differences were found.[11–16]

Harms: The placebo controlled RCT reported minor adverse events in 4.2% of people using norfloxacin and 7.1% using placebo (no statistical analysis available).[5] Placebo contained higher proportions of benzalkonium chloride (0.01% v 0.0025% in the norfloxacin solution). One non-systematic review described complications of topical antibiotics.[17] These included four reported cases of idiosyncratic aplastic anaemia associated with topical chloramphenicol and three cases of Stevens–Johnson syndrome associated with topical sulphonamides, but the review gave no figures on the number of people using these drugs.

Comment: The placebo controlled RCT did not address the effect of using topical antibiotics on antibiotic resistance, which would be of interest given the self limiting nature of the disease.[5] None of the trials specified their methods for selecting participants. The findings may not be generaliseable to primary care populations. Most trials included children as well as adults, and the ratio of children to adults was usually not specified. The comparisons of lomefloxacin versus chloramphenicol and fusidic acid, and the comparison of norfloxacin versus fusidic acid, were single blind. Lomefloxacin and fusidic acid are not available in the USA, and chloramphenicol is rarely used in the USA because of reports of idiosyncratic aplastic anaemia.

QUESTION **What are the effects of topical antibiotics in adults and children with culture positive conjunctivitis?**

RCTs in people with bacterial conjunctivitis proved on culture found faster clinical and microbiological improvement with ciprofloxacin, ofloxacin, or polymyxin–bacitracin than with placebo. Ofloxacin was associated with reduced relapse rates. Comparative RCTs found no significant difference between tobramycin and ciprofloxacin or between trimethoprim–polymyxin B, and sulfacetamide in clinical and microbiological cure rates. One RCT found greater clinical efficacy and less microbiological resistance with fusidic acid than chloramphenicol.

Benefits: **Versus placebo:** We found one systematic review (updated in 1999), which identified three placebo controlled RCTs evaluating polymyxin–bacitracin, ciprofloxacin, and ofloxacin in bacterial conjunctivitis proved by culture. The review identified no trials of gentamicin that included only culture proved conjunctivitis.[8] One RCT was in children (n = 84).[18] It found that in culture proved *H influenzae* and *S pneumoniae* bacterial conjunctivitis, there was a higher clinical cure rate at days 3–5 with polymyxin–bacitracin than placebo, although by days 8–10 the difference was not significant (62% v 28% at days 3–5, P < 0.02; 91% v 72% at days 8–10, P > 0.05). The microbiological cure rate was significantly higher with antibiotics both at days 3–5 and days 8–10. When systemic antibiotics were given for concurrent problems, there was no significant difference between groups, but the numbers were too small to rule out a clinically important effect (see table on website; http://www.clinicalevidence.org). Two other trials identified in the review did not specify the age of participants. One did not evaluate clinical outcome but found significantly greater microbiological improvement at day 3 in people treated with ciprofloxacin (n = 177).[19] One RCT was published as an abstract only; it found significantly greater clinical and microbiological improvement at day 2 in people treated with ofloxacin (n = 132, 64% v 22% improved at day 2, P < 0.001). It also found a lower relapse rate in people treated with ofloxacin 2 days after treatment stopped.[20] A fourth was published in Japanese and was not reviewed.[21] **Versus each other:** We found no systematic review which met our quality criteria. We found one RCT that did not specify the age of participants, three RCTs in children only, and one small RCT in children and adults. The RCT that did not specify age found no significant difference in microbiological eradication or improvement between ciprofloxacin (n = 140) and tobramycin (n = 111); eradication or improvement occurred in 94.3% v 91.9% (P > 0.5, no CI available).[19] Clinical cure was not evaluated. Of the three RCTs in children, two found no significant difference in clinical or overall microbiological efficacy between ciprofloxacin and tobramycin (n = 70 v 71, eradication 90% v 84%, P = 0.29; cure 87% v 90%, P = 0.6) or between trimethoprim–polymyxin B, gentamicin, and sulfacetamide (n = 53 v 57 v 46, eradication 83% v 68% v 72%, P > 0.1; cure 84% v 88% v 89%, P > 0.1).[22–23] The third (non-blinded) RCT found more clinical efficacy and less microbiological resistance with fusidic acid than chloramphenicol (n = 114 v 25, cure 85% v 48%, P < 0.0001; resistance 16% v 55%, statistical analysis not provided).[24] The RCT in children and adults (ratio not specified) found no difference between lomefloxacin and ofloxacin (n = 40, resolution of symptoms and signs at day 7: 88% v 75%, P < 0.08).[25]

Harms: Of the 116 children initially enrolled in the first RCT described above, one was excluded because of possible allergic reaction to the ointment; the other exclusions were unrelated to adverse effects[18] In RCTs that included people with both culture proved and suspected bacterial conjunctivitis, minor adverse events were reported with antibiotics: burning, bitter taste, pruritus, or punctate epithelial erosions (35% with tobramycin v 20% with ciprofloxacin; no statistical detail available from abstract),[26] bad taste (20% with norfloxacin v 6% with fusidic acid),[27] stinging (50% with norfloxacin v 37% with fusidic acid)[27] and burning (33% with gentamicin v 20% with lomefloxacin).[13]

Comment: None of the RCTs addressed the effect on antibiotic resistance of using topical antibiotics in bacterial conjunctivitis, which would be of interest given the self limiting nature of the disease. Furthermore, they did not report on patient oriented outcomes or look at rates of reinfection.

REFERENCES

1. Wishart PK, James C, Wishart MS, Darougar S. Prevalence of acute conjunctivitis caused by chlamydia, adenovirus, and herpes simplex virus in an ophthalmic casualty department. *Br J Ophthalmol* 1984;68:653–655.

2. Fitch CP, Rapoza PA, Owens S, et al. Epidemiology and diagnosis of acute conjunctivitis at an inner-city hospital. *Ophthalmology* 1989;96:1215–1220.

3. Woodland RM, Darougar S, Thaker U, et al. Causes of conjunctivitis and keratoconjunctivitis in Karachi, Pakistan. *Trans R Soc Trop Med Hygiene* 1992;86:317–320.

4. Seal DV, Barrett SP, McGill JI. Aetiology and treatment of acute bacterial infection of the external eye. *Br J Ophthalmol* 1982;66:357–360.

5. Miller IM, Wittreich J, Vogel R, Cook TJ, for the Norfloxacin-Placebo Ocular Study Group. The safety and efficacy of topical norfloxacin compared with placebo in the treatment of acute bacterial conjunctivitis. *Eur J Ophthalmol* 1992;2:58–66.

6. Gigliotti F, Williams WT, Hayden FG, et al. Etiology of acute conjunctivitis in children. *J Pediatr* 1981; 98:531–536.

7. Weiss A, Brinser JH, Nazar-Stewart V. Acute conjunctivitis in childhood. *J Pediatr* 1993;122: 10–14.

8. Sheikh A, Hurwitz B, Cave J. Antibiotics for acute bacterial conjunctivitis. In: The Cochrane Library, Issue 4, 1999. Oxford: Update Software. Updated April 1999, search date September 1998 primary sources Cochrane Controlled Trial Register 1998 issue, Medline 1994 to September 1998, bibliographies of identified trials, Science Citation Index, and personal contacts with investigators and pharmaceutical companies.

9. Bodor FF. Conjunctivitis-otitis media syndrome: more than meets the eye. *Contemp Pediatr* 1989; 6:55–60.

10. Barquet N, Gasser I, Domingo P, et al. Primary meningococcal conjunctivitis: report of 21 patients and review. *Rev Infect Dis* 1990;12:838–847.

11. Kettenmeyer A, Jauch A, Boscher M, et al. A double-blind double-dummy multicenter equivalence study comparing topical lomefloxacin 0.3% twice daily with norfloxacin 0.3% four times daily in the treatment of acute bacterial conjunctivitis. *J Clin Res* 1998;1:75–86.

12. Agius-Fernandez A, Patterson A, Fsadni M, et al. Topical lomefloxacin versus topical chloramphenicol in the treatment of acute bacterial conjunctivitis. *Clin Drug Invest* 1998;15: 263–269.

13. Montero J, Casado A, Perea E, et al. A double-blind double-dummy comparison of topical lomefloxacin 0.3% twice daily with topical gentamicin 0.3% four times daily in the treatment of acute bacterial conjunctivitis. *J Clin Res* 1998; 1:29–39.

14. Adenis JP, Arrata M, Gastaud P, et al. Etude randomisee multicentrique acide fusidique gel ophtalmique et rifamycine collyre dans les conjonctivites aigues. *J Fr Ophtalmol* 1989;12: 317–322.

15. Huerva V, Ascaso FJ, Latre B, et al. Tolerancia y eficacia de la tobramicina topica vs cloranfenicol en el tratamiento de las conjunctivitis bacterianas. *Ciencia Pharmaceutica* 1991;1:221–224.

16. Gallenga PE, Lobefalo L, Colangelo L, et al. Topical lomefloxacin 0.3% twice daily versus tobramycin 0.3% in acute bacterial conjunctivitis: a multicenter double-blind phase III study. *Ophthalmologica* 1999;213:250–257.

17. Stern GA, Killingsworth DW. Complications of topical antimicrobial agents. *Int Ophthalmol Clin* 1989;29:137–142.

18. Gigliotti G, Hendley JO, Morgan J, et al. Efficacy of topical antibiotic therapy in acute conjunctivitis in children. *J Pediatr* 1984;104:623–626.

19. Leibowitz HM. Antibacterial effectiveness of ciprofloxacin 0.3% ophthalmic solution in the treatment of bacterial conjunctivitis. *Am J Ophthalmol* 1991;112:29S–33S.

20. Ofloxacin Study Group III. A placebo-controlled clinical study of the fluoroquinolone ofloxacin in patients with external infection. *Invest Ophthalmol Vis Sci* 1990;31:572.

21. Mitsui Y, Matsuda H, Miyajima T, et al. Therapeutic effects of ofloxacin eye drops (DE-055) on external infection of the eye: multicentral double blind test. *J Rev Clin Ophthalmol* 1986;80:1813–1828.

22. Gross RD, Hoffman RO, Lindsay RN. A comparison of ciprofloxacin and tobramycin in bacterial conjunctivitis is children. *Clin Pediatr* 1997;36: 435–444.

23. Lohr JA, Austin RD, Grossman M, et al. Comparison of three topical antimicrobials for acute bacterial conjunctivitis. *Pediatr Infect Dis J* 1988;7:626–629.

24. Van Bijsterveld OP, el Batawi Y, Sobhi FS, et al. Fusidic acid in infections of the external eye. *Infection* 1987;15:16–19.

25. Tabbara KF, El-Sheik HF, Monowarul Islam SM, Hammouda E. Treatment of acute bacterial conjunctivitis with topical lomefloxacin 0.3% compared to topical ofloxacin 0.3%. *Eur J Ophthalmol* 1999; 9:269–275.

26. Alves MR, Kara JN. Evaluation of the clinical and microbiological efficacy of 0.3% ciprofloxacin drops and 0.3% tobramycin drops in the treatment of acute bacterial conjunctivitis. *Revista Brasiliera de Oftalmol* 1993;52:371–377.

27. Wall AR, Sinclair N, Adenis JP. Comparison of Fucithalmic (fusidic acid viscous eye drops 1%) and Noroxin (norfloxacin ophthalmic solution 0.3%) in the treatment of acute bacterial conjunctivitis. *J Clin Res* 1998;1:316–325.

28. The Trimethoprim-Polymyxin B Sulphate Ophthalmic Ointment Study Group. Trimethoprim-polymyxin B sulphate ophthalmic ointment versus chloramphenicol ophthalmic ointment in the treatment of bacterial conjunctivitis—a review of

four clinical studies. *J Antimicrob Chemother* 1989;23:261–266.

29. Behrens-Baumann W, Quentin CD, Gibson JR, et al. Trimethoprim-polymyxin B sulphate ophthalmic ointment in the treatment of bacterial conjunctivitis: a double-blind study versus chloramphenicol ophthalmic ointment. *Curr Med Res Opin* 1988;11:227–231.

30. van-Rensburg SF, Gibson JR, Harvey SG, Burke CA. Trimethoprim-polymyxin ophthalmic solution versus chloramphenicol ophthalmic solution in the treatment of bacterial conjunctivitis. *Pharmatherapeutica* 1982;3:274–277.

31. Gibson JR. Trimethoprim-polymyxin B ophthalmic solution in the treatment of presumptive bacterial conjunctivitis—a multicentre trial of its efficacy versus neomycin-polymyxin B-gramicidin and chloramphenicol ophthalmic solutions. *J Antimicrob Chemother* 1983;11:217–221.

32. Genee E, Schlechtweg C, Bauerreiss P, Gibson JR. Trimethoprim-polymyxin eye drops versus neomycin-polymyxin-gramicidin eye drops in the treatment of presumptive bacterial conjunctivitis—a double-blind study.

Ophthalmologica 1982;184:92–96.

33. Malminiemi K, Kari O, Latvala M-L, et al. Topical lomefloxacin twice daily compared with fucidic acid in acute bacterial conjunctivitis. *Acta Ophthalmol Scand* 1996;74:280–284.

34. Carr WD. Comparison of Fucithalmic (fusidic acid viscous eye drops 1%) and Chloromycetin Redidrops (chloramphenicol eye drops 0.5%) in the treatment of acute bacterial conjunctivitis. *J Clin Res* 1998;1:403–411.

35. Horven I. Acute conjunctivitis. A comparison of fusidic acid viscous eye drops and chloramphenicol. *Acta Ophthalmol* 1993;71:165–168.

36. Hvidberg J. Fusidic acid in acute conjunctivitis. Single-blind, randomized comparison of fusidic acid and chloramphenicol viscous eye drops. *Acta Ophthalmol* 1987;65:43–47.

37. Uchida Y. Clinical efficacy of topical lomefloxacin (NY-198) in bacterial infections of the external eye. *Folia Ophthalmologica* 1991;42:59–70.

38. References 28 to 37 relate to the table, which appears on the clinical evidence website: www.clinicalevidence.org.

Christine Chung
Cornea Fellow

Elisabeth Cohen
Director

Cornea Service, Wills Eye Hospital
Jefferson Medical College
Philadelphia
USA

Competing interests: None declared.

Glaucoma

Search date November 2000: expanded this issue

Colm O'Brien and Jeremy Diamond

QUESTIONS

INTERVENTIONS

PRIMARY OPEN ANGLE GLAUCOMA

Likely to be beneficial

Topical medical treatment (β blockers, miotics, adrenergic agonists, prostaglandin analogues, carbonic anhydrase inhibitors) 443

Laser trabeculoplasty. 444

Trade off between benefits and harms

Surgical trabeculectomy 444

NORMAL PRESSURE GLAUCOMA

Likely to be beneficial

Lowering intraocular pressure in normal pressure glaucoma . .445

ACUTE ANGLE CLOSURE GLAUCOMA

Unknown effectiveness

Medical treatments of acute angle closure glaucoma* New . . .446

Surgical treatments of acute angle closure glaucoma* New . . .446

To be covered in future issues of Clinical Evidence

Treating ocular hypertension in people without established glaucoma

Early detection of glaucoma (opportunistic case finding, population screening)

* No placebo controlled RCTs but strong consensus that treatments are effective

Key Messages

- RCTs have found that topical medical treatments reduce raised intraocular pressure in people with primary open angle glaucoma, but their protective effect on visual fields is uncertain.

- We found limited evidence suggesting that laser trabeculoplasty and surgical trabeculectomy provide greater protection of visual fields than medical treatment. However, trabeculectomy is associated with morbidity, including cataract formation and loss of visual acuity.

- One RCT has found that reducing intraocular pressure slows progression of visual field loss in normal pressure glaucoma.

- We found no RCTs of pilocarpine versus placebo in acute angle closure glaucoma. One RCT has found that topical medical treatment with intensive versus low dose pilocarpine reduces intraocular pressure after 2 hours. We found no other evidence from RCTs for medical treatments for acute angle closure glaucoma.

- We found no RCTs of surgical or laser iridectomy versus placebo. Two small RCTs found no significant difference with surgical iridectomy versus laser iridotomy in visual acuity or intraocular pressure. Two other small RCTs found no significant difference between different types of laser iridotomy.

DEFINITION	Glaucoma is a group of diseases characterised by progressive optic neuropathy. It is usually bilateral but asymmetric. All forms of glaucoma show optic nerve cupping with pallor, and peripheral visual field loss. In primary open angle glaucoma the level of intraocular pressure is greater than 21 mmHg. In low tension or normal pressure glaucoma the intraocular pressure is less than 22 mmHg. Acute angle closure glaucoma is a rapid and severe rise in intraocular pressure caused by physical obstruction of the anterior chamber drainage angle.
INCIDENCE/ PREVALENCE	Glaucoma occurs in 1–2% of white people aged over 40 years, rising to 5% at 70 years. Primary open angle glaucoma accounts for two thirds and normal pressure glaucoma for about a quarter of those affected.[1,2] In black people, glaucoma is more prevalent, presents earlier with higher pressures, is more difficult to control, and results in more frequent blindness.[1] Glaucoma blindness is responsible for 8% of new blind registrations in the UK.[3]
AETIOLOGY/ RISK FACTORS	The major risk factor for developing primary open angle glaucoma is raised intraocular pressure. Lesser risk factors include family history, myopia, and ethnic origin. Additional risk factors for normal pressure glaucoma include peripheral vascular diseases such as Raynaud's syndrome. Risk factors for angle closure glaucoma include family history, female sex, being long sighted, and cataract.
PROGNOSIS	Advanced field loss is found in 20% of people with glaucoma at diagnosis.[4] As the disease progresses, people with glaucoma have difficulty moving from a bright room to a darker room and judging steps and kerbs. Blindness results from gross loss of visual field or loss of central vision. Once early field defects have appeared, and where the intraocular pressure is greater than 30 mmHg, untreated people may lose the remainder of the visual field in 3 years or less.[5] Progression of visual field loss is often slower in normal pressure glaucoma. Acute angle glaucoma leads to rapid loss of vision, initially from corneal oedema and subsequently from ischaemic optic neuropathy.
AIMS	To prevent progression of visual field loss; to minimise adverse effects from treatment.
OUTCOMES	Visual acuity; visual fields. Optic disc cupping and intraocular pressure are intermediate outcomes.
METHODS	*Clinical Evidence* update search and appraisal November 2000.

QUESTION	What are the effects of treatments for established primary open angle glaucoma?

OPTION	TOPICAL MEDICAL TREATMENT

RCTs have found that topical medical treatment reduces intraocular pressure compared with placebo, but the few trials with long term follow up found no benefit in terms of protection against loss of visual field.

Benefits: We found one systematic review (search date 1991, 16 placebo controlled RCTs, 86 comparative RCTs in people with primary open angle glaucoma).[6] **Intraocular pressure:** Pooled analysis of the 16 placebo controlled trials found significant reduction in mean intraocular pressure of 4.9 mmHg (95% CI 2.5 mmHg to 7.3 mmHg). **Visual field loss:** Long term visual field changes were reported by only three RCTs (302 people), which found no significant benefit of medical treatment versus placebo on visual field loss (pooled OR for any worsening of visual field loss 0.75, 95% CI 0.42 to 1.35).

Harms: Systemic adverse effects of topical treatments are uncommon but may be serious, including exacerbation of chronic obstructive airways disease after use of non-selective topical β blockers. Non-selective topical β blockers can also cause systemic hypotension and reduction in resting heart rate, and are contraindicated in people with cardiac failure.[7]

Comment: We could not identify the types of participants or topical treatments from the systematic review.[6] Four RCTs sponsored by the US National Institutes of Health are underway: the early manifest glaucoma study, the ocular hypertension treatment study, the collaborative initial glaucoma treatment study, and the advanced glaucoma intervention study.

OPTION   LASER TRABECULOPLASTY

One RCT found greater long term improvement in intraocular pressure and visual fields with laser trabeculoplasty plus medical treatment than with medical treatment alone.

Benefits: We found no systematic review but found one RCT (203 people selected from 271 with newly diagnosed primary open angle glaucoma), which compared initial laser trabeculoplasty followed by medical treatment versus medical treatment alone.[8] After a mean follow up of 7 years, those treated initially with laser surgery had a 1.2 mmHg greater reduction in intraocular pressure (P = 0.001), a 0.6 dB greater improvement in visual field (P < 0.001), and significantly less deterioration in optic disc appearance (P = 0.005) compared with those given only medical treatment.

Harms: Adverse effects of laser trabeculoplasty are mild and include a transient rise in intraocular pressure (> 5 mmHg in 91 of 271 participants) and formation of peripheral anterior synechiae (in 93 of 271 participants).[8]

Comment: The RCT was a multicentre trial with multiple observers.[8] It does not state whether the observers were blind to the intervention.

OPTION   SURGICAL TRABECULECTOMY

Two RCTs have found that early surgical trabeculectomy versus medical treatment reduces the loss of visual field. Surgical drainage was associated with a reduction in central visual activity. One RCT found that initial surgical trabeculectomy followed by laser trabeculoplasty was followed by greater benefit than initial laser trabeculoplasty followed by surgical trabeculectomy, but the response depended on ethnic origin.

Benefits: We found no systematic review. **Versus medical treatment:** We found two RCTs.[9,10] One RCT (116 people with newly diagnosed primary open angle glaucoma) compared trabeculectomy (followed by medical treatment when indicated) versus medical treatment (followed by trabeculectomy when medical treatment failed).[9] It found that after a mean of 4.6 years there was no significant difference in visual acuity between the groups, but the medical treatment group had significantly greater loss of visual field. The second RCT (186 people with glaucoma) found that after 5 years there was major deterioration in visual fields in people on medical and laser treatment but not in those receiving early trabeculectomy surgery.[10] There was no significant difference in visual acuity between the three groups. **Versus initial laser trabeculoplasty:** One RCT (776 eyes with advanced glaucoma; 451 African–American, 325 white) compared surgical trabeculectomy versus laser trabeculoplasty as initial treatment. Initial trabeculectomy was followed by laser trabeculoplasty and repeat trabeculectomy as required; initial laser trabeculoplasty was followed by trabeculectomy as required. Initial surgical trabeculectomy was associated with the greatest reduction in intraocular pressure. The response to treatment differed according to ethnic origin. In black people, vision (both field and acuity) was best preserved in the group receiving initial laser trabeculoplasty, and this benefit continued for 7 years. In white patients, the greater protection of visual fields switched after 1 year of follow up to the group receiving initial surgical trabeculectomy.[11]

Harms: Surgical trabeculectomy is associated with a reduction in central vision. In one study, 83% of participants lost two lines of Snellen visual acuity.[12]

Comment: It was not possible to extract numerical data from either report.

QUESTION What are the effects of lowering intraocular pressure in people with normal pressure glaucoma?

One RCT has found that reducing intraocular pressure slows progression of visual field loss in normal pressure glaucoma.

Benefits: We found no systematic review. We found one RCT (144 eyes in 140 people with normal pressure glaucoma), which compared a treatment to reduce pressure by 30% (with drugs or surgical drainage, or both, 61 eyes) versus no treatment (79 eyes).[13] Progression of visual field loss was defined in terms of deepening of an existing scotoma, a new or expanded "threat to fixation," or a fresh scotoma in a previously normal part of the visual field. Optic disc changes were photographed and independently assessed by two ophthalmologists. Progression occurred in seven (12%) of the treated eyes and 28 (35%) of the control eyes ($P < 0.0001$). Mean time from baseline to progression was 2688 days for the treated group and 1695 days for the control group.[13]

Harms: There was a significantly higher rate of cataract formation in the treated group than in the control group (34 cataracts reported, 23

[38%] in the treatment group and 11 [14%] in the control group, P = 0.001); the excess risk was confined to those treated surgically (P = 0.0001).

Comment: A companion paper[14] to the RCT[13] suggests that the favourable effect of pressure lowering over no treatment is evident only when the cataract inducing effect of drainage surgery is removed. Not all cases of normal pressure glaucoma progress when untreated (40% at 5 years).[14]

| QUESTION | What are the effects of treatment for acute angle closure glaucoma   New |

| OPTION | MEDICAL TREATMENTS |

We found no RCTs of pilocarpine versus placebo in acute angle closure glaucoma. One RCT has found that topical medical treatment with intensive versus low dose pilocarpine reduces intraocular pressure after 2 hours. We found no RCTs about other medical treatments of acute angle closure glaucoma.

Benefits: **Pilocarpine versus placebo:** We found no RCTs. RCTs of pilocarpine versus placebo alone would be considered unethical. **Low dose pilocarpine versus intensive pilocarpine:** We found no systematic review but found one RCT comparing initial treatment of angle closure glaucoma with low dose pilocarpine versus intensive pilocarpine or ocular inserts (depo-pilocarpine) in people who were also treated with intravenous acetazolamide.[15] There was no significant difference between groups in the intraocular pressures after 2 hours.

Harms: We found no RCTs that reported harms. Acute glaucoma may recur if treatment is discontinued. Aqueous suppressants are usually not tolerated in the long term.

Comment: Intensive pilocarpine involved applying drops to the eye every 5 minutes for 1 hour or more. Low dose and depo-pilocarpine are easier to administer. There is a strong consensus that medical treatments are effective in acute angle closure glaucoma, but we found no good evidence from RCTs.

| OPTION | SURGICAL IRIDECTOMY AND LASER IRIDOTOMY   New |

Two small RCTs found no significant difference with surgical iridectomy versus laser iridotomy in visual acuity or intraocular pressure. Two other small RCTs found no significant difference between different types of laser iridotomy.

Benefits: **Surgical or laser procedure versus placebo:** We found no RCTs. **Surgical peripheral iridectomy versus Nd:YAG laser iridotomy:** We found no systematic review but found two RCTs.[16,17] The first RCT (48 people presenting consecutively with uniocular acute angle closure glaucoma over a 2 year period) compared peripheral iridectomy versus Nd:YAG laser iridotomy. It found that, after 3 years, there was no significant difference in visual acuity (0.30 logMAR units for peripheral iridectomy eyes v 0.57 for laser iridotomy eyes), or in intraocular pressure (intraocular pressure under 21 mmHg: 15/21 [70%] with peripheral iridectomy eyes v 19/27 [72%] with laser iridotomy eyes).[16] The second RCT (30 people in Germany) found no differences between the treatments in visual acuity or in intraocular pressure after 1 year. The only significant difference was improved patient acceptability in favour of laser treatment. **Laser iridotomy using Nd:YAG and argon lasers:** We found two RCTs.[18,19] The first RCT (43 people with bilateral chronic pupillary block glaucoma randomly assigned one eye to argon and one eye to Nd:YAG laser iridotomy) found that, after 20–42 months, more iridotomies closed after argon laser treatment than after Nd:YAG treatment (9 eyes [21%] v 0 eyes [0%]). A small number of eyes developed chronic glaucoma requiring surgical intervention (trabeculectomy), but the difference between groups was not significant.[18] The second RCT (38 people having bilateral laser iridotomy with Nd:YAG laser for right eyes and argon laser for left eyes)[19] found that, after a minimum of 8 months, visual acuity, post operative intraocular pressure, corneal change, and pigment dispersion were similar between groups.

Harms: Surgical iridotomy involves opening the eye with risk of serious complications, including intraocular infection or haemorrhage. We found no published evidence quantifying these risks. Nd:YAG laser iridotomy is associated with haemorrhage from the iris, pressure spikes, and corneal oedema.[20] Nd:YAG and argon laser iridotomy can produce focal, non-progressive lens opacity.[21] In one RCT, iris haemorrhage was more common with the Nd:YAG laser, but pupil distortion, iritis, and late blockage were more common with the argon laser.[19]

Comment: Management of acute angle closure glaucoma is aimed at restoring flow of aqueous humour to the anterior chamber angle and adjacent trabecular meshwork. Surgical iridectomy involves opening the eye at the corneal limbus and removing a triangle of tissue from the base of the iris. Laser iridotomy involves making a hole in the base of the iris (without opening the eye) using either an argon or Nd:YAG laser. In one of the RCTs, the mean number of burns required to penetrate the iris was six with the Nd:YAG and 73 with the argon laser.[19]

REFERENCES

1. Sommer A, Tielsch JM, Katz J, et al. Relationship between intraocular pressure and primary open angle glaucoma among white and black Americans. *Arch Ophthalmol* 1991;109:1090–1095.

2. Coffey M, Reidy A, Wormald R, Xian WX, Wright L, Courtney P. The prevalence of glaucoma in the west of Ireland. *Br J Ophthalmol* 1993;77:17–21.

3. Government Statistical Service. *Causes of blindness and partial sight amongst adults.* London: HMSO, 1988.

4. Sheldrick JH, Ng C, Austin DJ, Rosenthal AR. An analysis of referral routes and diagnostic accuracy in cases of suspected glaucoma. *Ophthal Epidemiol* 1994;1:31–38.

5. Jay JL, Murdoch JR. The rates of visual field loss in untreated primary open angle glaucoma. *Br J Ophthalmol* 1993;77:176–178.

6. Rossetti L, Marchetti I, Orzalesi N, Scorpiglione N, Torri V, Liberati A. Randomised clinical trials on medical treatment of glaucoma: are they appropriate to guide clinical practice? *Arch Ophthalmol* 1993;111:96–103. Search date 1991; primary source Medline.

7. Diamond JP. Systemic adverse effects of topical ophthalmic agents: implications for older patients. *Drugs Aging* 1997;11:352–360.

8. Glaucoma Laser Trial Group. The glaucoma laser trial (GLT) and glaucoma laser trial follow-up study: results. *Am J Ophthalmol* 1995;120:718–731.

9. Jay JL, Allan D. The benefit of early trabeculectomy versus conventional management in primary open angle glaucoma relative to severity of disease. *Eye* 1989;3:528–535.

10. Migdal C, Gregory W, Hitchins R, Kolker AE. Long-term functional outcome after early surgery compared with laser and medicine in open angle glaucoma. *Ophthalmology* 1994;101:1651–1657.

11. The Advanced Glaucoma Intervention Study (AGIS): 4. Comparison of treatment outcomes within race. Seven year results. *Ophthalmology* 1998;105:1146–1164.

12. Costas UP, Smith M, Spaeth GL, Gondham S, Markovitz B. Loss of vision after trabeculectomy. *Ophthalmology* 1993;100:599–612.

13. Anonymous. Comparison of glaucomatous progression between untreated patients with normal-tension glaucoma and patients with therapeutically reduced intraocular pressure. *Am J Ophthalmol* 1998;126:487–497.

14. Anonymous. The effectiveness of intraocular pressure reduction in the treatment of normal-tension glaucoma. *Am J Ophthalmol* 1998;126: 498–505.

15. Edwards RS. A comparative study of Ocusert Pilo 40, intensive pilocarpine and low-dose pilocarpine in the initial treatment of primary acute angle-closure glaucoma. *Curr Med Res Opin* 1997;13: 501–509.

16. Fleck BW, Wright E, Fairley EA. A randomised prospective comparison of operative peripheral iridectomy and Nd:YAG laser iridotomy treatment

of acute angle closure glaucoma: 3 year visual acuity and intraocular pressure control outcome. *Br J Ophthalmol* 1997;81:884–888.

17. Schwenn O, Sell F, Pfeiffer N, Grehn F. Prophylactic Nd:YAG-laser iridotomy versus surgical iridectomy: a randomized, prospective study. *Ger J Ophthalmol* 1995;4:374–379.

18. Del Priore LV, Robin AL, Pollack IP. Neodymium: YAG and argon laser iridotomy. Long-term follow-up in a prospective, randomized clinical trial. *Ophthalmology* 1988;95:1207–1211.

19. Moster MR, Schwartz LW, Spaeeth GL, Wilson RP, McAllister JA, Poryzees EM. Laser iridotomy. A controlled study comparing argon and neodymium: YAG. *Ophthalmology* 1986;93:20–24.

20. Fleck BW, Dhillon B, Khanna V, Fairley E, McGlynn C. A randomised, prospective comparison of Nd:YAG laser iridotomy and operative peripheral iridectomy in fellow eyes. *Eye* 1991;5:315–321.

21. Pollack IP, Robin AL, Dragon DM, et al. Use of neodymium:YAG laser to create iridotomies in monkeys and humans. *Trans Am Ophthalmol Soc* 1984;82:307–328.

Colm O'Brien
Consultant Ophthalmic Surgeon
Mater Hospital
Dublin
Republic of Ireland

Jeremy Diamond
Consultant Ophthalmic Surgeon
Bristol Eye Hospital
Bristol
UK

Competing interests: None declared.

Search date July 200: new for this issue

Nigel Barker

QUESTIONS

INTERVENTIONS

Key Messages

Treating epithelial disease

- We found no good evidence of any differences between topical antiviral agents.
- Two small RCTs found conflicting evidence for the role of debridement.
- RCTs have found that topical antiviral agents plus interferon are better than antiviral agents alone.

Treating stromal keratitits

- One RCT has found that topical corticosteroid reduces the progression and shortens the duration of stromal keratitis.
- We found no evidence that oral aciclovir is beneficial in stromal keratitis.
- One large RCT has found that long term oral aciclovir is effective in preventing recurrence of ocular herpes in people with at least one previous episode of epithelial or stromal keratitis.

Preventing ocular herpes simplex

- One RCT found no evidence that short term prophylaxis with oral aciclovir plus topical trifluorothymidine prevented stromal keratitis or iritis in people with epithelial keratitis.

© *Clinical Evidence* 2001;5:449–458.

Preventing ocular herpes simplex in people with corneal grafts

- One small RCT found limited evidence that prophylactic use of oral aciclovir reduced recurrences and improved graft survival after corneal transplantation performed for herpes simplex virus (HSV) infection.

DEFINITION	Ocular herpes simplex is usually caused by herpes simplex virus (HSV) type 1 (HSV-1) but occasionally by type 2 (HSV-2). Ocular manifestations of HSV are varied and include blepharitis, canalicular obstruction, conjunctivitis, keratitis, uveitis, and retinitis. HSV infections are classified as neonatal, primary (HSV in a person with no previous viral exposure), and recurrent (previous viral exposure with humoral and cellular immunity present).
INCIDENCE/ PREVALENCE	Infections with the HSV are usually acquired in early life. A US study found antibodies against HSV-1 in about 50% of people with high socioeconomic status and 80% of people with low socioeconomic status by the age of 30.[1] However, only about 20–25% of people with HSV antibodies had any history of clinical manifestations of ocular or cutaneous herpetic disease.[2] Ocular HSV is the most common cause of corneal blindness in high income countries and the most common cause of unilateral corneal blindness in the world.[3] A 33 year study of the population of Rochester, Minnesota, found the annual incidence of new cases of ocular herpes simplex to be 8.4 per 100 000 (95% CI 6.9 to 9.9), and the annual incidence of all episodes (new and recurrent) to be 20.7 per 100 000 (95% CI 18.3 to 23.1). The prevalence of ocular herpes was 149 cases per 100 000 population (95% CI 115 to 183). Twelve per cent had bilateral disease.[4]
AETIOLOGY/ RISK FACTORS	Epithelial keratitis results from productive, lytic viral infection of the corneal epithelial cells. Stromal keratitis and iritis are thought to result from a combination of viral infection and compromised immune mechanisms. We found no quantified measures of risk.
PROGNOSIS	HSV epithelial keratitis tends to resolve in 1–2 weeks. In a trial of 271 people treated with topical trifluorothymidine and randomly assigned to receive either oral aciclovir or placebo, the epithelial lesion had resolved completely or was at least less than 1 mm after 1 week of treatment with placebo in 89% of people, and after 2 weeks in 99% of people.[5] Stromal keratitis or iritis occurs in about 25% of people following epithelial keratitis.[6] The effects of HSV stromal keratitis include scarring, tissue destruction, neovascularisation, glaucoma, and persistent epithelial defects. Rate of recurrence of ocular herpes for people with one episode is 9.6% at 1 year, 22.9% at 2 years, and 49.5% at 10 years.[7] Five per cent of corneal grafts performed in Australia over a 10 year period were in people with visual disability or with actual or impending corneal perforation, following stromal ocular herpes simplex. The recurrence of HSV in a corneal graft has a major effect on graft survival. The Australian Corneal Graft Registry has found that, in corneal grafts performed for HSV keratitis, there was at least one HSV recurrence in 58% of corneal grafts that failed over a follow up period of 9 years.[8]

AIMS	To reduce the morbidity of HSV keratitis and iritis; to reduce the risk of recurrent disease after a first episode; to reduce the risk of recurrent disease; and to improve corneal graft survival after penetrating keratoplasty.
OUTCOMES	Healing time; severity and duration of symptoms; severity of complications; rates of recurrence; corneal graft survival.
METHODS	*Clinical Evidence* search and appraisal July 2000.

QUESTION   What are the effects of treatments for epithelial ocular herpes simplex?

OPTION   TOPICAL ANTIVIRAL AGENTS

Two RCTs have found that antivirals improve cure rates and reduce recurrences versus placebo. We found no good evidence of differences between topical antiviral agents.

Benefits: **Versus placebo:** We found no systematic review. We identified one small RCT, which compared 0.1% idoxuridine eye drops (hourly by day and two hourly by night) versus placebo.[9] It found a significantly higher cure rate with idoxuridine (73.7%, 99% CI 44% to 93% with idoxuridine v 15.4% with placebo [no confidence interval given]). We found one double blind RCT (25 men) comparing 3% aciclovir ointment (5 times daily for 7 days) versus placebo.[10] It found significantly fewer recurrences within 1 week of debridement among people receiving aciclovir (1 participant allocated to aciclovir was lost to follow up, intention to treat analysis with person lost to follow up recorded as recurrence: 1/12 [8.3%] with aciclovir v 7/12 [58.3%] with placebo; RR 0.15, 95% CI 0.01 to 0.84). **Versus each other:** We found no systematic review. We found 17 small RCTs comparing one topical antiviral agent with another topical antiviral (see table 1, p 457). Four RCTs compared 3% aciclovir ointment versus either 0.5% or 1% idoxuridine ointment. In two trials (0.5% idoxuridine was used in 1 trial and 1% in the other), aciclovir was found to be more effective. No difference was found in the other two trials. Seven RCTs compared adenine arabinoside (ara-A or vira-A) versus another antiviral (5 with aciclovir and 1 each with idoxuridine and trifluorothymidine). One RCT found aciclovir was more effective; the other six found no significant difference. No significant differences were reported for other comparisons.

Harms: Punctate epitheliopathy (see glossary, p 454) and stinging on application were reported with the use of topical antiviral agents with varying frequency.

Comment: Most of the trials were too small to detect a clinically significant difference.

OPTION DEBRIDEMENT

Three small RCTs found conflicting evidence about the role of debridement in epithelial disease.

Benefits: We found three RCTs, which compared debridement plus a topical antiviral versus an antiviral alone.[28–30] One RCT (50 people) found that the combination of debridement and aciclovir produced significantly more rapid healing than aciclovir alone (P < 0.025; no RR or confidence intervals available).[28] The second RCT (42 people) found that the healing rates in people treated with aciclovir alone were not significantly different from those treated with aciclovir plus debridement (P > 0.1).[29] The third RCT (34 people) found no significant difference between debridement plus trifluorothymidine versus trifluorothymidine alone (mean healing time 7.7 days v 6.8 days; no P value or confidence intervals available).[30]

Harms: No adverse effects were recorded for debridement.

Comment: None.

OPTION TOPICAL ANTIVIRAL AGENTS PLUS INTERFERONS

RCTs have found that a combination of topical antiviral agents and human interferon in different forms are more effective than an antiviral alone.

Benefits: We found no systematic review. We found five RCTs comparing a combination of topical antiviral agent and interferon with antiviral agent alone (see table 2, p 458). All found epithelial lesions healed faster with antiviral plus interferon treatment versus antiviral alone.

Harms: No significant adverse effects were reported.

Comment: None.

QUESTION What are the effects of treatments for stromal ocular herpes simplex?

OPTION TOPICAL CORTICOSTEROIDS

One RCT has found that topical corticosteroids reduce the progression and shorten the duration of stromal keratitis (see glossary, p 455).

Benefits: We found one RCT (106 people) comparing topical prednisolone sodium phosphate (in decreasing concentrations over 10 weeks) versus placebo.[35] All participants received topical trifluorothymidine. It found that prednisolone significantly reduced the persistence or progression of stromal inflammation and shortened the duration of stromal keratitis (see glossary, p 455) (corticosteroid group median 26 days v placebo group median 72 days; difference in medians 46 days; 95% CI 14 to 58 days).[35]

Harms: Adverse events were recorded in nine people given steroids. Four people developed dendritic epithelial keratitis (see glossary, p 454) and were removed from the trial. Four people developed toxic responses to trifluorothymidine after week 5. These people were not withdrawn but the trifluorothymidine was stopped. One person developed an epithelial defect and was withdrawn. Adverse events were reported in six people receiving placebo. All six were withdrawn from the study (1 developed dendritic keratitis, 3 developed an epithelial defect, and 2 developed allergic conjunctivitis attributed to trifluorothymidine within the first 9 days of the trial).

Comment: The trial did not specify whether intention to treat analysis was performed or if people who withdrew from the trial were excluded from the analysis.

OPTION ORAL ACICLOVIR

We found no evidence of benefit of oral aciclovir in the treatment of stromal keratitis.

Benefits: We found one RCT (104 people) of oral aciclovir for HSV stromal keratitis in people receiving concomitant topical corticosteroids and trifluorothymidine.[36] The primary outcome was time to treatment failure (assessed by 8 criteria). It found no significant effect of oral aciclovir (median time to treatment failure 84 days with aciclovir v 62 days with placebo; P = 0.46). There was no significant difference in reported rates of treatment failure by week 16 (38/51 [75%] with aciclovir v 39/53 [74%] with placebo; RR 1.01, 95% CI 0.78 to 1.24).

Harms: In the placebo group, two people developed adverse effects attributed to trifluorothymidine (epithelial keratopathy in one and an allergic reaction in the other). Other adverse effects were pneumonia with possible pulmonary embolus (1 person), congestive heart failure (1 person), diarrhoea (1 person), oedema of the lower extremities (1 person), and anaemia (1 person). Adverse reactions reported in the aciclovir group included toxicity to trifluorothymidine (1 person) and headache (1 person).

Comment: None.

QUESTION What are the effects of interventions used as prophylaxis?

OPTION ORAL ACICLOVIR

One large RCT found that long term oral aciclovir prevented recurrences of ocular herpes in people with at least one previous episode of epithelial or stromal keratitis. One RCT found that short term prophylaxis with oral aciclovir plus topical trifluorothymidine did not prevent stromal keratitis or iritis in people with epithelial keratitis.

Benefits: We found no systematic review. We found two RCTs. The first compared aciclovir (400 mg, orally twice daily) versus placebo in 703 immunocompetent people aged 12 years or older who had epithelial or stromal ocular HSV (in one or both eyes) within the preceding 12 months.[37] One year of aciclovir treatment reduced the probability of any type of recurrence (AR of recurrence 19% with aciclovir v 32% with placebo; RR 0.55, 95% CI 0.41 to 0.75). Prespecified subgroup analysis (337 people) found aciclovir reduced the risk of stromal keratitis only in people who had had at

Ocular herpes simplex

least one prior episode. Aciclovir significantly reduced the recurrence rate of HSV stromal keratitis (AR of recurrence 14% with aciclovir v 28% with placebo; RR 0.48, 95% CI 0.29 to 0.80). There was no rebound in the rate of ocular HSV in the 6 months after stopping treatment with aciclovir. The second RCT (287 people with epithelial keratitis all treated with topical trifluorothymidine) compared a 3 week course of oral aciclovir versus placebo.[38] It found no significant difference in the rate of stromal keratitis or iritis (11% with aciclovir v 10% with placebo; RR 1.04, 95% CI 0.52 to 2.10). The cumulative probability of developing stromal keratitis or iritis by 1 year of follow up was 12% with aciclovir and 11% with placebo (P = 0.92).

Harms: Adverse effects (mostly gastrointestinal problems) were uncommon and occurred with similar frequency in both groups. Thirty two people (15 aciclovir v 17 placebo) discontinued treatment because of adverse effects. The most common adverse effects reported were gastrointestinal upset (7 aciclovir v 9 placebo).

Comment: None.

QUESTION   What are the effects of antiviral prophylaxis on corneal graft survival?

OPTION   ORAL ACICLOVIR

One small RCT found limited evidence that prophylactic use of oral aciclovir reduced recurrences and improved graft survival following corneal transplantation performed for HSV infection.

Benefits: We found no systematic review. We found one small non-blinded RCT in people who had received keratoplasty (see glossary, p 454), which compared oral aciclovir (800 or 1000 mg, 4 or 5 times orally daily, tapered during the first 12 months, for a maximum of 15 months) versus usual care.[39] Oral aciclovir was given orally beginning before surgery or on the first day after surgery. It found no recurrence of ocular herpes simplex in 13 people receiving aciclovir (14 eyes, mean follow up 17 months) compared with recurrence in four out of nine people not taking aciclovir (9 eyes, mean follow up 21 months), (0% with aciclovir v 44% with placebo, P < 0.01). Graft failure occurred in 14% of aciclovir treated eyes compared with 56% without aciclovir (P < 0.05).

Harms: None reported.

Comment: None.

GLOSSARY

Epithelial keratitis Inflammation of the cells that form the surface layer of the cornea.

Keratoplasty A procedure in which diseased corneal tissue is removed and replaced by donor corneal material.

Punctate epitheliopathy Fine lesions of the cornea that stain brilliantly with rose bengal or fluorescein. These lesions are areas without normal surface epithelium, with exposure of underlying immature cells. They represent a non-specific response to injury.

Stromal keratitis Inflammation of the middle layer of the cornea. The stroma forms 90% of the corneal substance. It lies between the epithelium and Bowmans membrane anteriorly and Desçemet's membrane and the endothelium posteriorly.

REFERENCES

1. Nahmias AJ, Lee FK, Beckman-Nahmias S. Sero-epidemiological and sociological patterns of herpes simplex virus infection in the world. *Scand J Infect Dis Suppl* 1990;69:19–36.

2. Kaufman HE, Rayfield MA, Gebhardt BM. Herpes simplex viral infections. In: Kaufman HE, Baron BA, McDonald MB, eds. *The Cornea*. 2nd ed. Butterworth-Heinemann, 1997.

3. Dawson CR, Togni B. Herpes simplex eye infections: clinical manifestations, pathogenesis, and management. *Surv Ophthalmol* 1976;21:121–135.

4. Liesegang TJ, Melton LJ III, Daly PJ, et al. Epidemiology of ocular herpes simplex. Incidence in Rochester, Minnesota, 1950 through 1982. *Arch Ophthalmol* 1989;107:1155–1159.

5. The Herpetic Eye Disease Study Group. A controlled trial of oral acyclovir for the prevention of stromal keratitis or iritis in patients with herpes simplex virus epithelial keratitis. The Epithelial Keratitis Trial. *Arch Ophthalmol* 1997;115:703–712.

6. Wilhelmus KR, Coster DJ, Donovan HC, Falcon MG, Jones BR. Prognosis indicators of herpetic keratitis. Analysis of a five-year observation period after corneal ulceration. *Arch Ophthalmol* 1981;99:1578–1582.

7. Liesegang TJ. Epidemiology of ocular herpes simplex. Natural history in Rochester, Minnesota, 1950 through 1982. *Arch Ophthalmol* 1989;107:1160–1165.

8. Williams KA, Muehlberg SM, Lewis RF, Giles LC, Coster DJ. *The Australian Corneal Graft Registry: 1996 Report*. Adelaide: Mercury press, 1997.

9. Hart DR, Brightman VJ, Readshaw GG, Porter GT, Tully MJ. Treatment of human herpes simplex keratitis with idoxuridine: A sequential double-blind controlled study. *Arch Ophthalmol* 1965;73:623–634.

10. Jones BR, Coster DJ, Fison PN, Thompson GM, Cobo LM, Falcon MG. Efficacy of acycloguanosine (Wellcome 248U) against herpes-simplex corneal ulcers. *Lancet* 1979;1:243–244.

11. Coster DJ, Wilhelmus KR, Michaud R, Jones BR. A comparison of acyclovir and idoxuridine as treatment for ulcerative herpetic keratitis. *Br J Ophthalmol* 1980;64:763–765.

12. Collum LM, Benedict-Smith A, Hillary IB. Randomised double-blind trial of acyclovir and idoxuridine in dendritic corneal ulceration. *Br J Ophthalmol* 1980;64:766–769.

13. McCulley JP, Binder PS, Kaufman HE, O'Day DM, Poirier RH. A double-blind, multicenter clinical trial of acyclovir vs idoxuridine for treatment of epithelial herpes simplex keratitis. *Ophthalmology* 1982;89:1195–1200.

14. Klauber A, Ottovay E. Acyclovir and idoxiuridine treatment of herpes simplex keratitis – a double blind clinical study. *Acta Ophthalmol (Copenh)* 1982;60:838–844.

15. Wellings PC, Awdry PN, Bors FH, Jones BR, Brown DC, Kaufman HE. Clinical evaluation of trifluorothymidine in the treatment of herpes simplex corneal ulcers. *Am J Ophthalmol* 1972;73:932–942.

16. Sugar J, Stark W, Binder PS, et al. Trifluorothymidine treatment of Herpes simplex epithelial keratitis and comparison with idoxuridine. *Ann Ophthalmol* 1980;12:611–615.

17. Markham RH, Carter C, Scobie MA, et al. Double-blind clinical trial of adenine arabinoside and idoxuridine in herpetic corneal ulcers. *Trans Ophthalmol Soc UK* 1977;97:333–340.

18. Hovding G. A comparison between acyclovir and trifluorothymidine ophthalmic ointment in treatment of epithelial dendritic keratitis. A double blind, randomized parallel group trial. *Acta Ophthalmol (Copenh)* 1989;67:51–54.

19. La Lau C, Oosterhuis JA, Versteeg J, et al. Multicenter trial of acyclovir and trifluorothymidine in herpetic keratitis. *Am J Med* 1982;73:305–306.

20. Laibson PR, Pavan-Langston D, Yeakley WR, et al. Acyclovir and vidarabine for the treatment of herpes simplex keratitis. *Am J Med* 1982;73:281–285.

21. Young B, Patterson A, Ravenscroft T. A randomised double-blind clinical trial of acyclovir (Zovirax) and adenine arabinoside in herpes simplex corneal ulceration. *Br J Ophthalmol* 1982;66:361–363.

22. Pavan-Langston D, Lass J, Hettinger M, Udell I. Acyclovir and vidarabine in the treatment of ulcerative herpes simplex keratitis. *Am J Ophthalmol* 1981;92:829–835.

23. Collum LM, Logan P, McAuliffe-Curtin D, et al. Randomised double-blind trial of acyclovir (Zovirax) and adenine arabinoside in herpes simplex amoeboid corneal ulceration. *Br J Ophthalmol* 1985;69:847–850.

24. McGill J, Tormey P, Walker CB. Comparative trial of acyclovir and adenine arabinoside in the treatment of herpes simplex corneal ulcers. *Br J Ophthalmol* 1981;65:610–613.

25. Coster DJ, McKinnon JR, McGill JI, et al. Clinical evaluation of adenine arabinoside and trifluorothymidine in the treatment of corneal ulcers caused by herpes simplex virus. *J Infect Dis* 1976;133 (Suppl A):173–177.

26. Power WJ, Benedict-Smith A, Hillery M, et al. Randomised double-blind trial of bromovinyldeoxyuridine (BVDU) and trifluorothymidine (TFT) in dendritic corneal ulceration. *Br J Ophthalmol* 1991;75:649–651.

27. Panda A, Das GK, Khokhar S, et al. Efficacy of four antiviral agents in the treatment of uncomplicated herpetic keratitis. *Can J Ophthalmol* 1995;30:256–258.

28. Wilhelmus KR, Coster DJ, Jones BR. Acyclovir and debridement in the treatment of ulcerative herpetic keratitis. *Am J Ophthalmol* 1981;91:323–327.

29. Jensen KB, Nissen SH, Jessen F. Acyclovir in the treatment of herpetic keratitis. *Acta Ophthalmol (Copenh)* 1982;60:557–563.

30. Parlato CJ, Cohen EJ, Sakauye CM, Dreizen NG, Galentine PG, Laibson PR. Role of debridement and trifluridine (trifluorothymidine) in herpes simplex dendritic keratitis. *Arch Ophthalmol* 1985;103:673–675.

31. van Bijsterveld OP, Meurs PJ, de Clercq E, Maudgal PC. Bromovinyldeoxyuridine and interferon treatment in ulcerative herpetic keratitis: a double masked study. *Br J Ophthalmol* 1989;73:604–607.

32. Colin J, Chastel C, Renard G, Cantell K. Combination therapy for dendritic keratitis with human leukocyte interferon and acyclovir. *Am J Ophthalmol* 1983;95:346–348.

33. de Koning EW, van Bijsterveld OP, Cantell K. Combination therapy for dendritic keratitis with

human leucocyte interferon and trifluorothymidine. *Br J Ophthalmol* 1982;66:509–512.

34. de Koning EW, van Bijsterveld OP, Cantell K. Combination therapy for dendritic keratitis with acyclovir and α-interferon. *Arch Ophthalmol* 1983; 101:1866–1868.

35. Meurs PJ, van Bijsterveld OP. Combination therapy of recombinant human $α_2$ interferon and acyclovir in the treatment of herpes simplex keratitis. *Antiviral Res* 1985;Suppl 1:225–228.

36. Wilhelmus KR, Gee L, Hauck WW, et al. Herpetic Eye Disease Study. A controlled trial of topical corticosteroids for herpes simplex stromal keratitis. *Ophthalmology* 1994;101:1883–1895.

37. Barron BA, Gee L, Hauck WW, et al. Herpetic Eye Disease Study. A controlled trial of oral acyclovir for herpes simplex stromal keratitis. *Ophthalmology* 1994;101:1871–1882.

38. Herpetic Eye Disease Study Group. Acyclovir for the prevention of recurrent herpes simplex virus eye disease. *N Engl J Med* 1998;339:300–306.

39. Barney NP, Foster CS. A prospective randomized trial of oral acyclovir after penetrating keratoplasty for herpes simplex keratitis. *Cornea* 1994;13: 232–236.

Nigel Barker
Consultant Ophthalmologist
Specialist Eye Centre
Christ Church
Barbados

Competing interests: None declared.

TABLE 1 Interventions to treat HSV epithelial keratitis: comparison of topical antiviral agents with (see text, p 451).

Reference	People	Treatment	Composition	Comparison	Outcome	Comments
11	60	ACV	Ointment	1% IDU	NS	
12	60	ACV	Ointment	0.5% IDU	Mean healing rate (days): 4.4 v 9.2; ACV v IDU; P < 0.01	
13	64	ACV	Ointment	0.5% IDU	Mean healing rate (days): 5.9 v 7.2; ACV v IDU; NS	
14	38	ACV	Ointment	0.5% IDU	Cure rate 94% ACV v 70% IDU; P < 0.025	
15	78	1% TFT (9 x daily)	Drops (5 x daily)	0.1% IDU	Mean healing rate (days): 6.3 v 8.2; TFT v IDU; P < 0.005	Considered dendritic and geographic ulcers separately
16	61	1% TFT	Drops	0.1% IDU (19 x daily)	NS	
17	60	3% Ara-A	Ointment (4 x daily)	0.5% IDU	Mean healing rate (days): 8.1 v 9.9; Ara-A v IDU; NS	
18	55	ACV	Ointment	2% TFT	Mean healing rate (days): 5.9 v 6.7; TFT v ACV; NS	
19	59	ACV	Ointment	2% TFT	Cure rate 90% ACV v 75% TFT; NS	
20	73	ACV	Ointment	3% Vira-A	Mean healing rate (days): 3.9 v 5.0; ACV v Vira-A; NS	
21	93	ACV	Ointment	3% Ara-A	Cure rate 94% ACV v 82% Ara-A; P < 0.01	
22	41	ACV	Ointment	3% Vira-A	Mean healing rate (days): 3.8 v 5.2; ACV v Vira-A; NS	
23	51	ACV	Ointment	3% Ara-A	Mean healing rate (days): 12.2 v 11.0; ACV v Vira-A; NS	Only geographic ulcers studied
24	57	ACV	Ointment	3% Ara-A	Mean healing rate (days): 4.2 v 6.3; ACV v Ara-A; NS	
25	102	1% TFT	Drops/ointment (5 x daily)	3.3% Ara-A ointment	Mean healing rate (days): 5.75 v 5.13; TFT v Ara-A; NS	
26	60	0.1% BVDU	Drops (5 x daily)	1% TFT	Mean healing rate (days): 8.5 v 7.2; BVDU v TFT; P = 0.065; NS	
27	80	3% ACV	Ointment (5 x daily)	1% IDU; 2% TFT; 1% BVDU	Mean healing rate (days): 13.4 v 8.9 v 8.5 v 7.5; IDU v TFT v ACV v BVDU. No statistical analysis but concluded that BVDU was more effective than others	

ACV, aciclovir; Ara-A, adenosine arabinoside; BVDU, bromovinyldeoxyuridine; IDU, idoxuridine; NS, no significant difference; TFT, trifluorothymidine; Vira-A, vidarabine. Adenosine arabinoside and vidarabine are the same antiviral. Aciclovir and idoxuridine were administered 5 times daily unless stated otherwise. Aciclovir is used as 3% ointment unless stated otherwise.

TABLE 2 Interventions to treat HSV epithelial keratitis: topical antiviral agent plus interferon versus topical antiviral alone (see text, p 452).

Reference	People	Antiviral	Interferon	Dose	Outcome	Comments
31	41	BVDU	IF2C	1.5×10^6 IU	Average healing rate (days): 8.5 BVDU v 4–6 BVDU + IF	No toxic effects
32	43	ACV	HLI	30×10^6 IU/ml daily	Average healing rate (days): 3.9 ACV + HLI v 7 ACV + placebo; $P < 0.001$	
33	60	TFT	HLI	10×10^6 IU/ml	Average healing rate (days): 6.6 TFT + HLI v 11.3 TFT + placebo; $P < 0.001$	
34	59	ACV	IFα	30×10^6 IU/ml daily	Healing time significantly faster for ACV + IF	Minor toxic effects
35	93	ACV	IFα2		Significant reduction in both partial and complete healing time with ACV + IFN v ACV + placebo	

ACV, aciclovir; Ara-A, adenosine arabinoside; BVDU, bromovinyldeoxyuridine; HLI, human leukocyte interferon; IDU, idoxuridine; IFN, interferon; TFT, trifluorothymidine; Vira-A, vidarabine.

Search date March 2000

Denise Mabey and Nicole Fraser-Hurt

QUESTIONS

INTERVENTIONS

INTERVENTIONS TO PREVENT SCARRING TRACHOMA BY REDUCING ACTIVE TRACHOMA

Likely to be beneficial

Promotion of face washing. . . .461
Children having a sustained clean face 461
Fly control using insecticide . . .461
Antibiotics (versus placebo or no treatment). 461
Oral azithromycin (versus topical tetracycline) 461

TREATMENT OF SCARRING TRACHOMA

Likely to be beneficial

Bilamellar tarsal rotation (versus other eyelid surgery), when performed by an experienced operator 463

See glossary, p 463

Key Messages

Prevention of scarring trachoma by reducing active trachoma

- One RCT has found that promotion of face washing versus no promotion significantly reduces the rate of severe trachoma. It found no significant reduction of the overall rate of trachoma but the study was too small to rule out a clinically important effect.

- In a single pilot study for an RCT, the number of new cases of trachoma was reduced by fly control using insecticide versus no intervention.

- One unpublished systematic review found limited evidence from small RCTs that antibiotics may reduce active trachoma compared with placebo at 3 and 12 months follow up. The same review found limited evidence from three RCTs that oral azithromycin may reduce active trachoma compared with topical tetracycline after 3 months. These RCTs were small or of unusual design, and at 12 months the difference between treatments disappeared.

Treatment of scarring trachoma

- In people with trichiasis who have six or more lashes in contact with the globe, we found limited evidence from two RCTs that bilamellar tarsal rotation may relieve entropion and trichiasis more often than tarsal advance and rotation.

- In people with trichiasis who have five lashes or fewer in contact with the globe, one RCT found that tarsal rotation relieved entropion and trichiasis more often than electrolysis or cryoablation. In these trials, one experienced surgeon performed most of the operations.

Eye disorders

DEFINITION	Active trachoma is chronic inflammation of the conjunctiva caused by infection with *Chlamydia trachomatis*. The World Health Organization (WHO) classification for acute trachoma defines mild trachoma (grade TF) as the presence of five or more follicles in the upper tarsal conjunctiva of at least 0.5 mm diameter. Severe trachoma (grade TI) is defined as pronounced inflammatory thickening of the upper tarsal conjunctiva that obscures more than half of the normal deep vessels. Repeated infection causes scarring trachoma, in which the upper eyelid is shortened and distorted (entropion), and the lashes abrade the eye (trichiasis). Blindness results from corneal opacification, which is related to the degree of entropion/trichiasis.
INCIDENCE/ PREVALENCE	Trachoma is the world's leading cause of preventable blindness and is second only to cataract as an overall cause of blindness.[1] Globally, active trachoma affects an estimated 150 million people, most of them children. About 5.5 million people are blind or at risk of blindness as a consequence of trachoma. Trachoma is a disease of poverty regardless of geographical regions. Scarring trachoma is prevalent in large regions of Africa, the Middle East, South-West Asia, the Indian subcontinent, and Aboriginal communities in Australia, and there are small focuses in Central and South America.[1] In areas where trachoma is constantly present at high prevalence, active disease is found in more than 50% of preschool children and may have a prevalence of 60–90%.[2] As many as 75% of women and 50% of men over the age of 45 may show signs of scarring disease.[3] The prevalence of active trachoma decreases with increasing age, with less than 5% of adults showing signs of active disease.[2] Although similar rates of active disease are observed in male and female children, the later sequelae of trichiasis, entropion, and corneal opacification are more common in women than men.[2]
AETIOLOGY/ RISK FACTORS	Active trachoma is associated with young age and where there is close contact between people. Discharge from the eyes and nose may be a source of further reinfection.[4] Sharing a bedroom with someone who has active trachoma is a risk factor for infection.[5] Facial contact with flies is held to be associated with active trachoma, but studies reporting this relationship had weak methods.[6]
PROGNOSIS	Corneal damage from trachoma is caused by multiple processes. Scarring may cause an inadequate tear film, and a dry eye may be more susceptible to damage from inturned lashes, leading to corneal opacification. The prevalence of scarring and consequent blindness increases with age and is most commonly seen in older adults.[7]
AIMS	To prevent active trachoma; to reduce the rate of progression to scarring; and to relieve entropion and trichiasis in people with scarring trachoma, with minimal side effects of treatment.
OUTCOMES	Rates of active trachoma; clinical signs of active trachoma using the WHO grading scale; laboratory evidence of *Chlamydia trachomatis* infection; eyelid position; and degree of entropion/trichiasis.
METHODS	*Clinical Evidence* search and appraisal March 2000.

| QUESTION | What are the effects of interventions to prevent scarring trachoma by reducing active trachoma? |

| OPTION | PUBLIC HEALTH INTERVENTIONS |

One RCT has found that promotion of face washing compared with no advice significantly reduces the rate of severe trachoma. It found no significant reduction of the overall rate of trachoma, but the study was not powered to exclude a clinically important effect. One small RCT found that the number of new cases of trachoma was reduced by fly control using insecticide compared with no intervention.

Benefits:
: **Promotion of face washing:** We found no systematic review but found one RCT that randomised six villages to either promotion of face washing plus 30 days of daily topical tetracycline ointment or 30 days of daily topical tetracycline ointment only.[8] It found that, in 1417 children aged 1–7 years, promotion of face washing increased the likelihood of children having a clean face on at least two of three follow up visits, but the result was not significant (OR for having a clean face with intervention v control 1.6, 95% CI 0.94 to 2.74). After 1 year, promotion of face washing plus topical tetracycline compared with topical tetracycline reduced the risk of severe trachoma (OR for severe trachoma 0.62, 95% CI 0.40 to 0.97), but the reduction was not significant for all grades of trachoma (OR for mild and severe trachoma 0.81, 95% CI 0.42 to 1.59). When all participants from intervention and control villages were pooled, children who had a sustained clean face were less likely to have active trachoma than those who ever had a dirty face (OR 0.58, 95% CI 0.47 to 0.72). **Fly control using insecticide:** We found no systematic review and no completed RCTs. We found one pilot study for an RCT comparing spraying of deltamethrin for 3 months compared with no intervention in two pairs of villages.[6] One pair received the intervention or none in the wet season, one pair received the intervention or none in the dry season. There were a total of 191 children under 10 years in the control villages and 223 children in the intervention villages. The number of new cases of trachoma (WHO classification) at 3 months was 75% lower in the children living in the intervention villages than in the comparison group (RR 0.25, 95% CI 0.09 to 0.64).

Harms:
: None were identified.

Comment:
: The cluster randomisation used in both RCTs limits the power to detect differences between groups, and makes difficult interpretation of the results for individual children.[8]

| OPTION | ANTIBIOTICS |

One unpublished systematic review has found limited evidence from low powered RCTs that antibiotics reduce active trachoma at 3 and 12 months compared with no treatment. The same review found limited evidence from three RCTs that oral azithromycin may reduce active trachoma compared with topical tetracycline after 3 months. These RCTs were low powered or of unusual design and at 12 months the difference between treatments disappeared.

Benefits: **Versus placebo or no treatment:** We found one unpublished systematic review (search date 1999).[9] It identified eight RCTs that compared topical and oral antibiotics with no treatment, placebo, or a monthly vitamin tablet in people with active trachoma. All reported outcomes at 3 months. Five trials reported outcomes at 12 months (999 people in the treatment group, 76% completed the study; 832 people in the control group, 71% completed the study) (see table 1, p 465). The review found that antibiotics reduced active trachoma months (OR for active trachoma based on clinical assessment, antibiotics v control 0.43, 95% CI 0.35 to 0.52) and at 12 months (OR 0.47, 95% CI 0.38 to 0.60). It also found that antibiotics reduced *Chlamydia trachomatis* infection rates based on bacteriological testing compared with control at 12 months (1 RCT; OR 0.27 95% CI 0.11 to 0.67). At 3 months the infection rate was also reduced but not significantly (3 RCTs; OR for infection, antibiotic v control 0.63, 95% CI 0.38 to 1.05). **Oral versus topical antibiotics:** We found one unpublished systematic review of three RCTs comparing rates of active trachoma and bacteriological infection following oral azithromycin or topical tetracycline.[9] (see table 2, p 466) All trials had problems with methods that limit the results (see comment below). At 3 months, oral azithromycin compared with topical tetracycline reduced active trachoma (3 RCTs, n = 6226; OR 0.82, 95% CI 0.71 to 0.94) and infection rates (OR 0.49, 95% CI 0.39 to 0.62). At 12 months, the review found no significant difference between treatments for active trachoma (1 RCT, n = 5573; OR 0.88, 95% CI 0.77 to 1.01), but found that oral azithromycin reduced bacteriologically defined infection compared with topical tetracycline (OR 0.70, 95% CI 0.57 to 0.87).

Harms: None were reported.

Comment: **Versus placebo or no treatment:** The trials were undertaken in various settings; most were in children attending boarding schools. Several unusual study designs were used, for example family based treatment. The trials were all of moderate or poor quality and many had no intention to treat analysis. Antibiotic treatments included topical and oral doses. **Oral versus topical treatment:** Two of the RCTs were small (total n = 224) and low powered. The third trial compared mass treatment, in which people were treated irrespective of disease status, and were randomly allocated by village (cluster randomisation). Correlation analysis found some similarity between individuals within a cluster, so limiting the validity of results. We found no evidence about the development of bacterial resistance.

QUESTION   **Effects of surgical treatments for scarring trachoma (entropion and trichiasis)**

We found no good evidence on the effects of surgery to improve visual acuity in people with scarring trachoma. In people with trichiasis who have six or more lashes in contact with the globe, we found limited evidence from two RCTs that bilamellar tarsal rotation may relieve entropion and trichiasis more often than tarsal advance and rotation. In people with trichiasis who have five lashes or fewer in contact with the globe, one RCT found that tarsal rotation relieves entropion and trichiasis

more often than electrolysis or cryoablation. In these trials, one experienced surgeon performed most of the operations.

Benefits: We found no systematic review but found two RCTs comparing surgical interventions for entropion and trichiasis.[10,11] In both trials, one experienced surgeon performed most of the operations. Both trials defined operative success as no lashes in contact with the globe in primary position of gaze, and complete lid closure with gentle voluntary effort. **Major trichiasis:** See glossary, p 464. The trial compared five surgical techniques (bilamellar tarsal rotation, eversion splinting, tarsal advance, tarsal grooving, and tarsal advance and rotation (see glossary, p 464) in 165 Omani villagers major trichiasis (as defined for these trials). There were a total of 165 eyelids.[10] The trial found very limited evidence that bilamellar tarsal rotation was more successful than other surgical treatments. However, analysis was not by intention to treat, and the power of the trial was very low. The second RCT compared tarsal rotation with tarsal advance and rotation in Omani villagers with major trichiasis (total of 200 eyelids).[11] It found that bilamellar tarsal rotation was more successful than tarsal advance and rotation, after 25 months' follow up (HR for failure following tarsal advance and rotation v bilamellar tarsal rotation 3.1, 95% CI 1.9 to 5.2). **Minor trichiasis:** See glossary, p 464. The second RCT compared tarsal rotation versus cryoablation versus electrolysis in people with minor trichiasis (as defined for this trial) (total of 172 eyelids).[11] It found that tarsal rotation was more successful than the other treatments after 25 months' follow up (HR of failure, electrolysis v tarsal rotation 6.1, 95% CI 2.9 to 12.8; HR of failure, cryoablation v tarsal rotation 7.5, 95% CI 3.6 to 15.4).

Harms: Adverse outcomes of interventions were corneal exposure, ulceration, phthisis bulbi (see glossary, p 464), and severe recurrent trichiasis.[10,12] In these two trials, major trichiasis and defective closure after surgical procedures for scarring trachoma were more common after eversion splinting, tarsal advance, and tarsal grooving than after bilamellar tarsal rotation and tarsal advance and rotation. Cryoablation of the eyelashes can cause necrosis of the lid margin, corneal ulcers, and in the RCT in which cryoablation was used[11] it was the only procedure associated with onset of phthisis (2 cases out of 57). Further details of harms are summarised in table 3, p 467.

Comment: The pragmatic definitions of major and minor trichiasis are limited to use in these trials. The first RCT was very low powered, and was not analysed by intention to treat.[10] In both RCTs, one experienced operator performed most of the surgery. The evidence of both benefits and harms may not be applicable to different operators, or where the quality of surgical equipment does not match those in the trials.

GLOSSARY

Bilamellar tarsal rotation The upper lid is cut full thickness horizontally in a line parallel and 3 mm from the eyelid margin and running from just lateral to the lacrimal punctum to the lateral canthus. Everting sutures are then placed through all layers of the lid to prevent the margin from turning inwards.
Eversion splinting The lid margin is split posterior to the lashes, the eversion of the

anterior section is maintained by sutures tied over a roll of paraffin gauze.

Major trichiasis Lid closure complete; six or more lashes in contact with eyeball.

Minor trichiasis Lid closure complete; one to five lashes in contact with eyeball.

Phthisis bulbi A disorganised, shrunken eye which has no perception of light.

Tarsal advance The lid margin is split posterior to the lashes. The skin, lashes, and orbicularis are freed from the tarsal plate and retracted away from the cornea and are sutured back on to the tarsal plate leaving a bare area of tarsus to act as the lid margin.

Tarsal advance and rotation The upper lid is everted over a speculum. The tarsal plate is fractured parallel to and 3 mm from the lid margin. In this operation the skin and orbicularis are not cut. The short portion of tarsal plate attached to the lid margin is then rotated through 180 degrees and sutured into place to form the new lid margin.

Tarsal grooving A wedge of skin, orbicularis, and tarsus is removed parallel to the lid margin. Sutures through all layers act to evert the lid margin.

REFERENCES

1. Thylefors B, Negrel AD, Pararajasegaram R, et al.. Global data on blindness. *Bull World Health Organ* 1995;73:115–121.

2. West SK, Munoz B, Turner VM, et al. The epidemiology of trachoma in central Tanzania. *Int J Epidemiol* 1991;20:1088–1092.

3. Courtright P, Sheppard J, Schachter J, et al. Trachoma and blindness in the Nile Delta: current patterns and projections for the future in the rural Egyptian population. *Br J Ophthalmol* 1989;73: 536–540.

4. Bobo L, Munoz B, Viscidi R, et al. Diagnosis of Chlamydia trachomatis eye infection in Tanzania by polymerase chain reaction/enzyme immunoassay. *Lancet* 1991;338:847–850.

5. Bailey R, Osmond C, Mabey DCW, et al. Analysis of the household pattern of trachoma in a Gambian village using a Monte Carlo simulation procedure. *Int J Epidemiol* 1989;18:944–951.

6. Emerson PM, Lindsay SW, Walraven GE, et al. Effect of fly control on trachoma and diarrhoea. *Lancet* 1999;353:1401–1403.

7. Munoz B, West SK. The forgotten cause of blindness. *Epidemiol Rev* 1997;19:205–217.

8. West S, Munoz B, Lynch M, et al. Impact of facewashing on trachoma in Kongwa, Tanzania. *Lancet* 1995;345:155–158.

9. Mabey D, Fraser-Hurt N. Antibiotics for trachoma (Protocol for a Cochrane Review). In: The Cochrane Library, Issue 2, 2000. Oxford: Update software. Search date 1999; primary sources Medline, Embase, Cinalh, Science Citation Index, and personal contacts.

10. Reacher MH, Huber MJE, Canagaratnam R, et al. A trial of surgery for trichiasis of the upper lid from trachoma. *Br J Ophthalmol* 1990;74:109–113.

11. Reacher MH, Munoz B, Alghassany A, et al. A controlled trial of surgery for trachomatous trichiasis of the upper lid. *Arch Ophthalmol* 1992; 110:667–674.

12. Reacher MH, Taylor HR. The management of trachomatous trichiasis. *Rev Int Trach Pathol Ocul Trop Subtrop Sante Publique* 1990;67:233–262.

13. Attiah MA, el Kohly AM. Clinical assessment of the comparative effect of terramycin and GS 2989 in the mass treatment of trachoma. *Rev Int Trach Pathol Ocul Trop Subtrop Sante Publique* 1973; 50:11–20.

14. Darougar S, Jones BR, Viswalingam N, et al. Family-based suppressive intermittent therapy of hyperendemic trachoma with topical oxytetracycline or oral doxycycline. *Br J Ophthalmol* 1980;64:291–295.

15. Dawson CR, Hanna L, Wood TR, et al. Controlled trials with trisulphapyrimidines in the treatment of chronic trachoma. *J Infect Dis* 1969;119:581–590.

16. Foster SO, Powers DK, Thygeson P. Trachoma therapy: a controlled study. *Am J Ophthalmol* 1966;61:451–455.

17. Hoshiwara I, Ostler HB, Hanna L, et al. Doxycycline treatment of chronic trachoma. *JAMA* 1973;224:220–223.

18. Shukla BR, Nema HV, Mathur JS, et al. Gantrisin and madribon in trachoma. *Br J Ophthalmol* 1966;50:218–221.

19. Tabbara KF, Summanen P, Taylor PB, et al. Minocycline effects in patients with active trachoma. *Int Ophthalmol* 1988;12:59–63.

20. Woolridge RL, Cheng KH, Chang IH, et al. Failure of trachoma treatment with ophthalmic antibiotics and systemic sulphonamides used alone or in combination with trachoma vaccine. *Am J Ophthalmol* 1967;63(suppl):1577–1586.

21. Dawson CR, Schachter J, Sallam S, et al. A comparison of oral azithromycin with topical oxytetracycline/polymyxin for the treatment of trachoma in children. *Clin Infect Dis* 1997;24: 363–368.

22. Schachter J, West SK, Mabey D, et al. Azithromycin in control of trachoma. *Lancet* 1999; 354:630–635.

23. Tabbara KF, Abu el Asrar A, al Omar O, et al. Single-dose azithromycin in the treatment of trachoma. A randomized, controlled study. *Ophthalmology* 1996;103:842–846.

Denise Mabey
Guy's and St Thomas' Hospital Trust
London
UK

Nicole Fraser-Hurt
Epiconsult Ltd.
Nhlangano
Swaziland

Competing interests: None declared.

TABLE 1 Interventions to prevent scarring trachoma by reducing active trachoma: results of randomised controlled trials of antibiotics compared with no treatment placebo, or a monthly vitamin tablet in people with active trachoma (see text, p 462).

Study	Treatment	Route	Dose	Duration	Comparison
13	Tetracycline derivative GS2989	Topical	0.25%	Once every school day for 11 weeks	No treatment
13	Terramycin	Topical	Not stated	Once every school day for 11 weeks	No treatment
14	Oxytetracycline	Topical	1%	Twice daily for 7 consecutive days every month for 12 months	Vitamin pills, orally, 1 dose per month for 12 months
14	Doxycycline	Oral	5 mg/kg	1 dose per month for 12 months	Vitamin pills, orally, 1 dose per month for 12 months
15	Trisulfapyrimidine	Oral	3.5 g/day	3 daily during 3 consecutive weeks	Lactose, orally, 3 daily for 3 consecutive weeks
15	Trisulfapyrimidine	Oral	3.5 g/day	3 daily during 3 consecutive weeks	Lactose, orally, 3 daily for 3 consecutive weeks
16	Sulfametopyridazine	Oral	0.5 g	Once daily for 5 consecutive days every week for 3 weeks	No treatment
16	Tetracycline	Topical	1%	3 times daily on 5 consecutive days every week for 6 weeks	No treatment
17	Doxycycline	Oral	2.5–4.0 mg/kg	Once daily for 5 consecutive days every week up to 28 doses in 40 days	Placebo once daily for 5 consecutive days every week up to 28 doses in 40 days
18	Sulfafurazole + Sulfadimetoxine	Topical + oral	15%/100 mg/kg	Twice daily for 5 consecutive days every month for 5 months/bi-weekly for 5 months	No treatment
18	Sulfadimethoxine	Oral	100 mg/kg	Twice weekly or weekly dose for 5 months	No treatment
18	Sulfafurazole	Topical	15%	Twice daily for 5 consecutive days every month for 5 months	No treatment
19	Minocycline	Oral	100 mg	Once daily on 5 consecutive days every week for 5 weeks	Placebo topically twice daily on 5 consecutive days every week for 5 weeks
19	Tetracycline	Topical	1%	Twice daily on 5 consecutive days every week for 5 weeks	Placebo topically twice daily on 5 consecutive days every week for 5 weeks
20	Tetracycline	Topical	1%	Twice daily for 6 consecutive days per week for 6 weeks	No treatment

TABLE 2 Interventions to prevent scarring trachoma by reducing active trachoma: results of randomised controlled trials comparing rates of active trachoma and bacteriological infection following oral azithromycin or topical tetracycline (see text, p 462).

Study	Treatment	Dose	Duration	Comparison	Dose/duration
21	Azithromycin orally	20 mg/kg	1 dose, or 3 times 1 dose at weekly intervals, or 6 times 1 dose at 28 day intervals	1% topical oxytet/polymyxin + oral placebo	Ointment once daily for 5 consecutive days monthly for 6 months
22	Azithromycin orally	20 mg/kg up to 1 g	Once a week for 3 weeks	1% topical oxytetracycline	Once daily for 6 weeks
	Women of childbearing age erythromycin	500 mg bd or 250 mg qds	14 days		
23	Azithromycin orally	20 mg/kg	1 dose	1% topical tetracycline	Twice daily for 5 consecutive days per week for 6 weeks

bd, to be taken twice a day; qds, to be taken four times a day.

TABLE 3	Summary of harms following surgery for scarring trachoma (see text, p 463).				
	Bilamellar tarsal rotation	Tarsal advance and rotation	Eversion splinting	Tarsal advance	Tarsal grooving
Major trichiasis[11]	4/150	4/101	—*	—*	—*
Defective closure[11]	2/150	1/101	—*	—*	—*
Major trichiasis[12]	1/44	1/23	7/25	10/41	11/32
Defective closure[12]	2/44	0/23	0/25	0/41	5/32

*no data collected.

Congenital toxoplasmosis

Search date November 2000

Piero Olliaro

QUESTIONS
Treating toxoplasmosis in pregnancy 470

INTERVENTIONS	
Unknown effectiveness Spiramycin and other antiparasitic drugs 470	**To be covered in future issues of** ***Clinical Evidence*** Pregnancy termination Screening

Key Messages

- We found insufficient evidence to determine the effects on mother or baby of current antiparasitic treatment for women who seroconvert during pregnancy.

DEFINITION Toxoplasmosis is caused by the parasite *Toxoplasma gondii*. Infection is asymptomatic or unremarkable in immunocompetent individuals, but leads to a lifelong antibody response. During pregnancy, toxoplasmosis can be transmitted across the placenta and cause intrauterine death, neonatal growth retardation, mental retardation, ocular defects, and blindness in later life. Congenital toxoplasmosis (confirmed infection of the fetus or newborn) can present at birth, either as subclinical disease, which may evolve with neurological or ophthalmological disease later in life, or as a disease of varying severity, ranging from mild ocular damage to severe mental retardation.

INCIDENCE/ PREVALENCE We found few prospective population surveys of toxoplasma seroprevalence. Reported rates vary across and within countries, as well as over time. The risk of primary infection is highest in young people, including young women during pregnancy. We found no cohort studies describing annual seroconversion rates in women of childbearing age nor incidence of primary infection. One systematic review identified 15 studies that reported rates of seroconversion ranging from 2.4–16/1000 in Europe and from 2–6/1000 in the USA.[1] France began screening for congenital toxoplasmosis in 1978, and during the period 1980–1995 the seroconversion rate during pregnancy was 4–5/1000.[2]

AETIOLOGY/ RISK FACTORS Toxoplasma infection is usually acquired by ingesting either sporocysts (from unwashed fruit or vegetables contaminated by cat faeces) or tissue cysts (from raw or undercooked meat). The risk of contracting toxoplasma infection varies with eating habits, contact with cats and other pets, and occupational exposure. Infection can also be acquired congenitally.

PROGNOSIS One systematic review of studies conducted from 1983–1996 found no population based prospective studies of the natural history of toxoplasma infection during pregnancy.[1] One systematic review reported nine controlled, non-randomised studies, and found that untreated toxoplasmosis acquired during pregnancy was associated with infection rates in children of between 10–100%.[3] We found two European studies that correlated gestation at time of seroconversion with risk of transmission and severity of disease at birth.[4,5] Risk of transmission increased with gestational age at maternal seroconversion, reaching 70–90% for infections acquired after 30 weeks' gestation. In contrast, the risk of the infected infant developing clinical disease was highest when infection occurred early in pregnancy. The highest risk of early signs of disease (including chorioretinitis and hydrocephaly) was about 10%, and occurred with infection between 24 and 30 weeks' gestation.[5] Infants with untreated congenital toxoplasmosis and generalised neurological abnormalities at birth develop mental retardation, growth retardation, blindness or visual defects, seizures, and spasticity. Children with untreated subclinical infection at birth may develop cognitive and motor deficits and visual defects or blindness up to the age of 20. One case control study in 845 school children in Brazil found mental retardation and retinochoroiditis to be significantly associated with positive toxoplasma serology (population attributable risk 6–9%).[6]

Congenital toxoplasmosis

AIMS	To prevent fetal transmission, congenital infection, ocular defects, and mental retardation in neonates and in later life, with minimum adverse effects.
OUTCOMES	Incidence of spontaneous abortion, fetal infection, and overt neonatal disease (mental retardation and ocular defects); serological positivity in the newborn; adverse effects of treatment.
METHODS	*Clinical Evidence* update search and appraisal November 2000.

QUESTION What are the effects on mother and baby of antiparasitic treatment in women found to be seropositive for toxoplasma during pregnancy?

We found no reliable evidence on the effects of treating women who seroconvert during pregnancy.

Benefits: We found two systematic reviews (search dates 1998). The first identified no RCTs.[3] The second review identified nine small cohort studies comparing treatments (spiramycin alone, pyrimethamine-sulphonamides, or a combination of the two treatments) versus no treatment.[7] One study of case series of women treated with spiramycin or spiramycin plus pyrimethamine/sulphonamide found no evidence of difference in outcomes (fetal infection, overt neonatal disease) associated with treatment.[8] Comparing data from these studies was difficult because of different follow up periods.

Harms: Spiramycin and pyrimethamine-sulphonamides are reportedly well tolerated and non-teratogenic.[9] Sulpha drugs are known to carry a risk of kernicterus in the newborn and should be avoided if possible in the third trimester; there is also a risk of bone marrow suppression, which can be reduced through concomitant use of folic acid.[9]

Comment: We found that the quality of evidence was poor, so we are uncertain whether antiparasitic drugs are more beneficial than harmful. Studies included in the systematic review were small, groups were not directly comparable, only two studies provided information about the control group, congenital infection was common in the treatment groups, and treatment was associated with reduced transmission in only five out of nine of the included studies.[7] One decision analysis on screening for and treating intrauterine toxoplasma infection has suggested a theoretical risk that treatment may save the pregnancy without preventing infection in the neonate, leading to a net increase in congenital cases.[10] Drug regimens of cotrimoxazole (trimethoprim plus sulphamethoxazole), atovaquone, or fluoroquinolones, which are either used or are being tested for secondary prophylaxis of toxoplasmosis in immunocompromised people (particularly those with HIV infection), have not been studied in pregnancy because their reproductive toxicity has not been properly documented. Finally, optimal duration of follow up is not established, although the longer the children are observed, the higher the incidence of sequelae.

REFERENCES

1. Eskild A, Oxman A, Magnus P, et al. Screening for toxoplasmosis in pregnancy: what is the evidence of reducing a health problem? *J Med Screen* 1996;3:188–194. Search date February 1996; primary sources Medline 1983 to February 1996; Cochrane Pregnancy and Childbirth Database, and hand searched references.

2. Carme B, Tirard-Fleury V. Toxoplasmosis among pregnant women in France: seroprevalence, seroconversion and knowledge levels: trends 1965–1995. *Med Malad Infect* 1996;26:431–436.

3. Wallon M, Liou C, Garner P, et al. Congenital toxoplasmosis: systematic review of evidence of efficacy of treatment in pregnancy. *BMJ* 1999; 318:1511–1514. Search date 1997; primary sources Medline, Embase, Pascal, Biological Abstracts, and personal communications.

4. Foulon W, Villena I, Stray-Pedersen B, et al. Treatment of toxoplasmosis during pregnancy: a multicenter study of impact on fetal transmission and children's sequelae at age 1 year. *Am J Obstet Gynecol* 1999;180:410–415.

5. Dunn D, Wallon M, Peyron F, et al. Mother-to-child transmission of toxoplasmosis: risk estimates for clinical counselling. *Lancet* 1999;353:1829–1833.

6. Caiaffa WT, Chiari CA, Figueiredo AR, et al. Toxoplasmosis and mental retardation – report of a case-control study. *Mem Inst Oswaldo Cruz* 1993; 88:253–261.

7. Peyron F, Wallon M, Liou C, et al. Treatments for toxoplasmosis in pregnancy. In: The Cochrane Library, Issue 2, 2000. Oxford: Update Software. Search date 1997; primary sources Medline, Embase, Pascal, Biological Abstracts, and the Cochrane Controlled Trials Register.

8. Vergani P, Ghidini A, Ceruti P, et al. Congenital toxoplasmosis: efficacy of maternal treatment with spiramycin alone. *Am J Reprod Immunol* 1998; 39:335–340.

9. Garland SM, O'Reilly MA. The risks and benefits of antimicrobial therapy in pregnancy. *Drug Saf* 1995;13:188–205.

10. Bader TJ, Macones GA, Asch DA. Prenatal screening for toxoplasmosis. *Obstet Gynecol* 1997;90:457–464.

Piero Olliaro
Scientist/Manager
UNDP/World Bank/WHO Special
Programme for Research and Training in
Tropical Diseases, CDS/CRD
World Health Organization
Geneva
Switzerland

Competing interests: None declared.

Search date September 2000: expanded this issue

Guy de Bruyn

Key Messages

- One systematic review and one additional RCT have found that empirical use of antibiotics in travellers' diarrhoea significantly increases the cure rate of diarrhoea. Treatment was associated in some people with prolonged excretion of bacterial pathogens in the stool and development of resistant strains.

- RCTs have found that ciprofloxacin reduces the duration of community acquired diarrhoea by 1–2 days. Trials of other antibiotics found no evidence of benefit or have not reported time to cure.

- One small RCT found no significant difference in the volume or duration of diarrhoea between rehydration intravenously or by nasogastric tube.

- Small RCTs have found that amino acid oral rehydration solutions (ORS) compared with standard ORS (see glossary, p 478) reduce the total volume and duration of diarrhoea. ORS in which bicarbonate was replaced by chloride or citrate were of similar effectiveness to standard ORS.

- Three RCTs found a small and inconsistent effect of reduced osmolarity ORS compared with standard ORS.

- One systematic review has found that rice based ORS compared with standard ORS reduces the 24 hour stool volume.

- RCTs have found that loperamide and loperamide oxide significantly reduce the time to relief of symptoms, but frequently cause constipation. We found insufficient evidence about the effects of other antimotility agents.

Infectious diseases

DEFINITION Diarrhoea is watery or liquid stools, usually with an increase in stool weight above 200 g a day and an increase in daily stool frequency.

INCIDENCE/ PREVALENCE An estimated 4000 million cases of diarrhoea occurred worldwide in 1996, resulting in 2.5 million deaths.[1] In developing countries, diarrhoea is reported to cause more deaths in children under 5 years than any other condition.[1] In the USA, which has a low incidence, the estimated incidence for infectious intestinal disease is 0.44 episodes per person a year, or one episode per person every 2.3 years, resulting in about one consultation with a doctor per person every 28 years.[2] A recent community study in the UK reported an incidence of 19 cases per 100 person years, of which 3.3 cases per 100 person years resulted in consultation with a general practitioner.[3] The epidemiology of travellers' diarrhoea (in people who have crossed a national boundary) is not well understood. Incidence is higher in travellers visiting developing countries, but it varies widely by location and season of travel.[4]

AETIOLOGY/ RISK FACTORS The cause depends on geographic location, standards of food hygiene, sanitation, water supply, and season. Commonly identified causes of sporadic diarrhoea in adults in developed countries include *Campylobacter*, *Salmonella*, *Shigella*, *Escherichia coli*, *Yersinia*, protozoa, and viruses. No pathogens are identified in more than half of people with diarrhoea. In returning travellers, about 80% of episodes are caused by bacteria, such as enterotoxigenic *E coli*, *Salmonella*, *Shigella*, *Campylobacter*, *Vibrio*, enteroadherent *E coli*, *Yersinia*, and *Aeromonas*.

PROGNOSIS Few studies have examined which factors predict poor outcome in adults. In developed countries, death from infectious diarrhoea is rare, although serious complications causing admission to hospital sometimes occur, such as severe dehydration and renal failure. Elderly people and those in long term care have an increased risk of death.[5]

AIMS To reduce the infectious period; length of illness; risk of dehydration; risk of transmission to others; and rates of severe illness; and to prevent complications and death.

OUTCOMES Time from start of treatment to last loose stool; number of loose stools a day; stool volume; time to first formed stool; duration of diarrhoea; duration of excretion of organisms; presence of bacterial resistance; relief of cramps, nausea and vomiting; incidence of vomiting; incidence of severe illness; and rate of hospital admission.

METHODS *Clinical Evidence* update search and appraisal September 2000. Trial quality was assessed on allocation concealment and inclusion of all randomised participants. Most trial participants had moderate to severe diarrhoea, usually defined as acute diarrhoea lasting less than 1 week, more than three loose stools in 24 hours or more than two loose stools in 8 hours, and symptoms of an enteric illness such as nausea, vomiting, and abdominal cramps.

QUESTION What are the effects of empirical antibiotic treatment in travellers' diarrhoea?

One systematic review and one additional RCT have found that empirical use of antibiotics significantly increases the cure rate of travellers' diarrhoea. Treatment was associated in some people with prolonged presence of bacterial pathogens in the stool and development of resistant strains.

Benefits: We found one systematic review[6] and one additional RCT.[7] The review (search date 1999, 12 RCTs, 1474 people with travellers' diarrhoea, including students, package tourists, military personnel, and volunteers)[6] compared empirical use of antibiotics versus placebo. Antibiotics evaluated included aztreonam, bicozamycin, ciprofloxacin, co-trimoxazole, fleroxacin, norfloxacin, ofloxacin, and trimethoprim, which were given for durations varying from a single dose to 5 days. The review found that antibiotics significantly increased the cure rate at 72 hours (defined as cessation of unformed stools, or less than 1 unformed stool/24 hours without additional symptoms; OR 5.9, 95% CI 4.1 to 8.6).[6] The additional RCT (598 people, 70% of whom had travelled recently) comparing norfloxacin versus placebo found that norfloxacin significantly increased the number of people cured after 6 days (34/46 [74%] v 18/48 [38%]; RR 1.97, 95% CI 1.32 to 2.95).[7]

Harms: The review found that adverse effects varied with each antibiotic, and ranged from 2% to 18%. Gastrointestinal symptoms (cramps, nausea, anorexia), dermatological symptoms (rash), and respiratory symptoms (cough, sore throat) were most frequently reported.[6] One small RCT included in the review found that significantly more people taking ciprofloxacin developed resistant isolates at 48 hours (ciprofloxacin v placebo; ARI 50%, 95% CI 15% to 85%).[6] Another RCT reported three cases of continued excretion of Shigella in people taking trimethoprim–sulfamethoxazole versus one person taking placebo.[8] Two of these isolates became resistant to the drug, although the participants were clinically well.[6] Other RCTs found no post-treatment resistance, or did not report it.[6] The additional trial found that people with salmonella infection treated with norfloxacin versus placebo had significantly prolonged excretion of Salmonella species (median time to clearance of Salmonella species from stool: norfloxacin v placebo 50 days v 23 days, CI not available).[7] In addition, six of nine Campylobacter isolates obtained after treatment had developed resistance to norfloxacin.

Comment: Only three of 10 trials using the duration of diarrhoea as an outcome reported adequate statistical data for the duration of diarrhoea after initiation of treatment.[6] This limits the generalisability of the results.

QUESTION What are the effects of empirical antibiotic treatment in community acquired diarrhoea?

RCTs have found that ciprofloxacin reduces duration of diarrhoea developed in the community by 1–2 days. Trials of other empirical treatments with antibiotics either found no effect or did not report time to cure.

Benefits: We found no systematic review. We found nine RCTs in eight reports[9–16] (1760 people) comparing one or more antibiotics with placebo (see table 1, p 480).[9–14] Trials were conducted in 12 sites in 11 countries. Four trials were conducted in developed countries, and the others took place in developing countries. The largest study included 332 adults in hospital in a multicentre trial of fleroxacin.[9] Eight trials evaluated quinolones, four evaluated co-trimoxazole, and one evaluated cloquinol.[9–16] Entry criteria varied between trials, and treatment duration ranged from a single dose to 5 days. Three trials found that antibiotics reduced illness duration or decreased number of liquid stools at 48 hours, whereas five found no benefit in reducing illness duration.[9–13,15,16] One trial found reduced duration for ciprofloxacin but not for co-trimoxazole.[12]

Harms: Adverse effects varied by agent. In one RCT of lomefloxacin, 33% of treated people reported adverse effects compared with 2.7% taking placebo (ARI 31%, 95% CI 17% to 46%). Two people were withdrawn from the trial after developing anaphylactic reactions.[12] In the same trial, 18% of treated people developed isolates resistant to lomefloxacin.[12] In the multicentre trial of ciprofloxacin and co-trimoxazole, five people with *Campylobacter* isolated from stool (2 treated with ciprofloxacin, 3 treated with co-trimoxazole) developed isolates resistant to the treatment antibiotic.[14] In the largest trial, three deaths occurred (2 with fleroxacin v 1 with placebo). Two of the deaths occurred from hypovolaemic shock (1 with fleroxacin v 1 with placebo).[15]

Comment: The main pathogenic organisms found in each study varied and may partly explain variations in effect. Reported outcomes varied between trials, which precludes direct comparisons or summaries of treatment effect.

QUESTION What are the effects of oral rehydration for severe diarrhoea?

We found no direct studies of oral rehydration compared with placebo or no treatment. Numerous RCTs compared one type of rehydration with another. One small RCT found no difference in duration or volume of diarrhoea following rehydration intravenously or by nasogastric tube. Two RCTs have found that amino acid ORS compared with standard ORS reduces the total volume and duration of diarrhoea. One small RCT found no significant effect of replacing bicarbonate with chloride, and three RCTs found no effect of replacing bicarbonate with citrate. Three RCTs found a small and inconsistent effect of reduced osmolarity ORS compared with standard ORS. One systematic review has found that rice based ORS compared with standard ORS reduces the 24 hour stool volume.

Benefits: Results of the studies are summarised in Table 2 on the *Clinical Evidence* website (www.clinicalevidence.org) **Versus no rehydration:** We found no systematic review or RCTs. Such studies would be unethical. **Versus intravenous rehydration:** We found no systematic review. We found one small RCT (20 adults with cholera and severe dehydration) of enteral rehydration through a nasogastric tube compared with intravenous rehydration.[17] Both groups received initial intravenous fluids. The trial found no significant difference in the total duration of diarrhoea (44 hours v 37 hours; difference + 7 hours, 95% CI –6 to +20 hours), total volume of stool passed (8.2 litres v 11 litres; difference –2.8 litres, 95% CI –8 litres to +3 litres), or duration of Vibrio excretion (1.1 days v 1.4 days; difference 0.3 days, 95% CI 0 days to 1 day). **Amino acid ORS:** We found no systematic review. We found three RCTs.[18–20] In the two RCTs where intravenous rehydration was given, the amino acid ORS compared with the standard ORS reduced the total duration of diarrhoea and the total volume of stool.[18,19] **Bicarbonate free ORS:** We found no systematic review. We found one small RCT (60 people with cholera and severe dehydration) comparing standard ORS plus bicarbonate versus an otherwise identical ORS in which the bicarbonate was replaced with chloride.[21] The trial found no significant difference in total stool output or duration of diarrhoea. **Citrate ORS:** We found no systematic review. We found three RCTs (367 people).[22–24] None of the trials found a significant difference between citrate and standard/bicarbonate ORS in the duration or volume of diarrhoea. **Reduced osmolarity ORS:** We found no systematic review. We found three RCTs,[25–27] which found a small and inconsistent effect on total volume of stool and duration of diarrhoea. **Rice based ORS:** We found one systematic review (search date 1998, 22 RCTs) in people with cholera and non-cholera diarrhoea.[28] The review found that in adults and children with cholera, rice based ORS versus standard ORS significantly reduced the 24 hour stool volume (adults: 4 RCTs, WMD –51 ml/kg, 95% CI –66 ml/kg to –35 ml/kg; children: 5 RCTs, WMD –67 ml/kg, 95% CI –94 ml/kg to –41 ml/kg). One RCT found that both rice based ORS and low sodium rice based ORS reduced stool output compared with standard ORS (4 litres for rice based ORS v 5 litres for standard ORS, P < 0.02; 3 litres for low sodium rice based ORS v 5 litres for standard ORS, P < 0.05).[27]

Harms: **Versus amino acid ORS:** One RCT reported no episodes of hypernatraemia or hyponatraemia in people taking a modified ORS or standard ORS.[20] **Citrate versus bicarbonate ORS:** One RCT reported that more people taking citrate ORS had an unpleasant taste than those taking bicarbonate ORS (29% v 13%).[23] In another trial, two of 115 people taking an effervescent citrate ORS had an unpleasant taste (results not reported for bicarbonate ORS).[24] **Versus reduced osmolarity ORS:** Reduced osmolarity ORS significantly increased the risk of non-symptomatic hyponatraemia (OR 2.1, 95% CI 1.1 to 4.1).[25] In RCTs evaluating symptomatic hyponatraemia, no cases were reported.[25,26]

Comment: All people with cholera received antibiotic therapy in addition to fluid therapy. Oral tetracycline or doxycycline were widely used, and were initiated at varying intervals after the start of oral fluid therapy. Response to ORS in people with cholera may not be comparable to those with less severe forms of diarrhoea.

Infectious diseases

RCTs have found that in people with acute diarrhoea, loperamide and loperamide oxide significantly reduce the time to relief of symptoms, but may cause constipation. We found insufficient evidence about the effects of other antimotility agents.

Benefits: We found no systematic review. **Difenoxin:** We found no RCTs of sufficient quality. **Diphenoxylate:** One RCT (152 adults with acute diarrhoea for < 24 hours) comparing diphenoxylate–atropine versus placebo found that diphenoxylate significantly reduced the number of bowel actions in the 24 hours after treatment (P = 0.05).[29] The trial found no significant difference between in median time to last loose stool (25 v 30 hour, P = 0.29). **Lidamidine:** We found two RCTs (30 adults[30] and 105 adults[31] with acute diarrhoea), comparing lidamidine (loading dose of 2–4 mg, then subsequent doses 6-hourly or as required) versus placebo.[30,31] The first RCT found that lidamidine reduced the stool weight after 29 hours (lidamidine 4 mg v 2 mg v placebo; 435 g v 364 g v 576 g).[30] The second RCT found that lidamidine reduced the number of loose stools after 72 hours (8.5 v 3.9, significance not stated).[31] **Loperamide:** We found four RCTs comparing loperamide (loading dose of 4 mg, then 2 mg with each loose stool) versus placebo.[31–34] Two of the RCTs (409 people[32] and 261 people[33] with acute diarrhoea) found that loperamide significantly reduced the median time to complete relief of symptoms, which was defined as the time between taking the first two tablets and the time after which one pasty, watery, or loose stool was passed (189 people: loperamide v placebo, 27 v 45 hours, P = 0.006;[32] 123 people: loperamide v placebo, 18 v 37 hours, P = 0.007).[33] The third RCT (50 people) found that loperamide versus placebo significantly reduced the number of stools for the first 2 days, but subsequently the difference was not significant.[34] The fourth RCT found no significant difference in the number of stools passed within 72 hours.[31] **Loperamide oxide:** We found four RCTs (409 people,[32] 261 people,[33] 230 people,[35] 242 people[35] with acute diarrhoea) comparing loperamide oxide (loading dose varying between 1 and 4 mg, followed by 0.5–2 mg with each loose stool) versus placebo.[32,33,35,36] All RCTs found that loperamide oxide significantly reduced the time to complete relief of symptoms.

Harms: **Lidamidine:** Constipation occurred in one of 35 (2.8%) people taking lidamidine versus none of 35 (0%) people taking placebo.[31] **Loperamide:** Two RCTs found that constipation was significantly more frequent in people taking loperamide versus placebo (25% v 7%; ARI 18%, 95% CI 8% to 28%; NNH 5, 95% CI 3 to 12;[32] 22% v 10.3%; ARI 12%, 95% CI 5% to 29%; NNH 5, 95% CI 3 to 18).[33] **Loperamide oxide:** One RCT found that significantly more people taking loperamide oxide had constipation (loperamide oxide v placebo, 24% v 7%; ARI 17%, 95% CI 7% to 27%; NNH 5, 95% CI 3 to 14).[32] Another RCT found that symptom scores for tiredness and sleepiness were significantly higher in people taking loperamide oxide 1 mg versus placebo (P = 0.01).[35]

Comment: The RCTs used different outcome measures, making it difficult to summarise and compare results.

GLOSSARY

Standard ORS A solution that includes citrate 10 mmol/litre and glucose 111 mmol/litre, and has an osmolarity of 311 mmol/litre.

Substantive changes since last issue

Travellers' diarrhoea New systematic review;[6] conclusion unchanged.

REFERENCES

1. *The World Health Report 1997.* Geneva: World Health Organization, 1997:14–22.
2. Garthwright WE, Archer DL, Kvenberg JE. Estimates of incidence and costs of intestinal infectious diseases in the United States. *Public Health Rep* 1988;103:107–115.
3. Wheeler JG, Sethi D, Cowden JM, et al. Study of infectious intestinal disease in England: rates in the community, presenting to general practice, and reported to national surveillance. *BMJ* 1999; 318:1046–1050.
4. Cartwright RY, Chahed M. Foodborne diseases in travellers. *World Health Stat Q* 1997;50:102–110.
5. Lew JF, Glass RI, Gangarosa RE, et al. Diarrheal deaths in the United States 1979 through 1987. *JAMA* 1991;265:3280–3284.
6. De Bruyn G, Hahn S, Borwick A. Antibiotic treatment for travellers' diarrhoea (Cochrane Review). In: The Cochrane Library, Issue 3, 2000. Oxford: Update Software. Search date 1999; primary sources Medline, Embase, Cochrane Collaboration Trials Register, plus hand searching to identify additional trials.
7. Wistrom J, Jertborn M, Ekwall E, et al. Empiric treatment of acute diarrheal disease with norfloxacin: a randomized, placebo-controlled study. Swedish Study Group. *Ann Intern Med* 1992;117:202–208.
8. Ericsson CD, Johnson PC, DuPont HL, Morgan DR, Bitsura JM, De la Cabada FJ. Ciprofloxacin or trimethoprim–sulfamethoxazole as initial therapy for travelers' diarrhea. *Ann Intern Med* 1987;106: 216–220.
9. De la Cabada FJ, DuPont HL, Gyr K, et al. Antimicrobial therapy of bacterial diarrhea in adult residents of Mexico – lack of an effect. *Digestion* 1992;53:134–141.
10. Ellis-Pegler RB, Hyman LK, Ingram RJ, et al. A placebo controlled evaluation of lomefloxacin in the treatment of bacterial diarrhoea in the community. *J Antimicrob Chemother* 1995;36: 259–263.
11. Pichler HE, Diridl G, Stickler K, et al. Clinical efficacy of ciprofloxacin compared with placebo in bacterial diarrhea. *Am J Med* 1987;82(suppl 4A): 329–332.
12. Goodman LJ, Trenholme GM, Kaplan RL, et al. Empiric antimicrobial therapy of domestically acquired acute diarrhea in urban adults. *Arch Intern Med* 1990;150:541–546.
13. Noguerado A, Garcia-Polo I, Isasia T, et al. Early single dose therapy with ofloxacin for empirical treatment of acute gastroenteritis: a randomised, placebo-controlled double-blind clinical trial. *J Antimicrob Chemother* 1995;36:665–672.
14. Dryden MS, Gabb RJ, Wright SK. Empirical treatment of severe acute community-acquired gastroenteritis with ciprofloxacin. *Clin Infect Dis* 1996;22:1019–1025.
15. Butler T, Lolekha S, Rasidi C, et al. Treatment of acute bacterial diarrhea: a multicenter international trial comparing placebo with fleroxacin given as a single dose or once daily for 3 days. *Am J Med* 1993;94(3A):187–194.
16. Lolekha S, Patanachareon S, Thanangkul B, et al. Norfloxacin versus co-trimoxazole in the treatment of acute bacterial diarrhoea: a placebo controlled study. *Scand J Infect Dis* 1988;56(suppl):35–45.
17. Pierce NF, Sack RB, Mitra RC, et al. Replacement of water and electrolyte losses in cholera by an oral glucose-electrolyte solution. *Ann Intern Med* 1969;70:1173–1181.
18. Nalin DR, Cash RA, Rahman M, Yunus MD. Effect of glycine and glucose on sodium and water absorption in patients with cholera. *Gut* 1970;11: 768–772.
19. Patra FC, Sack DA, Islam A, Alam AN, Mazumder RN. Oral rehydration formula containing alanine and glucose for treatment of diarrhoea: a controlled trial. *BMJ* 1989;298:1353–1356.
20. Khin-Maung-U, Myo-Khin, Nyunt-Nyunt-Wai, Tin-U. Comparison of glucose/electrolyte and maltodextrin/glycine/glycyl-glycine/electrolyte oral rehydration solutions in cholera and watery diarrhoea in adults. *Ann Trop Med Parasitol* 1991; 85:645–650.
21. Sarker SA, Mahalanabis D. The presence of bicarbonate in oral rehydration solution does not influence fluid absorption in cholera. *Scand J Gastroenterol* 1995;30:242–245.
22. Mazumder RN, Nath SK, Ashraf H, Patra FC, Alam AN. Oral rehydration solution containing trisodium citrate for treating severe diarrhoea: controlled clinical trial. *BMJ* 1991;302:88–89.
23. Hoffman SL, Moechtar MA, Simanjuntak CH, et al. Rehydration and maintenance therapy of cholera patients in Jakarta: citrate-based versus bicarbonate-based oral rehydration salt solution. *J Infect Dis* 1985;152:1159–1165.
24. Ahmed SM, Islam MR, Butler T. Effective treatment of diarrhoeal dehydration with an oral rehydration solution containing citrate. *Scand J Infect Dis* 1986;18:65–70.
25. Alam NH, Majumder RN, Fuchs GJ, et al. Efficacy and safety of oral rehydration solution with reduced osmolarity in adults with cholera: a randomised double-blind clinical trial. *Lancet* 1999;354:296–299.
26. Faruque ASG, Mahalanabis D, Hamadani JD, Zetterstrom R. Reduced osmolarity oral rehydration salt in cholera. *Scand J Infect Dis* 1996;28:87–90.
27. Bhattacharya MK, Bhattacharya SK, Dutta D, et al. Efficacy of oral hyposmolar glucose-based and rice-based oral rehydration salt solutions in the treatment of cholera in adults. *Scand J Gastroenterol* 1998;33:159–163.
28. Fontaine O, Gore SM, Pierce NF. Rice-based oral rehydration solution for treating diarrhoea. In: The Cochrane Library, Issue 3, 2000. Oxford: Update Software. Search date 1998; primary sources Medline, Embase, Lilacs, Cochrane Controlled Trials Register, Cochrane Infectious Diseases Group.

29. Lustman F, Walters EG, Shroff NE, Akbar FA. Diphenoxylate hydrochloride (Lomotil®) in the treatment of acute diarrhoea. *Br J Clin Pract* 1987;41:648–651.

30. Heredia Diaz JG, Alcantara I, Solis A. Evaluation of the safety and effectiveness of WHR-1142A in the treatment of non-specific acute diarrhea. *Rev Gastroenterol Mex* 1979;44:167–73 [in Spanish].

31. Heredia Diaz JG, Kajeyama Escobar ML. Double-blind evaluation of the effectiveness of lidamidine hydrochloride (WHR-1142A) vs loperamide vs. placebo in the treatment of acute diarrhea. *Salud Publica Mex* 1981;23:483–491 [in Spanish].

32. Hughes IW. First line treatment in acute non-dysenteric diarrhoea: clinical comparison of loperamide oxide, loperamide and placebo. *Br J Clin Pract* 1995;49:181–185.

33. Van den Eynden B, Spaepen W. New approaches to the treatment of patients with acute, nonspecific diarrhea: a comparison of the effects of loperamide and loperamide oxide. *Curr Ther Res* 1995;56:1132–1141.

34. Van Loon FPL, Bennish ML, Speelman P, Butler C. Double blind trial of loperamide for treating acute watery diarrhoea in expatriates in Bangladesh. *Gut* 1989;30:492–495.

35. Dettmer A. Loperamide oxide in the treatment of acute diarrhea in adults. *Clin Ther* 1994;16:972–980.

36. Dreverman JWM, Van der Poel AJM. Loperamide oxide in acute diarrhoea: a double-blind, placebo-controlled trial. *Aliment Pharmacol Ther* 1995;9:441–446.

Guy de Bruyn
Resident in Internal Medicine
Baylor College of Medicine
Houston, Texas
USA

Competing interests: None declared.

TABLE 1   Effects of empirical antibiotic treatment of community acquired diarrhoea: results of placebo controlled RCTs (see text, p 475).

Intervention	Total number of participants	Mean duration of diarrhoea from start of treatment		Difference between means (95% CI)*
		Placebo group	Intervention group	
Lomefloxacin 400 mg daily for 5 days[10]	84	3.2 days	4.4 days	+ 1.2 days (0.1 day to 2.5 days)
Ofloxacin 400 mg single dose[13]	117	3.4 days	2.5 days	−0.9 days (−1.8 days to 0.0 days)
Cotrimoxazole 800/160 mg bd for 3 days[9]	287	30.2 h	24.4 h	−5.8 h
Cloquinol 250 mg tid for 3 days[9]	287	30.2 h	25.5 h	−4.7 h
Enoxacin 400 mg bd for 5 days[9]	137	44.9 h	38.9 h	−6 h
Cotrimoxazole 160/800 mg bd for 5 days[9]	137	44.9 h	42.3 h	−2.6 h
Ciprofloxacin 500 mg bd for 5 days[11]	162	2.9 days	1.5 days	−1.4 days
Ciprofloxacin 500 mg bd for 5 days[12]	173	3.4 days	2.4 days	−1 day
Cotrimoxazole 160/800 mg bd for 5 days[12]	173	3.4 days	NA	NA
Ciprofloxacin 500 mg bd for 5 days[14]	85	4.6 days	2.2 days	−2.4 days

*If available from published data; bd, twice daily; h, hours; NA, not available from published data; tid, three times daily.

Search date November 2000

David Wilkinson, Andrew Phillips and Margaret Johnson

INTERVENTIONS

Key Messages

Prevention

- One RCT has found that effective treatment of symptomatic sexually transmitted diseases (STDs) reduces the incidence of HIV infection.

- One RCT found no evidence of benefit from presumptive, mass treatment for STDs.

- We found limited evidence from one observational study suggesting that improving STD prevention and treatment services, and targeting them at high risk groups such as sex workers, reduces the incidence of HIV infection.

- We found limited evidence from one case control study suggesting that postexposure prophylaxis with zidovudine may reduce the risk of HIV infection. Evidence from other settings suggests that combining several antiretroviral drugs is likely to be more effective than zidovudine alone.

Treatment

- Two large RCTs have found that triple therapy (combining two nucleoside analogue drugs and a protease inhibitor) halves the risk of AIDS and death over about 1 year compared with double therapy.

HIV infection

- Large RCTs found no evidence that the overall risk of serious adverse effects is significantly greater on triple than on double therapy. Triple therapy is likely to reduce the risk of drug resistance compared with double therapy.
- One systematic review of RCTs of zidovudine monotherapy found no significant difference between early versus deferred treatment in the long term risk of AIDS free survival or overall survival. We found no RCTs evaluating delayed versus early treatment with two or three drug regimens.

DEFINITION	HIV infection refers to infection with the human immunodeficiency virus type 1 or type 2. Clinically, this is characterised by a variable period (average around 8–10 years) of asymptomatic infection, followed by repeated episodes of illness of varying and increasing severity as immune function deteriorates. The type of illness varies greatly by country, availability of specific treatment for HIV, and prophylaxis for opportunistic infections.
INCIDENCE/ PREVALENCE	Worldwide estimates suggest that, by December 1999, around 50 million people had been infected with HIV, about 16 million people had died as a result, and about 16 000 new HIV infections were occurring each day.[1] About 90% of HIV infections occur in the developing world.[1] Occupationally acquired HIV infection in health-care workers has been documented in 95 definite and 191 possible cases, although this is likely to be an underestimate.[2]
AETIOLOGY/ RISK FACTORS	The major risk factor for transmission of HIV is unprotected hetero-sexual or homosexual intercourse. Other risk factors include needle-stick injury, sharing drug injecting equipment, and blood transfu-sion. An HIV infected woman may also transmit the virus to her baby. This has been reported in 15–30% of pregnant women with HIV infection. Not everyone who is exposed to HIV will become infected, although risk increases if exposure is repeated, at high dose, or through blood. There is at least a 2–5 times greater risk of HIV infection among people with STDs.[3]
PROGNOSIS	Without treatment, about half of people infected with HIV will become ill and die from AIDS over about 10 years.
AIMS	To reduce transmission of HIV; to prevent or delay the onset of AIDS, as manifested by opportunistic infections and cancers; to increase survival; to minimise loss of quality of life caused by inconvenience of current regimens and adverse effects of interventions.
OUTCOMES	Incidence of HIV infection, new AIDS diseases, and adverse events; mortality; quality of life.
METHODS	*Clinical Evidence* update search and appraisal November 2000. In addition, we contacted experts in the field, and reviewed abstract books and CDs for conferences held since 1995. Trials were included if they were designed to detect differences in clinical end points. We have included data on single and two drug antiretroviral regimens, because the evidence may be useful in countries where three drug treatment is not currently widely available.

OPTION   EARLY DETECTION AND TREATMENT OF STDS

One RCT has found that effective treatment of symptomatic STDs reduces the incidence of HIV infection.

Benefits: We found no systematic review. One trial randomised 12 communities in Tanzania (about 12 000 people) to intervention or no intervention. Intervention consisted of providing effective drugs for STDs and healthcare workers trained in STD case management.[4] Intervention reduced the risk of acquiring HIV over 2 years (RRR 42%, 95% CI 21% to 58%).

Harms: Syndromic case management (treating people for the most likely causes of their symptoms and signs) may result in wrong or unnecessary treatment. The RCT gave no information on this.[4]

Comment: There is a clear biological mechanism for the synergistic effect of STDs on HIV transmission, and for STD control as an HIV control strategy. The inflammation associated with STDs increases HIV shedding in genital secretions, and treating STDs reduces this inflammation.[5] Syndromic management of STDs is more commonly used in developing countries. In developed countries, a microbiological diagnosis is usually made, allowing specific treatment. The trial, randomised by the community and analysed by the individual, uses regression analysis in an attempt to overcome the associated cluster bias, but it is unclear if this is successful.

OPTION   PRESUMPTIVE STD TREATMENT

One RCT found no evidence of benefit from presumptive, mass treatment for STDs.

Benefits: We found no systematic review. One RCT randomised 10 communities in Uganda (about 12 000 people) to intervention or no intervention.[6] Intervention consisted of treating all adults with several drugs for STDs every 10 months. Although prevalence of some STDs fell in intervention communities, there was no significant difference in the incidence of HIV between intervention and control communities over 20 months of follow up (incidence of HIV in both groups about 1.5 per 100 person years; RR intervention v control 0.97, 95% CI 0.81 to 1.16).[6]

Harms: Mass treatment means that many uninfected people will be unnecessarily treated for STDs, exposing them to risks of adverse drug reactions and drug resistance. The RCT gave no information on these.

Comment: The trials' negative finding has several possible explanations other than ineffectiveness of the intervention: a high incidence of symptomatic STDs between rounds of mass treatment; a low population attributable risk for treatable STDs; or intense exposure to HIV. The trial, randomised by the community and analysed by the individual, uses regression analysis in an attempt to overcome the associated cluster bias, but it is unclear if this is successful. As many as 80% of STDs are unrecognised or asymptomatic.[7]

OPTION IMPROVING AND TARGETING PREVENTIVE SERVICES

One observational study has found that improving STD prevention and treatment services and targeting them at high risk groups, such as sex workers, reduces the incidence of HIV infection.

Benefits: We found no systematic review and no RCTs. One observational study (531 sex workers in Zaire) found that promotion of condoms, improvement of STD treatment services, and monthly screening of women for STDs significantly reduced the incidence of HIV infection (3 year follow up; incidence of HIV reduced from 11.7% to 4.4%, $P = 0.003$).[8]

Harms: None reported.

Comment: This non-randomised study is subject to selection bias and confounding. For example, over time the number of uninfected sex workers, and therefore the pool of people susceptible to infection, will fall, which may partly explain the fall in HIV incidence.

QUESTION What are the effects of postexposure prophylaxis in healthcare workers?

One case control study found that, in people exposed to HIV, those who became infected were less likely to have received postexposure prophylaxis with zidovudine. Evidence from other settings suggests that combined treatment with several antiretroviral drugs is likely to be more effective than treatment with zidovudine alone.

Benefits: We found no systematic review or RCTs. **Zidovudine alone:** One case control study from the USA and France evaluated outcomes in 31 health workers who acquired HIV infection after occupational exposure, and outcomes in 679 controls who did not acquire HIV infection despite occupational exposure.[9] This study included people followed up for at least 6 months after exposure. HIV infection was less likely in people who received postexposure prophylaxis compared with those who did not (reduction in OR by 81%, 95% CI 43% to 94%). It found that that the risk of seroconversion increased with severity of exposure; for example, a penetrating injury with a hollow, bloody needle carried the greatest risk.[9] **Zidovudine plus other antiretroviral drugs:** We found no studies of postexposure prophylaxis using combinations of antiretroviral drugs.

Harms: Short term toxicity (including fatigue, nausea, and vomiting) and gastrointestinal discomfort have been reported by 50–75% of people taking zidovudine and caused 30% to discontinue postexposure prophylaxis.[10] Treatment studies suggest that frequency of adverse effects is higher in people taking a combination of antiretroviral drugs (reported in 50–90%), which may reduce adherence to postexposure prophylaxis (24–36% discontinued). The risk of drug interactions is also increased. Severe adverse effects, including hepatitis and pancytopenia, have been reported in people taking combination postexposure prophylaxis, but the incidence is not known.

Comment: Case control studies are considered sufficient because experimental studies are hard to justify ethically, and are logistically difficult because of the low rate of seroconversion in those exposed. A summary of 25 studies (22 seroconversions in 6955 exposed people) found that the risk of HIV transmission after percutaneous exposure was 0.32% (95% CI 0.18% to 0.45%) and the risk after mucocutaneous exposure was 0.03% (95% CI 0.006% to 0.19%).[2] Indirect evidence for postexposure prophylaxis comes from animal studies[9] and from a placebo controlled RCT of zidovudine in pregnant women, which found reduced frequency of mother to child HIV transmission, presumed to be caused in part by postexposure prophylaxis.[11] RCTs have found that combinations of two, three, or more antiretroviral drugs are more effective than single drug regimens in suppressing viral replication. There is also an unquantified risk that zidovudine alone may not prevent transmission of zidovudine resistant strains of HIV. This constitutes the rationale for combining antiretroviral drugs for postexposure prophylaxis.

QUESTION   What are the effects of different antiretroviral treatment regimens?

OPTION   TWO DRUG VERSUS ONE DRUG ANTIRETROVIRAL REGIMENS

Large RCTs, with an average follow up of 3.5 years, have found that two drug regimens (zidovudine plus another nucleoside analogue drug) reduce the risk of new AIDS defining illnesses and death compared with zidovudine alone. Adverse events were more common with two drug regimens.

Benefits: We found one systematic review (search date not stated, 6 RCTs, 7700 people) comparing zidovudine/didanosine or zidovudine/zalcitabine versus zidovudine alone.[12] Participants entered the trials with various stages of infection and were followed for an average of 29 months, during which time 2904 progressed and 1850 died. The combined drug regimens versus single drugs were associated with both delayed progression (RR with addition of didanosine 0.74, 95% CI 0.67 to 0.82; RR with addition of zalcitabine 0.86, 95% CI 0.78 to 0.94), and death (RR with addition of didanosine 0.72, 95% CI 0.64 to 0.82; RR with addition of zalcitabine 0.87, 95% CI 0.77 to 0.98). After 3 years, the estimated percentages of people who were alive and without a new AIDS event were 53% for zidovudine plus didanosine v 49% for zidovudine plus zalcitabine v 44% for zidovudine alone; the percentages alive were 68% v 63% v 59%. One trial (940 people) of zalcitabine plus saquinavir (a protease inhibitor) versus either drug as monotherapy found significantly fewer cases of clinical disease or death (RR 0.51, 95% CI 0.36 to 0.72).[13] Another large trial found that, in people with low CD4 positive T cell counts (25–250/mm³), adding lamivudine (a nucleoside analogue) to regimens containing zidovudine (zidovudine alone in 62%, zidovudine plus didanosine or zalcitabine in the rest) significantly reduced the risk of AIDS or death over about a year (HR 0.42, 95% CI 0.32 to 0.57).[14]

Harms: Adverse effects such as anaemia and neutropenia were common in all groups in these trials. Up to a third of participants experienced a serious adverse event, with the highest rates in those with lower CD4 counts. Adverse events led to cessation of blind treatment in about a third of participants. The addition of didanosine to zidovudine versus zidovudine alone increased the risk of nausea (RR 1.8, 95% CI 1.1 to 2.9), abdominal pain (RR 1.6, 95% CI 1.0 to 2.7), and pancreatitis (RR 4.6, 95% CI 1.0 to 22.0). Addition of zalcitabine increased the risk of neuropathy (RR 2.2, 95% CI 1.4 to 3.6).[12] Addition of lamivudine did not significantly increase the rate of adverse events.[14]

Comment: Two drug regimens, using two nucleoside analogue reverse transcriptase inhibitors, allow substantial residual viral replication in an environment where drug resistant variants have selective advantage. Resistance to these drugs tends to develop over several months to years.[15] The relevance of this is not fully understood but prior use of, and measurable resistance to, nucleoside analogue reverse transcriptase inhibitors tends to be associated with poorer virological response to new regimens that include drugs of this class.[16–18]

OPTION   **THREE DRUG REGIMENS CONTAINING PROTEASE INHIBITOR VERSUS TWO DRUG REGIMENS**

Two RCTs have found that using a protease inhibitor with two nucleoside analogue drugs halves the risk of new AIDS diseases or death over about 1 year compared with two nucleoside analogue drugs alone. The risk of serious adverse effects was not significantly increased over this time period.

Benefits: We found no systematic review. We found two large RCTs with less than 2 years' follow up. The first RCT compared zidovudine/lamivudine/indinavir versus zidovudine/lamivudine in people who had previously been treated with zidovudine (CD4 counts < 200/mm^3).[19] It found a significant difference in rates of AIDS or death in favour of triple therapy (RR 0.50, 95% CI 0.33 to 0.76; ARR 5%). The second RCT, published only in abstract form, compared zidovudine/zalcitabine/saquinavir versus zidovudine/zalcitabine or zidovudine/saquinavir in people with CD4 counts of 50–350/mm^3, who had no previous experience of zidovudine (HJ Stellbrink, Sixth European Conference on Clinical Aspects and Treatment of HIV Infection, Hamburg, 1997). It also found significantly greater benefit with triple therapy (RR of AIDS or death 0.5, P = 0.0001). This RCT found that health related quality of life did not change significantly over 48 weeks for those in the triple therapy group (change from baseline –0.4 points for physical health summary and +1.4 for mental health summary); a deterioration occurred in both dual therapy groups (–2.5 and +0.1, respectively, for zalcitabine/saquinavir and –2.2 and +0.3, respectively, for zidovudine/saquinavir).[20]

Harms: In the first RCT, about a fifth of participants in both groups experienced serious adverse events.[17] The most common were non-specific discomfort, malaise, fever, headache, nausea, and vomiting. The addition of indinavir reduced the risk of neutropenia (5% v 15%; P < 0.001) but increased the risk of hyperbilirubinaemia (6% v 1%; P < 0.001) and renal colic/nephrolithiasis (4% v 1%; P = 0.001).

Comment: Longer term follow up of patients taking protease inhibitors has found abnormal fat distribution, hyperglycaemia, and raised triglyceride and cholesterol concentrations. The clinical significance of these changes is uncertain. Many drugs interact with protease inhibitors because of inhibition of cytochrome P450.

OPTION   EARLY VERSUS DEFERRED ANTIRETROVIRAL TREATMENT

One systematic review of RCTs compared early with deferred antiretroviral treatment, but the RCTs were all started when zidovudine was the only drug available. Overall, they found no significant difference in the risk of AIDS free survival or overall survival with extended follow up. We found no RCTs exploring this question with two or three drug regimens.

Benefits: We found one systematic review (published 2000, search date not stated, 5 RCTs, 7722 people with asymptomatic HIV mainly with CD4 counts > 200/mm^3) comparing zidovudine given immediately versus zidovudine deferred until the early signs of AIDS.[21] It found that immediate versus deferred treatment significantly increased AIDS free survival at 1 year (78/4431 [1.76%] with immediate zidovudine v 131/3291 [3.98%] with deferred zidovudine; OR 0.52, 95% CI 0.39 to 0.68), but the difference was not significant at the end of the RCTs (median follow up 50 months; 1026/4431 [23.2%] with immediate zidovudine v 882/3291 [26.8%] with deferred zidovudine; OR 0.96, 95% CI 0.87 to 1.05). Overall survival was similar in the two groups at 1 year (24/4431 [5.4%] with immediate zidovudine v 18/3291 [5.5%] with deferred zidovudine; OR 1.22, 95% CI 0.67 to 2.25) and at the end of the RCTs (734/4431 [16.6%] with immediate zidovudine v 617/3291 [18.7%] with deferred zidovudine; OR 1.04, 95% CI 0.93 to 1.16).

Harms: A meta-analysis presented pooled toxicity data in terms of events per 100 patient years.[22] In asymptomatic people, early treatment conferred a significant but small increase in the risk of anaemia (RR of haemoglobin < 8.0 g/dl, early v deferred treatment 2.1, 95% CI 1.1 to 4.1; AR 0.4 events per 100 person years). There was also a small increase in risk of neutropenia with early treatment (AR 1.1 events per 100 person years; P = 0.07). In symptomatic people, the excess incidence of severe anaemia probably reflected the high doses of zidovudine (1200–1500 mg/day; RR of severe anaemia, high v low dose 3.6, 95% CI 1.3 to 10). The authors advised that the toxicity results should be interpreted cautiously, as the data varied considerably.

Comment: No new trials on this question are ongoing. With three drug regimens, rates of AIDS and death are currently low and treatment is known to be beneficial up to and over a 2 year period (see three drug regimens, p 486). Many feel sufficiently certain about when to start treatment — based on data on HIV pathogenesis, resistance, immune regeneration with treatment, and long term adverse effects — and so would not consider randomisation to immediate versus deferred treatment. Decisions on when to initiate multidrug treatment are currently based on our understanding of how HIV induces immune damage, the capacity for immune regeneration while on treatment, the toxicity and inconvenience of treatment, and the risk of resistance, rather than on results of RCTs.

Substantive changes since last issue

Early versus deferred antiretrovirals New systematic review;[22] conclusion unchanged.

REFERENCES

1. United Nations AIDS website: http://www.unaids.org.
2. Public Health Laboratory Services. *Occupational transmission of HIV. Summary of published reports.* London: PHLS, December 1997.
3. Centres for Disease Control and Prevention. HIV prevention through early detection and treatment of other sexually transmitted diseases – United States. *MMWR Morb Mortal Wkly Rep* 1998;47: RR12.
4. Grosskurth H, Mosha F, Todd J, et al. Impact of improved treatment of sexually transmitted diseases on HIV infection in rural Tanzania: randomised controlled trial. *Lancet* 1995;346: 530–536.
5. Cohen MS, Hoffman IF, Royce RA, et al. Reduction of concentration of HIV-1 in semen after treatment of urethritis: implications for prevention of sexual transmission of HIV-1. *Lancet* 1997;349:1868–1873.
6. Wawer MJ, Sewankambo NK, Serwadda D, et al. Control of sexually transmitted diseases for AIDS prevention in Uganda: a randomised community trial. *Lancet* 1999;353:525–535.
7. Wilkinson D, Abdool Karim SS, Harrison A, et al. Unrecognised sexually transmitted infections in rural South African women: a hidden epidemic. *Bull World Health Organ* 1999;77:22–28.
8. Laga M, Alary M, Nzila N, et al. Condom promotion, sexually transmitted diseases treatment, and declining incidence of HIV-1 infection in female Zairian sex workers. *Lancet* 1994;344:246–248.
9. Centers for Disease Control and Prevention. Public health service guidelines for the management of health-care worker exposures to HIV and recommendations for post exposure prophylaxis. *MMWR Morb Mortal Wkly Rep* 1998;47:RR7.
10. Cardo DM, Culver DH, Ciesielski CA, et al. Case-control study of HIV seroconversion in health care workers after percutaneous exposure. *N Engl J Med* 1997;337:1485–1490.
11. Connor EM, Sperling RS, Gelber R, et al. Reduction of maternal–infant transmission of human immunodeficiency virus type 1 with zidovudine treatment: paediatric AIDS clinical trials group protocol 076 study group. *N Engl J Med* 1994;331:1173–1180.
12. HIV Trialists' Collaborative Group. Zidovudine, didanosine, and zalcitabine in the treatment of HIV infection: meta-analyses of the randomised evidence. *Lancet* 1999;353:2014–2015. Search date not stated; primary sources Medline, hand searches of conference proceedings, and personal contact with investigators and pharmaceutical companies.
13. Haubrich R, Lalezari J, Follansbee SE, et al.

Improved survival and reduced clinical progression in HIV-infected patients with advanced disease treated with saquinavir plus zalcitabine. *Antivir Ther* 1998;3:33–42.
14. CAESAR Co-ordinating Committee. Randomized trial of addition of lamivudine or lamivudine plus loviride to zidovudine-containing regimens for patients with HIV-1 infection: the CAESAR trial. *Lancet* 1997;349:1413–1421.
15. Brun-Vezinet F, Boucher C, Loveday C, et al. HIV-1 viral load, phenotype, and resistance in a subset of drug-naïve participants from the Delta trial. *Lancet* 1997;350:983–990.
16. D'Aquila RT, Johnson VA, Welles SL, et al. Zidovudine resistance and HIV-1 disease progression during antiretroviral therapy. *Ann Intern Med* 1995;122:401–408.
17. Ledergerber B, Egger M, Opravil M, et al. Clinical progression and virological failure on highly active antiretroviral therapy in HIV-1 patients: a prospective cohort study. *Lancet* 1999;353:863–868.
18. Staszewski S, Miller V, Sabin CA, et al. Virological response to protease inhibitor therapy in an HIV clinic cohort. *AIDS* 1999;13:367–373.
19. Hammer SM, Squires KE, Hughes MD, et al. A controlled trial of two nucleoside analogues plus indinavir in persons with HIV infection and CD4 cell counts of 200/mm^3 or less. *N Engl J Med* 1997;337:725–733.
20. Revicki DA, Moyle G, Stellbrink HJ, Barker C. Quality of life outcomes of combination zalcitabine–zidovudine, saquinavir–zidovudine, and saquinavir–zalcitabine–zidovudine therapy for HIV-infected adults with CD4 cell counts between 50 and 350/mm^3. *AIDS* 1999;13:851–858.
21. Darbyshire J, Foulkes M, Peto R, et al. Immediate versus deferred zidovudine (AZT) in asymptomatic or mildly symptomatic HIV infected adults. In: The Cochrane Library, Issue 4, 2000. Oxford: Update Software. Search date not stated; primary sources Medline, hand searches of conference abstracts, and contact with investigators and pharmaceutical companies.s
22. Ioannidis JP, Cappelleri JC, Lau J, et al. Early or deferred zidovudine therapy in HIV-infected patients without an AIDS-defining illness: a meta-analysis. *Ann Intern Med* 1995;122:856–866. Search date 1994; primary sources Medline, AIDSLine, AIDSTrials, AIDSDrugs, CHEMID, hand searches of current contents, and international conferences on AIDS.

David Wilkinson
Professor
South Australian Centre
for Rural and Remote Health University
of Adelaide and University of South
Australia
Whyalla
Australia

Andrew Phillips
Professor
Royal Free Centre for HIV Medicine
and Department of Primary Care
and Population Sciences
Royal Free and University College
Medical School
London
UK

Margaret Johnson
Consultant in HIV Medicine
Royal Free Hospital
London
UK

Competing interests: DW and MJ, none declared. AP has received reimbursement for attending and speaking at symposia, funds for research and members of staff, and fees for consulting from various pharmaceutical companies producing antiretroviral drugs, including Abbott, Boehringer Ingleheim, Agouron, GlaxoSmithKline, Bristol-Myers Squibb, Roche, and DuPont.

Infectious diseases

Search date November 2000: new for this issue

Timothy Uyeki and Andrea Winquist

INTERVENTIONS

Key Messages

- One systematic review and four additional RCTs have found that oral amantadine versus placebo reduces the duration of influenza A symptoms by about 1 day. We found insufficient evidence about adverse effects in this setting.
- One systematic review has found that oral rimantadine versus placebo reduces the duration of influenza A symptoms by about 1 day. We found insufficient evidence about adverse effects in this setting
- One systematic review and three additional RCTs have found that orally inhaled zanamivir versus placebo reduces the duration of influenza symptoms by about 1 day. Adverse effects were similar in people taking zanamivir versus placebo.
- Two RCTs have found that oral oseltamivir versus placebo reduces the duration of influenza symptoms by about 1 day. Oral oseltamivir versus placebo increases the incidence of nausea and vomiting.
- We found insufficient evidence about the effects of antiviral agents on reducing serious complications of influenza, but we found strong evidence that influenza immunisation reduces the risk of complications and death in people at high risk for complications from influenza, including elderly people (see influenza vaccine under community acquired pneumonia, p 1040).
- We found no good evidence of benefit if treatment is started more than 2 days after symptom onset for amantadine, rimantadine, or zanamivir versus placebo, or if treatment is started more than 1.5 days after symptom onset with oseltamivir versus placebo.

DEFINITION	Influenza is caused by infection with influenza viruses. Uncomplicated influenza is characterised by the abrupt onset of fever, chills, non-productive cough, myalgias, headache, nasal congestion, sore throat, and fatigue.[1] Influenza is usually diagnosed clinically. Not all people infected with influenza viruses become symptomatic. People infected with other pathogens may have symptoms identical to those of influenza.[2] The percentage of infections resulting in clinical illness can vary from approximately 40–85%, depending on age and pre-existing immunity to the virus.[3] Influenza can be confirmed by viral culture, immunofluorescence staining, enzyme immunoassay, or rapid diagnostic testing of nasopharyngeal, nasal or throat swab specimens, or by serologic testing of paired sera. Some rapid tests detect influenza A only, some detect and distinguish between influenza A and B, whereas others detect but do not distinguish between influenza A and B.
INCIDENCE/ PREVALENCE	In temperate areas of the Northern Hemisphere, influenza activity typically peaks between late December and early March whereas, in temperate areas of the Southern Hemisphere, influenza activity typically peaks between May and September. In tropical areas, influenza can occur throughout the year.[2] The annual incidence of influenza varies yearly, and depends partly on the underlying level of population immunity to circulating influenza viruses.[1] One localised study in the USA found that serological conversion with or without symptoms occurred in 10–20% a year, with the highest infection rates in people aged under 20 years.[4] Attack rates are higher in institutions and in areas of overcrowding.[5]
AETIOLOGY/ RISK FACTORS	Influenza viruses are transmitted primarily from person to person through respiratory droplets disseminated during sneezing, coughing, and talking.[1,6]
PROGNOSIS	The incubation period of influenza is 1–4 days and infected adults are usually contagious from the day before symptom onset until 5 days after symptom onset. The signs and symptoms of uncomplicated influenza usually resolve within a week, although cough and fatigue may persist.[1] Complications include otitis media, bacterial sinusitis, secondary bacterial pneumonia, and less commonly, viral pneumonia and respiratory failure. Complications are also caused by exacerbation of underlying disease.[1,2] In the USA each year, over 110 000 admissions to hospital and about 20 000 deaths are related to influenza.[2] The risk of hospitalisation is highest in people 65 years or older, in very young children, and in those with chronic medical conditions.[1,7,8] Over 90% of influenza related deaths during recent seasonal epidemics in the USA have been in people 65 years or older.[1] During influenza pandemics, morbidity and mortality may be high in younger age groups.[1] Severe illness is more common with influenza A infections than influenza B infections.[1]
AIMS	To reduce the duration and severity of influenza signs and symptoms, the risk of complications, and to minimise adverse effects of treatment.
OUTCOMES	Severity and duration of symptoms; frequency and severity of complications of influenza; adverse effects of treatment.
METHODS	*Clinical Evidence* search and appraisal November 2000. The

authors searched Medline (1966 to 2000; major MeSH topics: amantadine and influenza, rimantidine and influenza; keywords: zanamivir, 4-guanidino-Neu5Ac2en, GG167, oseltamivir, GS4104, and Ro64-0796). Meeting abstracts were used to identify unpublished studies of zanamivir and oseltamivir. We included only systematic reviews and double blind RCTs of treatment versus placebo for naturally occurring influenza. We excluded RCTs and reviews of chemoprophylaxis of influenza, experimentally induced influenza, and reviews that combined RCTs of more than one agent. For amantadine and rimantadine, we included only RCTs of influenza A. For zanamivir and oseltamivir, we included studies of influenza A or B. For zanamivir, we included only RCTs of orally inhaled drug and excluded intranasal drops plus oral inhalation unless oral inhalation results were reported separately. For amantadine, rimantadine, and oseltamivir, we included only RCTs of oral administration. We excluded RCTs primarily on children younger than 18 years, those that used an antipyretic rather than a placebo as control, RCTs in which the delay from symptom onset to starting treatment was unclear, and RCTs without quantitative measures of clinical effectiveness.

| QUESTION | What are the effects of antiviral treatment of influenza in adults? |

| OPTION | ORAL AMANTADINE |

One systematic review and three additional RCTs have found that oral amantadine versus placebo reduces the duration of influenza A symptoms by about 1 day. We found insufficient evidence to assess adverse effects in this setting.

Benefits: We found one systematic review (search date 1997, 7 RCTs, 531 otherwise healthy people)[9] and three additional RCTs[10-12] of oral amantadine (usually started within 48 hours of symptom onset) versus placebo for the treatment of influenza A (see table 1 on website: www.clinicalevidence.org). The review found that amantadine significantly reduced the duration of fever (temperature > 37.0 °C reduced by 1 day, 95% CI 0.7 to 1.3). We found no RCTs of the effect of amantadine in preventing serious complications of influenza, such as pneumonia or exacerbation of chronic diseases. We found no RCTs of amantadine for treatment of influenza A in pregnant women, those with chronic disease, or in immunised people.

Harms: The review found no difference in the frequency of adverse effects between amantadine and placebo groups. However, the included RCTs contained little information about the relative adverse effects of amantadine compared with placebo when used for treatment of influenza A[13-15] (see table 1 on website: www.clinicalevidence.org). We found insufficient evidence to assess adverse effects in this setting. More evidence is available about the harms of amantadine when used for prophylaxis of influenza A (see comment below).

Comment: In vitro studies have found that amantadine has specific antiviral activity against influenza A, but not influenza B viruses.[16] The RCTs

Infectious diseases

used different outcome measures, so summarising results is difficult. Only one RCT examined amantadine in elderly people.[12] All RCTs considered only people with laboratory confirmed influenza A, so the analyses were not by intention to treat. The percentage of influenza isolates from the general population exhibiting resistance to amantadine has remained low.[17,18] Amantadine resistant influenza A viruses have not been found to be more virulent than non-resistant viruses.[2] The limited evidence from elderly and high risk groups makes it difficult to generalise results to these populations. A systematic review found that use of amantadine versus placebo for prophylaxis of influenza A is associated with an increased incidence of gastrointestinal and central nervous system adverse effects.[9]

| OPTION | ORAL RIMANTADINE |

One systematic review has found that oral rimantadine versus placebo reduces the duration of influenza A symptoms by about 1 day. We found insufficient evidence about adverse effects in this setting.

Benefits: We found one systematic review (search date 1997, 3 RCTs, 104 otherwise healthy adults)[9] and one small additional RCT[19] of rimantadine (usually started within 48 hours of symptom onset) versus placebo for the treatment of influenza A (see table 1 on website: www.clinicalevidence.org). The review found that rimantadine versus placebo significantly reduced the duration of fever (temperature > 37.0 °C reduced by 1.3 days, 95% CI 0.8 to 1.8). We found no RCTs of rimantadine for treatment of influenza A in people over 65 years of age, in pregnant women, in those with chronic disease, or in immunised people. We found no RCTs of the effect of rimantadine in preventing serious complications of influenza, such as pneumonia or exacerbation of chronic diseases.

Harms: The review found insufficient evidence about the adverse effects of rimantadine versus placebo in people with influenza A.[9] One non-systematic review (340 adults) of rimantadine treatment versus placebo found that more people taking rimantidine had central nervous system symptoms, most commonly insomnia (10.8% v 8.6%, P value not stated), and gastrointestinal symptoms, most commonly abdominal pain and nausea (6.0% v 2.3%, P value not stated).[20] Additional evidence is available about adverse effects of rimantadine when used for prophylaxis of influenza A (see comment below).

Comment: In vitro studies have found that rimantadine has specific antiviral activity against influenza A, but not influenza B viruses.[16] The RCTs used different outcome measures so summarizing results is difficult. Additional studies of rimantadine have been performed in Russia, but information in English is limited.[21] Viruses that are resistant to rimantadine show cross resistance to amantadine, and vice versa.[17] Influenza A viruses resistant to rimantadine have not been found to be more virulent than non-resistant viruses.[2] The proportion of influenza isolates from the general population exhibiting resistance to rimantadine (or amantadine) has remained low.[17,18] The limited evidence from elderly

Infectious diseases

and high risk groups makes it difficult to generalise results to these populations. A systematic review found that use of rimantadine versus placebo for prophylaxis of influenza A is associated with an increased incidence of gastrointestinal adverse effects.[9]

OPTION   ORALLY INHALED ZANAMIVIR

One systematic review and three additional RCTs have found that orally inhaled zanamivir versus placebo reduces the duration of influenza symptoms by about 1 day. Adverse effects are similar in people taking zanamivir versus placebo.

Benefits: We found one systematic review (search date 1999, 3 RCTs, 1588 people)[22] and three additional RCTs (387 people),[23–25] which compared inhaled zanamivir (usually started within 48 hours of symptom onset) versus placebo for the treatment of naturally occurring influenza (see table 2 on website: www.clinicalevidence.org). The review found that zanamivir versus placebo significantly reduced the time to alleviation of symptoms (median time reduced by 1.0 day, 95% CI 0.5 to 1.5 days). The results of the three additional RCTs have not yet been integrated into the systematic review but appear to find similar results (see table 2 on website: www.clinicalevidence.org).[23–25] Some of the RCTs included small numbers of people 65 years or older, and people with chronic cardiac or respiratory illness. We found no RCTs of the effect of zanamivir in preventing serious complications of influenza, such as pneumonia, or exacerbation of chronic diseases.

Harms: Adverse effects were similar in people taking zanamivir compared with placebo (the inhaled lactose vehicle alone) (see table 2 on website: www.clinicalevidence.org).[23–28] Use of zanamivir has been associated with bronchospasm and worsening of underlying respiratory disease (see comment below).[29]

Comment: Zanamivir is administered as an orally inhaled powder. In vitro studies have found that zanamivir has antiviral activity against both influenza A and B viruses.[30] RCTs have included predominantly people with influenza A (≥ 85%). Some of the RCTs included small numbers of people at high risk for complications from influenza (e.g. people aged 65 years and older, people with chronic cardiac or respiratory disease).[25–28] Because of the short period that zanamivir has been available, and the lack of optimal assays to detect resistant strains, we found insufficient evidence to comment on the development of viral resistance to zanamivir.[2,31,32] The observational evidence that zanamivir is associated with bronchospasm and worsening of underlying respiratory disease suggests that zanamivir should not usually be recommended for people with underlying airways disease because of the risk of serious events.[29]

| OPTION | ORAL OSELTAMIVIR |

Two RCTs have found that oral oseltamivir versus placebo reduces the duration of influenza symptoms by about one day but increases the incidence of nausea and vomiting.

Benefits: We found no systematic review of oseltamivir used to treat influenza. We found two RCTs of oseltamivir versus placebo.[33,34] People in both RCTs were selected with a temperature of 38.0°C or greater. Both RCTs found that oseltamivir (started within 36 hours of symptom onset) versus placebo significantly reduced the duration of influenza symptoms by about 1 day (see table 1 on website: www.clinicalevidence.org). We found no RCTs of oseltamivir for influenza in people 65 years or older, in pregnant women, in people with chronic disease, or in vaccinated people. We found no RCTs of the effect of oseltamivir in preventing serious complications of influenza, such as pneumonia, or exacerbation of chronic diseases.

Harms: Nausea and vomiting were significantly more common in people receiving oseltamivir versus placebo.[33,34]

Comment: Studies in mice and ferrets have found that oseltamivir has in vitro activity against both influenza A and B viruses.[35] The RCTs predominantly included people with influenza A (97%).[33,34] Because of the short period that oseltamivir has been available, and the lack of optimal assays to detect resistant strains, we found insufficient evidence to comment on the development of viral resistance to oseltamivir.[2,32]

REFERENCES

1. Cox NJ, Fukuda K. Influenza. Infect Dis Clin North Am 1998;12:27–38.
2. CDC. Prevention and control of influenza: recommendations of the Advisory Committee on Immunization Practices (ACIP). MMWR 2000; 49(No. RR-3).
3. Fox JP, Cooney MK, Hall CE, Foy HM. Influenza virus infections in Seattle families, 1975–1979. II. Pattern of infection in invaded households and relation of age and prior antibody to occurrence of infection and related illness. Am J Epidemiol 1982;116:228–242.
4. Sullivan KM, Monto AS, Longini IM. Estimates of the US health impact of influenza. Am J Public Health 1993;83:1712–1716.
5. Kilbourne ED. Influenza. New York: Plenum Medical Book Co, 1987:269–270.
6. Tablan OC, Anderson LJ, Arden NH, Breiman RF, Butler JC, McNeil MM. Hospital Infection Control Practices Advisory Committee. Guideline for prevention of nosocomial pneumonia. Infect Control Hosp Epidemiol 1994;15:587–604.
7. Neuzil KM, Mellen BG, Wright PF, Mitchel EF, Griffin MR. The effect of influenza on hospitalizations, outpatient visits, and courses of antibiotics in children. N Engl J Med 2000;342: 225–231.
8. Izurieta HS, Thompson WW, Kramarz P, et al. Influenza and the rates of hospitalization for respiratory disease among infants and young children. N Engl J Med 2000;342:232–239.
9. Jefferson TO, Demicheli V, Deeks JJ, Rivetti D. Amantadine and rimantadine for preventing and treating influenza A in adults. In: The Cochrane Library, Issue 3, 2000. Oxford: Update Software.

Search date 1997; primary sources Medline, Cochrane Controlled Trials Register, Embase, reviews of references of identified trials, and letters to manufacturers and authors.
10. Baker LM, Shock MP, Iezzoni DG. The therapeutic efficacy of Symmetrel (amantadine hydrochloride) in naturally occurring influenza A2 respiratory illness. J Am Osteopath Assoc 1969;68:1244–1250.
11. Galbraith AW, Schild AW, Schild GC, Potter CW, Watson GI. The therapeutic effect of amantadine in influenza occurring during the winter of 1971–1972 assessed by double-blind study. J R Coll Gen Pract 1973;23:34–37.
12. Walters HE, Paulshock M. Therapeutic efficacy of amantadine HCl. Mo Med 1970;67:176–179.
13. Kitamoto O. Therapeutic effectiveness of amantadine hydrochloride in influenza A2: double-blind studies. Jpn J Tuberc Chest Dis 1968;15: 17–26.
14. Kitamoto O. Therapeutic effectiveness of amantadine hydrochloride in naturally occurring Hong Kong influenza: double-blinded studies. Jpn J Tuberc Chest Dis 1971;17:1–7.
15. Van Voris LP, Betts RF, Hayden FG, Christmas WA, Douglas RG. Successful treatment of naturally occurring influenza A/USSR/77 H1N1. JAMA 1981;245:1128–1131.
16. Tominack RL, Hayden FG. Rimantadine hydrochloride and amantadine hydrochloride use in influenza A virus infections. Infect Dis Clin North Am 1987;1:459–478.
17. Belshe RB, Burk B, Newman F, Cerruti RL, Sim IS. Resistance of influenza A viruses to amantadine and rimantadine: results of one decade of

surveillance. *J Infect Dis* 1989;159:430–435.

18. Ziegler T, Hemphill ML, Ziegler M-L, et al. Low incidence of rimantadine resistance in field isolates of influenza A viruses. *J Infect Dis* 1999; 180:935–939.

19. Rabinovich S, Baldini JT, Bannister R. Treatment of influenza: the therapeutic efficacy of rimantadine HCl in a naturally occurring influenza A2 outbreak. *Am J Med Sci* 1969;257:328–335.

20. Soo W. Adverse effects of rimantadine: summary from clinical trials. *J Respir Dis* 1989;10 (suppl): S26–S31.

21. Zlydnikov DM, Kubar OI, Kovaleva TP, Kamforin LE. Study of rimantadine in the USSR: a review of the literature. *Rev Infect Dis* 1981;3:408–421.

22. National Institute of Clinical Excellence. Fast track appraisal of zanamivir (Relenza): summary of evidence. Available at: http://www.nice.org.uk/appraisals/appraisals.htm. Accessed December 23, 1999. Search date 1999; primary sources Cochrane library, Health Star, PharmLine, Medline, Embase, and National Research Register. Information was also solicited from drug manufacturer.

23. Hayden FG, Osterhaus ADME, Treanor JJ, et al. Efficacy and safety of the neuraminidase inhibitor zanamivir in the treatment of influenza virus infections. *N Engl J Med* 1997;337:874–880.

24. Matsumoto K, Ogawa N, Nerome K, et al. Safety and efficacy of the neuraminidase inhibitor zanamivir in treating influenza virus infection in adults: results from Japan. *Antiviral Ther* 1999;4: 61–68.

25. Bovin G, Goyette N, Hardy I, Aoki F, Wagner A, Trottier S. Rapid antiviral effect of inhaled zanamivir in the treatment of naturally occurring influenza in otherwise healthy adults. *J Infect Dis* 2000;181:1471–1474.

26. The MIST (Management of Influenza in the Southern Hemisphere Trialists) Study Group. Randomized trial of efficacy and safety of inhaled zanamivir in treatment of influenza A and B infections. *Lancet* 1998;352:1877–1881.

27. Lalezari J, Klein T, Stapleton J, Elliott M, Flack N, Keene O. The efficacy and safety of inhaled zanamivir in the treatment of influenza in otherwise healthy and 'high risk' individuals in North America [abstract]. *J Antimicrob Chemother* 1999;44(suppl A):42.

28. Makela MJ, Pauksens K, Rostila T, et al. Clinical efficacy and safety of the orally inhaled neuraminidase inhibitor zanamivir in the treatment of influenza: a randomized, double-blind, placebo-controlled European study. *J Infect* 2000;40:42–48.

29. Henney JE. Revised labeling for zanamivir. *JAMA* 2000;284:1234.

30. Woods JM, Bethell RC, Coates JAV, et al. 4-guanidino-2,4-dideoxy-2,3-dehydro-N-acetylneuraminic acid is a highly effective inhibitor of both the sialidase (neuraminidase) and growth of a wide range of influenza A and B viruses *in vitro*. *Antimicrob Agents Chemother* 1993;37: 1473–1479

31. Read RC. Letter to the Editor. *Lancet* 1999;353: 668–669.

32. Tisdale M. Monitoring of viral susceptibility: new challenges with the development of influenza NA inhibitors. *Rev Med Virol* 2000;10:45–55.

33. Treanor JJ, Hayden FG, Vrooman PS, et al. Efficacy and safety of the oral neuraminidase inhibitor oseltamivir in treating acute influenza: a randomized controlled trial. *JAMA* 2000;283: 1016–1024.

34. Nicholson KG, Aoki FY, Osterhaus ADME, et al. Efficacy and safety of oseltamivir in treatment of acute influenza: a randomized controlled trial. *Lancet* 2000;355:1845–1850.

35. Mendel DB, Tai CY, Escarpe PA, et al. Oral administration of a prodrug of the influenza virus neuraminidase inhibitor GS4071 protects mice and ferrets against influenza infection. *Antimicrob Agents Chemother* 1998;42:640–646.

Timothy Uyeki
Medical Epidemiologist
Centers for Disease Control and
Prevention
National Center for Infectious Diseases
Division of Viral and Rickettsial Diseases
Influenza Branch
Atlanta
Georgia
USA

Andrea Winquist
Medical Epidemiologist
Centers for Disease Control and
Prevention
Epidemiology Program Office
Division of Applied Public Health Training
State Branch
Atlanta
Georgia
USA

Competing interests: None declared.

Search date May 2000: new for this issue

Edward Hayes

QUESTIONS

INTERVENTIONS

Beneficial
Three doses of recombinant Osp–A Lyme disease vaccine with adjuvant in immunocompetent people aged 15–70 years exposed to North American strains of *Borrelia burgdorferi* 499

Likely to be beneficial
Penicillin (better than placebo for Lyme arthritis) 501
Doxycycline (as effective as amoxycillin and probenecid for Lyme arthritis) 501
*Ceftriaxone (more effective than penicillin for Lyme arthritis) . .501
*Cefotaxime (more effective than penicillin for Lyme arthritis) . .501
*Cefotaxime (more effective than penicillin for late neurological Lyme disease) 503

Unknown effectiveness
Lyme disease vaccine in Europe or Asia 499
Ceftriaxone (in late neurological Lyme disease) 503

Likely to be ineffective or harmful
Oral antibiotic treatment of people with Lyme arthritis plus neuroborreliosis 501

To be covered in future issues of *Clinical Evidence*
Effects of Lyme disease vaccine in children
Effects of prophylactic treatment of tick bite

* Based on subgroup analysis of RCTs
See glossary, p 504

Key Messages

Administration of Lyme disease vaccine

- One RCT has found that a vaccine (consisting of recombinant outer surface protein A [Osp–A] of *Borrelia burgdorferi* combined with adjuvant) reduces the incidence of Lyme disease in people at high risk of developing Lyme disease within North America. The vaccine does not appear to cause serious adverse effects. The commonest adverse effect is a local reaction at the injection site. Two large RCTs have found no evidence of arthritis after vaccination.

- We found no evidence about the effectiveness of recombinant Osp–A vaccine in European or Asian populations. There is heterogeneity of the species that cause Lyme disease in Europe and Asia. The vaccine may not be as effective in Europe or Asian populations as it is in North America.

- We found no evidence about the effectiveness of the vaccine in children.

© *Clinical Evidence* 2001;5:497–504.

Treatment of Lyme arthritis

- One RCT of people with Lyme arthritis has found that penicillin is significantly more effective than saline placebo in resolving Lyme arthritis.

- One RCT of people with Lyme arthritis has found that doxycycline is as effective as amoxicillin plus probenicid in resolving Lyme arthritis.

- Other RCTs have reported results for subgroups of people with Lyme arthritis and have found weak evidence that ceftriaxone and cefotaxime may both be more effective than penicillin at improving Lyme arthritis.

- We found limited evidence that some people may be at risk of developing symptoms of neuroborreliosis after oral antibiotic treatment of Lyme arthritis.

Treatment of late neurological Lyme disease

- We found no RCTs specifically in people with late neurological Lyme disease.

- Weak evidence from two small RCTs reporting results for subgroups of people with late neurological Lyme disease suggests that cefotaxime and ceftriaxone may be more effective than other antibiotics in eliminating neurological symptoms.

DEFINITION Lyme disease is an inflammatory illness resulting from infection with spirochetes of the *Borrelia burgdorferi* genospecies transmitted to humans by ticks. Some infected people have no symptoms. The characteristic manifestation of early Lyme disease is erythema migrans, a circular rash at the site of the infectious tick attachment that expands over a period of days to weeks in 80–90% of people with Lyme disease. Early disseminated infection may cause secondary erythema migrans, disease of the nervous system (facial palsy or other cranial neuropathies, meningitis, and radiculoneuritis), musculoskeletal disease (arthralgia) and, rarely, cardiac disease (myocarditis or transient atrioventricular block). Untreated or inadequately treated Lyme disease can cause late disseminated manifestations weeks to months after infection. These late manifestations include arthritis, polyneuropathy, and encephalopathy. Diagnosis of Lyme disease is based primarily on clinical findings and a high likelihood of exposure to infected ticks. Serologic testing may be helpful in people with endemic exposure who have clinical findings consistent with later stage disseminated Lyme disease.

INCIDENCE/ PREVALENCE Lyme disease occurs in temperate regions of North America, Europe, and Asia. It is the most commonly reported vector borne disease in the USA, with over 16 000 cases reported a year.[1] Most cases occur in the northeastern and northcentral states, with a reported annual incidence in endemic states as high as 67.9 of 100 000 people.[1] In highly endemic communities, the incidence of Lyme disease may exceed 1000 of 100 000 persons a year.[2] In some countries of Europe, the incidence of Lyme disease has been estimated to be over 100 of 100 000 persons a year.[3] Foci of Lyme disease have been described in northern forested regions of Russia, in China, and in Japan.[4] Transmission cycles of *B burgdorferi* have not been described in tropical areas or in the Southern hemisphere.[4]

AETIOLOGY/ RISK FACTORS Lyme disease is caused by infection with any of the *B burgdorferi* sensu lato genospecies. Virtually all cases of Lyme disease in North America are the result of infection with *B burgdorferi*. In Europe, Lyme disease may be caused by *B burgdorferi*, *B garinii*, and

B afzelii. The infectious spirochetes are transmitted to humans through the bite of certain *Ixodes* ticks.[4] Humans who have frequent or prolonged exposure to the habitats of infected *Ixodes* ticks are at highest risk of acquiring Lyme disease. Individual risk depends on the likelihood of being bitten by infected tick vectors, which varies with the density of vector ticks in the environment, the prevalence of infection in ticks, and the extent of a person's contact with infected ticks. The risk of Lyme disease is often concentrated in focal areas. In the USA, risk is highest in certain counties within northeastern and northcentral states during the months of April to July.[2] People become infected when they engage in activities in wooded or brushy areas that are favourable habitats for ticks, deer, and rodent hosts.

PROGNOSIS	Lyme disease is rarely fatal. Untreated Lyme arthritis resolves at a rate of 10–20% a year; over 90% of facial palsies due to Lyme disease resolve spontaneously, and most cases of Lyme carditis resolve without sequelae.[5] However, untreated Lyme disease can result in arthritis (50% of untreated patients), meningitis or neuropathies (15% of untreated patients), carditis (5–10% of untreated patients with erythema migrans) and, rarely, encephalopathy.
AIMS	To prevent Lyme disease; to ameliorate or eliminate the symptoms of established Lyme disease; to reduce sequelae, with minimal adverse effects.
OUTCOMES	For prophylaxis: incidence of Lyme disease, adverse events. For treatment: incidence, prevalence, or severity of symptoms and signs of short term manifestations; long term sequelae of infection; quality of life.
METHODS	*Clinical Evidence* search and appraisal May 2000. Additional searches of author's files.

QUESTION   What are the effects of measures to prevent Lyme disease?

OPTION   LYME DISEASE VACCINE

One RCT has found that the currently commercially available recombinant Osp–A vaccine significantly reduces the incidence of Lyme disease in immunocompetent adults 15 years or older in North America who are at high risk of Lyme disease. We found no evidence about the effectiveness of this vaccine in Europe or Asia, where a greater variety of *B burgdorferi* genospecies cause Lyme disease.

Benefits: We found no systematic review but found one RCT (10 936 people, aged 15–70 years, living in endemic areas in the USA), which compared a vaccine made of recombinant outer surface lipoprotein A (Osp–A) plus adjuvant (see glossary, p 504) versus placebo.[6] People in the RCT were self selected and were at high risk of Lyme disease. The RCT found that, compared with placebo, the vaccine significantly reduced laboratory confirmed Lyme disease after two doses in the first year (absolute risk of developing Lyme disease, AR 22/5469 [0.4%] with vaccine *v* 43/5467 [0.8%] with placebo; RR 0.51, 95% CI 0.31 to 0.85; NNT 260, 95% CI 146 to 1046). After a third dose 1 year later, there was a greater reduction of the incidence of laboratory confirmed Lyme disease (AR 16/5469 [0.3%] with vaccine v 66/5467 [1.2%] with placebo; RR 0.24, 95% CI 0.14 to 0.42; NNT 110, 95% CI 80 to 167); asymptomatic infection was prevented completely (AR 0/5469 [0%] with vaccine v 15/5467 [0.3%] with placebo; NNT 365, 95% CI 222 to 687).

Harms: We found five RCTs evaluating adverse events of Osp–A vaccines.[6–10] No serious adverse events were found to be causally related to the vaccine in any of these trials. The RCT comparing a commercially available 30 µg vaccine versus placebo[6] found that of 9998 people asked to report any adverse events after each dose, the commonest local adverse event was soreness at the injection site (RR 3.2, 95% CI 2.9 to 3.5; NNH 6). Redness and swelling were significantly more frequent in the vaccine group, although they occurred in under 2% of vaccinated people. Early systemic side effects were significantly higher in vaccinated people (RR 1.3, 95% CI 1.2 to 1.4; NNH 23, 95% CI 17 to 35). Systemic effects that had higher incidence in vaccinated people in the first month after injection were myalgias (RR 1.8, 95% CI 1.4 to 2.3; NNH 71), achiness (RR 1.4, 95% CI 1.1 to 1.9; NNH 166), influenza-like illness (RR 1.8, 95% CI 1.3 to 2.5; NNH 111), fever (RR 2.5, 95% CI 1.7 to 3.6; NNH 83), and chills (RR 3.6, 95% CI 2.3 to 5.6; NNH 76). Arthralgia during the 30 days following vaccination, headache, fatigue, upper respiratory tract infections, and arthralgias occurring more than 30 days after vaccination seldom occurred and were similar in both groups. Late effects (> 30 days after vaccination) were similar in both groups (RR 1.2, 95% CI 1.0 to 1.5). One RCT (250 children aged 5–15 years) compared two different doses of recombinant Osp–A vaccine (30 µg v 15 µg) with adjuvant.[8] Doses of vaccine were given at 0, 1, and 2 months. All participants completed and returned diary cards recording adverse events for 3 days after each vaccination. Soreness at the injection site was reported by 72% of those receiving the first 30 µg dose, and redness at the injection site by 43% of vaccine recipients after any given dose. Headache and malaise were the commonest systemic symptoms, particularly after the first 15 µg dose (18% reported headache and 20% reported malaise). All general symptoms resolved within 6 days of vaccination. No significant differences were found for duration of side effects with 15 µg versus 30 µg vaccines. One RCT (240 people) compared three formulations of vaccine (given at 0, 1, 2 months). Local redness and swelling occurred in around a quarter of people after the third dose of vaccine.[10] We found no evidence to evaluate the risk of adverse events of Lyme disease vaccine that might occur more than 2 years after vaccine administration.

Comment: **Applicability of the evidence:** The absolute benefit of vaccination in the RCT[6] was high (1 case of Lyme disease prevented for every 110 people vaccinated), partly because the people recruited into the RCT were self selected and had a very high incidence of Lyme disease in the untreated group. If the risk of Lyme disease in the unvaccinated population was 100 of 100 000 persons a year (comparable to the reported Lyme disease incidence in many endemic areas)[1,3] then about 1316 people would need to be vaccinated to prevent one case of Lyme disease. We found no evidence about the effectiveness of this vaccine in Europe or Asia, and no evidence of efficacy in children. **Other RCTs:** One RCT evaluated the efficacy of recombinant Osp–A vaccine without adjuvant.[7] It found that the vaccine reduced the incidence of Lyme disease by 68% (95% CI 36% to 85%) after two doses in the first year. However, the criteria for confirming the diagnosis of Lyme disease were not clearly defined. Of 1734 suspected cases of Lyme disease in 2 years, only 499 were reviewed "in depth" by the data and safety monitoring board. The RCT reported an estimate of vaccine efficacy after a third dose of vaccine, but this dose was not part of the original RCT protocol, was given only to a subset of participants, and the criteria for selection of the subset who received the third dose were not specified. This RCT found that the efficacy of vaccine was highest in people aged under 60 years, but results for this subgroup were not presented.[7] A large RCT of Lyme disease vaccine in children (aged 4 years or older in the USA) is in progress.[8]

QUESTION   **What are the effects of antibiotic treatment for Lyme disease arthritis?**

One RCT has found that penicillin is significantly more effective in resolving Lyme arthritis than saline placebo. Another RCT has found that doxycycline is as effective in resolving Lyme arthritis as amoxicillin plus probenicid. Other RCTs have reported results for subgroups of people with Lyme arthritis and have found that ceftriaxone and cefotaxime may both be more effective than penicillin at improving Lyme arthritis. Some people have developed symptoms of neuroborreliosis (see glossary, p 504) after oral antibiotic treatment of arthritis.

Benefits: We found no systematic review. **People with Lyme arthritis:** We found two RCTs[11,12] that selected people with Lyme disease arthritis and randomised them to different treatments. The first RCT (40 people with Lyme disease arthritis) compared intramuscular benzathine penicillin (7.3 million units once a week for 3 weeks) versus saline placebo.[11] It found that penicillin versus saline increased the number of people having complete resolution of the arthritis (AR 7/20 [35%] with penicillin v 0/20 [0%] with placebo; NNT 2, 95% CI 1 to 8). The second RCT (48 people with Lyme arthritis) compared oral doxycycline (100 mg twice daily for 30 days) versus oral amoxicillin (500 mg) plus probenicid (4 times daily for 30 days).[12] After 3 months, an intention to treat analysis found similar rates of arthritis resolution in both groups (AR 18/25 [72%] with doxycyline v 16/23 [70%] with amoxicillin plus probenicid; RR 1.04, 95% CI 0.72 to 1.49). In the doxycycline group, one person had recurrence of arthritis and another developed polyneuropathy after treatment. In the amoxicillin plus probenicid group, one person had recurrent arthritis, two developed polyneuropathy, and two developed encephalopathy. **Subgroup analyses:** We found three other RCTs that recruited people with a variety of forms of late Lyme disease (including Lyme arthritis).[13–15] The first RCT (23 people with late Lyme disease, 70% with arthritis) compared ceftriaxone (2 g intravenously every 12 hours for 14 days) versus penicillin (4 million units intravenously every 4 hours for 10 days).[13] Ceftriaxone appeared to be more effective than penicillin, but the differences in

Infectious diseases

rates of clinical improvement after 3 months were not significant (absolute risk of improvement, AR 12/13 [92%] with ceftriaxone v 5/10 [50%] with penicillin; RR 1.85, 95% CI 0.97 to 3.50). More of the subgroup of people with arthritis improved with ceftriaxone (AR 9/9 [100%] with ceftriaxone v 2/7 [29%] with penicillin; NNT 2, 95% CI 1 to 4). The second RCT (135 people with late Lyme disease, 73 with arthritis) compared cefotaxime (6 g/day for 8–10 days) versus penicillin G (20 million units/day for 8–19 days).[14] Two years after treatment, full recovery was more frequent with cefotaxime (AR 44/69 [64%] with cefotaxime v 25/66 [38%] with penicillin; RR 1.68, 95% CI 1.18 to 2.41; NNT 3, 95% CI 2 to 11). In the subgroup with arthritis, recovery was also increased by cefotaxime (17/39 [44%] with cefotaxime v 4/34 [12%] with penicillin; RR 3.7, 95% CI 1.4 to 9.9; NNT 4). The third RCT (62 people with disseminated Lyme disease, 13 people with Lyme arthritis) did not report separate results for the subgroup with arthritis. It compared intravenous ceftriaxone followed by oral amoxicillin plus probenicid versus oral cefixime plus probenicid.[15]

Harms: Some people have developed symptoms of neuroborreliosis after oral antibiotic treatment of arthritis. Jarisch-Herxheimer reactions (see glossary, p 504) have been described in people treated for late Lyme disease. This reaction was reported in 11 (25%) of 44 people treated with ceftriaxone,[13] in 10 (15%) of 66 treated with penicillin, and 19 (28%) of 69 treated with cefotaxime (RR with cefotaxime v with penicillin: 1.8, 95% CI 0.9 to 3.6; NNH 8).[14] Possible "Herxheimer-like" reactions, including fever, transient rash, and worsening of symptoms or cardiac arrhythmia were reported in an unspecified number of people treated with cefixime and probenicid, and with ceftriaxone followed by amoxicillin.[15] No significant differences were found in the risk of developing a prolonged form of such reactions for people receiving ceftriaxone plus amoxicillin versus cefixime plus probenecid (AR 18/30 [60%] with ceftriaxone and amoxicillin therapy v 12/30 [40%] with cefixime and probenicid; RR 1.50, 95% CI 0.88 to 2.54). Other harms include those expected from the antibiotics. In RCTs including people with Lyme arthritis, the following adverse effects were reported: diarrhoea and skin rash with ceftriaxone;[13] shock and colitis with penicillin; anaphylaxis and colitis with cefotaxime;[14] rash and gastrointestinal effects with amoxicillin and probenicid;[12] diarrhoea and rash with cefixime; and nausea, diarrhoea, and rash with ceftriaxone followed by amoxicillin.[15]

Comment: Results of the RCTs that presented results for subgroups of people with Lyme arthritis should be interpreted with caution as people with arthritis were not randomly assigned to treatment groups. The RCTs were small, and the type, dose, and regimen of antibiotics used, varied between trials. The enrolment criteria also varied between trials. Only one RCT had a placebo control. The proportion of people who respond in comparative RCTs is difficult to interpret because, without a placebo comparison, it is unclear how many people would have responded without treatment.

QUESTION **What are the effects of antibiotic treatments for late neurological Lyme disease?**

We found no RCTs that randomised people with late neurological Lyme disease to different treatments. One small RCT that reported results for a subgroup of people with late neurological Lyme disease found weak evidence that cefotaxime may be more effective than penicillin in eliminating neurological symptoms. A small RCT of people with neuroborreliosis of varying durations found no significant difference between cefotaxime and ceftriaxone.

Benefits: We found no systematic review. **People with late neurological Lyme disease:** We found no RCT that randomised only people with late neurological Lyme disease. **Subgroup analyses:** We found no placebo controlled RCTs, but found two comparative RCTs that reported results for people with late neurological Lyme disease.[14–16] The first RCT (135 people with late Lyme disease, 93 with neuropathy) compared cefotaxime (6 g/day for 8–10 days) versus penicillin G (20 million units/day for 8–19 days).[14] Two years after treatment, complete recovery was increased by cefotaxime (AR 44/69 [64%] with cefotaxime v 25/66 [38%] with penicillin; RR 1.68, 95% CI 1.18 to 2.41; NNT 4). Similar results were reported for the subgroup with neuropathy (AR 35/49 [71%] with cefotaxime v 20/44 [46%] with penicillin; RR 1.57, 95% CI 1.09 to 2.27; NNT 4). The second RCT (33 people with Lyme neuroborreliosis of varying duration) compared ceftriaxone (2 g intravenously daily for 10 days) versus cefotaxime (2 g intravenously every 8 hours for 10 days).[16] Some of the people treated with ceftriaxone were asymptomatic prior to treatment, and so were excluded from analysis (3 of 17). Of the remaining people, most (17/30) had disease duration of over 30 days at study entry, and some (8/30) had a duration over 60 days. The RCT found no significant difference in the proportion of people who were asymptomatic after 8 months (8/14 [57%] with ceftriaxone v 9/16 [56%] with cefotaxime; RR 1.02, 95% CI 0.54 to 1.90).

Harms: See harms under treatments for Lyme disease arthritis, p 501. In the clinical trials involving late neurological Lyme disease reported above, the following adverse effects were reported: shock and colitis with penicillin, and anaphylaxis and colitis with cefotaxime;[13] rash with cefotaxime and fever, diarrhoea, and elevated liver enzymes with ceftriaxone.[16] One case control study found an association between biliary disease and ceftriaxone treatment of suspected late Lyme disease.[17]

Comment: The RCTs either recruited people with late Lyme disease, some of whom had neurological manifestations, or people with Lyme neuroborreliosis, some of whom had late disease. Results presented for these subsets of study participants may be subject to undetected biases, because patients with late neurological disease were not randomly assigned to treatment groups. None of the RCTs had a placebo treated control group. The antibiotics used in RCTs, as well as doses and schedules, varied between trials. The enrolment criteria also varied between trials.

Infectious diseases

GLOSSARY

Adjuvant A substance such as aluminium hydroxide included in a vaccine to enhance its effectiveness.

Jarisch-Herxheimer reaction An inflammatory reaction in tissues induced by antibiotic treatment of spirochetal diseases, and believed to be caused by an immunologic reaction to the release of spirochetal antigens.

Neuroborreliosis Central or peripheral neuropathy resulting from infection with *Borrelia sp.* spirochetes.

REFERENCES

1. Orloski KA, Hayes EB, Campbell GL, Dennis DT. Surveillance for Lyme Disease – United States, 1992–1998. *MMWR* 2000;49(SS-3):1–11.
2. CDC. Recommendations for the use of Lyme disease vaccine: recommendations of the Advisory Committee on Immunization Practices (ACIP). *MMWR* 1999;48(no. RR-7).
3. O'Connel S, Granstorm M, Gray JS, Stanek G. Epidemiology of European Lyme borreliosis. *Zent. Bl Bakteriol* 1998;287:229–240.
4. Dennis DT. Epidemiology, ecology, and prevention of Lyme disease. In: Rahn DW, Evans J, eds. *Lyme Disease*, Philadelphia, PA, USA: American College of Physicians, 1998.
5. Rahn DW, Evans J, eds. *Lyme Disease*. Philadelphia, PA, USA, American College of Physicians, 1998:35–45, 79, 108–109.
6. Steere AC, Sikand VJ, Meurice F, et al. Vaccination against Lyme disease with recombinant Borrelia burgdorferi outer-surface lipoprotein A with adjuvant. *N Eng J Med* 1998;339:209–215.
7. Sigal LH, Zahradnik JM, Lavin P, et al. A vaccine consisting of recombinant Borrelia burgorferi outer-surface protein A to prevent Lyme disease. *N Engl J Med* 1998;339:216–222.
8. Feder HM, Beran J, Van Hoecke C, et al. Immunogenicity of a recombinant Borrelia burgdorferi outer surface protein A vaccine against Lyme disease in children. *J Pediatr* 1999;135: 575–579.
9. Keller D, Koster FT, Marks DH, et al. Safety and Immunogenicity of a recombinant outer surface protein A Lyme vaccine. *JAMA* 1994;271:1764–1768.
10. Van Hoecke C, Comberbach M, De Grave D, et al. Evaluation of the saftey, reactogenicity and immonogenicity of three recombinant outer surface protein (OspA) lyme vaccines in healthy adults. *Vaccine* 1996;14 (17–18):1620–1626
11. Steere AC, Green J, Schoen RT, et al. Succesful parenteral penicillin therapy of established Lyme arthritis. *N Engl J Med* 1985;312:869–874.
12. Steere AC, Levin RE, Molloy PJ, et. al. Treatment of Lyme arthritis. *Arthr Rheum* 1994;37:878–888.
13. Dattwyler RJ, Halperin JJ, Volkman DJ, et al. Treatment of late Lyme borreliosis — randomized comparison of ceftriaxone and penicillin. *Lancet* 1998;1:1191–1194.
14. Hassler D, Zoller M, Haude H-D, et al. Cefotaxime versus penicillin in the late stage of Lyme disease — prospective, randomized therapeutic study. *Infection* 1990;18:16–20.
15. Oksi J, Nikoskelainen J, Vijanen MK. Comparison of oral cefixime and intravenous ceftriaxone followed by oral amoxicillin in disseminated Lyme borreliosis. *Eur J Clin Microbiol Infect Dis* 1998; 17:715–719.
16. Pfister H-W, Preac-Mursic V, Wilske B, et al. Randomized comparison of ceftriaxone and cefotaxime in Lyme neuroborreliosis. *J Infect Dis* 1991;163:311–318.
17. Ettestad PJ, Campbell GL, Welbel SF, et al. Biliary complications in the treatment of unsubstantiated Lyme disease. *J Infect Dis* 1995;171:356–361.

Edward Hayes
Chief, Epidemiology Section
BZB, DVBID, NCID
US Centers for Disease
Control and Prevention
Fort Collins
Colorado
USA

Competing interests: None declared.

Search date November 2000

Ashley Croft

INTERVENTIONS

Key Messages

Non-drug preventive interventions

■ One systematic review in residents of an endemic malaria area has found that nets treated with insecticide reduce both the number of mild episodes of malaria and child mortality.

■ One RCT has found that wraps and top sheets treated with insecticide significantly reduces the number of episodes of malaria.

■ Observational studies that used clinical malaria as an outcome have found that air conditioning and wearing trousers and long sleeved shirts, reduces the incidence of malaria, but we found no evidence of an effect of aerosol insecticides.

- Several other interventions (mainly in observational studies) have been found to reduce the risk of being bitten. These include insecticide treated clothing, electric fans, mosquito coils, vaporising mats, smoke, insect repellent soap, and topical diethyltoluamide (DEET).

Drug prophylaxis

- Single RCTs in soldiers have found that doxycycline and mefloquine reduce the risk of malaria. We found insufficient evidence on the effects of other antimalaria drugs.

- We found little good evidence on the adverse effects of antimalaria drugs, particularly mefloquine. Observational studies have associated DEET and doxycycline with severe adverse effects in children.

Vaccines

- We found insufficient evidence on the effects of antimalaria vaccines in travellers.

DEFINITION	Malaria is caused by a protozoan infection of red blood cells with one of four species of the genus *Plasmodium*: *P falciparum*, *P vivax*, *P ovale*, and *P malariae*.[1] Clinically, malaria may present in different ways, but is usually characterised by fever (which may be swinging), tachycardia, rigors, and sweating. Anaemia, hepatosplenomegaly, cerebral involvement, renal failure, and shock may occur.
INCIDENCE/ PREVALENCE	Each year there are 300–500 million clinical cases of malaria. About 40% of the world's population is at risk of acquiring the disease.[2,3] Each year 25–30 million people from non-tropical countries visit malaria endemic areas, of whom 10 000–30 000 contract malaria.[4,5] Most RCTs of malaria prevention have been carried out on western travellers and soldiers. The results of these trials may not be applicable to people such as refugees and migrants, who are likely to differ in their health status and their susceptibility to disease and adverse drug reactions.
AETIOLOGY/ RISK FACTORS	Malaria is mainly a rural disease, requiring nearby standing water. It is transmitted by bites of infected female anopheline mosquitoes, mainly at dusk and during the night.[1,6–8] In cities, mosquito bites are usually from female culicine mosquitoes, which are not vectors of malaria.[9] Malaria is resurgent in most tropical countries and risk to travellers is increasing.[10] The sickle cell trait has been shown to convey some protection against malaria in non-immune carriers of that trait. Non-immune adults with the sickle cell trait who develop severe malaria have lower parasite densities, fewer complications (e.g. cerebral malaria), and a reduced mortality compared with adults without the trait.[11] There is little good evidence on the degree of protection afforded by the sickle cell trait.[12]
PROGNOSIS	Ninety per cent of tourists and business travellers who contract malaria do not become ill until after they return home.[5] "Imported malaria" is easily treated if diagnosed promptly, and follows a serious course in only about 12% of people.[13,14] The most severe form is cerebral malaria, with a case fatality rate in adult travellers of 2–6%, mainly because of delays in diagnosis.[3,15]
AIMS	To reduce the risk of infection; to prevent illness and death, with minimal adverse effects of treatment.

OUTCOMES	Rates of clinical malaria and death, and adverse effects of treatment. Proxy measures include numbers of mosquito bites and rates of mosquito catches in indoor areas. We found limited evidence linking numbers of mosquito bites and risk of malaria.[16]
METHODS	*Clinical Evidence* update search and appraisal November 2000.

QUESTION What are the effects of non-drug preventive interventions in adult travellers?

OPTION AEROSOL INSECTICIDES

We found insufficient evidence on the effects of aerosol insecticides in travellers.

Benefits:	We found no systematic review or RCTs. We found one questionnaire survey of 89 617 European tourists returning from East Africa, which found that commercially available personal aerosol insecticides alone did not significantly reduce the incidence of malaria (P = 0.55).[17]
Harms:	We found no reports of adverse effects.
Comment:	Two community RCTs found that indoor residual spraying of synthetic pyrethroids reduces clinical malaria in lifelong residents of malaria endemic areas.[18,19] Historically, indoor residual spraying has not been recommended for short stay travellers, but we found no evidence to support this.

OPTION BIOLOGICAL CONTROL MEASURES

We found no good evidence for the effectiveness of biological control measures in preventing malaria, nor evidence of harm.

Benefits:	We found no systematic review or RCTs. Cohort studies based on mosquito counts have found no evidence that growing the citrosa plant and encouraging natural predation of insects by erecting bird or bat houses reduce bites to humans from infected anopheline mosquitoes.[20]
Harms:	We found no evidence of harms.
Comment:	The only known way to reduce mosquitoes naturally is to eliminate sources of standing water, such as tree stump holes, discarded tyres, cans, and bottles.[20]

OPTION AIR CONDITIONING AND ELECTRIC FANS

One large observational study in travellers has found that air conditioning reduces the incidence of malaria. One small observational study has found that electric fans reduces numbers of mosquitoes in indoor spaces.

Benefits:	We found no systematic review or RCTs. One questionnaire survey of 89 617 European tourists returning from East Africa found that sleeping in an air conditioned room significantly reduced the incidence of malaria (P = 0.04).[17] One cohort study of various anti-mosquito interventions (in 6 experimental huts in Pakistan villages)

found that fans significantly reduced catches of culicine mosquitoes ($P < 0.05$) but did not significantly reduce catches of blood fed anopheline mosquitoes.[21]

Harms: We found no evidence of harms.

Comment: These studies support the finding that mosquitoes are reluctant to fly in windy conditions.[22]

OPTION   INSECT BUZZERS AND ELECTROCUTERS

We found no evidence for the effectiveness of insect electrocuters and ultrasonic buzzers in preventing malaria.

Benefits: We found no systematic review and no RCTs with clinical malaria as an outcome.

Harms: We found no evidence of harms.

Comment: We found one non-randomised controlled trial (18 houses in Gabon) of a commercially available ultrasound emitting device. The trial lasted 6 weeks and used total mosquito catches as a proxy outcome.[23] Most mosquitoes were culicine. It found no significant difference in mosquito catches between the ultrasound emitting device and a sham device ($P = 0.48$).[23] See comment under biological control measures, p 507.

OPTION   MOSQUITO COILS AND VAPORISING MATS

One RCT of coils and one observational study of pyrethroid vaporising mats has found that these devices reduce numbers of mosquitoes in indoor spaces.

Benefits: We found no systematic review and no RCTs that used clinical malaria as an outcome. We found one RCT (18 houses in Malaysia) of various mosquito coil formulations that found coils reduced populations of culicine mosquitoes by 75%.[24]

Harms: We found no evidence of harms.

Comment: One observational study of pyrethroid vaporising mats in six experimental huts in a Pakistan village setting found that the mats reduced total catches of blood fed mosquitoes by 56%.[20]

OPTION   SMOKE

One controlled trial has found that smoke acts as a cheap and effective means of repelling mosquitoes during the evening.

Benefits: We found no systematic review and no RCTs that used clinical malaria as an outcome. One controlled trial, in which five small fires were tended on five successive evenings in a village in Papua New Guinea, found a smoke specific and species specific effect from different types of smoke. Catches of one anopheline species were reduced by 84% through burning betelnut (95% CI 62% to 94%), by 69% through burning ginger (95% CI 25% to 87%), and by 66% through burning coconut husks (95% CI 17% to 86%).[25]

Harms: There may be an irritant and toxic effect of smoke on the eyes and respiratory system, but this effect was not quantified.[25]

Comment: None.

One systematic review of RCTs has found that insecticide treated nets prevent malaria and reduce overall mortality.

Benefits: We found one systematic review (search date not stated), which identified 18 RCTs in malaria endemic settings (non-traveller participants).[26] It found that nets sprayed or impregnated with permethrin reduced the number of mild episodes of malaria (ARR 39%, 95% CI 27% to 48%) and child mortality (RR of death compared with no nets or untreated nets 0.83, 95% CI 0.77 to 0.90; NNT 180).

Harms: We found no evidence of harms.

Comment: Permethrin remains active for about 4 months.[6]

One RCT has found that insecticide treated wraps and top sheets significantly reduce the risk of contracting malaria.

Benefits: We found no systematic review. One RCT (102 refugee households in north western Pakistan) found that permethrin-treated wraps and top sheets significantly reduced the unadjusted risk of falciparum malaria (RR 0.56, 95% CI 0.41 to 0.78) compared with placebo.[27]

Harms: **Permethrin:** We found no evidence of harms. **DEET:** See harms of topical insect repellents, p 510.

Comment: None.

One observational study in travellers has found that wearing trousers and long sleeved shirts reduces the incidence of malaria.

Benefits: We found no systematic review or RCTs. **Clothing:** We found one questionnaire survey of 89 617 European tourists returning from East Africa, which found that wearing long sleeved shirts and trousers significantly reduced the incidence of malaria (P = 0.02).[17] **Other lifestyle changes:** We found no studies (see comment below).

Harms: None.

Comment: Lifestyle change implies not travelling to malaria endemic regions during the rainy season (when most malaria transmission occurs), and not going outdoors in the evening or at night. Travellers who take day trips from a malaria free city to a malarious region may be at minimal risk if they return to the city before dusk.[28] It would seem

Infectious diseases

sensible to wear long sleeved shirts and trousers at dusk, and to wear light rather than dark colours, as insects prefer landing on dark surfaces.[9,28]

OPTION **TOPICAL INSECT REPELLENTS**

One RCT has found that an insect repellent soap reduces insect bites. No RCTs have examined whether topical insect repellents prevent malaria. One very small crossover RCT has found that DEET preparations protects against mosquito bites.

Benefits: We found no systematic review and no RCTs using clinical malaria as an outcome. One small RCT (8 people in a Colombian forest setting) compared repellent soap (20% DEET and 0.5% permethrin) with placebo soap and found repellent soap reduced the numbers of sandfly bites at 4 and 8 hours (P < 0.05).[29] One small crossover RCT (4 people) involving successive random exposure to *Aedes aegyptii* mosquitos compared six different controlled release preparations of DEET. It found that all gave at least 95% protection against mosquito bites.[30] **Combined with insecticide treated clothing:** See insecticide treated clothing, p 509.

Harms: We found a case series of systemic toxic reactions (confusion, irritability, insomnia) in US national park employees after repeated and prolonged use of DEET.[31] We found 14 case reports of contact urticaria and of irritant contact dermatitis (mostly in soldiers) as a result of DEET.[17] The risk of absorption is especially high if DEET is left in the antecubital fossa overnight.[32] DEET may be harmful to children under 8 years if applied in excessive amounts (see insect repellents containing DEET in children, p 514). It also attacks certain plastics, such as spectacle frames.[33]

Comment: DEET is a broad spectrum repellent effective against mosquitoes, biting flies, chiggers, fleas, and ticks,[20] which has been used for 40 years. Although most authorities would recommend the use of topical repellents in malaria endemic areas, the only evidence comes from small RCTs with non-clinical outcomes. Larger RCTs are needed to compare DEET with other topical repellents and placebo in preventing malaria.

QUESTION **What are the effects of drug prophylaxis in adult travellers?**

OPTION **CHLOROQUINE**

We found insufficient evidence on the effects of chloroquine prophylaxis in travellers.

Benefits: We found no systematic review. We found one RCT (173 Austrian industrial workers based in Nigeria) comparing chloroquine with sulfadoxine plus pyrimethamine.[34] It found no evidence of a difference in the incidence of malaria.

Harms: We found no large cohort studies in travellers. In one RCT, the commonest reported symptom with chloroquine was insomnia, occurring in 3% of people.[34] Retrospective questionnaire surveys suggest that severe adverse effects are rare at prophylactic dosages.[35]

Comment: Most drug trials have been in soldiers, and their results may not be generalisable to tourists or business travellers.[36,37] Alcohol consumption, other medication, and comorbidities can modify the effects of antimalaria drugs.[38,39]

OPTION   CHLOROQUINE PLUS PROGUANIL

RCTs found no evidence that chloroquine plus proguanil is more effective than proguanil alone or than chloroquine plus other antimalaria drugs.

Benefits: We found no systematic review. We found two RCTs in travellers. One open label RCT (767 Scandinavian travellers to East Africa) compared chloroquine plus proguanil versus chloroquine plus sulfadoxine-pyrimethamine. It found no significant difference in rates of *P falciparum* infection between groups (4/384 [1%] v 3/383 [0.7%] travellers; RR 1.3, 95% CI 0.3 to 5.9).[40] **Versus proguanil alone:** The second RCT in Dutch travellers to Africa found no significant difference in incidence of *P falciparum* malaria with chloroquine 300 mg weekly plus proguanil 200 mg daily compared with proguanil alone (risk per 100 person months: cholorquine plus proguanil 2.8, 95% CI 0.9 to 10.1 v proguanil 6.0, 95% CI 2.6 to 14.0).[41]

Harms: In the RCT in Scandinavian travellers, adverse effects associated with chloroquine plus proguanil were nausea (3%), diarrhoea (2%), and dizziness (1%).[40] One cohort study in 470 British soldiers in Belize found that the risk of mouth ulcers almost doubled with chloroquine plus proguanil compared with proguanil alone (RR 1.9, P = 0.025).[42]

Comment: The rates of confirmed *P falciparum* infection in both trials were small and so a clinically important effect cannot be excluded.

OPTION   DOXYCYCLINE IN ADULTS

One RCT in soldiers has found doxycycline reduces the risk of malaria. Short term adverse effects, including skin reactions and nausea and vomiting, were reported in up to 40% of people. We found no evidence on long term safety.

Benefits: We found no systematic review. One RCT (136 Indonesian soldiers) found that doxycycline reduced the risk of malaria compared with placebo (AR 1/67 [2%] with doxycycline v 53/69 [77%] with placebo; ARR 75%; RR 0.02, 95% CI 0.003 to 0.14; NNT 1, 95% CI 1 to 2).[43] One RCT (300 Indonesian adults with limited immunity) found two out of 75 cases of *P falciparum* malaria versus 29 out of 77 on placebo (96% protective efficacy, 95% CI 85% to 99.6%), and one out of 75 cases of *P vivax* malaria versus 27 out of 75 on placebo (98% protective efficacy, 95% CI 88% to 99.9%).[44]

Harms: In one RCT in soldiers, commonly reported adverse effects were unspecified dermatological problems (33%), cough (31%), and headache (16%).[43] One questionnaire survey (383 returned

Infectious diseases

Australian travellers) found that 40% reported nausea or vomiting, 12% reported diarrhoea, and 9% of female travellers reported vaginitis.[45] Evidence from case reports suggests that, in sunny conditions, up to 50% of travellers using doxycycline may experience photoallergic skin rash.[46]

Comment: Trials in soldiers may not be generalisable to other travellers. The first trial was a three arm parallel RCT. It compared mefloquine (68 people), doxycycline (67 people), and placebo (69 people). Only the comparison of doxycycline and placebo is included here.[42]

OPTION   MEFLOQUINE IN ADULTS

One systematic review of RCTs has found that mefloquine is effective in preventing malaria. We found no good evidence that reliably attributes serious adverse reactions to mefloquine.

Benefits: We found one systematic review (search date 2000), which identified five RCTs in travellers (all soldiers).[47] Only one, a placebo controlled trial in 137 Indonesian soldiers, assessed the protective efficacy of mefloquine in a malaria endemic setting.[43] It found that in an area of drug resistance, mefloquine had a protective efficacy of 100% (95% CI 93% to 100%).

Harms: The review found no significant difference in the rate of withdrawals from mefloquine compared with other drug treatments.[47] Commonly reported adverse effects associated with mefloquine were headache (16%), insomnia (15%), and fatigue (8%).[47] Retrospective questionnaire surveys in tourists and business travellers found that sleep disturbance and psychosis were common.[48,49] One review of 74 dermatological case reports found that up to 30% of mefloquine users developed a maculopapular rash, and 4–10% had pruritus.[50] Nine cohort studies in tourists found that women tolerated mefloquine less well than men.[45,48,49,51–56] One retrospective questionnaire survey of 93 668 European travellers to East Africa found that elderly travellers tolerated mefloquine better than younger travellers (P < 0.05).[57] There is evidence from over 500 case reports that mefloquine is a potentially harmful drug for tourists and business travellers and requires more careful evaluation through an RCT in these groups.[47]

Comment: Trials in soldiers may not be generalisable to other travellers. The trial in Indonesian soldiers was a three arm parallel RCT. It compared mefloquine (68 people), doxycycline (67 people), and placebo (69 people). Only the comparison of mefloquine and placebo is included here.[43]

OPTION   ATOVAQUONE PLUS PROGUANIL

We found insufficient evidence on the effects of atovaquone plus proguanil prophylaxis for travellers.

Benefits: We found no systematic review and no placebo controlled RCTs. We found one multicentre RCT (in 1083 non-immune travellers), which compared atovaquone plus proguanil versus chloroquine plus proguanil.[58] It found no significant difference in malaria acquisition rates (1/511 [0.2%] cases of P ovale malaria v 3/511 [0.6%] cases of P falciparum malaria; ARR 0.4%, RR 0.33, 95% CI 0.03 to 3.16).

Harms: In one RCT in non-immune travellers, 311 of 351 (61%) atovaquone-proguanil users reported one or more adverse events compared with 329 of 511 (64%) chloroquine-proguanil users (ARR 3.5%; RR 0.95, 95% CI 0.85 to 1.04).[58] Common adverse effects were mainly gastrointestinal (diarrhoea 5% v 7%, mouth ulcers 4% v 5%, abdominal pain 3% v 6%, nausea 2% v 7%) and neuropsychiatric (strange/vivid dreams 4% v 3%, dizziness 3% v 4%, insomnia 2% v 2%), and visual difficulties (2% v 2%).[58]

Comment: None.

OPTION   OTHER ANTIMALARIA DRUGS

We found insufficient evidence on the effects of other antimalaria drugs in travellers.

Benefits: We found no systematic review. **Sulfadoxine plus pyrimethamine:** See benefits of cholorquine plus proguanil, p 511. **Amodiaquine:** We found no RCTs in travellers. **Pyrimethamine plus dapsone:** We found no RCTs in travellers. One RCT in Thai soldiers comparing pyrimethamine/dapsone with proguanil/dapsone found no significant differences in P falciparum infection rates over 40 days.[59]

Harms: **Sulfadoxine plus pyrimethamine:** One retrospective cohort study in 182 300 US travellers taking prophylactic sulfadoxine plus pyrimethamine reported severe cutaneous reactions (erythema multiforme, Stevens-Johnson syndrome, toxic epidermal necrolysis) in one of 5000–8000 users, with a mortality of about one of 11 000–25 000 users.[60] **Amodiaquine:** One retrospective cohort study in 10 000 British travellers taking prophylactic amodiaquine reported severe neutropenia in about one of 2000 users.[61] We found 28 case reports describing liver damage or hepatitis in travellers who had taken amodiaquine to treat or prevent malaria.[62–67] **Atovaquone plus proguanil:** We found no evidence of adverse effects in travellers. **Pyrimethamine plus dapsone:** One RCT in Thai soldiers found that fewer than 2% reported any drug related symptoms from pyrimethamine plus dapsone.[59] One retrospective cohort study in 15 000 Swedish travellers taking pyrimethamine plus dapsone reported agranulocytosis in about one of 2000 users.[60]

Comment: None.

QUESTION   What are the effects of antimalaria vaccines in travellers?

We found insufficient evidence on the effects of antimalaria vaccines in travellers.

Benefits: We found no systematic review or RCTs of antimalaria vaccines in travellers.

Malaria: prevention in travellers

Harms:
One systematic review (search date 1999) identified 13 RCTs in residents of malaria endemic areas. It found that, in all but one of the trials of the SPf66 vaccine, fewer than 10% of recipients reported a systemic reaction (fever, headache, gastric symptoms, muscle pain, dizziness), and fewer than 35% reported a local reaction (inflammation, nodules, pain, erythema, pruritis, induration, injection site warmth).[68] The remaining RCT found a larger proportion of local cutaneous reactions, although these resolved within 24 hours with symptomatic treatment. It also reported higher systemic reaction rates after vaccination (11–16%), although rates after placebo were also higher (10–13%). Surveillance was also more intense than in the other trials.

Comment:
The review found only the SPf66 vaccine reduced first attacks of *P falciparum* malaria (OR 0.80, 95% CI 0.71 to 0.90).[68]

QUESTION What are the effects of antimalaria interventions in child travellers?

OPTION INSECT REPELLENTS CONTAINING DEET IN CHILDREN

We found insufficient evidence on the effects of DEET in child travellers. Case reports in young children found serious adverse effects with DEET when used excessively.

Benefits:
We found no systematic review or RCTs in child travellers.

Harms:
We found 13 case reports of encephalopathic toxicity in children aged under 8 years after excessive use of topical insect repellents containing DEET.[69,70]

Comment:
Infants and young children have thinner skin and greater surface area to mass ratio.[71] Some authors advise that ethylhexanediol should be used as a topical insect repellent in preference to DEET in children aged 1–8 years and that in infants only plant based topical repellents such as citronella oil are safe.[72] However, we found insufficient evidence about the effects of these alternative repellents.

OPTION DOXYCYCLINE IN CHILDREN

We found no good evidence on the use of doxycycline in child travellers. Case reports in young children found adverse effects with doxycycline.

Benefits:
We found no systematic reviews or RCTs on the effects of doxycycline in child travellers.

Harms:
Case reports have found that doxycycline inhibits bone growth and discolours teeth in children aged under 12 years.[9,35]

Comment:
Infants and young children have thinner skin and greater surface area to mass ratio.[71]

| OPTION | MEFLOQUINE IN CHILDREN |

We found no good evidence.

Benefits: We found no RCTs or systematic reviews.

Harms: Three RCTs of mefloquine found children tolerate higher doses compared with adults.[73–75]

Comment: None.

| QUESTION | What are the effects of antimalaria interventions in pregnant travellers? |

| OPTION | INSECTICIDE TREATED NETS IN PREGNANT TRAVELLERS |

We found insufficient evidence on the effects of antimalaria interventions in pregnant travellers. It is unclear which topical insect repellents are safe in pregnancy.

Benefits: We found no systematic review or RCTs in pregnant travellers. We found one RCT of permethrin treated nets versus non-treated nets versus usual practice in three sites with 341 pregnant women living in Thailand.[76] Two sites found no significant difference in malaria rates, whereas the third found significantly lower rates with treated nets.

Harms: We found little evidence relating to pregnant travellers. The trial of permethrin treated nets in Thailand found no evidence of toxic effects to mother or fetus.[76]

Comment: Pregnant women are relatively immunosuppressed and are at greater risk of malaria than non-pregnant women.[77] Contracting malaria significantly increases the likelihood of losing the fetus.[78]

| OPTION | INSECTICIDE TREATED CLOTHING IN PREGNANT TRAVELLERS |

We found insufficient evidence on the effects of antimalaria interventions in pregnant travellers.

Benefits: We found no systematic review or RCTs in pregnant travellers.

Harms: We found little evidence relating to pregnant travellers. **Permethrin:** A trial of permethrin treated nets in Thailand found no evidence of toxic effects to mother or fetus.[76] **DEET:** We found little evidence relating to pregnant travellers. Some, but not all, animal studies have found that DEET crosses the placental barrier.[79] Animal studies of reproductive effects of DEET are conflicting.[78,80] We found one case report indicating an adverse fetal outcome (mental retardation, impaired sensorimotor coordination, craniofacial dysmorphology) in a child whose mother had applied DEET daily throughout her pregnancy.[81]

Comment: Pregnant women are relatively immunosuppressed and are at greater risk of malaria than non-pregnant women.[77] Contracting malaria significantly increases the likelihood of losing the fetus.[78]

| OPTION | TOPICAL INSECT REPELLENTS IN PREGNANT TRAVELLERS |

We found insufficient evidence. It is unclear which topical insect repellents are safe in pregnancy.

Benefits: We found no systematic review or RCTs in pregnant travellers.

Harms: We found little evidence relating to pregnant travellers. Some, but not all, animal studies have found that DEET crosses the placental barrier.[79] Animal studies of reproductive effects of DEET are conflicting.[78,80] We found one case report indicating an adverse fetal outcome (mental retardation, impaired sensorimotor coordination, craniofacial dysmorphology) in a child whose mother had applied DEET daily throughout her pregnancy.[81]

Comment: Pregnant women are relatively immunosuppressed and are at greater risk of malaria than non-pregnant women.[77] Contracting malaria significantly increases the likelihood of losing the fetus.[78] Because of a theoretical risk of mutagenicity from DEET, some authors advise that only plant based topical insect repellents such as citronella oil are safe in pregnancy.[72] However, we found insufficient evidence on the effects of this alternative repellent.

| OPTION | ANTIMALARIA DRUGS IN PREGNANT TRAVELLERS |

We found insufficient evidence on the effects of antimalaria drugs in pregnant travellers. One RCT found chloroquine to be safe in pregnancy. The safety of mefloquine in pregnancy has not been established.

Benefits: We found one systematic review (search date not stated), which identified no good evidence in pregnant travellers. It identified 15 RCTs of antimalaria drugs in pregnancy, all in residents of malaria endemic settings.[82] It found no significant difference in the number of perinatal deaths or preterm births. However, it found fewer episodes of fever during the first pregnancy (OR 0.36, 95% CI 0.15 to 0.86) and higher birth weight in the infant (OR 0.53, 95% CI 0.32 to 0.81).[82]

Harms: **Chloroquine:** One RCT (1464 long term residents of Burkina Faso) found no adverse effects in pregnant women.[83] **Doxycycline:** Case reports have found that doxycycline taken in pregnancy or while breastfeeding may damage fetal or infant bones or teeth.[9,35] **Mefloquine:** One placebo controlled RCT (339 long term Thai residents) found more reports of dizziness with mefloquine (28% v 14%, P < 0.005) but no other significant adverse effects on the mother, the pregnancy, or on infant survival or development over 2 years of follow up.[84]

Comment: Pregnant women are relatively immunosuppressed and are at greater risk of malaria than non-pregnant women.[77] Contracting malaria significantly increases the likelihood of losing the fetus.[78] Mefloquine is secreted in small quantities in breast milk, but it is believed that levels are too low to harm infants.[35]

QUESTION   What are the effects of antimalaria interventions in airline pilots?

OPTION   INSECTICIDES IN AIRLINE PILOTS

We found no good evidence on the use of insecticides in airline pilots.

Benefits: We found no systematic review or RCTs.

Harms: We found no good evidence of harms of insecticides in airline pilots.

Comment: None.

OPTION   ANTIMALARIA DRUGS IN AIRLINE PILOTS

We found insufficient evidence about the effects of antimalaria drugs in airline pilots.

Benefits: We found no systematic review or RCTs.

Harms: **Doxycycline:** One retrospective questionnaire survey of 28 Israeli pilots found that 39% experienced adverse effects from doxycycline (abdominal pain 7/28, fatigue 5/28).[85] **Mefloquine:** One placebo controlled RCT (23 trainee commercial pilots) found no evidence that mefloquine significantly affected flying performance (mean total number of errors recorded by the instrument coordination analyser 12.6 with mefloquine v 11.7 with placebo).[86] One retrospective questionnaire survey of 15 Israeli non-aviator aircrew found that 13% experienced adverse effects from mefloquine (dizziness, nausea, and abdominal pain in 2/15, abdominal discomfort in 1/15).[85]

Comment: None.

Substantive changes since last issue

Drug prophylaxis New RCT;[58] conclusion unchanged.

REFERENCES

1. White NJ. Malaria. In: Cook GC, ed. *Manson's tropical diseases.* 20th ed. London: WB Saunders, 1996:1087–1164.
2. World Health Organization. *The world health report 1997. Conquering suffering, enriching humanity.* Geneva: WHO Office of Information, 1997.
3. Murphy GS, Oldfield EC. Falciparum malaria. *Infect Dis Clin North Am* 1996;10:747–755.
4. Kain KC, Keystone JS. Malaria in travelers. Epidemiology, disease and prevention. *Infect Dis Clin North Am* 1998;12:267–284.
5. World Health Organization. *International Travel and Health.* Geneva: WHO, 1999.
6. Winstanley P. Malaria: treatment. *J R Coll Physicians Lond* 1998;32:203–207.
7. Baudon D, Martet G. Paludisme et voyageurs: protection et information [in French]. *Med Trop (Mars)* 1997;57:497–500.
8. *Health information for international travel, 1996–97.* Atlanta: US Department of Health and Human Services, Public Health Service, Centers for Disease Control and Prevention, National Center for Infectious Diseases, Division of Quarantine; 1997 HHS Publication No 95:8280.
9. Bradley DJ, Warhurst DC. Guidelines for the prevention of malaria in travellers from the United Kingdom. *Commun Dis Rep CDR Rev* 1997;7: R137–152.
10. Krogstad DJ. Malaria as a reemerging disease. *Epidemiol Rev* 1996;18:77–89.
11. Hill AVS. Malaria resistance genes: a natural selection. *Trans R Soc Trop Med Hyg* 1992;86: 225–232.
12. Fleming AF. Haematological diseases in the tropics. In: Cook GC, ed. *Manson's tropical diseases.* 20th ed. London: WB Saunders, 1996: 101–173.
13. Olsen VV. Basic considerations in connection with malaria prophylaxis [in Danish]. *Ugeskr Læger* 1998;160:2410–2411.
14. Miller SA, Bergman BP, Croft AM. Epidemiology of malaria in the British Army from 1982–1986. *J R Army Med Corps* 1999;145:20–22.
15. Dolmans WMV, van der Kaay HJ, Leentvaar-Kuijpers A, et al. Malariaprofylaxe: adviezen wederom aangepast. *Ned Tijdschr Geneeskd* 1996;140:892–893.
16. Beier JC, Oster CN, Onyango FK, et al. *Plasmodium falciparum* incidence relative to entomological inoculation rates at a site proposed for testing malaria vaccines in western Kenya. *Am J Trop Med Hyg* 1994;50:529–536.

17. Schoepke A, Steffen R, Gratz N. Effectiveness of personal protection measures against mosquito bites for malaria prophylaxis in travelers. *J Travel Med* 1998;128:931–940.

18. Misra SP, Webber R, Lines J, et al. Spray versus treated nets using deltamethrin–a community randomized trial in India. *Trans R Soc Trop Med Hyg* 1999;93:456–457.

19. Rowland M, Mahmood P, Iqbal J, et al. Indoor residual spraying with alphacypermethrin controls malaria in Pakistan: a community-randomized trial. *Trop Med Int Health* 2000;5:472–481.

20. Fradin MS. Mosquitoes and mosquito repellents: a clinician's guide. *Ann Intern Med* 1998;128:931–940.

21. Hewitt SE, Farhan M, Urhaman H, et al. Self-protection from malaria vectors in Pakistan: an evaluation of popular existing methods and appropriate new techniques in Afghan refugee communities. *Ann Trop Med Parasitol* 1996;90:337–344.

22. Service MW. *Mosquito ecology: field sampling methods*. 2nd ed. London: Chapman and Hall, 1993.

23. Sylla el-HK, Lell B, Krsmsner PG. A blinded, controlled trial of an ultrasound device as mosquito repellent. *Wein Klin Wochenschr* 2000;112:448–450.

24. Yap HH, Tan HT, Yahaya AM, et al. Field efficacy of mosquito coil formulations containing d-allethrin and d-transallethrin against indoor mosquitoes especially *Culex quinquefasciatus* Say. *Southeast Asian J Trop Med Public Health* 1990;21:558–563.

25. Vernéde R, van Meer MMM, Aplers MP. Smoke as a form of personal protection against mosquitoes, a field study in Papua New Guinea. *Southeast Asian J Trop Med Public Health* 1994;25:771–775.

26. Lengeler C. Insecticide treated bednets and curtains for preventing malaria. In: The *Cochrane Library*, Issue 4, 2000. Oxford: Update Software. Search date not given; primary sources Cochrane Infectious Diseases Group Trial Register, Medline, Embase, and hand searches of reference lists, relevant journals and personal contact with funding agencies and manufacturers.

27. Rowland M, Durrani N, Hewitt S, et al. Permethrin-treated *chaddars* and top-sheets: appropriate technology for protection against malaria in Afghanistan and other complex emergencies. *Trans R Soc Trop Med Hyg* 1999;93:465–472.

28. Juckett G. Malaria prevention in travelers. *Am Fam Physician* 1999;59:2523–2530.

29. Alexander B, Cadena H, Usma MC, et al. Laboratory and field evaluations of a repellent soap containing diethyl toluamide (DEET) and permethrin against phlebotomine sand flies (Diptera: Psychodidae) in Valle del Cauca, Colombia. *Am J Trop Med Hyg* 1995;52:169–173.

30. Gupta RK, Rutledge LC. Laboratory evaluation of controlled-release repellent formulations on human volunteers under three climatic regimens. *J Am Mosq Control Assoc* 1989;5:52–55.

31. McConnell R, Fidler AT, Chrislip D. Everglades National Park health hazard evaluation report. Cincinatti, Ohio: US Department of Health and Human Services, Public Health Service, 1986. NIOSH Health Hazard Evaluation Report No. HETA-83-085-1757.

32. Lamberg SI, Mulrennan JA. Bullous reaction to diethyl toluamide (DEET) resembling a blistering insect eruption. *Arch Dermatol* 1969;100:582–586.

33. Curtis CF, Townson H. Malaria: existing methods of vector control and molecular entomology. *Br Med Bull* 1998;54:311–325.

34. Stemberger H, Leimer R, Widermann G. Tolerability of long-term prophylaxis with Fansidar: a randomized double-blind study in Nigeria. *Acta Trop* 1984;41:391–399.

35. Petersen E. Malariaprofylakse. *Ugeskr Læger* 1997;159:2723–2730.

36. Croft A, Garner P. Mefloquine to prevent malaria: a systematic review of trials. *BMJ* 1997;315:1412–1416.

37. Anonymous. Mefloquine and malaria prophylaxis [letter]. *Drug Ther Bull* 1998;36:20–22.

38. Gherardin T. Mefloquine as malaria prophylaxis. *Aust Fam Physician* 1999;28:310.

39. Schlagenhauf P. Mefloquine for malaria chemoprophylaxis 1992–1998: a review. *J Travel Med* 1999;6:122–133.

40. Fogh S, Schapira A, Bygbjerg IC, et al. Malaria chemoprophylaxis in travellers to east Africa: a comparative prospective study of chloroquine plus proguanil with chloroquine plus sulfadoxine-pyrimethamine. *BMJ* 1988;296:820–822.

41. Wetsteyn JCFM, de Geus A. Comparison of three regimens for malaria prophylaxis in travellers to east, central, and southern Africa. *BMJ* 1993;307:1041–1043.

42. Drysdale SF, Phillips-Howard PA, Behrens RH. Proguanil, chloroquine, and mouth ulcers. *Lancet* 1990;335:164.

43. Ohrt C, Richie TL, Widjaja H, et al. Mefloquine compared with doxycycline for the prophylaxis of malaria in Indonesian soldiers. A randomized, double-blind, placebo-controlled trial. *Ann Intern Med* 1997;126:963–972.

44. Taylor WR, Richie TL, Fryauff DJ, et al. Malaria prophylaxis using azithromycin: a double-blind, placebo-controlled trial in Irian Jaya, Indonesia. *Clin Infect Dis* 1999;28:74–81.

45. Phillips MA, Kass RB. User acceptability patterns for mefloquine and doxycycline malaria chemoprophylaxis. *J Travel Med* 1996;3:40–45.

46. Leutscher PDC. Malariaprofylakse. *Ugeskr Læger* 1997;159:4866–4867.

47. Croft AMJ, Garner P. Mefloquine for preventing malaria in non-immune adult travellers. In: The *Cochrane Library*, Issue 4, 2000. Oxford: Update Software. Search date July 2000; primary sources Cochrane Infectious Diseases Group trials register, Medline, Embase, Lilacs, Science Citation Index, hand searches of reference lists of articles, and personal contact with researchers in the subject of malaria chemoprophylaxis, and drug companies.

48. Barrett PJ, Emmins PD, Clarke PD, Bradley DJ. Comparison of adverse events associated with use of mefloquine and combinations of chloroquine and proguanil as antimalarial prophylaxis: postal and telephone survey of travellers. *BMJ* 1996;313:525–528.

49. Weinke T, Trautmann M, Held T, et al. Neuropsychiatric side effects after the use of mefloquine. *Am J Trop Med Hyg* 1991;45:86–91.

50. Smith HR, Croft AM, Black MM. Dermatological adverse effects with the antimalarial drug mefloquine: a review of 74 published case reports. *Clin Exp Dermatol* 1999;24:249–254.

51. Bem L, Kerr L, Stuerchler D. Mefloquine prophylaxis: an overview of spontaneous reports of severe psychiatric reactions and convulsions. *J Trop Med Hyg* 1992;95:167–169.

52. Huzly D, Schönfeld C, Beurle W, et al. Malaria chemoprophylaxis in German tourists: a prospective study on compliance and adverse reactions. *J Travel Med* 1996;3:148–155.

53. Schlagenhauf P, Steffen R, Lobel H, et al. Mefloquine tolerability during chemoprophylaxis: focus on adverse event assessments, stereochemistry and compliance. *Trop Med Int Health* 1996;1:485–494.

54. Handschin JC, Wall M, Steffen R, et al. Tolerability and effectiveness of malaria chemoprophylaxis with mefloquine or chloroquine with or without co-medication. *J Travel Med* 1997;4:121–127.

55. Van Riemsdijk MM, van der Klauw MM, van Heest JAC, et al. Neuro-psychiatric effects of antimalarials. *Eur J Clin Pharmacol* 1997;52:1–6.

56. Micheo C, Arias C, Rovira A. Adverse effects and compliance with mefloquine or chloroquine + proguanil malaria chemoprophylaxis. *Proceedings of the Second European Conference on Travel Medicine,* Venice, Italy;2000:29–31.

57. Mittelholzer ML, Wall M, Steffen R, et al. Malaria prophylaxis in different age groups. *J Travel Med* 1996;4:219–223.

58. Hogh B, Clarke PD, Camus D, et al. Atovaquone-proguanil versus chloroquine-proguanil for malaria prophylaxis in non-immune travellers: a randomised, double-blind study. *Lancet* 2000; 356:1888–1894.

59. Shanks GD, Edstein MD, Suriyamongkol V, et al. Malaria chemoprophylaxis using proguanil/dapsone combinations on the Thai-Cambodian border. *Am J Trop Med Hyg* 1992;46:643–648.

60. Miller KD, Lobel HO, Satriale RF, et al. Severe cutaneous reactions among American travelers using pyrimethamine-sulfadoxine for malaria prophylaxis. *Am J Trop Med Hyg* 1986;35:451–458.

61. Hatton CSR, Peto TEA, Bunch C, et al. Frequency of severe neutropenia associated with amodiaquine prophylaxis against malaria. *Lancet* 1986;1:411–414.

62. Neftel K, Woodtly W, Schmid M, et al. Amodiaquine induced agranulocytosis and liver damage. *BMJ* 1986;292:721–723.

63. Larrey D, Castot A, Pessayre D, et al. Amodiaquine-induced hepatitis. A report of seven cases. *Ann Intern Med* 1986;104:801–803.

64. Woodtli W, Vonmoos P, Siegrist P, et al. Amodiaquin-induzierte hepatitis mit leukopenie. *Schweiz Med Wochenschr* 1986;116:966–968.

65. Bernuau J, Larrey D, Campillo B, et al. Amodiaquine-induced fulminant hepatitis. *J Hepatol* 1988;6:109–112.

66. Charmot G, Goujon C. Hépatites mineures pouvant être dues à l'amodiaquine. *Bull Soc Pathol Exot* 1987;80:266–270.

67. Raymond JM, Dumas F, Baldit C, et al. Fatal acute hepatitis due to amodiaquine. *J Clin Gastroenterol* 1989;11:602–603.

68. Graves P, Gelband H. Vaccines for preventing malaria. In: The Cochrane Library, Issue 4, 2000. Oxford: Update Software. Search date November 1999; primary sources Cochrane Infectious Diseases Group Trials Register; Cochrane Controlled Trials Register; Medline; Embase, and hand searches of reference lists; and personal contact with organisations and researchers in the field.

69. Osimitz TG, Murphy JV. Neurological effects associated with use of the insect repellent *N,N*-diethyl-*m*-toluamide (DEET). *J Toxicol Clin Toxicol* 1997;35:435–441.

70. De Garbino JP, Laborde A. Toxicity of an insect repellent: N,N-diethyl-m-toluamide. *Vet Hum Toxicol* 1983;25:422–423.

71. Are insect repellents safe [editorial]? *Lancet* 1988;2:610–611.

72. Bouchaud O, Longuet C, Coulaud JP. Prophylaxie du paludisme. *Rev Prat* 1998;48:279–286.

73. Smithuis FM, van Woensel JBM, Nordlander E, et al. Comparison of two mefloquine regimens for treatment of *Plasmodium falciparum* malaria on the northeastern Thai-Cambodian border. *Antimicrob Agents Chemother* 1993;37:1977–1981.

74. Ter Kuile FO, Dolan G, Nosten F, et al. Halofantrine versus mefloquine in treatment of multidrug-resistant falciparum malaria. *Lancet* 1993;341:1044–1049.

75. Luxemburger C, Price RN, Nosten F, et al. Mefloquine in infants and young children. *Ann Trop Paediatr* 1996;16:281–286.

76. Dolan G, ter Kuile FO, Jacoutot V, et al. Bed nets for the prevention of malaria and anaemia in pregnancy. *Trans R Soc Trop Med Hyg* 1993;87:620–626.

77. Suh KN, Keystone JS. Malaria prophylaxis in pregnancy and children. *Infect Dis Clin Pract* 1996;5:541–546.

78. Osimitz TG, Grothaus RH. The present safety assessment of DEET. *J Am Mosq Control Assoc* 1995;11:274–278.

79. Blomquist L, Thorsell W. Distribution and fate of the insect repellent 14C-N, N-diethyl-m-toluamide in the animal body. II. Distribution and excretion after cutaneous application. *Acta Pharmacol Toxicol (Copenh)* 1977;41:235–243.

80. Samuel BU, Barry M. The pregnant traveler. *Infect Dis Clin North Am* 1998;12:325–354.

81. Schaefer C, Peters PW. Intrauterine diethyltoluamide exposure and fetal outcome. *Reprod Toxicol* 1992;6:175–176.

82. Garner PGü, Imezoglu AM. Prevention versus treatment for malaria in pregnant women. In: The Cochrane Library, Issue 4, 2000. Oxford: Update Software. Search date not given; primary sources Cochrane Infectious Diseases Group Trials Register; Cochrane Controlled Trials' Register; Medline; Embase; and hand searches of reference lists and personal contact with researchers.

83. Cot M, Roisin A, Barro D, et al. Effect of chloroquine chemoprophylaxis during pregnancy on birth weight: results of a randomized trial. *Am J Trop Med Hyg* 1992;46:21–27.

84. Nosten F, texr Kuile F, Maelankiri L, et al. Mefloquine prophylaxis prevents malaria during pregnancy: a double-blind, placebo-controlled study. *J Infect Dis* 1994;169:595–603.

85. Shamiss A, Atar E, Zohar L, Cain Y. Mefloquine versus doxycycline for malaria prophylaxis in intermittent exposure of Israeli Air Force aircrew in Rwanda. *Aviat Space Environ Med* 1996;67:872–873.

86. Schlagenhauf P, Lobel H, Steffen R, et al. Tolerance of mefloquine by Swissair trainee pilots. *Am J Trop Med Hyg* 1997;56:235–240.

Ashley Croft
Consultant in Public Health Medicine
Ministry of Defence
London
UK

Competing interests: None declared.

Infectious diseases

Meningococcal disease

Search date January 2001

C Hart

QUESTIONS

INTERVENTIONS

Likely to be beneficial
Prophylactic antibiotics in

Unknown effectiveness
Antibiotics for throat carriage
(reduce carriage but unknown

To be covered in future issues of Clinical Evidence
Vaccines (monovalent/multivalent,
polysaccharide alone, or
conjugate)
Empirical treatment of suspected
meningococcal disease
Treatment of meningococcal
disease

Key Messages

- We found no randomised evidence about the effects of prophylactic antibiotics on the incidence of meningococcal disease among contacts. Observational evidence suggests that antibiotics reduce the risk of disease. We found no good evidence to address the question of which contacts should be treated.

- RCTs have found that antibiotics reduce throat carriage of the meningococcus. We found no evidence that eradicating throat carriage reduces the risk of meningococcal disease.

DEFINITION   Meningococcal disease is any clinical condition caused by *Neisseria meningitidis* (the meningococcus) groups A, B, C, or other serogroups. These conditions include purulent conjunctivitis, septic arthritis, meningitis, and septicaemia with or without meningitis.

INCIDENCE/ PREVALENCE   Meningococcal disease is sporadic in temperate countries, and is most commonly caused by group B or C meningococci. The incidence in the UK varies from 2–8 cases per 100 000 people a year,[1] and in the USA from 0.6–1.5 per 100 000 people.[2] Occasional outbreaks occur among close family contacts, secondary school pupils, and students living in halls of residence. Sub-Saharan Africa has regular epidemics due to serogroup A, particularly in countries lying between Gambia in the west and Ethiopia in the east (the "meningitis belt"), where incidence during epidemics reaches 500 per 100 000 people.[3]

AETIOLOGY/ RISK FACTORS   Meningococcus infects healthy people and is transmitted by close contact, probably by exchange of upper respiratory tract secretions (see table 1, p 525). Risk of transmission is greatest in the first week of contact.[4] Risk factors include crowding and exposure to cigarette smoke.[5] Children younger than 2 years have the highest incidence, with a second peak between ages 15–24. There is currently an increased incidence of meningococcal disease among university students, especially among those in their first term and living in catered accommodation,[6] although we found no accurate numerical estimate of risk from close contact in, for example, halls of residence. Close contacts of an index case have a much higher risk of infection than people in the general population.[4,7,8] The risk of epidemic spread is higher with group A and C meningococci than with group B meningococci.[9–12] It is not known what makes a meningococcus virulent, but certain clones tend to predominate at different times and in different groups. Carriage of meningococcus in the throat has been reported in 10–15% of people; recent acquisition of a virulent meningococcus is more likely to be associated with invasive disease.

PROGNOSIS   Mortality is highest in infants and adolescents, and is related to disease presentation: case fatality rates are 19–25% in septicaemia, 10–12% in meningitis plus septicaemia, and less than 1% in meningitis alone.[13–15]

AIMS   To prevent disease in contacts.

OUTCOMES   Rates of infection; rates of eradication of throat carriage; adverse effects of treatment.

METHODS   *Clinical Evidence* update search and appraisal January 2001. In addition, the author drew from a collection of references from the pre-electronic data era.

QUESTION What are the effects of prophylactic antibiotics on risk of disease in people exposed to someone with meningococcal disease?

We found no randomised evidence on the effects of prophylactic antibiotics on the incidence of meningococcal disease among contacts. Observational studies suggest that antibiotics reduce the risk of disease. We found no good evidence to address the question of which contacts should be treated.

Benefits: We found no systematic review and no RCTs examining the effect of prophylactic antibiotics in people who have been in contact with someone with meningococcal disease. **Rifampicin:** We found only anecdotal data. **Phenoxymethylpenicillin:** We found one retrospective study whose results cannot be generalised beyond the sample tested.[16] **Sulfadiazine:** One observational cohort study of soldiers in temporary troop camps in the 1940s compared the incidence of meningococcal disease in camps where sulfadiazine was given to everyone after a meningococcal outbreak, versus incidence in camps where no prophylaxis was given. The study reported a higher incidence of meningococcal disease in soldiers not given prophylaxis (approximate figures 17/9500 [0.2%] v 2/7000 [0.03%] over 8 weeks).[17]

Harms: **Rifampicin:** No excess adverse effects compared with placebo were found in RCTs on throat carriage of meningococcal disease.[18,19] However, rifampicin is known to turn urine and contact lenses orange, and to induce hepatic microsomal enzymes, potentially rendering oral contraception ineffective. Rifampicin prophylaxis may be associated with emergence of resistant strains.[20] **Sulfadiazine:** One in 10 soldiers experienced minor adverse events, including headache, dizziness, tinnitus, and nausea.[17]

Comment: RCTs addressing this question are unlikely to be performed, because the intervention has few associated risks whereas meningitis has high associated risks. RCTs would also need to be large to find a difference in incidence of meningococcal disease. In the sulfadiazine cohort study, the two infected people in the treatment group only became infected after leaving the camp.[17]

QUESTION What are the effects of antibiotics in people with throat carriage of meningococcal disease?

RCTs have found that antibiotics reduce throat carriage of meningococcus. We found no evidence that eradicating throat carriage reduces the risk of meningococcal disease.

Benefits: We found no systematic review. **Incidence of disease:** We found no RCTs or observational studies examining whether eradicating throat carriage of meningococcus reduces the risk of meningococcal disease. **Throat carriage:** We found five placebo controlled RCTs examining the effect of antibiotics on carriage of meningococcus in the throat (see table 2, p 526).[18,19,21–23] All trials reported that antibiotics (rifampicin, minocycline, or ciprofloxacin) achieved high rates of eradication (ranging from 90–97%), except one trial of rifampicin in students with heavy growth on culture, where the rate of eradication was 73%. Eradication rates on placebo ranged from 9–29%. We found seven RCTs comparing different antibiotic regimens (see table 3, p 527).[24–30] Three RCTs found no significant difference between rifampicin and either minocycline, ciprofloxacin, or intramuscular ceftriaxone.[25,28,30] A fourth RCT randomised households to different treatments and found that intramuscular ceftriaxone achieved higher eradication rates than rifampicin.[27] However, the trial used cluster randomisation, and therefore the results should be interpreted with caution. In another trial, oral azithromycin proved as effective as rifampicin in eradicating meningococcal throat carriage.[29]

Harms: **Minocycline:** One RCT reported adverse effects (1 or more of nausea, anorexia, dizziness, and abdominal cramps) in 36% of participants.[21] **Rifampicin:** See harms of postexposure antibiotic prophylaxis, p 522. **Ciprofloxacin:** Trials of single dose prophylactic regimens reported no more adverse effects than comparators or placebo.[22,23,28] Ciprofloxacin is contraindicated in pregnancy and in children because animal studies have indicated a possibility of articular cartilage damage in developing joints.[31] **Ceftriaxone:** Two trials of ceftriaxone found no significant adverse effects.[27,28] In one trial, 12% of participants complained of headache.[29] Ceftriaxone is given as a single intramuscular injection. **Azithromycin:** No serious or moderate adverse effects were reported, but nausea, abdominal pain, and headache of short duration were reported equally in the azithromycin and rifampicin treated groups.[27]

Comment: Eradication of meningococcal throat carriage is a well accepted surrogate for prevention of meningococcal disease. It is unlikely that any RCT will be conducted on the efficacy of prophylactic antibiotics in preventing secondary community acquired meningococcal disease in household contacts, because the number of participants required would be large.

REFERENCES

1. http://www.phls.co.uk/facts/meni.htm. Disease Facts: Meningococcal Disease.
2. Centers for Disease Control. Summary of notifiable diseases United States, 1997. *Morbid Mortal Wkly Rtn* 1998;46:1–87.
3. Hart CA, Cuevas LE. Meningococcal disease in Africa. *Ann Trop Med Parasitol* 1997;91:777–785.
4. De Wals P, Herthoge L, Borlée-Grimée I, et al. Meningococcal disease in Belgium. Secondary attack rate among household, day-care nursery and pre-elementary school contacts. *J Infect* 1981;3(suppl 1):53–61.
5. Stanwell-Smith RE, Stuart JM, Hughes AO, et al. Smoking, the environment and meningococcal disease: a case control study. *Epidemiol Infect* 1994;112:315–328.
6. Communicable Disease Surveillance Centre. Meningococcal disease in university students. *Commun Dis Rep CDR Wkly* 1998;8:49.
7. The Meningococcal Disease Surveillance Group. Meningococcal disease secondary attack rate and chemoprophylaxis in the United States. *JAMA* 1976;235:261–265.
8. Olcen P, Kjellander J, Danielson D, Linquist BC. Epidemiology of *Neisseria meningitidis*: prevalence and symptoms from the upper respiratory tract in family members to patients with meningococcal

disease. *Scand J Infect Dis* 1981;13:105–109.
9. French MR. Epidemiological study of 383 cases of meningococcus meningitis in the city of Milwaukee, 1927–1928 and 1929. *Am J Public Health* 1931;21:130–137.
10. Pizzi M. A severe epidemic of meningococcus meningitis in 1941–1942, Chile. *Am J Public Health* 1944;34:231–239.
11. Lee WW. Epidemic meningitis in Indianapolis 1929–1930. *J Prev Med* 1931;5:203–210.
12. Kaiser AB, Hennekens CH, Saslaw MS, Hayes PS, Bennett JV. Seroepidemiology and chemoprophylaxis of disease due to sulphonamide resistant *Neisseria meningitidis* in a civilian population. *J Infect Dis* 1974;130:217–221.
13. Andersen BM. Mortality in meningococcal infections. *Scand J Infect Dis* 1978;10:277–282.
14. Thomson APJ, Sills JA, Hart CA. Validation of the Glasgow meningococcal septicaemia prognostic score: a 10 year retrospective survey. *Crit Care Med* 1991;19:26–30.
15. Riordan FAI, Marzouk O, Thomson APJ, Sills JA, Hart CA. The changing presentation of meningococcal disease. *Eur J Pediatr* 1995;154:472–474.
16. Hoiby EA, Moe PJ, Lystad A, Froholm LO, Bovre K. Phenoxymethyl-penicillin treatment of household contacts of meningococcal disease patients.

Antonie Van Leeuwenhoek 1986;52:255–257.

17. Kuhns DW, Nelson CT, Feldman HA, Kuhns LR. The prophylactic value of sulfadiazine in the control of meningococcic meningitis. *JAMA* 1943;123:335–339.

18. Deal WB, Sanders E. Efficacy of rifampicin in treatment of meningococcal carriers. *N Engl J Med* 1969;281:641–645.

19. Eickhoff TC. In vitro and in vivo studies of resistance to rifampicin in meningococci. *J Infect Dis* 1971;123:414–420.

20. Weidmer CE, Dunkel TB, Pettyjohn FS, Smith CD, Leibowitz A. Effectiveness of rifampin in eradicating the meningococcal carrier state in a relatively closed population: emergence of resistant strains. *J Infect Dis* 1971;124:172–178.

21. Devine LF, Johnson DP, Hagerman CR, Pierce WE, Rhode SL, Peckinpaugh RO. The effect of minocycline on meningococcal nasopharyngeal carrier state in naval personnel. *Am J Epidemiol* 1971;93:337–345.

22. Renkonen OV, Sivonen A, Visakorpi R. Effect of ciprofloxacin on carrier rate of *Neisseria meningitidis* in army recruits in Finland. *Antimicrob Agents Chemother* 1987;31:962–963.

23. Dworzack DL, Sanders CC, Horowitz EA, et al. Evaluation of single dose ciprofloxacin in the eradication of *Neisseria meningitidis* from nasopharyngeal carriers. *Antimicrob Agents Chemother* 1988;32:1740–1741.

24. Artenstein MS, Lamson TH, Evans JR. Attempted prophylaxis against meningococcal infection using intramuscular penicillin. *Mil Med* 1967;132:1009–1011.

25. Guttler RB, Counts GW, Avent CK, Beaty HN. Effect of rifampicin and minocycline on meningococcal carrier rates. *J Infect Dis* 1971;124:199–205.

26. Blakebrough IS, Gilles HM. The effect of rifampicin on meningococcal carriage in family contacts in northern Nigeria. *J Infect* 1980;2:137–143.

27. Schwartz B, Al-Tobaiqi A, Al-Ruwais A, et al. Comparative efficacy of ceftriaxone and rifampicin in eradicating pharyngeal carriage of Group A *Neisseria meningitidis*. *Lancet* 1988;i:1239–1242.

28. Cuevas LE, Kazembe P, Mughogho GK, Tillotson GS, Hart CA. Eradication of nasopharyngeal carriage of *Neisseria meningitidis* in children and adults in rural Africa: A comparison of ciprofloxacin and rifampicin. *J Infect Dis* 1995;171:728–731.

29. Girgis N, Sultan Y, Frenck RW Jr, et al. Azithromycin compared with rifampin for eradication of masopharyngeal colonization by *Neisseria meningitidis*. *Pediatr Infect Dis J* 1998;17:816–819.

30. Simmons G, Jones N, Calder L. Equivalence of ceftriaxone and rifampicin in eliminating nasopharyngeal carriage of serogroup B *Neisseria meningitidis*. *J Antimicrob Chemother* 2000;45:909–911.

31. Schulter G. Ciprofloxacin: a review of its potential toxicologic effects. *Am J Med* 1987(suppl 4A):82;91–93.

32. Zangwill KM, Schuchat A, Riedo FX, et al. School-based clusters of meningococcal disease in the United States. *JAMA* 1997;277:389–395.

33. Hudson, PJ, Vogt PL, Heun EM, et al. Evidence for school transmission of *Neisseria meningitidis* during a Vermont outbreak. *Pediatr Infect Dis* 1986;5:213–217.

C Hart
Professor
Department of Medical Microbiology
and Genitourinary Medicine
University of Liverpool
Liverpool
UK

Competing interests: None declared.

TABLE 1 Risk of infection among contacts (see text, p 521).

Group of Meningococcus	Setting	Risk
A	Household contacts in Milwaukee, USA[9]	AR 1100/100 000; RR not possible to estimate.
	General population in Santiago province, Chile. Household contacts[10]	Attack rate in general population 23–262/100 000 (1941 and 1942). Attack rate in household contacts 250/100 000 (2.5%) over both years.
	General population in Indianapolis, USA[11]	AR 4500/100 000; RR not possible to estimate.
B	Household contacts in Belgium[4]	RR 1245*
	Nursery schools[4]	RR 23*
	Day care centres[4]	RR 76*
C	Household contacts from two lower socioeconomic groups Dade County, Florida, USA[12]	Attack rate in two communities 13/100 000 population. Attack rate in household contacts 5/85 (582/100 000).
Unspecified	School based clusters in USA. Predominant meningococcal types: 13 clusters of Gp C, 7 Gp B, 1 Gp Y, 1 GpC/W135 (impossible to distinguish)[32]	RR 2.3*
	Household contacts from several states in USA, meningococcus types B and C predominantly[7]	RR 500–800*
	Household contact in Norway. Meningococcus types A, B, and C predominantly[8]	RR up to 4000*
	Schools. Predominant meningococcus type C[33]	OR 14.1 (95% CI 1.6 to 127)

*Compared with the risk in the general population.

TABLE 2 Effect of antibiotics on throat carriage: results of placebo controlled RCTs (see text, p 522).

Antibiotic	Group of Meningococcus	Participants	Treatment (%)	Placebo (%)	RR (95% CI)
			Eradication		
Rifampicin (oral)[18]	B, X, Z	30 students with heavy growth on culture	11/15 (73)	2/15 (13)	5.5 (1.5 to 21)
Rifampicin (oral)[19]	B, C, Y, Z29 E, W 135, NT	76 airforce recruits	36/38* (95)	3/22‡ (14)	7.0 (5.8 to 8.1)
Minocycline (oral)[21]	Predominantly Y (63%)	149 naval recruits	37/41 (90)†	14/48 (29)§	3.1 (2.6 to 3.6)
Ciprofloxacin (oral)[22]	Non-groupable (61%), B (17.5%)	120 army recruits in Finland	54/56 (97) 5 second samples missing	7/53 (13) 6 second samples missing or not a carrier	7.3 (6.5 to 8.1)
Ciprofloxacin (oral)[23]	B (41%), Z (33%)	46 healthy volunteers	22/23 (96) (one did not adhere to treatment)	2/22 (9)	10.5 (8.9 to 12.1)

*9 lost to follow up. †37 either did not have meningococci prior to therapy or did not provide a full set of cultures. ‡7 lost to follow up. §23 either did not have meningococci prior to therapy or did not provide a full set of cultures.

TABLE 3	Effects of antibiotics on throat carriage: results of comparative RCTs (see text, p 523).			
Antibiotic	**Group of meningococcus**	**Participants**	**Rate of eradication (%)**	**RR (95% CI)**
Phenoxymethylpenicillin (im)[24]	C (49%), B (33%), NG (17%)	Adults	41/118 (35)	No data
Erythromycin (oral)[24]	C	Adults	0/7 (0)	No data
Rifampicin (oral)[25]	B + C (31%), NG (69%)	Adults	43/51 (84)	0.89 (0.76 to 1.02)
Minocycline (oral)[25]	B + C (31%), NG (69%)	Adults	36/38 (95)	No data
Rifampicin (oral)[25]	A	Children	37/48 (77)	No data
Sulfadimidine (oral)[26]	A	Children	0/34 (0)	No data
Ceftriaxone (im)[27]	A	Adults and children	66/68 (97)	1.29 (1.10 to 1.49)
Rifampicin (oral)[27]	A	Adults and children	27/36 (75)	No data
Ceftriaxone (im)[28]	A	Adults and children	39/41 (95)	No data
Ciprofloxacin (oral)[28]	A	Adults and children	70/79 (89)	No data
Rifampicin (oral)[28]	A	Adults and children	85/88 (97)	No data
Azithromycin (oral)[29]	B (63%), A (37%)	Adults	56/60 (93)	No data
Rifampicin (oral)[29]	B (63%), A (37%)	Adults	56/59 (95)	No data
Ceftriaxone (im)[30]	B (54%), other serogroups (46%)	Adults and children	97/100 (97)	No data
Rifampicin (oral)[30]	B (51%), other serogroups (49%)	Adults and children	78/82 (95.1)	No data

Im, intramuscular.

Search date July 2000: new for this issue

Jimmy Volmink

INTERVENTIONS

Key Messages

- One systematic review has found that, in mothers with human immunodeficiency virus (HIV), zidovudine versus placebo given to mothers significantly reduces the incidence of HIV in infants.

- One RCT found that nevirapine versus zidovudine given to mothers with HIV and to their newborns significantly reduced the incidence of HIV in infants.

- One RCT found limited evidence that elective caesarean section versus vaginal delivery in women with HIV reduced the incidence of HIV in infants.

- One RCT in women with HIV who had access to clean water and health education found that formula feeding versus breast feeding significantly reduced the incidence of HIV in infants, without increasing infant mortality. However, in countries with high infant mortality, avoiding breast feeding may increase infant morbidity and mortality.

- We found insufficient evidence about the effects of vaginal microbicides on the transmission of HIV to infants.

- One RCT found no significant difference in the incidence of HIV in infants of mothers taking hyperimmune globulin (HIVIG) versus immunoglobulin without HIV antibody (IVIG), in addition to a standard zidovudine regimen.

- RCTs found no significant difference in the incidence of HIV in the infants of pregnant women given vitamin A or multivitamins versus placebo.

DEFINITION Mother to child transmission of HIV type 1 (see glossary, p 533) infection can occur during pregnancy, in the intrapartum period, or postnatally through breast feeding.[1] In contrast, HIV type 2 (see glossary, p 533) is rarely transmitted from mother to child.[2] Infected children usually have no symptoms and signs of HIV at birth, but develop them over subsequent months or years.[3]

INCIDENCE/ A review of 13 cohorts found that the risk of mother to child
PREVALENCE transmission of HIV is about 15–20% in Europe, 15–30% in the USA, and 25–35% in Africa.[4] One global report estimated that 620 000 children below the age of 15 years were infected with HIV during 1999, bringing the total number of children with HIV/AIDS to 1.3 million worldwide.[5] Most of these children were infected from their mother, and 90% live in sub-Saharan Africa. An estimated 3.8 million children have died of HIV since the start of the epidemic.

AETIOLOGY/ Transmission of HIV to children is more likely if the mother has a
RISK FACTORS high viral load.[1,6,7] Women with detectable viraemia (by p24 antigen or culture) have double the risk of transmitting HIV-1 to their babies than those who do not.[1] Breast feeding has also been shown in prospective studies to be a risk factor.[8,9] Other risk factors include sexually transmitted diseases, chorioamnionitis, prolonged rupture of membranes, and vaginal mode of delivery.[5,10–13]

PROGNOSIS About 25% of babies infected with HIV progress rapidly to AIDS or death in the first year. Some survive beyond 12 years of age.[3] One European study found a mortality of 15% in the first year of life, and a mortality of 28% by the age of 5 years.[14]

AIMS To reduce mother to child transmission of HIV and improve infant survival, with minimal adverse effects.

OUTCOMES HIV infection status of the child; infant morbidity and mortality; maternal morbidity and mortality; adverse effects of treatment.

METHODS *Clinical Evidence* search and appraisal July 2000.

QUESTION **What are the effects of measures to reduce mother to child transmission of HIV?**

OPTION **ANTIRETROVIRAL DRUGS**

One systematic review has found that zidovudine versus placebo significantly reduces mother to child transmission of HIV. Preliminary results of an RCT in progress suggested that zidovudine plus lamivudine versus placebo significantly reduces mother to child transmission of HIV. One RCT found that nevirapine versus zidovudine given to the mother and to her newborn significantly reduced the risk of HIV transmission.

Benefits: **Versus placebo:** We found one systematic review (search date not stated, 4 RCTs, 1585 women), which compared zidovudine versus placebo given to the mother before, during, or after labour (see table 1, p 534).[15] In one of the included RCTs, infants of mothers receiving zidovudine were also given zidovudine for 6 weeks after birth.[16] Overall, zidovudine versus placebo significantly reduced the incidence of HIV in infants (AR 79/616 [13%] with zidovudine v 150/634 [24%]; RR 0.54, 95% CI 0.42 to 0.69; NNT 9, 95% CI 7 to 14). The results were still significant when the RCT of zidovudine which used the most intensive regimen[16] was excluded from the analysis (combined results for less intensive regimens versus placebo: AR 70/495 [14%] v 119/507 [23%]; RR 0.60, 95% CI 0.46 to 0.79; NNT 11, 95% CI 8 to 20).[17–19] The effect of zidovudine versus placebo was similar in reducing the incidence of HIV in infants from breast feeding and non-breast feeding mothers (breast feeding RR 0.62, 95% CI 0.46 to 0.85; non-breast feeding RR 0.50, 95% CI 0.30 to 0.85). The review[15] also identified one RCT of combination antiretroviral therapy versus placebo currently in progress in South Africa, Uganda, and Tanzania. Preliminary results suggest that zidovudine plus lamivudine versus placebo reduces the risk of HIV transmission at 6 weeks of age when administered in the antenatal, intrapartum, and postpartum period (RR 0.52, 95% CI 0.35 to 0.76), and during the intrapartum and postpartum period (RR 0.66, 95% CI 0.46 to 0.94). The trial found that lamivudine given during the intrapartum period alone did not significantly reduce the risk of transmission (RR 1.01, 95% CI 0.74 to 1.38). **Versus each other:** The systematic review[15] identified one unblinded RCT (626 women from a predominantly breast feeding population in Uganda), which compared nevirapine versus zidovudine.[20] It found that nevirapine given to mothers as a single oral dose at the onset of labour and to babies as a single dose within 72 hours of birth, versus zidovudine given orally to women during labour, and to their newborns for 7 days after birth significantly reduced the number of infants with HIV at 14 to 16 weeks (RR 0.58, 95% CI 0.40 to 0.83).

Harms: The review found that intensive zidovudine versus placebo significantly increased the risk of neonatal haematological toxicity (RR 1.86, 95% CI 1.18 to 2.94, specific effects undefined); whereas no significant difference was found for less intensive regimens versus placebo (RR 0.77, 95% CI 0.44 to 1.35).[15] Infants who received the most intensive regimen who were followed for 18 months had mild reversible anaemia, which resolved by 12 weeks of age.[21] The same trial in uninfected infants followed for a median of 4.2 years found no significant difference between zidovudine versus placebo in growth patterns, immunological parameters, or the occurrence of childhood cancers.[22] The RCT of combination antiretroviral therapy has reported no serious adverse drug reactions to date.[15] **Versus each other:** The RCT of zidovudine versus nevirapine found no significant difference in serious adverse effects in mothers and infants (4.0% v 4.7% in mothers; 19.8% v 20.5% in infants up to 18 months of age).[22]

Comment: RCTs evaluating alternative antiretroviral drug regimens, including one comparing different lengths of zidovudine treatment, are currently in progress and will be reported in future issues of *Clinical Evidence*.

OPTION   **ELECTIVE CAESAREAN SECTION**

One RCT found limited evidence that elective caesarean section versus vaginal delivery significantly reduced the incidence of HIV in children.

Benefits: We found one systematic review (search date not stated, 1 RCT, 436 women), which compared elective caesarean section at 38 weeks versus vaginal delivery.[15] It found that caesarean section significantly reduced the number of infants with HIV at 18 months (AR 3/170 [2%]

with caesarean section v 21/200 [11%] with vaginal delivery; RR 0.16, 95% CI 0.05 to 0.55; NNT 11, 95% CI 10 to 21).

Harms: No serious adverse effects were reported in either group. Postpartum fever was significantly more common in women with caesarean section versus vaginal delivery (AR 2/183 [1%] v 15/225 [7%]; RRI 6.1, 95% CI 1.45 to 22; NNH 18, 95% CI 16 to 50). Postpartum bleeding, intravascular coagulation, or severe anaemia occurred rarely in either group.

Comment: A total of 85% of the randomised women were included in the analysis. None of the women analysed breast fed. More women who gave birth by caesarean section versus vaginal delivery had received zidovudine during pregnancy (70% v 58%); this means that the observed difference between groups may not have been due exclusively to the different delivery methods.

OPTION AVOIDING BREAST FEEDING

One RCT in women with HIV who had access to clean water and health education found that formula feeding versus breast feeding significantly reduced the incidence of HIV in infants, without increasing mortality.

Benefits: We found no systematic review. We found one RCT (425 HIV-1 seropositive women with access to clean water and health education in Kenya), which found that breast feeding versus formula feeding significantly increased the number of infants with HIV at 24 months (AR 61/197 [31%] with breast feeding v 31/205 [15%]; RR 2.0, 95% CI 1.4 to 3.0; NNT 6, 95% CI 4 to 13).[23] Although infants were breast fed throughout the trial duration, the greatest exposure to breast milk occurred during the first 6 months of life. The trial found no significant difference in the mortality rate at 24 months with breast feeding versus formula feeding (AR 45/197 [23%] with breast feeding v 39/204 [19%] with formula feeding; RR 1.2, 95% CI 0.82 to 1.75).[23]

Harms: The RCT did not report on adverse effects.

Comment: In countries with high infant mortality, avoiding breast feeding may increase infant morbidity and mortality through its effect on nutrition, immunity, maternal fertility, and birth spacing. Access to clean water and education when using formula feeds may explain the similar mortality rates in breast fed and formula fed infants.

OPTION VAGINAL MICROBICIDES

We found insufficient evidence about the effects of vaginal microbicides on the incidence of HIV in infants.

Benefits: We found no systematic review or RCTs.

Harms: One non-randomised trial (see comment) reported no adverse effects in mothers or in infants.

Comment: We found one non-randomised trial (2094 women), which compared vaginal cleansing (with 0.25% chlorhexidine) from admission in labour to delivery versus no vaginal cleansing.[24] Women were allocated to the treatment or control group on the basis of months of the year. The trial found no significant difference in the transmission of

HIV after vaginal cleansing versus no cleansing (AR 136/505 [26.9%] v 133/477 [27.9%]; RR 0.95, 95% CI 0.8 to 1.2). The results should be interpreted with caution since HIV status was not determined in the 41% of infants who were lost to follow up, and the trial was not randomised and was therefore potentially biased.

OPTION   IMMUNOTHERAPY

One RCT found no significant difference in the incidence of HIV in infants of mothers taking HIVIG versus IVIG in addition to a standard zidovudine regimen.

Benefits: We found one systematic review (search date not stated, 1 RCT, 501 women),[15] which compared intravenous HIVIG versus IVIG given to women during pregnancy, the intrapartum period, and to their babies at birth. Women in both groups received a standard course of zidovudine and no babies breast fed. The RCT found no significant difference in transmission of HIV between HIVIG versus IVIG regimens at 6 months of age (4.1% v 6.0%, 95% CI for difference not provided, P = 0.36).

Harms: The trial reported no significant adverse effects.

Comment: The low overall transmission rate (5%) in this study was much lower than the anticipated rate of greater than 15% used to calculate the appropriate sample size. The trial is unable to exclude a clinically important effect of HIVIG on the number of children with HIV.

OPTION   VITAMIN SUPPLEMENTS

Two RCTs found that vitamin supplements versus placebo given to pregnant women had no significant effect on the incidence of HIV in their infants.

Benefits: We found no systematic review but found two RCTs.[25,26] The first RCT (1083 women with HIV-1 between 12 and 27 weeks gestation in Tanzania) compared vitamin A and/or multivitamin supplements (excluding vitamin A) versus placebo, using a factorial design.[25] It found no significant difference in the risk of transmission of HIV in women taking multivitamins or vitamin A versus placebo at birth (multivitamins v placebo: AR 38/376 [10%] v 24/363 [7%]; RR 1.54, 95% CI 0.94 to 2.51. Vitamin A v placebo: AR 38/380 [10%] v 24/358 [6.7%]; RR 1.49, 95% CI 0.91 to 2.43), or at 6 weeks among babies free of infection at birth (multivitamins v placebo: 31/191 [16%] v 28/179 [16%]; RR 1.04, 95% CI 0.65 to 1.66. Vitamin A v placebo: 35/196 [18%] v 24/174 [14%]; RR 1.30, 95% CI 0.80 to 2.09).[25] The second RCT (728 pregnant women with HIV in South Africa) compared vitamin A with placebo.[26] It found no significant difference in the risk of HIV infection at 3 months (20.3% with vitamin A v 22.3% with placebo, 95% CI for difference not provided). Mortality rates were similar in vitamin A and placebo groups at 1 month, 3 months, and 13 months of age.

Harms: Neither RCT reported adverse effects.[25,26]

Comment: The RCTs were performed because observational studies have found an association in pregnant women between transmission of HIV and low serum levels of vitamin A.[27]

GLOSSARY

Human immunodeficiency virus type 1 (HIV-1) is the most common cause of HIV disease throughout the world.

Human immunodeficiency virus type 2 (HIV-2) is predominantly found in West Africa and is more closely related to the simian immunodeficiency virus than to HIV-1.

REFERENCES

1. John GC, Kreiss J. Mother-to-child transmission of human immunodeficiency virus type 1. *Epidemiol Rev* 1996;18:149–157.
2. Adjorlolo-Johnson G, De Cock KM, Ekpini E, et al. Prospective comparison of mother-to-child transmission of HIV-1 and HIV-2 in Abidjan, Ivory Coast. *JAMA* 1994;272:462–466.
3. Peckham C, Gibb D. Mother-to-child transmission of the human immunodeficiency virus. *N Engl J Med* 1995;333:298–302.
4. The Working Group on MTCT of HIV. Rates of mother-to-child transmission of HIV-1 in Africa, America and Europe: results of 13 perinatal studies. *J Acquir Immune Defic Syndr* 1995;8:506–510.
5. UNAIDS (Joint United Nations Programme on HIV/AIDS). *Report of the global HIV/AIDS epidemic.* June 2000. Geneva: UNAIDS; 2000. UNAIDS/00.13E.
6. Mofenson LM. Epidemiology and determinants of vertical HIV transmission. *Semin Pediatr Infect Dis* 1994;5:252–256.
7. Khouri YF, McIntosh K, Cavacini L, et al. Vertical transmission of HIV-1: correlation with maternal viral load and plasma levels of CD4 binding site anti-gp 120 antibodies. *J Clin Invest* 1995;95:732–737.
8. Dunn DT, Newell ML, Ades AE, Peckham CS. Risk of human immunodeficiency virus type-1 transmission through breastfeeding. *Lancet* 1992;240:585–588.
9. Miotti PG, Taha ET, Newton I, et al. HIV transmission through breastfeeding: a study in Malawi. *JAMA* 1999;282:744–749.
10. Nair P, Alger L, Hines S, Seiden S, Hebel R, Johnson JP. Maternal and neonatal characteristics associated with HIV infection in infants of seropositive women. *J Acquir Immune Defic Syndr* 1993;6:298–302.
11. Minkoff H, Burns DN, Landesman S, et al. The relationship of the duration of ruptured membranes to vertical transmission of human immunodeficiency virus. *Am J Obstet Gynecol* 1995;173:585–589.
12. European Collaborative Study. Risk factors for mother-to-child transmission of HIV-1. *Lancet* 1992;339:1007–1012.
13. Mofenson LM. A critical review of studies evaluating the relationship of mode of delivery to perinatal transmission of human immunodeficiency virus. *Pediatr Infect Dis J* 1995;14:169–176.
14. The European Collaborative Study. Natural history of vertically acquired human immunodeficiency virus-1 infection. *Pediatrics* 1994;94:815–819.
15. Brocklehurst P. Interventions aimed at decreasing the risk of mother-to-child transmission of HIV infection. In: The Cochrane Library, Issue 3, 2000. Oxford: Update Software. Search date not stated; primary sources Cochrane Pregnancy and Childbirth Group Trials Register; Cochrane Controlled Trials Register.
16. Connor EM, Sperling RS, Gelber RD, et al. Reduction of maternal-infant transmission of human immunodeficiency virus type 1 with zidovudine treatment. *N Engl J Med* 1994;311:1173–1180.
17. Shaffer N, Chuachoowong R, Mock PA, et al. Short-course zidovudine for perinatal HIV-1 transmission in Bangkok, Thailand: a randomised controlled trial. Bangkok Collaborative Perinatal HIV Transmission Study Group. *Lancet* 1999;353:773–780.
18. Wiktor SZ, Ekpini E, Karon JM, et al. Short-course oral zidovudine for prevention of mother-to-child transmission of HIV-1 in Abidjan, Cote d'Ivoire: a randomised trial. *Lancet* 1999;353:781–785.
19. Dabis F, Msellati P, Meda N, et al. Six-month efficacy, tolerance, and acceptability of a short regimen of oral zidovudine to reduce vertical transmission of HIV in breastfed children in Cote d'Ivoire and Burkina Faso: a double-blind placebo-controlled multicentre trial. DITRAME Study Group. Diminution de la Transmission Mere-Enfant. *Lancet* 1999;353:786–792.
20. Guay LA, Musoke P, Fleming T, et al. Intrapartum and neonatal single-dose nevirapine compared with zidovudine for prevention of mother-to-child transmission of HIV-1 in Kampala, Uganda: HIVNET 012 randomised trial. *Lancet* 1999;354:795–802.
21. Sperling RS, Shapiro DE, McSherry GD, et al. Safety of the maternal-infant zidovudine regimen utilized in the Pediatric AIDS Clinical Trial Group 076 Study. *AIDS* 1998;12:1805–1813.
22. Culnane M, Fowler MG, Lee S, et al. Lack of long term effects of in utero exposure to zidovudine among uninfected children born to HIV-infected women. *JAMA* 1999;281:151–157.
23. Nduati R, John G, Mbori-Ngacha D, et al. Effect of breastfeeding and formula feeding on transmission of HIV-1: a randomized clinical trial. *JAMA* 2000;283:1167–1174.
24. Biggar RJ, Miotti PG, Taha TE, et al. Perinatal intervention trial in Africa: effect of a birth canal cleansing intervention to prevent HIV transmission. *Lancet* 1996;347:1647–1650.
25. Fawzi WW, Msamanga G, Hunter D, et al. Randomized trial of vitamin supplements in relation to vertical transmission of HIV-1 in Tanzania. *J Acquir Immune Defic Syndr* 2000;23:246–254.
26. Coutsoudis A, Pillay K, Spooner E, Kuhn L, Coovadia HM. Randomized trial testing the effect of vitamin A supplementation on pregnancy outcomes and early, mother-to-child HIV-1 transmission in Durban, South Africa. *AIDS* 1999;13:1517–1524.
27. Fawzi WW, Hunter DJ. Vitamins in HIV disease progression and vertical transmission. *Epidemiology* 1998;9:457–466.

Jimmy Volmink

South African Cochrane Centre, Medical Research Council
Cape Town, South Africa
Competing interests: None declared.

Infectious diseases

TABLE 1   Placebo controlled trials of zidovudine to reduce mother to child transmission of HIV (see text, p 529).

Reference	Participants	Maternal treatment	Infant treatment	Transmission rate	RRR (95% CI)
Infants not breast fed					
16	477 women with confirmed HIV (60 centres in USA and France)	*Antepartum* Orally 1 mg 5 times daily starting at 14–34 weeks gestation *Intrapartum* 2 mg/kg IV over 1 hour then 1 mg/kg/h until delivery	Orally 2 mg/kg 6 hourly for 6 weeks (given only to babies of mothers treated with ZDV)	At 18 months: placebo 26% ZDV 8%	70% (39% to 85%)
17	397 women with confirmed HIV-1 (2 gcentres in Bangkok, Thailand)	*Antepartum* Orally 3 mg twice daily from 36 weeks gestation *Intrapartum* Orally 300 mg every 3 hours until delivery	Nil	At 6 months: placebo 19% ZDV 9%	50% (15% to 70%)
Infants breast fed					
18	280 women with confirmed HIV-1 (1 hospital in Cote d'Ivoire)	*Antepartum* Orally 3 mg twice daily from 36 weeks gestation *Intrapartum* Orally 300 mg every 3 hours until delivery	Nil	At 3 months: placebo 25% ZDV 16%	37% (−6% to +62%)
19	431 women with confirmed HIV-1 (Cote d'Ivoire and Burkina Faso)	*Antepartum* Orally 250 or 3 mg twice daily from 36 to 38 weeks gestation *Intrapartum* Orally single dose of 500 or 600 mg at onset of labour *Postpartum* Orally 250 or 3 mg twice daily for 7 days	Nil	At 6 months: placebo 28% ZDV 18%	35% (4% to 56%)

ZDV, zidovudine.

INTERVENTIONS

Opportunistic infections and HIV

Key Messages

- Systematic reviews have found that TMP/SMX is more effective than pentamidine or placebo at reducing the incidence of *Pneumocystis carinii* pneumonia (PCP) or toxoplasmosis.

- One systematic review found no significant difference between high and low dose TMP/SMX for PCP, although adverse effects were more common with the higher dose.

- Systematic reviews have found that TMP/SMX compared with dapsone/pyrimethamine reduces the incidence of PCP, but does not reduce the incidence of toxoplasmosis.

- Two systematic reviews of RCTs have found that antituberculosis prophylaxis reduces the rate of tuberculosis and death in the short term in people who are human immunodeficiency virus (HIV) and tuberculin skin test positive. We found insufficient evidence about the long term effects on rates of tuberculosis and death. The reviews found no evidence of benefit in people who are HIV positive but tuberculin skin test negative.

- We found evidence from RCTs that
  - Dapsone or aerosolised pentamidine have similar effectiveness to atovaquone at preventing PCP in TMP/SMX intolerant people.
  - Azithromycin, either alone or in combination with rifabutin, reduces the risk of PCP compared with rifabutin alone in people receiving standard PCP prophylaxis.
  - Regimens using combinations of tuberculosis drugs for 2–3 months have similar effectiveness as those using isoniazid alone for 6–12 months. One RCT found that adverse reactions causing cessation of treatment are more common with multidrug regimens.
  - Azithromycin and clarithromycin reduce the incidence of *Mycobacterium avium* complex (MAC) more than placebo.
  - Clarithromycin alone, and clarithromycin plus rifabutin, both reduce the incidence of MAC compared with rifabutin alone. Azithromycin plus rifabutin reduce the incidence of MAC compared with azithromycin alone.
  - Clarithromycin plus ethambutol, with or without rifabutin, reduces the incidence of MAC in people with previous MAC disease. Clofazimine and high dose clarithromycin are associated with increased mortality.
  - Oral ganciclovir may reduce the incidence of cytomegalovirus (CMV) in people with severe CD4 depletion compared with placebo, but one RCT found important side effects.
  - Valaciclovir reduces the incidence of CMV more than aciclovir, but is associated with increased mortality. One systematic review found that aciclovir did not reduce the incidence of CMV compared with placebo, but significantly reduced herpes simplex virus (HSV) and varicella zoster virus (VZV) infection and overall mortality in people at different stages of HIV infection.
  - Famciclovir compared with placebo reduces the rate of HSV shedding, but we found insufficient evidence on the effect of famciclovir on HSV recurrence.
  - Fluconazole and itraconazole reduce the incidence of invasive fungal infections compared with placebo in people with advanced HIV disease. Fluconazole reduces the incidence of invasive fungal disease and mucocutaneous candidiasis more than clotrimazole. There was no significant difference between high and low dose fluconazole.

- Itraconazole reduces the incidence of relapse of *Penicillium marneffei* infection, and is more effective than fluconazole in reducing the relapse of cryptococcal meningitis.
- In people with adequate increases in CD4 cell count while on potent antiretroviral therapy, stopping prophylaxis does not increase the incidence of PCP, toxoplasmosis, or MAC disease.
- We found insufficient evidence on the effects of stopping maintenance therapy for CMV retinitis or other end organ disease.

DEFINITION   Opportunistic infections are intercurrent infections that occur in people infected with HIV. Prophylaxis aims to avoid either the first occurrence of these infections (primary prophylaxis) or their recurrence (secondary prophylaxis, maintenance therapy). This review includes *Pneumocystis carinii* pneumonia (PCP), *Toxoplasma gondii* encephalitis, *Mycobacterium tuberculosis*, *Mycobacterium avium* complex (MAC) disease, cytomegalovirus (CMV) disease (most often retinitis), infections from other herpes viruses (herpes simplex virus [HSV] and varicella zoster virus [VZV]), and invasive fungal disease (*Cryptococcus neoformans*, *Histoplasma capsulatum* and Penicillium marneffei).

AETIOLOGY/   Opportunistic infections are caused by a wide array of pathogens
RISK FACTORS and result from immune defects induced by HIV. The risk of developing opportunistic infections increases dramatically with progressive impairment of the immune system. Each opportunistic infection has a different threshold of immune impairment, beyond which the risk increases substantially.[1] Opportunistic pathogens may infect the immunocompromised host *de novo*, but usually they are simply reactivations of latent pathogens in such hosts.

PROGNOSIS   Prognosis depends on the type of opportunistic infection. Even with treatment they may cause serious morbidity and mortality. Most deaths due to HIV infection are caused by opportunistic infections.

AIMS   To prevent the occurrence and relapse of opportunistic infections; to discontinue unnecessary prophylaxis; to minimise adverse effects of prophylaxis, and loss of quality of life.

OUTCOMES   First occurrence and relapse of opportunistic infections and adverse effects of treatments. We have not considered neoplastic diseases associated with specific opportunistic infections.

METHODS   *Clinical Evidence* search and appraisal March 2000. We also reviewed abstract books/CDs for the following conferences held between 1995 and early 2000: European Clinical AIDS, HIV Drug Therapy, Interscience Conferences on Antimicrobial Agents and Chemotherapy, National Conferences on Human Retroviruses and Opportunistic Infections, North American Retrovirus and Oppportunistic Infection (Washington/Chicago, USA), and World AIDS Conference. We placed emphasis on systematic reviews and RCTs published after 1993. We considered observational evidence if no RCTs were available or if it covered a broader spectrum than randomised evidence.

Infectious diseases

John Ioannidis

OPTION TMP/SMX

Systematic reviews have found that TMP/SMX is more effective than
pentamidine or placebo at reducing the incidence of PCP or
toxoplasmosis. Two systematic reviews found that TMP/SMX compared
with dapsone (with or without pyrimethamine) reduced the incidence of
PCP, but found no difference in the incidence of toxoplasmosis. One
systematic review and one subsequent RCT found no significant
difference between high and low dose TMP/SMX for PCP prophylaxis,
although adverse effects were more common with the higher dose.

Benefits: **TMP/SMX versus placebo:** We found one systematic review (39
RCTs, search date 1995) in people with either CD4 < 200/mm^3, or
a prior history of PCP, of prophylaxis for PCP (39 RCTs, n = 6583),
and toxoplasmosis (15 RCTs, n = 3641).[2] People with oropharyngeal candidiasis were often also considered for prophylaxis. Overall,
it found that prophylaxis with TMP/SMX reduced the incidence of
PCP more than placebo (RR 0.32, 95% CI 0.23 to 0.46). There
were no placebo controlled data on the incidence of toxoplasmosis.
One subsequent RCT (n = 545) in sub-Saharan Africa compared
TMP/SMX against placebo in 545 people with symptomatic disease
(2nd or 3rd clinical stage disease in the WHO staging system (see
glossary, p 549) regardless of CD4 cell count.[3] It found no significant difference in incidence of PCP or toxoplasmosis. **TMP/SMX
versus pentamidine:** We found two systematic reviews.[2,4] The first
review (search date 1995) found that TMP/SMX was significantly
more effective at preventing PCP than aerosolised pentamidine (RR
0.58, 95% CI 0.45 to 0.75).[2] The second (22 RCTs, search date
1995) found similar results.[4] TMP/SMX was also more effective
than aerosolised pentamidine at preventing toxoplasmosis.[4] **TMP/
SMX versus dapsone (with or without pyrimethamine):** The first
systematic review found that TMP/SMX compared with dapsone
(with or without pyrimethamine) reduced the incidence of PCP, but
the result did not reach significance (RR 0.61, 95% CI 0.34 to
1.10).[2] The second review found that TMP/SMX was significantly
more effective in preventing PCP than dapsone/pyrimethamine (RR
0.49, 95% CI 0.26 to 0.92).[4] It found no significant difference
between TMP/SMX and dapsone/pyrimethamine in preventing toxoplasmosis (RR 1.17, 95% CI 0.68 to 2.04). **High versus low dose
TMP/SMX:** The first systematic review found no significant difference between lower dose TMP/SMX 160/800 mg three times
weekly or 80/400 mg daily, and higher dose TMP/SMX, 160/800 mg
daily (failure rate per 100 person years was 1.6, 95% CI 0.9 to 2.5
with lower dose v 0.5, 95% CI 0% to 2.9% with higher dose).[2] A
subsequent RCT (n = 2625) also found no significant difference in
the rate of PCP infection in people receiving daily compared with
thrice weekly TMP/SMX 160/800 mg (3.5 v 4.1 per 100 person
years; P = 0.16).[5]

Harms: One systematic review found that adverse effects (predominantly
rash, fever, and haematological side effects) severe enough to lead

to discontinuation within 1 year occurred in more people taking higher doses of TMP/SMX than taking lower doses (25% v 15%).[2] The RCT comparing high dose with low dose TMP/SMX found that discontinuation due to adverse effects was significantly more common in people taking high doses of TMP/SMX (RR 2.14; P < 0.001).[5] Adverse effects occurred in more people taking high doses than low doses of dapsone (29% v 12%).[2] The RCT in sub-Saharan Africa found that people on TMP/SMX were less likely to suffer a serious event (death or hospital admission, irrespective of the cause) than those on placebo regardless of their initial CD4 cell count (84 v 124; hazard ratio 0.57, 95% CI 0.43 to 0.75; P < 0.001). Moderate neutropenia occurred more frequently with TMP/SMX (neutropenia AR 62/271 [23%] with TMP/SMX versus 26/244 [10%] with placebo; RR 2.1, 95% 1.4 to 3.3; NNH 8, 95% CI 5 to 14).[3] Two RCTs (abstract only; largest n = 377) found that gradual initiation of TMP/SMX may improve tolerance of the regimen.[6,7] Two RCTs (n = 238, n = 50) found no significant benefit from acetylcysteine in preventing TMP/SMX hypersensitivity reactions in HIV infected people.[8,9] Bronchospasm occurred in 2.5% of people taking aerosolised pentamidine 300 mg monthly.[2]

Comment: **Concomitant coverage for toxoplasmosis:** Standard TMP/SMX prophylaxis or dapsone should offer adequate coverage for toxoplasmosis. Pentamidine has no intrinsic activity against *T gondii*. Toxoplasmosis risk is probably clinically meaningful only with CD4 < 100/mm^3 and positive toxoplasma serology.[1] **Role of HAART:** We found more than 50 RCTs on the prophylaxis of PCP and/or toxoplasmosis, but their results should be interpreted with caution since they were conducted mostly before the advent and widespread use of highly active antiretroviral regimens. Although this is unlikely to affect the comparative results, HAART has resulted in a large decrease in the rate of PCP, toxoplasmosis and other opportunistic infections. Therefore, the absolute benefits of these prophylactic regimens are probably smaller when used with HAART. **Prophylaxis in Africa:** Beneficial effects of TMP/SMX in Africa are mostly due to coverage for bacterial infections rather than PCP.

| OPTION | ATOVAQUONE IN TMP/SMX INTOLERANT PEOPLE |

RCTs found no significant difference between atovaquone, dapsone, or aerosolised pentamidine in preventing PCP. None of the interventions were compared to placebo.

Benefits: We found no systematic review. **Versus placebo:** We found no RCTs. **Versus dapsone:** One RCT in 1057 people, of whom 298 had a history of PCP, found no significant difference between atovaquone (1500 mg daily) compared with dapsone (100 mg daily) in people intolerant of TMP/SMX (15.7 v 18.4 cases of PCP per 100 person years; P = 0.20).[10] **Versus pentamidine:** One RCT in 549 people intolerant of TMP/SMX compared high dose with low dose atovaquone (1500 mg daily v 750 mg daily) with monthly aerosolised pentamidine (300 mg). It found no significant difference between the groups in the incidence of PCP (26% v 22% v

17%) or mortality (20% *v* 13% *v* 18%) after a median follow up of 11.3 months.[11]

Harms: The RCT comparing atovaquone with dapsone found that the overall risk of stopping treatment owing to adverse effects was similar in the two arms (RR 0.94, 95% CI 0.74 to 1.19).[10] Atovaquone was stopped more frequently than dapsone in people who were receiving dapsone at baseline (RR 3.78, 95% CI 2.37 to 6.01; P < 0.001), and less frequently in people not receiving dapsone at baseline (RR 0.42, 95% CI 0.30 to 0.58; P < 0.001).

Comment: See role of HAART in comment under TMP/SMX, p 539.

OPTION   AZITHROMYCIN

One RCT found that azithromycin, either alone or in combination with rifabutin, reduced the risk of PCP compared with rifabutin alone in people receiving standard PCP prophylaxis.

Benefits: We found no systematic review. **Versus placebo:** We found no RCTs. **Versus other drugs:** We found one RCT (n = 693), which compared azithromycin, rifabutin, and both drugs in combination, in people who were already receiving standard PCP prophylaxis. It found that azithromycin, either alone or in combination with rifabutin, reduced the risk of developing PCP by 45% when compared with rifabutin alone (P = 0.008).[12]

Harms: Gastrointestinal side effects are common with azithromycin, but they are usually mild and do not lead to stopping treatment. The addition of rifabutin significantly increased the risk of stopping treatment (RR 1.67; P = 0.03).[13]

Comment: See role of HAART in comment under TMP/SMX, p 539. The low incidence of PCP infection in people taking HAART means that the benefit of prophylaxis is smaller.

QUESTION   What are the effects of antituberculosis prophylaxis in people with HIV infection?

Margaret Johnson, Andrew Phillips, and David Wilkinson

OPTION   ANTITUBERCULOSIS PROPHYLACTIC REGIMENS VERSUS PLACEBO

Two systematic reviews of RCTs have found that in people who are HIV and tuberculin skin test positive antituberculosis prophylaxis reduces frequency of tuberculosis in the short term. Long term effects on rates of tuberculosis and death are unknown. The reviews found no evidence of benefit in people who are HIV positive but tuberculin skin test negative.

Benefits: We found two systematic reviews; one (updated in 1999)[14] identified six well conducted RCTs in 4652 HIV positive adults from Haiti, Kenya, USA, Zambia, and Uganda. All compared isoniazid (6–12 months) or combination therapy (3 months) with placebo. Mean follow up was 2–3 years, and the main outcomes, stratified by tuberculin skin test positivity, were tuberculosis (either microbiological or clinical) and death. Among tuberculin skin test positive adults, antituberculosis prophylaxis significantly reduced the incidence of tuberculosis (RR compared with placebo 0.24, 95% CI 0.14 to 0.40) and was associated with a trend towards reducing the risk of death (RR compared with placebo 0.77, 95% CI 0.58 to 1.03). Among tuberculin skin test negative adults, there was no significant difference in risk of tuberculosis (RR compared with placebo 0.87, 95% CI 0.56 to 1.36) or death (RR compared with placebo 1.07, 95% CI 0.88 to 1.30). The second review included seven trials comprising 4529 participants and compared isoniazid with placebo only. Among tuberculin skin test positive participants the incidence of tuberculosis was significantly reduced (RR compared with placebo 0.40, 95% CI 0.24 to 0.65), but this was not so among tuberculin skin test negative participants (RR compared with placebo 0.84, 95% CI 0.54 to 1.30). There was no evidence of any impact on mortality in this review.[15]

Harms: Data on adverse drug reactions were not always stratified by tuberculin skin test positivity. In the first review there was a significant increase in adverse drug reactions requiring cessation of treatment on isoniazid compared with placebo (RR 1.75, 95% CI 1.23 to 2.47).[14] In the second review, the estimated RR was 1.36 (95% CI 1.00 to 1.86).[15]

Comment: Without prophylaxis, people who are HIV and tuberculin skin test positive have a 50% or more lifetime risk of developing tuberculosis, compared with a 10% lifetime risk in people who are HIV positive but tuberculin skin test negative.[16] Clinical features of tuberculosis may be atypical in people with HIV infection, and diagnosis may be more difficult, disease progression more rapid, and outcome worse.

OPTION	DIFFERENT ANTITUBERCULOSIS PROPHYLACTIC REGIMENS

RCTs have found no evidence of a difference in effectiveness between regimens using combinations of tuberculosis drugs for 2–3 months and those using isoniazid alone for 6–12 months. Adverse reactions causing cessation of treatment are more common with multidrug regimens.

Benefits: We found no systematic review. We found four published RCTs. Three compared isoniazid with rifampicin/pyrazinamide in people who were HIV and tuberculin skin test positive (n = 750, n = 1583, and n = 393).[17–19] All found no significant difference in rates of tuberculosis. The fourth RCT included 1564 HIV and tuberculin skin test positive people from Uganda.[20] It found that the risk of tuberculosis was reduced with isoniazid alone (RR compared with placebo 0.33, 95% CI 0.14 to 0.77), and with isoniazid and rifampicin combined (RR compared with placebo 0.40, 95% CI 0.18 to 0.86), and showed a trend towards reduction with isoniazid, rifampicin, and pyrazinamide combined (RR compared with placebo 0.51, 95% CI 0.24 to 1.08).

Harms: The proportion of people discontinuing treatment increased with the number of drugs given: isoniazid 0.6%, isoniazid plus rifampicin 2.3%, and all three drugs 5.6%.[20]

Comment: There is concern about emergence of rifampicin resistance if this drug is used in antituberculosis prophylaxis, although we found no reports of this. On the other hand, there is a theoretical risk that widespread, unsupervised use of isoniazid alone could promote resistance to this drug, although there is no evidence that this has happened. We found no adequate comparison of the long term effects of single drug compared with combination drug antituberculosis prophylaxis.

| QUESTION | What are the effects of prophylaxis for disseminated MAC disease for people without previous MAC disease? |

John Ioannidis

| OPTION | AZITHROMYCIN |

One RCT found that azithromycin reduced the incidence of MAC more than placebo.

Benefits: We found no systematic review. One RCT (174 people with AIDS and CD4 $< 100/mm^3$) found that azithromycin reduced the incidence of MAC more than placebo (10.6% v 24.7%; P = 0.004).[21]

Harms: Gastrointestinal side effects were more likely with azithromycin than with placebo (71/90 [79%] v 25/91 [28%]), but they were rarely severe enough to cause discontinuation of treatment (8% v 2.3% in the two arms; P = 0.14).[21]

Comment: Prospective cohort studies have found that the risk of disseminated MAC disease increases substantially with a lower CD4 count and is clinically important only for CD4 $< 50/mm^3$.[1] **Role of HAART:** Most of the RCTs of MAC prophylaxis were conducted before the widespread use of HAART. HAART reduces the absolute risk of MAC infection. The absolute risk reduction of prophylactic regimens may be smaller when used in people treated with HAART.

| OPTION | CLARITHROMYCIN |

One RCT found that clarithromycin reduced the incidence of MAC compared with placebo.

Benefits: We found one systematic review of prophylaxis and treatment of MAC (search date 1997).[22] It identified one RCT in 682 people with advanced AIDS, which found that clarithromycin compared with placebo significantly reduced the incidence of MAC (6% v 16%; hazard ratio 0.31; 95% CI 0.18 to 0.53). It found no significant difference in the death rate (32% v 41%; hazard ratio 0.75; P = 0.026).[23]

Harms: Adverse effects led to discontinuation of treatment in more people taking clarithromycin than placebo (8% v 6%; P = 0.45). More people taking clarithromycin suffered taste perversion (11% v 2%) or rectal disorders (8% v 3%).[23]

Comment: Prospective cohort studies found that the risk of disseminated MAC disease increased substantially with a lower CD4 count and was clinically important only for CD4 $< 50/mm^3$.[1] See role of HAART in comment under azithromycin, p 540.

| OPTION | COMBINATION THERAPY |

RCTs have found that clarithromycin alone, and clarithromycin plus rifabutin, both reduce the incidence of MAC compared with rifabutin alone. Azithromycin plus rifabutin reduced the incidence of MAC compared with azithromycin alone.

Benefits: **Clarithromycin plus rifabutin:** We found no systematic review. One RCT in 1178 people with AIDS compared rifabutin with clarithromycin, and rifabutin with clarithromycin and rifabutin combined.[24] It found that the risk of MAC was significantly reduced in the clarithromycin alone group (RRR 44% for clarithromycin v rifabutin; P = 0.005) and the combination group when compared with rifabutin alone (RRR 57% for combination v rifabutin; P = 0.0003). There was no significant difference in the risk of MAC between the combination and clarithromycin arms (P = 0.36). **Azithromycin plus rifabutin:** We found one systematic review of prophylaxis and treatment of MAC (search date 1997).[22] It identified one RCT (n = 693), found the combination of azithromycin and rifabutin was more effective than azithromycin alone (1 year incidence of MAC: 15.3% with rifabutin, 7.6% for azithromycin, 2.8% for rifabutin plus azithromycin: P = 0.008 for rifabutin v azithromycin, P = 0.03 for combination v azithromycin).[13]

Harms: In one RCT, dose limiting toxicity was more likely with azithromycin plus rifabutin than with azithromycin alone (hazard ratio 1.67; P = 0.03).[13] In another RCT adverse events occurred in 31% of people receiving the combination of clarithromycin and rifabutin compared with 16% on clarithromycin alone and 18% on rifabutin alone (P < 0.001).[24] Uveitis occurred in 42 people: 33 were on clarithromycin plus rifabutin, seven were on rifabutin alone, and two were on clarithromycin alone. **Uveitis:** We found one systematic review in 54 people with rifabutin associated uveitis (search date December 1996).[25] It found that uveitis was dose dependent. It occurred from 2 weeks to more than 7 months after initiation of rifabutin therapy, and was more likely in people taking rifabutin and clarithromycin. In most cases uveitis resolved 1–2 months after discontinuation of rifabutin.

Comment: Prospective cohort studies have found that the risk of disseminated MAC disease increased substantially with a lower CD4 count and was clinically important only for CD4 < 50/mm^3.[1] Clarithromycin may inhibit rifabutin metabolism; rifabutin may decrease levels of delavirdine and saquinavir. See role of HAART in comment under azithromycin, p 540.

| QUESTION | What are the effects of prophylaxis for disseminated MAC disease for people with previous MAC disease? |

John Ioannidis

| OPTION | COMBINATION THERAPY |

RCTs found that clarithromycin and ethambutol, with or without rifabutin, reduced the incidence of MAC. Clofazimine and high dose clarithromycin were associated with increased mortality.

Benefits: We found no systematic review but found four RCTs. The first RCT in 95 people found that the combination of clarithromycin (1000 mg daily), clofazimine and ethambutol was associated with significantly fewer relapses of MAC than the combination of clarithromycin plus clofazimine without ethambutol (12% relapsed in three-drug regimen v 68% in two-drug regimen at 36 weeks; P = 0.004).[26] The second RCT (n = 106) found that the addition of clofazimine to clarithromycin and ethambutol did not improve clinical response and was associated with higher mortality.[27] The third RCT (n = 144) found that the combination of clarithromycin, rifabutin, and ethambutol reduced the relapse rate of MAC compared with clarithromycin plus clofazimine.[28] The fourth RCT found no difference in survival between people taking clarithromycin plus ethambutol and people taking clarithromycin plus ethambutol plus rifabutin.[29]

Harms: The second RCT, which added clofazimine to clarithromycin plus rifabutin, found a higher mortality in the clofazimine arm (62% with clofazimine v 38% without clofazimine; P = 0.012).[27] High doses of clarithromycin (1000 mg twice daily)[30,31] and clofazimine[27] were associated with increased mortality. One RCT of clarithromycin 500 mg bd compared with 1000 mg bd found that after a median follow up of 4.5 months, more people died with the higher dose (17/40 [43%] with 1000 mg bd v 10/45 [22%] with 500 mg bd; ARI 20%, 95% CI 0.2% to 33%; NNH 5, 95% CI 3 to 470).[30] A similar difference was seen in another RCT (n = 154).[31] Combinations of drugs may lead to increased toxicity. Optic neuropathy may occur with ethambutol, but has not been reported in RCTs in people with HIV where the dose and symptoms were carefully monitored.

Comment: The observed increased mortality associated with high doses of clarithromycin and clofazimine has led to avoidance of these drugs.

QUESTION What are the effects of prophylaxis for CMV, HSV and VZV?

John Ioannidis

OPTION GANCICLOVIR

One RCT found that oral ganciclovir reduced the incidence of CMV in people with severe CD4 depletion compared with placebo. It found that 25% of people who did not develop CMV developed severe neutropenia. A subsequent RCT found no significant differences.

Benefits: We found no systematic review. **Versus placebo:** We found two RCTs. The first RCT in 725 people with a median CD4 count of 22/mm^3 found that oral ganciclovir halved the incidence of CMV compared with placebo (event rate 16% v 30%; P = 0.001).[32] The second RCT in 994 HIV-1 infected people with CD4 < 100/mm^3 and CMV seropositivity found no difference in the rate of CMV in people taking oral ganciclovir compared with placebo (event rates 13.1 v 14.6 per 100 person years; hazard ratio 0.92, 95% CI 0.65 to 1.27).[33] Both RCTs found no significant difference in overall mortality.

Harms: In the first RCT, 25% of people who did not develop CMV developed severe neutropenia (and were then treated with granulocyte colony stimulating factor).[32]

Comment: Differences in the results of RCTs may have arisen by chance or protocol variability; for example, no baseline ophthalmologic examinations were performed in the second trial.[33] The low incidence of CMV disease in people taking HAART, and the high rates of adverse events, means that the clinical value of oral ganciclovir in people who have not had active CMV disease is unclear.

OPTION   **ACICLOVIR AND VALACICLOVIR**

A systematic review found that aciclovir did not reduce the incidence of CMV compared with placebo, but significantly reduced HSV and VZV infection and overall mortality in people at different clinical stages of HIV infection. One RCT found that valaciclovir reduced the incidence of CMV more than aciclovir, but was associated with increased mortality.

Benefits: We found one systematic review of individual data (8 RCTs, search date not stated) in people with asymptomatic HIV infection to full-blown AIDS. It found no difference in protection against CMV disease between aciclovir compared with no therapy or placebo. However, aciclovir significantly reduced overall mortality (RR 0.81; $P = 0.04$), HSV, and VZV infections ($P < 0.001$ for both).[34] One RCT in 1227 CMV seropositive people with CD4 $< 100/mm^3$ compared valaciclovir, high dose aciclovir, and low dose aciclovir. It found increased mortality in the valaciclovir group, which did not reach statistical significance ($P = 0.06$).[35] The CMV rate was lower in the valaciclovir group than the aciclovir groups (11.7% v 17.5%; $P = 0.03$).

Harms: In the RCT, toxicity and early medication discontinuations were significantly more frequent in the valaciclovir arm (1 year discontinuation rate: 51% for valaciclovir v 46% for high dose aciclovir v 41% for low dose aciclovir).[35]

Comment: The survival benefit with aciclovir is unclear. The absolute risk reduction may be higher in people who have frequent HSV or VZV infections.

OPTION   **FAMCICLOVIR**

One small RCT found that famciclovir compared with placebo reduced the rate of viral shedding, but provided insufficient evidence on the effect of famciclovir on HSV recurrence.

Benefits: We found no systematic review. One small crossover placebo controlled RCT (n = 48) found that famciclovir suppressed HSV in people with frequent recurrences (HSV was isolated in 9/1071 famciclovir days v 122/1114 placebo days; $P < 0.001$).[36] Breakthrough reactivations on famciclovir were shortlived and often asymptomatic.

Harms: Famciclovir was well tolerated, and the incidence of adverse effects was similar in both groups.

Infectious diseases

Comment: The conclusions of this study are difficult to interpret. The randomisation process allocated participants to groups, but the intention to treat analysis involved the number of days with symptoms rather than the number of participants who improved. There was no assessment of statistical significance of clinical outcomes. The trials' completer analysis is impeded by a high dropout rate.

QUESTION What are the effects of prophylaxis for invasive fungal disease in people without previous fungal disease?

John Ioannidis

OPTION AZOLES

RCTs have found that both fluconazole and itraconazole reduce the incidence of invasive fungal infections compared with placebo in people with advanced HIV disease. One RCT found that fluconazole reduced the incidence of invasive fungal disease and mucocutaneous candidiasis more than clotrimazole. One RCT found no difference between high and low dose fluconazole.

Benefits: We found no systematic review. **Fluconazole versus placebo:** One RCT in 323 women with CD4 $\leq 300/mm^3$ found that fluconazole was more effective in reducing the incidence of candidiasis than placebo (44% v 58% suffered at least one episode of candidiasis; RR 0.56, 95% CI 0.41 to 0.77).[37] **Itraconazole versus placebo:** One RCT in 295 people with advanced HIV disease found that itraconazole reduced the incidence of invasive fungal infections (6 v 19; P = 0.0007).[38] It found no significant effect on recurrent or refractory candidiasis.[39] **High dose versus low dose fluconazole:** One RCT (n = 636) compared fluconazole 200 mg daily with 400 mg once weekly and found no difference in the rate of invasive fungal infections over a follow up of 74 weeks (7.7% v 5.5%; ARR 2.2%, 95% CI −1.7% to +6.%). However the incidence of thrush was twice as common in people taking the weekly dose.[40] **Fluconazole versus clotrimazole:** One RCT found that fluconazole reduced the incidence of invasive fungal disease and mucocutaneous candidal infections compared with clotrimazole (4.1% v 10.9%; relative hazard 3.3, 95% CI 1.5 to 7.6).[39] None of the above RCTs found any difference in mortality.

Harms: Congenital anomalies have occurred in a few children born to mothers receiving fluconazole. Itraconazole is embryotoxic and teratogenic in animals. Azoles may interact with antiretroviral regimens.[41] Azole drugs inhibit the metabolism of terfenadine, astemizole, or cisapride. Theoretically they may increase the risk of sudden death due to ventricular tachycardia.

Comment: Azoles effectively reduce invasive fungal disease. Any absolute benefit is probably even lower in people treated with HAART. Lack of evidence of any survival benefit, potential for complex drug interactions with current antiretroviral regimens, and potential for developing resistant fungal isolates, means that there is doubt about routine anti-fungal prophylaxis in HIV infected people without previous invasive fungal disease.

Infectious diseases

John Ioannidis

OPTION AZOLES

One RCT found that itraconazole reduced the incidence of relapse of Penicillium marneffei (see glossary, p 549) infection. One RCT found itraconazole was more effective in reducing the relapse of cryptococcal meningitis compared with fluconazole.

Benefits: We found no systematic review. **Itraconazole versus placebo:** One RCT in 71 people with AIDS in Asia found that itraconazole reduced the relapse of Penicillium marneffei infection compared with placebo (0/36 [0%] v 20/35 [57%] relapsed within 1 year; P < 0.001).[42] **Itraconazole versus fluconazole:** One RCT in 108 people with HIV infection found that itraconazole reduced relapses of successfully treated cryptococcal meningitis more than fluconazole (13/57 [23%] v 2/51 [4%]; ARR 19%, 95% CI 6.2 to 31.7; RR 0.17, 95% CI 0.04 to 0.71; NNT 5, 95% CI 3 to 16).[43] The trial was stopped early, because of the higher rate of relapse with fluconazole.

Harms: In the second RCT, discontinuation of itraconazole occurred in two people because of skin rashes, one due to severe anaemia and one due to gastrointestinal effects compared with none taking fluconazole.[43]

Comment: In addition to these studies, one open label uncontrolled study (n = 44) found that itraconazole may be effective in preventing the relapse of histoplasmosis.[44] Recurrent infection is common in people with previous C neoformans, H capsulatum, and Penicillium marneffei infections. Maintenance for life may be needed in the presence of immune impairment.

John Ioannidis

OPTION DISCONTINUATION OF PROPHYLAXIS FOR PCP AND TOXOPLASMOSIS IN PEOPLE WITH CD4 > 200/MM^3 ON HAART

Two unblinded RCTs found that discontinuation of prophylaxis did not increase the incidence of PCP or toxoplasmosis.

Benefits: We found no systematic review. We found two unblinded RCTs. The first RCT (abstract only) in 332 people with a satisfactory response to HAART (CD4 > 200/mm^3 and viral load < 5000 copies/mm3 for > 3 months) compared discontinuation with continuation of PCP prophylaxis.[45] It found no PCP episodes in either group over a mean follow up of 6.6 months. The second RCT, in 302 people with a satisfactory response to HAART, compared discontinuation with continuation of toxoplasma prophylaxis.[46] It found no episodes of toxoplasmic encephalitis in either group over a median of 10 months. A new trial related to discontinuation of primary prophylaxis for Pneumocystis carinii pneumonia and toxoplasmic encephlitis in human immunodeficiencey virus type I-infected people has been recently published and will be considered in future issues.[47]

Harms: The trials found no direct harms from discontinuing prophylaxis.

Comment: We found a number of retrospective and prospective cohort studies (see table 1, p 553).[48-56] They all found that discontinuation of prophylaxis was safe in people with adequate response to antiretroviral therapy and appropriate recovery of the CD4 cell count. The risk of PCP may increase again in people who do not respond to antiretroviral therapy. We found no direct evidence on the effects of different HAART regimens on the risk of PCP or toxoplasmosis. Antiretroviral regimens with different mechanisms of action may have different clinical effects on opportunistic infections and HIV disease progression, despite inducing satisfactory suppression of HIV-1 replication and adequate CD4 responses. Also, CD4 cell count is an incomplete marker of immune reconstitution. It is theoretically conceivable that people with the same CD4 count may have different immune deficits regarding control of PCP and other opportunistic pathogens. An extensive amount of research is being conducted on other parameters of immune reconstitution, but the clinical implications are uncertain at present.

OPTION DISCONTINUATION OF PROPHYLAXIS FOR MAC DISEASE IN PEOPLE WITH CD4 > 100/MM^3 ON HAART

One RCT found that discontinuation of prophylaxis for MAC disease did not increase the incidence of MAC disease.

Benefits: We found no systematic review. We found one RCT in 520 people without previous MAC disease, with CD4 > 100/mm^3 in response to HAART, which compared azithromycin with placebo.[57] There were no episodes of confirmed MAC disease in either group over a median follow up of 12 months.

Harms: Adverse effects leading to discontinuation of therapy were more common with azithromycin than with placebo (7.4% v 1.1%; $P = 0.002$).

Comment: It is not clear whether different antiretroviral regimens may have different clinical effects on opportunistic infections and the need for specific prophylaxis.

OPTION DISCONTINUATION OF MAINTENANCE THERAPY FOR CMV IN PEOPLE WITH A CD4 > 100/MM^3 ON HAART

We found insufficient evidence on the effects of discontinuation of maintenance therapy for CMV retinitis or other end organ disease.

Benefits: We found no systematic review or RCTs.

Harms: We found no evidence from systematic reviews or RCTs.

Comment: We found several small case series (see table 2, p 553).[58-64] No cases of CMV retinitis reactivation or progression were recorded in the six studies with average follow up less than 1 year. The study with longer follow up (mean 14.5 months) found five relapses among 17 participants who withdrew from maintenance; all of them occurred after the CD4 cell count had dropped again to below $50/mm^3$ (8 days to 10 months after this event).[59] In one observational series 12/14 participants had evidence of immune reconstitution retinitis even before starting withdrawal of prophylaxis.[58] Worsening uveitis was associated with a substantial vision loss (> 3 lines) in three participants. It is difficult to conduct an RCT of adequate sample size to exclude modest differences in relapse rates. The observational evidence suggests that withdrawal of CMV maintenance therapy may be considered in selected people in whom CMV disease is in remission, CD4 > $100mm^3$, and HIV replication remains suppressed. We found no clear data on whether quantification of CMV viraemia should be considered in the decision to withdraw from maintenance. One small case series found that relapses were associated with a drop in the CD4 cell count.[59] However, we found no randomised or other reliable data of when CMV maintenance therapy should be reinstituted.

GLOSSARY

Immune reconstitution related syndromes are due to excess inflammation when the immune system is recovering on antiretroviral therapy.

Penicillium marneffei infection is a common opportunistic infection in Southeast Asia.

The WHO staging system for HIV infection and disease consists of a "clinical axis" which is represented by a sequential list of clinical conditions believed to have prognostic significance, which subdivides the course of HIV infection into four clinical stages; and a "laboratory axis" which subdivides each clinical stage into three strata according to CD4 cell count or total lymphocyte count.

REFERENCES

1. Gallant JE, Moore RD, Chaisson RE. Prophylaxis for opportunistic infections in patients with HIV infection. *Ann Intern Med* 1994;120:932–44.

2. Ioannidis JPA, Cappelleri JC, Skolnik PR, Lau J, Sacks HS. A meta-analysis of the relative efficacy and toxicity of *Pneumocystis carinii* prophylactic regimens. *Arch Intern Med* 1996;156:177–88. search date to late 1995; primary sources MEDLINE and conference abstracts.

3. Anglaret X, Chene G, Attia A, et al. Early chemoprophylaxis with trimethroprim-sulphamethoxazole for HIV-1-infected adults in Abidjan, cote d'Ivoire: a randomized trial. *Lancet* 1999;353:1463–1468.

4. Bucher HC, Griffith L, Guyatt GH, Opravil M. Meta-analysis of prophylactic treatments against *Pneumocystis carinii* pneumonia and toxoplasma encephalitis in HIV-infected patients. *J Acquir Immune Defic Syndr Hum Retrovirol* 1997;15:104–114.

5. El-Sadr W, Luskin-Hawk R, Yurik TM, et al. A randomized trial of daily and thrice weekly trimethoprim-sulfamethoxazole for the prevention of *Pneumocystis carinii* pneumonia in HIV-infected individuals. *Clin Infect Dis* 1999;29:775–783.

6. Leoung G, Stanford J, Giordano M, et al. A randomized, double-blind trial of TMP/SMX dose escalation v direct challenge in HIV+ persons at risk for PCP and with prior treatment-limiting rash or fever. In: Abstracts of the 37th Interscience Conference on Antimicrobial Agents and Chemotherapy. Washington, DC: American Society for Microbiology, 1997. Abstract no. LB10.

7. Para MF, Dolin M, Frame P, et al for the ACTG 268 Study Team. ACTG 268 Trial – gradual initiation of trimethoprim/sulfamethoxazole (T/S) as primary prophylaxis for *Pneumocystis carinii* pneumonia (PCP). In: Program and abstracts: 4th Conference on Retroviruses and Opportunistic Infections. Alexandria, Virginia: Westover Management Group, 1997. Abstract no. 2.

8. Walmsley SL, Khorasheh S, Singer J, Djurdjev O. A randomized trial of N-acetylcysteine for prevention of trimethoprim-sulfamehtoxazole hypersensitivity reactions in *Pneumocystis carinii* pneumonia prophylaxis (CTN057). Canadian HIV Trials Network 057 Study Group. *J Acquir Immune Defic Syndr Hum Retrovirol* 1998;19:498–505.

9. Akerlund B, Tynell E, Bratt G, Bielenstein M, Lidman C. N-acetylcysteine treatment and the risk of toxic reactions to trimethoprim-sulphamethoxazole in primary *Pneumocystis carinii* prophylaxis in HIV-infected patients. *J Infect* 1997;35:143–147.

10. El Sadr WM, Murphy RL, Yurik TM, et al. Atovaquone compared with dapsone for the prevention of *Pneumocystis carinii* pneumonia in patients with HIV infection who cannot tolerate

trimethoprim, sulfonamides, or both. Community Programs for clinical Research on AIDS and the AIDS Clinical Trials Group. *N Engl J Med* 1998; 339:1889–1895.

11. Chan C, Montaner J, Lefebre EA, et al. Atovaquone suspension compared with aerosolized pentamidine for prevention of *Pneumocystis carinii* in human immunodeficiency virus-infected subjects intolerant of trimethoprim or sulfonamides. *J Infect Dis* 1999;180:369–376.

12. Dunne MW, Bozzette S, McCutchan JA, et al. Efficacy of azithromycin in prevention of *Pneumocystis carinii* pneumonia: a randomized trial. California Collaborative Treatment Group. *Lancet* 1999;354:891–895.

13. Havlir DV, Dube MP, Sattler FR, et al. Prophylaxis against disseminated *Mycobacterium avium* complex with weekly azithromycin, daily rifabutin, or both. California Collaborative Treatment Group. *N Engl J Med* 1996;335:392–398.

14. Wilkinson D. Drugs for preventing tuberculosis in HIV infected persons. In: The Cochrane Library, Issue 4, 1999. Oxford: Update software. Search date July/August 1998; primary sources Cochrane Infectious Diseases Group Trials Register; Cochrane Controlled Trials Register Issue 3, 1998; Medline 1982 to 1998, Embase 1980 to 1998, and hand searched references.

15. Bucher HC, Griffith LE, Guyatt GH, et al. Isoniazid prophylaxis for tuberculosis in HIV infection: a meta-analysis of randomised controlled trials. *AIDS* 1999;13:501–507. Search date not given; primary sources Medline, Embase, CAB Health, Biosis, Health Star, IDIS Drug File, DHSS-Data, Medical Toxicology and Health, Drug Information, AIDSLINE, AIDSTRIAL, AIDSDRUG, Cochrane Controlled Trials Register, hand search references, and conference proceedings.

16. Selwyn PA, Hartel D, Lewis VA, et al. A prospective study of the risk of tuberculosis among intravenous drug users with human immunodeficiency virus infection. *N Engl J Med* 1989;320:545–550.

17. Halsey NA, Coberly JS, Desmormeaux J, et al. Randomised trial of isoniazid versus rifampicin and pyrazinamide for prevention of tuberculosis in HIV-1 infection. *Lancet* 1998;351:786–792.

18. Mwinga A, Hosp M, Godfrey-Fausset P, et al. Twice weekly tuberculosis preventive therapy in HIV infection in Zambia. *AIDS* 1998;12:2447–2457.

19. Gordin F, Chaisson RE, Matts JP, et al. Rifampin and Pyrazinamide vs Isoniazid for Prevention of Tuberculosis in HIV-Infected Persons: An International Randomized Trial. *JAMA* 2000;283: 1445–1450.

20. Whalen CC, Johson JL, Okwera A, et al. A trial of threee regimens to prevent tuberculosis in Ugandan adults with the human immunodeficiency virus. *N Engl J Med* 1997;337:801–808.

21. Oldfield EC, Fessel WJ, Dunne MW, et al. Once weekly azithromycin therapy for prevention of *Mycobacterium avium* complex infection in patients with AIDS: a randomized, double-blind, placebo-controlled multicenter trial. *Clin Infect Dis* 1998;26:611–619.

22. Faris MA, Raasch RH, Hopfer RL, Butts JD. Treatment and prophylaxis of disseminated *Mycobacterium avium* complex in HIV-infected individuals. *Ann Pharmacother* 1998;32:564–573. Search date 1997; primary sources Medline 1966 to 1997, Aidsline 1980 to 1997.

23. Pierce M, Crampton S, Henry D, et al. A randomized trial of clarithromycin as prophylaxis against disseminated *Mycobacterium avium* complex infection in patients with advanced immunodeficiency syndrome. *N Engl J Med* 1996; 335:384–391.

24. Benson CA, Williams PL, Cohn DL, et al. Clarithromycin or rifabutin alone or in combination for primary prophylaxis of *Mycobacterium avium* complex disease in patients with AIDS: a randomized, double-blind, placebo-controlled trial. *J Infect Dis* 2000;181:1289–1297.

25. Tseng AL, Walmsley SL. Rifabutin-associated uveitis. *Ann Pharmacother* 1995;29:1149–1155.

26. Dube MP, Sattler FR, Torriani FJ, et al. A randomized evaluation of ethambutol for prevention of relapse and drug resistance during treatment of *Mycobacterium avium* complex bacteremia with clarithromycin-based combination therapy. *J Infect Dis* 1997;176:1225–1232.

27. Chaisson RE, Keiser P, Pierce M, et al. Clarithromycin and ethambutol with or without clofazimine for the treatment of bacteremic *Mycobacterium avium* complex disease in patients with HIV infection. *AIDS* 1997;11:311–317.

28. May T, Brel F, Beuscart C, et al. Comparison of combination therapy regimens for the treatment of human immunodeficiency virus-infected patients with disseminated bacteremia due to *Mycobacterium avium*. ANRS Trial 033 Curavium Group. Agence Nationale de Reserche sur le Sida. *Clin Infect Dis* 1997;25:621–629.

29. Gordin F, Sullam P, Shafran S, et al. A placebo-controlled trial of rifabutin added to a regimen of clarithromycin and ethambutol in the treatment of *M. avium* complex bacteremia. *Clin Infect Dis* 1999;28:1080–1085.

30. Cohn DL, Fisher EJ, Peng GT, et al. A prospective randomized trial of four three-drug regimens in the treatment of disseminated *Mycobacterium avium* complex disease in AIDS patients: excess mortality associated with high-dose clarithromycin. Terry Beirn Programs for Clinical Research on AIDS. *Clin Infect Dis* 1999;29:125–133.

31. Chaisson RE, Benson CA, Dube MP, et al. Clarithromycin therapy for bacteremic *Mycobacterium avium* complex disease: a randomized, double-blind, dose-ranging study in patients with AIDS. *Ann Intern Med* 1994;121: 905–911.

32. Spector SA, McKinley GF, Lalezari JP, et al. Oral ganciclovir for the prevention of cytomegalovirus disease in persons with AIDS. Roche Cooperative Oral Ganciclovir Study Group. *N Engl J Med* 1996; 334:1491–1497.

33. Brosgart CL, Louis TA, Hillman DW, et al. A randomized, placebo-controlled trial of the safety and efficacy of oral ganciclovir for prophylaxis of cytomegalovirus disease in HIV-infected individuals. Terry Beirn Community Programs for Clinical Research on AIDS. *AIDS* 1998;12:269–277.

34. Ioannidis JPA, Collier AC, Cooper DA, et al. Clinical efficacy of high-dose acyclovir in patients with human immunodeficiency virus infection: a meta-analysis of randomized individual patient data. *J Infect Dis* 1998;178:349–359. Search date not stated; primary sources Medline; abstract searching from major meetings; trial directories; and communication with experts, investigators of the identified trials, and industry researchers.

35. Feinberg JE, Hurwitz S, Cooper D, et al. A randomized, double-blind trial of valaciclovir prophylaxis for cytomegalovirus disease in patients with advanced human immunodeficiency virus infection. AIDS Clinical Trials Group Protocol 204/ Glaxo Wellcome 123–014 International CMV Prophylaxis Study Group. *J Infect Dis* 1998;177: 48–56.

36. Schacker T, Hu HL, Koelle DM, et al. Famciclovir for the suppression of symptomatic and asymptomatic herpes simplex virus reactivation in HIV-infected persons: a double-blind, placebo-

controlled trial. *Ann Intern Med* 1998;128:21–28.

37. Schuman P, Capps L, Peng G, et al. Weekly fluconazole for the prevention of mucosal candidiasis in women with HIV infection: a randomized, double-blind, placebo-controlled trial. *Ann Intern Med* 1997;126:689–696.

38. McKinsey DS, Wheat LJ, Cloud GA, et al. Itraconazole prophylaxis for fungal infections in patients with advanced human immunodeficiency virus infection: randomized, placebo-controlled, double-blind study. National Institute of Allergy and Infectious diseases Mycoses Study Group. *Clin Infect Dis* 1999;28:1049–1056.

39. Powderly WG, Finkelstein DM, Feinberg J, et al. A randomized trial comparing fluconazole with clotrimazole troches for the prevention of fungal infections in patients with advanced human immunodeficiency virus infection. *N Engl J Med* 1995;332:700–705.

40. Havlir DV, Dube MP, McCutchan JA, et al. Prophylaxis with weekly versus daily fluconazole for fungal infections in patients with AIDS. *Clin Infect Dis* 1998;27:253–256.

41. Tseng AL, Foisy MM. Management of drug interactions in patients with HIV. *Ann Pharmacother* 1997;31:1040–1058.

42. Supparatpinyo K, Perriens J, Nelson KE, Sirisanthana T. A controlled trial of itraconazole to prevent relapse of *Penicillium marneffei* infection in patients with the human immunodeficiency virus. *New Engl J Med* 1998;339:1739–1743.

43. Saag MS, Cloud GA, Graybill JR, et al. A comparison of itraconazole versus fluconazole as maintenance therapy for AIDS-associated cryptococcal meningitis. *Clin Infect Dis* 1999;28:291–296.

44. Wheat J, Hafner R, Wulfsohn M, et al. Prevention of relapse of histoplasmosis with itraconazole in patients with the acquired immunodeficiency syndrome. *Ann Intern Med* 1993;118:610–616.

45. Lopez JC, Pena JM, Miro JM, Podzamczer D, and the GESIDA 04/98 study group. Discontinuation of PCP prophylaxis (PRO) is safe in HIV-infected patients (PTS) with immunological recovery with HAART. Preliminary results of an open, randomized and multicentric clinical trial (GESIDA 04/98). In: Abstracts of the 6th Conference on Retroviruses and Opportunistic Infections, Alexandria, Virginia: Foundation for Retrovirology and Human Health, 1999. Abstract no. LB7.

46. Mussinin C, Pezzotti P, Govoni A, Borghi V, Antinori A, D'Arminio Monforte A, De Luca A, Mongiardo N, Cerri MC, Chiodo F,Conica E, Bonazzi L, Moroni M, Ortona L, Esposito R, Cossarizza A, De Rienzo B. Discontinuation of primary prophylaxis for Pneumocystis carinii pneumonia and toxoplasmic encephalitis in human immunodeficiency virus type I-infected patients: the changes in opportunistic prphylaxis study. *J Infect Dis* 2000; 181:1635–42.

47. Miro JM, Lopez JC, Podzamcer D, et al, and the GESIDA 04/98B study group. Discontinuation of toxoplasmic encephalitis prophylaxis is safe in HIV-1 and *T. gondii* co-infected patients after immunological recovery with HAART. Preliminary results of the GESIDA 04/98-B study. In: Abstracts of the 7th Conference on Retroviruses and Opportunistic Infections, Alexandria, Virginia: Foundation for Retrovirology and Human Health. Abstract no. 230.

48. Koletar SL, Heald AE, Murphy RL, et al. Discontinuation primary and secondary PCP prophylaxis in patients who have increased CD4 counts in response to antiretroviral therapy: preliminary results – ACTG 888. In: Abstracts of the 7th Conference on Retroviruses and Opportunistic Infections, Alexandria, Virginia:

49. Foundation for Retrovirology and Human Health. Abstract no. 243.

49. Lederberger B, Mocroft A, Reiss P, et al. Is it safe to discontinue secondary prophylaxis for PCP in HIV-infected patients treated with HAART: results from eight prospective European cohorts. In: Abstracts of the 7th Conference on Retroviruses and Opportunistic Infections, Alexandria, Virginia: Foundation for Retrovirology and Human Health. Abstract no. LB5.

50. Yangco BG, Von Bargen JC, Moorman AC, Holmberg SD. Discontinuation of chemoprophylaxis against *Pneumocystis carinii* pneumonia in patients with HIV infection. HIV outpatient study (HOPS) investigators. *Ann Intern Med* 2000;132:201–205.

51. Kirk O, Lundgren JD, Pedersen C, Nielsen H, Gerstoft J. Can chemoprophylaxis against opportunistic infections be discontinued after an increase in CD4 cells induced by highly active antiretroviral therapy? *AIDS* 1999;13:1647–1651.

52. Furrer H, Egger M, Opravil M, et al. Discontinuation of primary prophylaxis against *Pneumocystis carinii* pneumonia in HIV-1 infected adults treated with combination antiretroviral therapy. Swiss HIV cohort Study. *N Engl J Med* 1999;340:1301–1306.

53. Furrer H, Opravil M, Rossi M, et al. The Swiss StopCox study: is it safe to discontinue PCP prophylaxis in patients with detectable viremia, low nadir CD4 count or *T. gondii* seropositivity? In: Abstracts of the 7th Conference on Retroviruses and Opportunistic Infections, Alexandria, Virginia: Foundation for Retrovirology and Human Health. Abstract no. 244.

54. Weverling GJ, Mocroft A, Lederberger B, et al. Discontinuation of *Pneumocystis carinii* pneumonia prophylaxis after start of highly active antiretroviral therapy in HIV-1 infection. EuroSIDA Study Group. *Lancet* 1999;353:1293–1298.

55. Schneider MM, Borleffs JC, Stolk RP, Jaspers CA, Hoepelman AI. Discontinuation of prophylaxis for *Pneumocystis carinii* pneumonia in HIV-1-infected patients treated with highly active antiretroviral therapy. *Lancet* 1999;353:201–203.

56. Garcia Vazquez E, de Gorgolas Hernandez M, Garcia Delgado R, Fernandez Guerrero ML. Withdrawal of *Pneumocystis carinii* pneumonia prophylaxis in patients receiving efficacious combined antiretroviral treatment. Study of 85 cases. *Med Clin (Barc)* 1999;113:89–90.

57. El-Sadr WM, Burman WJ, Grant LB, et al. Discontinuation of prophylaxis for *Mycobacterium avium* complex disease in HIV-infected patients who have a response to antiretroviral therapy. *N Engl J Med* 2000;342:1085–1092.

58. Whitcup SM, Fortin E, Lindblad AS, et al. Discontinuation of anticytomegalovirus therapy in patients with HIV infection and cytomegalovirus retinitis. *JAMA* 1999;282:1633–1637.

59. Torriani FJ, Freeman WR, MacDonald JC, et al. CMV retinitis recurs after stopping treatment in virological and immunological failure of potent antiretroviral therapy. *AIDS* 2000;14:173–180.

60. Postelmans L, Gerald M, Sommereijns B, Caspers-Velu L. Discontinuation of maintenance therapy for CMV retinitis in AIDS patients on highly active antiretroviral therapy. *Ocul Immunol Inflamm* 1999;7:199–203.

61. Jabs DA, Bolton SG, Dunn JP, Palestine AG. Discontinuing anticytomegalovirus therapy in patients with immune reconstitution after combination therapy. *Am J Opthalmol* 1998;126:817–822.

62. Vrabec TR, Baldassano VF, Whitcup SM. Discontinuation of maintenance therapy in

Infectious diseases

patients with quiescent cytomegalovirus retinitis and elevated CD4+ counts. *Ophthalmology* 1998; 105:1259–1264.

63. McDonald JC, Torriani FJ, Morse LS, Karavellas MP, Reed JB, Freeman WR. Lack of reactivation of cytomegalovirus (CMV) retinitis after stopping CMV maintenance therapy in AIDS patients with sustained elevations in CD4 T cells in response to highly active antiretroviral therapy. *J Infect Dis* 1998;177:1182–1187.

64. Tural C, Romeu J, Sirera G, et al. Long-lasting remission of cytomegalovirus retinitis without maintenance therapy in human immunodeficiency virus-infected patients. *J Infect Dis* 1998;177: 1080–1083.

John Ioannidis
Chairman
Department of Hygiene and
Epidemiology, University of Ioannina
School of Medicine
Ioannina
Greece

Margaret Johnson
Consultant in HIV Medicine
Royal Free Hospital
London
UK

Andrew Phillips
Professor
Royal Free Centre for HIV Medicine and
Department of Primary Care and
Population Sciences, Royal Free and
University College Medical School
London
UK

David Wilkinson
Professor
South Australian Centre for Rural and
Remote Health University of Adelaide
and University of South Australia
Whyalla
Australia

Competing interests: None declared.

TABLE 1	Observational studies of discontinuation of PCP prophylaxis (see text, p 548).

Author	Criteria for discontinuation	Participants (prior PCP)	Person (years)	PCP events
Koletar[48]	CD4 > 200 sustained	269 (125)	186	0
Lederberger*[49]	CD4 277–371 (8 cohorts)	246 (246)	236	0
Yangco[50]	CD4 > 200 sustained	146 (0)	221	0
Kirk[51]	Increased CD4 for ≥ 6 months	219 (26)	174	1
Furrer[52,53]	CD4 > 200 and > 14% for ≥ 12 weeks	381 (0)	473	1
Weverling[54]	CD4 274 median	378 (59)	247	0
Schneider[55]	CD4 > 200 twice, 1 month apart	78 (16)	83	0
Vazquez[56]	CD4 > 200	85 (6)	84	0

Studies with at least 80 person years of follow up are included in the table.*Combined analysis from eight cohorts of prophylaxis discontinuations among people with previous PCP; it may include prophylaxis discontinuations from Schneider et al,[55] Weverling et al,[54] and Kirk et al.[50] CD4 count is measured in cells/mm^3. PCP, Pneumocystis carinii pneumonia.

TABLE 2	Observational studies of discontinuation of CMV maintenance therapy in people with previous CMV disease (see text, p 549).

Author	Criteria for discontinuation	Participants	Follow up (months)	Relapses
Torriani*[59]	CD4 > 70	17	14.5 (mean)	5
Postelmans[60]	CD4 ≥ 75	8	8 (median)	0
Whitcup[58]	CD4 > 150	14	16.4 (mean)	0
Jabs[61]	CD4 297 median	15	8 (median)	0
Vrabec[62]	CD4 > 100	8	11.4 (mean)	0
McDonald*[63]	(183 median)	11	5 (median)	0
Tural[64]	CD4 > 150, VL < 200/ml –ve CMV by PCR	7	9 (median)	0

Studies with more than five people are included. CD4 count is measured in cells/mm^3; CMV, cytomegalovirus; PCR, polymerase chain reaction; VL, viral load (HIV-1 RNA in plasma).*McDonald et al is an early report of the same study followed by the Torriani et al report. All relapses in the latter report occurred in people who had already experienced a decrease of CD4 to < 50 cells/mm^3.

Postherpetic neuralgia

Search date October 2000

John Yaphe and Tim Lancaster

QUESTIONS

INTERVENTIONS

Key Messages

Preventing postherpetic neuralgia

- Systematic reviews have found that daily aciclovir versus placebo reduces the risk of postherpetic pain at 6 months. One systematic review of one RCT found that famciclovir significantly reduced pain duration after acute herpes zoster. One systematic review of one RCT found that valaciclovir compared with aciclovir was associated with a slightly decreased prevalence of postherpetic neuralgia. One RCT found no advantage of netivudine over aciclovir. One RCT found no advantage of valaciclovir over famciclovir.

- One systematic review found idoxuridine to be associated with short term pain relief in acute herpes zoster, but no evidence that it reduced the risk of postherpetic neuralgia.

- Systematic reviews found conflicting evidence from RCTs about the effects of corticosteroids alone on postherpetic neuralgia. We found limited evidence that high dose steroids added to antiviral agents may speed healing of acute herpes zoster, but we found no evidence that it reduces the risk of postherpetic neuralgia. RCTs have found that corticosteroids may disseminate herpes zoster.

- One systematic review of one small RCT found that amitriptyline, started during the acute episode, is associated with a non-significantly reduced postherpetic neuralgia prevalence at 6 months.

- We found insufficient evidence on the effects of other drug treatments in acute herpes zoster.

Treating established postherpetic neuralgia

- One systematic review has found that tricyclic antidepressants are associated with pain relief from postherpetic neuralgia.
- RCTs have found that topical counterirritants such as capsaicin are associated with relief of postherpetic neuralgia but can also cause painful skin reactions.
- One small RCT of lignocaine patches found short term pain relief in postherpetic neuralgia.
- One RCT has found that gabapentin relieves postherpetic neuralgia.
- One crossover RCT found oral oxycodone to be associated with relief from postherpetic neuralgia. One small RCT found that epidural morphine was poorly tolerated and of little benefit. One RCT of dextromethorphan found no evidence of benefit.

DEFINITION Postherpetic neuralgia is pain that sometimes follows resolution of acute herpes zoster and healing of the zoster rash. It can be severe, accompanied by itching, and follows the distribution of the original infection. Herpes zoster is an acute infection caused by activation of latent varicella zoster virus (human herpes virus 3) in people who have been rendered partially immune by a previous attack of chickenpox. Herpes zoster infects the sensory ganglia and their areas of innervation. It is characterised by pain along the distribution of the affected nerve, and crops of clustered vesicles over the area.

INCIDENCE/ PREVALENCE In a UK general practice survey of 321 cases, the annual incidence of herpes zoster was 3.4/1000.[1] Incidence varied with age. Herpes zoster was relatively uncommon in people under the age of 50 years (< 2/1000 a year), but rose to 5–7/1000 a year in people aged 50–79 years, and 11/1000 in people aged 80 years or older. In a population based study of 590 cases in Rochester, Minnesota, USA, the overall incidence was lower (1.5/1000) but with similar increases in incidence with age.[2] Prevalence of postherpetic neuralgia depends on when it is measured after acute infection, and there is no agreed time point.

AETIOLOGY/ RISK FACTORS The main risk factor for postherpetic neuralgia is increasing age. In a UK general practice study (involving 3600–3800 people, 321 cases of acute herpes zoster) there was little risk in those under the age of 50 years, but postherpetic neuralgia developed in over 20% of people who had had acute herpes zoster aged 60–65 years and in 34% aged over 80 years.[1] No other risk factor has been found to predict consistently which people with herpes zoster will experience continued pain. In a general practice study in Iceland (421 people followed for up to 7 years after an initial episode of herpes zoster), the risk of postherpetic neuralgia was 1.8% (95% CI 0.59% to 4.2%) for people under 60 years of age and the pain was mild in all cases.[2] The risk of severe pain after 3 months in people aged over 60 years was 1.7% (95% CI 0% to 6.2%).

PROGNOSIS About 2% of people with acute herpes zoster in the UK general practice survey had pain for more than 5 years.[1] Prevalence of pain falls as time elapses after the initial episode. Among 183 people aged over 60 years in the placebo arm of a UK trial, the prevalence

Infectious diseases

of pain was 61% at 1 month, 24% at 3 months, and 13% at 6 months after acute infection.[3] In a more recent RCT, the prevalence of postherpetic pain at 6 months was 35% in 72 people over 60 years of age in the placebo arm.[4]

AIMS   To prevent or reduce postherpetic neuralgia by intervention during acute attack; to reduce the severity and duration of established postherpetic neuralgia, with minimal adverse effects of treatment.

OUTCOMES   Prevalence of persistent pain 6 months after resolution of acute infection and healing of rash. We did not consider short term outcomes such as rash healing or pain reduction during the acute episode. It is difficult to assess the clinical significance of reported changes in "average pain". Therefore we present data as dichotomous outcomes where possible (pain absent or greatly reduced, or pain persistent).

METHODS   Our initial search was part of two systematic reviews of RCTs of treatments for acute herpes zoster and postherpetic neuralgia on the basis of comprehensive searches of published and unpublished studies to 1993.[5,6] The details of the searches are described in the published reports. This search was updated by a *Clinical Evidence* search and appraisal from 1993 to October 2000. Where meta-analytic estimates from systematic reviews were available, these were taken to be the most reliable estimates of treatment effectiveness. In trials, the most common time point chosen for assessing the prevalence of persistent pain was 6 months, which we use in this review unless otherwise specified.

QUESTION   What are the effects of interventions during an acute attack of herpes zoster aimed at preventing postherpetic neuralgia?

OPTION   ORAL ANTIVIRAL AGENTS (ACICLOVIR, FAMCICLOVIR, VALACICLOVIR, NETIVUDINE)

Systematic reviews of five RCTs have found that daily aciclovir reduces the relative risk of postherpetic pain at 6 months by about 50% compared with placebo. One systematic review of one RCT found that famciclovir significantly reduced pain duration after acute herpes zoster. One systematic review of one RCT found that valaciclovir was associated with slightly decreased prevalence of postherpetic neuralgia versus aciclovir. One RCT found no advantage of netivudine over aciclovir. One RCT found no significant difference between valaciclovir and famciclovir in the resolution of postherpetic neuralgia and a similar safety profile.

Benefits: **Aciclovir versus placebo:** We found three systematic reviews.[7,5,8] The most recent review (search date 1998) reported the results of older reviews.[7] The oldest review (search date 1993) pooled estimates from eight placebo controlled RCTs of aciclovir in both inpatient and general practice settings (932 people).[5] It found no significant pain reduction from aciclovir at 6 months (OR 0.70, 95% CI 0.47 to 1.06). The second systematic review (search date 1997) identified five placebo controlled RCTs (792 people) of oral aciclovir, including one not published at the time of the earlier systematic review.[8] Taking a minimum of 4 g aciclovir daily for at least 7 days was associated with a significant reduction in prevalence of postherpetic neuralgia at 6 months (OR for presence of pain 0.54, 95% CI 0.36 to 0.81; ARR 0.16; NNT 7, 95% CI not available). **Famciclovir versus placebo:** We found one systematic review (search date 1998, 1 RCT, 419 people).[7] The multicentre RCT of famciclovir (2 doses) in immunocompetent adults (age > 18 years) defined duration of postherpetic neuralgia as time to pain resolution. The RCT found a significant reduction in duration of pain after acute herpes zoster on both doses of famciclovir versus placebo (median duration of pain with 500 mg [138 people] 63 days, with 750 mg [135 people] 61 days, with placebo [146 people] 119 days; P values not given). **Aciclovir versus other antivirals:** We found one systematic review (search date 1998, 1 RCT, 1141 people).[7] The RCT (1141 people) compared valaciclovir (a precursor of aciclovir) given three times daily for 7 or 14 days versus 7 days of aciclovir. When the results from the two valaciclovir regimens were combined, those treated with valaciclovir had a lower prevalence of pain at 6 months (AR 19.3% v 25.3%; RR 92%; NNT 16, 95% CI 9 to 100). We found one double blind RCT of netivudine versus aciclovir (511 people), which found no difference in effectiveness between the two.[9] **Addition of amitriptyline:** We found no systematic review or RCTs. **Valaciclovir versus famciclovir:** We found no systematic review. One RCT (597 immunocompetent people aged 50 years and over) compared valaciclovir (1 g 3 times daily) versus famciclovir (500 mg 3 times daily) given within 72 hours of appearance of the rash for 7 days.[10] It found no significant difference in postherpetic neuralgia (hazard ratio 1.01, 95% CI 0.82 to 1.24).

Harms: The reviews found that the most common adverse events reported with aciclovir were headache and nausea. In placebo controlled trials, these effects occurred with similar frequency with treatment and placebo (headache 37% v 43%, nausea 13% v 14%). There were no major adverse events reported in the RCTs included in the systematic review.[5] In the RCTs, famciclovir, valaciclovir, and netivudine had similar safety profiles to aciclovir.[9,11,12] In the RCT comparing valaciclovir versus famciclovir the two drugs had similar safety profiles.[10]

Comment: We found no evidence on adherence, but it has been suggested that adherence to treatment may be better with the newer antiviral drugs because they are given one to three times daily compared with five times daily for aciclovir.

OPTION **TOPICAL ANTIVIRAL AGENTS (IDOXURIDINE) FOR RELIEF OF ACUTE PAIN ONLY**

One systematic review of RCTs has found idoxuridine to be associated with short term pain relief in acute herpes zoster but found no evidence that idoxuridine reduced the risk of postherpetic neuralgia.

Benefits: We found one systematic review (search date 1993, 3 RCTs, 242 people).[5] Two RCTs found treatment during acute attack to be associated with significant pain relief at 1 month but not at 6 months. However, pooled results were not reported because of heterogeneity and poor quality of the trials. The other RCT compared topical idoxuridine versus oral aciclovir. It found idoxuridine to be associated with greater pain relief at 1 month (OR 0.41, 95% CI 0.15 to 1.11), but no significant difference in prevalence of pain at 6 months (RR 0.38, 95% CI 0.13 to 1.00).[13]

Harms: We found no reports of significant adverse effects from idoxuridine. Application beneath dressings may be cumbersome.

Comment: None.

OPTION   CORTICOSTEROIDS

Systematic reviews have found conflicting evidence from RCTs about the effects of corticosteroids alone on postherpetic neuralgia. We found limited evidence that high dose steroids added to antiviral agents may speed healing of acute herpes zoster, but we found no evidence that high dose steroids reduce the risk of postherpetic neuralgia.

Benefits: **Corticosteroids alone:** We found two systematic reviews (search dates 1998 and 1993).[5,7] The earlier review (search date 1993) included RCTs of corticosteroids with conflicting results and concluded that it was not possible to assess the effect of corticosteroids.[5] The more recent review (search date 1998) identified one RCT (201 people) subsequent to the earlier review.[7] The RCT found no significant differences in pain at 3 or 6 months. **Corticosteroids plus aciclovir:** We found one systematic review (search date 1998, 2 RCTs, 608 people). The first RCT (400 people) randomised people into four active treatment groups: 7 days of aciclovir (101 people); 7 days of aciclovir plus 21 days of prednisolone (99 people); 21 days of aciclovir (101 people); or 21 days of aciclovir plus prednisolone (99 people).[14] It found no significant differences in relief of postherpetic neuralgia. The second RCT (208 people) had a factorial design, randomising people to 21 days of aciclovir plus prednisone (60 mg initially, tapered over 3 weeks), prednisone plus placebo, aciclovir plus placebo, or two placebos. Although there was evidence of short term benefit from prednisone, there was no significant effect on pain prevalence at 6 months after disease onset.[15]

Harms: It is feared that corticosteroids might cause dissemination of herpes zoster. This effect was not reported in the RCT of prednisolone.[5] In the aciclovir plus prednisone RCT, two people receiving prednisone plus aciclovir placebo and one receiving aciclovir plus prednisone placebo developed cutaneous dissemination of lesions[15] (see harms of corticosteroids under rheumatoid arthritis, p 832).

Comment: None.

| OPTION | TRICYCLIC ANTIDEPRESSANTS (AMITRIPTYLINE) |

One systematic review of one small RCT has found that amitriptyline started during the acute episode is associated with a non-significantly reduced prevalence of postherpetic neuralgia at 6 months.

Benefits: We found one systematic review (search date 1998, 1 RCT, 90 people).[7] The double blind RCT (72 people aged over 60 years) compared amitriptyline 25 mg taken within 48 hours of rash onset and continued for 90 days versus placebo.[4] Amitriptyline was associated with a non-significantly reduced prevalence of postherpetic neuralgia at 6 months (AR 16% v AR 35%; RR 0.45; ARR +0.19, 95% CI –0.003 to +0.39).

Harms: The RCT did not report adverse effects.[4] In another RCT, amitriptyline was associated with adverse anticholinergic effects such as dry mouth, sedation, and urinary difficulties.[5]

Comment: Interpretation of the RCT is complicated because practitioners were allowed to decide whether an antiviral agent was prescribed as well as amitriptyline.[4] Blinding may also have been inadequate.

| OPTION | OTHER DRUG TREATMENTS |

We found insufficient evidence on the effects of other drug treatments in acute herpes zoster.

Benefits: We found one systematic review (search date 1993), which identified small, single RCTs of adenosine monophosphate, amantadine, and levodopa.[5] The RCTs found some short term benefit in treating herpes zoster. No benefit was found in small studies of cimetidine and isoprinosine.[5]

Harms: We found no evidence.

Comment: None.

| QUESTION | What are the effects of interventions after the rash has healed to relieve established postherpetic neuralgia? |

| OPTION | TRICYCLIC ANTIDEPRESSANTS |

One systematic review of RCTs has found that tricyclic antidepressants are associated with pain relief from postherpetic neuralgia.

Benefits: We found one systematic review (search date 1993, 3 RCTs, 216 people).[6] Two RCTs compared amitriptyline versus placebo, one RCT compared desipramine versus placebo. In pooled analysis, taking tricyclic antidepressants for 3–6 weeks significantly improved pain relief from postherpetic neuralgia at the end of the treatment period (OR for complete or large reduction in pain at end of treatment period 0.15, 95% CI 0.08 to 0.27).

Harms: Tricyclic antidepressants are associated with anticholinergic adverse effects. In one RCT, amitriptyline versus placebo was associated with more adverse effects: dry mouth (AR 62% v 40%), sedation (AR 62% v 40%), and urinary difficulties (AR 12% v less than 5%).[16] Syncope and heart block were encountered in one person in a trial of desipramine in people with postherpetic neuralgia.[17]

Comment: The adverse effects of tricyclic antidepressants are dose related. They may therefore be less pronounced when used to treat postherpetic neuralgia, because lower doses are used compared with treating depression.

OPTION   **TOPICAL COUNTERIRRITANTS**

RCTs have found that topical counterirritants such as capsaicin are associated with relief of postherpetic neuralgia but can also cause painful skin reactions.

Benefits: We found one systematic review (search date 1993, 2 placebo controlled RCTs, 205 people) of capsaicin. Pooled analysis found capsaicin to be associated with pain relief (total 205 people; OR for complete or greatly reduced pain 0.29, 95% CI 0.16 to 0.54).[5]

Harms: Reported local skin reactions included burning, stinging, and erythema. These effects tended to subside with time and frequency of use.[18]

Comment: The difficulty in blinding studies with capsaicin because of skin burning may have caused overestimation of its benefit.

OPTION   **TOPICAL ANAESTHESIA**

One small RCT of lignocaine patches found short term pain relief in postherpetic neuralgia.

Benefits: We found no systematic review. We found one small, placebo controlled RCT of lignocaine patches (35 people).[19] Active patches reduced average pain scores on a visual analogue scale over 12 hours.

Harms: No systemic adverse effects were noted with lignocaine patches, and systemic absorption as determined by blood concentrations was minimal.[19]

Comment: None.

OPTION   **GABAPENTIN**

One RCT has found that gabapentin relieves postherpetic neuralgia.

Benefits: We found no systematic review. We found one multicentre, double blind, placebo controlled RCT (229 people) of the anticonvulsant drug gabapentin in people who remained on tricyclic antidepressants or opiates during the trial.[20] At the end of the 8 week treatment period, gabapentin was associated with a significant reduction in reported pain (much or moderately reduced; RR 0.73; ARR 0.20; NNT 5, 95% CI 3 to 13).

Harms: Gabapentin was associated with somnolence, dizziness, ataxia, and peripheral oedema more frequently than placebo.[20] However, withdrawal rates were not significantly different.

Comment: None.

| OPTION | NARCOTIC ANALGESICS |

One small crossover RCT found oral oxycodone to be associated with relief from postherpetic neuralgia but was associated with more adverse effects. One small RCT found that epidural morphine was poorly tolerated and of little benefit. One RCT of the non-opioid dextromethorphan found no evidence of benefit.

Benefits: We found no systematic review. We found one double blind, placebo controlled, crossover RCT of oxycodone (50 people, 4 weeks on each treatment). Oxycodone was associated with significant pain reduction on a visual analogue scale, but the data could not be converted into a dichotomous outcome. However, it found that 67% of people had a masked preference for oxycodone versus 11% for placebo.[21] In a small, single blinded, placebo controlled RCT, epidural morphine led to pain reduction of more than 50% in two of 11 people, but this could not be sustained beyond 36 hours.[22] A third, small, double blind, crossover placebo controlled RCT (18 people) found no evidence of pain relief from 6 weeks' treatment with dextromethorphan (a codeine analogue).[23]

Harms: Oxycodone was reported to produce adverse effects such as constipation, nausea, and sedation with greater frequency than placebo (76% v 49%; RR 1.4, 95% CI 0.5 to 3.4).[20] Epidural morphine produced intolerable opioid effects in six of eight people treated.[22] High dose dextromethorphan produced sedation and ataxia, causing treatment to stop in five of 18 people.[23]

Comment: None.

Substantive changes since last issue

Aciclovir versus placebo New systematic review;[7] conclusion unchanged.

Famciclovir versus placebo New systematic review;[7] conclusion unchanged.

Aciclovir versus other antivirals New systematic review;[7] conclusion unchanged. New RCT of netivudine versus aciclovir;[9] it found no difference in effectiveness between the two.

Valaciclovir versus famciclovir We found no systematic review.[10] New RCT found no significant difference in postherpetic neuralgia.

Steroids versus placebo One new systematic review identified one RCT (201 people) subsequent to the earlier review.[7] It found no significant differences in pain at 3 or 6 months.

Amitriptyline One new systematic review;[7] conclusion unchanged.

REFERENCES

1. Hope-Simpson RE. Postherpetic neuralgia. *J R Coll Gen Pract* 1975;25:571–575.
2. Ragozzino MW, Melton J III, Kurland LT, et al. Population based study of herpes zoster and its sequelae. *Medicine* 1982;61:310–316.
3. Mckendrick MW, McGill JI, Wood MJ. Lack of effect of aciclovir on postherpetic neuralgia. *BMJ* 1989;298:431.
4. Bowsher D. The effects of pre-emptive treatment of postherpetic neuralgia with amitriptyline: a randomised, double-blind, placebo-controlled trial. *J Pain Symptom Manage* 1997;13:327–331.
5. Lancaster T, Silagy C, Gray S. Primary care management of acute herpes zoster: systematic review of evidence from randomised controlled trials. *Br J Gen Pract* 1995;45:39–45. Search

date 1993; primary sources Medline, hand searched primary care journals, references from books, specialists and makers of drugs in identified trials for published and unpublished data.
6. Volmink J, Lancaster T, Gray S, et al. Treatments for postherpetic neuralgia—a systematic review of randomised controlled trials. *Fam Pract* 1996;13:84–91. Search date December 1993; primary sources Medline, and Embase.
7. Alper BS, Lewis R. Does treatment of acute herpes zoster prevent or shorten postherpetic neuralgia? A systematic review of the literature. *J Fam Pract* 2000;49:255–264. Search date December 1998; primary sources Medline, Cochrane Controlled Trials Register, hand searched

reference lists and web based searches.

8. Jackson JL, Gibbons R, Meyer G, et al. The effect of treating herpes zoster with oral aciclovir in preventing postherpetic neuralgia. A meta-analysis. *Arch Intern Med* 1997;157:909–912. Search date 1996; primary sources Medline, National Institute of Health database of funded studies, Cochrane Controlled Trials Register.

9. Soltz-Szots J, Tyring S, Andersen PL, et al. A randomised controlled trial of aciclovir versus netivudine for treatment of herpes zoster. International zoster study group. *J Antimicrob Chemother* 1998;41:549–556.

10. Tyring SK, Beutner KR, Tucker BA, Anderson WC, Crooks RJ. Antiviral therapy for herpes zoster: Randomised, controlled clinical trial of valaciclovir and famciclovir therapy in immunocompetent patients aged 50 years and older. *Arch Fam Med* 2000;9:863–869.

11. Tyring S, Barbarash RA, Nahlik JE, et al. Famciclovir for the treatment of acute herpes zoster: effects on acute disease and postherpetic neuralgia. A randomised, double-blind, placebo-controlled trial. Collaborative famciclovir herpes zoster study group. *Ann Intern Med* 1995;123: 89–96.

12. Beutner KR, Friedman DJ, Forszpaniak C, et al. Valaciclovir compared with aciclovir for improved therapy for herpes zoster in immunocompetent adults. *Antimicrob Agents Chemother* 1995;39: 1546–1553.

13. Aliaga A, Armijo M, Camacho F, et al. A topical solution of 40% idoxuridine in dimethyl sulfoxide compared to oral aciclovir in the treatment of herpes zoster. A double-blind multicenter clinical trial [in Spanish]. *Med Clin (Barc)* 1992;98:245–249.

14. Wood MJ, Johnson RW, McKendrick MW, et al. A randomised trial of aciclovir for 7 days or 21 days with and without prednisolone for treatment of acute herpes zoster. *N Engl J Med* 1994;330: 896–900.

15. Whitley RJ, Weiss H, Gnann JW Jr, et al. Aciclovir with and without prednisone for the treatment of herpes zoster. A randomized, placebo-controlled trial. The National Institute of Allergy and Infectious Diseases Collaborative Antiviral Study Group. *Ann Intern Med* 1996;125:376–383.

16. Max MB, Schafer SC, Culnane M, et al. Amitriptyline, but not lorazepam, relieves postherpetic neuralgia. *Neurology* 1988;38: 1427–1432.

17. Kishore-Kumar R, Max MB, Schafer SC, et al. Desipramine relieves postherpetic neuralgia. *Clin Pharmacol Ther* 1990;47:305–312.

18. Bernstein JE, Korman NJ, Bickers DR, et al. Topical capsaicin treatment of chronic postherpetic neuralgia. *J Am Acad Dermatol* 1989; 21:265–270.

19. Rowbotham MC, Davies PS, Verkempinck C, et al. Lidocaine patch: double-blind controlled study of a new treatment method for postherpetic neuralgia. *Pain* 1996;65:39–44.

20. Rowbotham M, Harden N, Stacey B, et al. Gabapentin for the treatment of postherpetic neuralgia: a randomised controlled trial. *JAMA* 1998;280:1837–1842.

21. Watson CP, Babul N. Efficacy of oxycodone in neuropathic pain: a randomised trial in postherpetic neuralgia. *Neurology* 1998;50: 1837–1841.

22. Watt JW, Wiles JR, Bowsher DR. Epidural morphine for postherpetic neuralgia. *Anaesthesia* 1996;51: 647–651.

23. Nelson KA, Park KM, Robinovitz E, et al. High-dose oral dextromethorphan versus placebo in painful diabetic neuropathy and postherpetic neuralgia. *Neurology* 1997;48:1212–1218.

John Yaphe
Department of Family Medicine
Rabin Medical Centre
Petach Tikvah
Israel

Tim Lancaster
Reader in General Practice
Department of Primary Health Care
University of Oxford
Oxford
UK

Competing interests: None declared.

Search date December 2000

Alison Holmes and Paul Garner

INTERVENTIONS

© *Clinical Evidence* 2001;5:563–571.

Treating newly diagnosed tuberculosis

- RCTs found no evidence of a difference in relapse rates between standard short course (6 months) and longer term (8–9 months) chemotherapy in people with pulmonary tuberculosis. RCTs suggest that taking pyrazinamide in the first 2 months speeds up sputum clearance but that there is conflicting evidence relating to its effect on relapse rates.
- Limited evidence from two RCTs found no significant difference between daily versus twice or thrice weekly short course regimens.
- One systematic review of RCTs found evidence that reducing treatment from 6 to 4 months results in significantly higher relapse rates.
- We found no good evidence comparing regimens containing quinolones versus existing regimens.

Treating multidrug resistant tuberculosis

- We found no good evidence comparing different drug regimens for multidrug resistant tuberculosis.

Improving adherence and reattendance

- We found insufficient evidence on the effects of training health staff, health education by a doctor, routine prompts to attend, or sanctions if failed to attend.
- We found limited evidence suggesting that adherence to treatment may be improved by defaulter actions, cash incentives, and health education by a nurse.
- We found conflicting evidence from three RCTs on the effects of direct observation on treatment adherence.
- Two RCTs found conflicting evidence on the effects of prompts and contracts on reattendance for Mantoux test reading.

DEFINITION Tuberculosis is caused by *Mycobacterium tuberculosis* and can affect many organs. Specific symptoms relate to site of infection and are generally accompanied by fever, sweats, and weight loss.

INCIDENCE/ PREVALENCE About a third of the world's population is infected with *M tuberculosis*. The organism kills more people than any other infectious agent. The World Health Organization estimates that 95% of cases are in developing countries, and that 25% of avoidable deaths in developing countries are caused by tuberculosis.[1]

AETIOLOGY/ RISK FACTORS Social factors include poverty, overcrowding, homelessness, and inadequate health services. Medical factors include HIV and immunosuppression.

PROGNOSIS Prognosis varies widely and depends on treatment.[2]

AIMS To cure tuberculosis; eliminate risk of relapse; reduce infectivity; avoid emergence of drug resistance; and prevent death.

OUTCOMES *M tuberculosis* in sputum (smear examination and culture), symptoms, weight, and relapse rates.

METHODS *Clinical Evidence* update search and appraisal December 2000. Search terms: tuberculosis, pulmonary; isoniazid, pyrazinamide, rifampicin. We included all Cochrane systematic reviews and studies that were randomised or used alternate allocation, and had at least 1 year follow up after completion of treatment.

Infectious diseases

What are the effects of different drug regimens in people with newly diagnosed pulmonary tuberculosis?

OPTION **SHORT COURSE CHEMOTHERAPY (6 MONTHS)**

RCTs found no evidence of a difference in relapse rates between standard short course (6 months) and longer term (8–9 months) chemotherapy in people with pulmonary tuberculosis. RCTs suggest that use of pyrazinamide in the first 2 months speeds up sputum clearance, but the evidence relating to its effect on relapse rates is conflicting.

Benefits: We found no systematic review. **Versus longer courses:** We found two RCTs (published in the mid 1980s, 1295 people with untreated, culture/smear positive pulmonary tuberculosis), which compared 6 versus 8 or 9 months' chemotherapy.[3,4] Participants were followed up for at least 1 year after treatment was completed. The trials were performed in the UK and in East and Central Africa, and used different combinations of isoniazid, rifampicin, ethambutol, streptomycin, and pyrazinamide for initial (first 2 months) and continuation treatment. Overall, there was no significant difference between short course and longer regimens. **Different short course regimens:** The second RCT found no significant difference between regimens using ethambutol or streptomycin as the fourth drug in the initial phase.[4] A 6 month regimen using rifampicin and isoniazid throughout was highly effective (relapse rate 2%) and significantly better than isoniazid alone in the 4 month continuation phase (relapse rate 9%). When use of isoniazid alone was prolonged in a 6 month continuation phase, the relapse rate was not significantly better than with 4 months' continuation.[3] **Pyrazinamide:** The second RCT found that sputum conversion was faster with regimens containing pyrazinamide for the first 2 months, but there was no significant difference in relapse rates at 3 years' follow up.[4] A third RCT (833 people) compared four different 6 month regimens and found that bacterial relapse in the 12 months after chemotherapy was higher for those not receiving pyrazinamide (12/160 v 8/625).[5] A fourth RCT (497 people) of ongoing pyrazinamide found that relapse at 18 months was more likely in those not receiving pyrazinamide, but the difference was not significant (3.1% v 1%).[6]

Harms: In the largest trial, possible adverse reactions were reported in 24 of 851 people (3%), with six requiring modification of treatment.[3] Two people in the trial developed jaundice, one of whom died. **Pyrazinamide:** Adding pyrazinamide did not increase the incidence of hepatitis (4% with and without pyrazinamide).[4] However, mild adverse effects were more common, including arthralgia, skin rashes, flu like symptoms, mild gastrointestinal disturbance, vestibular disturbance, peripheral neuropathy, and confusion. Arthralgia was the most common adverse effect, reported in about 0.7% of people on pyrazinamide, but was mild and never required modification of treatment.[3,4]

Comment: In people treated previously, the organisms may have acquired drug resistance, so short course chemotherapy may not be effective.

Two RCTs found no significant difference in cure rates between daily versus twice or thrice weekly short course regimens, but the limited data available did not exclude a clinically important difference.

Benefits: We found one systematic review (search date 1999, 1 RCT, 399 people)[7] and one subsequent RCT.[8] The review compared thrice weekly versus daily chemotherapy for 6 months in people with newly diagnosed pulmonary tuberculosis. One month after treatment was completed, there was no significant difference in rates of bacteriological cure (defined as negative sputum culture, 99.9% v 100%) or relapse (5/186 people v 1/192 people; RR 4.0, 95% CI 0.7 to 24.1). The subsequent RCT (206 children) comparing twice weekly versus daily chemotherapy found no significant difference in cure rates (85/89 v 114/117; RR 0.98, 95% CI 0.84 to 1.02).[8] At least 12 cohort studies have found cure rates of 80–100% with thrice weekly regimens taken over 6–9 months.[7]

Harms: Intermittent treatment has the potential to contribute to drug resistance, but this was not shown in the studies.[7]

Comment: The RCTs had low event rates and therefore were too small to exclude a clinically significant difference between the dosing regimens.

One systematic review found limited evidence suggesting that reducing duration of treatment to less than 6 months significantly increased relapse rates.

Benefits: We found one systematic review (search date 1999, 7 RCTs published between 1979 and 1989, 2248 outpatients with newly diagnosed pulmonary tuberculosis), which compared a variety of shorter (minimum 2 months) and longer (maximum 12 months) drug regimens.[9] The trials included people in India, Hong Kong, Singapore, and Germany. The review found that a 3 month versus a 12 month regimen significantly increased relapse rates (5 RCTs; RR 3.03, 95% CI 2.08 to 4.4). One of the RCTs found that people given a 2 month regimen were significantly less likely to change or discontinue drugs than those given a 12 month regimen (6/299 v 17/299; RR 0.35; RRR 0.65, 95% CI 0.12 to 0.86).[9]

Harms: The review found similar rates of adverse events or toxicity.

Comment: The treatments were given under optimal conditions. In clinical practice, adherence is likely to be lower, so relapse rates associated with the shorter regimens are likely to be higher than those in clinical trials.

We found insufficient evidence on regimens containing quinolones.

Benefits: We found no systematic review. We found two RCTs.[10,11] One RCT in Tanzania (200 people) comparing a regimen containing ciprofloxacin versus a regimen not containing a quinolone found that more people relapsed following the ciprofloxacin regimen, but the difference was not significant (RR of relapse at 6 months 16, 95% CI 0.94 to 278).[10] A relatively low dosage of ciprofloxacin was used (750 mg daily). The second RCT (160 people) compared a regimen containing ciprofloxacin versus a regimen without, and focused only on adverse effects (see harms below).[11]

Harms: Adverse effects, which were mild and responsive to symptomatic treatment, were similar in people taking quinolone regimens versus controls.[11]

Comment: Quinolones have good bactericidal activity *in vitro*. Some of the newer quinolones have enhanced antimycobacterial activity compared with ciprofloxacin.

> **QUESTION** What are the effects of different drug regimens in people with multidrug resistant tuberculosis?

We found insufficient evidence comparing different drug regimens for multidrug resistant tuberculosis.

Benefits: We found no systematic review and no RCTs comparing different regimens in people with multidrug resistant tuberculosis.

Harms: We found insufficient data.

Comment: Current clinical practice in multidrug resistant tuberculosis is to include at least three drugs to which the particular strain of tuberculosis is sensitive, using as many bactericidal agents as possible. People are directly observed and managed by a specialised clinician.

> **QUESTION** Which interventions improve adherence to treatment?

> **OPTION** STAFF TRAINING

We found insufficient evidence on the effects of training of health staff on adherence to treatment.

Benefits: We found one systematic review (search date 1999, 1 poorly randomised RCT, see comment below) comparing intensive staff supervision versus routine supervision at centres in Korea performing tuberculosis extension activities.[12] Centres were paired and randomised, and supervision was carried out by senior doctors. The review found that higher completion rates were achieved with intensive supervision (RR 1.2, CIs not estimated because of cluster design).

Harms: None reported.

Comment: The trial used cluster randomisation, but the unit of analysis was the individual.

PROMPTS

We found no good evidence.

Benefits: We found one systematic review (search date 1999), which found no RCTs of prompts to return for treatment.

Harms: None.

Comment: None.

OPTION   **DEFAULTER ACTIONS**

One systematic review has found that intensive action for defaulters improves completion of treatment (see glossary, p 570).

Benefits: We found one systematic review (search date 1999, 2 RCTs conducted in India).[12] The first RCT found that up to four home visits to defaulters improved completion of treatment compared with routine policy of a reminder letter followed by one home visit (RR 1.32, 95% CI 1.02 to 1.71). The second RCT found that up to two reminder letters improved completion of treatment (RR 1.21, 95% CI 1.05 to 1.39), even in people who were illiterate.

Harms: None reported.

Comment: None.

OPTION   **CASH INCENTIVES**

One systematic review has found that cash incentives improve adherence among people living in deprived circumstances.

Benefits: We found one systematic review (search date 1999, 2 RCTs conducted in the USA).[12] The first RCT found that, in homeless men, money ($5) versus usual care improved attendance at the first appointment (RR 1.6, 95% CI 1.3 to 2.0). The second RCT, in migrants, found that combining cash ($10) with health education versus usual care improved attendance (RR 2.4, 95% CI 1.5 to 3.7).

Harms: None measured.

Comment: None.

OPTION   **HEALTH EDUCATION**

One RCT found that health education by a nurse improved treatment completion, with no evidence of benefit from health education by a doctor. One RCT in drug users found no significant effect of health education.

Benefits: We found one systematic review (search date 1999, 2 RCTs conducted in the USA).[12] The first RCT in the review compared three methods of health education versus an educational leaflet. Health education consisted of telephoning by a nurse, visiting by a nurse, or consultation by the clinic doctor. The trial found that, compared with the leaflet, treatment completion was significantly increased by the nurse phone call (75/80 v 55/77; RR 1.3, 95% CI 1.18% to 1.37%) and by the nurse visit (75/79 v 55/77; RR 1.33, 95% CI 1.20% to 1.38%). However, consultation by the clinic doctor was not significantly better than the education leaflet (64/82 v 55/77; RR 1.09, 9%, 95% CI 0.89% to 1.23%). The second RCT in drug users found that 5–10 minutes of health education had no significant effect on whether people kept a scheduled appointment (RR 1.04, 95% CI 0.70 to 1.54).

Harms: None measured.

Comment: Education is often part of a package of care that includes prompts and incentives, which makes it difficult to evaluate the independent effects of education.

OPTION   SANCTIONS

We found insufficient evidence on the effects of sanctions for failure to adhere to treatment.

Benefits: We found one systematic review (search date 1999), which identified no RCTs of sanctions.[12]

Harms: The use of sanctions may be ethically dubious.

Comment: In New York, incarcerating people who failed to comply with treatment was thought to increase compliance with the Department of Health's community tuberculosis treatment programme.[13]

OPTION   COMMUNITY HEALTH WORKERS

One RCT has found that health advisors recruited from the community increase attendance for treatment.

Benefits: We found one systematic review (search date 1999, 1 RCT in homeless people).[12] It found that health advisors recruited from the community helped people keep their appointments (62/83 attended v 42/79; RR 1.4, 95% CI 1.1 to 1.8).

Harms: None reported.

Comment: None.

OPTION   DIRECT PATIENT OBSERVATION

We found conflicting evidence from three RCTs on the effects of direct observation on treatment adherence.

Benefits: We found one systematic review (search date 2000, 2 RCTs, 1052 people)[12] and one subsequent RCT.[14] The two RCTs in the review compared direct observation of people as they took their drugs versus self administered treatment at home. The first (216 people) conducted in South Africa found no significant difference between the two strategies, although overall adherence in the study was low.[15] The second RCT (836 people) conducted in Thailand compared self treatment with direct observation (either from health centre staff, community members, or a family member). It found that direct observation versus self treatment improved treatment completion (347/414 [84%] v 320/422 [76%]; RR 1.11, 95% CI 1.04 to 1.16; NNT 13, 95% CI 8 to 36) and cure rate (RR 1.64, 95% CI 1.17 to 2.3).[16] The subsequent RCT (156 people) conducted in South Africa compared direct observation by lay health workers versus direct observation by clinic nurse versus self treatment. It found no significant difference in cure rates.[14]

Harms: Potential harms include reduced co-operation between patient and doctor, removal of individual responsibility, detriment to long term sustainability of antituberculosis programmes, and increased burden on health services to the detriment of care for other diseases. None of these have been adequately investigated.

Comment: Numerous observational studies have evaluated interventions described as directly observed treatment, but all were packages of interventions that included specific investment in antituberculosis programmes, such as strengthened drug supplies, improved microscopy services, and numerous incentives, sanctions, and other co-interventions that were likely to influence adherence.[17,18] One recently published RCT subsequent to the search date will be reported in future issues of *Clinical Evidence*.[19]

QUESTION Which interventions improve reattendance for Mantoux test reading?

OPTION PROMPTS AND CONTRACTS TO IMPROVE REATTENDANCE FOR MANTOUX TEST READING

Two RCTs found conflicting evidence on the effects of prompts and contracts on reattendance for Mantoux test reading.

Benefits: **Prompts:** We found one systematic review (search date 1999, 1 RCT in 701 healthy people).[12] The RCT compared an automatic telephone message prompt to return for Mantoux reading versus no prompt. People were slightly more likely to return in the intervention group, but the difference was not significant (93% v 88%; RR 1.05, 95% CI 1.0 to 1.10). **Contracts:** We found no systematic review. One RCT in healthy students in the USA found that, compared with no commitment, reattendance for Mantoux reading was improved by verbal commitments (RR 1.1, 95% CI 1.03 to 1.18) and by written commitments (RR 1.12, 95% CI 1.05 to 1.19).[20]

Harms: None reported.

Comment: None.

GLOSSARY

Defaulter actions Actions taken by health workers when people fail to attend for treatment of their tuberculosis.

Substantive changes since last issue

Intermittent short course chemotherapy New RCT;[8] conclusion unchanged.

Direct patient observation New RCT;[14] conclusion unchanged.

REFERENCES

1. Global Tuberculosis Programme. *Treatment of tuberculosis*. Geneva: World Health Organization, 1997:WHO/TB/97.220.

2. Enarson D, Rouillon A. Epidemiological basis of tuberculosis control. In: Davis PD, ed. *Clinical tuberculosis*. 2nd ed. London: Chapman and Hall Medical, 1998.

3. East and Central African/British Medical Research Council Fifth Collaborative Study. Controlled clinical trial of 4 short-course regimens of chemotherapy (three 6-month and one 8-month) for pulmonary tuberculosis. *Tubercle* 1983;64: 153–166.

4. British Thoracic Society. A controlled trial of 6 months chemotherapy in pulmonary tuberculosis, final report: results during the 36 months after the end of chemotherapy and beyond. *Br J Dis Chest* 1984;78:330–336.

5. Hong Kong Chest Service/British Medical Research Council. Controlled trial of four thrice weekly regimens and a daily regimen given for 6 months for pulmonary tuberculosis. *Lancet* 1981;1:171–174.

6. Farga V, Valenzuela M, et al. Short-term chemotherapy of tuberculosis with 5-month regimens with and without pyraxinamide in the second phase (TA-82) [in Spanish]. *Rev Med Chil* 1986;114:701–705.

7. Mwandumba HC, Squire SB. Fully intermittent dosing with drugs for tuberculosis. In: The Cochrane Library, Issue 4, 2000. Oxford: Update Software. Search date June 2000; primary sources Cochrane Infectious Diseases Group Trials Register; Cochrane Controlled Trials Register; Medline 1996 to 1999; Embase 1988–1999; reference lists of article; researchers contacted for unpublished trials.

8. Naude JMTW, Donald PR, Huseey GD, et al. Twice weekly vs. daily chemotherapy for childhood tuberculosis. *Pediatr Infect Dis* 2000;19:405–410.

9. Gelband H. Regimens of less than six months treatment for TB. In: The Cochrane Library, Issue 4, 2000. Oxford: Update Software. Search date 1999; primary sources Medline; Cochrane Parasitic Diseases Trials Register; contact with researchers, and hand searched references.

10. Kennedy N, Berger L, Curran J, et al. Randomized controlled trial of a drug regimen that includes ciprofloxacin for the treatment of pulmonary tuberculosis. *Clin Infect Dis* 1996;22:827–833.

11. Kennedy N, Fox R, Uiso L, Ngowi FI, Gillespie SH. Safety profile of ciprofloxacin during long-term therapy for pulmonary tuberculosis. *J Antimicrob Chemother* 1993;32:897–902.

12. Volmink J, Garner P. Interventions for prompting adherence to tuberculosis treatment. In: The Cochrane Library, Issue 4, 2000. Oxford: Update Software. Search date 2000; primary sources Medline; Embase; Cochrane Controlled Trials Register 1998, Issue 3; Cochrane Collaboration Effective Professional Practice (CCEPP) Registry Trials to 14 October 1996; LILACS to 2000; hand searched journals, references, and contact with authors.

13. Fujiwara PI, Larkin C, Frieden TR. Directly observed therapy in New York history, implementation, results and challenges. *Tuberculosis* 1997;18: 135–148.

14. Zwarenstein M, Schoeman JH, Vundule C, Lombard CJ, Tatley M. A randomised controlled trial of lay health workers as direct observers of tuberculosis. *Int J Tuberc Lung Dis* 2000;4:550–554.

15. Zwarenstein M, Schoeman JH, Vundule C, Lombard C, Tatley M. Randomised controlled trial of self-supervised and directly observed treatment of tuberculosis. *Lancet* 1998;352:1340–1343.

16. Kamolratanakul P, Sawert H, Lertmaharit S, et al. Randomized controlled trial of directly observed treatment (DOT) for patients with pulmonary tuberculosis in Thailand. *Trans R Soc Trop Med Hyg* 1999;93:552–557.

17. Garner P. What makes DOT work? *Lancet* 1998; 352:1326.

18. Volmink J, Matchaba P, Garner P. Directly observed therapy and treatment adherence. *Lancet* 2000; 355:1345–1350. Search date 1999; primary sources Medline, Embase, Cochrane Controlled Trials Register and hand searches of reference lists.

19. Walley JD, Khan MA, Newell JN, Hussain Khan M. Effectiveness of the direct observation component of DOTS for tuberculosis: a randomised controlled trial in Pakistan. *Lancet* 2001;357:664–669.

20. Wurtele SK, Galanos AN, Roberts MC. Increasing return compliance in a tuberculosis detection drive. *J Behav Med* 1980;3:311–318.

Alison Holmes
Senior Lecturer
Hammersmith Hospital
Imperial College
London
UK

Paul Garner
Senior Lecturer
Liverpool School of Tropical Medicine
Liverpool
UK

Competing interests: None declared.

Acute renal failure

Search date December 2000: expanded this issue

John A Kellum and Martine Leblanc

QUESTIONS

INTERVENTIONS

IN ACUTE RENAL FAILURE PREVENTION

TREATMENTS FOR ACUTE RENAL FAILURE IN CRITICALLY ILL PEOPLE

To be covered in future issues of *Clinical Evidence*
Endothelin receptor antagonists
Antibodies against adhesion
molecules
Growth factors
Noradrenaline
Antioxidants
Nutritional management

* We found insufficient evidence of
effectiveness, but failure or delay
in hydration results in harm

See glossary, p 584

Key Messages

Acute renal failure prevention

- We found no RCTs evaluating the use of fluids in the prevention of acute renal failure (ARF). However, dehydration is an important risk factor for ARF and recommended volumes of fluid have little potential for harm.

- One systematic review found no evidence that diuretics or dopamine reduce the risk of ARF from various causes. A subsequent RCT found no evidence that dopamine reduces the risk of ARF in people with sepsis.

- Two RCTs have found that diuretics appear to worsen outcome in acute tubular necrosis induced by contrast media and following cardiac surgery.

- We found insufficient evidence from low powered RCTs on the effects of mannitol on the development of ARF in people with traumatic rhabdomyolysis, or undergoing coronary artery bypass surgery, or vascular or biliary tract surgery.

- We found no evidence that natriuretic peptides, adenosine antagonists, or calcium channel blockers were effective in reducing the risk of ARF.

- We found insufficient evidence from one low powered RCT on the effects of acetylcysteine on preventing ARF induced by contrast media.

- We found limited evidence that lipid formulations of amphotericin and single daily dosing of aminoglycosides cause less nephrotoxicity compared with standard preparations and dosing.

- One systematic review comparing low osmolality with standard contrast media, found that the development of ARF or need for dialysis were rare events. However, there was less nephrotoxicity with low osmolality contrast media. The overall benefit was small and was greatest in people with underlying renal impairment, especially those with diabetes mellitus.

Acute renal failure in critically ill people

- One systematic review found insufficient evidence from small observational studies to compare continuous and intermittent renal replacement therapy.

- Limited evidence from RCTs suggests that, compared with non-biocompatible membranes, biocompatible membranes reduce mortality.

- We found insufficient evidence from low powered RCTs on the effects of diuretics.

- We found no good evidence on the effects of dopamine, bolus versus continuous loop diuretics, or combined albumin and diuretics.

DEFINITION ARF is characterised by abrupt and sustained decline in glomerular filtration rate (see glossary, p 584),[1] which leads to accumulation of urea and other chemicals in the blood. There is no clear consensus on a biochemical definition,[2] but most studies define it as a serum creatinine of 2–3 mg/dl (200–250 µmol/l), an elevation of more than 0.5 mg/dl (45 µmol/l) over a baseline creatinine below 2 mg/dl (170 µmol/l), or a twofold increase of baseline creatinine. "Severe" ARF has been defined as a serum concentration of creatinine above 5.5 mg/dl (500 µmol/l) or as requiring renal replacement therapy. ARF is usually classified according to the location of the predominant primary pathology (prerenal, intrarenal, and postrenal failure — see glossary, p 584). People who are critically ill are those who are unstable and at imminent risk of death, which usually implies that they are people who need to be in, or have been admitted to, the intensive care unit (ICU).

INCIDENCE/ PREVALENCE	Two prospective observational studies (2576 people) have found that established ARF affects nearly 5% of people in hospital and as many as 15% of critically ill people depending on the definitions used.[3,4]
AETIOLOGY/ RISK FACTORS	**For acute renal failure prevention:** Risk factors for ARF that are consistent across multiple aetiologies include hypovolemia, hypotension, sepsis, pre-existing renal, hepatic, or cardiac dysfunction, diabetes mellitus, and exposure to nephrotoxins (e.g. aminoglycosides, amphotericin, immunosuppressive agents, nonsteroidal anti-inflammatory drugs, angiotensin converting enzyme inhibitors, intravenous contrast media) (see table 1, p 587). Isolated episodes of ARF are rarely seen in critically ill people, but are usually part of multiple organ dysfunction syndromes (see glossary, p 584). ARF requiring dialysis is rarely seen in isolation (under 5% of people). The kidneys are often the first organs to fail.[5] In the perioperative setting, ARF risk factors include prolonged aortic clamping, emergency rather than elective surgery, and use of higher volumes (> 100 ml) of intravenous contrast media. One study (3695 people) using multiple logistic regression identified these independent risk factors: baseline creatinine clearance below 47 ml a minute (OR 1.20, 95% CI 1.12 to 1.30), diabetes (OR 5.5, 95% CI 1.4 to 21), and identified a marginal effect for doses of contrast media above 100 ml (OR 1.01, 95% CI 1.00 to 1.01). The mortality rate of people with ARF requiring dialysis was 36% during hospitalisation.[6] **For acute renal failure in critically ill people:** Prerenal ARF is caused by reduced blood flow to the kidney from renal artery disease, systematic hypotension, or maldistribution of blood flow. Intrarenal ARF is caused by parenchymal injury (acute tubular necrosis, interstitial nephritis, embolic disease, glomerulonephritis, vasculitis, or small vessel disease). Postrenal ARF is caused by urinary tract obstruction. Observational studies (in several hundred people from Europe, North America, and West Africa with ARF) found a prerenal cause in 40–80%, an intrarenal cause in 10–50%, and a postrenal cause in the remaining 10%.[7–11] Prerenal ARF is the commonest type of ARF in people who are critically ill,[7,12] but ARF in this context is usually part of multisystem failure, and most frequently due to acute tubular necrosis resulting from ischaemic or nephrotoxic injury, or both.[13,14]
PROGNOSIS	One retrospective study (1347 people with ARF) found that mortality was less than 15% in people with isolated ARF.[15] One recent prospective study (over 700 people) found that, in people with ARF, overall mortality and the need for dialysis was higher in an ICU than in a non-ICU setting, despite no significant difference between the groups in mean maximal serum creatinine (need for dialysis 71% in ICU v 18%, P < 0.001; mortality 72% in ICU v 32%, P = 0.001).[16]
AIMS	**Prevention:** To preserve renal function. **Critically ill people:** To prevent death; to prevent complications of ARF (volume overload, acid base disturbance, and electrolyte abnormalities); and to prevent the need for chronic dialysis, with minimum adverse effects.
OUTCOMES	**Prevention:** Rates of ARF and/or nephrotoxicity (see glossary, p 584). Surrogate outcomes were limited to measurements of biochemical evidence of organ function (serum creatinine or

creatinine clearance) following the intervention. Surrogate markers such as urine output or renal blood flow were not considered as evidence of effectiveness. **Critically ill people:** Rate of death; rate of renal recovery; adverse effects of treatment. Extent of natriuresis is a proxy outcome.

METHODS
Clinical Evidence update search and appraisal December 2000. **Prevention:** Studies were identified through Medline using the following search terms: kidney failure acute; diuretics/therapeutic use; dopamine/therapeutic use; mannitol/therapeutic use; contrast media/adverse events; rhabdomyolysis/complications, drug therapy; amphotericin; fat emulsions/administration; antibiotics, aminoglycosides/adverse effects, administration and dosing; iatrogenic disease/epidemiology. We identified aditional studies from the bibliographies of review articles and from personal files. **Critically ill people:** The following search terms were used: kidney failure acute/epidemiology, aetiology, therapy; diuretics; dopamine; haemodialysis membranes; albumin/therapeutic uses. We identified additional studies from the bibliographies of review articles and from personal files.

QUESTION   **What are the effects of interventions to prevent ARF in people at high risk?**   New

---

OPTION   **FLUIDS**

We found insufficient evidence on the effect of fluids in the prevention of ARF.

Benefits:
We found no RCTs comparing fluids with placebo. RCTs have combined fluids (especially 0.45% saline) with other active treatments. Comparisons between outcomes in these trials and historical untreated controls are difficult but suggest benefit from fluids.[17] In certain settings, such as traumatic rhabdomyolysis, early and aggressive fluid resuscitation has had dramatic benefits compared with historical controls.[18]

Harms:
The volumes of fluids recommended, such as 1 litre, and the rates of infusion (generally < 500 ml/hour) have very little potential for harm in the vast majority of people.

Comment:
Hypovolemia is a significant risk factor for ARF. The provision of adequate maintenance fluids is considered very important in preventing ARF. Additional fluid loading may be useful because it assures adequate intravascular volume. It also stimulates urine output, theoretically limiting renal exposure time to higher concentrations of nephrotoxins.

OPTION   **LOOP DIURETICS**

We found evidence that loop diuretics are not effective and may be harmful in the prevention of ARF.

Benefits:
We found one systematic review (search date not stated, 7 RCTs) comparing fluids alone versus diuretics in people at risk of ARF from various causes.[19] It found no evidence of benefit associated with diuretics.

Kidney disorders

Harms: Diuretics appear to worsen outcomes in acute tubular necrosis induced by contrast media,[17] and following cardiac surgery.[20] We found two RCTs addressing harms. The first RCT (78 people with chronic renal insufficiency who underwent cardiac angiography, mean serum creatinine 2.1 ± 0.6 mg/dl or 186 ± 53 µmol/l) found that ARF (defined as an increase in serum creatinine ≥ 0.5 mg/dl or 44 µmol/l at 48 h) was significantly more likely to occur when people were treated with furosemide (AR 10/25 [40%] v 3/28 [11%] with saline; RR 3.73, 95% CI 1.16 to 12.05; NNH 4, 95% CI 2 to 17).[17] The second RCT found that furosemide was associated with the development of postcardiac surgery ARF (AR 6/41 [15%] with furosemide v 0/40 [0%] with placebo; NNH 6, 95% CI 3 to 34).[20]

Comment: The trials addressing harms[17,20] provided a three way comparison showing significant differences among the three groups, $P < 0.05$. Although they seem to have used the same control group for both comparisons, no adjustment for multiple comparisons was carried out.

OPTION	MANNITOL

We found insufficient evidence to address the effect of mannitol in prevention of ARF.

Benefits: We found no systematic review. Several small RCTs found no decrease in the incidence of ARF with mannitol over hydration alone in a variety of conditions, including coronary artery bypass surgery,[21] traumatic rhabdomyolysis,[22] vascular,[23] or biliary tract surgery.[24] One trial comparing the use of saline, furosemide, and mannitol (78 people with chronic renal insufficiency who underwent cardiac angiography, mean serum creatinine 2.1 ± 0.6 mg/dl or 186 ± 53 µmol/l) found that ARF (defined as an increase in serum creatinine ≥ 0.5 mg/dl or 44 µmol/l at 48 h) was more likely to occur, although this difference was not significant, when people were treated with mannitol rather than with saline fluids (see harms below).[17]

Harms: In ARF induced by contrast media, mannitol was not associated with a statistically significant increased risk of ARF compared with saline fluids (AR 7/25 [28%] with mannitol v 3/28 [11%] with saline; RR 2.61, 95% CI 0.76 to 9.03), but the sample size was small and it was not possible to exclude harms.[17]

Comment: Mannitol is an intravascular volume expander and may also function as a free radical scavenger, as well as an osmotic diuretic. A trial addressing the effect of mannitol[17] provided a three way comparison showing significant differences among the three groups, $P < 0.05$. Although they seem to have used the same control group to compare both interventions, no adjustment for multiple comparisons was carried out.

OPTION	DOPAMINE (AND OTHER DOPAMINE RECEPTOR AGONISTS)

We found good evidence that dopamine is not effective in the prevention of ARF.

Benefits: We found one systematic review using dopamine (18 RCTs, > 700 people at risk of ARF from various causes),[19] and one subsequent large RCT.[25] The systematic review found no evidence of benefit associated with dopamine. The subsequent RCT (328 critically ill people with signs of sepsis) of dopamine in early renal dysfunction (see glossary, p 584) found that dopamine had no significant effect on the development of ARF, the requirement for dialysis, ICU length of stay, hospital length of stay, or mortality.[25]

Harms: One systematic review[19] and a large RCT in people with sepsis[25] found no evidence that dopamine caused harm. However, dopamine may worsen renal medullary ischaemia by increasing oxygen demand without increasing oxygen delivery.[26,27] Dopamine has recognised adverse effects, but we found no data on actual incidence/prevalence of harms in people with critical illness.

Comment: The increase in urine output associated with dopamine is often thought to be caused exclusively by the increase in renal blood flow and, therefore, it may be confused with evidence of benefit. However, dopamine also has a significant diuretic effect. Fenoldopam, a selective dopamine-1 receptor agonist, appears to increase renal blood flow in humans.[28] We found no RCTs evaluating this agent with clinically significant outcomes.

OPTION   NATRIURETIC PEPTIDES

We found evidence that atrial natriuretic peptide is ineffective in reducing the incidence of ARF induced by contrast media. We found insufficient evidence to evaluate the effect of natriuretic peptides for other forms of ARF.

Benefits: We found one large RCT (247 people) evaluating atrial natriuretic peptide versus placebo in the prevention of ARF induced by contrast media.[29] It found no difference in the incidence of ARF between groups.

Harms: Theoretically, natriuretic peptides might worsen renal medullary oxygenation by increasing glomerular filtration in a state of low medullary blood flow. We found one RCT in 504 people with early ARF. It found worse dialysis free survival in a subgroup of people (378 non-oliguric people) when treated with atrial natriuretic peptide versus placebo (survival rates AR 88/183 [48%] with atrial natriuretic peptide v 116/195 [60%] with placebo; RR 1.24, 95% CI 1.02 to 1.50; NNH 8, 95% CI 4 to 36).[30]

Comment: Natriuretic peptides (atrial natriuretic peptide and urodilantin) have also been evaluated in the treatment of ARF (see benefits of natriuretic peptides, p 583).

OPTION   ADENOSINE ANTAGONISTS (THEOPHYLLINE)

We found no evidence that adenosine antagonists are effective in preventing ARF.

Benefits: We found one systematic review (3 RCTs, 177 people) of theophylline, a non-selective adenosine antagonist, for prevention of ARF induced by contrast media.[31] It found that theophylline provided no protection against ARF when people are adequately hydrated. We found no RCTs evaluating selective adenosine antagonists or non-selective adenosine antagonists for other forms of ARF.

Harms: Theophylline has a narrow therapeutic index and known adverse effects (see harms of theophyllines under chronic obstructive pulmonary disease, p 1028).

Comment: None.

OPTION CALCIUM CHANNEL BLOCKERS

One RCT found that calcium channel blockers are ineffective in reducing early allograft dysfunction (see glossary, p 584) in renal transplantation. There is no evidence that calcium channel blockers are effective in reducing other forms of ARF.

Benefits: We found one large RCT (210 people) evaluating the effect of isradipine on renal allograft function after transplantation.[32] Median serum creatinine levels at 3 months and 12 months were significantly better in the isradipine group. However, there was no significant difference in the incidence of graft dysfunction (34/98 [35%] with isradipine v 44/112 [39%] with placebo; RR 1.13, 95% CI 0.79 to 1.62) or in the severity or duration (isradipine 9.1, SD±8.7 days v placebo 9.3, SD±8.1 days) of graft dysfunction.

Harms: As a class, calcium channel blockers are associated with hypotension and bradycardia as well as numerous, less serious adverse effects. The incidence and nature of adverse effects varies between individual drugs (see harms of antihypertensive drug treatment under primary prevention, p 63).

Comment: None.

OPTION ACETYLCYSTEINE

We found insufficient evidence to evaluate the effectiveness of acetylcysteine in the prevention of ARF due to exposure to contrast media or other aetiologies.

Benefits: We found one small, low-powered RCT (83 people with chronic renal insufficiency) examining the effect of acetylcysteine on the prevention of ARF induced by contrast media.[33] It found that the incidence of ARF (defined as an increase in serum creatinine ≥ 0.5 mg/dl or 44 μmol/l at 48 h) was significantly reduced (AR 1/41 [2%] with acetylcysteine v 9/42 [21%] with placebo; RR 0.11, 95% CI 0.02 to 0.86; NNT 6, 95% CI 3 to 21).

Harms: Acetylcysteine has been widely used to treat people with acetaminophen overdose, and has virtually no toxicity at therapeutic levels (see harms of paracetamol [acetaminophen] poisoning, p 953).

Comment: The clinical relevance of a rise in serum creatinine of 0.5 mg/dl at 48 hours, the study end point, is unclear. Long term follow up was not done and the study was far too small to evaluate either dialysis or mortality as end points.

SINGLE VERSUS MULTIPLE DOSES OF AMINOGLYCOSIDES

We found insufficient evidence. Single daily dosing may reduce the incidence of nephrotoxicity in people with normal renal function, but data are inconclusive.

Benefits: We found one systematic review (not limited to people in intensive care units).[34] It found equal antimicrobial efficacy and no difference in nephrotoxicity with single doses versus multiple doses of aminoglycosides (RR 0.78, 95% CI 0.31 to 1.94). One of the RCTs included in the review (85 people), which was highlighted for its methodological rigour, compared once daily versus three times daily dosing of gentamicin. It found equal efficacy but significantly less incidence of nephrotoxicity with single dosing (AR 2/40 [5%] with single dosing v 11/45 [24%]; RR 0.21, 95% CI 0.05 to 0.87; NNT 5, 95% CI 2 to 24).[35] Nephrotoxicity was defined as an increase in serum creatinine of 45 µmol/litre (0.5 mg/dl) or more.

Harms: The review found no evidence of greater harm from once daily aminoglycoside dosing.

Comment: The risk from aminoglycosides is highest in people with volume depletion, underlying renal, cardiac, or hepatic disease, or when combined with diuretics or other nephrotoxic agents (see glossary, p 584).

LIPID FORMULATIONS OF AMPHOTERICIN VERSUS STANDARD FORMULATIONS

We found insufficient evidence. Lipid formulations of amphotericin (see glossary, p 584) appear to cause less nephrotoxicity compared with standard formulations, but direct comparisons of long term safety are lacking.

Benefits: We found no systematic reviews and no RCTs.

Harms: There is no evidence of greater harms from lipid formulations of amphotericin. However, these formulations are still nephrotoxic and should be used with great care.

Comment: A phase II trial of a lipid formulation of amphotericin (556 people) found an incidence of renal toxicity (defined by any increase in serum creatinine) of 24% (v over 60–80% with standard formulation of amphotericin). People with baseline serum creatinine in excess of 2.5 mg/dl (221 µmol/l) on standard amphotericin showed a significant decrease in serum creatinine when transferred to the lipid formulation (P < 0.001).[36] One trial found that simply infusing amphotericin in a lipid solution designed for parenteral nutrition does not result in any benefit and may be associated with pulmonary side effects.[37] Fluid loading may be useful in reducing the risk of ARF from all nephrotoxins. Considerable variability may exist between individual lipid formulations of amphotericin in terms of efficacy and safety.

OPTION　LOW OSMOLALITY VERSUS STANDARD CONTRAST MEDIA

One systematic review found that low osmolality contrast media (see glossary, p 584) are associated with less renal toxicity. It found no evidence of benefit in people without underlying renal disease, or risk factors in people in whom ARF induced by contrast media is rare.

Benefits:　We found one systematic review (31 RCTs, 5146 people) comparing low osmolality contrast media with standard contrast media.[38] Overall, low osmolality contrast media did not influence the development of ARF or need for dialysis (these are rare events), but there was less nephrotoxicity with low osmolality contrast media, measured by serum creatinine. The overall benefit was small for people without prior renal failure (OR 0.75, 95% CI 0.52 to 1.1), and was greatest in people with underlying renal impairment (OR 0.5, 95% CI 0.36 to 0.68).

Harms:　We found no evidence of increased harms with low osmolality contrast media.

Comment:　Low osmolality contrast media are much more expensive than standard contrast media, and their use may be less cost effective in the general population. The use of low osmolality contrast media may be cost effective in high risk populations, but this has not been formally established. ARF induced by contrast media occurs most commonly in people with diabetic nephropathy (incidence nearly 50%, varies with the degree of baseline renal function).

QUESTION　What are effects of treatments for critically ill people with acute renal failure?

OPTION　CONTINUOUS VERSUS INTERMITTENT RENAL REPLACEMENT THERAPY

One systematic review found insufficient evidence to compare continuous renal replacement therapy (see glossary, p 584) versus intermittant renal replacement therapy (see glossary, p 584) in this setting.

Benefits:　**Versus placebo:** We found one systematic review, which found no RCTs.[39] **High dose versus low dose:** We found one RCT (425 people), which compared three doses of continuous renal replacement therapy (20, 35, and 45 ml/kg/h of haemofiltration).[40] Mortality was the same for the two high dose arms (AR 60/139 [43%] with 35 ml/kg/h v 59/140 [42%] with 45 ml/kg/hour, but was significantly higher in the low dose arm (AR 86/146 [59%] with 20 ml). Survival time analysis was adjusted for three way comparison (combined RR 1.38, 95% CI 1.14 to 1.67; NNT 7, 95% CI 4 to 16). Although standard methods of comparing dialysis dosage between continuous and intermittent renal replacement therapies do not exist, urea-kinetic modelling predicts that the doses used in this study would be impossible to achieve without continuous renal replacement therapy.[41]

Harms:　We found no good studies comparing the adverse effects of continuous renal replacement therapy and intermittent renal replacement therapy. Heparin is often used with both intermittent and continuous renal replacement therapy, and this can have adverse effects (see thromboembolism, p 158).[42]

Comment: The systematic review (search date 1994, 15 observational studies, 1173 people) found mostly small retrospective and prospective observational studies.[39] Eleven of these studies reported mortality. The review found no overall evidence of a significant difference in survival to hospital discharge between people treated with continuous renal replacement therapy and intermittent renal replacement therapy (survival to discharge 31% with continuous renal replacement therapy v 26% with intermittent renal replacement therapy; RR continuous renal replacement therapy v intermittent renal replacement therapy 1.07, 95% CI 0.99 to 1.16; P = 0.10; calculated by authors using the Mantel-Haenzel method and the true sample of 1006 people after correction for double counting). Biocompatible membranes were used in continuous renal replacement therapy more than in intermittent renal replacement therapy; this could confound the results.

| OPTION | BIOCOMPATIBLE VERSUS NON-BIOCOMPATIBLE DIALYSIS MEMBRANES |

We found limited evidence from three out of four RCTs that biocompatible membranes (see glossary, p 584) versus non-biocompatible membranes may reduce mortality in critically ill people with ARF.

Benefits: We found no systematic review, but found four RCTs (491 people)[43–47] comparing biocompatible (synthetic) versus non-biocompatible (cellulose based) dialysis membranes in critically ill people with all cause ARF; despite being described as randomised, two of the RCTs had important methodological problems. The first quasi randomised RCT (alternate assignment),[44] found that when recruitment from the original sample of 72 people with ARF[43] was extended to 153,[44] there was a significant difference in survival to discharge (57% with biocompatible membranes v 46% with non-biocompatible membranes; P = 0.03) and recovery of renal function (64% v 43%; P = 0.001).[43,44] This RCT found that mortality due to sepsis (by time of discharge) was lower with biocompatible membranes (12% v 46%; P = 0.016). The second RCT (52 people) found a better survival rate with biocompatible membranes (62% v 35%; P = 0.05) and a higher incidence of renal recovery at time of discharge with biocompatible membranes (AR for survival 23/37 [62%] with biocompatible membranes v 13/35 [37%] with non-biocompatible membranes; RR 1.67, 95% CI 1.02 to 2.76; NNT 4, 95% CI 3 to 51).[45] The third RCT (180 people) found 60% survival with biocompatible membranes versus 58% with bio-incompatible membranes (OR 1.07, 95% CI 0.54 to 2.11; P = 0.87), and identical rates of recovery of renal function between groups (57%).[46] However, the RCT was not analysed by intention to treat, and 12% of people were excluded after randomisation. It was funded by makers of bio-incompatible membranes. A recent RCT (106 people) compared two types of synthetic membranes to a semi-synthetic cellulose based membrane, and found no significant difference in survival at 80 days.[47]

Acute renal failure

Harms: Severe anaphylactoid reactions in people taking angiotensin converting enzyme inhibitors have been reported occasionally with certain synthetic biocompatible membranes (exact frequency unknown).[48]

Comment: One prospective observational cohort study (2410 people with chronic renal failure) found a 25% relative increase in mortality in people using non-biocompatible (cellulose based) versus biocompatible (synthetic) membranes (P < 0.001).[49] The ability of the membrane to cause immune activation depends on the structure of the material used.[50] We found no evidence that the results comparing synthetic and cellulose based materials can be extrapolated to highly substituted cellulose based ("semi-biocompatible") membranes.

OPTION   **DOPAMINE**

We found insufficient evidence on the effects of dopamine in critically ill people with ARF.

Benefits: We found no good systematic reviews or RCTs.

Harms: Dopamine has recognised adverse effects. We found no good data on harms in this setting.

Comment: None.

OPTION   **LOOP DIURETICS**

Two small RCTs found that loop diuretics versus placebo had no significant effect on renal recovery, the number of days spent on dialysis, and mortality. The RCT lacked power to exclude a clinically important effect, and included people from a non-ICU setting.

Benefits: We found no systematic review, but found two RCTs (66 and 58 people; some in ICUs, proportion unknown) comparing intravenous furosemide with placebo in people with oliguric ARF of various causes.[51,52] In the second RCT, all people received one dose of furosemide 1 g and were then randomised to continued treatment or placebo. Neither RCT found significant differences in renal recovery (first RCT 19/33 [58%] with furosemide v 22/33 [67%] with placebo; ARR 9%, 95% CI –12% to +33%;[51] second RCT 10/28 [36%] with furosemide v 12/28 [43%] with placebo; ARR 7%, 95% –19% to +27%)[52] or mortality, although the RCTs lacked power to exclude a clinically important effect of loop diuretics on these outcomes.

Harms: Ototoxicity can occur with high dose loop diuretics. No adverse effects were reported in the first trial.[51] Deafness occurred in two people in the second trial; both were randomised to furosemide. Hearing loss was permanent in one of these people.[52] Diuretics may reduce renal perfusion and add a prerenal component to the renal failure, but the frequency of this event is uncertain.[53] See harms of loop diuretics, p 576.

Comment: None.

OPTION | CONTINUOUS INFUSION VERSUS BOLUS INJECTION OF LOOP DIURETICS

We found insufficient evidence to compare continuous infusion versus bolus injection of loop diuretics.

Benefits: We found no systematic review and no RCTs in critically ill people with ARF.

Harms: One small, crossover RCT (8 people with acute deterioration of chronic renal failure, mean creatinine clearance 0.28 ml/s) foundthat fewer people experienced myalgia when treated with continuous infusion than with bolus dosing of bumetanide (3/8 people had myalgias with bolus dosing v none with continuous infusion).[54]

Comment: The small crossover trial found that continuous infusion resulted in a net increase in sodium excretion over a 24 hour period (mean increase in sodium excretion 48 mmol/day, 95% CI 16 to 60 mmol/day, P = 0.01).

OPTION | INTRAVENOUS ALBUMIN SUPPLEMENTATION PLUS LOOP DIURETICS

We found insufficient evidence on the effects of adding intravenous albumin to loop diuretic treatment in critically ill people with ARF.

Benefits: We found no systematic review and no RCTs assessing clinical outcomes in critically ill people with ARF.

Harms: We found insufficient evidence in people with ARF. One systematic review of 30 RCTs (1419 people, most without ARF) found that albumin increased the risk of death in unselected critically ill people (mortality 14% with albumin v 8% with control; RR 1.68, CI 1.26 to 2.23). All of the included trials were small and combined highly heterogeneous populations.[55]

Comment: One crossover RCT (9 people with nephrotic syndrome) compared furosemide alone versus furosemide plus albumin versus albumin alone.[56] It found that furosemide was superior to albumin alone, and furosemide plus albumin resulted in the greatest urine and sodium excretion. The clinical significance of this finding is unclear.

OPTION | NATRIURETIC PEPTIDES   New

We found evidence that both atrial natriuretic peptide and urodilantin are ineffective in treating ARF in oliguric (see glossary, p 584) and non-oliguric people. In addition, atrial natriuretic peptide is possibly harmful in non-oliguric people.

Benefits: One large RCT (504 people) showed no overall difference in dialysis free survival in people with ARF.[30] Pre-planned subgroup analysis suggested a possible benefit to people with oliguria, and lower survival rates in non-oliguric people. However, a follow up RCT (250 people) just in ARF with oliguria was halted after an interim ananlysis found there was no benefit.[57] Urodilantin, a natriuretic peptide with less system hemodynamic effects, was evaluated in a dose-finding, placebo-controlled RCT (176 people) but did not reduce the requirement for dialysis.[58]

Harms: See harms of natururetic peptides, p 577.

Comment: None.

GLOSSARY

Biocompatibility Artificial materials may induce an inflammatory response. This response may be humoral (including complement) or cellular. Materials are classified as biocompatible if they are less likely to induce an immune response or induce a less severe response compared with bio-incompatible materials. We found no standards by which this comparison can be made. Biocompatible dialysis membranes are made from synthetic materials, whereas bio-incompatible membranes are cellulose based.

Continuous renal replacement therapy Any extracorporeal blood purification therapy intended to substitute for impaired renal function over an extended period of time and applied for, or aimed at being applied for, 24 hours a day.

Early allograft dysfunction Renal dysfunction that occurs following renal transplantation, and which is usually secondary to ischaemic injury.

Early renal dysfunction An acute derangement in renal function that is still evolving.

Glomerular filtration rate The most basic aspect of renal function, glomerular filtration rate is the rate of elaboration of protein-free plasma filtrate (ultrafiltration) across the walls of the glomerular capillaries.

Intermittent renal replacement therapy Renal support that is not, nor intended to be, continuous; usually prescribed for a period of 12 hours or less.

Intrarenal ARF Caused by parenchymal injury, most commonly acute tubular necrosis, but also interstitial nephritis, embolic disease, glomerulonephritis, vasculitis, or small vessel disease.

Lipid formulations of amphotericin Complexes of amphotericin and phospholipids or sterols. This reduces the toxicity of amphotericin while preserving its antifungal activity.

Low osmolality contrast media Contrast media with osmolality less than 300 mOsm/litre.

Multiple organ dysfunction syndrome A syndrome of progressive organ failure, affecting one organ after another and believed to be the result of persistent or recurrent infection or inflammation.

Nephrotoxic agents Any agent that has the potential to produce nephrotoxicity.

Nephrotoxicity Renal parenchymal damage manifested by a decline in glomerular filtration rate, tubular dysfunction, or both.

Oliguria Urine output less than 5 ml/kg/day.

Postrenal (obstructive) ARF Caused by urinary tract obstruction.

Prerenal (functional) ARF Caused by renal hypoperfusion, secondary to renal artery disease, systemic hypotension, or maldistribution of blood flow.

REFERENCES

1. Nissenson AR. Acute renal failure: definition and pathogenesis. *Kidney Int Suppl* 1998;66:7–10.
2. Bellomo R, Ronco C. The changing pattern of severe acute renal failure. *Nephrology* 1991;2: 602–610.
3. Hou SH, Bushinsky DA, Wish JB, Cohen JJ, Harrington JT. Hospital-acquired renal insufficiency: a prospective study. *Am J Med* 1983;74:243–248.
4. Brivet FG, Kleinknecht DJ, Loirat P, Landais PJM, on behalf of the French Study Group on Acute Renal Failure. Acute renal failure in intensive care units–causes, outcomes and prognostic factors of hospital mortality: a prospective multicenter study. *Crit Care Med* 1996;24:192–198.
5. Tran DD, Oe PL, De Fijter CWH, Van der Meulen J, Cuesta MA. Acute renal failure in patients with acute pancreatitis: prevalence, risk factors, and outcome. *Nephrol Dial Transplant* 1993;8:1079–1084.
6. McCullough PA, Wolyn R, Rocher LL, Levin RN, O'Neil WW. Acute renal failure after coronary intervention: incidence, risk factors, and

relationship to mortality. *Am J Med* 1997;103: 368–375.

7. Thadhani R, Pascual M, Bonventre JV. Acute renal failure. *N Engl J Med* 1996;334:1448–1460.

8. Kleinknecht D. Epidemiology in acute renal failure in France today. In: Biari D, Neild G, eds. *Acute renal failure in intensive therapy unit*. Berlin: Springer–Verlag, 1990:13–21.

9. Coar D. Obstructive nephropathy. *Del Med J* 1991; 63:743–749.

10. Kaufman J, Dhakal M, Patel B, Hamburger R. Community acquired acute renal failure. *Am J Kidney Dis* 1991;17:191–198.

11. Bamgboye EL, Mabayoje MO, Odutala TA, Mabadeje AF. Acute renal failure at the Lagos University Teaching Hospital. *Ren Fail* 1993;15: 77–80.

12. Cantarovich F, Bodin L. Functional acute renal failure. In: Cantarovich F, Rangoonwala B, Verho M, eds. *Progress in acute renal failure 1998*. Paris: Hoechst Marion Roussel, 1998:55–65.

13. Brezis M, Rosen S. Hypoxia of the renal medulla. Its implication for disease. *N Engl J Med* 1995; 332:647–655.

14. Bonventre JV. Mechanisms of ischemic acute renal failure. *Kidney Int* 1993;43:1160–1178.

15. Turney JH, Marshall DH, Brownjohn AM, Ellis CM, Parsons FM. The evolution of acute renal failure, 1956–1988. *QJM* 1990;74:83–104.

16. Liano F, Junco E, Pascual J, Madero R, Verde E. The spectrum of acute renal failure in the intensive care unit compared to that seen in other settings. The Madrid Acute Renal Failure Study Group. *Kidney Int Suppl* 1998;53:16–24.

17. Solomon R, Werner C, Mann D, D'Elia J, Silva P. Effects of saline, mannitol, and furosemide to prevent acute decreases in renal function induced by radiocontrast agents. *N Engl J Med* 1994;331: 1416–1420.

18. Better OS, Stein JH. Early management of shock and prophylaxis of acute renal failure in traumatic rhabdomyolysis. *N Engl J Med* 1990;322:825–829.

19. Kellum JA. The use of diuretics and dopamine in acute renal failure: a systematic review of the evidence. *Crit Care* 1997;1:53–59. Search date not available; primary sources Medline and hand searches of bibliographies of relevant articles.

20. Lassnigg A, Donner E, Grubhofer G, Presterl E, Druml W, Hiesmayr M. Lack of renoprotective effects of dopamine and furosemide during cardiac surgery. *J Am Soc Nephrol* 2000;11:97–104.

21. Ip-Yam PC, Murphy S, Baines M, et al. Renal function and proteinuria after cardiopulmonary bypass: the effects of temperature and mannitol. *Anesth Analg* 1994;78:842–847.

22. Homsi E, Barreiro MF, Orlando JM, et al. Prophylaxis of acute renal failure in patients with rhabdomyolysis. *Ren Fail* 1997;19:283–288.

23. Beall AC, Holman MR, Morris GC, et al. Mannitol-induced osmotic diuresis during vascular surgery. *Arch Surg* 1963;86:34–42.

24. Gubern JM, Sancho JJ, Simo J, et al. A randomized trial on the effect of mannitol on postoperative renal function in patients with obstructive jaundice. *Surgery* 1988;103:39–44.

25. Australian and New Zealand Intensive Care Society Clinical Trials Group: a multicenter, randomized, double-blind, placebo-controlled trial of low-dose dopamine in critically ill patients with early renal dysfunction. *Lancet* 2000;356:2139–2143.

26. Olsen NV, Hansen JM, Ladefoged SD, Fogh-Andersen N, Leyssac PP. Renal tubular reabsorption of sodium and water during infusion of low-dose dopamine in normal man. *Clin Sci (Colch)* 1990;78:503–507.

27. Weisberg LS, Kurnik PB, Kurnik BR. Risk of radiocontrast nephropathy in patients with and without diabetes mellitus. *Kidney Int* 1994;45: 259–265.

28. Mathur VS, Swan SK, Lambrecht LJ, et al. The effects of fenoldopam, a selective dopamine receptor agonist, on systemic and renal hemodynamics in normotensive subjects. *Crit Care Med* 1999;27:1832–1837.

29. Kurnik BR, Allgren RL, Genter FC, et al. Prospective study of atrial natriuretic peptide for the prevention of radiocontrast-induced nephropathy. *Am J Kidney Dis* 1998;31:674–680.

30. Allgren RL, Marbury TC, Rahman SN, et al. Anaritide in ATN. Auriculin anaritide ARF study group. *N Engl J Med* 1997;336:828–834.

31. Venkataraman R, Kellum JA. Novel approaches to the treatment of acute renal failure. *Expert Opin Invest Drugs* 2000;9:2579–2592.

32. Van Riemsdijk IC, Mulder PG, De Fijter JW, et al. Addition of Isradipine (lomir) results in a better renal function after kidney transplantation: a double-blind, randomized, placebo-controlled, multi-center study. *Transplantation* 2000;70:122–126.

33. Tepel M, Van der Giet M, Schwarzfeld C, Laufer U, Liermann D, Zidek W. Prevention of radiographic-contrast-agent-induced reductions in renal function by acetylcysteine. *N Engl J Med* 2000; 343:180–184.

34. Hatala R, Dinh TT, Cook DJ. Single daily dosing of aminoglycosides in immunocompromised adults: a systematic review. *Clin Infect Dis* 1997;24:810–815. Search date April 1995; primary sources Medline, hand searches of selected infectious diseases journals, bibliographies of relevant articles, and personal contact with primary investigators of selected studies.

35. Prins JM, Buller HR, Kuijper EJ, Tange RA, Speelman P. Once versus thrice daily gentamicin in patients with serious infections. *Lancet* 1993; 341:335–339.

36. Walsh TJ, Hiemenz JW, Seibel NL, et al. Amphotericin B lipid complex for invasive fungal infections: analysis of safety and efficacy in 556 cases. *Clin Infect Dis* 1998;26:383–396.

37. Schoffski P, Freund M, Wunder R, et al. Safety and toxicity of amphotericin B in glucose 5% or intralipid 20% in neutropenic patients with pneumonia or fever of unknown origin: randomised study. *BMJ* 1998;317:379–384.

38. Barrett BJ, Carlisle EJ. Metaanalysis of the relative nephrotoxicity of high and low-osmolality iodinated contrast media. *Radiology* 1993;188:171–178. Search date 1991; primary sources Medline, Embase, hand searches of reference lists of selected articles, personal contact with authors of selected primary studies, and pharmaceutical companies manufacturing contrast media.

39. Jakob SM, Frey FJ, Uehlinger DE. Does continuous renal replacement therapy favourably influence the outcome of the patients? *Nephrol Dial Transplant* 1996;11:1250–1255. Search date 1986–1994; primary sources not available.

40. Ronco C, Bellomo R, Homel P, et al. Effects of different doses in continuous veno–venous haemofiltration on outcomes of acute renal failure: a prospective randomised trial. *Lancet* 2000;356:26–30.

41. Gotch FA, Sargent JA, Keen ML. Whither goest Kt/V? *Kidney Int* 2000;58(suppl 76):3–18.

42. Ronco C. Continuous renal replacement therapies for the treatment of acute renal failure in intensive care patients. *Clin Nephrol* 1993;40:187–198.

43. Hakim RM, Wingard RL, Parker RA. Effect of the dialysis membrane in the treatment of patients

with acute renal failure. *N Engl J Med* 1994;331: 1338–1342.

44. Himmelfarb J, Tolkoff RN, Chandran P, Parker RA, Wingard RL, Hakim RM. A multicenter comparison of dialysis membranes in the treatment of acute renal failure requiring dialysis. *J Am Soc Nephrol* 1998;9:257–266.

45. Schiffl H, Lang SM, Konig A, Strasser T, Haider MC, Held E. Biocompatible membranes in acute renal failure: prospective case-controlled study. *Lancet* 1994;344:570–572.

46. Jorres A, Gahl GM, Dobis C, et al. Haemodialysis-membrane biocompatibility and mortality of patients with dialysis-dependent acute renal failure: a prospective randomised multicentre trial. International Multicentre Study Group. *Lancet* 1999;354:1337–1341.

47. Gastaldello K, Melot C, Kahn RJ, Vanherweghem JL, Vincent JL, Tielemans C. Comparison of cellulose diacetate and polysulfone membranes in the outcome of acute renal failure. A prospective randomized study. *Nephrol Dial Transplant* 2000; 15:224–230.

48. Kammerl MC, Schaefer RM, Schweda F, Schreiber M, Riegger GA, Kramer BK. Extracorporal therapy with AN69 membranes in combination with ACE inhibition causing severe anaphylactoid reactions: still a current problem? *Clin Nephrol* 2000;53: 486–488.

49. Hakim RM, Held PJ, Stannard DC, et al. Effect of the dialysis membrane on mortality of chronic hemodialysis patients. *Kidney Int* 1996;50:566–570.

50. Kellum JA. Primum non nocere and the meaning of modern critical care. *Curr Opin Critical Care* 1998;4:400–405.

51. Kleinknecht D, Ganeval D, Gonzales-Duque LA, Fermanian J. Furosemide in acute oliguric renal failure. A controlled trial. *Nephron* 1976;17:51–58.

52. Brown CB, Ogg CS, Cameron JS. High dose furosemide in acute renal failure: a controlled trial. *Clin Nephrol* 1981;15:90–96.

53. Kellum JA. Use of diuretics in the acute care setting. *Kidney Int* 1998;53(suppl 66):67–70.

54. Rudy DW, Voelker JR, Greene PK, et al. Loop diuretics for chronic renal insufficiency: a continuous infusion is more efficacious than bolus therapy. *Ann Intern Med* 1991;115:360–366.

55. The Albumin Reviewers. Human albumin solution for resuscitation and volume expansion in critically ill patients. In: The Cochrane Library, Issue 1, 2000. Oxford: Update Software. Search date 1998; primary sources The Cochrane Injuries Group Register, Cochrane Library, Medline, Embase, BIDS, Index to Scientific and Technical Proceedings, and hand searched references.

56. Fliser D, Zurbruggen I, Mutschler E, et al. Coadministration of albumin and furosemide in patients with the nephrotic syndrome. *Kidney Int* 1999;55:629–634.

57. Allgren RL. Update on clinical trials with atrial natriuretic peptide in acute tubular necrosis. *Ren Fail* 1998;20:691–695.

58. Meyer M, Pfarr E, Schirmer G, et al. Therapeutic use of natriuretic peptide ularitide in acute renal failure. *Ren Fail* 1999;21:85–100.

59. Wiecek A, Zeier M, Ritz E. Role of infection in the genesis of acute renal failure. *Nephrol Dial Transplant* 1994;9(suppl 4):40–44.

60. Myers BD, Moran SM. Hemodynamically mediated acute renal failure. *N Engl J Med* 1986;314:97–100.

61. Ward MM. Factors predictive of acute renal failure in rhabdomyolysis. *Arch Intern Med* 1988;148: 1553–1557.

62. Kahlmeter G, Dahlager JI. Aminoglycoside toxicity–a review of clinical studies published between 1975 and 1982. *J Antimicrob Chemother* 1984;13(suppl A):9–22. Search date 1982; primary sources Medline, Toxline, and personal contact with pharmaceutical companies.

63. Butler WT, Bennett JE, Alling DW, Wertlake PT, Utz JP. Nephrotoxicity of amphotericin B, early and late events in 81 patients. *Ann Intern Med* 1964;61: 175–187.

John A Kellum
Associate Professor of
Anesthesiology/Critical Care Medicine
and Medicine
University of Pittsburgh
Pittsburgh
USA

Martine Leblanc
Assistant Professor of Nephrology and
Critical Care
Maisonneuve–Rosemont Hospital
University of Montreal
Montreal
Canada

Competing interests: JK has been paid by Gambro Healthcare Inc. for lecturing and running educational programmes on acute renal failure; ML, none declared.

TABLE 1	Selected risk factors for ARF (see text, p 574).	
Risk factor	**Incidence of ARF**	**Comments**
Sepsis	Unknown	Sepsis seems to be a contributing factor in as many as 43% of ARF cases[59]
Aortic clamping	Approaches 100% when > 60 minutes[60]	Refers to cross-clamping (no flow) above the renal arteries
Rhabdomyolysis	16.5%[61]	
Aminoglycosides	8–26%[62]	
Amphotericin	88% with > 5 g total dose[63]	60% overall incidence of nephrotoxicity
ARF, acute renal failure.		

Search date August 2000: expanded this issue

Michael Barry and Claus Roehrborn

INTERVENTIONS

To be covered in future issues of
Clinical Evidence
Open prostatectomy
Other alternative/complementary
  treatments

Key Messages

- Two systematic reviews of RCTs have found that α blockers are more effective than placebo for improving lower urinary tract symptoms in men with benign prostatic hyperplasia. Two RCTs found limited evidence that α blockers were more effective than 5α reductase inhibitors for reducing symptoms. We found no direct comparisons of these drugs versus surgical treatment.

- One systematic review has found that 5α reductase inhibitors reduce symptoms compared with placebo.

- Two RCTs have found that transurethral resection (TURP) is more effective than watchful waiting for improving symptoms and reducing complications, but found no evidence that it was associated with an increase in the risk of erectile dysfunction or incontinence.

- We found no good comparison of TURP with medical treatments or with newer, less invasive techniques.

- RCTs have found that transurethral microwave thermotherapy (TUMT) versus sham treatment significantly reduces symptoms. Weaker evidence found no significant difference in short term symptom relief between TURP and TUMT, but one RCT found that TURP was more effective at reducing symptoms than transurethral needle ablation (TUNA).

- One systematic review has found that self rated improvement is better in men taking saw palmetto compared with placebo. It found no significant difference in symptom scores between saw palmetto and finasteride.

- One systematic review has found that β–sitosterol plant extracts versus placebo reduce lower urinary tract symptoms in the short term.

- One systematic review has found limited evidence that rye grass pollen extract versus placebo increases self rated improvement and reduces nocturia in the short term.

DEFINITION Benign prostatic hyperplasia (BPH) is defined histologically. Clinically, it is characterised by lower urinary tract symptoms (urinary frequency, urgency, a weak and intermittent stream, needing to strain, a sense of incomplete emptying, and nocturia), and can lead to complications, including acute urinary retention.

INCIDENCE/ PREVALENCE Estimates of the prevalence of symptomatic BPH range from 10–30% for men in their early 70s, depending on how BPH is defined.[1]

AETIOLOGY/ RISK FACTORS The mechanisms by which BPH causes symptoms and complications are unclear, although bladder outlet obstruction is an important factor.[2] The best documented risk factors are increasing age and functioning testes.[3]

PROGNOSIS Community and practice based studies suggest that men with lower urinary tract symptoms can expect slow progression of the symptoms.[4,5] However, symptoms can wax and wane without treatment. In men with symptoms of BPH, rates of acute urinary retention range from 1–2% a year.[5–7]

AIMS To reduce or alleviate lower urinary tract symptoms; to prevent complications; and to minimise adverse effects of treatment.

OUTCOMES Burden of lower urinary tract symptoms; rates of acute urinary retention and prostatectomy; rates of adverse effects of treatment. Symptoms are measured using the validated International Prostate Symptom Score (IPSS), which includes seven questions quantifying symptoms on an overall scale from 0–35, with higher scores representing more frequent symptoms.[8] Older studies used a variety of symptom assessment instruments, which makes comparisons difficult.

METHODS This review was originally based on ongoing Medline searches and prospective journal hand searches by the Patient Outcomes Research Team for Prostatic Diseases (Agency for Health Care Policy and Research grant number HS0837). *Clinical Evidence* update search and appraisal August 2000.

QUESTION What are the effects of medical treatments?

OPTION α BLOCKERS

Two systematic reviews have found that α blockers are more effective than placebo for improving lower urinary tract symptoms in men with BPH. Two RCTs found limited evidence that α blockers were more effective in improving symptoms than 5α reductase inhibitors. We found no direct comparison of α blockers with surgical treatment.

Benefits: **Versus placebo:** We found two systematic reviews (search date 1998, 21 RCTs,[9] and 1999, 24 RCTs[10]). Most RCTs found a greater improvement in symptoms with α blockers than with placebo (results presented graphically or in tabular form; overall significance not stated). The largest RCT (2084 men with BPH) compared terazosin at doses of up to 10 mg daily for 1 year versus placebo. Treatment achieved significantly greater mean improvement in International Prostate Symptom Score (IPSS) (–7.6 points from baseline with terazosin v –3.7 with placebo; mean change, terazosin v placebo –3.9 points, 95% CI –5.5 points to –3.3 points).[11] We found insufficient evidence on the effect of α blockers on complications of BPH. One small RCT found sustained release alfuzosin (5 mg twice daily) for 48 hours increased the ability to pass urine after catheter removal in men catheterised for acute retention, from 5% to 29% (NNT 4).[12] **Versus each other:** The first systematic review[9] identified three head to head comparisons that reported clinical outcomes, and we found three subsequent RCTs of limited quality.[13–15] The largest RCT in the review (256 men) compared tamsulosin versus alfuzosin.[12] The second RCT (103 men) compared alfuzosin versus prazosin, and the third trial (98 men) compared tamsulosin versus terazosin. The RCTs found no significant difference in symptom score among α blockers. The first subsequent RCT (212 men) found that tamsulosin improved total IPSS compared with terazosin (9.7% change from baseline with tamsulosin v 8.5% with terazosin; P < 0.05).[13] The second subsequent RCT (61 men) compared terazosin versus tamsulosin and found no significant difference in IPSS score.[14] The third RCT comparing terazosin versus alfuzosin also found no significant difference in IPSS score.[15] **Versus 5α reductase inhibitors:** We found no systematic review. We found two RCTs of limited quality (see comment below). One RCT (1229 men with a diagnosis of BPH) compared finasteride versus an α blocker or versus both treatments combined.[16] Terazosin was associated with a greater reduction in symptoms than finasteride, regardless of prostate size. The difference in mean IPSS scores at 1 year was 2.9 points. There was no significant difference between treatment with both agents versus terazosin alone. The second RCT (1051 men) compared alfuzosin versus finasteride versus both drugs combined over 6 months. It found that alfuzosin versus finasteride significantly decreased the mean IPSS score from baseline, and found no significant difference between alfuzosin alone versus combination therapy.[17] **Versus TUMT:** See TUMT, p 593.

Harms: The first systematic review found that withdrawals attributed to adverse events were similar for alfuzosin, tamsulosin (0.4 mg dose), and placebo (results were presented graphically; significance not stated).[9] However, a higher withdrawal rate was found with doxazosin, terazosin, and tamsulosin (0.8 mg dose). There was little observable difference between the number of men experiencing dizziness with alfuzosin or tamsulosin compared with placebo (results were presented graphically; significance not stated). However, more men experienced dizziness after terazosin and doxazosin than placebo (results were presented graphically; significance not stated). One large RCT included in the systematic review compared tamsulosin versus a less selective α blocker, alfuzosin. It found that adverse effects were similar: dizziness occurred in 7%, asthenia in 2%, and postural hypotension in 2%.[9] One RCT from China compared low dose terazosin (2 mg daily) and tamsulosin (0.2 mg daily). It found dizziness (32% v 10%) and hypotension limiting therapy (9% v 1%) were more common with terazosin.[13] Both selective and less selective α blockers may be associated with abnormal ejaculation: the risk of abnormal ejaculation was higher with tamsulosin than placebo (4.5% v 1%) but similar with tamsulosin versus alfuzosin (0.8% v 0%).[18] **Versus 5α reductase inhibitors:** In the trial comparing terazosin versus finasteride, dizziness was seen in about 25% of men on terazosin, generalised weakness in 15%, rhinitis in 8%, and postural hypotension in 8%, whereas sexual dysfunction was more common in men taking finasteride.[16]

Comment: Men with severe symptoms can expect the largest absolute fall in their symptom scores with medical treatment.[11,19] Prazosin, alfuzosin, terazosin, and doxazosin lower blood pressure and may be used to treat both hypertension and BPH.[20] The three subsequent RCTs comparing α blockers are limited by their small sample sizes, short duration (4,[13] 4[14] and 16[15] weeks), low drug doses, and unclear methods of randomisation and blinding.

OPTION	5α REDUCTASE INHIBITORS

One systematic review has found that 5α reductase inhibitors are more effective than placebo for improving lower urinary tract symptoms and reducing complications in men with BPH, especially in men with larger prostates. Two RCTs found limited evidence that 5α reductase inhibitors were less effective at improving symptoms than α blockers. We found no direct comparison with surgical treatment.

Benefits: **Versus placebo:** We found one systematic review (search date 1999, 12 RCTs),[10] two non-systematic reviews,[21,22] and one subsequent RCT (published numerous times).[7,23–26] The systematic review found that finasteride versus placebo significantly reduced symptom scores (10 RCTs, results presented in tabular form; overall significance not stated).[10] The first non-systematic review (meta-analysis, published in 1996) combined the results of six RCTs of finasteride.[21] Treatment versus placebo was associated with a significantly greater reduction in symptom scores (difference in symptom score −0.9 points, 95% CI −1.2 to −0.6 [range of score 0–30 points]). The benefit over placebo was greatest in men with larger prostates (≥ 40 g). The second non-systematic review (meta-analysis, published in 1997) combined the results of three placebo controlled RCTs of finasteride.[22] Finasteride reduced the 2 year risk of acute urinary retention requiring catheterisation from 2.7% to 1.1% (NNT 62), of progression to prostatectomy from 6.5% to 4.2% (NNT 44), and of either event from 7.5% to 4.9% (NNT 38). The subsequent RCT (3040 men with enlarged prostates and symptoms of BPH) compared finasteride 5 mg daily versus placebo.[7] After 4 years of treatment, finasteride versus placebo significantly reduced symptoms (difference in symptom score −1.6 points, 95% CI −2.5 to −0.7 [range of score 0–34 points]). Finasteride versus placebo significantly reduced the risk of acute urinary retention (6.6% v 2.8%; NNT 26, 95% CI 22 to 38), of prostatectomy (8.3% v 4.2%; NNT 24, 95% CI 19 to 37), and of the risk of either event (13.2% v 6.6%; NNT 15, 95% CI 12 to 20). There was a greater effect among men with higher concentrations of prostate specific antigen (PSA) at baseline (3.3–12.0 ng/ml), reflecting larger prostates (risk of either acute urinary retention or of needing prostatectomy was 19.9% with placebo v 8.3% with finasteride; NNT 8, 95% CI 7 to 11).[24] This RCT also found that, after 4 years, finasteride versus placebo produced a larger fall in IPSS score. The fall was greater for men with PSAs greater than 1.3 ng/ml than with men with PSAs ≤ 1.3 ng/ml.[23] **Versus α blockers:** See α blockers, p 589. We found two RCTs. Neither trial selected men on the basis of prostate size.[16,17]

Harms: The most common adverse events associated with finasteride in the first year were decreased libido (6%), impotence (8%), and decreased ejaculation (4%). After the first year of treatment, there was no significant difference in adverse effects between finasteride and placebo.[7] Although finasteride reduced concentrations of PSA by an average of 50% (individual responses were highly variable), its use for up to 4 years did not change the rate of detection of prostate cancer compared with placebo.[7] **Versus α blockers:** See α blockers, p 589.

Comment: The meta-analysis of finasteride's impact on symptoms at 1–2 years found that finasteride was significantly more effective than placebo in men with larger prostates.[21] However, the absolute difference in mean decrease of symptom score from baseline between men with the smallest and largest prostates was only about one point. The relative effectiveness of finasteride versus placebo also seemed higher in men with slightly raised PSA,[23] and it is assumed that the higher PSA is a proxy for a larger prostate.

QUESTION What are the effects of surgical treatments?

OPTION TRANSURETHRAL RESECTION (TURP)

We found limited evidence from two RCTs that TURP is more effective than watchful waiting for improving symptoms and reducing complications, and does not increase the risk of erectile dysfunction or incontinence. We found no good long term comparisons of TURP with medical treatments or with newer, less invasive techniques such as transurethral incision, laser ablation, and electrovaporisation.

Benefits: We found no recently updated systematic reviews. **Versus watchful waiting:** We found two RCTs comparing TURP versus conservative treatment.[27,28] The first RCT (556 men with moderate symptoms of BPH) compared TURP versus watchful waiting.[27] More men receiving TURP improved (90% v 39%), and had reduced symptoms compared with watchful waiting. After 5 years, the treatment failure rate was 21% with TURP versus 10% with watchful waiting (NNT 9, 95% CI 7 to 17), and 36% of men assigned to watchful waiting had crossed over to surgery.[29] Treatment failure was defined as death, acute urinary retention, high residual urine volume, renal azotaemia, bladder stones, persistent incontinence, or a high symptom score. The major categories of treatment failure reduced by TURP were acute urinary retention, development of a large bladder residual (> 350 ml), and deterioration to a severe symptom level.

The second RCT (223 men) had a shorter duration of follow up (7.5 months).[28] It found that TURP versus conservative treatment significantly improved the IPSS score (difference in IPSS 10.4 points, 95% CI 8.5 to 12.3). **Versus less invasive techniques:** Numerous small RCTs have found similar symptomatic outcomes with TURP and with transurethral incision of the prostate (TUIP) in men with smaller prostates. In the RCT with the longest follow up (120 men, mean follow up 34 months), symptomatic outcomes were similar for TURP and TUIP.[30] Long term symptom relief and effect on the incidence of complications of BPH have not yet been adequately evaluated. Two recently reported trials of older laser techniques versus TURP found higher surgical retreatment rates after laser therapy (38% v 16% at 5 years with a side firing laser,[31] and 18% v 9% at 3 years with a contact laser.[32] Several small short term RCTs (maximum 2 years) found either no significant difference between TURP and laser ablation or electrovapourisation,[28,33–42] or that TURP achieved better symptom relief. **Versus TUMT and TUNA:** See TUMT below, and TUNA, p 594.

Harms: Analysis of administrative data found that mortality in the 30 days after TURP for BPH ranged from 0.4% for men aged 65–69 years to 1.9% for men aged 80–84 years, and has fallen in recent years.[43] In one review of observational studies, TURP for BPH was associated with immediate surgical complications in 12% of men, bleeding requiring intervention in 2%, erectile dysfunction in 14%, retrograde ejaculation in 74%, and incontinence in about 5%.[44–46] Analysis of claims data found a reoperation rate, implying need for retreatment, of about 1% a year.[43] However, in the only comparative trial, men randomised to prostatectomy did not seem to have a greater rate of erectile dysfunction or incontinence than men assigned to watchful waiting.[27,29] Laser prostatectomy and electrovaporisation require less hospital time and may cause fewer short term adverse effects and less bleeding than TURP.[28,33–38,42,47,48]

Comment: Rapid changes in techniques and few controlled trials with adequate follow up make comparisons between TURP and newer surgical techniques difficult.

OPTION	TRANSURETHRAL MICROWAVE THERMOTHERAPY (TUMT)

RCTs have found that TUMT versus sham treatment significantly reduces symptoms of BPH. We found conflicting evidence about whether TUMT relieves short term symptoms as effectively as TURP. One RCT found limited evidence that TUMT was more effective than α blockers over 6 months.

Benefits: We found no systematic review. **Versus sham treatment:** Several small to medium sized RCTs compared TUMT versus sham treatment. In the largest trial (220 men), TUMT improved the IPSS significantly more than sham treatment (5.0 points lower, $P < 0.05$).[49] **Versus TURP:** Two small trials with follow up to 2.5 years found no difference in symptom relief between TUMT and TURP.[50,51] A third trial found better symptomatic outcomes with TURP (significance not stated).[52] **Versus α blockers:** One RCT (103 men) compared TUMT versus terazosin (up to 10 mg daily) and found significantly better improvement in IPSS after TUMT at 6 months.[53]

Harms: Adverse events associated with TUMT varied among trials, but included the need for catheterisation for more than a week (8% with TUMT v 2% with sham treatment),[54] persistent irritative symptoms (22% v 8%),[49] haematuria (14% v 1%),[49] and sexual dysfunction (mostly haematospermia and other ejaculatory abnormalities, 29% v 1%).[49] In one trial, retrograde ejaculation was substantially less common after TUMT versus TURP (27% v 74%).[52]

Comment: TUMT can be performed in an outpatient setting, and uses heat generated by a microwave antennae in the urethra to coagulate prostate tissue. The long term effects of TUMT have not been adequately evaluated in controlled studies.

OPTION   TRANSURETHRAL NEEDLE ABLATION (TUNA)

We found limited evidence from one RCT that TURP versus TUNA reduced symptoms of BPH, although TUNA caused fewer adverse effects.

Benefits: We found no systematic review. **Versus TURP:** We found one RCT (121 men) comparing TUNA versus TURP.[55] The mean IPSS fell from 24.7 to 11.1 points at 1 year with TUNA, 2.4 points less than the decrease following TURP. Benefit at 1 year was significantly greater with TURP than TUNA (IPSS 11.1 with TUNA v 8.3 with TURP, P = 0.04).

Harms: Compared with TURP, TUNA was associated with less retrograde ejaculation (38% v 0%) and bleeding (100% v 32%).[55]

Comment: TUNA can be performed in an outpatient setting, and uses radio-frequency energy through two intraprostatic electrodes to generate heat to coagulate prostate tissue. Anaesthesia requirements vary in reported studies. The long term effects of treatment have not been adequately evaluated.

QUESTION   What are the effects of non-medical treatments?

OPTION   SAW PALMETTO PLANT EXTRACTS

One systematic review has found that self rated improvement is better in men taking saw palmetto compared with placebo. It found no significant difference in symptom scores between saw palmetto and finasteride.

Benefits: We found one systematic and one non-systematic review. The systematic review (search date 1997, 18 RCTs, 2939 men) included all saw palmetto preparations;[56] the non-systematic review (11 RCTs) included only one pure saw palmetto preparation.[57] **Versus placebo:** The systematic review found that patient rated improvement was better in men taking saw palmetto compared with placebo (6 RCTs, RR 1.7, 95% CI 1.2 to 2.4). It found a significant difference in nocturia in men receiving saw palmetto compared with placebo (10 RCTs, WMD of 0.76 episodes per night, 95% CI 0.32 to 1.21). The non-systematic review focused only on nocturia and found similar results.[57] **Versus finasteride:** The systematic review found similar symptom scores with saw palmetto and finasteride.[56]

Harms: In the systematic review, withdrawal rates were significantly higher with saw palmetto versus placebo (9% v 7%, P = 0.02), and not signicantly different versus finasteride (9% v 11%, P = 0.87). The risk of erectile dysfunction was similar with saw palmetto versus placebo (1.1% v 0.7%, P = 0.58), but was significantly lower versus finasteride (1.1% v 4.9%, P < 0.001).[56]

Comment: The RCTs were brief and few used a validated symptom score. Different preparations, which may not be equivalent, are available directly to consumers without prescription in many countries.

OPTION β–SITOSTEROL PLANT EXTRACT New

One systematic review found that β–sitosterol plant extract versus placebo significantly improved lower urinary tract symptoms in the short term.

Benefits: **Versus placebo:** We found one systematic review (search date 1998, 4 RCTs, 519 men), which compared β–sitosterol versus placebo.[58] Trials lasted for 4–26 weeks. It found that β–sitosterol significantly reduced the IPSS (2 RCTs, WMD –4.9 points, 95% CI –6.3 to –3.5).

Harms: Gastrointestinal adverse effects occurred in more men taking β–sitosterol than placebo (1.6% v 0%, significance not stated). Impotence was also more common in men taking β–sitosterol (0.5% v 0%, significance not stated). Withdrawal rates were similar in both groups (7.8% in men taking β–sitosterol v 8.0% taking placebo, significance not stated).[58]

Comment: The RCTs were limited by a short follow up period (maximum 26 weeks). Different preparations are available, which may be of variable content, making it difficult to generalise results.

OPTION RYE GRASS POLLEN EXTRACT New

One systematic review found limited evidence that rye grass pollen extract versus placebo increased self rated improvement and reduced nocturia in the short term.

Benefits: **Versus placebo:** We found one systematic review (search date 1998, 2 RCTs, 163 men), which compared rye grass pollen extract versus placebo.[59] It found that pollen extract versus placebo significantly increased self rated improvement (1 RCT, 60 men; 69% v 29%; RR 2.40, 95% CI 1.21 to 4.75), and significantly reduced nocturia (2 RCTs; AR 50/79 [63%] with pollen extract v 23/74 [31%] with placebo; RR 2.05, 95% CI 1.41 to 3.99). However, the results should be interpreted with caution; see comment below.

Harms: The review found that nausea occurred in one man taking pollen extract (number in placebo group not stated). Withdrawal rates were not significantly different (4.8% with pollen extract v 2.7% with placebo, P = 0.26).[59]

Comment: Both RCTs were limited by small sample sizes and a short follow up period (12 and 24 weeks). Concealment of treatment allocation was unclear. The composition of the preparations was unknown, making it difficult to generalise results.

Benign prostatic hyperplasia

Men's health

Substantive changes since last issue

α Blockers versus placebo New systematic review;[10] conclusion unchanged.
α Blockers versus each other Two new RCTs;[14,15] conclusion unchanged.
5α Reductase inhibitors versus placebo New systematic review;[10] conclusion unchanged.
TURP versus watchful waiting One new RCT;[28] conclusion unchanged.

REFERENCES

1. Bosch JL, Hop WC, Kirkels WJ, Schroder FH. Natural history of benign prostatic hyperplasia: appropriate case definition and estimation of its prevalence in the community. *Urology* 1995; 46(suppl A):34–40.

2. Barry MJ, Adolfsson J, Batista JE, et al. Committee 6: measuring the symptoms and health impact of benign prostatic hyperplasia and its treatments. In: Denis L, Griffiths K, Khoury S, et al, eds. *Fourth International Consultation on BPH, Proceedings*. Plymouth, UK: Health Publication Ltd, 1998:265–321.

3. Oishi K, Boyle P, Barry MJ, et al. Committee 1: Epidemiology and natural history of benign prostatic hyperplasia. In: Denis L, Griffiths K, Khoury S, et al, eds. *Fourth International Consultation on BPH, Proceedings*. Plymouth, UK: Health Publication Ltd, 1998:23–59.

4. Jacobsen SJ, Girman CJ, Guess HA, Rhodes T, Oesterling JE, Lieber MM. Natural history of prostatism: longitudinal changes in voiding symptoms in community dwelling men. *J Urol* 1996;155:595–600.

5. Barry MJ, Fowler FJ, Bin L, Pitts JC, Harris CJ, Mulley AG. The natural history of patients with benign prostatic hyperplasia as diagnosed by North American urologists. *J Urol* 1997;157:10–15.

6. Jacobsen S, Jacobson D, Girman C, et al. Natural history of prostatism: risk factors for acute urinary retention. *J Urol* 1997;158:481–487.

7. McConnell J, Bruskewitz R, Walsh P, et al. The effect of finasteride on the risk of acute urinary retention and the need for surgical treatment among men with benign prostatic hyperplasia. *N Engl J Med* 1998;338:557–563.

8. Barry MJ, Fowler FJ Jr, O'Leary MP, et al. The American Urological Association symptom index for benign prostatic hyperplasia. *J Urol* 1992;148:1549–1557.

9. Djavan B, Marberger M. A meta-analysis on the efficacy and tolerability of α1–adrenoceptor antagonists in patients with lower urinary tract symptoms suggestive of benign prostatic obstruction. *Eur Urol* 1999;36:1–13. Search date October 1998; primary source Medline.

10. Clifford GM, Farmer RDT. Medical therapy for benign prostatic hyperplasia: a review of the literature. *Eur Urol* 2000;38:2–19. Search date 1999; primary sources Medline, Embase,and the Cochrane Library.

11. Roehrborn CG, Oesterling JE, Auerbach S, et al. The Hytrin community assessment trial study: a one–year study of terazosin versus placebo in the treatment of men with symptomatic benign prostatic hyperplasia. *Urology* 1996;47:159–168.

12. McNeil SA, Daruwala PD, Mitchell IDC, Shearer MG, Hargreave TB. Sustained-release alfuzosin and trial without catheter after acute urinary retention: a prospective placebo-controlled trial. *BJU Int* 1999;84:622–627.

13. Na YJ, Guo YL, Gu F-L, et al. Clinical comparison of selective and non-selective alpha 1A-adreno receptor antagonists for bladder outlet obstruction associated with benign prostatic hyperplasia: studies on tamsulosin and terazosin in Chinese patients. *J Med* 1998;29:289–303.

14. Okada H, Kamidono S, Yoshioka T, et al. A comparative study of terazosin and tamsulosin for symptomatic benign hyperplasia in Japanese patients. *BJU Int* 2000;85:676–681.

15. Fourcade RO. Efficiency and tolerance of terazosine in ambutory patients with benign prostatic hyperthrophy: comparative randomized and double-blind trial versus alfuzosin. *Prog Urol* 2000;10:246–253.

16. Lepor H, Williford WO, Barry MJ, et al. The efficacy of terazosin, finasteride, or both in benign prostatic hyperplasia. Veterans' Affairs cooperative studies benign prostatic hyperplasia study group. *N Engl J Med* 1996;335:533–539.

17. Debruyne FMJ, Jardin A, Colloi D, et al. Sustained-release alfuzosin, finasteride and the combination of both in the treatment of benign prostatic hyperplasia. *Eur Urol* 1998;34:169–175.

18. Hofner K, Claes H, De Reijke TM, et al. Tamsulosin 0.4 mg once daily: effect on sexual function in patients with lower urinary tract symptoms suggestive of benign prostatic obstruction. *Eur Urol* 1999;36:335–341.

19. Mobley D, Dias N, Levenstein M. Effects of doxazosin in patients with mild, intermediate, and severe benign prostatic hyperplasia. *Clin Ther* 1998;20:101–109.

20. Kaplan S, Kaplan N. Alpha–blockade: monotherapy for hypertension and benign prostatic hyperplasia. *Urology* 1996;48:541–550.

21. Boyle P, Gould AL, Roehrborn CG. Prostate volume predicts outcome of treatment of benign prostatic hyperplasia with finasteride: meta-analysis of randomized clinical trials. *Urology* 1996;48:398–405.

22. Andersen J, Nickel J, Marshall V, Schulman C, Boyle P. Finasteride significantly reduces acute urinary retention and need for surgery in patients with symptomatic benign prostatic hyperplasia. *Urology* 1997;49:839–845.

23. Roehrborn CG, Boyle P, Bergner D, et al. Serum prostate specific antigen and prostate volume predict long-term changes in symptoms and flow rate: results of a four-year, randomised trial comparing finasteride and placebo. *Urology* 1999: 54;663–669.

24. Roehrborn CG, McConnell JD, Lieber M, et al. Serum prostate-specific antigen concentration is a powerful predictor of acute urinary retention and the need for surgery in men with clinical benign prostatic hypoplasia. *Urology* 1999;53:473–480.

25. Roehrborn CG, Bruskewitz R, Nickel GC, et al. Urinary retention in patients with BPH treated with finasteride or placebo over 4 years. *Eur Urol* 2000;37:528–536.

26. Kaplan S, Garvin D, Gilhooly P, et al. Impact of baseline symptom severity on future risk of benign prostatic hyperplasia-related outcomes and long-term response to finasteride. *Urology* 2000;56: 610–616.

27. Wasson J, Reda D, Bruskewitz R, et al. A comparison of transurethral surgery with watchful waiting for moderate symptoms of benign prostatic hyperplasia. *N Engl J Med* 1995;332:75–79.

28. Donovan JL, Peters T, Neal DE, et al. A randomized trial comparing transurethral resection

of the prostate, laser therapy and conservative treatment of men with symptoms associated with benign prostatic enlargement: the ClasP study. *J Urol* 2000;164:65–70.

29. Flanigan RC, Reda DC, Wasson JH, Anderson RJ, Abdellatif M, Bruskewitz RC. Five year outcome of surgical resection and watchful waiting for men with moderately symptomatic benign prostatic hyperplasia: a Department of Veterans' Affairs cooperative study. *J Urol* 1998;160:12–17.

30. Riehmann M, Knes JM, Heisey D, Madsen PO, Bruskewitz RC. Transurethral resection versus incision of the prostate: a randomized, prospective study. *Urology* 1995;45:768–775.

31. McAllister WJ, Absalom MJ, Mir K, et al. Does endoscopic laser ablation of the prostate stand the test of time? Five-year results test results from a multicentre randomised controlled trial of endoscopic laser ablation against transurethral resection of the prostate. *BJU Int* 2000;85:437–439.

32. Keoghane SR, Lawrence KC, Gray AM, et al. A double-blind randomized controlled trial and economic evaluation of transurethral resection vs contact laser vaporization for benign prostatic enlargement: a 3-year follow-up. *BJU Int* 2000; 85:74–78.

33. Shokeir A, Al-Sisi H, Farage Y, El-Maaboud M, Saeed M, Mutabagani H. Transurethral prostatectomy: a prospective randomized study of conventional resection and electrovaporisation in benign prostatic hyperplasia. *Br J Urol* 1997;80: 570–574.

34. Kaplan S, Laor E, Fatal M, Te A. Transurethral resection of the prostate versus transurethral electrovaporization of the prostate: a blinded, prospective comparative study with 1-year follow up. *J Urol* 1998;159:454–458.

35. Kupeli S, Baltaci S, Aytac S, Yulmaz E, Budak M. A prospective randomized study of transurethral resection of the prostate and transurethral vaporization of the prostate as a therapeutic alternative in the management of men with BPH. *Eur Urol* 1998;34:15–18.

36. Hammadeh MY, Madaan S, Singh M, Philp T. Two year follow-up of a prospective randomised trial of electrovaporization versus resection of prostate. *Eur Urol* 1998;34:188–192.

37. Gallucci M, Puppo P, Perachino M, et al. Transurethral electrovaporation of the prostate vs. Transurethral resection. *Eur Urol* 1998;33: 359–364.

38. Kupeli B, Yalcinkaya F, Topaloglu H, Karabacak O, Gunlusoy B, Unal S. Efficacy of transurethral electrovaporization of the prostate with respect to transurethral resection. *J Endourol* 1998;12:591–594.

39. Tuhkaren K, Heino A, Ala-Opas M. Contact laser prostatectomy compared to TURP in prostatic hyperplasia smaller than 40 ml. *Scand J Urol Nephrol* 1999;33:31–34.

40. Carter A, Sells H, Speakman M, Ewings P, MacDonagh R, O'Boyle P. A prospective randomized controlled trial of hybrid laser treatment or transurethral resection of the prostate, with a 1-year follow-up. *BJU Int* 1999; 83:254–259.

41. Shingleton WB, Terrell F, Renfoe DL, Kolski JM, Fowler JE. A randomised prospective study of laser ablation of the prostate versus transurethral resection of the prostate in men with benign prostatic hyperplasia. *Urology* 1999;54:1017–1021.

42. Gujral S, Abrams P, Donovan JL, et al. A prospective randomized trial comparing transurethral resection of the prostate and laser therapy in men with chronic urinary retention: the

ClasP study. *J Urol* 2000;164:59–64.

43. Lu-Yao GL, Barry MJ, Chang CH, Wasson JH, Wennberg JE, and the Prostate PORT. Transurethral resection of the prostate among Medicare beneficiaries in the United States: time trends and outcomes. *Urology* 1994;44:692–698.

44. McConnell JD, Barry MJ, Bruskewitz RC, et al. Direct treatment outcomes–complications. Benign prostatic hyperplasia: diagnosis and treatment. Clinical Practice Guideline, Number 8. Rockville, Maryland: Agency for Health Care Policy and Research, Public Health Service, US Department of Health and Human Services, 1994:91–98.

45. McConnell JD, Barry MJ, Bruskewitz RC, et al. Direct treatment outcomes – sexual dysfunction. Benign prostatic hyperplasia: diagnosis and treatment. Clinical Practice Guideline, Number 8. Rockville, Maryland: Agency for Health Care Policy and Research, Public Health Service, US Department of Health and Human Services, 1994: 99–103.

46. McConnell JD, Barry MJ, Bruskewitz RC, et al. Direct treatment outcomes – urinary incontinence. Benign prostatic hyperplasia: diagnosis and treatment. Clinical Practice Guideline, Number 8. Rockville, Maryland: Agency for Health Care Policy and Research, Public Health Service, US Department of Health and Human Services, 1994: 105–106.

47. Cowles RS III, Kabalin JN, Childs S, et al. A prospective randomized comparison of transurethral resection to visual laser ablation of the prostate for the treatment of benign prostatic hyperplasia. *Urology* 1995;46:155–160.

48. Kabalin JN, Gill HS, Bite G, Wolfe V. Comparative study of laser versus electrocautery prostatic resection: 18-month follow up with complex urodynamic assessment. *J Urol* 1995;153:94–97.

49. Roehrborn C, Preminger G, Newhall P, et al. Microwave thermotherapy for benign prostatic hyperplasia with the Dornier Urowave: results of a randomized, double-blind, multicenter, sham-controlled trial. *Urology* 1998;51:19–28.

50. Ahmed M, Bell T, Lawrence WT, Ward JP, Watson GM. Transurethral microwave thermotherapy (Prostatron version 2.5) compared with transurethral resection of the prostate for the treatment of benign prostatic hyperplasia: a randomized, controlled, parallel study. *Br J Urol* 1997;79:181–185.

51. D'Ancona FCH, Francisca EAE, Witjes WPJ, Welling L, Debruyne FMJ, De La Rosette JJMCH. Transurethral resection of the prostate vs high energy Thermotherapy of the prostate in patients with benign prostatic hyperplasia: long term results. *Br J Urol* 1998;81:259–264.

52. Francisca EA, D'Ancona FCH, Meuleman EJ, Debruyne FM, DeLaRosette JJ. Sexual function following high energy microwave thermotherapy: results of a randomized controlled study comparing transurethral microwave thermotherapy to transurethral prostatic resection. *J Urol* 1999; 161:486–490.

53. Djavan B, Roehrborn CG, Shariat S, Ghawidel K, Marberger M. Prospective randomized comparison of high energy transurethral microwave thermotherapy versus alpha blocker treatment of patients with benign prostatic hyperplasia. *J Urol* 1999;161:139–143.

54. Larson T, Blute M, Bruskewitz R, Mayer R, Ugarte R, Utz W. A high-efficiency microwave thermoablation system for the treatment of benign prostatic hyperplasia: results of a randomized, sham-controlled, prospective, double-blind, multicenter clinical trial. *Urology* 1998;51:731–742.

Men's health

55. Bruskewitz R, Issa M, Roehrborn C, et al. A prospective, randomized 1-year clinical trial comparing transurethral needle ablation to transurethral resection of the prostate for the treatment of symptomatic benign prostatic hyperplasia. *J Urol* 1998;159:1588–1594.

56. Wilt T, Ishani A, Stark G, Mac Donald R, Mulrow C, Lau J. Serenoa repens for benign prostatic hyperplasia. In: The Cochrane Library, Issue 3, 2000. Oxford: Update Software. Search date 1997; primary sources Medline, Embase, Phytodok, The Cochrane Library.

57. Boyle P, Robertson C, Lowe F, Roehrborn C. Meta-analysis of clinical trials of Permixon in the treatment of benign prostatic hyperplasia. *Urology* 2000;55:533–539.

58. Wilt TJ, Macdonald R, Ishani A. Beta–sitosterol for the treatment of benign prostatic hyperplasia: a systematic review. *BJU Int* 1999;83:976–983. Search date 1998; primary sources Medline, Embase, Phytodok, The Cochrane Library.

59. Macdonald R, Ishani A, Rutks I, Wilt TJ. A systematic review of Cernilton for the treatment of benign prostatic hyperplasia. *BJU Int* 2000;85: 836–841. Search date 1998; primary source Medline. Search date 1997; primary sources Embase and The Cochrane Library.

Michael Barry
General Medicine Unit
Massachusetts General Hospital
Boston
Massachusetts
USA

Claus Roehrborn
Associate Professor
Department of Urology
The University of Texas
Southwestern Medical Center
Dallas
Texas
USA

Competing interests: MB, none declared. CR has received a fee for consulting, speaking, research, and/or running educational programs for Merck, Sharpe & Dohme Inc., Glaxo Wellcome, Sanofi-Synthelabo, and Urologix.

Search date May 2000

Jeffrey Stern and Anthony Schaeffer

INTERVENTIONS

Key Messages

In men with chronic bacterial prostatitis

■ Antimicrobial drugs have not been adequately evaluated. Retrospective cohort studies report cure rates of 0%–90% depending on the drug used and the duration of treatment.

■ We found no good evidence that local injection of antimicrobial agents is more effective than oral or parenteral antimicrobial treatment.

■ Limited evidence from one RCT suggests that adding α blockers to antimicrobial treatment may improve outcome and reduce recurrence.

■ We found that transurethral resection and radical prostatectomy have not yet been adequately evaluated.

In men with chronic abacterial prostatitis

■ Limited evidence from one RCT suggests that α blockers may improve symptoms.

■ Limited evidence from one RCT suggests that transurethral microwave thermotherapy may improve symptoms; we found no evidence on cure or recurrence rate.

■ Allopurinol thermotherapy, prostatic massage, Sitz baths, and biofeedback have not yet been adequately evaluated.

Chronic prostatitis

DEFINITION	**Chronic bacterial prostatitis** is characterised by a positive culture of expressed prostatic secretions. It can be symptomatic (recurrent urinary tract infection, suprapubic, lower back, or perineal pain), asymptomatic, or associated with minimal urgency, frequency, and dysuria. **Chronic abacterial prostatitis** is characterised by pelvic or perineal pain, often associated with urinary urgency, nocturia, weak urinary stream, frequency, dysuria, hesitancy, dribbling after micturition, interrupted flow, and inflammation (white cells) in prostatic secretions. Symptoms can also include suprapubic, scrotal, testicular, penile, or lower back pain or discomfort, known as prostodynia in the absence of inflammation in prostatic secretions
INCIDENCE/ PREVALENCE	One community based study estimated that 9% of men have a diagnosis of chronic prostatitis at any one time.[1] Another study found that, of men with genitourinary symptoms, 8% presenting to urologists and 1% presenting to primary care physicians are diagnosed with chronic prostatitis.[2] Most cases of chronic prostatitis are abacterial. Acute bacterial prostatitis, while easy to diagnose and treat, is rare.
AETIOLOGY/ RISK FACTORS	Organisms commonly implicated in bacterial prostatitis include *Escherichia coli*, other Gram negative *Enterobacteriaciae*, occasionally *Pseudomonas* species, and rarely Gram positive enterococci. The cause of abacterial prostatitis is unclear, but autoimmunity may be involved.[3]
PROGNOSIS	One recent study found that chronic abacterial prostatitis had an impact on quality of life similar to that from angina, Crohn's disease, or a previous myocardial infarction.[4]
AIMS	To relieve symptoms and eliminate infection where present, with minimum adverse effects.
OUTCOMES	Symptom improvement (symptom scores, bother scores); quality of life; urodynamics; rates of bacteriological cure (clearance of previously documented organisms from prostatic secretions).
METHODS	We searched Medline up to July 1998. A full update *Clinical Evidence* search and appraisal was performed in May 2000. No systematic reviews were identified. We reviewed all relevant RCTs identified.

QUESTION What are the effects of treatments for chronic bacterial prostatitis?

OPTION ORAL ANTIMICROBIAL DRUGS

We found that oral antimicrobial drugs have not been adequately evaluated in men with chronic bacterial prostatitis. Retrospective cohort studies report cure rates (clearing prostatic secretions of previously documented organisms) of 0%–90% depending on the drug used and the duration of treatment. Limited evidence from retrospective studies suggests that quinolones may be more effective than trimethoprim-sulfamethoxazole (TMP-SMZ).

Benefits: We found no systematic review and no RCTs. **TMP-SMZ:** One non-systematic review identified 10 retrospective cohort studies in

135 men with bacteriologically confirmed prostatitis treated with TMP-SMZ 160 mg/800 mg twice daily for 10–140 days.[5] The studies reported bacteriological cure rates of 0%–67%. Over 30% of men were cured when treated for at least 90 days. **Quinolones:** One review summarised three retrospective cohort studies in 106 men treated with norfloxacin 400 mg twice daily for 10, 28, and 174 days.[6] The studies reported cure rates of 64%–88%. We also found six retrospective cohort studies in 141 men treated with ciprofloxacin 250–500 mg twice daily for 14–259 days, with cure rates of 60%–75%. **Amoxicillin/clavulanic acid and clindamycin:** One cohort study included 50 men who were resistant to empirical treatment with quinolone. The expressed prostatic secretions from 24 of these men exhibited high colony counts of Gram positive and Gram negative anaerobic bacteria, either alone (18 men) or in combination with aerobic bacteria (6 men). After treatment with either amoxicillin/clavulanic acid or clindamycin for 3–6 weeks, all patients had a decrease or total elimination of symptoms, and no anaerobic bacteria were detected in prostatic secretions.[7]

Harms: The studies of TMP-SMZ did not report adverse effects. In the other studies, toxicity from quinolones was rare. Late relapse (6–12 months after treatment) was common.

Comment: Higher cure rates with quinolones may be explained by greater penetration into the prostate.[8] We reviewed only studies that used standard methods to localise infection to the prostate.[9]

OPTION   LOCAL INJECTION OF ANTIMICROBIALS

We found no good evidence that local injection of antimicrobial agents is more effective than oral or parenteral antimicrobial treatment.

Benefits: We found no systematic review and no RCTs. One small cohort study of 24 men with refractory chronic bacterial prostatitis found that eradication of infection was eventually achieved after an unstated period in 15 men with 160 mg gentamicin plus 3 g cefazolin injected directly into the prostate via the perineum.[10]

Harms: Although not reported in this study, infection is a potential risk of this invasive procedure.

Comment: None.

OPTION   α BLOCKERS

We found limited evidence from one RCT suggesting that adding α blockers to antimicrobial treatment may improve outcome and reduce recurrence in men with chronic bacterial prostatitis.

Benefits: We found no systematic review. We found one RCT of α blockers (either 1–2 mg terazosin daily or 2.5 mg terazosin daily or 2.5 mg alfuzosin once or twice daily) in 270 men with bacterial or abacterial prostatitis or prostadynia.[11] Antimicrobials were given to all men with positive culture of expressed prostatic secretions and to half of those with inflammatory expressed prostatic secretions. Of men with bacterial prostatitis, those given α blockers and antimicrobials had significantly higher rates of clinical improvement and significantly lower rates of recurrence (assessed by culture of expressed prostatic secretions) compared with those given antimicrobials alone (P = 0.019, no RR or CI given).

Harms: No adverse effects of α blockers were reported in this study.[11]

Comment: None.

OPTION TRANSURETHRAL RESECTION

We found insufficient evidence on the effects of transurethral resection of the prostate in men with chronic bacterial prostatitis.

Benefits: We found no systematic review, RCTs, or prospective cohort studies.

Harms: One trial in men with benign prostatic hypertrophy found no difference in the incidence of impotence or urinary incontinence with transurethral resection or watchful waiting.[12]

Comment: One retrospective cohort study reported 40%–50% cure rates in 50 men with chronic prostatitis treated with transurethral resection. However, proof of bacterial prostatitis was not shown in many cases.[13]

OPTION RADICAL PROSTATECTOMY

Radical prostatectomy is associated with impotence, stress incontinence, and complications of open surgery. We found that its use in men with chronic prostatitis has not been adequately evaluated.

Benefits: We found no RCTs. We found one report of radical prostatectomy in two young men whose refractory bacterial prostatitis caused relapsing haemolytic crises.[14]

Harms: Radical prostactectomy can cause impotence (9–75% depending upon age)[15] and varying degrees of urinary stress incontinence (8%).[16] Other potential harms include those associated with any open surgery.

Comment: None.

QUESTION What are the effects of treatments for chronic abacterial prostatitis?

OPTION α BLOCKERS

Limited evidence from one RCT suggests that α blockers may relieve symptoms in men with abacterial prostatitis.

Benefits: We found no systematic review. We found one RCT of α blockers (either 1–2 mg terazosin daily or 2.5 mg terazosin daily or 2.5 mg alfuzosin once or twice daily) in 270 men with bacterial or abacterial prostatitis or prostadynia.[11] Antimicrobials were given to all men with positive culture of expressed prostatic secretions and to half of those with inflammatory expressed prostatic secretions. Of men with abacterial prostatitis, those given α blockers had significantly lower rates of symptomatic recurrence compared with those given either no treatment or antimicrobials (P < 0.001, no RR or CI given).

Harms: No adverse effects of α blockers were reported.[11]

Comment: None.

OPTION TRANSURETHRAL MICROWAVE THERMOTHERAPY

We found insufficient evidence on the effects of thermotherapy in abacterial prostatitis for cure or recurrence rate. One small RCT found that it relieved symptoms compared with sham treatment.

Benefits: We found no systematic review. We found one small double blind RCT comparing transurethral microwave thermotherapy versus sham treatment in 20 men.[17] Outcomes were assessed using a symptom severity index and symptom frequency questionnaire. Seven of 10 men in the treatment group improved significantly over a mean of 21 months' follow up, compared with one of the 10 men in the sham group (no CI or P value reported).

Harms: Four men complained of transient (resolved in 3 weeks) adverse reactions, including haematuria (2 men), urinary tract infection, impotence, urinary retention, urinary incontinence, and premature ejaculation (each occurring in one man).[17]

Comment: The trial measured changes in clinical symptoms to determine efficacy. Thermotherapy caused persistent elevation of leukcocytes in the prostatic fluid, which could indicate tissue damage.

OPTION ALLOPURINOL

We found no good evidence on the effects of allopurinol in men with chronic abacterial prostatitis.

Benefits: We found one systemic review,[18] which identified one RCT. Fifty four men were initially enrolled in the study and divided into three groups: treatment with 600 mg allopurinol daily, treatment with 300 mg allopurinol daily, and placebo. Thirty four men completed the study, which lasted 240 days. The trial found that there was a significant effect of allopurinol on urate concentration in expressed prostatic secretion; men in treatment groups had a far lower ratio of urate to creatinine in their expressed prostatic secretions than did the placebo group. Moreover, the "degree of discomfort" score was lower among the allopurinol groups than the placebo group (P = 0.019).

Harms: No men receiving allopurinol reported any significant adverse effects.

Comment: From the data presented, it is not clear that the decreases in urate concentration in expressed prostatic secretion led directly to symptom relief. The symptom score was not validated.[18]

OPTION OTHER INTERVENTIONS

We found that prostatic massage, Sitz baths, and biofeedback (training the patient to contract and relax the pelvic floor muscles to interrupt the myofascial pain attacks) have not yet been formally evaluated in men with chronic abacterial prostatitis.

Chronic prostatitis

Benefits: We found no systematic review or RCTs.

Harms: Insufficient data.

Comment: None.

REFERENCES

1. Roberts RO, Lieber MM, Rhodes T, et al. Prevalence of a physician-assigned diagnosis of prostatitis: the Olmsted County study of urinary symptoms and health status among men. *Urology* 1998;51:578–584.

2. Collins MM, Stafford, RS, O'Leary MP, Barry MJ. How common is prostatitis? A national survey of physician visits. *J Urol* 1998;159:1224–1228.

3. Alexander RB, Brady F, Ponniah S. Autoimmune prostatitis: evidence of T cell reactivity with normal prostatic proteins. *Urology* 1997;50:893–899.

4. Wenninger K, Heiman JR, Rothman I, Berghuis JP, Berger RE. Sickness impact of chronic nonbacterial prostatitis and its correlates. *J Urol* 1996;155:965–968.

5. Hanus PM, Danzinger LH. Treatment of chronic bacterial prostatitis. *Clin Pharm* 1984;3:49–55.

6. Naber KG, Sorgel F, Kees F, et al. Norfloxacin concentration in prostatic adenoma tissue (patients) and in prostatic fluid in patients and volunteers. 15th International Congress of Chemotherapy, Landsberg. In: Weidner N, Madsen PO, Schiefer HG, eds. *Prostatitis: etiopathology, diagnosis and therapy.* New York: Springer Verlag, 1987.

7. Szoke I, Torok L, Dosa E, et al. The possible role of anaerobic bacteria in chronic prostatitis. *Int J Androl* 1998;21:163–168.

8. Cox CE. Ofloxacin in the management of complicated urinary tract infections, including prostatitis. *Am J Med* 1980;87(suppl 6c):61–68.

9. Meares EM, Stamey TA. Bacteriologic localization patterns in bacterial prostatitis and urethritis. *Invest Urol* 1968;5:492–518.

10. Baret L, Leonare A. Chronic bacterial prostatitis: 10 years of experience with local antibiotics. *J Urol* 1998;140:755–757.

11. Barbalias GA, Nikiforidis G, Liatsikos EN. Alpha-blockers for the treatment of chronic prostatitis in combination with antibiotics. *J Urol* 1998;159:883–887.

12. Wasson JH, Reda DJ, Bruskewitz RC, et al. A comparison of transurethral surgery with watchful waiting for moderate symptoms of benign prostatic hyperplasia. *N Engl J Med* 1995;332:75–79.

13. Smart CJ, Jenkins JD, Lloyd RS. The painful prostate. *Br J Urol* 1975;47:861–869.

14. Davis BE, Weigel JW. Adenocarcinoma of the prostate discovered in 2 young patients following total prostatovesiculectomy for refractory prostatitis. *J Urol* 1990;144:744–745.

15. Quinlan DM, Epstein JI, Carter BS, Walsh PC. Sexual function following radical prostatectomy: influence of preservation of neurovascular bundles. *J Urol* 1991;145:998–1002.

16. Steiner MS, Morton RA, Walsh PC. Impact of radical prostatectomy on urinary continence. *J Urol* 1991;145:512–515.

17. Nickel J, Sorensen R. Transurethral microwave thermotherapy for nonbacterial prostatitis: a randomized double-blind sham controlled study using new prostatitis specific assessment questionnaires. *J Urol* 1996;155:1950–1955.

18. Persson B, Ronquist G, Ekblom M. Ameliorative effect of allopurinol on nonbacterial prostatitis: a parallel double-blind controlled study. *J Urol* 1996;155:961–964.

Jeffrey Stern

Anthony Schaeffer

Northwestern University Medical School
Chicago
USA

Competing interests: AS has been reimbursed by Ortho McNeil for attending and speaking at several conferences. He has also received consulting fees from Bayer Corp. and Johnson and Johnson.

Search date December 2000

Michael O'Leary

INTERVENTIONS

To be covered in future issues of
Clinical Evidence
Vascular bypass procedures
Psychological counselling

Key Messages

- We found good evidence from well conducted RCTs that yohimbine and sildenafil are effective and well tolerated compared with placebo. We found no trials comparing one directly with the other. Limited evidence from indirect comparison of data from placebo controlled trials suggests that yohimbine may be less effective but safer.

- Small RCTs found no evidence that L-arginine or trazodone were more effective than placebo, although the trials were not adequately powered to rule out a clinically important difference.

- RCTs have found that prostaglandin E1 (alprostadil) is effective in about 30–80% of men, and more effective when administered by intracavernosal injection than intraurethrally. For both methods, adherence to treatment in the long term is poor. One small RCT found that topical prostaglandin E1 was significantly more effective than placebo, but sequential allocation of men to each group may mean that groups were not comparable.

- Neither vacuum devices nor penile prostheses have been adequately evaluated in RCTs.

© *Clinical Evidence* 2001;5:605–611.

DEFINITION	Erectile dysfunction has largely replaced the term "impotence". It is defined as the persistent inability to obtain or maintain sufficient rigidity of the penis to allow satisfactory sexual performance.
INCIDENCE/ PREVALENCE	There is little good epidemiological information, but current normative data suggest that age is the variable most strongly associated with erectile dysfunction, and that up to 30 million men in the USA may be affected.[1] Even among men in their 40s, nearly 40% report at least occasional difficulty obtaining or maintaining erection, whereas this approaches 70% in 70 year olds.
AETIOLOGY/ RISK FACTORS	It is now believed that about 80% of cases of erectile dysfunction have an organic cause, the rest being psychogenic in origin. Risk factors include increasing age, smoking, and obesity. Erectile problems fall into three categories: failure to initiate; failure to fill, caused by insufficient arterial inflow into the penis to allow engorgement and tumescence, owing to vascular insufficiency; and failure to store, owing to veno-occlusive dysfunction.
PROGNOSIS	In erectile dysfunction of organic cause, treatment is almost always symptomatic. We found no good evidence on prognosis in untreated organic erectile dysfunction.
AIMS	To restore satisfactory erections, with minimal adverse effects.
OUTCOMES	Patient and partner self reports of satisfaction and sexual function; objective tests of penile rigidity; adverse effects of treatment.
METHODS	*Clinical Evidence* update search and appraisal December 2000.

QUESTION   What are the effects of treatments?

OPTION   YOHIMBINE

RCTs have found that yohimbine is significantly more effective than placebo. Yohimbine has not yet been compared directly with other oral or local treatments. Mild, transient adverse effects are reported in up to a third of men.

Benefits: We found one systematic review (search date 1997, 7 RCTs, 11–100 men with erectile dysfunction, defined variously as organic, psychogenic, and of unknown cause) comparing the α blocker, yohimbine, versus placebo.[2] Duration of treatment ranged from 2–10 weeks, and outcomes varied from self reported improvement in sexual function to objective tests of penile rigidity. The RCTs found positive responses in significantly more men taking yohimbine versus placebo (34–73% v 9–28%; RR 3.85, 95% CI 2.22 to 6.67). One subsequent placebo controlled, crossover trial (22 men, randomisation not mentioned) comparing yohimbine (single daily dose 100 mg for 30 days) versus placebo found no significant difference in the promotion of erections.[3]

Harms: Adverse events were reported in 10–30% of men receiving yohimbine and were generally mild, including agitation, anxiety, headache, mild increase in blood pressure, increased urinary output, and gastrointestinal upset. However, in at least one study, no men discontinued treatment.[3]

Comment: The end points in some of these trials were subjective and of questionable validity.

RCTs have found that sildenafil is effective compared with placebo and well tolerated in men with and without diabetes. It has not yet been compared directly with other treatments for erectile dysfunction. Mild transient adverse effects are reported in up to a fifth of men, and deaths have been reported in men on concomitant treatment with oral nitrates. Long term safety is unknown.

Benefits: We found no systematic review. We found six RCTs. **In men with any cause of erectile dysfunction:** Three RCTs evaluated sildenafil in 1496 men with erectile dysfunction from a variety of causes. They all found that sildenafil improved outcomes compared with placebo.[4-6] The largest trial comparing sildenafil versus placebo (861 men, age 20–87 years) involved two different evaluations in men with 3–5 years of erectile dysfunction from all causes.[4] In the first evaluation, 532 men were randomised to receive either placebo or 25 mg, 50 mg, or 100 mg sildenafil about 1 hour before planned sexual activity, but not more than once per day, for 24 weeks. In the second, 329 different men were randomised to placebo or sildenafil in an escalating dose up to 100 mg for 12 weeks, followed by open label treatment for a further 32 weeks. Significantly more men taking sildenafil versus placebo had successful attempts at sexual intercourse (69% v 22%, P < 0.001; CI values not quoted in report). Efficacy increased with increasing dose and did not vary according to the cause of erectile dysfunction. **In men with diabetes:** One double blind multicentre RCT in 268 men with erectile dysfunction and diabetes found that sildenafil versus placebo significantly improved erections at 12 weeks (AR 56% v 10%; ARI 46%, 95% CI 30% to 62%; RR 5.5, 95% CI 3.9 to 7.0; NNT 2, 95% CI 2 to 3).[7] **In men with spinal cord injury:** We found two RCTs. The first compared sildenafil with placebo in 26 men with spinal cord injury (T6 to L5). It found that sildenafil significantly improved erections (9/12 in treatment group v 1/14 in placebo group, P = 0.004). At 28 days, significantly more men in the treatment group reported improvements in quality of sex life (P = 0.001) and wished to continue treatment (P = 0.02).[8] The second RCT (111 men with erectile dysfunction secondary to spinal trauma) was a double blind crossover comparison of oral sildenafil versus placebo. It found that sildenafil improved sexual intercourse more than placebo (80% reported improved sexual intercourse with sildenafil v 10% with placebo).[6]

Harms: In the first RCT, headache, flushing, and dyspepsia were reported in 6–18% of men taking sildenafil.[3,4] In the RCT in men with diabetes, comparable cardiovascular events were similar in the two groups (3% sildenafil v 5% placebo).[7] In one RCT, none of the 12 men with spinal cord injury discontinued treatment.[8] Another article reported specifically on adverse effects of sildenafil. It summarised results from a series of double blind placebo controlled RCTs in a total of 4274 men aged 19–87 years with erectile dysfunction owing to a range of causes for more than 6 months and a mean of 5 years. All men were treated for up to 6 months, and 2199 received open label treatment for up to a further year.[9] Headache, flushing, and dyspepsia were reported in 7–16% of men taking sildenafil compared with 1–4% taking placebo. Similar proportions in both groups discontinued treatment (about 2.4%). An important contraindication to prescribing sildenafil is concomitant use of oral nitrates. This combination results in precipitous hypotension. To date, about 60 deaths have been reported to the US Food and Drug Administration in men who had been given prescriptions for sildenafil. However, it is not known whether any were directly attributable to the drug. Long term (> 1 year) safety of sildenafil is unknown.

Comment: None.

OPTION **L-ARGININE**

One small RCT found no evidence that L-arginine improved sexual function compared with placebo, although the trial was too small to rule out a clinically important difference.

Benefits: We found no systematic review. We found one small double blind RCT (50 men with erectile dysfunction) comparing high dose L-arginine (5 g per day given orally) versus placebo.[10] It found no significant difference in sexual function between L-arginine and placebo, although the power of the study was not adequate to rule out a clinically important difference (sexual function improved in 9/29 men with L-arginine v 2/17 with placebo, P = NS, 4 men not included in analysis).

Harms: The trial reported decreases in systolic or diastolic blood pressure, or both, although this caused no systemic effects and required no drug interruptions. The trial found some "fluctuation in heart rate", which was described as clinically insignificant. Nausea, vomiting, diarrhoea, headache, flushing, and numbness have been reported after the administration of L-arginine, although none of the men in this study reported any such complaints.

Comment: None.

OPTION **TRAZODONE**

One small RCT found no evidence that trazodone was more effective than placebo in men with erectile dysfunction, although the trial was too small to rule out a clinically important effect.

Benefits: We found no systematic review. One small two way, crossover RCT (48 men with erectile dysfunction, washout period 3 weeks) compared trazodone versus placebo.[11] Men were treated with either trazodone 50 mg or placebo at bedtime for 3 months. It found no evidence that trazodone improved erections or libido (improved erections reported by 19% v 24% receiving placebo, P < 0.50; improved libido reported by 35% v 20% with placebo, P < 0.36).

Harms: The trial reported drowsiness (31% of men), dry mouth (1%), and fatigue (19%, comparative rates for trazodone v placebo not available).

Comment: None.

| OPTION | INTRAURETHRAL PROSTAGLANDIN E1 |

RCTs have found that intraurethral administration of prostaglandin E1 (alprostadil) leads to satisfactory erection in about 40% of men. About a third of men suffered penile ache, which caused many to discontinue treatment. Intraurethral prostaglandin E1 has not yet been directly compared with either intracavernosal or oral drug treatment.

Benefits: We found no systematic review. One double blind RCT began by testing the response to intraurethral alprostadil in 1511 men aged 27–88 years who had erectile dysfunction of organic cause for at least 3 months. In clinic testing, 66% had erections sufficient for intercourse. These 996 men were randomised to intraurethral alprostadil or placebo for use at home.[12] Over 3 months, those given alprostadil were more likely to report having successful sexual intercourse (64.9% v 18.6% on placebo, P < 0.001) and at least one orgasm (63.6% v 23.6% on placebo, P < 0.001). Subsequent RCTs, published only in abstract form, found slightly lower efficacies of 30–48% on alprostadil.

Harms: The most common adverse effect was mild to moderate penile ache, occurring in about a third of men.[12] This caused many men to discontinue treatment. We found no reports of priapism, penile fibrosis, or other serious adverse events.

Comment: The trial preselected men who had a good response to alprostadil before randomisation. This limits the generaliseability of results.

| OPTION | INTRACAVERNOSAL PROSTAGLANDIN E1 |

RCTs have found that intracavernosal injection of prostaglandin E1 (alprostadil) leads to satisfactory erection in about 80% of men, but long term adherence is poor. Intracavernosal prostaglandin E1 has not yet been directly compared with either intraurethral or oral drug treatment.

Benefits: We found no systematic review. The largest study was a multicentre trial in 1128 men aged 20–79 years with all causes of erectile dysfunction.[13] Heavy smokers and men with uncontrolled hypertension or diabetes were excluded. Nearly 300 men were randomly assigned to double blind doses of placebo or 2.5 µg, 5 µg, 10 µg, or 20 µg of alprostadil. Injections were given, and outcome was assessed by an investigator or research nurse. None of the 59 men who received placebo had a response. There were significant differences in response between all doses versus placebo, and a significant dose response relationship. The remaining 884 men, including 52 who had taken part in the dose response study, were enrolled in a single blind, dose escalation study (201 men) and an uncontrolled open label flexible dose study to assess efficacy, safety, and feasibility of self injection at home (683 men). Of the 13 762 injections for which men recorded their response, nearly 90% were followed by satisfactory sexual activity. **Versus vacuum devices:** One crossover RCT (50 men with erectile dysfunction, 44 of whom completed the study) compared intracavernosal self injections versus vacuum devices.[14] Outcome was assessed by a questionnaire to men and their partners after 15 uses for each device, and couples were followed for 18–24 months. There was no significant difference in the ability to achieve an erection suitable for intercourse. However, the ability to attain orgasm was significantly better with injection (P < 0.05). On a scale of 1 to 10, overall satisfaction was significantly better when using injections, both for men (6.5 v 5.4, P < 0.05) and partners (6.5 v 5.1, P < 0.05). Younger men (< 60 years), and those with shorter duration of erectile dysfunction (< 12 months), favoured injections (P < 0.05).

Harms: Penile pain was reported by half of the men in the study of efficacy and safety of alprostadil injection, and priapism (prolonged erection for > 4 hours) by 1%.[13] There was no significant difference in the frequency of adverse events between vacuum devices and injections.[14]

Comment: Most men can be taught to inject themselves using small gauge needles. In the RCT comparing injections and vacuum devices, 80% of the 44 couples who completed the study were still using one or other treatment after 18–24 months.[14]

OPTION   TOPICAL PROSTAGLANDIN E1

One small, single blind RCT found that topical prostaglandin E1 was significantly more effective than placebo, but sequential allocation of men to each group may mean that groups were not comparable.

Benefits: We found no systematic review. We found one single blind trial (48 men with erectile dysfunction owing to organic, psychogenic, or mixed causes) comparing topical prostaglandin E1 versus placebo.[15] Men were assigned in sequential order to either 0.5 mg, 1 mg, or 2.5 mg prostaglandin gel (36 men), or placebo (12 men). One dose of prostaglandin or placebo gel was applied to the glans and shaft of the penis and washed off after 3 hours. Significantly more men achieved an erection sufficient for intercourse with any dose of prostaglandin E1 versus placebo (25/36 [69%] with prostaglandin E1 v 2/12 [17%] with placebo; ARI 53%, 95% CI 13% to 76%; RR 4.2, 95% CI 1.8 to 5.5; NNT 2, 95% CI 1 to 8).

Harms: Men receiving prostaglandin were significantly more likely to have skin irritation than those on placebo (100% on 0.5 mg dose v 67%, no P value provided). Irritation was more severe with prostaglandin than with placebo (measured by mean irritation score ranging from 0–2; 1.75 with 0.5 mg dose v 0.67 with placebo, P < 0.0013).[15]

Comment: Allocation of men to each group was sequential and may mean that the groups were not comparable; the characteristics of each group were not reported. The study was too small to exclude a clinically important dose response effect.

OPTION   VACUUM DEVICES

Vacuum devices have not been adequately evaluated in RCTs. One small RCT found that they were as effective as intracavernosal prostaglandin E1 injections.

Benefits: We found no systematic review. **Versus intracavernosal injections:** See benefits of intracavernosal prostaglandin E1, p 609.

Harms: We found insufficient evidence.

Comment: Vacuum devices may be less popular than injections because only the distal portion of the penis becomes firm, but they are presumed to be safe.[14]

OPTION   PENILE PROSTHESES

Penile prostheses have not been formally evaluated in RCTs. They are usually considered only after less invasive treatments have failed.

Benefits: We found no RCTs. Anecdotal evidence suggests that patient satisfaction may be high, but we found no good studies.

Harms: One recent study found the morbidity of penile prostheses to be 9% (surgical revision 7%, mechanical failure 2.5%). Infection rates were between 2% and 7%.[16]

Comment: None.

REFERENCES

1. Feldman HA, Goldstein I, Dimitrios GH, Krane RJ, McKinlay JB. Impotence and its medical and psychosocial correlates: results of the Massachusetts male aging study. J Urol 1994; 151:54–61.
2. Ernst E, Pittler MH. Yohimbine for erectile dysfunction: a systemic review and meta-analysis of randomized clinical trials. J Urol 1998;159: 433–436. Search date 1997, primary sources Medline, Embase, Cochrane Library, Issue 4, 1999, and hand searched references.
3. Teloken C, Rhoden EL, Sogari P, Dambros M, Souto CA. Therapeutic effects of high dose yohimbine hydrochloride on organic erectile dysfunction. J Urol 1998;159:122–124.
4. Goldstein I, Lue TF, Harin PN, Rosen RC, Steers WD, Wicker PA, for the Sildenafil Study Group. Oral sildenafil in the treatment of erectile dysfunction. N Engl J Med 1998;338:1397–1404.
5. Montorsi F, McDermott PED, Morgan R, et al. Efficacy and safety of fixed dose oral sildenafil in the treatment of erectile dysfunction of various etiologies. Urology 1999;53:1011–1018.
6. Dinsmore WW, Hodges M, Hargreaves C, et al. Sildenafil citrate in erectile dysfunction: near normalization in men with broad spectrum erectile dysfunction compared with age-matched healthy control subjects. Urology 1999;53:800–805.
7. Rendell MS, Rajfer J, Wicker PA, Smith MD. Sildenafil for treatment of erectile dysfunction in men with diabetes: A randomized controlled trial. JAMA 1999;281:421–426.
8. Derry FA, Dinsmore WW, Fraser M, et al. Efficacy and safety of oral sildenafil in men with erectile dysfunction caused by spinal cord injury. Neurology 1998;51:1629–1633.
9. Morales A, Gingell C, Collins M, Wicker PA, Osterloh IH. Clinical safety of oral sildenafil citrate (Viagra) in the treatment of erectile dysfunction. Int J Impot Res 1998;10:69–74.
10. Chen J, Wollman Y, Chernichovsky T, et al: Effect of oral administration of high-dose nitric oxide donor L-Arginine in men with organic erectile dysfunction: results of a double-blind randomized placebo-controlled study. BJU Int 1999;83:269–273.
11. Costabile RA, Spevak M. Oral trazodone is not effective therapy for erectile dysfunction: a double blind placebo-controlled trial. J Urol 1999;161: 1819–1822.
12. Padma-Nathan H, Hellstrom WJ, Kaiser FE, et al, for the Medicated Urethral System for Erection (MUSE) Study Group. Treatment of men with erectile dysfunction with transurethral alprostadil. N Engl J Med 1997;336:1–7.
13. PGE1 Study Group. Prospective, multicenter trials of efficacy and safety of intracavernosal alprostadil (prostaglandin E1) sterile powder in men with erectile dysfunction. N Engl J Med 1996;334: 873–877.
14. Soderdahl DW, Thrasher JB, Hansberry KL, et al. Intracavernosal drug induced erection therapy vs external vacuum device in the treatment of erectile dysfunction. Br J Urol 1997;79:952–957.
15. McVary KT, Polepalle S, Riggi S, Pelham RW. Topical prostaglandin E1 SEPA gel for the treatment of erectile dysfunction. J Urol 1999; 162:726–730.
16. Goldstein I, Newman L, Baum N, et al. Safety and efficacy outcome of Mentor α 1 inflatable penile prosthesis implantation for impotence treatment. J Urol 1997;157:833–839.

Michael O'Leary
Associate Professor
Department of Surgery
Harvard Medical School
Boston, USA

Competing interests: The author has received honoraria from Pfizer for educational programmes on sildenafil, and has received research support to study this agent.

Search date September 2000

Matthew Smith, Philip Kantoff and James Talcott

INTERVENTIONS

Key Messages

In men with metastatic prostate cancer

- We found limited data from RCTs suggesting that androgen deprivation reduced mortality.

- One non-systematic review of RCTs has found that androgen deprivation initially improves symptoms and objective signs of disease in most men, but found no evidence of a difference between different methods of androgen deprivation (orchiectomy, diethylstilboestrol, luteinising hormone-releasing hormone [LHRH] agonists).

- In men with metastatic disease, one small RCT has found a survival benefit from immediate treatment versus deferring androgen deprivation until disease progression becomes apparent in men with stage D1 prostate cancer. Subgroup analysis from a larger RCT found a survival benefit from immediate treatment in men with stage C prostate cancer but not stage D. Without surveillance, deferred androgen deprivation resulted in higher rates of complications.

- One systematic review of RCTs found no overall benefit from adding androgen blockade to androgen deprivation versus androgen deprivation alone. However, it did find an additional benefit from combined androgen blockade if only RCTs using non-steroidal antiandrogens were considered.

- We found no trials evaluating the long term effects of intermittent androgen deprivation on mortality, morbidity, or quality of life.

In men with symptomatic androgen independent prostate cancer

- RCTs have found that chemotherapy has palliative benefit, but found no evidence that it prolongs survival.
- One systematic review of trials comparing different schedules of external beam radiation found that pain was reduced in some men. We found no comparison of external beam radiation with other palliative treatments.
- We found limited evidence suggesting that radionuclides with selective bone localisation decrease pain in some men.
- We found insufficient evidence to evaluate bisphosphonates.

DEFINITION	See non-metastatic prostate cancer, p 620. Androgen independent metastatic disease is defined as disease that progresses despite androgen deprivation.
INCIDENCE/ PREVALENCE	See non-metastatic prostate cancer, p 620.
AETIOLOGY/ RISK FACTORS	See non-metastatic prostate cancer, p 620.
PROGNOSIS	Prostate cancer metastasises predominantly to bone. Metastatic prostate cancer can result in pain, weakness, paralysis, and death.
AIMS	To prevent premature death and disability; control symptoms and maximise quality of life; and to minimise adverse effects of treatment.
OUTCOMES	Survival, response in terms of symptoms and signs, quality of life, adverse effects of treatment.
METHODS	*Clinical Evidence* update search and appraisal September 2000.

QUESTION What are the effects of treatment in men with metastatic prostate cancer?

OPTION ANDROGEN DEPRIVATION

We found limited evidence from RCTs suggesting that androgen deprivation reduces mortality in men with metastatic prostate cancer. One non-systematic review and one subsequent RCT have found that androgen deprivation initially improves symptoms and objective signs of disease in most men, but it found no evidence of a difference in effectiveness between different methods of androgen deprivation (orchiectomy, diethylstilboestrol, LHRH agonists).

Benefits: **Versus no initial treatment:** We found no systematic review and no recent RCTs. Three RCTs (about 4000 men with all stages of prostate cancer) performed between 1959 and 1975 compared androgen deprivation (diethylstilboestrol, orchiectomy, or oestrogens) versus no initial treatment. They found no difference in overall survival. Re-analysis of updated data from these RCTs found a modest survival advantage with androgen deprivation.[1] The report did not provide statistical details. **Different types of androgen deprivation:** We found one non-systematic review, which identified 25 RCTs comparing different types of androgen deprivation (orchiectomy, diethylstilboestrol, LHRH agonist) in men with meta-static disease.[2] Disease related symptoms and objective criteria, including radiographic findings and laboratory tests, improved in most men (symptomatic and objective response seen in 22–90% of people). There were no significant differences in response rates, time to progression, or survival. For all forms of androgen deprivation, duration of response was 12–18 months, and overall survival was 24–36 months. One large subsequent RCT (915 men) compared parenteral oestrogen versus total androgen ablation (orchiectomy or triptorelin). It found no significant difference in survival at follow up (mortality at 18 months median follow up; 266/458 [58.1%] with oestrogen v 269/457 [58.9%] with total androgen ablation).[3]

Harms: All forms of androgen deprivation are known to be associated with vasomotor flushing, loss of libido, gynaecomastia, weight gain, osteoporosis, and loss of muscle mass; we found insufficient prospective frequency data for these adverse effects. **Diethylstilboestrol** is associated with an increased risk of cardiovascular events, gastric irritation, and allergic reactions, and for these reasons is not routinely used. **Orchiectomy** has cosmetic and potential psychological consequences. **LHRH agonists** may cause an initial clinical flare owing to transient increases in androgen levels.

Comment: The high cardiovascular event rate with high dose diethylstilboestrol in the early RCTs[1] may have masked any survival benefit of androgen deprivation.

OPTION	IMMEDIATE VERSUS DEFERRED ANDROGEN DEPRIVATION

In men with metastatic disease, one small RCT has found a survival benefit from immediate treatment versus deferring androgen deprivation until disease progression becomes apparent in men with stage D1 prostate cancer. Subgroup analysis from a larger RCT found a survival benefit from immediate treatment in men with stage C prostate cancer but not stage D. However, without surveillance, deferred androgen deprivation resulted in higher rates of complications.

Benefits: We found no systematic review. We found two RCTs.[4,5] The first RCT in 938 men with stage C (locally advanced) and D (asymptomatic metastatic) prostate cancer (see table 1 in non-metastatic prostate cancer, p 620) compared immediate versus deferred androgen deprivation (orchiectomy or LHRH antagonist). Immediate androgen deprivation was initiated at diagnosis of prostate cancer; deferred androgen deprivation was initiated at the time of clinical disease progression. The RCTs had no formal surveillance requirements or criteria for starting androgen deprivation in the deferred treatment group.[4] It found no overall reduction in mortality. However, in the subgroup of men with stage C prostate cancer it found a reduction in mortality ($P = 0.02$) and disease related mortality with immediate treatment (62% of deaths were from prostate cancer compared with 71% in the deferred treatment arm, $P = 0.001$), but this was limited to men with stage C disease.[4] Immediate androgen deprivation therapy almost halved the risk of major complications such as pathological fractures (AR 2.3% with immediate treatment v 4.5% with deferred treatment), spinal cord compression (AR 1.9% v 4.9%), ureteric obstruction (AR 7% v 11.8%), and extraskeletal metastases (AR 7.9% v 11.8%). The report did not provide confidence intervals nor make clear the time interval over which outcomes were recorded, although this seemed to be at least 10 years. The second smaller RCT (98 men after radical prostatectomy and pelvic lymphadenectomy for nodal metastases) evaluated immediate androgen deprivation versus androgen deprivation deferred until disease progression.[5] It found that androgen deprivation therapy reduced mortality in the long term (median follow up 7.1 years, mortality 7/47 [14.9%] with antiandrogen v 18/51[35.3%] with watchful waiting, ARR 20.4%, P < 0.01), and resulted in a higher proportion of men with undetectable prostate specfic antigen (PSA) (see glossary, p 618) (P < 0.001).

Harms: The second RCT found that, compared with deferred androgen deprivation, immediate androgen deprivation caused more haemotological effects (15% v 4%), gastrointestinal effects (25% v 6%), non-specific genitourinary effects (48% v 12%), hot flushes (56% v 0%), and weight gain (18% v 2%).[5]

Comment: The high rate of complications in the deferred treatment group in the first RCT suggests that men with advanced prostate cancer in whom hormonal treatment is deferred require careful surveillance for disease progression. About 10% of men assigned to deferred hormonal treatment were not treated until they developed a pathological fracture or spinal cord compression.[6]

OPTION **COMBINED ANDROGEN BLOCKADE (ANDROGEN DEPRIVATION AND ANTIANDROGEN)**

One systematic review found no overall evidence of additional benefit from combined androgen blockade (androgen deprivation plus an antiandrogen) compared with androgen deprivation alone. However, it did find an additional benefit from combined androgen blockade if only RCTs using non-steroidal antiandrogens were considered.

Benefits: We found one recent systematic review (search date not stated), which identified 27 RCTs, 8215 men, most of whom had stage D2 disease (see table 1 in non-metastatic prostate cancer, p 620).[7] Individual patient data were obtained. Interventions were androgen deprivation (orchiectomy or LHRH agonist) with or without an antiandrogen. The review found no clear significant difference in 5 year survival among treatments (AR of dying within 5 years with androgen deprivation alone 76.4 v 74.6% with combined blockade; ARR 1.8%, P = 0.11). Seven of the 22 RCTs used cyproterone acetate, a steroidal antiandrogen with intrinsic androgenic activity and lower antiandrogenic activity than non-steroidal antiandrogens. Exclusion of these seven RCTs produced a significant reduction in mortality at 5 years (AR of dying with androgen deprivation alone 75.3% v 72.4% combined with non-steroidal antiandrogens, ARR 2.9%, P = 0.005).

Harms: The first RCT found that combined androgen blockade using flutamide, a non-steroidal antiandrogen, was associated with significantly higher rates of diarrhoea (6.3% v 2.7%, P = 0.002) and anaemia (8.5% v 5.4%, P = 0.024) than androgen deprivation alone.[4]

Comment: None.

OPTION   INTERMITTENT VERSUS CONTINUOUS ANDROGEN
          DEPRIVATION

We found insufficient evidence on the effects of intermittent androgen deprivation in men with metastatic prostate cancer.

Benefits: We found no systematic review and no RCTs evaluating the long term effects of intermittent androgen deprivation on mortality, morbidity, or quality of life.

Harms: Insufficient data.

Comment: None.

QUESTION   Are there any effective treatments for men with symptomatic androgen independent metastatic disease?

OPTION   CHEMOTHERAPY

RCTs have found that chemotherapy decreases pain and prolongs palliation in some men with symptomatic androgen independent prostate cancer. We found no evidence that chemotherapy prolongs survival.

Benefits: We found no systematic review. We found three RCTs, all using crossover designs, only one of which has been published in full. This RCT (161 men with symptomatic androgen independent metastatic prostate cancer) compared mitoxantrone plus prednisone versus prednisone alone.[8] It found that men receiving chemotherapy were more likely to experience pain reduction (29% with chemotherapy plus steroids v 12% with steroids alone, P = 0.01), enjoyed longer palliation (43 v 18 weeks, P < 0.0001), and showed improvements in quality of life. There was no significant difference in overall survival. Two other RCTs are published only in abstract form. One (242 men) compared mitoxantrone plus prednisone versus prednisone alone. Pain and analgesic use were reduced after chemotherapy.[9] The other RCT (458 men) compared suramin plus hydrocortisone versus hydrocortisone alone.[10] Chemotherapy improved pain and duration of palliation.

Harms: The RCTs reported no treatment related deaths. There were nine episodes of febrile neutropenia (World Health Organization [WHO] grade 3 or 4) among 130 men treated with 796 courses of mitoxantrone. Five men experienced cardiac arrhythmias or decreased left ventricular ejection fraction, including two who developed congestive heart failure.[8]

Comment: The crossover design of these RCTs precludes reliable conclusions about the effect of chemotherapy on survival, because men who died while in one arm of the study were not available for evaluation in the other.

OPTION   EXTERNAL BEAM RADIATION

One systematic review found no evidence of a difference in survival benefit between external beam radiation, strontium-89, or both treatments combined. However, strontium-89 seems to reduce the number of new pain sites. One systematic review of RCTs comparing different radiation schedules has found that external beam radiation provides effective pain relief in some men. We found no comparisons of external beam radiation with other palliative treatments.

Benefits: **Versus other palliative treatments:** We found no systematic reviews or RCTs. **Versus or as an adjunct to radionuclides:** We found one systematic review (search date not stated), which identified two RCTs in men with prostate cancer and symptomatic bone metastases.[11] The first (126 men who had received external beam radiation) compared strontium-89 versus placebo. It found no significant difference in median survival (27 v 34 weeks) or symptom relief (clinical response rate 80% v 60%). However, strontium-89 significantly reduced the number of new pain sites (P < 0.02), the requirement for analgesia (17% stopped taking analgesics with radionuclide v 2% on placebo, P < 0.05), and subsequent radiotherapy (median time to radiotherapy 35 weeks v 20 weeks on placebo, P = 0.06). The second RCT (305 men) compared external beam radiation versus strontium-89. Strontium-89 was associated with significantly fewer new sites of pain (P < 0.05), and reduced need for additional radiotherapy (P < 0.04). Effect on survival was not reported. **Different schedules and doses:** We found one systematic review (search date 1994, 9 RCTs, 1486 men with symptomatic bone metastases from a variety of malignancies). The trials compared different radiation treatment fractionation schedules and doses of external beam radiation.[12] There were minimal differences in effectiveness between different fractionation schedules and doses. External beam radiation produced greater than 50% pain relief in 42% of men and complete pain relief in 27%.

Harms: External beam radiation was associated with a 10% higher rate of gastrointestinal adverse effects.[11] Thrombocytopenia occurred twice as often with strontium-89 (6.9% v 3.4% with external beam radiation) and 3% of men receiving strontium-89 developed leukopenia.[11] There was no significant difference between treatment schedules and doses in rates of nausea, vomiting, or diarrhoea.[12]

Comment: The systematic review of different radiation treatment schedules provides no direct information on effectiveness of external beam radiation in men with bone metastasis, because all participants in the trials received radiation treatment.[12]

Prostate cancer: metastatic

OPTION   RADIONUCLIDE TREATMENT

We found limited evidence from one RCT that radionuclides with selective bone localisation may reduce pain in men with symptomatic bone metastases. One systematic review of RCTs found no difference in survival between radionuclides and external beam radiation, and no effect of radionuclides on survival. However, radionuclides seem to reduce the number of new pain sites.

Benefits: **Versus placebo:** We found no systematic review. We found one very small RCT (9 men with prostate cancer and symptomatic bone metastases) comparing rhenium-186 with placebo.[13] Treatment with rhenium-186 resulted in significantly better pain control than placebo (no RR or CI reported). **Versus or as an adjunct to external beam radiation:** See option, p 617.[11]

Harms: Strontium-89 resulted in thrombocytopenia (WHO grade 3 or 4) in 7–33% of men, and leukopenia (WHO grade 3 or 4) in 3–12%.[11,13] Other radionuclides with selective bone localisation have similar rates of haematological toxicity.

Comment: None.

OPTION   BISPHOSPHONATES

We found insufficient evidence on the effects of bisphosphonates in men with prostate cancer.

Benefits: We found one systematic review (search date not stated 2 RCTs, 156 men with prostate cancer and symptomatic bone metastases).[14] The trials found no significant reduction in bone pain with bisphosphonates. Both RCTs were flawed. One did not use a pain scale. The other evaluated etidronate, a bisphosphonate that is pharmacologically unsuitable for treating bone metastases.

Harms: The systematic review identified a total of 18 RCTs of bisphosphonates in men with bone metastases from a variety of cancers.[14] No RCT reported major toxicity. Treatment with pamidronate was associated with increased frequency of anterior uveitis and episcleritis.

Comment: None.

GLOSSARY

Prostate specific antigen (PSA) A protein released into the blood stream from the prostate, which can be measured by laboratory analysis of a blood sample. The level of PSA in the blood is increased in some forms of prostate cancer, as well as in some other abnormalities of the prostate.

Substantive changes since last issue

Combined androgen blockade New RCT;[7] conclusions unchanged.
Combined androgen blockade New systematic review;[7] it found a survival benefit with combined androgen blockade using non-steroidal antiandrogens.
Immediate versus deferred androgen deprivation New RCT;[3] it found a survival benefit with immediate androgen deprivation in men with stage D1 prostate cancer.

REFERENCES

1. Byar DP, Corle DK. Hormone therapy for prostate cancer: results of the Veterans Administration cooperative urologic research group studies. *NCI Monogr* 1988;7:165–170.

2. Robson M, Dawson N. How is androgen-dependent metastatic prostate cancer best treated? *Hematol Oncol Clin North Am* 1996;10:727–747. Search dates and primary sources not given.

3. Hedlund PO, Henriksson P. Parenteral estrogen versus total androgen ablation in the treatment of advanced prostate carcinoma: effects on overall survival and cardiovascular mortality. *Urology* 2000;55:328–332.

4. Eisenberger MA, Blumenstein BA, Crawford ED, et al. Bilateral orchiectomy with or without flutamide for metastatic prostate cancer. *N Engl J Med* 1998;339:1036–1042.

5. Messing EM, Manola J, Sarodsy M, Wilding G, Crawford ED, Trump D. Immediate hormonal therapy compared with observation after radical prostatectomy and pelvic lymphadenectomy in men with node-positive prostate cancer. *N Engl J Med* 1999;341:1781–1789.

6. Medical Research Council Prostate Cancer Working Party Investigators Group. Immediate versus deferred treatment for advanced prostatic cancer: initial results of the Medical Research Council trial. *Br J Urol* 1997;79:235–246.

7. Prostate Cancer Clinical Trialists' Collaborative Group. Maximum androgen blockade in advanced prostate cancer: an overview of the randomized trials. *Lancet* 2000;355:1491–1498. Search date not given; primary sources computerised literature search, proceedings of congresses, contacts with authors, trial groups, and pharmaceutical industry.

8. Tannock IF, Osoba D, Stockler MR, et al. Chemotherapy with mitoxantrone plus prednisone or prednisone alone for symptomatic hormone-resistant prostate cancer: a Canadian randomized trial with palliative end points. *J Clin Oncol* 1996;14:1756–1764.

9. Kantoff PW, Halabi S, Conaway M, et al. Hydrocortisone with or without mitoxantrone in men with hormone-refractory prostate cancer: results of the Cancer and Leukemia Group B 9182 Study. *J Clin Oncol* 1999;17:2506–2513.

10. Small EJ, Marshall E, Reyno L, et al. Superiority of suramin + hydrocortisone over placebo + hydrocortisone: results of a multicenter double-blind phase III study in patients with hormone refractory prostate cancer [abstract]. *Proc Am Soc Clin Oncol* 1998;17:1187.

11. McQuay HJ, Carroll D, Moore RA. Radiotherapy for painful bone metastases: a systematic review. *Clin Oncol (R Coll Radiol)* 1997;9:150–154. Search date not given; primary sources Medline 1966 to March 1996; The Oxford Pain Relief database 1950 to 1994; Embase; The Cochrane Library; and reference lists.

12. Robinson RG, Preston DF, Schiefelbein M, et al. Strontium 89 therapy for the palliation of pain due to osseous metastases. *JAMA* 1995;274:420–424. Search date December 1994; primary source Medline.

13. Maxon HR, Schroder LE, Hertzberg VS, et al. Rhenium-186(Sn)HEDP for treatment of painful osseous metastases: results of a double-blind crossover comparison with placebo. *J Nucl Med* 1991;32:1877–1881.

14. Bloomfield DJ. Should bisphosphonates be part of the standard therapy of patients with multiple myeloma or bone metastases from other cancers? An evidence-based review. *J Clin Oncol* 1998;16:1218–1225. Search date not given; primary sources Medline from 1976; hand search of major cancer journals; reference lists; and contact with experts.

Matthew Smith
Assistant Professor
Massachusetts General Hospital
Boston
USA

Philip Kantoff
Director
Lank Center for
Genitourinary Oncology
Dana Farber Cancer Institute
Boston
USA

James Talcott
Assistant Professor of Medicine
Harvard Medical School
Boston
USA

Competing interests: None declared.

Prostate cancer: non-metastatic

Search date May 2000

Timothy Wilt and Michael Brawer

QUESTIONS

INTERVENTIONS

Key Messages

In men with clinically localised disease

- We found no clear evidence for the superiority of any one treatment, including androgen deprivation. Limited evidence from one RCT suggests that radical prostatectomy may reduce recurrence compared with radiation treatment.

- Limited data from RCTs provide no evidence that radical prostatectomy or external beam radiation improve survival or reduce the risk of metastatic disease or need for palliative treatment compared with watchful waiting.

- We found no RCTs comparing external beam radiation, brachytherapy, and cryosurgery versus watchful waiting.

- We found no RCTs examining whether androgen deprivation should be offered to asymptomatic men in whom raised concentrations of prostate specific antigen (PSA) are detected after primary treatment or during watchful waiting.

In men with locally advanced disease

- We found limited evidence from RCTs suggesting that treatment with androgen deprivation from time of diagnosis (compared with deferral to disease progression) improves survival and reduces the risk of major complications.

- One RCT has found that immediate antiandrogen treatment after radical prostatectomy and pelvic lymphadenectomy reduces mortality compared with radical prostatectomy and deferred androgen suppression in men with node-positive prostate cancer and local node metastasis.

- One systematic review has found that adding androgen deprivation to radiation treatment improves survival compared with radiation alone. A subsequent RCT found no difference in overall survival or disease control after orchiectomy, whether or not it was combined with radiotherapy.

- We found no good evidence that radiation alone improves survival.

DEFINITION Prostatic cancer is staged according to two systems: the tumour, node, metastasis (TNM) classification system and the American Urologic Staging system (see table 1, p 629). Non-metastatic prostate cancer can be divided into clinically localised disease and advanced disease.

INCIDENCE/ PREVALENCE Prostate cancer is the most common non-dermatological malignancy worldwide and the second commonest cause of cancer death in men in the USA.[1] There were an estimated 180 400 new cases and 31 900 deaths in the USA in 2000.[2] For a 50 year old man with a life expectancy of 25 years, the lifetime risk of microscopic prostate cancer is about 42%, the risk of clinically evident prostate cancer is 10%, and that of fatal prostate cancer is 3%.[3]

AETIOLOGY/ RISK FACTORS Risk factors include age, family history of prostate cancer, black race, and possibly higher dietary fat and calcium intake.

PROGNOSIS The chance that men with well to moderately differentiated, palpable, clinically localised prostate cancer will remain free of symptomatic progression is 70% at 5 years and 40% at 10 years.[4] The risk of symptomatic disease progression is higher in men with poorly differentiated prostate cancer.[5] One retrospective analysis of a large surgical series in men with clinically localised prostate cancer found that the median time from the increase in PSA concentration to the development of metastatic disease was 8 years. Time to PSA progression, PSA doubling time, and Gleason score (see glossary, p 628) were predictive of the probability and time to development of metastatic disease. Once men developed metastatic disease, the median actuarial time to death was 5 years.[6] Morbidity from local or regional disease progression includes haematuria, bladder obstruction, and lower extremity oedema. In the USA, population based studies found that rates of death from prostate cancer have declined by only about 1/100 000 men since 1992, despite widespread testing for PSA and increased rates of radical prostatectomy and radiotherapy.[7,8] Regions of the USA with the greatest decreases in mortality are those with the lowest rates of testing for PSA and treatment with radical prostatectomy or radiation.[8] Countries with low rates of testing and treatment do not have consistently higher age adjusted rates of death from prostate cancer than countries with high rates of testing and treatment such as the USA.

AIMS To prevent premature death and disability while minimising adverse effects of treatment.

OUTCOMES Survival; time to progression; response in terms of symptoms and signs; quality of life; adverse effects of treatment. Where clinical outcomes are not available, surrogate outcome have been used (PSA concentration; Gleason score for histological grade).

METHODS We searched the Cochrane Library and Medline to May 2000 for systematic reviews and RCTs, using the search strategy of the Department of Veterans' Affairs Coordinating Centre for the Cochrane Review Group on Prostatic Diseases.

QUESTION What are the effects of treatment in men with clinically localised prostate cancer?

OPTION WATCHFUL WAITING

Limited data from RCTs suggest that watchful waiting provides similar length of life in men with clinically localised prostate cancer compared with other management strategies. We found no information from RCTs on quality of life.

Benefits: We found no recent systematic reviews, but found one overview that did not itemise the studies included (search date 1993, 165 articles),[1] and one non-systematic decision analysis (search date not stated, published in 1993).[9] We found two more recent, large cohort studies, which found that, in men managed with watchful waiting 15 years disease specific survival was 80%, ranging from 95% for well differentiated to 30% for poorly differentiated cancers.[10,11] **Versus early androgen deprivation:** We found no RCTs. **Versus radical prostatectomy:** See glossary, p 628. We found one RCT (see benefits of radical prostatectomy, below).[12]

Harms: Watchful waiting may avoid the risks of surgery but does not remove a cancer that is potentially curable that may progress to cause death and disability. However, we found insufficient evidence to comment on whether early intervention reduces the risk of disease specific death and disability compared with watchful waiting.

Comment: There is about a 10 year lead time between the detection of cancers by raised PSA concentrations and detection by digital rectal examination or the development of symptoms. This means that outcomes are likely to be similar in men with palpable tumours who are followed for 15 years and men whose tumours are detected because of raised PSA concentrations who are followed for 25 years (lead time bias).

OPTION RADICAL PROSTATECTOMY

Limited data from one RCT provided no evidence that radical prostatectomy may not improve survival compared with watchful waiting. Radical prostatectomy may reduce the risk of metastases compared with external beam radiation. Radical prostatectomy carries the risks of major surgery and of sexual and urinary dysfunction.

Benefits: We found no recent systematic reviews. **Versus watchful waiting:** One RCT compared radical prostatectomy versus watchful waiting in 142 men with clinically localised prostate cancer. After a median follow up of 23 years (range 19–27 years), it found no difference in survival between the two groups (median survival 10.6 years with prostatectomy v 8 years with watchful waiting, no 95% CI quoted).[12] **Versus external beam radiation:** One RCT compared radical prostatectomy versus external beam radiation in 97 men with clinically localised prostate cancer. Men receiving radiation had an increased risk of metastases (4 "treatment failures" with prostatectomy v 17 with radiation).[13]

Harms: Fatal complications have been reported in 0.5–1% of men treated with radical prostatectomy and may exceed 2% in men aged 75 years and older.[14] Nearly 8% of men older than 65 years suffered major cardiopulmonary complications within 30 days of operation. The incidence of other adverse effects of surgery was over 80% for sexual dysfunction, 30% for urinary incontinence requiring pads or clamps to control wetness, 18% for urethral stricture, 3% for total urinary incontinence, 5% for faecal incontinence, and 1% for bowel injury requiring surgical repair.[1,15–17]

Comment: Both RCTs of radical prostatectomy took place before the advent of tests for PSA and were too small to rule out a clinically important difference between groups. Radical prostatectomy may benefit selected groups of men with localised prostate cancer, particularly younger men with higher grade tumours, but the studies did not look for this effect. The available data suggest that in most men the benefits in quality adjusted life expectancy are at best small and sensitive to patients' preferences.[9] No differences have been found in the general health related quality of life among non-randomised groups treated with radical prostatectomy, radiation, or watchful waiting.[18] Two ongoing trials are comparing radical prostatectomy versus watchful waiting.[19,20]

OPTION   EXTERNAL BEAM RADIATION

We found limited evidence from one small RCT that, compared with radical prostatectomy, external beam radiation increased the risk of metastases in men with clinically localised prostate cancer. External beam radiation has not been compared directly with watchful waiting. One RCT found that conformal radiation therapy (see glossary, p 628) reduces rates of radiation proctitis and rectal bleeding compared with conventional radiotherapy. We found no evidence of a difference in survival between conventional and conformal radiation therapy.

Benefits: **Versus watchful waiting:** We found no RCTs. **Versus radical prostatectomy:** We found one RCT (see benefits of radical prostatectomy above).[13] **Conformal versus conventional radiotherapy:** One RCT in 225 men with non-metastatic prostate cancer (T1–T4, N0 or M0) compared conformal versus conventional radiotherapy.[21] Primary outcomes were adverse effects (see harms below). It did not report on survival, but found no significant difference in tumour control (by PSA level) between treatments after a median follow up of 3.6 years.

Harms: The RCT of radiotherapy versus radical prostatectomy made no mention of adverse effects.[13] One survey of men treated with external beam radiation reported that 7% wore pads to control wetness, 23–32% were impotent, and 10% reported problems with bowel dysfunction.[22] Treatment related mortality was less than 0.5%.[1] External beam radiation requires that men return for daily outpatient treatment for up to 6 weeks. **Conventional versus conformal radiotherapy:** The RCT found that significantly fewer men treated with conformal radiation developed radiation induced proctitis and rectal bleeding. It found no differences between groups for adverse effects on the bladder.[21]

Comment: Up to 30% of men with clinically localised prostate cancer treated with radiotherapy still have positive biopsies 2–3 years after treatment.[23] One retrospective, non-randomised, multicentre pooled analysis found 5 year estimates of overall survival, disease specific survival, and freedom from biochemical failure (as defined by raised PSA) to be 85%, 95%, and 66%. Estimated 5 year rates of no biochemical recurrence according to PSA concentrations before treatment and Gleason histological scores ranged from 81% for pretreatment PSA < 10 ng/ml to 29% for PSA ≥ 20 ng/ml, and a Gleason score from 7 to 10.[24]

OPTION	BRACHYTHERAPY

One systematic review found no direct evidence from RCTs that brachytherapy (see glossary, p 628) improves length or quality of life in men with clinically localised prostate cancer.

Benefits: We found one systematic review (published in 1997), which identified no RCTs comparing brachytherapy alone or in combination with other treatments (androgen deprivation or radiation).[25]

Harms: Complications reported in case series include urinary retention (6–8%), incontinence (13–18%), cystitis/urethritis (4–7%), proctitis (6–14%), and impotence (6–50%).[26] Long term outcomes from a representative national sampling of men have not been reported.

Comment: One retrospective cohort study (1872 men) found that in low risk men (see table 1, p 629) (stage T1c, stage T2a, PSA concentration ≤ 10 ng/ml, and Gleason score ≤ 6) the chance of a high PSA concentration at 5 years was similar whether they were treated with radiation or brachytherapy implant (with or without preceding androgen deprivation) or with radical prostatectomy. Men at intermediate or high risk (Gleason score > 6 or PSA > 10 ng/ml) were more likely to have high PSA concentration at 5 years with brachytherapy than with radical prostatectomy (RR of high PSA in men at intermediate risk 3.1, 95% CI 1.5 to 6.1; RR in men at high risk 3.0, 95% CI 1.8 to 5.0).[27] The study used proxy outcomes (PSA concentrations) rather than clinical outcomes. RCTs comparing brachytherapy versus radical prostatectomy are planned.

OPTION	CRYOSURGERY

We found no direct evidence from RCTs that cryosurgery improves length or quality of life in men with clinically localised prostate cancer.

Benefits: We found no systematic review or RCTs.

Harms: Complications reported in case series include impotence (65%), transient scrotal oedema (10%), sloughed urethral tissue (3%), urethral stricture (1%), incontinence, urethrorectal fistula, and prostatic abscess (1%).[28]

Comment: One ongoing trial is comparing cryosurgery with radiation.

OPTION	ANDROGEN DEPRIVATION

We found no direct evidence from RCTs that primary treatment with early androgen deprivation in the absence of symptoms improves length or quality of life in men with clinically localised prostate cancer.

Benefits: We found no systematic review or RCTs.

Harms: See harms of androgen deprivation for the treatment of men with locally advanced prostate cancer, p 626.

Comment: None.

QUESTION	In men who have received primary treatment and remain asymptomatic, should androgen deprivation be offered when raised concentrations of PSA are detected?

We found insufficient evidence on the effects of initiating androgen suppression when PSA rises or persists after primary treatment.

Benefits: We found one systematic review, which identified no RCTs.[29]

Harms: See harms of androgen deprivation for the treatment of men with locally advanced prostate cancer, p 626.

Comment: In the USA, clinicians often monitor blood concentrations of PSA and offer androgen suppression when these rise. Consequently, more men with persistent disease are considered for androgen suppression and treatment initiated earlier in the natural course of the disease. RCTs are needed to evaluate the effectiveness of this approach and of intermittent treatment, where androgen suppression is initiated when PSA rises after primary treatment and discontinued when the antigen concentrations return to nadir.[29]

QUESTION	What are the effects of treatment in men with locally advanced prostate cancer?

OPTION	ANDROGEN DEPRIVATION

RCTs have found limited evidence that, in men with locally advanced disease, androgen deprivation initiated at diagnosis reduces complications and may improve survival.

Benefits: **Versus no initial treatment:** We found no recent RCTs. Three RCTs performed between 1960 and 1975 compared androgen deprivation (stilboestrol, orchiectomy, or oestrogens) versus no initial treatment in about 4000 men with all stages of prostate cancer. They found no difference in overall survival. Reanalysis of updated data from these RCTs provided tentative evidence of a modest survival advantage with androgen deprivation.[30] **Immediate (initiated at diagnosis) versus deferred androgen deprivation:** We found one systematic review, which identified three RCTs (n = 2143), two of which were conducted in the 1960s.[29] None had a uniform protocol for initiating deferred treatment, so deferred treatment in these trials reflects the varied practices of the treating clinicians. Men in the deferred hormonal therapy group were not closely monitored with PSA testing. The systematic review found no significant survival difference at 5 years between immediate compared with deferred androgen deprivation (HR 0.91, 95% CI 0.81 to 1.03).[30] The more recent trial, which included 938 men with stage C (locally advanced) and D (asymptomatic metastatic) disease, reported a survival benefit from immediate treatment (62% of deaths were from prostate cancer compared with 71% in the deferred treatment arm, P < 0.001). The survival benefit was limited to men with stage C disease.[31] Immediate androgen deprivation almost halved the risk of major complications, such as pathological fractures (AR 2.3% v 4.5% with deferred treatment), spinal cord compression (AR 1.9% v 4.9%), ureteric obstruction (AR 7% v 11.8%), and extraskeletal metastases (AR 7.9% v 11.8%). The report did not quote CIs, nor make clear the time interval over which outcomes were recorded, though this seemed to be at least 10 years. The lower incidence of complications was more apparent in men presenting with stage C disease.

Harms: Adverse events were not well reported in the review. Earlier initiation of androgen deprivation means longer exposure to adverse effects, which include osteoporosis, weight gain, hot flushes (10–60%), loss of muscle mass, gynaecomastia (5–10%), impotence (10–30%), and loss of libido (5–30%).[29] These adverse effects are particularly important in the treatment of men with long life expectancy or younger men with lower grade cancers.

Comment: The RCTs conducted in the 1960s[29] included men who were older and had more advanced cancers than those in the more recent RCT.[31] RCTs are needed to evaluate the effectiveness of androgen deprivation before surgery when disease extends beyond the capsule.

| OPTION | EXTERNAL BEAM RADIATION IN ADDITION TO ANDROGEN DEPRIVATION |

Androgen deprivation improves survival in men with locally advanced disease treated with radiotherapy. One RCT found no difference in overall survival or local disease control after orchiectomy, whether or not it was combined with radiotherapy.

Benefits: **External beam radiation versus or in addition to androgen deprivation:** We found one systematic review,[29] and one additional RCT.[32] The review (4 RCTs, 1565 men) compared early versus deferred androgen deprivation in men receiving external beam radiation.[29] Early androgen deprivation was initiated at the same time as radiation treatment for locally advanced, or asymptomatic but clinically evident metastatic prostate cancer, and continued until the development of hormone refractory disease. The deferred group received radiation treatment alone, with androgen deprivation initiated only in those in whom the disease progressed. The systematic review found that early androgen deprivation improved overall 5 year survival compared with deferred treatment (percentage surviving at 5 years 76.5% v 68.2%; ARR 8.3%; HR 0.63, 95% CI 0.48 to 0.83; NNT at 5 years 12).[29] The additional RCT compared orchiectomy alone versus radiotherapy alone, versus radiotherapy in addition to orchiectomy in 277 men with advanced localised prostate cancer (T2–T4, M0, with and without nodal disease).[32] It found no significant differences between the three treatment groups for overall survival or need for further treatment for local disease progression (data presented as a diagram, no P value given).

Harms: The review reported adverse effects of androgen deprivation.[29] In the additional RCT, adverse effects attributable to radiotherapy included bowel symptoms (19%), urinary symptoms excluding transient frequency (8%), bowel and urinary complications (1%), rectal bleeding necessitating blood transfusion (2%), and radiation proctitis (1%), which was a contributory factor in the two patients that died. After orchiectomy, hot flushes (15%) were the predominant adverse effect.

Comment: We found no evidence from RCTs about the effectiveness of external beam radiation alone versus no treatment in men with locally advanced prostate cancer.

OPTION   **ANDROGEN DEPRIVATION PLUS RADICAL PROSTATECTOMY AND PELVIC LYMPHADENECTOMY**

One RCT has found that immediate androgen deprivation after radical prostatectomy and pelvic lymphadenectomy improves survival and reduces the risk of recurrence in men with node-positive prostate cancer compared with radical prostatectomy, pelvic lymphadenectomy, and deferred androgen deprivation.

Benefits: **Radical prostatectomy and pelvic lymphadenectomy plus androgen deprivation:** We found one RCT (98 men after radical prostatectomy and pelvic lymphadenectomy for nodal metastases) of immediate androgen deprivation (with either goserelin or bilateral orchiectomy) versus androgen deprivation deferred until disease progression.[33] It found that antiandrogens decreased mortality in the long term (median follow up 7.1 years, mortality 7/47 [14.9%] with antiandrogen v 18/51 [35.3%] with watchful waiting, ARR 20.4%, P < 0.01) and resulted in a higher proportion of men with undetectable PSA (P < 0.001).

Harms: The RCT found that, compared with deferred androgen deprivation, immediate androgen deprivation caused more haematological effects (15% v 4%), gastrointestinal effects (25% v 6%), non-specific genitourinary effects (48% v 12%), hot flushes (56% v 0%), and weight gain (18% v 2%).

Comment: None.

Prostate cancer: non-metastatic

GLOSSARY

Brachytherapy Radiotherapy, where the source of ionising radiation is applied by permanently inserting many radioactive implants directly into the prostate gland.

Conformal radiation therapy 3D radiotherapy planning systems and methods to match the radiation treatment to irregular tumour volumes.

Gleason score A number from 1–10 with 1 being the most well differentiated and 10 being the most poorly differentiated.

Radical prostatectomy Surgical removal of the prostate with its capsule, seminal vesicles, ductus deferens, some pelvic fasciae, and sometimes pelvic lymph nodes; performed via either the retropubic or the perineal route.

REFERENCES

1. Middleton RG, Thompson IM, Austenfeld MS, et al. Prostate cancer clinical guidelines panel summary report on the management of clinically localized prostate cancer. *J Urol* 1995;154:2144–2148. Search date December 1993; primary source Medline 1966 to December 1993.
2. Landis SH, Murray T, Bolden S, et al. Cancer statistics. *CA Cancer J Clin* 2000;50:12–13.
3. Whitmore WF. Localized prostatic cancer: management and detection issues. *Lancet* 1994; 343:1263–1267.
4. Adolfsson J, Steineck G, Hedund P. Deferred treatment of clinically localized low-grade prostate cancer: actual 10-year and projected 15-year follow-up of the Karolinska series. *Urology* 1997; 50:722–726.
5. Johansson J-E, Holmberg L, Johansson S, et al. Fifteen-year survival in prostate cancer: prospective, population-based study in Sweden. *JAMA* 1997;277:467–471.
6. Pound CR, Partin AW, Eisenberger MA, et al. Natural history of progression after PSA elevation following radical prostatectomy. *JAMA* 1999;281: 1591–1597.
7. Brawley OW. Prostate carcinoma incidence and patient mortality. *Cancer* 1997;80:1857–1863.
8. Wingo PA, Ries LAG, Rosenberg HM, et al. Cancer incidence and mortality, 1973–1995. *Cancer* 1998;82:1197–1207.
9. Fleming C, Wasson J, Albertsen PC, et al. A decision analysis of alternative strategies for clinically localized prostate cancer. *JAMA* 1993; 269:2650–2658.
10. Albertsen PC, Hanley JA, Gleason DF, Barry MJ. Competing risk analysis of men aged 55 to 74 years at diagnosis managed conservatively for clinically localized prostate cancer. *JAMA* 1998; 280:975–980.
11. Lu-Yao GL, Yao S. Population-based study of long-term survival in patients with clinically localised prostate cancer. *Lancet* 1997;349:906–910.
12. Iversen P, Madsen PO, Corle DK. Radical prostatectomy versus expectant treatment for early carcinoma of the prostate: 23 year follow-up of a prospective randomized study. *Scand J Urol Nephrol Suppl* 1995;172(suppl):65–72.
13. Paulsen DF, Lin GH, Hinshaw W, et al. The uro-oncology group: radical surgery versus radiotherapy for adenocarcinoma of the prostate. *J Urol* 1982;128:502–504.
14. Lu-Yao GL, McLerran D, Wasson JH. An assessment of radical prostatectomy: time trends, geographic variation, and outcomes. *JAMA* 1993; 269:2633–2636.
15. Anonymous. Screening for prostate cancer. *Ann Intern Med* 1997;126:480–484.
16. Fowler FJ, Barry MJ, Lu-Yao G, et al. Patient-reported complications and follow-up treatment after radical prostatectomy: the national Medicare experience 1988–1990 (updated June 1993).

17. Bishoff JT, Motley G, Optenberg SA, et al. Incidence of fecal and urinary incontinence following radical perineal and retropubic prostatectomy in a national population. *J Urol* 1998;160:454–458.
18. Litwin MS, Hays RD, Fink A, et al. Quality-of-life outcomes in men treated for localized prostate cancer. *JAMA* 1995;273:129–135.
19. Wilt TJ, Brawer MK. The prostate cancer intervention versus observation trial. *Oncology* 1997;11:1133–1139.
20. Norlen BJ. Swedish randomized trial of radical prostatectomy versus watchful waiting. *Can J Oncol* 1994;4(suppl 1):38–42.
21. Dearnaley DP, Khoo VS, Norman AR, et al. Comparison of radiation side-effects of conformal and conventional radiotherapy in prostate cancer: a randomized trial. *Lancet* 1999;353:267–272.
22. Fowler FJ, Barry MJ, Lu-Yao G, et al. Outcomes of external beam radiation therapy for prostate cancer: a study of Medicare beneficiaries in three surveillance, epidemiology, and end results areas. *J Clin Oncol* 1996;14:2258–2265.
23. Crook J, Perry G, Robertson S, Esche B. Routine prostate biopsies: results for 225 patients. *Urology* 1995;45:624–632.
24. Shipley WU, Thames HD, Sandler HM, et al. Radiation therapy for clinically localized prostate cancer. A multi-institutional pooled analysis. *JAMA* 1999;281:1598–1604.
25. Brachytherapy for prostate cancer. Tec assessment program. *Blue Cross Blue Shield Assoc* 1997;12:1–27. Primary sources Medline; 1980–May 1997; Current Contents; bibliographies; and abstracts of proceedings of scientific meetings. Talcott JA, Clark JC, Stark P, Nadir B, Ragde N. Long term complications of brachytherapy for early prostate cancer: A survey of treated patients. American Society of Clinical Oncology Annual Meeting 1999; Abstract 1196.
26. D'Amico AV, Whittington R, Malkowicz SB, et al. Biochemical outcome after radical prostatectomy, external beam radiation therapy, or interstitial radiation therapy for clinically localized prostate cancer. *JAMA* 1998;280:969–974.
27. Talcott JA, Clark JC, Stark P, Nadir B, Ragde N. long term complications of brachytherapy for early prostate cancer. A survey of treated patients. American Society of Clinical Oncology Annual Meeting 1999; Abstract 1196.
28. Littrup PJ, Mody A, Sparschu RA. Prostate cryosurgery complications. *Semin Int Radiol* 1994; 11:226–230.
29. Agency for Health Care Policy and Research. Relative effectiveness and cost-effectiveness of methods of androgen suppression in the treatment of advanced prostatic cancer. Summary. Rockville, MD: Agency for Health Care Policy and Research, 1999. (Evidence Report/Technology

Assessment: No 4.) http://www.ahcpr.gov/clinic/prossumm.htm. Search date 1998; primary sources Medline; Cancerlit; Embase; Current Contents on Diskette, and Cochrane Library.

30. Byar DP, Corle DK. Hormone treatment for prostate cancer: results of the Veterans' Administration cooperative urologic research group studies. *NCI Monograph* 1988;7:165–170.

31. The Medical Research Council Prostate Cancer Working Party Investigators Group. Immediate versus deferred treatment for advanced prostatic cancer: initial results of the Medical Research Council trial. *Br J Urol* 1997;79:235–246.

32. Fellows GJ, Clark PB, Beynon, LL, et al. Treatment of advanced localised prostatic cancer by orchiectomy, radiotherapy, or combined treatment. *Br J Urol* 1992:70;304–309.

33. Messing EM, Manola J, Sarodsy M, Wilding G, Crawford ED, Trump D. Immediate hormonal therapy compared with observation after radical prostatectomy and pelvic lymphadenectomy in men with node-positive prostate cancer. *N Engl J Med* 1999;341:1781–1789.

Timothy Wilt
Associate Professor of Medicine
VA Coordinating Center for the
Cochrane Review Group in Prostate
Diseases and Urologic Malignancies
Center for Chronic Diseases Outcomes
Research Minneapolis VA Hospital
Minneapolis
USA

Michael Brawer
Director
Northwest Prostate Institute
Seattle
USA

Competing interests: None declared.

TABLE 1	Prostatic cancer staging systems (see text, p 621).

Tumour, node, metastasis (TNM) classification system

Tumour

T0	Clinically unsuspected
T1	Clinically inapparent (not palpable or visible by imaging)
T2	Tumour confined within prostate
T3	Tumour outside capsule or extension into vesicle
T4	Tumour fixed to other tissue

Nodes

N0	No evidence of involvement of regional nodes
N1	Involvement of regional node

Metastases

M0	No evidence of distant metastases
M1	Evidence of distant metastases

American urologic staging system

Stage A	No palpable tumour
Stage B	Tumour confined to the prostate gland
Stage C	Extracapsular extension
Stage D	Metastatic prostate cancer
Stage D1	Pelvic lymph node metastases
Stage D2	Distant metastases

Alzheimer's disease

Search date September 2000: expanded this issue

James Warner and Rob Butler

QUESTIONS

INTERVENTIONS

Key Messages

- Most RCTs used proxy outcome measures, such as cognitive function, rather than clinical outcomes likely to be important to people with Alzheimer's disease and their carers, such as quality of life.
- Systematic reviews of RCTs have found:
  - Improved cognitive function and global clinical state with donepezil 10 mg versus placebo. Treatment is well tolerated.
  - Limited evidence that tacrine improves cognitive function or behaviour. In trials, tacrine is associated with hepatotoxicity.
  - Improved cognitive function but frequent nausea with rivastigmine 6–12 mg.
  - Reduced anxiety with short term thioridazine, but no evidence of an effect on clinical global state and a suggestion of rare but serious cardiac arrhythmias.
  - Risperidone reduces psychotic symptoms and aggression in people with dementia.
  - No evidence of benefit from oestrogen (in women).
  - Selegiline versus placebo improves cognitive function, behaviour, and mood but no evidence of an effect on clinical global state. Selegiline is well tolerated with no serious adverse events.
  - No evidence of benefit from vitamin E.
  - No evidence about aspirin in people with vascular dementia.
  - Ginkgo biloba improves cognitive function and is well tolerated.
  - Insufficient evidence about reminisence therapy.

- Reality orientation versus no treatment improves cognitive function.
- Weak evidence that music therapy may be beneficial in people with dementia.
- Two RCTs have found that galantamine is associated with improved cognition.
- One small RCT found no benefit from diclofenac versus placebo.
- We found no long term evidence about the effects of any treatment on the progression of Alzheimers disease.

DEFINITION	**Dementia** is characterised by global non-reversible impairment of cerebral function with preservation of clear consciousness. It usually results in loss of memory (initially of recent events), loss of executive function (such as the ability to make decisions or sequence complex tasks), and changes in personality. **Alzheimer's disease** is characterised by an insidious onset and slow deterioration, and may be diagnosed after other systemic and neurological causes of dementia have been excluded clinically and by laboratory investigation.
INCIDENCE/ PREVALENCE	About 5% of people aged over 65 years and 20% of people aged over 80 years have some form of dementia.[1] Dementia is rare before the age of 60 years. The most common type of dementia is Alzheimer's disease, accounting for about 60% of cases in the UK.[2] The rest comprise mainly vascular dementia, mixed vascular and Alzheimer's disease, and cortical Lewy body dementia.[3]
AETIOLOGY/ RISK FACTORS	The cause of Alzheimer's disease is unclear. A key pathological process is deposition of abnormal amyloid in the central nervous system.[4] Most people with the relatively rare condition of early onset dementia (before age 60) show autosomal dominance. Later onset dementia is sometimes clustered in families. Vascular dementia is related to cardiovascular risk factors, such as smoking, hypertension, and diabetes.
PROGNOSIS	Alzheimer's disease usually has an insidious onset when it can be difficult to diagnose. There is progressive reduction in cerebral function, with an average life expectancy after diagnosis of 7–10 years.[3] Behavioural problems, depression, and psychosis occur in most people at some stage.[5,6] Eventually, most people with dementia find it difficult to perform simple tasks without help.
AIMS	To improve cognitive function (memory, orientation, attention, and concentration); to reduce behavioural and psychological symptoms (wandering, aggression, anxiety, depression, psychosis); to improve quality of life, with minimum adverse effects.
OUTCOMES	Quality of life both of the person with dementia and their carer (rarely used in clinical trials). Comprehensive scales of cognitive function such as the Alzheimer's disease assessment scale cognitive subscale (ADAS-cog, where lower scores signify improving function)[7] are more sensitive than briefer scales such as the Mini Mental State Examination (MMSE),[8] but both are proxy measures that may not reflect outcomes important to people with dementia or their careers. A seven point change in the ADAS-cog may be regarded as clinically important. Overall condition is reflected in scales such as global clinical state. One measure of global state is the clinician interview-based impression of change with caregiver

input (CIBIC-Plus) scale. Psychiatric symptoms are assessed using scales such as the dementia mood assessment scale (DMAS), the brief psychiatric rating scale (BPRS) (both of which use lower scores to signify improved symptoms), and the Behave-AD scale. Other outcomes include time to institutionalisation or death.

METHODS   *Clinical Evidence* update search and appraisal September 2000.

QUESTION   What are the effects of drug treatments?

OPTION   CHOLINESTERASE INHIBITORS

One systematic review of RCTs has found evidence that donepezil is well tolerated and is better than placebo in improving cognitive function and global clinical state. One systematic review of RCTs has found no evidence of benefit from tacrine in terms of improved cognitive function or behaviour. Tacrine has also been associated with hepatotoxicity. One systematic review has found that rivastigmine is associated with improved cognitive function in older people with Alzheimer's disease but that nausea was common. We found no evidence that any of the drugs significantly improved quality of life. Two RCTs have found that galantamine (a cholinesterase inhibitor with nicotinic agonist properties) is associated with improved cognition and functioning in older people with Alzheimer's disease.

Benefits: **Donepezil:** We found one systematic review of donepezil (search date 2000, 8 RCTs of 12, 24, and 52 weeks duration, 2264 people with mild or moderate Alzheimer's disease)[9] and one subsequent RCT.[10] Five studies reported results using the ADAS-cog; three of 12 weeks duration and two were 24 week studies. The review found that, over 12 or 24 weeks, donepezil improved cognitive function, measured by the ADAS-cog score (see table 1, p 641) and significantly improved global clinical state (OR 0.47, 95% CI 0.33 to 0.67 for 10 mg donepezil for 24 weeks). It found no evidence of an effect on quality of life. The first RCT (24 weeks, double blind, 473 people with mild to moderate Alzheimer's disease) compared 10 mg donezepil versus placebo. It found that for a four point improvement in ADAS-cog the number needed to treat was 4, and for a seven point improvement in ADAS-cog the number needed to treat was 6.[14] The subsequent RCT (818 people with Alzheimer's disease, 30 weeks) compared donepezil 10 mg versus donepezil 5 mg versus placebo. It found improved global state with both donepezil treatments (NNT 10, 95% CI 6 to 25 with donepezil 10 mg *v* placebo for a 3 point improvement in CIBIC score). It found no evidence of any effect on quality of life.[10] **Tacrine:** We found one systematic review (search date 1998, 5 RCTs, 1434 people) comparing tacrine versus placebo.[15] Various dosages of tacrine were given for 1–39 weeks. The review found no significant difference in overall clinical improvement (OR 0.87, 95% CI 0.61 to 1.23), a significant (but probably clinically unimportant) improvement in cognition (WMD in ADAS-cog −0.22, 95% CI −0.32 to −0.12), and no significant difference in MMSE (SMD 0.14, 95% CI −0.02 to +0.3). It found no evidence of improved behaviour (SMD in behavioural disturbance on the non-cognitive subscale of ADAS −0.04, 95% CI −0.52 to +0.43). **Rivastigmine:** We found one systematic review (search date 2000, 7 RCTs).[11] The review found that rivastigmine (6–12 mg) versus placebo improved ADAS-cog (1917 people, for a 4 point change in the ADAS-cog; NNT 17, 95% CI 12 to 34). It found no significant difference between 1–4 mg rivastigmine and placebo. **Galantamine:** We found no systematic review but found two multicentre RCTs.[12,13] One RCT (636 people with probable Alzheimer's disease) compared galantamine (24 or 32 mg/day for 24 weeks) versus placebo.[13] The second RCT (978 people with probable Alzheimer's disease) compared galantamine (6, 16, or 24 mg/day for 20 weeks) versus placebo.[12] Both RCTs found that galantamine versus placebo significantly improves ADAS-cog scores (see table 1, p 641).

Harms: **Donepezil:** Donepezil was well tolerated in the RCTs. Common adverse effects were mild and transient nausea, vomiting, and diarrhoea. Hepatotoxicity was reported as non-significant. More people withdrew with donepezil 10 mg than with placebo.[9] **Tacrine:** Inconsistencies in reporting make it hard to give an overall withdrawal figure. Withdrawals were common (for 2 studies, 812 people, OR for withdrawal 5.7, 95% CI 4.1 to 7.9). Withdrawals were more likely at higher doses. In one high dose study, 72% of people taking tacrine 160 mg withdrew, and reversible hepatotoxicity was reported in about 50%.[16] Diarrhoea, anorexia, and abdominal pain were common. **Rivastigmine:** Commonly reported adverse effects with rivastigmine were nausea (50%), vomiting (34%), dizziness (20%), headache (19%), and diarrhoea (17%).[15] **Galantamine:** Adverse effects of galantamine were infrequent in two RCTs.[12,13] Common adverse effects were nausea (44% with higher dose galantamine v 13% with placebo) and vomiting (20% v 8%). Discontinuations because of adverse events occurred in 32% with 32 mg galantamine, 23% with 24 mg galantamine, and 13% with placebo.[13]

Comment: The trials all used proxy outcomes (cognitive scores) rather than outcomes likely to be important to people with Alzheimer's disease and their carers. All trials of donepezil used reliable methods, but participants were highly selected and may not be representative. Quality of life of carers was not assessed.[9] The quality of tacrine trials was generally poor. The longest RCT lasted 30 weeks[16] and doses varied considerably among trials. Rivastigmine is the only cholinesterase inhibitor we found to have been studied in a routine clinical (pragmatic) setting,[17] although the NNT was higher than that for donepezil. A significant issue with dementia trials is the way missing data are managed. Many trials show much higher dropout rates (30% or more) at doses where the drug is effective than in the placebo arm. In these studies, missing data are often managed using "last observation carried forward". In people with dementia, the likely trend over the course of the trial will be to get worse. If people drop out of the trial, relatively better scores are carried forward to end point than if the person completed. If more people drop out of the intervention arm, an artificially better score, compared with the placebo arm, will result. There are only two RCTs evaluating galantamine but they suggest it has a similar efficacy to donepezil.

| OPTION | THIORIDAZINE |

One systematic review has found that short term treatment with thioridazine reduces anxiety but found no evidence of an effect on clinical global state. We found only limited data on adverse effects. Recent observational evidence suggests thioridazine is associated with cardiotoxicity and should be used with caution in the elderly.

Benefits: We found one systematic review (search date not stated, 7 RCTs).[18] Six RCTs lasted 3–4 weeks and one lasted 8 weeks. Of the seven RCTs, two were placebo controlled.[18] The review found that thioridazine reduced symptoms of anxiety (v placebo OR 4.91, 95% CI 3.12 to 7.50; v diazepam OR 1.8, 95% CI 1.04 to 3.10) but did not significantly affect clinical global state (v placebo OR 1.58, 95% CI 0.42 to 5.96).

Harms: The RCTs included in the review did not report harms systematically.[18] Adverse effects were no more common with thioridazine than with placebo (OR 0.41, 95% CI 0.09 to 1.86) or diazepam (OR 0.84, 95% CI 0.25 to 2.82). One RCT included in the review (60 people) found that people taking thioridazine were significantly less alert than people taking chlormethiazole (OR for alertness 0.31, 95% CI 0.11 to 0.89) and significantly less likely to be continent of urine (OR 0.24, 95% CI 0.07 to 0.69). Observational studies have suggested a link between thioridazine and cardiac arrhythmias.[19]

Comment: The dose of thioridazine varied from 10–200 mg. Doses of comparator drugs also varied. The review identified 51 studies.[18] However, all but seven were excluded because of poor quality methods or lack of usable data. All RCTs were brief. The limited evidence suggests that any benefits are offset by possibile harms.

| OPTION | RISPERIDONE | New |

One RCT has found that risperidone versus placebo reduces psychotic symptoms and aggression in people with dementia.

Benefits: We found no systematic review but found two RCTs.[20,21] One RCT (double blind, 625 people with moderate–severe dementia and behavioural and psychological symptoms, 73% with Alzheimer's disease, mean age 83 years, 68% women) compared risperidone versus placebo over 12 weeks.[20] Risperidone 1 mg and 2 mg significantly reduced behavioural and psychological symptoms measured on the Behave-AD scale. Gender and the type of dementia did not significantly affect the results. Reduction of 50% or more in baseline scores of a symptom scale (Behave-AD) was defined as a response, and was found in 33% of people with placebo, 45% with risperidone 1 mg (NNT 9, 95% CI 5 to 100) and 50% with risperidone 2 mg (NNT 6, 95% CI 4 to 17). The second RCT (344 people with severe dementia, mean age 81 years, 56% women) compared adusted doses of risperidone (mean dose 1.1 mg, 115 people) versus haloperidol (mean dose 1.2 mg, 115 people) versus placebo (114 people) over 13 weeks for the treatment of behavioural symptoms and aggression.[21] Reduction of 30% or more in baseline scores of the Behave-AD scale was defined as a response. Risperidone had no significant effect on the number of responders compared with placebo (37/68 [54%] with risperidone v 35/74 [47%] with placebo; ARI +7%, 95% CI –9% to +23%). Haloperidol increased the number of responders compared with placebo (51/81 [62%] with placebo; ARI 15%, 95% CI 0% to 31%; P = 0.05), but the difference between risperidone and haloperidol was not significant (see comment below).

Harms: Parkinsonism was more common in people receiving 2 mg risperidone than placebo.[20] Total numbers of reported adverse events were similar with placebo (85% of people receiving placebo), and risperidone (84% with 0.5 mg, 82% with 1 mg, 89% with 2 mg). Discontinuation because of adverse events was more common with high dose risperidone (12% with placebo, 8% with 0.5 mg, 16% with 1 mg, 24% with 2 mg).[20] In the second RCT, about 18% of people withdrew because of adverse effects from each of the three arms.[21]

Comment: The first RCT found that risperidone 1 mg and 2 mg compared with placebo increased the number of people with improved behavioural and psychological symptoms. The second RCT[21] is difficult to interpret because 35% of people randomised did not complete the study, and the proportion dropping out varied among the groups (47/115 [41%] with risperidone v 34/115 [30%] with haloperidol v 40/114 [35%] with placebo). The results of the study depend critically on what assumptions are made about the people who left the RCT.

OPTION	OESTROGEN	New

We found one systematic review of one very small RCT of oestrogen therapy in women with Alzheimer's disease from which no conclusions could be drawn. Three subsequent RCTs failed to find evidence that oestrogen therapy is effective.

Benefits: We found one systematic review (search date 1997, 1 RCT, 14 women with Alzheimer's disease)[22] and three subsequent RCTs.[23–25] The systematic review found that the very small RCT of oestrogen (1.25 mg/day) versus placebo for 3 weeks was inadequate to make conclusions. The first subsequent RCT (120 women with mild to moderate Alzheimer's disease) found that oestrogen (0.625 mg/day) versus placebo for 52 weeks produced no significant difference in the Clinical Global Impression of Change 7 point scale or in secondary outcome measures.[23] The second subsequent RCT (42 women) found that oestrogen (1.25 mg/day) versus placebo for 16 weeks produced no significant benefits.[24] The third subsequent RCT (50 women) also found that oestrogen (1.25 mg) versus placebo for 12 weeks produced no significant differences in outcome measures.[25]

Harms: There is concern that oestrogen therapy may increase the risk of developing breast cancer (see harms of hormone replacement therapy under secondary prevention of ischaemic cardiac events, p 95).

Comment: The evidence we found does not suggest that oestrogen is helpful for treating Alzheimer's disease in women.

OPTION   VITAMIN E   New

One RCT of vitamin E versus placebo in Alzheimer's disease found no convincing evidence of benefit.

Benefits: We found one systematic review (search date 1997, 1 RCT, 341 people with moderately severe Alzheimer's disease).[26] The multicentre RCT[27] compared high dose α-tocopherol versus placebo and selegilene versus placebo. It found that high dose α-tocopherol (2000 IU/day) versus placebo for 2 years did not significantly affect the cognitive portion of the Alzheimer's Disease Assessment Scale.

Harms: The RCT found no significant differences in adverse effects between placebo and α-tocopherol.[27] Other studies have found weak evidence of associations between high dose α-tocopherol and bowel irritation, headache, muscular weakness, visual complaints, vaginal bleeding, bruising, thrombophlebitis, deterioration of angina pectoris, worsening of diabetes, syncope, and dizziness.[28] A few case reports have created concern that vitamin E may increase the risk of haemorrhagic stroke.

Comment: The groups in the RCT[27] were not matched evenly at baseline: the placebo group had a higher mean MMSE score, and these baseline scores were a significant predictor of outcome. Attempts to correct for this imbalance suggested that α-tocopherol might increase mean survival, but the need for statistical adjustments weakens the strength of this conclusion. Further RCTs are needed before conclusions about the efficacy of vitamin E can be made.

OPTION   ASPIRIN   New

We found no good evidence about the effects of aspirin in people with dementia.

Benefits: We found one systematic review of aspirin for vascular dementia that found no RCTs (see comment below).[29]

Harms: The RCT did not report adverse effects or dropout rates. (see harms of antiplatelet treatment under secondary prevention of ischaemic cardiac events, p 95).

Comment: Earlier versions of the systematic review included one RCT (70 people with vascular dementia) with many flaws, including a lack of placebo control. In August 2000 this RCT was removed from the systematic review because of the RCT's low quality score. We found no good evidence about the effects of aspirin in people with dementia.

OPTION   SELEGILINE

One systematic review has found that in people with Alzheimer's disease, selegiline is better than placebo at improving cognitive function, behavioural disturbance, and mood. It found no evidence of an effect on clinical global state. Selegiline was well tolerated and no serious adverse events were reported.

Benefits: We found one systematic review (search date 2000, 15 RCTs)[30] comparing selegiline versus placebo (average number of people 50, typical duration of treatment 3 months). Analysis of pooled results found that selegiline improved several outcome measures: cognitive function scores (as measured by several parameters, SMD −0.56, 95% CI −0.88 to −0.24); mood score (DMAS, SMD −1.14, 95% CI −2.11 to −0.18); and behavioural symptom score (BPRS, SMD −0.53, 95% CI −0.94 to −0.12). However, the review found no evidence of an effect on global rating scales (SMD −0.11, 95% CI −0.49 to +0.27).

Harms: Withdrawal rates were low and, except in one study, no significant difference was found between groups.[31] The RCTs reported no major adverse events.

Comment: The trials all used proxy outcomes (cognitive function) rather than clinical outcomes likely to be important to people with Alzheimer's disease and their carers.

OPTION GINKGO BILOBA

One systematic review of RCTs has found good evidence that Ginkgo biloba improves cognitive function and is well tolerated.

Benefits: One systematic review (search date 1998, 9 double blind RCTs in people with Alzheimer's disease, vascular or mixed Alzheimer/vascular dementia)[32] found that in eight RCTs Ginkgo biloba was superior to placebo for a variety of outcomes. The largest and longest trial (52 weeks, 309 people of which 236 had Alzheimer's disease) found that, in people with Alzheimer's disease, Ginkgo biloba versus placebo significantly improved cognition (change in ADAS-cog score −1.7, 95% CI −3.2 to −0.2; NNT for 4 point change in ADAS-cog, completer analysis for people with Alzheimer's disease or vascular dementia: 8, 95% CI 5 to 50), care giver assessed improvement (change in GERRI score −0.19, 95% CI −0.28 to −0.08), but not in mean Clinician's Global Impression of Change score (change in score: 0, 95% CI −0.2 to +0.2).[32] The RCT had a high withdrawal rate (137 people [44%] withdrew).

Harms: The largest RCT reported adverse events in 31% with Ginkgo biloba versus 31% with placebo.[33] No specific pattern of adverse events was reported.

Comment: Most of these RCTs were brief and used different entry criteria, outcomes, and doses. In the UK Ginkgo biloba is classified as a foodstuff, and can be purchased freely. Manufacturers of Ginkgo biloba sponsored all trials identified in the review. The high withdrawal rate of the largest RCT weakens its conclusions, although the authors did conduct both completer and intention to treat analyses.[33]

OPTION DICLOFENAC PLUS MISOPROSTOL

One small RCT found no benefit from diclofenac compared with placebo.

Benefits: We found no systematic review but found one RCT (41 people) that found diclofenac plus misoprostol versus placebo for 25 weeks produced no significant difference in ADAS-cog scores (mean difference +1.14, 95% CI −2.9 to +5.2) or Clinician Global Impression of Change scores (+0.24, 95% CI −0.26 to +0.74).[34]

Alzheimer's disease

Harms: More people withdrew by week 25 with diclofenac plus misoprostol versus placebo (12 [50%] v 2 [12%]). No serious drug related adverse events were reported.[34]

Comment: We found no good evidence that non-steroidal anti-inflammatory drugs are beneficial in people with Alzheimer's disease.

QUESTION   What are the effects of non-drug treatments?

OPTION   REMINISCENCE THERAPY

We found insufficient evidence on the effects of reminiscence therapy (see glossary, p 639) in people with dementia.

Benefits: We found one systematic review of reminiscence therapy (search date 1998, 2 RCTs).[35] Analysis of pooled data was compromised by poor trial methods and diverse outcomes.[35]

Harms: We found no evidence.

Comment: None.

OPTION   REALITY ORIENTATION

One systematic review of small RCTs has found that reality orientation (see glossary, p 639) improves cognitive function and behaviour compared with no treatment. We found no evidence about harms.

Benefits: We found one systematic review (search date 1997, 6 RCTs, 125 people).[36] The RCTs compared reality orientation versus no treatment and used different measures of cognition. The review found that reality orientation improved cognitive function score (SMD −0.59, 95% CI −0.95 to −0.22) and behavioural symptom score (SMD −0.66, 95% CI −1.27 to −0.05).

Harms: The RCTs gave no information on adverse effects.[36]

Comment: The RCTs did not use standardised interventions or outcomes.[36]

OPTION   MUSIC THERAPY   New

One systematic review found no good evidence of music therapy to include in a meta-analysis. Another systematic review found limited evidence that music therapy versus control therapy significantly improved pooled outcomes. No adverse effects were reported.

Benefits: We found two systematic reviews of music therapy.[37,38] The first systematic review (search date 2000)[37] found no good evidence about music therapy to include in a meta-analysis. The second review (search date 1998, 21 studies, 336 people)[38] included studies with weak methods and found in a meta-analysis that music therapy versus control interventions significantly improved reported outcomes (mean effect size 0.79, 95% CI 0.62 to 0.95). Significant effects were noted with different types of music therapy (active v passive, taped v live).[38]

Harms: Harms were not reported.

Comment: The primary studies lacked adequate controls, had potential for bias, used diverse interventions, and used inadequate outcome measures. Although one meta-analysis found significant benefits for music therapy on pooling the results of many studies, further high quality studies are needed to clarify whether the results are explained by a true effect or by bias.

GLOSSARY

Reality orientation Involves presenting information that is designed to reorient a person in time, place, or person. It may range in intensity from a board giving details of the day, date, and season, to staff reorienting a patient at each contact.

Reminiscence therapy Involves encouraging people to talk about the past in order to enable past experiences to be brought into consciousness. It relies on remote memory, which is relatively well preserved in mild to moderate dementia.

Substantive changes since last issue

Cholinesterase inhibitors Two new RCTs;[12,13] conclusions unchanged.

REFERENCES

1. Livingston G. The scale of the problem. In: Burns A, Levy R, eds. *Dementia.* 1st ed. London: Chapman and Hall, 1994:21–35.
2. Panisset M, Stern Y, Gauthier S, eds. *Clinical diagnosis and management of Alzheimer's disease.* 1st ed. London: Dunitz, 1996:129–139.
3. McKeith I. The differential diagnosis of dementia. In: Burns A, Levy R, eds. *Dementia.* 1st ed. London: Chapman and Hall, 1994:39–57.
4. Hardy J. Molecular classification of Alzheimer's disease. *Lancet* 1991;i:1342–1343.
5. Eastwood R, Reisberg B. Mood and behaviour. In: Panisset M, Stern Y, Gauthier S, eds. *Clinical diagnosis and management of Alzheimer's disease.* 1st ed. London: Dunitz, 1996:175–189.
6. Absher JR, Cummings JL. Cognitive and noncognitive aspects of dementia syndromes. In: Burns A, Levy R, eds. *Dementia.* 1st ed. London: Chapman and Hall, 1994:59–76.
7. Rosen WG, Mohs RC, Davis KL. A new rating scale for Alzheimer's disease. *Am J Psychiatry* 1984; 141:1356–1364.
8. Folstein MF, Folstein SE, McHugh PR. Mini Mental State: a practical method for grading the cognitive state of patients for the clinician. *J Psychiatr Res* 1975;12:189–198.
9. Birks JS, Melzer D. Donepezil for mild and moderate Alzheimer's disease. In: The Cochrane Library, Issue 3, 2000. Oxford: Update Software. Search date 1998; primary sources Cochrane Dementia and Cognitive Impairment Group Register of Clinical Trials, Medline, Psychlit, Embase and general contact with members of the Donepezil Study Group and Eisai Inc.
10. Burns A, Rossor M, Gauthier S, et al. The effects of donepezil in Alzheimer's disease – results from a multinational trial. *Dementia Geriatr Disord* 1999;10:237–244.
11. Birks, J Iakovidou V, Tsolaki M. Rivastigmine for Alzheimer's disease. In: The Cochrane Library, Issue 3, 2000. Oxford, Update Software. Search date 1999; primary sources Cochrane Controlled Trials Register, Cochrane Dementia Group Register of Clinical Trials, Medline, Embase, Psychlit, Cinahl, and hand searches of geriatric and dementia journals and conference abstracts.
12. Tariot PN, Solomon PR, Morris JC, Kershaw P, Lilienfeld S, Ding C. A 5-month, randomized, placebo-controlled trial of galantamine in AD. The Galantamine USA-10 Study Group. *Neurology* 2000;54:2269–2276.
13. Raskind MA, Peskind ER, Wessel T, Yuan W. Galantamine in AD: A 6-month randomized, placebo-controlled trial with a 6-month extension. The Galantamine USA-1 Study Group. *Neurology* 2000;54:2261–2268.
14. Rogers SL, Farlow MR, Doody RS, et al. A 24-week double blind placebo controlled trial of donepezil in patients with Alzheimer's disease. *Neurology* 1998;50:136–145.
15. Qizilbash N, Birks J, Lopez Arrieta J, et al. Tacrine in Alzheimer's disease. In: The Cochrane Library, Issue 3, 2000. Oxford: Update Software. Search date November 1998; primary sources the Cochrane Dementia Group Register of Clinical Trials.
16. Knapp MJ, Knopman DS, Soloman PR, et al. A 30-week randomized controlled trial of high-dose tacrine in patients with Alzheimer's disease. *JAMA* 1994;271:985–991.
17. Rosler M, Anand R, Cicin-Sain A. Efficacy and safety of rivastigmine in patients with Alzheimer's disease: international randomised controlled trial. *BMJ* 1999;318:633–640.
18. Kirchner V, Kelly C, Harvey R. Thioridazine for dementia. In: The Cochrane Library, Issue 3, 2000. Oxford: Update Software. Search date not stated, amended August 1998; primary sources Medline, Embase, Psychlit, Cinahl, and Novartis, the pharmaceutical company that develops and markets thioridazine was approached and asked to release any published or unpublished data they had on file.
19. Reilly JG, Ayis SA, Ferrier IN, et al. QT interval abnormalities and psychotropic drug therapy in psychiatric patients. *Lancet* 2000;355:1048–1052.
20. Katz IR, Jeste DV, Mintzer JE, et al. Comparison of risperidone and placebo for psychosis and behavioural disturbances associated with dementia: a randomized double-blind trial. *J Clin Psychiatry* 1999;60:107–115.
21. De Deyn PP, Rabheru K, Rasmussen A, et al. A randomized trial of risperidone, placebo and haloperidol for behavioural symptoms of dementia. *Neurology* 1999;53:946–955.
22. Yaffe K, Sawaya G, Lieberburg I, Grady D. Estrogen therapy in postmenopausal women: effects on cognitive function and dementia. *JAMA* 1998;279: 688–695. Search date June 1997; primary sources Medline 1966 to June 1997.

23. Mulnard RA, Cotman CW, Kawas C, et al. Estrogen replacement therapy for treatment of mild to moderate Alzheimer disease: a randomized controlled trial. Alzheimer's Disease Cooperative Study. *JAMA* 2000;283:1007–1015.

24. Henderson VW, Paganini-Hill A, Miller BL, et al. Estrogen for Alzheimer's disease in women: randomized, double-blind, placebo-controlled trial. *Neurology* 2000;54:295–301.

25. Wang PN, Liao SQ, Liu RS, et al. Effects of estrogen on cognition, mood, and cerebral blood flow in AD: a controlled study. *Neurology* 2000; 54:2061–2066.

26. Flynn BL, Ranno AE. Pharmacologic management of Alzheimer disease. Part II: Antioxidants, antihypertensives, and ergoloid derivatives. *Ann Pharmacother* 1999;33:188–197. Search date 1997; primary sources medline 1989–1997 and hand searched reference lists.

27. Sano M, Ernesto C, Thomas RG, et al. A controlled trial of selegiline, α-tocopherol, or both as treatment for Alzheimer's disease. *N Engl J Med* 1997;336:1216–1222.

28. Myers DG, Maloley PA, Weeks D. Safety of antioxidant vitamins. *Arch Intern Med* 1996;156: 925–935.

29. Williams PS, Spector A, Orrell M, Rands G. Aspirin for vascular dementia. In: The Cochrane Library, Issue 3, 2000. Oxford: Update Software. Search date February 2000; primary sources Medline 1966 to February 2000; Cochrane Library Trials Register, last edition October 1999; Embase 1980 to January; Cinahl 1982 to 1999; Psychlit 1974 to December 1999; Amed; Sigle; National Research Register; hand searched reference lists and contact with specialists.

30. Birks J, Flicker L. Selegiline for Alzheimer's disease. In: The Cochrane Library, Issue 3, 2000. Oxford: Update Software. Search date not given, review amended August 1998; primary sources Cochrane Dementia and Cognitive Impairment Group Register of Clinical Trials.

31. Freedman M, Rewilak D, Xerri T, et al. L deprenyl in Alzheimer's disease. Cognitive and behavioural effects. *Neurology* 1998;50:660–668.

32. Ernst E, Pittler MH. Ginkgo biloba for dementia. *Clin Drug Invest* 1999;17:301–308. Search date 1998; primary sources Medline, Embase, Biosis, Cochrane Register of Controlled Clinical Trials, hand searches of bibliographies, and contact with manufacturers.

33. Le Bars P, Katz MM, Berman N, Itil T, Freedman A, Schatzberg. A placebo-controlled, double-blind, randomised trial of an extract of Ginkgo biloba for dementia. *JAMA* 1997;278:1327–1332.

34. Scharf S, Mander A, Ugoni A, Vajda F, Christophidis N. A double-blind, placebo-controlled trial of diclofenac/misoprostol in Alzheimer's disease. *Neurology* 1999;53:197–201.

35. Spector A, Orrell M. Reminiscence therapy for dementia. In: The Cochrane Library, Issue 3, 2000. Oxford: Update Software. Search date 1998; primary sources Cochrane Controlled Trials Register, Medline, Psychlit, Embase, Omni, Bids, Dissertation Abstracts International, Sigle, and reference lists of relevant articles, relevant internet sites, and hand searching of specialist journals.

36. Spector A, Orrell M, Davies S, et al. Reality orientation for dementia. In: The Cochrane Library, Issue 3, 2000. Oxford: Update Software. Search date 1997; primary sources Medline, Psychlit, Embase, Cochrane Database of Systematic Reviews, Omni, Bids, Dissertation Abstracts International, Sigle, plus Internet searching of HealthWeb, Mental Health Infosources, American Psychiatric Association, Internet Mental Health, Mental Health Net, NHS Confederation, and hand searching of specialist journals.

37. Koger SM, Brotons M. Music therapy for dementia symptoms. In: Cochrane Library Issue 3, 2000. Oxford: Update Software. Search date March 2000; primary sources Medline, Cochrane Dementia and Cognitive Improvement Group Trials Register, Embase, Cinahl and Psychlit 1987 to December 1999.

38. Koger SM, Chaplin K, Brotons M. Is music therapy an effective intervention for dementia? A meta-analytic review of the literature. *J Music Ther* 1999;36:2–15. Search date 1998; primary sources Medline, Psychlit and hand searched reference lists.

James Warner
Senior Lecturer/Consultant in Old Age
Psychiatry

Rob Butler
Lecturer in Old Age Psychiatry
Imperial College School of Medicine
London
UK

Competing interests: JW has been reimbursed by Novartis, the manufacturer of rivastigmine, for conference attendance and has received speaker fees from Janssen pharmaceuticals for educational events. RB, none declared.

TABLE 1 Effects of donepezil, rivastigmine, and galantamine on ADAS-cog scores (see text, p 332, 333).

Drug	Reference	Dose (mg)	Duration (weeks)	Number of people	Effect size difference in ADAS-cog between treatment and placebo arms (95% CI)	NNT (95% CI) 4 point change in ADAS-cog	OR (95% CI) for treatment withdrawal§
Donepezil	9	5	12	488	−2.3 (−3.2 to −1.5)	NA*	2.3 (1.0 to 5.3)
	9	5	24	831	−1.9 (−2.6 to −1.1)	NA*	0.9 (0.5 to 1.4)
	9	10	12	253	−3.1 (−4.2 to −1.9)	NA*	4.1 (1.6 to 10.4)
	9	10	24	821	−2.9 (−3.7 to −2.2)	4 (3 to 7)	1.6 (1.1 to 2.3)
Rivastigmine	11	1–4	12	1293	−0.3 (−0.9 to +0.3)	−†	2.7 (1.1 to 6.8)
	11	1–4	26	1293	−0.8 (−15 to −0.2)	100 (+15 to −20)‡	1.0 (0.7 to 1.5)
	11	6–12	12	1917	−1.5 (−2.0 to −1.0)	15 (10 to 25)	3.1 (1.3 to 7.6)
	11	6–12	26	1917	−2.1 (−2.7 to −1.5)	17 (12 to 34)	3.0 (2.3 to 3.8)
Galantamine	12	16	20	565	−3.3 (−4.5 to −2.2)	7 (5 to 13)	1.0 (0.51 to 1.9)
	12	24	20	559	−3.6 (−4.8 to −2.4)	7 (5 to 15)	1.5 (0.8 to 2.6)
	13	32	24	424	−3.8 (−5.4 to −2.2)	−†	4.7 (2.9 to 7.5)

All intention to treat analyses. A negative change in mean ADAS-cog scores (70 point scale) signifies improvement. NA, not applicable.
*NNTs for donepezil not calculable from systematic review and refer to one study.[14]
†NNTs shown only for significant effects.
‡Confidence intervals for an NNT that changes from positive to negative (i.e. cross infinity) is not significant.
§Odds ratio > 1 favours placebo.

Mental health

Search date December 2000

Phillipa Hay and Josue Bacaltchuk

Key Messages

Psychotherapy

- Two systematic reviews and one subsequent large RCT have found that cognitive behavioural therapy (CBT) versus remaining on a waiting list reduces specific symptoms of bulimia nervosa and also improves non-specific symptoms, such as depression. One RCT has found that CBT versus interpersonal psychotherapy significantly reduces binge eating in the short term, but not in the long term.

- One systematic review and one subsequent RCT have found that other psychotherapies versus waiting list controls improve the symptoms of bulimia nervosa.

- One well designed RCT found that CBT was more effective than interpersonal psychotherapy at 20 weeks, but the difference was not maintained 4 months later.

Antidepressants

- Two systematic reviews of RCTs have found that antidepressants reduce bulimic symptoms in the short term, but we found insufficient evidence about their role in maintenance treatment.

- We found insufficient evidence about the effects of different classes of antidepressants.

- One systematic review of RCTs comparing antidepressants with psychotherapy found no significant difference in bulimic symptoms.

Combinations of antidepressants and psychotherapy

- One systematic review of RCTs has found that combination treatment (antidepressants plus psychotherapy) versus antidepressants alone reduces binge frequency and depressive symptoms but not remission rates. It also found that combination treatment versus psychotherapy alone reduced short term remission and depressive symptoms but had no significant effect on binge eating.

DEFINITION   Bulimia nervosa (see glossary, p 648) is an intense preoccupation with body weight and shape, with regular episodes of uncontrolled overeating of large amounts of food (binge eating — see glossary, p 648) associated with use of extreme methods to counteract the feared effects of overeating. If a person also meets the diagnostic criteria for anorexia nervosa, then the diagnosis of anorexia nervosa takes precedence.[1] Bulimia nervosa can be difficult to identify because of extreme secrecy about binge eating and purgative behaviour. Weight may be normal but there is often a history of anorexia nervosa or restrictive dieting. Some people alternate between anorexia nervosa and bulimia nervosa.

INCIDENCE/   In community based studies, the prevalence of bulimia nervosa is
PREVALENCE   between 0.5% and 1.0%, with an even social class distribution.[2-4] About 90% of people diagnosed with bulimia nervosa are women. The numbers presenting with bulimia nervosa in industrialised countries increased during the decade that followed its recognition in the late 1970s and "a cohort effect" is reported in community surveys,[2,5,6] implying an increase in incidence. The prevalence of eating disorders such as bulimia nervosa is lower in non-industrialised populations,[7] and varies across ethnic groups. African-American women have a lower risk of restrictive dieting than white American women, but have a similar risk of recurrent binge eating.[8]

AETIOLOGY/   Young women from the developed world who restrict their dietary
RISK FACTORS   intake are at highest risk of developing bulimia nervosa and other eating disorders. One community based case control study compared 102 people with bulimia nervosa with 204 healthy controls and found higher rates of the following in people with the eating disorder: obesity, mood disorder, sexual and physical abuse, parental obesity, substance misuse, low self esteem, perfectionism, disturbed family dynamics, parental weight/shape concern, and early menarche.[9] Compared to a control group of 102 women with other psychiatric disorders, women with bulimia nervosa had higher rates of parental problems and obesity.

PROGNOSIS   A 10 year follow up study (50 people with bulimia nervosa from a former trial of mianserin treatment) found that 52% had fully recovered, and only 9% continued to experience symptoms of bulimia nervosa.[10] A larger study (222 people from a trial of antidepressants and structured intensive group psychotherapy) found that after a mean follow up of 11.5 years, 11% still met criteria for bulimia nervosa, whereas 70% were in full or partial remission.[11] Short term studies found similar results: about 50% of people made a full recovery, 30% made a partial recovery, and 20% continued to be symptomatic.[12] There are few consistent predictors of longer term outcome. Good prognosis has been associated with shorter illness duration, a younger age of onset, higher social class, and a family history of alcoholism.[10] Poor prognosis has been associated with a history of substance misuse,[11] premorbid and paternal obesity,[13] and, in some studies, personality disorder.[14-17] One study (102 people) of the natural course of bulimia nervosa found that 31% still had the disorder at 15 months, and 15% at 5 years.[18] Only 28% received treatment in the follow up period.

AIMS	To reduce symptoms of bulimia nervosa; to improve general psychiatric symptoms; to improve social functioning and quality of life.
OUTCOMES	Frequency of binge eating, abstinence from binge eating, frequency of behaviours to reduce weight and counter the effects of binge eating, severity of extreme weight and shape preoccupation, severity of general psychiatric symptoms, severity of depression, improvement in social and adaptive functioning, remission rates, relapse rates, and withdrawal rates.
METHODS	*Clinical Evidence* search and appraisal December 2000, and hand-search of reference lists of identified reviews. One systematic review was not included because it included uncontrolled studies.[19]

> **QUESTION** What are the effects of treatments for bulimia nervosa in adults?

> **OPTION** COGNITIVE BEHAVIOURAL THERAPY

Two systematic reviews and one subsequent large RCT have found that cognitive behavioural therapy (CBT) (see glossary, p 649) versus remaining on a waiting list reduces specific symptoms of bulimia nervosa, and improves non-specific symptoms, such as depression. One RCT has found that CBT versus interpersonal psychotherapy significantly reduces binge eating in the short term, but there was no significant difference in the long term.

Benefits:
We found three systematic reviews of RCTs of psychotherapy[20–22] and one subsequent RCT.[23] The third systematic review is in German and may be included in a future issue of *Clinical Evidence*.[22] The first systematic review (search date 2000, 27 RCTs) included RCTs of other binge eating disorders, although most studies were of people with bulimia nervosa (18 RCTs in people with bulimia nervosa characterised by purging behaviour).[20] The second review (search date 1998, 26 RCTs) used a broad definition of CBT, including exposure and response prevention, and included non-randomised trials.[21] **Versus waiting list controls:** The first review (individual analyses included a maximum of 10 RCTs and 668 people) found that CBT compared to remaining on a waiting list increased the proportion of people abstaining from binge eating at the end of the trial (7 RCTs; RR 0.64, 95% CI 0.53 to 0.78), and reduced depression scores (4 RCTs, 159 people) (see table 1, p 651).[20] Weight at the end of treatment was similar with CBT and remaining on the waiting list (3 RCTs). The review found insufficient evidence about other outcomes such as social functioning. The second systematic review (9 RCTs of specific CBT, 173 people) found that abstinence from binge eating at the end of treatment ranged from 33% to 92% (mean 55%).[21] Pooled effect sizes (weighted for sample size) ranged from 1.22 to 1.35 for reduction in binge eating frequency, purging frequency, depression, and disturbed eating attitudes. Tests for heterogeneity were not significant. In one RCT, the benefits of CBT were maintained for up to 5 years.[13] **Versus other psychotherapies:** The first review found that more people abstained from binge eating after CBT than after other psychotherapies, but the difference did not quite reach

significance (7 RCTs; RR 0.80, 95% CI 0.61 to 1.04).[20] CBT in a full or less intensive form was not significantly superior to CBT in a pure self help form (see glossary, p 649) (4 RCTs; RR 0.90, 95% CI 0.74 to 1.10). CBT was associated with significantly lower depression scores at the end of treatment compared with other psychotherapies (8 RCTs, 273 people; SMD −0.52, 95% CI −0.76 to −0.27). CBT plus exposure therapy was not significantly more effective than CBT alone (3 RCTs; RR abstinence from binge eating 0.87, 95% CI 0.65 to 1.16). Depression scores were significantly lower at the end of treatment with CBT plus exposure therapy versus CBT alone (3 RCTs, 122 people; SMD 0.54, 95% CI 0.17 to 0.91). One RCT included in the review (220 people) compared classic CBT versus interpersonal psychotherapy (see glossary, p 649) for bulimia nervosa that involved purging.[25] It found that CBT significantly improved abstinence from binge eating at the end of treatment (19 individual sessions conducted over 20 weeks; intention to treat analysis: 29% with CBT v 6% with interpersonal psychotherapy); however, the difference was not significant at 4, 8, and 12 months' follow up, although both groups were improved from baseline. The subsequent RCT (125 people with bulimia nervosa) compared four sessions of motivational enhancement therapy versus CBT. It found no significant differences between the treatments.[23] **Versus antidepressants:** See antidepressants, p 646.

Harms: The RCTs did not report details of adverse effects.[20,21,23,25] The first systematic review found no significant difference in completion rates between interventions,[20] suggesting no major difference in acceptability. However, neither review could exclude infrequent serious adverse effects. An observational study found that group psychotherapy offered very soon after presentation was sometimes perceived as threatening.[10]

Comment: The first review defined CBT as psychotherapy that uses specified techniques and models,[20] but it did not define the number of sessions or specialist expertise.[26] Effect sizes for CBT were large, but over 50% of people were still binge eating at the end of treatment.[20,21] Research is needed to evaluate the specific as well as non-specific effects of CBT and other psychotherapies to identify individual characteristics that may predict response, and to explore the long term effects of treatment. Rates of abstinence from binge eating were higher in all experimental groups, but the differences reached significance only when compared with those remaining on a waiting list. It is difficult to interpret the clinical importance of the statistically significant changes in depression scores. It is also difficult to interpret directly the clinical importance of the benefits reported as effect sizes, where the individual RCTs used different outcomes. Further limitations are that the quality of trials was variable (e.g. 57% were not blinded).[20] Sample sizes were often small. None of the studies measured harms rigorously. Waiting list or delayed treatment control groups are subject to bias as it is not possible to "blind" someone to the knowledge they are not in the active treatment group.

One systematic review and one additional RCT have found that non-CBT psychotherapy increases abstinence from binge eating compared with waiting list controls. One small RCT has found that self psychology therapy (see glossary, p 649) versus both cognitive orientation therapy and nutritional counselling increases the remission rate.

Benefits: **Versus waiting list controls:** We found one systematic review[20] and one additional RCT.[27] The review also included data from studies of other binge eating syndromes. It found that non-CBT psychotherapies (e.g. hypnobehavioural therapy and interpersonal psychotherapy — see glossary, p 649) versus waiting list controls significantly increased abstinence rates (3 RCTs, 131 people; RR 0.67, 95% CI 0.56 to 0.81) and reduced bulimia nervosa symptom severity measures (4 RCTs, 177 people; SMD −1.2, 95% CI −1.52 to −0.87). The additional small RCT (17 people with bulimia nervosa) compared structured, behaviour orientated group treatment versus a waiting list. It found that psychotherapy reduced binge eating frequency, depression, and other indices of eating disorder symptom severity.[27] **Versus a control therapy:** We found one three armed RCT (25 people with bulimia nervosa) comparing self psychology therapy versus cognitive orientation therapy (see glossary, p 649) versus a control nutritional counselling treatment group.[28] It found that the remission rate was higher after self psychology therapy compared with both cognitive orientation therapy and nutritional counselling (4/8 [50%] v 2/10 [20%] v 1/7 [14%]). **Versus CBT:** We found one systematic review and one subsequent RCT comparing other psychotherapies versus cognitive behavioural therapies (see option, p 644).

Harms: The RCTs did not report details of individual adverse events (see harms of CBT, p 645). Non-CBT psychotherapies include a large number of options, and it remains to be elucidated which therapies are most effective.

Comment: The quality of trials was variable, few were blinded, sample sizes were small, and none of the studies measured harms rigorously (see comment under CBT, p 645). Waiting list or delayed treatment control groups are subject to bias as it is not possible to "blind" someone to the knowledge they are not in the active treatment group.

Two systematic reviews of RCTs have found short term reduction of bulimic symptoms and a small reduction of depressive symptoms. We found insufficient evidence about the persistence of these effects or about the effects of different classes of antidepressants. One systematic review of RCTs comparing antidepressants versus psychotherapy found no significant difference in bulimic symptoms.

Benefits: We found two systematic reviews,[21,29] two additional RCTs,[30,31] and two subsequent RCTs.[32,33] **Versus placebo:** Both reviews found that antidepressants reduced bulimic symptoms. The first review (search date 1998, 9 RCTs) found that antidepressants versus placebo significantly reduced binge eating (5 RCTs, 163 people; at the end of the trials 16% not binge eating with antidepressants; effect size weighted for sample size 0.66, 95% CI 0.52 to 0.81).[21] Antidepressants versus placebo improved purging (6 RCTs, effect size 0.39, 95% CI 0.24 to 0.54), depression (effect size 0.73, 95% CI 0.58 to 0.88), and improved scales of eating attitudes. The second review (search date 1997, 8 RCTs) found more frequent remission of bulimic episodes with antidepressants (19% v 8% with placebo; pooled RR 0.88, 95% CI 0.83 to 0.94; NNT 9, 95% CI 6 to 16). The review found no significant difference in effect between different classes of antidepressants, but there were too few trials to exclude a clinically important difference (see table 2, p 651). Fluoxetine was the only selective serotonin reuptake inhibitor (SSRI) included in the review, and only one trial reported remission rates.[29] Two additional RCTs (not in either of the above reviews) found that significantly more improvement was maintained after withdrawal of antidepressant treatment that had been continued for 6 months.[34] However, relapse rates of symptoms (30–45%) over 4–6 months were high with both antidepressants and placebo.[30,31] The first subsequent RCT was double blinded and compared fluvoxamine versus placebo.[32] It found relapse rates during a 15 week maintenance period after successful psychotherapy treatment were significantly higher (intention to treat analysis) for placebo, but withdrawal rates were very high (19/33 people randomised to fluvoxamine). Fluvoxamine reduced relapses of general psychiatric symptoms and depression, but differences were not significant (P < 0.1).[35] The second subsequent RCT (22 people who relapsed following a trial of psychotherapy) compared fluoxetine versus placebo. It found that more people taking fluoxetine reported 1 months' abstinence from bingeing and purging (5/13 [39%] v 0/9 [0%] taking placebo, 95% CI not provided, P = 0.05).[33] **Cognitive behavioural therapy:** See option, p 644. **Versus psychotherapy:** We found one systematic review (search date 1997, 5 RCTs) of antidepressants versus psychotherapy (all CBT trials), which found no significant difference in remission rates (39% with psychotherapies, 20% with antidepressants; effect size 1.28; P = 0.07), bulimic symptom severity (3 RCTs), or depression symptom severity at the end of the trial (3 RCTs).[36] **Antidepressants plus psychotherapy:** See option, p 648.

Harms:
One systematic review found higher withdrawal rates with antidepressants than with psychotherapy (4 RCTs, 189 people; AR 40% v 18%, RR 2.18, 95% CI 1.09 to 4.35).[36] The second systematic review found significantly higher withdrawal rates in people taking antidepressants than with placebo (12 RCTs, 10.5% v 5.1%).[29] It found no significant difference in withdrawal rates due to adverse effects among and within classes of antidepressants. In pooled analysis, withdrawal due to any cause was more likely with tricyclic antidepressants than with placebo (6 RCTs, 29% v 14.4%, P = 0.01), but more likely with placebo than selective serotonine reuptake inhibitors (3 RCTs, 37% v 40%, P = 0.04). We found two RCTs examining specific adverse effects. One found significant increases in reclining and standing blood pulse rate, lying systolic and diastolic blood pressure, and greater orthostatic effects on blood pressure with desipramine than with placebo.[37] The cardiovascular changes were well tolerated, and few people

withdrew because of these effects. Meta-analysis of two double blind RCTs of fluoxetine versus placebo found no significant difference in the incidence of suicidal acts or ideation in people treated with fluoxetine versus placebo.[38] However, the overall incidence of events was low (suicide attempts 1.2%, none fatal; emergent suicidal ideation 3.1%).

Comment: We found no consistent predictors of response to treatment. Antidepressants included in the trials were imipramine, amitriptyline, desipramine, phenylzine, isocaboxazid, brofaramine, fluoxetine, mianserin, and buproprion. We found no good evidence on the effects of newer antidepressants, such as venlafaxine and moclobemide. Both reviews commented on the lack of follow up.[21,29]

OPTION **COMBINATION TREATMENT**

One systematic review of RCTs has found that combination treatment (antidepressants plus psychotherapy) versus antidepressants alone reduces binge frequency and depressive symptoms but not remission rates. It also found that combination treatment versus psychotherapy alone reduced short term remission and depressive symptoms but had no significant effect on binge frequency. Antidepressants alone or in combination with psychotherapy were associated with higher withdrawal rates.

Benefits: We found one systematic review (search date 1997, 7 RCTs, 343 people) comparing combination treatment (antidepressants plus psychotherapy) versus either treatment alone.[39] One meta-analysis found that combined treatment with antidepressants plus psychotherapy versus antidepressants alone significantly improved binge frequency and depressive symptoms (3 RCTs, effect size 0.47, P = 0.04), but found no significant difference in short term remission rates (4 RCTs, 141 people, 42% [with combined treatment] v 23% [with antidepressants alone]; RR 1.38, P = 0.06).[39] A second meta-analysis compared psychotherapy alone versus a combination of psychotherapy plus antidepressants.[39] Combination treatment was associated with significantly higher rates of short term remission (6 RCTs, 257 people, 49% v 36%; RR 1.21, P = 0.03) and greater improvement in depressive symptoms, but no significant difference in frequency of binge eating compared with psychotherapy alone.

Harms: Withdrawal rates were lower after psychotherapy plus antidepressants than with antidepressants alone (4 RCTs, 196 people, 34% v 41%; RR 1.19, 95% CI 0.69 to 2.05).[39] Withdrawal rates were significantly higher with psychotherapy plus antidepressants than with psychotherapy alone (6 RCTs, 295 people, 30% v 16%; RR 0.57, P = 0.01).[39]

Comment: None.

GLOSSARY

Binge eating Modified from DSM-IV.[1] Eating, in a discrete period (e.g. hours), a large amount of food, accompanied by a lack of control over eating during the episode.

Bulimia nervosa The American Psychiatric Association DSM-IV[1] criteria include recurrent episodes of binge eating; recurrent inappropriate compensatory behaviour to prevent weight gain; frequency of binge eating and inappropriate compensatory behaviour both, on average, at least twice a week for 3 months; self evaluation unduly influenced by body shape and weight; and disturbance occurring not exclusively during episodes of anorexia nervosa.

Types of bulimia nervosa, modified from DSM-IV[1]: purging: using self induced vomiting, laxatives, diuretics, or enemas. Non-purging: fasting, exercise, but not vomiting or other abuse as purging type.

Cognitive behavioural therapy (CBT) In bulimia nervosa this uses three overlapping phases. Phase one: aims to educate the person about bulimia nervosa. People are helped to increase regularity of eating, and resist urge to binge or purge. Phase two: introduces procedures to reduce dietary restraint (e.g. broadening food choices). In addition, cognitive procedures supplemented by behavioural experiments are used to identify and correct dysfunctional attitudes and beliefs, and avoidance behaviours. Phase three: maintenance. Relapse prevention strategies are used to prepare for possible future set backs.[25]

Cognitive orientation therapy The cognitive orientation theory aims to generate a systematic procedure for exploring the meaning of a behaviour around themes, such as avoidance of certain emotions. Therapy for modifying behaviour focuses on systematically changing beliefs related to themes, not beliefs referring directly to eating behaviour. No attempt is made to persuade the people that their beliefs are incorrect or maladaptive.[28]

Hypnobehavioural psychotherapy Uses a combination of behavioural techniques such as self-monitoring to change maladaptive eating disorders, and hypnotic techniques to reinforce and encourage behaviour change.

Interpersonal psychotherapy In bulimia nervosa this is a three phase treatment. Phase one analyses in detail the interpersonal context of the eating disorder. This leads to the formulation of an interpersonal problem area, which form the focus of the second stage aimed at helping the person make interpersonal changes. Phase three is devoted to the person's progress and an exploration of ways to handle future interpersonal difficulties. At no stage is attention paid to eating habits or body attitudes.[25]

Pure self help CBT A modified form of CBT, in which a treatment manual is provided for people to proceed with treatment on their own, or with support from a non-professional. "Guided self help" usually implies that the support person may or may not have some professional training, but is usually not a specialist in eating disorders.

Self psychology therapy This approaches bulimia nervosa as a specific case of the pathology of the self. The treated person cannot rely on people to fulfil their needs such as self esteem. They instead rely on a substance, food, to fulfill personal needs. Therapy progresses when the people move to rely on human beings, starting with the therapist.[28]

Substantive changes since last issue

Other psychotherapies versus a control therapy New RCT;[28] conclusion unchanged.

Antidepressants versus placebo New RCT;[33] conclusion unchanged.

REFERENCES

1. American Psychiatric Association. *Diagnostic and statistical manual of mental disorders* 4th ed. Washington DC: American Psychiatric Press, 1994.

2. Bushnell JA, Wells JE, Hornblow AR, Oakley-Brown MA, Joyce P. Prevalence of three bulimic syndromes in the general population. *Psychol Med* 1990;20:671–680.

3. Garfinkel PE, Lin B, Goering P, et al. Bulimia nervosa in a Canadian community sample: prevalence, co-morbidity, early experiences and psychosocial functioning. *Am J Psychiatry* 1995; 152:1052–1058.

4. Gard MCE, Freeman CP. The dismantling of a myth: a review of eating disorders and socioeconomic status. *Int J Eat Disord* 1996;20: 1–12.

5. Hall A, Hay PJ. Eating disorder patient referrals from a population region 1977–1986. *Psychol Med* 1991;21:697–701.

6. Kendler KS, Maclean C, Neale M, et al. The genetic epidemiology of bulimia nervosa. *Am J Psychiatry* 1991;148:1627–1637.

7. Choudry IY, Mumford DB. A pilot study of eating disorders in Mirpur (Pakistan) using an Urdu version of the Eating Attitude Test. *Int J Eat Disord* 1992;11:243–251.
8. Striegel-Moore RH, Wifley DE, Caldwell MB, Needham ML, Brownell KD. Weight-related attitudes and behaviors of women who diet to lose weight: a comparison for black dieters and white dieters. *Obes Res* 1996;4:109–116.
9. Fairburn CG, Welch SL, Doll HA, Davies BA, O'Connor ME. Risk factors for bulimia nervosa: a community-based case-control study. *Arch Gen Psychiatry* 1997;54:509–517.
10. Collings S, King M. Ten year follow-up of 50 patients with bulimia nervosa. *Br J Psychiatry* 1994;164:80–87.
11. Keel PK, Mitchell JE, Miller KB, Davis TL, Crow SJ. Long-term outcome of bulimia nervosa. *Arch Gen Psychiatry* 1999;56:63–69.
12. Keel PK, Mitchell JE. Outcome in bulimia nervosa. *Am J Psychiatry* 1997;154:313–321.
13. Fairburn CG, Norman PA, Welch SL, et al. A prospective study of outcome in bulimia nervosa and the long-term effects of three psychological treatments. *Arch Gen Psychiatry* 1995;52:304–312.
14. Coker S, Vize C, Wade T, Cooper PJ. Patients with bulimia nervosa who fail to engage in cognitive behaviour therapy. *Int J Eat Disord* 1993;13:35–40.
15. Fahy TA, Russell GFM. Outcome and prognostic variables in bulimia. *Int J Eat Disord* 1993;14:135–146.
16. Rossiter EM, Agras WS, Telch CF, Schneider JA. Cluster B personality disorder characteristics predict outcome in the treatment of bulimia nervosa. *Int J Eat Disord* 1993;13:349–358.
17. Johnson C, Tobin DL, Dennis A. Differences in treatment outcome between borderline and nonborderline bulimics at 1-year follow-up. *Int J Eat Disord* 1990;9:617–627.
18. Fairburn C, Cooper Z, Doll H, Norman P, O'Conner M. The natural course of bulimia nervosa and binge eating disorder in young women. *Arch Gen Psychiatry* 2000;57:659–665.
19. Lewandowski LM, Gebing TA, Anthony JL, O'Brien WH. Meta-analysis of cognitive behavioural treatment studies for bulimia. *Clin Psychol Rev* 1997;17:703–718. Search date 1995; primary sources Psychinfo, and hand searches of references lists.
20. Hay PJ, Bacaltchuk J. Psychotherapy for bulimia nervosa and binging. In: The Cochrane Library, Issue 4, 2000. Oxford: Update Software. Search date May 2000; primary sources Medline, Extramed, Embase, Psychlit, Current Contents, Lilacs, Scisearch up to 1998; The Cochrane Controlled Trials Register 1997; The Cochrane Collaboration Depression and Anxiety Trials Register up to May 2000; handsearch of *Int J Eat Disord* since its first issue and citation lists in identified studies and reviews, and personal contacts.
21. Whittal ML, Agras WS, Gould RA. Bulimia nervosa: a meta-analysis of psychosocial and pharmacological treatments. *Behav Ther* 1999;30:117–135. Search date 1998; primary sources Psychlit, Medline, and handsearch of *Int J Eat Disord* 1990–1998; handsearch other relevant (not specified) journals and identified studies. This was reviewed in Waller G. *Evidenced Based Medicine* (September/October 1999).
22. Jacobi C, Dahme B, Rustenbach S. Comparison of controlled pshco- and pharmacotherapy studies in bulimia anorexia nervosa.[in German] *Psychother Psychosom Med Psychol* 1997;47:346–364. Search date not stated; primary sources

Psychological Abstracts, Medline, Psychindex, Psychinfo from 1994.
23. Treasure JL, Katzman M, Schmidt U, et al. Engagement and outcome in the treatment of bulimia nervosa: first phase of a sequential design comparing motivation enhancement therapy and cognitive behavioural therapy. *Behav Res Ther* 1999;37:405–418.
24. Loeb KL, Wilson GT, Gilbert JS, Labouvie E. Guided and unguided self-help for binge eating. *Behav Res Ther* 2000;38:259–272.
25. Agras WS, Walsh BT, Fairburn CG, Wilson GT, Kraemer HC. A multicenter comparison of cognitive-behavioral therapy and interpersonal psychotherapy. *Arch Gen Psychiatry* 2000;54:459–465.
26. Wilson GT, Fairburn CG. Treatments for eating disorders. In: Nathan PE, Gorman JM, eds. *A Guide to Treatments that Work*. New York: Oxford University Press, 1998:501–530.
27. Laessle RG, Waadt S, Pirke KM. A structured behaviourally orientated group treatment for bulimia nervosa. *Psychother Psychosom* 1987;48:141–145.
28. Bachar E, Latzer Y, Kreitler S, Berry EM. Empirical comparison of two psychological therapies. Self psychology and cognitive orientation in the treatment of anorexia and bulimia. *J Psychother Pract Res* 1999;8:115–128.
29. Bacaltchuk J, Hay P, Mari JJ. Antidepressants versus placebo for the treatment of bulimia nervosa: a systematic review. *Aust N Z J Psychiatry* 2000;34:310–317. Search date 1997; primary sources Medline, Extramed, Embase, Psychlit, Current Contents, Lilacs, Scisearch, The Cochrane Controlled Trials Register, The Cochrane Collaboration Depression and Anxiety Trials Register, handsearch of citation lists in identified studies, and reviews and personal contact.
30. Walsh BT, Hadigan CM, Devlin MJ, Gladis M, Roose SP. Long-term outcome of antidepressant treatment for bulimia nervosa. *Am J Psychiatry* 1991;148:1206–1212.
31. Pyle RL, Mitchell JE, Eckert ED, et al. Maintenance treatment and 6-month outcome for bulimic patients who respond to initial treatment. *Am J Psychiatry* 1990;147:871–875.
32. Fichter MM, Krüger R, Rief W, Holland R, Döhne J. Fluvoxamine in prevention of relapse in bulimia nervosa: effects on eating specific psychopathology. *J Clin Psychopharmacol* 1996;16:9–18.
33. Walsh BT, Agras WS, Devlin MJ, et al. Fluoxetine for bulimia nervosa following poor response to psychotherapy. *Am J Psychiatry* 2000;157:1332–1334.
34. Agras WS, Rossiter EM, Arnow B, et al. One-year follow-up of psychosocial and pharmacologic treatments for bulimia nervosa *J Clin Psychiatry* 1994;55:179–183.
35. Fichter MM, Leibl C, Krüger R, Rief W. Effects of fluvoxamine on depression, anxiety, and other areas of general psychopathology in bulimia nervosa. *Pharmacopsychiatry* 1997;30:85–92.
36. Bacaltchuk J, Trefiglio RP, de Oliveira IR, Lima MS, Mari JJ. Antidepressants versus psychotherapy for bulimia nervosa: a systematic review. *J Clin Pharm Ther* 1999;24:23–31. Search date 1997; primary sources Medline, Extramed, Embase, Psychlit, Current Contents, Lilacs, Scisearch, Cochrane Controlled Trials Register, Cochrane Collaboration Depression and Anxiety Trials Register, handsearch of *Int J Eat Disord* since its first issue, citation lists of identified studies and reviews, and personal contacts.
37. Agras WS, Rossiter EM, Arnow B, et al. Pharmacologic and cognitive-behavioral treatment

for bulimia nervosa: a controlled comparison. *Am J Psychiatry* 1992;149:82–87.

38. Wheadon DE, Rampey AH, Thompson VL, et al. Lack of association between fluoxetine and suicidality in bulimia nervosa. *J Clin Psychiatry* 1992;53:235–241.

39. Bacaltchuk J, Trefiglio RP, Oliveira IR, et al. Combination of antidepressants and psychotherapy for bulimia nervosa: a systematic review. *Acta Psychiatr Scand* 2000;101:256–264. Search dates 1997; primary sources handsearch of *Int J Eat Disord* since its first issue; Medline 1966–1998; Extramed, Embase, Psychlit, Current Contents, Lilacs, Scisearch up to 1997; Cochrane Controlled Trials Register 1997 Internet version; Cochrane Collaboration Depression and Anxiety Trials Register; handsearch of all citation lists in identified studies, and reviews and personal contact.

40. Agras WS, Crow SJ, Halmi KA, Mitchell JE, Wilson GT, Kraemer HC. Outcome predictors for the cognitive behavior treatment of bulimia nervosa: data from a multisite study. *Am J Psychiatry* 2000; 157:1302–1308.

Phillipa Hay
Psychiatrist
University of Adelaide
Adelaide
Australia

Josue Bacaltchuk
Psychiatrist
Federal University of Sao Paulo
Sao Paulo
Brazil

Competing interests: PH has received reimbursement for attending symposia from Solvay Pharmaceuticals, Bristol-Myers Squibb and Pfizer Pharmaceuticals, and for educational training of family doctors from Bristol-Myers Squibb. JB has received fees from Janssen-Cilag Farmaceutica.

| TABLE 1 | Comparison of remission rates between cognitive behaviour therapy or other active psychotherapy and comparison group (see text, p 644).[20] |

Comparison	Number of RCTs	Number of people	Absolute remission rates	RR of not remitting (95% CI)
CBT v waiting list	7	300	42% v 6%	0.64 (0.53 to 0.78)
CBT v other psychotherapy	7	474*	40% v 21%	0.80 (0.61 to 1.04)
CBT v pure self help CBT	4	223	46% v 36%	0.90 (0.74 to 1.10)
Other psychotherapy v waiting list	3	131	36% v 3%	0.67 (0.56 to 0.813)

CBT, cognitive behavioural therapy. *Updated to include new trial;[24]

| TABLE 2 | Comparison of remission rates between active drug and placebo by class of antidepressant (see text, p 647).[29] |

Class: Drug(s)	Number of RCTs	Number of people	RR	95% CI
TCA: desipramine, imipramine	3	132	0.86	0.7 to 1.07
SSRI: fluoxetine	1	398	0.92	0.84 to 1.01
MAOI: phenylzine, brofaramine	2	98	0.81	0.68 to 0.96
Other: bupropion, trazodone	2	87	0.86	0.76 to 0.97

MAOI, monoamine oxidase inhibitor; N, number of participants; SSRI, selective serotonin reuptake inhibitor; TCA, tricyclic antidepressant.

Search date May 2000: expanded this issue

John Geddes and Rob Butler

INTERVENTIONS

Key Messages

- Systematic reviews of RCTs have found that antidepressant drugs are effective in acute treatment of all grades of depressive disorders in all common treatment settings and in people with or without coexistent physical illness. We found no evidence of a clinically significant difference in the benefits of different antidepressant drugs, although drugs vary in adverse effects.

- One systematic review of RCTs has found that cognitive therapy is effective and may be more effective than drug treatment for mild to moderate depression.

- One systematic review of mixed quality RCTs has found that St John's Wort is an effective treatment for mild to moderate depression.

- One large RCT has found that interpersonal therapy is effective treatment for mild to moderate depression. Less robust RCTs have found that problem solving therapy is also effective. Specific psychological treatments, such as cognitive and interpersonal therapy have been shown to be as effective as drugs.

- We found limited evidence suggesting that other treatments, including exercise, bibliotherapy, befriending, and non-directive counselling, may be effective.

- We found no reliable evidence to suggest that one type of treatment (drug or non-drug) is superior to another. Limited evidence suggests that combining drug and psychological treatments may be effective in severe but not mild to moderate depression.

- Of the interventions examined in this issue, prescription antidepressant drugs are the only treatment for which there is good evidence of effectiveness in severe and psychotic depressive disorders. We found no RCTs comparing drug and non-drug treatments in severe depressive disorder.

- RCTs have found that continuing antidepressant drug treatment for 4–6 months after recovery reduces risk of relapse.

- We found no evidence of a difference between treatments in terms of long term benefits.

DEFINITION   Depressive disorders are characterised by persistent low mood, loss of interest and enjoyment, and reduced energy. They often impair function. **Older adults:** Older adults are generally defined as people aged 65 years or more. The presentation of depression in older adults may be atypical; low mood may be masked and anxiety or memory impairment may be the principal presenting symptoms. Dementia should be considered in the differential diagnosis of depression in older adults.[1]

INCIDENCE/ PREVALENCE   **Younger adults:** Depressive disorders are common, with a prevalence of major depression between 5–10% of people seen in primary care settings.[2] Two to three times as many people may have depressive symptoms but do not meet criteria for major depression. Women are affected twice as often as men. Depressive disorders are the fourth most important cause of disability worldwide and are expected to become the second most important cause by 2020.[3,4] **Older adults:** 10–15% of older people have significant depressive symptomatology, although major depression is relatively rare in older adults.[5]

AETIOLOGY/ RISK FACTORS   The causes are uncertain but include both childhood events and current psychosocial adversity.

PROGNOSIS   About half of people suffering a first episode of major depressive disorder experience further symptoms in the next 10 years.[6] Different levels of severity[7,8] indicate different prognosis and treatment. **Mild to moderate depression** is characterised by depressive symptoms and some functional impairment. Many people recover in the short term but about half experience recurrent symptoms. **Severe depression** is characterised by additional agitation or psychomotor retardation with marked somatic symptoms. In this review, treatments are considered to have been evaluated in severe depression if the RCTs included inpatients. **Psychotic depression** is characterised by additional hallucinations, delusions, or both. **Older adults:** The prognosis may be especially poor in elderly people with a chronic or relapsing course.[9]

AIMS

To improve mood, social and occupational functioning, and quality of life; to reduce morbidity and mortality; to prevent recurrence of depressive disorder; and to minimise adverse effects of treatment. Depression should not be regarded as a natural concomitant of older age.

OUTCOMES

Depressive symptoms rated by the depressed person and clinician, social functioning, occupational functioning, quality of life, admission to hospital, rates of self harm, relapse of depressive symptoms, rates of adverse events. Trials often use continuous scales to measure depressive symptoms (such as the Hamilton Depression Rating Scale and the Beck Depression Inventory). Clinician reports and self reported global outcome measures are also used. Changes in continuous measures can be dealt with in two ways. They can be dichotomised in an arbitrary but clinically helpful manner (e.g. taking a reduction in depressive symptoms of more than 50% as an end point), which allows results to be expressed as relative risks and numbers needed to treat. Alternatively, they can be treated as continuous variables, as is done for systematic analysis. In this case, the pooled estimate of effect (the effect size) expresses the degree of overlap between the range of scores in the control and experimental groups. The effect size can be used to estimate the proportion of people in the control group who had a poorer outcome than the average person in the experimental group. **Older adults:** The Hamilton Depression Rating Scale is not ideal for older people because it includes a number of somatic items that may be positive in older people who are not depressed. It has been the most widely used scale, although specific scales for elderly people (such as the Geriatric Depression Scale) avoid somatic items.

METHODS

A validated search for systematic reviews and RCTs was conducted between May and September 1998 from the Cochrane Database of Systematic Reviews and the Database of Abstract of Reviews of Effectiveness, *Best Evidence* and *Evidence-Based Mental Health*, Medline, PsychLit, and Embase. Studies were included by using epidemiological criteria and relevance to the clinical question. A *Clinical Evidence* search and appraisal was conducted in May 2000 including a search for data on depression in older adults. To date, few studies have concentrated on older adults as a separate subgroup. Most published evidence for the efficacy of antidepressants includes all ages over 16 or is limited to people aged under 65.

QUESTION   What are the effects of treatments?

OPTION   PRESCRIPTION ANTIDEPRESSANT DRUGS

Younger adults: Systematic reviews of RCTs have found that antidepressant drugs are effective in acute treatment of all grades of depressive disorders. They have also found no clinically significant difference in effectiveness between different kinds of antidepressant drug. However, the drugs differ in their adverse event profiles. On average, people seem to tolerate selective serotonin reuptake inhibitors (SSRIs) a little more than older drugs, but this difference is too small to

be grounds for a policy of always choosing an SSRI as first line treatment. We found no strong evidence that fluoxetine is associated with increased risk of suicide. Abrupt withdrawal of SSRIs is associated with symptoms, including dizziness and rhinitis in some patients, and this is more likely and probably more severe with drugs with a short half life, such as paroxetine. **Older adults:** One systematic review has found that heterocyclic antidepressants and SSRIs are effective in older people with mild to moderate depression. However, overall treatment effects were modest. Limitations of this review include the variety of populations studied and the short duration of many studies. Future, high quality RCTs are unlikely for ethical reasons.

Benefits:
: **In younger adults: Versus placebo:** We found two systematic reviews.[10,11] The first review (published in 1996, search date not given, 49 RCTs in people with depressive disorder) included five trials of people admitted to hospital (probably more severely ill); 40 RCTs in a setting outside hospital; one in both settings; and three trials that did not specify the setting. Each RCT compared two antidepressant drugs and included a placebo control group. The review found a mean effect size of 0.50 for antidepressant drugs versus placebo, which means that 69% of those taking placebo did worse than the average person taking antidepressants. Drugs were more effective in those with depressive disorders diagnosed according to standard criteria (mainly *Diagnostic and Statistical Manual of Mental Disorders*, 3rd edition, revised [DSM-III-R]). The second systematic review (updated in 1998, 15 RCTs, 1871 people) compared antidepressant versus placebo in people with dysthymia (chronic mild depressive disorders).[11] Response to treatment was about twice as likely in the antidepressant group (RR versus placebo 1.9, 95% CI 1.6 to 2.3; NNT 4, 95% CI 3 to 5). **Tricyclic antidepressants (TCAs) versus SSRIs:** We found three systematic reviews comparing SSRIs with TCAs.[12–14] These found no significant difference in effectiveness overall. SSRIs seem to be slightly more acceptable overall as measured by the number of people who withdrew from clinical trials (RR 0.88, 95% CI 0.83 to 0.93; NNT 26).[12] The third systematic review (search date 1998, 28 RCTs, 5940 people) compared the efficacy in primary care of newer antidepressants versus placebo and versus older antidepressants.[14] The average response rate was 63% for newer agents, 35% for placebo, and 60% for TCAs (RR for SSRIs compared with placebo 1.6, 95% CI 1.2 to 2.1). One small RCT (152 people) compared adherence on dothiepin with fluoxetine over 12 weeks and found no significant difference between the drugs. However, the study was probably underpowered.[15] **Monoamine oxidase inhibitors (MAOIs) versus TCAs:** We found one systematic review (search date not given, 55 RCTs comparing MAOIs versus TCAs in several subgroups of people with depression).[16] It found that MAOIs were less effective in people with severe depressive disorders but may be more effective in atypical depressive disorders (depressive disorders with reversed biological features—for example, increased sleep, increased appetite, mood reactivity, and rejection sensitivity). **Older adults:** We identified one systematic review (search date 1998, 40 RCTs of pharmacological and psychological treatments of depression in people older than 55 years), in an outpatient or community setting. Of the trials, 26 were of pharmacological

treatments and 21 of these were placebo controlled. People were recruited mainly from outpatient clinics. There was significant heterogeneity in the study results (P = 0.03). Nine heterocyclic drug studies had a mean difference in Hamilton Depression Rating scores after treatment of −5.78 (95% CI −8.31 to −3.25). Significant benefits were also found for fluoxetine, trazodone, and phenelzine. Of the 17 drug versus drug comparisons (mainly involving heterocyclic drugs), none showed significant benefit above the others.[17] **In people with depression plus a physical illness versus placebo:** One systematic review (search date 1998, 18 RCTs, n = 838) found that antidepressants were more effective than placebo in people with depression and a physical illness (NNT 4, 95% CI 3 to 7). People allocated to antidepressants were more likely to withdraw from the study than those on placebo (NNH 10, 95% CI 5 to 43).[18]

Harms:

Common adverse events: One systematic review of RCTs (search date 1996) compared TCAs versus SSRIs in people with all severities of depression (see table 1, p 666).[19] There may also be differences between SSRIs. One large cohort study of people receiving four different SSRIs (fluvoxamine [n = 10 983], fluoxetine [n = 12 692], sertraline [n = 12 734], and paroxetine [n = 13 741]) in British primary care found that reports of common adverse events (nausea/vomiting, malaise/lassitude, dizziness, and headache/migraine) varied between SSRIs (fluvoxamine 78 per 1000 participant months; fluoxetine 23 per 1000 participant months; RR versus fluvoxamine 0.29, 95% CI 0.27 to 0.32; paroxetine 28 per 1000 participant months, RR 0.35, 95% CI 0.33 to 0.37; sertraline 21 per 1000 participant months, RR 0.26, 95% CI 0.25 to 0.28).[20] Only 52% of people responded to the questionnaire, although this response rate was similar for all four drugs. A study of spontaneous reports to the UK Committee on Safety of Medicines found no difference in safety profiles between the same four SSRIs.[21] **Suicide:** One systematic review (which included trials completed by December 1989) pooled data from 17 double blind RCTs in people with depressive disorder comparing fluoxetine (n = 1765) versus a TCA (n = 731) or placebo (n = 569).[22] There was no significant difference in the rate of suicidal acts between the groups (fluoxetine 0.3%, placebo 0.2%, TCAs 0.4%), whereas development of suicidal ideation was less frequent in the fluoxetine group (1.2% fluoxetine v 2.6% placebo, P = 0.042, and v 3.6% TCAs, P = 0.001). One historical cohort study followed 172 598 people who had at least one prescription for one of 10 antidepressants during the study period in general practice in the UK. The risk of suicide was higher in people who received fluoxetine (19 per 10 000 person years, 95% CI 9 to 34) than those receiving dothiepin (RR of suicide v dothiepin 2.1, 95% CI 1.1 to 4.1).[23] In a nested case controlled subanalysis in people with no history of suicidal behaviour or previous antidepressant prescription, the risk remained the same, although the confidence interval broadened to make the result indeterminate (RR 2.1, 95% CI 0.6 to 7.9). Although the apparent association may be due to residual confounding, there remains uncertainty about the possible association between fluoxetine and suicide. However, any absolute increase in risk is unlikely to be large. **Withdrawal effects:** We found one RCT comparing abrupt discontinuation of fluoxetine (n = 96) versus continued treatment (n = 299) in people who had been taking the drug for 12 weeks. Abrupt discontinuation was associated with increased dizziness (7% v 1%), dysmenorrhoea (3% v 0%), rhinitis (10% v 3%), and somnolence (4% v 0%). However, there was a high drop out rate in this study because of return of symptoms of depression (39%), so these may be underestimates of the true rate of withdrawal symptoms.[24] The rate of spontaneous reports of suspected withdrawal reactions per million defined daily doses to the World Health Organization Collaborating Centre for International Drug Monitoring between 1987 and 1995 was higher for paroxetine than for sertraline and fluoxetine.[25] The most common withdrawal effects were dizziness, nausea, paraesthesia, headache, and vertigo. **Older adults:** We found no specific evidence on adverse effects in older adults. **During pregnancy:** One systematic review of the risks of fetal harm of antidepressants in pregnancy found four small prospective studies published since 1993.[26] No evidence of increased risk was found, although the chances of adverse effects with a low incidence cannot be excluded. Decreased birth weights of infants exposed to fluoxetine in the third trimester were identified in one study and direct drug effects and withdrawal syndromes were identified in some neonates.

Comment: A systematic review is under way to examine the efficacy of antidepressants in older people, including data on adverse effects.[17] Metabolic and physical changes with age mean that older people may be more prone to adverse effects such as falls. As older people take more medications, they are at more risk of drug interactions. Suicide is a risk in elderly people.

| OPTION | CARE PATHWAYS |

We found limited evidence that effectiveness of drug treatment may be improved by collaborative working between primary care clinicians and psychiatrists, or by intensive patient education.

Benefits: We found no systematic review. We found four RCTs.[27–30] The first in 217 people with mild to moderate depressive disorders in primary care in the USA found that, compared with standard treatment, outcomes were improved by collaborative working between primary care physician and psychiatrist, and by intensive patient education. Clinical outcomes were improved only in the subgroup of people with major depressive disorder (n = 91; AR of clinical response of > 50% reduction on symptom checklist: 74% v 44% with standard treatment; NNT 4, 95% CI 3 to 10).[27] The second (613 people) in a Health Maintenance Organization (HMO) in Seattle compared usual care, feedback (in which doctors received a detailed report on each person at 8 and 16 weeks following randomisation), or feedback plus care management (in which the care manager assessed people with depression by telephone at 8 and 16 weeks, doctors received a detailed report, and care managers facilitated the follow up). The care management group were more likely than those treated with usual care to have a clinically significant reduction in depressive symptoms 6 months after randomisation (estimated event rates 40% of the control group v 56% of the care management group OR 2.22, 95% CI 1.31 to 3.75; NNT 7).[28] The third RCT (1356 people) in 46 primary care clinics in US HMOs compared a multifaceted quality improvement programme with usual care (including mailed practice guidelines). People in the intervention group improved on continuous rating scales. Among people initially employed, 89.7% of the intervention group worked at 12 months compared with 84.7% of the control group (P = 0.05). For people initially not working, there was no difference in employment rates between intervention and control groups at 12 months (17% v 18%).[29] The fourth, a cluster randomised RCT in UK primary care, compared the effects of a clinical practice guideline and practice based education with usual care and found that the intervention did not improve either detection or outcome of depression.[30]

Harms: None reported.

Comment: None.

OPTION   **ST JOHN'S WORT (*HYPERICUM PERFORATUM*)**

One systematic review of RCTs has found that St John's Wort (*Hypericum perforatum*) is more effective than placebo in mild to moderate depressive disorders and as effective as prescription antidepressant drugs. However, these findings have yet to be repeated in fully representative groups of people using standardised preparations.

Benefits: We found one systematic review (updated in 1998, 27 RCTs, 2291 people with mild to moderate depression).[31] Of these trials, 17 were placebo controlled (1168 participants). Ten trials (1123 participants) compared hypericum (8 trials used single preparations, 2 used combinations of hypericum and valeriana) versus other antidepressant or sedative drugs. Hypericum preparations were associated with significant clinical improvement compared with placebo (RR 2.47, 95% CI 1.69 to 3.61) but not compared with standard antidepressants (single preparations RR 1.01, 95% CI 0.87 to 1.16, combinations RR 1.52, 95% CI 0.78 to 2.94).

Harms: We found two systematic reviews (one cited above[31] and one other, search date 1997[32]). The review cited above found that adverse events were poorly reported in the trials. They were reported by 26% of people on hypericum compared with 45% of people on standard antidepressants (RR 0.57, 95% CI 0.47 to 0.69) and 15% on combinations of hypericum and valeriana compared with 27% on amitriptyline or desipramine (RR 0.49, 95% CI 0.23 to 1.04).[31] The second systematic review included RCTs and observational postmarketing surveillance studies of hypericum.[32] The commonest adverse effects of hypericum in the included trials were gastrointestinal symptoms, dizziness/confusion, tiredness/sedation, and dry mouth, although all occurred less frequently than on conventional drugs. Findings from observational studies were consistent with these findings. Photosensitivity is theoretically possible; however only two cases have been reported. Allergic skin reactions seem uncommon.

Comment: The evidence cited above must be interpreted cautiously for the following reasons: (1) it is unclear how closely participants in these trials match people in clinical practice; and (2) the preparations and doses of hypericum and types and doses of standard antidepressants varied. More studies are needed on clearly defined, clinically representative people using standardised preparations. Interactions with other drugs are possible and should be considered.

OPTION **ELECTROCONVULSIVE THERAPY**

One systematic review of RCTs has found that electroconvulsive therapy (ECT) is effective in the acute treatment of depressive illness.

Benefits: We found two systematic reviews. The first (search date not given) included six RCTs and a total of 205 people with depressive disorder that compared ECT versus simulated ECT (in which people received everything but electric stimulation).[33] People treated with real ECT were more likely to respond to treatment (pooled OR 3.7, 95% CI 2.1 to 6.5; NNT 3, 95% CI 2 to 5, calculated from data in the article). The more recent systematic review (search date 1998) included 11 additional RCTs published between 1987 and 1998, but it did not undertake quantitative analysis.[34]

Harms: We found no adequate systematic review of possible adverse cognitive effects of ECT. However, people often complain of memory impairment after ECT. One of the main difficulties in studying this is that depressive disorders also lead to cognitive impairments that usually improve during the course of treatment. For this reason most of the many small studies in this area find an average improvement in people treated with ECT. This does not rule out the possibility of more subtle, subjective memory impairment secondary to ECT. Adverse memory effects would probably vary according to the dose and electrode used.

Comment: The first review cited above[26] did not include several recent RCTs comparing real versus simulated ECT.[35–39] However, the results of these trials are consistent with the review's findings. A further systematic review is in progress.[40] As ECT may be unacceptable to some people and because it is a short term treatment, there is a consensus that it should normally be reserved for people who cannot tolerate or have not responded to drug treatment, although it may be useful when a rapid response is required.

OPTION **SPECIFIC PSYCHOLOGICAL TREATMENTS**

Younger adults: One systematic review of RCTs has found that cognitive therapy (see glossary, p 663) is effective, and may be more effective than drug treatment in people with mild to moderate depression. Weaker evidence from RCTs suggests that interpersonal psychotherapy, problem solving therapy and brief, non-directive counselling (see glossary, p 663) may be as effective as drug treatment in mild to moderate depression. We found limited evidence on the relative efficacy of drug and non-drug treatment in severe depression. Older adults: One systematic review of RCTs has found that rational psychological treatments (such as cognitive therapy or cognitive behaviour therapy) are effective for older people with mild to moderate depression. However, people receiving these treatments improved no more than controls who received similar but non-specific attention. This review was based on a small number of studies, the populations varied (although most were community samples), and many of the studies were short term.

Depressive disorders

Benefits: **Younger adults:** The evidence comparing psychological treatments versus drug or no treatment is summarised in table 2, p 667.[41–43]

Older adults: We identified one systematic review of 40 controlled trials of pharmacological and psychological treatments in people over the age of 55 in an outpatient or community setting.[44] The review found four comparisons in older adults of psychological treatments (such as psychotherapy) versus untreated controls. None of the trials found a significant difference between treatment and no treatment, measured on the Hamilton Depression Rating Scale. The review also identified six comparisons of different psychological treatments. None found significant differences in effectiveness. Five of six comparisons of "rational" treatments (such as cognitive therapy or cognitive behaviour therapy) versus no treatment in older adults found significant benefit with treatment. Combined, the rational treatments performed significantly better than no treatment, with a mean difference in the Hamilton Depression Rating score of −7.25 (95% CI, −10.1 to −4.4). However, neither of the two rational treatments performed significantly better than non-specific attention.

Harms: See table 2, p 667.

Comment: Large RCTs are needed in more representative people in a range of clinical settings, including primary care. Because of varying exclusion criteria, the generaliseability of the studies is questionable (see table 2, p 667). Other factors to be considered when psychological treatments are compared with drug treatment include whether serum concentrations of drugs reach therapeutic concentrations, whether changes in medication are allowed (reflecting standard clinical practice), and whether studies reflect the natural course of depressive disorders.

OPTION | **SPECIFIC PSYCHOLOGICAL TREATMENTS PLUS DRUG TREATMENT**

We found evidence from RCTs suggesting that, in severe depression, the addition of drug treatment to interpersonal or cognitive therapy is more effective than either psychological therapy alone. No such effect was observed in mild to moderate depression.

Benefits: We found no systematic review. A non-systematic meta-analysis of six RCTs (595 people) found no advantage in combining drug and specific psychological treatments in mild to moderate depressive disorders, but that in more severe depressive disorders, combining drug and interpersonal therapy or cognitive therapy was more effective than interpersonal therapy or cognitive therapy alone.[45] One recent RCT compared nefazodone or cognitive behavioural–analysis psychotherapy alone with combination treatment in 681 adults with chronic depressive disorder.[46] At 12 weeks, the combined treatment improved the rate of clinical response (at least 50% reduction on the Hamilton Depression Rating Scale and a score of 15 or less, combined therapy v both single interventions, NNT 5, 95% CI 3 to 6).

Harms: We found no evidence of adverse effects.

Comment: A systematic review is needed to address this question.

OPTION **EXERCISE**

RCTs have found that exercise, alone or combined with other treatments, improves mild to moderate depression.

Benefits: We found one systematic review (published in 1990, search date not given), which examined exercise in depressive disorders. However, it was difficult to interpret because it included non-randomised studies and did not clearly describe participants.[47] One small RCT (156 people) compared aerobic exercise, sertraline hydrochloride (an SSRI), and combined treatment for 16 weeks. It found that all groups improved on continuous rating scales, but there was no significant difference in overall improvement between treatments.[48]

Harms: None reported.

Comment: None.

OPTION **BIBLIOTHERAPY**

We found limited evidence from a systematic review of RCTs that bibliotherapy (see glossary, p 663) may reduce mild depressive symptoms.

Benefits: We found one systematic review (published in 1997). It identified six small short term RCTs of bibliotherapy in 273 participants recruited by advertisement through the media and probably only mildly ill.[49] The mean effect size of bibliotherapy was 0.82 (95% CI 0.50 to 1.15). This means that 79% of control people had a worse outcome than the average member of the group receiving bibliotherapy.

Harms: None reported.

Comment: Further studies are needed in clinically representative groups.

OPTION **BEFRIENDING** New

Limited evidence from one small RCT found that befriending reduced symptoms of depression.

Benefits: We found one small RCT (86 people) of befriending (see glossary, p 663) of women with chronic depression in London. Initial identification was by postal screening of women registered with but not attending primary care.[50] It found that the befriended group were more likely to experience remission of symptoms at 13 months (65% with befriending v 39% with control; P < 0.05; NNT 4, 95% CI 2 to 18).

Harms: None recorded.

Comment: Less than half of the women screened were interested in befriending as a treatment option.

Mental health

RCTs have found that continuation treatment (see glossary, p 663) with antidepressant drugs for 4–6 months after recovery reduces risk of relapse.

Benefits: **Continuation treatment:** We found one systematic review (published in 1991, 6 RCTs, 312 people).[51] Continuation of antidepressant medication for 4–6 months after acute treatment reduced the relapse rate by nearly half (RR 0.6, 95% CI 0.4 to 0.7). Several more recent RCTs confirm this reduction in risk of early relapse with continuing antidepressant treatment for 6–12 months after acute treatment. **Maintenance treatment:** We found no adequate systematic review, but several RCTs have found that maintenance treatment reduced the relapse rate compared with placebo in recurrent depressive disorder. However, they all have problems with their methods (e.g. high withdrawal rates[52]), and will be considered for the next issue of *Clinical Evidence*. **Older adults:** We found one RCT that compared dothiepin versus placebo in 69 older people who had recovered sufficiently and consented to enter a 2 year trial of continuation treatment.[53] Dothiepin reduced the risk of relapse by 55% (RR 0.45, 95% CI 0.22 to 0.96).

Harms: Adverse effects seem to be similar to those reported in trials of acute treatment.

Comment: A systematic review is in progress.[54]

We found no evidence of a difference between treatments in terms of long term benefits. We found limited evidence that cognitive therapy may be an alternative to drug maintenance therapy in preventing relapse.

Benefits: We found one systematic review (published in 1998, search date not given), which identified eight small RCTs examining long term (at least 1 year) recovery or relapse rates after treatment had stopped. The trials compared cognitive therapy versus antidepressants in people with mainly mild to moderate depressive disorders.[41] Overall, 30% of people[16] treated with cognitive therapy relapsed compared with 60% of those treated with antidepressants. However, the number of people in these trials was too small for this trend to be significant. We found one small additional RCT (40 people) comparing cognitive therapy with normal clinical management for residual depressive symptoms in people who had responded to antidepressants. It also found that at 2 years fewer people relapsed with cognitive therapy than with antidepressants.[55]

Harms: See harms of prescription antidepressant drugs, p 656 and see table 2, p 667.

Comment: The review did not present data on the proportion of people who recovered and remained well in the long term. The largest RCT found that only a fifth of participants remained well over 18 months' follow up, and that there were no significant differences between interpersonal psychotherapy, cognitive therapy, or drug treatment.[43] It is possible that different people respond to different treatments. Further large scale comparative studies are needed of the long term effectiveness of treatments in people with all severities of depressive disorders.

GLOSSARY

Befriending Consists of a befriender meeting the patient to talk and socialise for at least 1 hour per week, acting as a friend.

Bibliotherapy Consists of advising people to read written material such as *Feeling good: the new mood therapy* by David Burns (New York: New American Library 1980).

Brief, non-directive counselling Aims to help people to express feelings and clarify thoughts and difficulties; therapist suggests alternative understandings and does not give direct advice but tries to encourage people to solve their own problems.

Cognitive therapy Brief (20 sessions over 12–16 weeks) structured treatment aimed at changing the dysfunctional beliefs and negative automatic thoughts that characterise depressive disorders. It requires a high level of training in the therapist.[56]

Continuation treatment Continuation of treatment after successful resolution of a depressive episode to prevent relapse.

Interpersonal psychotherapy Standardised form of brief psychotherapy (usually 12–16 weekly sessions) primarily intended for outpatients with unipolar non-psychotic depressive disorders. It focuses on improving the patient's interpersonal functioning and identifying the problems associated with the onset of the depressive episode.[57]

Maintenance treatment Long term treatment of recurrent depressive disorder to prevent the recurrence of further depressive episodes.

Problem solving Consists of three stages: (1) identifying the main problems for the patient; (2) generating solutions; (3) trying out the solutions. Potentially briefer and simpler than cognitive therapy and may be feasible in primary care.[43]

REFERENCES

1. Rosenstein, Leslie D. Differential diagnosis of the major progressive dementias and depression in middle and late adulthood: a summary of the literature of the early 1990s. *Neuropsychol Rev* 1998;8:109–167.
2. Katon W, Schulberg H. Epidemiology of depression in primary care. *Gen Hosp Psychiatry* 1992;14: 237–247.
3. Murray CJ, Lopez AD. Regional patterns of disability-free life expectancy and disability-adjusted life expectancy: global burden of disease study. *Lancet* 1997;349:1347–1352.
4. Murray CJ, Lopez AD. Alternative projections of mortality and disability by cause 1990–2020: global burden of disease study. *Lancet* 1997;349: 1498–1504.
5. Beekman ATF, Copeland JRM, Prince MJ. Review of community prevalence of depression in later life. *Br J Psychiatry* 1999;174:307–11.
6. Judd LL, Akiskal HS, Maser JD, et al. A prospective 12 year study of subsyndromal and syndromal depressive symptoms in unipolar major depressive disorders. *Arch Gen Psychiatry* 1988; 55:694–700.
7. American Psychiatric Association. *Diagnostic and statistical manual of mental disorders*, 4th ed. Washington, DC: American Psychiatric Association, 1994.
8. World Health Organization. *The ICD-10 classification of mental and behavioural disorders*. Geneva: World Health Organization, 1992.
9. Cole MG, Bellavance F, Mansour A. Prognosis of depression in elderly community and primary care populations: a systematic review and meta-analysis. *Am J Psychiatry* 1999;156:1182–1189.
10. Joffe R, Sokolov S, Streiner D. Antidepressant treatment of depression: a meta-analysis. *Can J Psychiatry* 1996;41:613–616. Search date not given; primary source Medline 1966 to June 1995.
11. Lima MS, Moncrieff J. A comparison of drugs versus placebo for the treatment of dysthymia: a systematic review. In: Cochrane library, Issue 3, 1998. Oxford: Update Software. Search date 1997; primary sources Biological Abstracts 1984 to 1997; Medline 1966 to January 1997; Psychlit 1974 to January 1997; Embase 1980 to January 1997; Lilacs 1982 to January 1997; Cochrane library; personal communication; conference abstracts; unpublished trials from the pharmaceutical industry; and book chapters on the treatment of depression.
12. Geddes JR, Freemantle N, Mason J, Eccles MP, Boynton J SSRIs versus other antidepressants for depressive disorder. In: The Cochrane Library, Issue 3, 2000. Oxford: Update software. Search

date 1999; primary source Medline, Embase, Cochrane Group Register of Controlled Trials, hand searches of reference lists of all located studies, and contact with manufacturers.

13. Anderson IM. Selective serotonin reuptake inhibitors versus tricyclic antidepressants: a meta-analysis of efficacy and tolerability. *J Affect Disord* 2000;58:19–36. Search date 1997; primary sources Medline, and hand searches of reference lists of meta-analyses and reviews.

14. Mulrow CD, Williams JW, Chiqueete E, et al. Efficacy of newer medications for treating depression in primary care patients. *Am Med J* 2000;108:54–64. Search date 1998; primary source Cochrane Depression Anxiety and Neurosis Group Specialised Register of Clinical Trials, hand searches of trials and 46 pertinent meta-analyses and consultation with experts.

15. Thompson C, Peveler RC, Stephenson D, et al. Compliance with antidepressant medication in the treatment of major depressive disorder in primary care: a randomized comparison of fluoxetine and a tricyclic antidepressant. *Am J Psychiatry* 2000; 157:338–343.

16. Thase ME, Trivedi MH, Rush AJ. MAOIs in the contemporary treatment of depression. *Neuropsychopharmacology* 1995;12:185–219. Search date not given; primary sources Medline and Psychological Abstracts 1959–July 1992.

17. Wilson K, Mottram P, Sivanthan A. A review of antidepressant drug trials in the treatment of older depressed people (protocol for a Cochrane Review). In: The Cochrane Library. Issue 4, 1998. Oxford: Update software. Search date June 1998; primary sources Cochrane Depression, Neurosis and Anxiety Review Group; hand searched journals, and reference lists. Review not to be published until 2001.

18. Gill D, Hatcher S. Antidepressants for depression in people with physical illness. In: The Cochrane Library, Issue 3, 2000. Oxford: Update software. Search date 1998; primary sources Medline, Cochrane Library Trials Register, Cochrane Depression and Neurosis Group Trials Register, and hand searches of two journals and reference lists.

19. Trindade E, Menon D. Selective serotonin reuptake inhibitors differ from tricyclic antidepressants in adverse events [abstract]. *Selective serotonin reuptake inhibitors (SSRIs) for major depression. Part I. Evaluation of the clinical literature.* Ottawa: Canadian Coordinating Office for Health Technology Assessment, 1997 August Report 3E. *Evidence-Based Mental Health* 1998;1:50. Search date 1996; primary sources Medline; Embase; PsycINFO; International Pharmaceutical Abstracts; Pascal; Health Planning and Administration; Mental Health Abstracts; Pharmacoeconomics and Outcomes News; Current Contents databases; scanning bibliographies of retrieved articles; hand searching journals; consulting researchers.

20. Mackay FJ, Dunn NR, Wilton LV, et al. A comparison of fluvoxamine, fluoxetine, sertraline and paroxetine examined by observational cohort studies. *Pharmacoepidemiol Drug Safety* 1997;6: 235–246.

21. Price JS, Waller PC, Wood SM, et al. A comparison of the post marketing safety of four selective serotonin reuptake inhibitors including the investigation of symptoms occurring on withdrawal. *Br J Clin Pharmacol* 1996;42:757–763.

22. Beasley CM Jr, Dornseif BE, Bosomworth JC, et al. Fluoxetine and suicide: a meta-analysis of controlled trials of treatment for depression. *BMJ* 1991;303:685–692. Search date not given; but included trials that had been completed/analysed by December 1989; primary sources not given in detail but based on clinical report form data from trials and data from the Drug Experience Network Database.

23. Jick SS, Dean AD, Jick H. Antidepressants and suicide. *BMJ* 1995;310:215–218.

24. Zajecka J, Fawcett J, Amsterdam J, et al. Safety of abrupt discontinuation of fluoxetine: a randomised, placebo controlled study. *J Clin Psychopharmacol* 1998;18:193–197.

25. Stahl MM, Lindquist M, Pettersson M, et al. Withdrawal reactions with selective serotonin reuptake inhibitors as reported to the WHO system. *Eur J Clin Pharmacol* 1997;53:163–169.

26. Wisner KL, Gelenberg AJ, Leonard H, et al. Pharmacologic treatment of depression during pregnancy. *JAMA* 1999;282:1264–1269. Search date 1999; primary sources Medline, Healthstar, hand searches of bibliographies of review articles, and discussions with investigators in the field.

27. Katon W, Von Korff M, Lin E, et al. Collaborative management to achieve treatment guidelines: impact on depression in primary care. *JAMA* 1995;273:1026–1031.

28. Simon GE, Vonkorff M, Rutter C, et al. Randomised trial of monitoring, feedback, and management of care by telephone to improve treatment of depression in primary care. *BMJ* 2000;320:550–554.

29. Wells KB, Sherbourne C, Schoenbaum M, et al. Impact of disseminating quality improvement programs for depression in managed primary care: a randomized controlled trial. *JAMA* 2000;283: 212–220.

30. Thompson C, Kinmonth AL, Stevens L, et al. Effects of a clinical-practice guideline and practice-based education on detection and outcome of depression in primary care: Hampshire Depression Project randomised controlled trial. *Lancet* 2000;355:185–191.

31. Linde K, Mulrow CD. St John's Wort for depression. In: The Cochrane Library. Issue 4, 1998. Oxford: Update software. Search date 1998; primary sources Medline 1983 to 1997; Embase 1989 to 1997; PsychLit 1987 to 1997; Psychindex 1987 to 1997; specialised databases: Cochrane Complementary Medicine Field, Cochrane Depression and Neurosis CRG, Phytodok; bibliographies of pertinent articles; manufacturers and researchers.

32. Ernst E, Rand JI, Barnes J, et al. Adverse effects profile of the herbal antidepressant St John Wort (*Hypericum perforatum L*) *Eur J Clin Pharmacol* 1998;54:589–594. Search date September 1997; primary sources AMED 1985 to September 1997; Cochrane Library 1997 Issue 2; Embase 1980 to September 1997, Medline 1996 to September 1997; handsearched reference lists; contacted WHO Collaborating Centre for International Drug Monitoring; UK Committee on Safety of Medicines and German Bundesinstitut f r Arzneimittel und Medizinproducte plus 12 German manufacturers of hypericum products.

33. Janicak PG, Davis JM, Gibbons RD, et al. Efficacy of ECT: a meta-analysis. *Am J Psychiatry* 1985; 142:297–302. Search date not given; primary source Medline.

34. Wijeratne GS, Halliday GS, Lyndon RW. The present status of electroconvulsive therapy: a systematic review. *Med J Austr* 1999;171:250–254. Search date 1998; primary source Medline 1987 to 1998.

35. Johnstone EC, Deakin JF, Lawler P, et al. The Northwick Park electroconvulsive therapy trial. *Lancet* 1980;1:1317–1320.

36. Brandon S, Cowley P, McDonald C, et al. Electroconvulsive therapy: results in depressive illness from the Leicestershire trial. *BMJ* 1984; 288:22–25.

37. Gregory S, Shawcross CR, Gill D. The Nottingham ECT study. A double-blind comparison of bilateral, unilateral and simulated ECT in depressive illness. *Br J Psychiatry* 1985;146:520–524.

38. Vaughan McCall W, Reboussin DM, Weiner RD, et al Titrated moderately suprathreshold vs fixed high-dose right unilateral electroconvulsive therapy. *Arch Gen Psychiatry* 2000;57:438–444 .

39. Sackeim HA, Prudic J, Devanand DP, et al. A prospective, randomized, double-blind comparison of bilateral and right unilateral electroconvulsive therapy at different stimulus intensities. *Arch Gen Psychiatry* 2000;57:425–434.

40. Scott AIF, Doris AB. Electroconvulsive therapy for depression (protocol). In: The Cochrane Library. Issue 4, 1998. Oxford: Update software.

41. Gloaguen V, Cottraux J, Cucherat M, et al. A meta-analysis of the effects of cognitive therapy in depressed patients 1998. *J Affect Disord* 1998; 49:59–72. Search date not given; primary sources Medline 1966 to December 1996; Embase 1966 to December 1996; references in books and papers; previous reviews and meta-analyses; abstracts from congress presentations; preprints sent by authors.

42. Elkin I, Shea MT, Watkins JT, et al. National Institute of Mental Health treatment of depression collaborative research program: general effectiveness of treatments. *Arch Gen Psychiatry* 1989;46:971–982.

43. Mynors-Wallis LM, Gath DH, Lloyd-Thomas, AR, et al. Randomised controlled trial comparing problem solving treatment with amitriptyline and placebo for major depression in primary care. *BMJ* 1995; 310:441–445.

44. Churchill R, Dewey M, Gretton V, et al. Should general practitioners refer patients with major depression to counsellors? A review of current published evidence. *Br J Gen Pract* 1999;49: 738–743.

45. Thase ME, Greenhouse JB, Frank E, et al. Treatment of major depression with psychotherapy or psychotherapy—pharmacotherapy combinations. *Arch Gen Psychiatry* 1997;54: 1009–1015. Pooled results of six research protocols conducted 1982 to 1992 at the Mental Health Clinical Research Center, University of Pittsburgh School of Medicine.

46. Keller MB, McCullough JP, Klein DN, et al. A comparison of nefazodone, the cognitive behavioral-analysis system of psychotherapy, and their combination for the treatment of chronic depression. *N Engl J Med* 2000;342:1462–1470.

47. North TC, McCullagh P, Tran ZV. Effect of exercise on depression. *Exerc Sport Sci Rev* 1990;18:379–415. Search date not given; primary sources dissertation abstracts online, ERIC, PsychInfo, Medline, books, abstracts from meetings to June 1989.

48. Blumenthal JA, Babyak MA, Moore KA, et al. Effects of exercise training on older patients with major depression. *Arch Intern Med* 1999;159: 2349–2356.

49. Cuijpers P. Bibliotherapy in unipolar depression: a meta-analysis. *J Behav Ther Exp Psychiatry* 1997; 28:139–147. Search date not given; primary sources Psychlit; Psychinfo; Medline.

50. Harris T, Brown GW, Robinson R. Befriending as an intervention for chronic depression among women in an inner city: Randomised controlled trial. *Br J Psychiatry* 1999;174:219–224.

51. Loonen AJ, Peer PG, Zwanikken GJ. Continuation and maintenance therapy with antidepressive agents: meta-analysis of research. *Pharm Week Sci* 1991;13:167–175. Search date not given; primary sources references of textbooks and review articles; Medline 1977 to 1988; Embase 1977 to 1988; review of reference lists of primary studies.

52. Keller MB, Kocsis JH, Thase ME, et al. Maintenance phase efficacy of sertraline for chronic depression: a randomized controlled trial. *JAMA* 1998;280:1665–1672.

53. Old age depression interest group. How long should the elderly take antidepressants? A double-blind placebo-controlled study of continuation/prophylaxis therapy with dothiepin. *Br J Psychiatry* 1993;162:175–182.

54. Carney S, Geddes J, Davies D, Furukawa T, Kupfer D, Goodwin G. Duration of treatment with antidepressants in depressive disorder (protocol). In: The Cochrane Library, Issue 3 2000. Oxford: Update software.

55. Fava GA, Rafanelli C, Grandi S, et al. Prevention of recurrent depression with cognitive behavioral therapy: preliminary findings. *Arch Gen Psychiatry* 1998;55:816–820.

56. Haaga DAF, Beck AT. Cognitive therapy. In: Paykel ES, ed. *Handbook of affective disorders*. Edinburgh: Churchill Livingstone, 1992:511–523.

57. Klerman GL, Weissman H. Interpersonal psychotherapy. In: Paykel ES, ed. *Handbook of affective disorders*. Edinburgh: Churchill Livingstone, 1992:501–510.

John Geddes

Senior Clinical Research Fellow/Honorary Consultant Psychiatrist

University of Oxford

Oxford

UK

Rob Butler

Lecturer in Old Age Psychiatry

Imperial College School of Medicine

London

UK

Competing interests: None declared.

TABLE 1	Adverse events (% of patients) with selective serotonin reuptake inhibitors (SSRIs) versus tricyclic antidepressants (TCAs) (see text, p 656).[20]	

Adverse effects	SSRIs event rates (%)	TCAs event rates (%)
Dry mouth	21	55
Constipation	10	22
Dizziness	13	23
Nausea	22	12
Diarrhoea	13	5
Anxiety	13	7
Agitation	14	8
Insomnia	12	7
Nervousness	15	11
Headache	17	14

TABLE 2 Effects of specific psychological treatments for depressive disorders (see text, p 660).

Intervention	Evidence	Benefits	Harms/disadvantages
Cognitive therapy	One systematic review identified 48 RCTs of psychological therapies (n = 2765 people, mainly outpatients in secondary care therefore probably with mild to moderate depression; people with psychotic or bipolar symptoms were excluded). Twenty RCTs compared cognitive therapy with waiting list or placebo and 17 compared it with drug treatment.[41]	79% of people in the placebo control group were more symptomatic than the average person treated with cognitive therapy (effect size 0.82, 95% CI 0.81 to 0.83).[41] 65% of people treated with cognitive therapy were less symptomatic than the average person treated with antidepressant drugs (effect size −0.38, 95% CI −0.39 to −0.37).[41]	No harms reported. Requires extensive training. Limited availability. RCTs in primary care suggest limited acceptability to some people.
Interpersonal psychotherapy	No systematic reviews. One large RCT, including people with mild to moderate depressive disorders, compared interpersonal psychotherapy versus drug treatment, cognitive therapy, or placebo plus clinical management of 16 weeks' duration.[41]	Recovery rates were: placebo-clinical management (21%); interpersonal psychotherapy (43%, NNT 5, 95% CI 3 to 19), imipramine (42%, NNT 5, 95% CI 3 to 22).[41]	No harms reported. Requires extensive training. Limited availability.
Problem solving therapy	No systematic reviews. Several small RCTs comparing problem solving versus drug treatment in primary care in people with mild depressive disorders.[43,44]	Problem solving was as effective as drug treatment.	No harms reported. Requires some training. Limited availability.
Non-directive counselling	One systematic review identified five RCTs comparing counselling with routine GP management in UK primary care.[44] The RCTs included people with depressive disorders. There is also a protocol registered with the Cochrane database.	No quantitative results provided in review. No consistent improvement in main outcomes, although studies report higher levels of satisfaction with treatment in counselling.	No harms reported. Requires some training. Limited availability.

Mental health

Search date October 2000: expanded this issue

Christopher Gale and Mark Oakley-Browne

INTERVENTIONS

Key Messages

- Two systematic reviews of RCTs have found that cognitive therapy is more effective than remaining on the waiting list, anxiety management training alone, or non-directive therapy. We found no evidence of adverse effects.

- One systematic review of RCTs comparing psychological treatments has not established or excluded a clinically important difference in the effects of applied relaxation and cognitive therapy.

- Two systematic reviews of RCTs have found that, compared with placebo, benzodiazepines are an effective and rapid treatment for generalised anxiety disorder (GAD). They increase the risk of dependence, sedation, industrial accidents, and road traffic accidents. They have been associated with neonatal and infant morbidity when used late in pregnancy or while breast feeding.

- One systematic review has found that buspirone increases physician rated improvement. Limited evidence from RCTs found no significant difference in benefits between busipirone, benzodiazepines, or antidepressants. Buspirone had slower onset than benzodiazepines but fewer adverse effects.

- One non-systematic review found no benefit from hydroxyzine.

- One RCT found no significant difference between abecarnil and placebo.

- RCTs have found that imipramine, trazodone, venlafaxine, and paroxetine are effective treatments. One RCT has found that paroxetine is more effective than a benzodiazepine. Adverse effects of antidepressants include sedation, confusion, and falls.

© *Clinical Evidence* 2001;5:668–678.

- One RCT in people with GAD found that trifluoperazine, an antipsychotic, reduced anxiety more than placebo, but caused more adverse effects.
- We found that β blockers have not been adequately evaluated in generalised anxiety disorder.

DEFINITION GAD is defined as excessive worry and tension, on most days, for at least 6 months, together with the following symptoms and signs: increased motor tension (fatigability, trembling, restlessness, muscle tension); autonomic hyperactivity (shortness of breath, rapid heart rate, dry mouth, cold hands, and dizziness) but not panic attacks; and increased vigilance and scanning (feeling keyed up, increased startling, impaired concentration). One non-systematic review of epidemiological and clinical studies found marked reduction of quality of life and psychosocial functioning in people with anxiety disorder (including generalised anxiety disorder).[1] It also found that (using the Composite Diagnostic International Instrument) people with GAD have low overall life satisfaction and some impairment in ability to fulfil roles and/or social tasks.[1]

INCIDENCE/ PREVALENCE Assessment of the incidence and prevalence is difficult. There is a high rate of comorbidity with other anxiety and depressive disorders.[2] The reliability of the measures used in epidemiological studies is unsatisfactory.[3] One US study, with explicit diagnostic criteria (DSM-III-R), estimated that 5% of people will develop GAD at some time during their lives.[4] The reliability of measures used in cross sectional studies to diagnose GAD are unsatisfactory.[2] A recent cohort study that followed people with depressive and anxiety disorders over 2 years found the diagnosis was consistently maintained in 49% of those initially diagnosed with GAD.[5] One recent non-systematic review found that the incidence of GAD in men is only half the incidence in women.[6] One non-systematic review of seven studies found reduced prevalence of anxiety disorders in older people.[7]

AETIOLOGY/ RISK FACTORS One community study and a clinical study have found GAD is associated with an increase in the number of minor stressors, independent of demographic factors,[8] but this finding was common in people with other diagnoses in the clinical population.[5] One non-systematic review (5 case control studies) of psychological sequelae to civilian trauma found rates of GAD reported in four of the five studies were increased significantly compared with a control population (rate ratio 3.3, 95% CI 2.0 to 5.5).[9]

PROGNOSIS GAD is a long term condition. It often begins before or during young adulthood and can be a lifelong problem. Spontaneous remission is rare.[4]

AIMS To reduce anxiety; to minimise disruption of day to day functioning; and to improve quality of life, with minimum adverse effects.

OUTCOMES Severity of symptoms and effects on quality of life, as measured by symptom scores, usually the Hamilton Anxiety Scale (HAM-A), State-Trait Anxiety Inventory, or Clinical Global Impression Symptom Scores. Where numbers needed to treat are given, these represent the number of people requiring treatment within a given time period (usually 6–12 weeks) for one additional person to achieve a certain improvement in symptom score. The method for obtaining numbers needed to treat was not standardised across studies. Some used a reduction by, for example, 20 points in the HAM-A as a response, others defined a response as a reduction, for example, by 50% of the premorbid score. We have not attempted to standardise methods, but instead have used the response rates reported in each study to calculate numbers needed to treat. Similarly, we have calculated numbers needed to harm from original trial data.

METHODS *Clinical Evidence* update search and appraisal October 2000. Recent changes in diagnostic classification make it hard to compare older studies with more recent ones. In the earlier classification system, DSM-III-R, the diagnosis was made only in the absence of other psychiatric disorder. In current systems (DSM-IV and ICD-10), GAD can be diagnosed in the presence of any comorbid condition. All drug studies were short term, at most 12 weeks.

QUESTION   What are the effects of cognitive therapy?

Two systematic reviews of RCTs have found that cognitive therapy, using a combination of behavioural interventions such as exposure, relaxation, and cognitive restructuring, is more effective than remaining on a waiting list (no treatment), anxiety management training alone, or non-directive therapy. One small subsequent RCT found cognitive behaviour therapy was slightly better than applied relaxation. We found no evidence of adverse effects.

Benefits: We found two systematic reviews.[10,11] The first (search date 1996, 35 RCTs, 4002 people, 60% women) of medical treatment, cognitive therapy, or both.[9] Thirteen RCTs included 22 cognitive behavioural therapies, which involved (alone or in combination) cognitive restructuring, relaxation training, exposure, and systematic desensitisation. Combined results from these RCTs found significantly better results with active treatment compared with control treatments (effect size 0.70, 95% CI 0.57 to 0.83). Controls included remaining on a waiting list, anxiety management training, relaxation training, and non-directive psychotherapy. One year follow up of an RCT found that cognitive therapy was associated with better outcomes than analytic psychotherapy and anxiety management training.[10,12] The second systematic review (search date 1998, 8 RCTs, 404 people) found that more people given individual cognitive therapy maintained recovery after 6 months than those given other treatments (participants maintaining recovery at 6 months: individual cognitive therapy 41%, non-directive therapy 19%, group cognitive therapy 18%, group behaviour therapy 12%, individual behaviour therapy 18%, and analytical psychotherapy 0%; P values not reported).[11] **Versus applied relaxation:** We found one subsequent RCT (36 people) of 12 sessions of cognitive therapy versus applied relaxation. It found a small significant difference in response rates (response defined as improvement to score 3 or 4 on cognitive global impression score, cognitive therapy 10/18 [56%] v applied relaxation 8/18 [44%]; RR 1.25, 95% CI 1.10 to 1.42; NNT 9, 95% CI 4 to 118).[13]

Harms: We found no evidence of adverse effects.

Comment: None.

We found no RCTs of applied relaxation (see glossary, p 677) versus placebo treatment. One systematic review of RCTs comparing applied relaxation with cognitive therapy found no significant difference in the proportion of people with clinically important improvement of their anxiety scores over 6 months. One subsequent RCT found cognitive therapy was slightly better than applied relaxation.

Benefits: **Versus placebo:** We found no systematic review or RCT. **Versus other psychological treatments:** We found one systematic review (search date 1998, 6 RCTs, 404 people) of psychological therapy in GAD.[11] The six RCTs all used the State-Trait Anxiety Inventory. There was significant variation in the type of cognitive therapy (group or individual) and in the comparison therapies (applied relaxation, analytical psychotherapy, behaviour therapy, and non-directive therapy). Only one of the six RCTs included a placebo group, and that RCT did not examine applied relaxation. Two RCTs included individual applied relaxation (38 people) and four included individual cognitive behavioural therapy (87 people). The systematic review compared arms across RCTs and analysed the raw data from individual studies to calculate the proportion of people who experienced a clinically significant change after treatment and maintained that improvement until 6 months after treatment. Applied relaxation was more likely than individual cognitive behavioural therapy to improve the anxiety inventory after 6 months (52% with applied relaxation v 41%).[11] No statistical tests of significance were performed by the systematic review, but even if the figures presented are taken at face value (see comment below) then the difference between the effects of individual applied relaxation and individual cognitive behavioural therapy may have arisen by chance (recovery maintained to 6 months: AR 20/38 [52%] with applied relaxation v 41/87 [47%] with cognitive therapy; RR 1.1, 95% CI 0.8 to 1.6). We found one subsequent RCT (see cognitive therapy, p 670).

Harms: No evidence of harms was noted.

Comment: The State-Trait Anxiety Inventory covers only a restricted range of symptoms, and it may not satisfactorily reflect treatment outcomes in GAD. It is very difficult to interpret the results of the systematic review because the comparison involves arms from different RCTs. This removes the benefit of randomisation because the groups being compared may have different characteristics. The figures presented in the systematic review produce estimates of relative effectiveness with wide confidence intervals: a clinically important difference has not been established or excluded.

OPTION BENZODIAZEPINES

One systematic review of RCTs has found that, compared with placebo, benzodiazepines are an effective and rapid treatment for GAD. They increase the risk of dependence, sedation, industrial accidents, and road

Generalised anxiety disorder

traffic accidents. **If used in late pregnancy or while breast feeding, they can cause adverse effects in neonates. One RCT found no significant difference between sustained release alprazolam and bromazepam. One RCT found no evidence of a difference in effectiveness between benzodiazepines and buspirone. One systematic review of RCTs, which looked at long term treatment, found no good evidence that any short term benefit of benzodiazepines was sustained.**

Benefits:

Versus placebo: We found one systematic review (search date 1996, 24 RCTs, benzodiazepines [19 RCTs], buspirone [9 RCTs], antidepressants [ritanserin and imipramine, 3 RCTs], all in people with GAD).[10] Pooled analysis for benzodiazepines found a mean effect size of 0.70 (no 95% CIs available) compared with results from all RCTs of 0.60 (95% CI 0.50 to 0.70). The review found no significant differences in effect sizes between different benzodiazepines, although there was insufficient power to rule out a clinically important difference. **Versus each other:** One subsequent RCT (121 people) compared sustained release alprazolam with bromazepam and found no significant difference in effects (HAM-A scores).[14] **Versus buspirone:** See buspirone, p 673. **Versus abecarnil:** See abecarnil, p 674. **Long term treatment:** We found one systematic review (search date 1998, 8 RCTs, any benzodiazepine medication, greater than 2 months' duration, people with GAD). The weak methods of these RCTs prevent firm conclusions being made.[15]

Harms:

Sedation and dependence: Benzodiazepines have been found to cause impairment in attention, concentration, and short term memory. One RCT found an increased rate of drowsiness (71% with diazepam v 13% with placebo; P = 0.001) and dizziness (29% v 11%; P = 0.001).[10] Sedation can interfere with concomitant psychotherapy. Rebound anxiety on withdrawal has been reported in 15–30% of participants.[16] There is a high risk of substance abuse and dependence with benzodiazepines. **Memory:** Thirty one people with agoraphobia/panic disorder from an RCT of 8 weeks' alprazolam versus placebo were reviewed after 3.5 years. Five people were still taking benzodiazepines and had significant impairment in memory tasks.[17] There was no difference in memory performance between those who had been in the placebo group and those who had been given alprazolam but were no longer taking the drug. **Road traffic accidents:** We found one systematic review (search date 1997) examining the relation between benzodiazepines and road traffic accidents.[18] In the case control studies, the odds ratio for death or emergency medical treatment in those who had taken benzodiazepines compared with those who had not taken them ranged from 1.45 to 2.4. The odds ratio increased with higher doses and more recent intake. In the police and emergency ward studies, benzodiazepine use was a factor in 1–65% of accidents (usually 5–10%). In two studies in which participants had blood alcohol concentrations under the legal limit, benzodiazepines were found in 43% and 65%. For drivers over 65 years, the risk of being involved in reported road traffic accidents was higher if they had taken longer acting and larger quantities of benzodiazepines. These results are from case control studies and are therefore subject to confounding factors. **Pregnancy and breast feeding:** One systematic review (search date 1997) of 23 case series and reports found no association between cleft lip and palate and use of benzodiazepines in the first trimester of pregnancy.[19] However, one non-systematic review found that use of benzodiazepines in late pregnancy is associated with neonatal hypotonia and withdrawal syndrome.[20] Benzodiazepines are secreted in breast milk, and there have been reports of sedation and hypothermia in infants.[20]

Other: One non-systematic industry funded review of eight RCTs of benzodiazepines versus placebo or buspirone, found consistent improvement with benzodiazepines. However, recent use of benzodiazepines limited the effectiveness of buspirone.[21]

Comment: All the benzodiazepine studies were short term (at most 12 weeks). There was usually a significant improvement at 6 weeks, but response rates were given at the end of the RCTs.

OPTION	BUSPIRONE

RCTs have found that, compared with placebo, buspirone increases the proportion of people who improve clinically in the short term. Limited evidence from RCTs found no significant differences in the benefits of buspirone, benzodiazepines, or antidepressants. Buspirone had slower onset than benzodiazepines but had fewer adverse effects.

Benefits: **Versus placebo:** We found one systematic review of buspirone (search date 1996, 9 studies), but it did not report on effects as distinct from pharmacotherapy in general.[10] One of the included studies was itself a non-systematic industry funded meta-analysis of eight placebo controlled RCTs of buspirone in 520 people with GAD (see comment below). It found that, compared with placebo, buspirone was associated with a greater response rate, defined as the proportion of people much or very much improved as rated by their physician (54% v 28%, $P \leq 0.001$). A subsequent double blind RCT (162 people with GAD) of busprone versus placebo found similar results (buspirone 55% v placebo 35%, $P < 0.05$).[22] A non-systematic re-analysis by the manufacturer of pooled data from eight RCTs (735 people) found a differential response to buspirone depending on whether the participant had been exposed to benzodiazepines (no previous exposure to benzodiazepine: response rate 62% [buspirone] v 31% [placebo]; recent benzodiazepine use: response rate 41% [buspirone] v 21% [placebo]). The latter result was not significant.[21] **Versus benzodiazepines:** The systematic review did not directly compare buspirone with benzodiazepines. One large RCT (230 people) included in the review found no significant difference between buspirone and benzodiazepines.[11] A recent reanalysis of eight RCTs found no significant difference in the effects of buspirone compared with benzodiazepines.[21] **Versus antidepressants:** See antidepressants, p 675. **Versus hydroxyzine:** See hydroxyzine, p 674.

Harms: **Sedation and dependence:** The systematic review found that, compared with benzodiazepines, buspirone had a slower onset of action but fewer adverse effects.[10] The subsequent RCT found that, compared with placebo, buspirone caused significantly more nausea (34% v 13%), dizziness (64% v 12%), and somnolence (19% v

7%). We found no reports of dependency on buspirone. **Pregnancy and breast feeding:** We found no evidence.

Comment: All RCTs in the industry sponsored meta-analysis were sponsored by pharmaceutical companies and had been included in new drug applications for buspirone as an antidepressant. Other search criteria were not given. RCT methods were similar.[10]

| OPTION | HYDROXYZINE | New |

We found one non-systematic review, which found no benefit with hydroxyzine.

Benefits: **Versus placebo:** We found one non-systematic review (2 RCTs, 1344 people).[23] The first RCT (100 people) found a significantly greater reduction in HAM-A scores on hydroxyzine 50 mg daily versus placebo. The second RCT (244 people) compared hydroxyzine versus buspirone versus placebo. It found that hydroxyzine (50 mg daily) versus placebo had no significant effect on the number of people with a HAM-A reduction of 50% or greater (AR 42% with hydroxyzine v 29% with placebo; RR 1.4). **Versus buspirone:** It also found hydroxyzine versus busprione had no significant effect on the number of people with a HAM-A reduction of 50% or greater (AR 42% with hydroxyzine v 36% with buspirone; RR 1.2).

Harms: The second RCT (244 people) found significantly more somnolence (9.9% v 0%), and headaches (6.1% v 1.2%) in people taking hydroxyzine compared with placebo.[23] Overall adverse effects were reported in 39.5% of people taking hydroxyzine versus 37.5% taking buspirone versus 28.4% taking placebo.

Comment: None.

| OPTION | ABECARNIL | New |

One RCT found no significant difference between abecarnil and placebo.

Benefits: We found one multicentre RCT (310 people) comparing abecarnil (7.5–17.5 mg daily) versus diazepam (15–35 mg daily), and versus placebo.[24] No dichotomous outcomes were reported. At 6 weeks there was no significant difference between placebo and abecarnil in HAM-A scores or clinical improvement. However, diazepam was significantly better than placebo ($P < 0.05$) for clinical improvement.

Harms: Abecarnil was associated with significantly more drowsiness (47% v 14%; NNH 3), dizziness (16% v 3%; NNH 8), irritability (9% v 3%; NNH 16), equilibrium loss (5% v 0%; NNH 20); and decreased libido (5% v 0%; NNH 20).

Comment: None.

OPTION ANTIDEPRESSANTS

RCTs have found that imipramine, trazodone, venlafaxine, and paroxetine are effective treatments for GAD. Individual RCTs found that they were more effective than benzodiazepines, with no evidence of a difference in effectiveness compared with buspirone. There is a significant risk of sedation, confusion, and falls with these drugs.

Benefits: **Versus placebo:** We found one systematic review (search date 1996, 3 placebo controlled RCTs)[10] and two subsequent RCTs. The review found antidepressants to be significantly associated with a greater response than placebo (pooled effect size 0.57).[10] The review pooled results for trazodone, imipramine, and ritanserin, so limiting the conclusions that may be drawn for trazodone and imipramine alone.[10] In another placebo controlled RCT (230 people) the number needed to treat for moderate or pronounced improvement after 8 weeks of treatment with imipramine was 3 (completer analysis calculated from data by author; withdrawal rates unknown). With trazodone the number needed to treat was 4 (95% CI 3 to 4, calculated from data by author).[25] We found three RCTs comparing venlafaxine extended release versus placebo.[26–28] The first RCT (365 people) compared 75 mg daily and 150 mg daily versus buspirone 30 mg daily or placebo over 8 weeks. Treatment with both doses of venlafaxine found a significant improvement in adjusted HAM-A scores against placebo. Response was defined as a 50% reduction in HAM-A and "very much improved" or "much improved" on the Clinical Global Improvement Scale. There was no significant difference in response rate for 75 mg daily versus placebo (43/87 [49%] v 35/98 [36%]; RR 1.4, 95% CI 0.94 to 2.04) or 150 mg daily versus placebo (44/89 [49%]; RR 1.4, 95% CI 0.94 to 2.04). The second RCT compared three venlafaxine regimens (75 mg daily, 150 mg daily, and 225 mg daily) versus placebo over 8 weeks. It found significant improvements in HAM-A, and on the Hospital Anxiety and Depression scale. All doses were significantly better than placebo and were not significantly different from each other.[27] There was no significant difference in Clinical Global Impression Scale. Clinical response was not reported. The third RCT (261 people) compared venlafaxine 75–225 mg daily versus placebo over a 6 month period. Intention to treat analysis (last observation carried forward, 44/127 [35%] on placebo and 60/124 [48%] on venlafaxine completed) found a significant response in both HAM-A and Clinical Global Impression Scale, sustained over the 6 months (42% response with venlafaxine v 21% with placebo, response defined as a reduction of 40% on baseline HAM-A score). We were unable, because of the nature of the analysis and reporting, to calculate relative risk or number needed to treat with meaningful confidence intervals. **Versus benzodiazepines:** We found one RCT (81 people with GAD) comparing paroxetine, imipramine, and 2'-chlordesmethyldiazepam for 8 weeks.[29] Paroxetine and imipramine were significantly more effective than 2'-chlordesmethyldiazepam in improving anxiety scores (mean HAM-A after 8 weeks 11.1 for paroxetine, 10.8 for imipramine, 12.9 for 2'-chlordesmethyldiazepam; P = 0.05). **Versus buspirone:** We found no systematic review. We found one RCT (365 people) comparing venlafaxine 75 mg and 150 mg a day with buspirone 30 mg a day over 8 weeks, with a small placebo arm. All treatments were significantly better than placebo but there was no significant difference between them (venlafaxine 75 mg versus placebo, NNT 8, 95% CI 6 to 9; venlafaxine 150 mg versus placebo, NNT 7, 95% CI 6 to 9; buspirone 30 mg versus placebo, NNT 11, 95% CI 10 to 12).[26] **Sedating tricyclic antidepressants:** We found no systematic review or RCTs evaluating sedating tricyclics in people with GAD.

Harms: Sedation, confusion, dry mouth, and constipation have been reported with both imipramine and trazodone.[25] Nausea, somnolence, dry mouth, sweating, constipation, anorexia, and sexual dysfunction have been reported with venlafaxine. Most of the adverse effects (apart from dizziness and sexual dysfunction) decreased over 6 months in those who continued to take the medication, which (over 6 months) was the minority.[28] **Overdose:** In a series of 239 coroner directed necropsies from 1970 to 1989, tricyclic antidepressants were considered to be a causal factor in 12% of deaths and hypnosedatives (primarily benzodiazepines and excluding barbiturates) in 8% of deaths.[30] **Accidental poisoning:** Tricyclic antidepressants are a major cause of accidental poisoning.[31] A study estimated that there was one death for every 44 children admitted to hospital after ingestion of tricyclic antidepressants.[32] **Hyponatraemia:** One case series reported 736 incidents of hyponatraemia in people taking selective serotonin reuptake inhibitors (SSRIs); 83% of episodes were in hospital inpatients aged over 65 years.[33] It is not possible to establish causation from this type of data. **Nausea:** There have been case reports of nausea in people taking paroxetine.[29] **Falls:** One retrospective cohort study (2428 elderly residents of nursing homes) found an increased risk of falls in new users of antidepressants (adjusted RR for tricyclic antidepressants: 2.0, 95% CI 1.8 to 2.2, 665 people; for SSRIs: 1.8, 95% CI 1.6 to 2.0, 612 people; and for trazodone: 1.2, 95% CI 1.0 to 1.4, 304 people).[34] The increased rate of falls persisted through the first 180 days of treatment and beyond. One case control study (8239 people aged, 66 years or older, treated in hospital for hip fracture) found an increased risk of hip fracture in those taking antidepressants (adjusted odds ratio, SSRIs 2.4, 95% CI 2.0 to 2.7; secondary amine tricyclic antidepressants such as nortriptyline 2.2, 95% CI 1.8 to 2.8; and tertiary amine tricyclic antidepressants such as amitriptyline 1.5, 95% CI 1.3 to 1.7).[35] This study could not control for confounding factors; people taking antidepressants may be at increased risk of hip fracture for other reasons. **In pregnancy:** We found no reports of harmful effects in pregnancy. One case controlled study found no evidence that imipramine or fluoxetine increased the rate of malformations in pregnancy.[36]

Comment: None.

OPTION   **ANTIPSYCHOTIC DRUGS**

One RCT found that 4 weeks treatment with trifluoperazine lowered anxiety more than placebo but caused more adverse effects.

Benefits: We found no systematic review. We found one RCT (415 people) comparing 4 weeks of trifluoperazine treatment 2–6 mg a day versus placebo.[37] The RCT found that trifluoperazine versus placebo reduced the score on the total anxiety rating scale of HAM-A (difference 14 points; $P < 0.001$).

Harms: Cohort studies have found short term treatment with antipsychotic drugs increased sedation, acute dystonias, akathisia, and parkinsonism. Cohort studies found that in the longer term, rates of tardive dyskinesia are increased the more often treatment is interrupted.[38]

Comment: None.

OPTION β BLOCKERS

We found no good evidence of β blockers in people with GAD.

Benefits: We found no systematic review or good RCTs of β blockers in people with GAD.

Harms: We found no good evidence in people with GAD.

Comment: None.

GLOSSARY
Applied relaxation A technique involving imagination of relaxing situations to induce muscular and mental relaxation.

Substantive changes since last issue
Cognitive therapy versus applied relaxation One new small subsequent RCT found cognitive behaviour therapy was better than applied relaxation.[13]
Antidepressants Two new RCTs;[27,28] conclusions unchanged.

REFERENCES

1. Mendlowicz MV, Stein MB. Quality of life in individuals with anxiety disorders. *Am J Psychiatry* 2000;157:669–682.
2. Judd LL, Kessler RC, Paulus MP, et al. Comorbidity as a fundamental feature of generalised anxiety disorders: results from the national comorbidity study (NCS). *Acta Psychiatr Scand* 1998;98(suppl 393):6–11.
3. Andrews G, Peters L, Guzman AM, Bird K. A comparison of two structured diagnostic interviews: CIDI and SCAN. *Aust N Z J Psychiatry* 1995;29:124–132.
4. Jessker RC, McGonagle KA, Zhao S, et al. Lifetime and 12-month prevalence of DSM-III-R psychiatric disorders in the United States: results from the national comorbidity survey. *Arch Gen Psychiatry* 1992;51:8–19.
5. Seivewright N, Tyrer P, Ferguson B, Murphy S, Johnston T. Longitudinal study of the influence of life events and personality status on diagnostic change in three neurotic disorders. *Depression Anx* 2000;11:105–113.
6. Pigott T. Gender differences in the epidemiology and treatment of anxiety disorders. *J Clin Psychiatry* 1999;60(suppl 18):15–18.
7. Jorm AF. Does old age reduce the risk of anxiety and depression? A review of epidemiological studies across the adult life span. *Psychol Med* 2000;30:11–22.
8. Brantley PJ, Mehan DJ, Ames SC, Jones GN. Minor stressors and generalized anxiety disorders among low income patients attending primary care clinics. *J Nerv Ment Dis* 1999;187:435–440.
9. Brown ES, Fulton MK, Wilkeson A, Petty F. The psychiatric sequelae of civilian trauma. *Comp Psychiatry* 2000;41:19–23.
10. Gould RA, Otto MW, Pollack MH, Yap L. Cognitive behavioural and pharmacological treatment of generalised anxiety disorder: a preliminary meta-analysis. *Behav Res Ther* 1997;28:285–305. Search date January 1996; primary sources Psychlit 1974 to 1996; Medline 1966 to January 1996; examination of reference lists; and unpublished articles presented at national conferences.
11. Fisher PL, Durham RC. Recovery rates in generalized anxiety disorder following psychological therapy: an analysis of clinically significant change in the STAI-T across outcome studies since 1990. *Psychol Med* 1999;29:1425–1434. Search date: December 1998; primary sources Medline 1987 to December 1998; Psychlit 1987 to December 1998; and Cochrane Controlled Trials Register 1987 to December 1998.
12. Durham RC, Fisher PL, Trevling LR, Hau CM, Richard K, Stewart JB. One year follow-up of cognitive therapy, analytic psychotherapy and anxiety management training for generalised anxiety disorder: symptom change, medication usage and attitudes to treatment. *Behav Cogn Psychother* 1999;27:19–35.
13. Ost L, Breitholts E. Applied relaxation vs. cognitive therapy in the treatment of generalized anxiety disorder. *Behav Res Ther* 2000;38:777–790.
14. Figueira ML. Alprazolam SR in the treatment of generalised anxiety: a multicentre controlled study

with bromazepam. *Hum Psychother* 1999;14: 171–177.

15. Mahe V, Balogh A. Long-term pharmacological treatment of generalized anxiety disorder. *Int Clin Psychopharmacol* 2000;15:99–105. Search date 1998; primary sources Medline, Biosis, Embase.

16. Tyrer P. Current problems with the benzodiazepines. In: Wheatly D, ed. *The anxiolytic jungle: where next?* Chichester: J Wiley and Sons, 1990;23–60.

17. Kilic C, Curran HV, Noshirvani H, Marks IM, Basoglu MB. Long-term effects of alprazolam on memory: a 3.5 year follow-up of agoraphobia/panic patients. *Psychol Med* 1999;29:225–231.

18. Thomas RE. Benzodiazepine use and motor vehicle accidents. Systematic review of reported association. *Can Fam Physician* 1998;44:799–808. Search date 1997; primary sources Medline 1980 to 1997.

19. Dolovich LR, Addis A, Regis Vaillancourt JD, et al. Benzodiazepine use in pregnancy and major malformations of oral cleft: meta-analysis of cohort and case-control studies. *BMJ* 1998;317: 839–843. Search date December 1998; primary sources Medline 1966 to 1997; Embase 1980 to 1997; Reprotox, references of included studies and review articles.

20. Bernstein JG. *Handbook of drug therapy in psychiatry*, 3rd ed. St Louis, Missouri: Mosby Year Book, 1995;401.

21. DeMartinis N, Rynn M, Rickels K, Mandos L. Prior benzodiazepine use and buspirone response in the treatment of generalized anxiety disorder. *J Clin Psychiatry* 2000;61:91–94.

22. Sramek JJ, Transman M, Suri A, et al. Efficacy of buspirone in generalized anxiety disorder with coexisting mild depressive symptoms. *J Clin Psychiatry* 1996;57:287–291.

23. Lader M, Anxiolytic effect of hydroxyzine: A double-blind trial versus placebo and buspirone. *Hum Psychopharmacol Clin Exp* 1999;14;S94–S102.

24. Rickels K, DeMartinis N, Aufdembrinke B. A double-blind, placebo controlled trial of abecarnil and diazepam in the treatment of patients with generalized anxiety disorder. *J Clin Psychopharmacol* 2000:20:12–18.

25. Rickels K, Downing R, Schweizer E, Hassman H. Antidepressants for the treatment of generalized anxiety disorder: a placebo-controlled comparison of imipramine, trazodone and diazepam. *Arch Gen Psychiatry* 1993;50:884–895.

26. Davidson JR, DuPont RL, Hedges D, Haskins JT. Efficacy, safety and tolerability of venlafaxine extended release and busperone in outpatients with generalised anxiety disorder. *J Clin Psychiatry* 1999;60:528–535.

27. Rickels K, Plooack MH, Sheehan D, Haskins J. Efficacy of extended-release venlafaxine in nondepressed outpatients with generalized anxiety disorder. *Am J Psychiatry* 2000;157:968–974.

28. Gelenberg A, Lydiard R, Rudolph R, Aguiar L, Haskins J, Salinas E. Efficacy of venlafaxine extended releases capsules in nondepressed outpatients with generalized anxiety disorder: a 6-month randomized controlled trial. *JAMA* 2000; 283:3082–3088.

29. Rocca P, Fonzo V, Scotta M, Zanalda E, Ravizza L. Paroxetine efficacy in the treatment of generalized anxiety disorder. *Acta Psychiatr Scand* 1997;95: 444–450.

30. Dukes PD, Robinson GM, Thomson KJ, Robinson BJ. Wellington coroner autopsy cases 1970–89: acute deaths due to drugs, alcohol and poisons. *N Z Med J* 1992;105:25–27. (Published erratum appears in *N Z Med J* 1992;105:135.)

31. Fraser NC. Accidental poisoning deaths in British children 1958–77. *BMJ* 1980;280:1595–1598.

32. Pearn J, Nixon J, Ansford A, Corcoran A. Accidental poisoning in childhood: five year urban population study with 15 year analysis of fatality. *BMJ* 1984;288:44–46.

33. Lui BA, Mitmann N, Knowles SR, Shear NH. Hyponatraemia and the syndrome of inappropriate secretion of antidiuretic hormone associated with the use of selective serotonin reuptake inhibitors: a review of spontaneous reports. *Can Med Assoc J* 1995;155:519–527.

34. Thapa PB, Gideon P, Cost TW, Milam AB, Ray WA. Antidepressants and the risk of falls among nursing home residents. *N Engl J Med* 1998;339: 875–882.

35. Liu B, Anderson G, Mittmann N, To T, Axcell T, Shear N. Use of selective serotonin-reuptake inhibitors or tricyclic antidepressants and risk of hip fractures in elderly people. *Lancet* 1998;351: 1303–1307.

36. Kulin NA, Pastuszak A, Koren G. Are the new SSRIs safe for pregnant women? *Can Fam Physician* 1998;44;2081–2083.

37. Mendels J, Krajewski TF, Huffer V, et al. Effective short-term treatment of generalized anxiety with trifluoroperazine. *J Clin Psychiatry* 1986;47:170–174.

38. Van Harten PN, Hoek HW, Matroos GE, Koeter M, Kahn RS. Intermittent neuroleptic treatment and risk of tardive dyskinesia: Curacao extrapyramidal syndromes study III. *Am J Psychiatry* 1998;155: 565–567.

Christopher Gale
Psychiatrist

Mark Oakley-Browne
Associate Professor

Department of Psychiatry
University of Auckland
Auckland
New Zealand

Competing interests: CG has been paid by Eli Lilly, the manufacturer of Prozac, to attend one symposium. MOB has been reimbersed by Eli Lilly for attending a conference and for running an educational programme.

Search date January 2001: expanded this issue

G Mustafa Soomro

QUESTIONS

INTERVENTIONS

Beneficial

Likely to be beneficial

To be covered in future issues of *Clinical Evidence*
Other forms of psychotherapy
Other drug monotherapies
Adjuvant/augmentation drug treatment
Psychosurgery
Electroconvulsive treatment
Treatment in children and adolescents

See glossary, p 685

Key Messages

- Three systematic reviews have found that serotonin reuptake inhibitors improve symptoms more than placebo. One double blind placebo study found that most participants relapsed within weeks of stopping treatment.

- We found limited evidence from one RCT that sertraline is more effective than clomipramine at reducing symptoms. One systematic review and one RCT found no significant difference between clomipramine and other serotonin reuptake inhibitors. However, clomipramine has more adverse effects than selective serotonin reuptake inhibitors, particularly cholinergic and cardiac effects.

- One systematic review has found that behavioural therapy improves symptoms compared with relaxation. Two follow up studies found that improvement was maintained for up to 2 years.

- We found limited evidence from data pooling within a systematic review and one RCT that found that cognitive therapy is as effective as behavioural therapy.

- One systematic review found no evidence of a difference between serotonin reuptake inhibitors and behavioural therapy.

- We found limited evidence from RCTs that behavioural therapy plus fluvoxamine is more effective than behavioural therapy alone.

DEFINITION Obsessive compulsive disorder (OCD) is characterised by obsessions, compulsions, or both, which cause significant personal
distress or social dysfunction, but are not caused by drugs or
physical disorder. **Obsessions** are defined as recurrent and persistent ideas, images, or impulses that cause pronounced anxiety and
which the person perceives to be self produced. **Compulsions** are
intentional repetitive behaviours or mental acts performed in
response to obsessions or according to certain rules, and are aimed
at reducing distress or preventing certain imagined dreaded events.
Obsessions and compulsions are usually recognised as pointless
and are resisted by the person. There are minor differences in the
criteria for OCD between the third, revised third, and fourth editions
of the *Diagnostic and Statistical Manual* (DSM-III, DSM-III-R, and
DSM-IV).[1]

INCIDENCE/ One national, community based survey of OCD in the UK (1993,
PREVALENCE 10 000 people) found prevalence to be 1% in men and 1.5% in
women.[2] In the USA, the lifetime prevalence of OCD was found to
be between 1.9 and 3.3% in 1984 (18 500 people).[3] One international study found lifetime prevalence to be 3% in Canada, 3.1% in
Puerto Rico, 0.3–0.9% in Taiwan, and 2.2% in New Zealand.[2]

AETIOLOGY/ Aetiology is unknown. Behavioural, cognitive, genetic, and neuro-
RISK FACTORS biological factors are implicated.[4–10]

PROGNOSIS One study that followed 144 people for an average of 47 years
found that an episodic (see glossary, p 685) course was more
common during the initial years (about 1–9 years), whereas a
chronic (see glossary, p 685) course was more common afterwards.[11] Over time, the study found that 39–48% of people showed
symptomatic improvement. A 1 year prospective cohort study found
46% of people to have an episodic course and 54% to have a
chronic course.[12]

AIMS To improve symptoms and to reduce impact of illness on social
functioning and quality of life.

OUTCOMES Severity of symptoms; adverse effects of treatment; and social
functioning. The most commonly used instruments for measuring
symptoms are the Yale–Brown Obsessive Compulsive Scale and the
National Institute of Mental Health's Global Obsessive Compulsive
Scale, both of which are observer rated and well validated.[13–16]
Most trials use a 25% decrease in Yale–Brown Scale scores from
baseline as indicative of clinically significant improvement. Some
studies use a 35% reduction.[16]

METHODS *Clinical Evidence* update search and appraisal January 2001.

QUESTION What are the effects of treatments in adults?

OPTION SEROTONIN REUPTAKE INHIBITORS

Three systematic reviews and two subsequent RCTs have found good evidence that serotonin reuptake inhibitors are more effective than placebo in reducing symptoms. Apart from limited evidence from one RCT that sertraline is more effective than clomipramine, we found no evidence of different efficacy between serotonin reuptake inhibitors. One systematic review and two subsequent RCTs have found that serotonin reuptake inhibitors are more effective than other kinds of antidepressants. RCTs have found clomipramine to be associated with more adverse effects than selective serotonin reuptake inhibitors (see glossary, p 686). One follow up study found that most people relapsed within a few weeks of stopping drug treatment. Two small RCTs found reduced symptoms from combined antipsychotics with serotonin reuptake inhibitors in people who had not responded to serotonin reuptake inhibitors alone.

Benefits: **Serotonin reuptake inhibitors versus placebo:** We found three systematic reviews and two subsequent RCTs. All found overall benefit of treatment versus placebo.[17-21] The first review (search date 1994, 9 RCTs, 668 people, mean treatment duration 12 weeks) compared clomipramine (a non-selective serotonin reuptake inhibitor — see glossary, p 686) versus placebo. Two RCTs were in 73 children, but the review did not give separate effect sizes.[18] This review found treatment to be more effective than placebo at reducing symptoms (WMD 1.31, 95% CI 1.15 to 1.47). The first review found fluoxetine, fluvoxamine, and sertraline (selective serotonin reuptake inhibitors) to be more effective than placebo (fluoxetine: 1 RCT, 287 people, WMD 0.57, 95% CI 0.33 to 0.81; fluvoxamine: 3 RCTs, 395 people, WMD 0.57, 95% CI 0.37 to 0.77; sertraline: 3 RCTs, 270 people, WMD 0.52, 95% CI 0.27 to 0.77).[17] The second review (search date not stated) pooled data from eight placebo controlled RCTs of clomipramine (4 trials included in the first review; total of 1131 people with OCD).[18] It found clomipramine to be more effective than placebo (WMD 1.31, CI not given). The third review (search date 1997, 3 RCTs, 338 people) found paroxetine (a selective serotonin reuptake inhibitor) to be more effective than placebo over 12 weeks (WMD 0.48, 95% CI 0.24 to 0.72).[19] The first subsequent double blind RCT (350 people) compared fluoxetine 20 mg a day (87 people) versus 40 mg a day (89 people) versus 60 mg a day (90 people) versus placebo (84 people).[20] It found that people on all doses of fluoxetine improved significantly more than people on placebo (improvement on the Yale–Brown Scale: fluoxetine 20 mg 19.5%; 40 mg 22.1%; 60 mg 26.6%; placebo 3.3%; CI not given; all P values v placebo ≤0.001). It also found a significant dose related response (P < 0.001). The second subsequent double blind RCT (164 people) found that sertraline was significantly more effective than placebo in reducing symptoms (P < 0.01, mean reduction on the Yale–Brown Scale 9 points with sertraline and 4 points with placebo, CI not given).[21] **Serotonin reuptake inhibitors versus each other:** The first review (85 people, 3 RCTs) found no significant difference in the improvement of obsessive compulsive symptoms between clomipramine and selective serotonin reuptake inhibitors (fluoxetine or fluvoxamine; WMD −0.04, 95% CI −0.43 to +0.35).[17] One subsequent double blind RCT of clomipramine (82 people) versus sertraline (86 people) found sertraline to be more effective (associated with an 8% greater mean reduction in obsessive compulsive symptoms; P = 0.036).[22] A second subsequent double blind RCT (133 people) compared clomipramine with fluvoxamine.[23] It found no significant difference in mean improvement in symptoms (improvement on the Yale–Brown Scale clomipramine 50.2% v fluvoxamine 45.6%; CI and P value not given). **Serotonin reuptake inhibitors versus other antidepressants:** The first systematic review identified seven RCTs comparing clomipramine with non-serotonin reuptake inhibitor antidepressants (147 people with OCD; 2 trials [67 people] in children/adolescents without separate results).[17] This review found clomipramine to be more likely to reduce symptoms (WMD 0.65, 95% CI 0.36 to 0.92). One subsequent RCT of fluoxetine (17 people) versus phenelzine (19 people) versus placebo (18 people) found the largest effect from fluoxetine (WMD not given, mean reduction in symptoms was 15% fluoxetine, 9% phenelzine, and 1% placebo).[24] A second subsequent double blind RCT compared sertraline (79 people) with desipramine (85 people) in people with concurrent OCD and major depressive disorder.[25] It found sertraline to be more effective at reducing obsessive compulsive and depressive symptoms. The response rate for improvement in obsessive compulsive symptoms (≥ 40% improvement on Yale–Brown Scale) was 48% with sertraline versus 31% with desipramine (CI not given, P = 0.01). There was no significant difference in response rate for depressive symptoms (≥ 50% improvement on Hamilton Rating Scale for Depression), but the remission rate (defined as a score ≤ 7 on Hamilton Rating Scale for Depression) was significantly better with sertraline (49% v 35%, CI not given; P = 0.04). **Serotonin reuptake inhibitors versus behavioural therapy:** We found weak evidence from the third systematic review, which included mixed method studies (number of studies and people not stated).[19] This review found no significant difference between effect sizes of serotonin reuptake inhibitors and behavioural therapy (see glossary, p 685) when compared with placebo, but did not make direct comparisons.[19] **In people who do not respond to serotonin treatment alone:** We found two small RCTs that assessed combined antipsychotics and serotonin reuptake inhibitors in people who did not respond to serotonin treatment alone.[26,27] The first RCT (34 people) compared fluvoxamine plus haloperidol (maximum daily dose of haloperidol 10 mg) versus fluvoxamine plus placebo in people with OCD (with or without tic disorder or depression) who had not responded to 8-week treatment with fluvoxamine.[26] It found that those in the combined haloperidol plus fluvoxamine arm were significantly more likely to have met two out of three different response criteria (11/17 [65%] with combined haloperidol plus fluvoxamine v 0/17 [0%] with fluvoxamine plus placebo; NNT 2, 95% CI 2 to 3; P < 0.0002). The second RCT (36 people), comparing 6 weeks of serotonin reuptake inhibitor plus risperidone versus serotonin reuptake inhibitor plus placebo in people who did not respond to 12 weeks of serotonin reuptake inhibitor, found that those in the risperidone group had fewer symptoms of OCD (reduction in the Yale–Brown Scale 36% v 9%, P = 0.001) and depression and anxiety (reduction in the Hamilton Scale for depression 35% v 20%, P = 0.002; for anxiety 31% v 12%, P = 0.007).[27] As in the previous study, people in the combined risperidone arm were more likely to have met two of the response criteria (8/18 [44%] with risperidone plus serotonin reuptake inhibitor v 0/15 [0%] with placebo plus serotonin reuptake inhibitor; NNT 2, 95% CI 2 to 3; P < 0.005).

Harms: **Serotonin reuptake inhibitor adverse effects:** In the second review, 16 RCTs found a greater incidence of adverse effects with serotonin reuptake inhibitors than placebo (RRI 54% for clomipramine, 11% for fluoxetine, 19% for fluvoxamine, and 27% for sertraline).[18] The third systematic review of controlled and uncontrolled studies found the withdrawal rate due to adverse effects to be 11% for clomipramine, 10% for fluoxetine, 13% for fluvoxamine, 9% for sertraline, and 11% for paroxetine.[19] Anticholinergic adverse effects (dry mouth, blurred vision, constipation, and urinary retention), cardiac adverse effects, drowsiness, dizziness, and convulsions (convulsions usually at doses > 250 mg/day) have been reported to be most common with clomipramine,[28–30] whereas selective serotonin reuptake inhibitors are associated with fewer adverse effects but more nausea, diarrhoea, anxiety, agitation, insomnia, and headache.[27] Both clomipramine and selective serotonin reuptake inhibitors were associated with weight change and sexual dysfunction.[28,30] The subsequent RCT comparing sertraline (79 people) with desipramine (85 people) found more people discontinued because of adverse effects with desipramine (26% v 10%, P = 0.009).[25] One non-systematic review identified three prospective cohort studies and five surveys, which found fluoxetine during pregnancy did not significantly increase the risk of spontaneous abortion or major malformation (figures not provided).[31] It included one prospective cohort study (174 people) and three surveys, which suggested similar outcomes from other selective serotonin reuptake inhibitors (sertraline, paroxetine, or fluvoxamine). One prospective cohort study (55 people) found preschool age children exposed to fluoxetine *in utero* showed no significant differences from children not exposed in global IQ, language, or behaviour. It included no information on long term harms for the other selective serotonin reuptake inhibitors. **In people who do not respond to serotonin treatment alone:** The study assessing the effect of augmentation of serotonin reuptake inhibitors with risperidone found that common adverse effects were experienced by at least 10% people. Adverse effects included sedation, restlessness, increased appetite, dry mouth, and tinnitus.[27] Risperidone is also commonly associated with hypotension and prolactinaemia. Extrapyramidal adverse effects are more common with haloperidol, which can also cause prolactinaemia.

Comment: The first systematic review also identified two small RCTs, which found no difference in the effects of placebo and non-serotonin reuptake inhibitors (imipramine and nortriptyline).[17] One small, observer blinded RCT of fluvoxamine (10 people) versus paroxetine (9 people) versus citalopram (11 people) found no significant differences in the effects of these drugs, but the study was too small to exclude a clinically significant effect.[32] **Duration and discontinuation of treatment:** Most RCTs assessed efficacy over 10–12 weeks.[30,33] One prospective, 1 year study found that further significant improvement occurred in the 40-week open label extension, with some continuing adverse effects.[34] One placebo substitution study of clomipramine found that 16 (89%) of 18 people relapsed within 7 weeks of placebo treatment.[35] **Effects on people without depression:** The first systematic review found that serotonin reuptake inhibitors reduced symptoms in people without depression (5 RCTs including 594 people; WMD 1.37, 95% CI 1.19 to 1.55).[17] **Factors predicting outcome:** Four RCTs found that people who did not respond to treatment had younger age of onset, longer duration of the condition, higher frequency of symptoms, co-existing personality disorders, and a greater likelihood of previous hospital admission. Predictors of good response were older age of onset, history of remissions, no previous drug treatment, more severe OCD, and either high or low score on the Hamilton Depression Rating Scale.[36–39] Two cohort studies of people with OCD found that poor response to serotonin reuptake inhibitors was predicted by concomitant schizotypal personality disorder (see glossary, p 686), by tic disorder (see glossary, p 686), and also by severe OCD with cleaning rituals (OR 4.9, 95% CI 1.1 to 21.2).[40,41] The nonsystematic review of effects in pregnancy may have been systematic but did not make explicit how articles were selected.[31]

| OPTION | BEHAVIOURAL THERAPY AND COGNITIVE THERAPY |

One systematic review has found that behavioural therapy is associated with greater symptom reduction than relaxation. The review found limited evidence of no significant difference in symptom reduction between cognitive therapy and behavioural therapy (see glossary, p 685). We found limited evidence that behavioural therapy plus fluvoxamine is more effective than behavioural therapy alone. One RCT found no significant difference between cognitive therapy alone and cognitive therapy plus fluvoxamine. Two follow up studies found that after behavioural therapy, significant improvement was maintained for up to 2 years, but that some people required additional behavioural therapy.

Benefits: **Behavioural therapy versus relaxation:** We found one systematic review (search date not stated), which pooled results from two RCTs (121 people with OCD, further characteristics not specified).[18] It found that behavioural therapy reduced symptoms more than relaxation (WMD 1.18, P < 0.01, CI not given; 88% of people in the relaxation group did worse than the average improvement on behavioural therapy).[18] **Behavioural therapy versus cognitive therapy:** The same systematic review pooled results from four RCTs (92 people with OCD, further characteristics not specified). It found no significant difference in reduction of symptoms between behavioural therapy and cognitive therapy (WMD –0.19, CI not available).[18] **Combination treatment:** We found weak evidence from one systematic review (search date 1997).[19] It pooled data from mixed method studies (number of studies and people not given) and compared three different regimens with placebo: behavioural therapy plus serotonin reuptake inhibitors; behavioural therapy alone; and serotonin reuptake inhibitors alone. The review found similar reductions in symptoms, but did not make direct comparisons between treatments.[19] One RCT (99 people in an outpatient setting) compared behavioural therapy, cognitive therapy, behavioural therapy plus fluvoxamine, and cognitive therapy plus fluvoxamine.[42] It found no significant differences in outcomes on the Yale–Brown Scale (mean reduction in symptoms 32% with behavioural therapy, 47% with cognitive therapy, 49% with behavioural therapy plus fluvoxamine, 43% with cognitive therapy plus fluvoxamine). One double blind RCT (49 people in a hospital setting) found significantly greater improvement in symptoms with behavioural therapy plus fluvoxamine than with behavioural therapy plus pill placebo (88% v 60% achieved a ≥35% reduction on the Yale–Brown Scale; RR 0.3, 95% CI 0.1 to 0.96; NNT 3).[43] **Maintenance of improvement:** One prospective follow up of 20 people with OCD (specific diagnostic criteria not given) from a 6 month RCT of behavioural therapy found that 79% maintained improvement in obsessive compulsive symptoms at 2 year follow up.[44] One prospective non-inception cohort study of behavioural therapy in 21 people with OCD (specific diagnostic criteria not given) found that after the initial 2 weeks of treatment, 68–79% maintained complete or much improvement in symptoms at 3 months' follow up.[45] However, in both studies, some people required additional behavioural therapy during the follow up period.

Harms: We found no evidence from RCTs or cohort studies of adverse effects from behavioural or cognitive therapy. Case reports have described unbearable and unacceptable anxiety in some people receiving behavioural therapy.

Comment: **Factors predicting outcome:** We found two RCTs of behavioural therapy (total 96 people, duration 2.5 months and 32 weeks) and two retrospective cohort studies (total 346 people, duration 1 year and 11 weeks).[46–49] These found poorer outcome to be predicted by initial severity, depression, longer duration, poorer motivation, and dissatisfaction with the therapeutic relationship. Good outcome was predicted by early adherence to "exposure homework" (that is, tasks to be carried out outside regular therapy sessions involving contact with anxiety provoking situations), employment, living with one's family, no previous treatment, having fear of contamination, overt ritualistic behaviour, and absence of depression.[46–48] Good outcome for women was predicted by having a co-therapist (someone usually related to the person, who is enlisted to help with treatment outside regular therapy sessions; OR 19.5, 95% CI 2.7 to 139.3).[49] Two systematic reviews of drug, behavioural, cognitive, and combination treatments for OCD are being prepared.

GLOSSARY

Behavioural therapy Consists of exposure to the anxiety provoking stimuli and prevention of ritual performance.

Chronic Continuous course without periods of remission since first onset.

Cognitive therapy Aims to correct distorted thoughts (such as exaggerated sense of harm and personal responsibility) by Socratic questioning, logical reasoning, and hypothesis testing.

Episodic Episodic course with periods of remission since first onset.

Obsessive compulsive disorder

Non-selective serotonin reuptake inhibitor Clomipramine (also classed as a tricyclic antidepressant).

Schizotypal personality disorder Characterised by discomfort in close relationships, cognitive and perceptual distortions, and eccentric behaviour.

Selective serotonin reuptake inhibitors Fluoxetine, fluvoxamine, sertraline, paroxetine, citalopram.

Tic disorder Characterised by motor tics, vocal tics, or both.

Substantive changes since last issue

Serotonin reuptake inhibitors Two new RCTs[26,27] found limited evidence for combining antipsychotics and serotonin reuptake inhibitors in people who do not respond to serotonin reuptake inhibitor treatment alone.

REFERENCES

1. American Psychiatric Association. *Diagnostic and statistical manual of mental disorders*, 4th ed. Washington, DC: American Psychiatric Association, 1994.
2. Bebbington PE. Epidemiology of obsessive–compulsive disorder. *Br J Psychiatry* 1998; 35(suppl):2–6.
3. Karno M, Golding JM, Sorenson SB, Burnam MA. The epidemiology of obsessive–compulsive disorder in five US communities. *Arch Gen Psychiatry* 1988;45:1094–1099.
4. Baer L, Minichiello WE. Behavior therapy for obsessive–compulsive disorder. In: Jenike MA, Baer L, Minichiello WE, eds. *Obsessive–compulsive disorders*. St Louis: Mosby, 1998.
5. Steketee GS, Frost RO, Rheaume J, Wilhelm S. Cognitive theory and treatment of obsessive–compulsive disorder. In: Jenike MA, Baer L, Minichiello WE, eds. *Obsessive–compulsive disorders*. St Louis: Mosby, 1998.
6. Alsobrook JP, Pauls DL. The genetics of obsessive–compulsive disorder. In: Jenike MA, Baer L, Minichiello WE, eds. *Obsessive–compulsive disorders*. St Louis: Mosby, 1998.
7. Rauch SL, Whalen PJ, Dougherty D, Jenike MA. Neurobiologic models of obsessive compulsive disorder. In: Jenike MA, Baer L, Minichiello WE, eds. *Obsessive–compulsive disorders*. St Louis: Mosby, 1998.
8. Delgado PL, Moreno FA. Different roles for serotonin in anti-obsessional drug action and the pathophysiology of obsessive–compulsive disorder. *Br J Psychiatry* 1998;35(suppl):21–25.
9. Saxena S, Brody AL, Schwartz JM, Baxter LR. Neuroimaging and frontal–subcortical circuitry in obsessive–compulsive disorder. *Br J Psychiatry* 1998;35(suppl):26–37.
10. Rauch SL, Baxter LR Jr. Neuroimaging in obsessive–compulsive disorder and related disorders. In: Jenike MA, Baer L, Minichiello WE, eds. *Obsessive–compulsive disorders*. St Louis: Mosby, 1998.
11. Skoog G, Skoog I. A 40-year follow up of patients with obsessive–compulsive disorder. *Arch Gen Psychiatry* 1999;56:121–127.
12. Ravizza L, Maina G, Bogetto F. Episodic and chronic obsessive–compulsive disorder. *Depress Anxiety* 1997;6:154–158.
13. Goodman WK, Price LH, Rasmussen SA, et al. The Yale–Brown obsessive compulsive scale. I. Development, use, and reliability. *Arch Gen Psychiatry* 1989;46:1006–1011.
14. Insel TR, Murphy DL, Cohen RM, Alterman I, Kilts C, Linnoila M. Obsessive–compulsive disorder. A double-blind trial of clomipramine and clorgyline. *Arch Gen Psychiatry* 1983;40:605–612.
15. Goodman WK, Price LH, Rasmussen SA, et al. The Yale–Brown obsessive compulsive scale. II. Validity. *Arch Gen Psychiatry* 1989;46:1012–1016.
16. Goodman WK, Price LH. Rating scales for obsessive–compulsive disorder. In: Jenike MA, Baer L, Minichiello WE, eds. *Obsessive–compulsive disorders*. St Louis: Mosby, 1998.
17. Piccinelli M, Pini S, Bellantuono C, Wilkinson G. Efficacy of drug treatment in obsessive–compulsive disorder. A meta-analytic review. *Br J Psychiatry* 1995;166:424–443. Search dates 1975 to May 1994; primary sources Medline and Excerpta Medica-Psychiatry.
18. Abramowitz JS. Effectiveness of psychological and pharmacological treatments for obsessive–compulsive disorder: a quantitative review. *J Consult Clin Psychol* 1997;65:44–52. Search date not given; primary sources Medline and PsycLIT.
19. Kobak KA, Greist JH, Jefferson JW, Katzelnick DJ, Henk HJ. Behavioral versus pharmacological treatments of obsessive compulsive disorder: a meta-analysis. *Psychopharmacology (Berl)* 1998; 136:205–216. Search date May 1997; primary sources Medline, PsycINFO, Dissertations, and Abstracts International databases.
20. Tollefson GD, Rampey AH, Potvin JH, et al. A multicenter investigation of fixed-dose fluoxetine in the treatment of obsessive–compulsive disorder. *Arch Gen Psychiatry* 1994;51:559–567.
21. Kronig MH, Apter J, Asnis G, et al. Placebo controlled multicentre study of sertraline treatment for obsessive–compulsive disorder. *J Clin Psychopharmacol* 1999;19:172–176.
22. Bisserbe JC, Lane RM, Flament MF. A double blind comparison of sertraline and clomipramine in outpatients with obsessive–compulsive disorder. *Eur Psychiatry* 1997;12:82–93.
23. Mundo E, Maina G, Uslenghi C. Multicentre, double-blind, comparison of fluvoxamine and clomipramine in the treatment of obsessive–compulsive disorder. *Int Clin Psychopharmacol* 2000;15:69–76.
24. Jenike MA, Baer L, Minichiello WE, Rauch SL, Buttolph ML. Placebo-controlled trial of fluoxetine and phenelzine for obsessive–compulsive disorder. *Am J Psychiatry* 1997;154:1261–1264.
25. Hoehn-Saric R, Ninan P, Black DW, et al. Multicenter double-blind comparison of sertraline and desipramine for concurrent obsessive–compulsive and major depressive disorders. *Arch Gen Psychiatry* 2000;57:76–82.
26. McDougle CJ, Goodman WK, Leckman JF, et al. Haloperidol addition in fluvoxamine-refractory obsessive–compulsive disorder. A double-blind, placebo-controlled study in patients with and without tics. *Arch Gen Psychiatry* 1994;51(4):302–308.

27. McDougle CJ, Epperson CN, Pelton GH, Wasylink S, Price LH. A double-blind, placebo-controlled study of risperidone addition in serotonin reuptake inhibitor-refractory obsessive-compulsive disorder. Arch Gen Psychiatry 2000;57:794–801.

28. British National Formulary. London: British Medical Association and Royal Pharmaceutical Society of Great Britain, 1999.

29. Trindade E, Menon D. Selective serotonin reuptake inhibitors differ from tricyclics antidepressants in adverse events (Abstract). Selective serotonin reuptake inhibitors for major depression. Part 1. Evaluation of clinical literature. Ottawa: Canadian Coordinating Office for Health Technology Assessment, August 1997 Report 3E. Evid Based Ment Health 1998;1:50.

30. Jenike MA. Drug treatment of obsessive-compulsive disorders. In: Jenike MA, Baer L, Minichiello WE, eds. Obsessive-compulsive disorders. St Louis: Mosby, 1998:469–532.

31. Goldstein DJ, Sundell K. A review of safety of selective serotonin reuptake inhibitors during pregnancy. Hum Psychopharmacol Clin Exp 1999; 14:319–324.

32. Mundo E, Bianchi L, Bellodi L. Efficacy of fluvoxamine, paroxetine, and citalopram in the treatment of obsessive-compulsive disorder: a single-blind study. J Clin Psychopharmacol 1997; 17:267–271.

33. Rauch SL, Jenike MA. Pharmacological treatment of obsessive compulsive disorder. In: Nathan PE, Gorman JM, eds. Treatments that work. New York: Oxford University Press, 1998:359–376.

34. Rasmussen S, Hackett E, DuBoff E, et al. A 2-year study of sertraline in the treatment of obsessive-compulsive disorder. Int Clin Psychopharmacol 1997;12:309–316.

35. Pato MT, Zohar-Kadouch R, Zohar J, Murphy DL. Return of symptoms after discontinuation of clomipramine in patients with obsessive-compulsive disorder. Am J Psychiatry 1988;145: 1521–1525.

36. Ravizza L, Barzega G, Bellino S, Bogetto F, Maina G. Predictors of drug treatment response in obsessive-compulsive disorder. J Clin Psychiatry 1995;56:368–373.

37. Cavedini P, Erzegovesi S, Ronchi P, Bellodi L. Predictive value of obsessive-compulsive personality disorder in antiobsessional pharmacological treatment. Eur Neuropsychopharmacol 1997;7:45–49.

38. Ackerman DL, Greenland S, Bystritsky A. Clinical characteristics of response to fluoxetine treatment of obsessive-compulsive disorder. J Clin Psychopharmacol 1998;18:185–192.

39. Ackerman DL, Greenland S, Bystritsky A, Morgenstern H, Katz RJ. Predictors of treatment response in obsessive-compulsive disorder: multivariate analyses from a multicenter trial of clomipramine. J Clin Psychopharmacol 1994;14: 247–254.

40. Mundo E, Erzegovesi S, Bellodi L. Follow up of obsessive-compulsive patients treated with proserotonergic agents (letter). J Clin Psychopharmacol 1995;15:288–289.

41. Alarcon RD, Libb JW, Spitler D. A predictive study of obsessive-compulsive disorder response to clomipramine. J Clin Psychopharmacol 1993;13: 210–213.

42. van Balkom AJ, de Haan E, van Oppen P, et al. Cognitive and behavioral therapies alone versus in combination with fluvoxamine in the treatment of obsessive compulsive disorder. J Nerv Ment Dis 1998;186:492–499.

43. Hohagen F, Winkelmann G, Rasche-Ruchle H, et al. Combination of behaviour therapy with fluvoxamine in comparison with behaviour therapy and placebo. Results of a multicentre study. Br J Psychiatry 1998;35(suppl):71–78.

44. Marks IM, Hodgson R, Rachman S. Treatment of chronic obsessive-compulsive neurosis by in-vivo exposure. A two-year follow up and issues in treatment. Br J Psychiatry 1975;127:349–364.

45. Foa EB, Goldstein A. Continuous exposure and complete response prevention in obsessive-compulsive neurosis. Behav Ther 1978;9:821–829.

46. Keijsers GP, Hoogduin CA, Schaap CP. Predictors of treatment outcome in the behavioural treatment of obsessive-compulsive disorder. Br J Psychiatry 1994;165:781–786.

47. De Araujo LA, Ito LM, Marks IM. Early compliance and other factors predicting outcome of exposure for obsessive-compulsive disorder. Br J Psychiatry 1996;169:747–752.

48. Buchanan AW, Meng KS, Marks IM. What predicts improvement and compliance during the behavioral treatment of obsessive compulsive disorder? Anxiety 1996;2:22–27.

49. Castle DJ, Deale A, Marks IM, et al. Obsessive-compulsive disorder: prediction of outcome from behavioural psychotherapy. Acta Psychiatr Scand 1994;89:393–398.

G Mustafa Soomro
Honorary Research Fellow
Section of Community Psychiatry
St George's Hospital Medical School
London
UK

Competing interests: None declared.

Post-traumatic stress disorder

Search date September 2000

Jonathan Bisson

QUESTIONS

INTERVENTIONS

Key Messages

Prevention

- One systematic review of RCTs found no evidence that debriefing prevents post-traumatic stress disorder (PTSD), and one RCT found that it was associated with an increased risk of PTSD at 1 year.

- We found conflicting evidence on the effects of multiple episode intervention. One RCT found no evidence of benefit from multiple episode psychological intervention. Two small RCTs found that five sessions of either cognitive behavioural therapy or prolonged exposure are superior to supportive counselling for preventing PTSD in people with acute stress disorder after a traumatic event.

- One RCT found evidence of more benefit from one to six sessions of cognitive behavioural therapy than from standard care.

Treatment

- Evidence from mainly small RCTs suggests benefit from specific psychological treatments compared with supportive counselling, relaxation therapy, or no treatment.

- One systematic review of mainly small RCTs has found that antidepressants reduce symptoms more than placebo. We found insufficient evidence on the effects of antipsychotic drugs or carbamazepine.

- One RCT found sertraline to be more effective than placebo.

DEFINITION	PTSD occurs after a major traumatic event. Symptoms include upsetting thoughts and nightmares about the traumatic event, avoidance behaviour, numbing of general responsiveness, increased irritability, and hypervigilance.[1]
INCIDENCE/ PREVALENCE	One large cross sectional study in the USA found that one in 10 women and one in 20 men experience PTSD at some stage in their lives.[2]
AETIOLOGY/ RISK FACTORS	Risk factors include major trauma such as rape, a history of psychiatric disorders, acute distress and depression after the trauma, lack of social support, and personality factors (such as neuroticism).[3]
PROGNOSIS	One large cross sectional study in the USA found that over a third of sufferers continued to satisfy the criteria for a diagnosis of PTSD 6 years after diagnosis.[2] Cross sectional studies provide weak evidence about prognosis.
AIMS	To reduce initial distress after a traumatic event; to prevent PTSD and other psychiatric disorders; to reduce levels of distress in the long term; and to improve function and quality of life.
OUTCOMES	Presence or absence of PTSD and severity of symptoms. Scoring systems include impact of event scale and clinician administered PTSD scale.
METHODS	*Clinical Evidence* update search and appraisal September 2000.

QUESTION   **What are the effects of preventive psychological interventions?**

One systematic review of RCTs found no evidence that single episode interventions prevent PTSD, and one of these RCTs found an increased risk of PTSD at 1 year. We found conflicting evidence on the effects of multiple episode intervention from four RCTs. One RCT found no significant evidence of benefit, one found that five episodes of cognitive behavioural therapy (see glossary, p 692) were superior to supportive counselling (see glossary, p 693), and one found five episodes of prolonged exposure (see glossary, p 693) were superior to supportive counselling.

Benefits: **Single episode intervention ("debriefing"):** We found one systematic review (search date 1999), which identified eight RCTs comparing early single episode interventions ("debriefing") with no intervention in 607 people.[4] The trials used psychological debriefing (see glossary, p 693) or similar techniques. The review found that more people treated with debriefing still had PTSD at 3–5 months but the difference was not significant (OR [3–5 months] 1.2, 95% CI 0.7 to 2.1; OR [12 months] 2.0, 95% CI 0.9 to 4.5). One of the trials followed people for 1 year after debriefing and found that debriefing versus no treatment was associated with increased rates of PTSD (OR 2.9, 95% CI 1.1 to 7.5). **Multiple episode intervention:** We found no systematic review. We found four RCTs. The first RCT (151 people) compared three to six sessions of educational and cognitive behavioural techniques with no psychological intervention.[5] Intervention began at least 1 month after a road traffic accident. There were no significant differences in outcomes between groups. The second RCT (24 people) compared five sessions of cognitive behavioural therapy with five sessions of supportive counselling in people with acute stress disorder within 2 weeks of a road accident or industrial accident.[6] Cognitive behavioural therapy was associated with a large reduction in the number of people who met PTSD diagnostic criteria immediately after treatment (8% v 83% with supportive counselling, P < 0.001) and at 6 months (17% v 67% with supportive counselling, P < 0.05).[7] The third RCT (66 survivors of road accidents or non-sexual assault with acute stress disorder) evaluated five 90 minute sessions of prolonged exposure (see glossary, p 693) versus supportive counselling versus prolonged exposure plus anxiety management. Immediately after completion of treatment, significantly lower rates of PTSD were found in the prolonged exposure group (14%) and in the prolonged exposure plus anxiety management group (20%) compared with the supportive counselling group (56%). The differences were still significant at 6 months' follow up (15% v 23% v 67%).[8] The fourth RCT (132 French bus drivers who had been attacked)[9] compared one to six sessions of cognitive behavioural therapy with standard care. At 6 months' follow up, the reductions in anxiety (7.4 to 6.2 v 7.0 to 6.9) and intrusive symptoms (10.9 to 7.7 v 7.2 to 4.5) were significantly greater in the treatment group, but there were no statistically significant differences in depression (3.6 to 3.2 v 3.6 to 3.3) or avoidance symptoms (11.0 to 9.5 v 8.4 to 7.3).

Harms: Two trials of single episode intervention found an increased risk of subsequent psychological problems in people receiving the intervention. However, initial traumatic exposure had been higher in these people.[4]

Comment: The systematic review found that the overall quality of the RCTs was poor.[4] Problems included lack of blinding, failure to state loss to follow up, and lack of intention to treat analysis despite high withdrawal rates. There are also methodological problems with the multiple episode studies.

| QUESTION | What are the effects of psychological treatments? |

Mainly small RCTs found evidence of benefit from specific psychological treatments compared with supportive counselling, relaxation therapy (see glossary, p 693), or no treatment.

Benefits: We found one systematic review of psychological treatments for PTSD (search date not given, published in 1998, 17 RCTs, 690 people).[7] The RCTs compared a range of specific psychological treatments versus supportive treatment or no intervention. All trials found that psychological treatment was associated with a greater improvement in immediate outcome (using a composite score of PTSD symptoms, anxiety, and depression) compared with supportive counselling or no treatment (overall effect size immediately after treatment 0.54, 95% CI not stated). The difference was still evident at 1 year (overall effect size from 12 RCTs with long term follow up

0.53, CI not stated). **Cognitive behavioural treatments:** We found one systematic review (search date not given) and two subsequent RCTs.[7,10,11] The review identified 14 RCTs of cognitive behavioural treatments in people with PTSD. Although many were of poor quality, all described a positive effect compared with no treatment. One RCT (45 people) in the review evaluated three types of cognitive therapy and found that all were better than no treatment at 3 months (effect sizes compared with no treatment: stress inoculation 1.1, 95% CI 0.66 to 1.5; supportive counselling 0.55, 95% CI 0.17 to 0.94; prolonged exposure therapy 1.67, 95% CI 1.2 to 2.1).[12] One subsequent RCT (87 people) compared exposure, cognitive therapy, or both, with relaxation therapy.[10] The trial found that all cognitive behavioural treatments reduced symptoms of PTSD more than relaxation therapy, immediately and at 3 months (53 people assessed; no intention to treat analysis performed).[13] The second subsequent RCT (54 people) found that 39% of people continued to suffer from PTSD 1 year after 16 1 hour sessions of imaginal exposure therapy or cognitive therapy. There was no difference in the prevalence of PTSD between the two treatment groups.[11] **Eye movement desensitisation and reprocessing (EMDR):** We found one systematic review (search date 1999, 16 RCTs, 563 people).[14] Two RCTs found EMDR (see glossary, p 693) as effective as exposure therapy, three found that EMDR was more effective than relaxation therapy, and three found that EMDR was more effective than remaining on a waiting list. Five RCTs considered EMDR with and without eye movements. In two RCTs, eyes moving was more effective than eyes fixed. In three RCTs there was no difference. **Affect management:** We found one RCT comparing psychotherapy plus drug treatment with or without affect management (see glossary, p 692) in 48 women. The trial found that symptom control was greater with affect management.[15] The withdrawal rate was high (31%) and the analysis was not by intention to treat. **Other psychological treatments:** We found one RCT (112 people), which found no significant difference between psychodynamic psychotherapy (see glossary, p 693), exposure therapy, and hypnotherapy (see glossary, p 693). However, all were slightly better than remaining on the waiting list (no treatment control). The trial did not quantify results.[16] One RCT (42 police officers)[17] evaluated brief eclectic psychotherapy (which combines components of cognitive behavioural therapy and psychodynamic therapy) over 16 sessions of treatment. The treatment group fared better than a waiting list control after treatment (9% v 50% remained PTSD positive), and at 3 months' follow up (4% v 65% remained PTSD positive). **Inpatient treatment programme:** We found no RCTs. **Drama therapy:** See glossary, p 692. We found no RCTs.

Harms: The RCTs gave no information on harms. Overall, cognitive behavioural therapy seems well tolerated. However, there have been case reports in some people of imaginal flooding (a form of cognitive behavioural therapy) worsening symptoms, leading to calls for caution when assessing people for treatment.[18]

Comment: Most RCTs were of poor quality.

Post-traumatic stress disorder

QUESTION What are the effects of drug treatments?

One systematic review of mainly small RCTs has found that antidepressants versus placebo reduce symptoms more than placebo. One RCT found sertraline to be more effective than placebo.[19] One small RCT of alprazolam versus placebo found a small effect. We found insufficient evidence on the effects of antipsychotic drugs or carbamazepine.

Benefits: **Antidepressants and anxiolytics:** We found one systematic review of antidepressants and anxiolytics for PTSD and one subsequent RCT.[19] The review (search date July 1996) identified six placebo controlled trials in 242 people.[20] The effect size for PTSD from all trials and all drugs versus placebo was 0.41 (CI not available). Effect sizes for individual drugs (CI not available) were fluoxetine 0.77 (64 people, 1 trial), phenelzine 0.39 (63 people, 2 trials), tricyclic antidepressants 0.32 (149 people, 3 trials), and alprazolam 0.25 (16 people, 1 trial). The review also found that drug treatment reduced depression and anxiety. The subsequent RCT (187 people attending an outpatient clinic with PTSD from a variety of traumatic events) compared sertraline, a selective serotonin reuptake inhibitor, with placebo. Sertraline increased the response rate (53% with sertraline v 32% with placebo; P = 0.008), although the reduction in traumatic stress symptoms was not very large.[19] **Antipsychotic drugs:** We found no RCTs. **Carbamazepine:** We found no RCTs.

Harms: The trials gave no information on harms. Known adverse effects include possible hypertensive crisis with monoamine oxidase inhibitors (and also the need for dietary restriction), anticholinergic effects with tricyclic antidepressants, nausea and headache with SSRIs, and dependency with benzodiazepines.

Comment: Small trial sizes and different populations make it difficult to compare results. Other treatments or combinations of drug and psychological treatment await evaluation. It is difficult to interpret effect sizes in terms of clinical importance rather than statistical significance. Some categorise effect sizes of less than 0.5 as small; between 0.5 and 0.8 as medium; and greater than 0.8 as large.

GLOSSARY

Affect management Entails managing mood.

Cognitive behavioural therapy Covers a variety of techniques. *Imaginal exposure* entails exposure to a detailed account or image of what happened. *Real life exposure* involves confronting real life situations that have become associated with the trauma, and cause fear and distress. *Cognitive therapy* entails challenging distorted thoughts about the trauma, the self, and the world. *Stress inoculation* entails instruction in coping skills and some cognitive techniques such as restructuring.

Drama therapy Entails using drama as a form of expression and communication.

Eye movement desensitisation and reprocessing (EMDR) Entails asking the person to focus on the traumatic event, a negative cognition associated with it, and the associated emotions.[21] The person is then asked to follow the therapist's finger as it moves from side to side.

Hypnotherapy Entails hypnosis to allow people to work through the traumatic event.

Prolonged exposure A type of cognitive behavioural treatment that includes repeated exposure to memories of the trauma, and to non-dangerous real life situations that are avoided because of trauma related fear.

Psychodynamic psychotherapy Entails analysis of defence mechanisms, interpretations, and pre-trauma experiences.

Psychological debriefing A technique that entails detailed consideration of the traumatic event and the normalisation of psychological reactions.

Relaxation therapy A technique involving imagination of relaxing situations to induce muscular and mental relaxation.

Supportive counselling A non-directive intervention dealing with current issues rather than the trauma itself.

Substantive changes since last issue

Single episode intervention Systematic review updated,[4] and one additional RCT; conclusion unchanged.

Psychological management Updated with one systematic review;[14] conclusion unchanged.

REFERENCES

1. American Psychiatric Association. *Diagnostic and statistical manual of mental disorders.* 4th ed. Washington: APA, 1994.

2. Kessler RC, Sonnega A, Bromet E, et al. Posttraumatic stress disorder in the national comorbidity survey. *Arch Gen Psychiatry* 1995;52: 1048–1060.

3. O'Brien S. *Traumatic events and mental health.* Cambridge: Cambridge University Press, 1998.

4. Wessely S, Rose S, Bisson J. A systematic review of brief psychological interventions ('debriefing') for the treatment of immediate trauma related symptoms and the prevention of posttraumatic stress disorder. In: The Cochrane Library, issue 4, 1999. Oxford: Update Software. Search date 1996, primary sources Medline, Embase, Psychlit, Pilots, Biosis, Pascal, *Occup Health Saf*, CDSR and the Trials register of the Cochrane Depression, Anxiety and Neurosis Group; hand search of *J Trauma Stress*, and contact with experts.

5. Brom D, Kleber RJ, Hofman MC. Victims of traffic accidents: incidence and prevention of post-traumatic stress disorder. *J Clin Psychol* 1993;49: 131–140.

6. Bryant RA, Harvey AG, Basten C, Dang ST, Sackville T, Basten C. Treatment of acute stress disorder: a comparison of cognitive behavioural therapy and supportive counselling. *J Consult Clin Psychol* 1998;66:862–866.

7. Sherman JJ. Effects of psychotherapeutic treatments for PTSD: a meta-analysis of controlled clinical trials. *J Trauma Stress* 1998;11:413–436. Search date not given; primary sources Psychlit, ERIC, Medline, Cinahl, Dissertation Abstracts, Pilots Traumatic Stress Database.

8. Bryant RA, Sackville T, Dang ST, Moulds M, Guthrie R. Treating acute stress disorder: an evaluation of cognitive behavior therapy and

supportive counselling techniques. *Am J Psychiatry* 1999;156:1780–1786.

9. Andre C, Lelord F, Legeron P, Reigner A, Delattre A. Controlled study of outcomes after 6 months to early intervention of bus driver victims of aggression [in French]. *Encephale* 1997;23:65–71.

10. Rothbaum BO. A controlled study of eye movement desensitization and reprocessing in the treatment of posttraumatic stress disordered sexual assault victims. *Bull Menninger Clin* 1997; 61:317–334.

11. Tarrier N, Sommerfield C, Pilgrim H, Humphreys L. Cognitive therapy or imaginal exposure in the treatment of post-traumatic stress disorder. *Br J Psychiatry* 1999;175:571–575.

12. Foa EB, Rothbaum BO, Riggs DS, et al. Treatment of posttraumatic stress disorder in rape victims: a comparison between cognitive-behavioural procedures and counselling. *J Consult Clin Psychol* 1992;59:715–723.

13. Marks I, Lovell K, Noshirvani H, et al. Treatment of posttraumatic stress disorder by exposure and/or cognitive restructuring: a controlled study. *Arch Gen Psychiatry* 1998;55:317–325.

14. Shepherd J, Stein K, Milne R. Eye movement desensitization and reprocessing in the treatment of post-traumatic stress disorder: a review of an emerging therapy. *Psychological Med* 2000;30: 863–871. Search date 1999; primary sources Medline, Embase, Healthstar, Psyclit, Cochrane Library, Best Evidence, National Research Register, the Medical Research Council trials database, Internet sites on PTSD, hand searches of reference lists, and personal contact with experts in the field.

15. Zlotnick C, Shea T, Rosen K, et al. An affect-management group for women with posttraumatic stress disorder and histories of childhood sexual

abuse. *J Trauma Stress* 1997;10:425–436.

16. Brom D, Kleber RJ, Defares PB. Brief psychotherapy of posttraumatic stress disorders. *J Consult Clin Psychol* 1989;57:607–612.

17. Pitman RK, Altman B, Greenwald E, et al. Psychiatric complications during flooding therapy for posttraumatic stress disorder. *J Clin Psychiatry* 1991;52:17–20.

18. Gersons BPR, Carlier IVE, Lamberts RD, Van der Kolk BA. Randomised clinical trial of brief eclectic psychotherapy for police officers with posttraumatic stress disorder. *J Trauma Stress* 2000;13:333–348.

19. Brady K, Pearlstein T, Asnis GM, et al. Efficacy and safety of sertraline treatment of posttraumatic stress disorder: a randomized controlled trial. *JAMA* 2000;283:1837–1844.

20. Penava SJ, Otto MW, Pollack MH, et al. Current status of pharmacotherapy for PTSD: an effect size analysis of controlled studies. *Depress Anxiety* 1997;4:240–242. Search date July 1994; primary sources Psychlit, Medline.

21. Shapiro, F. Eye movement desensitisation: a new treatment for post-traumatic stress disorder. *J Behav Ther Exp Psychiatry* 1989;20:211–217.

Jonathan Bisson
Consultant Liaison Psychiatrist
Cardiff and Vale NHS Trust
Cardiff
UK

Competing interests: None declared.

Search date December 2000: expanded this issue

Andrew McIntosh and Stephen Lawrie

INTERVENTIONS

Key Messages

- Most evidence is from systematic reviews of small brief RCTs that report different outcomes. There is a need for larger trials, over longer periods, with well designed end points, including standardised, validated symptom scales.

Systematic reviews of RCTs have found:

- Chlorpromazine improves clinical outcomes, but adverse effects make it unacceptable to many people.

- There is limited evidence of benefit from depot haloperidol decanoate compared with placebo.

- The newer antipsychotic drugs loxapine, molindone, pimozide, olanzapine, quetiapine, risperidone, sulpiride, thioridazine, ziprasidone, and zotepine are as effective as standard antipsychotics and have different profiles of adverse effects.

- Clozapine is more effective than standard antipsychotics but is associated with potentially fatal blood dyscrasias.

- Relapse rates are significantly reduced by continuing antipsychotic medication for at least 6 months after an acute episode, by family interventions, and by psychoeducational interventions. Weaker evidence suggests that social skills training and cognitive behavioural therapy may also reduce relapse rates.

- No intervention has been consistently found to reduce negative symptoms.

RCTs have found:

- Limited evidence that compliance therapy, family therapy, behavioural therapy, and psychoeducational therapy may improve adherence with antipsychotic medication.

DEFINITION	Schizophrenia is characterised by the "positive symptoms" of auditory hallucinations, delusions, and thought disorder, and the "negative symptoms" of demotivation, self neglect, and reduced emotion[1] (see glossary, p 713).
INCIDENCE/ PREVALENCE	Onset of symptoms typically occurs in early adult life (average age 25 years) and is earlier in men than women. Prevalence worldwide is 2–4/1000. One in 100 people will develop schizophrenia in their lifetime.[2,3]
AETIOLOGY/ RISK FACTORS	Risk factors include a family history (although no major genes have been identified); obstetric complications; developmental difficulties; central nervous system infections in childhood; cannabis use; and acute life events.[2] The precise contributions of these factors and ways in which they may interact are unclear.
PROGNOSIS	About three quarters of people suffer recurrent relapse and continued disability, although outcomes were worse in the pretreatment era.[4] Outcome may be worse in people with insidious onset and delayed initial treatment, social isolation, or a strong family history; in people living in industrialised countries; in men; and in people who misuse drugs.[3] Drug treatment is generally successful in treating positive symptoms, but up to a third of people derive little benefit and negative symptoms are notoriously difficult to treat. About half of people with schizophrenia do not adhere to treatment in the short term. The figure is even higher in the longer term.[5]
AIMS	To relieve symptoms and to improve quality of life, with minimal adverse effects of treatment.
OUTCOMES	Severity of positive and negative symptoms; global clinical improvement; global clinical impression (a composite measure of symptoms and everyday functioning); rate of relapse; adherence to treatment; adverse effects of treatment.
METHODS	*Clinical Evidence* update search and appraisal December 2000. We also searched The Cochrane Library, Issue 2, 2000. Most of the trials we found were small, short term, with high withdrawal rates, and many different outcome measures.[6] There were a large number of high quality recent systematic reviews. Therefore, if possible we

focused primarily on systematic reviews at the expense of subsequent RCTs and included only the outcomes we thought were the most clinically relevant (because different treatments are associated with different benefits and harms, we used estimates of global effectiveness if they were available). We searched for placebo controlled studies for standard antipsychotic medication, and comparative studies for newer antipsychotics.

QUESTION What are the effects of drug treatments?

OPTION CHLORPROMAZINE

One systematic review of RCTs has found that chlorpromazine versus placebo produces global improvement in the short and medium term but adverse effects make it unacceptable to many people.

Benefits: **Versus placebo:** We found one systematic review (search date 1999, 45 RCTs, 3116 people, mean dose 511 mg/day, range 25–2000 mg/day).[7] Chlorpromazine was more effective than placebo in reducing psychiatrist rated global improvement by at least 50% (RR 1.3, 95% CI 1.1 to 1.4; NNT 7, 95% CI 5 to 10) and global severity (RR 1.5, 95% CI 1.1 to 2.0; NNT 5, 95% CI 4 to 8) in the short and medium term (up to 6 months).

Harms: **Versus placebo:** The systematic review found that chlorpromazine caused significantly higher rates of sedation (RR 2.4, 95% CI 1.7 to 3.3; NNH 6, 95% CI 4 to 8), acute dystonias (RR 3.1, 95% CI 1.3 to 7.6; NNH 24, 95% CI 14 to 77), parkinsonism (RR 2.6, 95% CI 1.2 to 5.4; NNH 10, 95% CI 8 to 16), weight gain (RR 4.4, 95% CI 2.1 to 9; NNH 3, 95% CI 2 to 5), skin photosensitivity (RR 5.2, 95% CI 3 to 10; NNH 7, 95% CI 6 to 10), dizziness caused by hypotension (RR 1.9, 95% CI 1.3 to 2.6; NNH 12, 95% CI 8 to 20), and dry mouth (RR 4, 95% CI 1.6 to 10; NNH 19, 95% CI 12 to 37).[7] Chlorpromazine was also associated with a non-significantly higher rate of seizures (RR 2.4, 95% CI 0.4 to 16) and blood dyscrasias (RR 2.0, 95% CI 0.7 to 6). We found no long term data on the risk of tardive dyskinesia or the rare but potentially fatal neuroleptic malignant syndrome. Despite the frequent adverse effects, people receiving active treatment were more likely to stay in trials than those receiving placebo in both the short and the medium term.

Comment: The review did not categorise symptoms as positive or negative as this information was rarely available from included trials. Relative risks and numbers needed to treat were based on 6 months' data.

OPTION DEPOT HALOPERIDOL DECANOATE

One systematic review found limited evidence from one RCT that depot haloperidol decanoate is more effective than placebo.

Benefits: **Versus placebo:** We found one systematic review (search date 1998, 2 RCTs, 78 people).[8] Both RCTs found that people on haloperidol were more likely to stay in the RCT (OR 11, 95% CI 5 to 33; NNT 2, 95% CI 1 to 3). One RCT (22 people) comparing intramuscular depot haloperidol decanoate (mean dose 150 mg monthly) versus placebo found that haloperidol decanoate was more likely to result in a "reduced need for medication" at 4 months (RR 2.6, 95% CI 1.1 to 5.6; NNT with 4 months' treatment 2, 95% CI 1 to 2).

Harms: Fewer people receiving haloperidol versus placebo left the trial early (RR 0.2, 95% CI 0.1 to 0.4; NNT 2, 95% CI 1 to 3).[8]

Comment: How "reduced need for medication" was measured was not described. Depot injection is believed to ensure adherence, but we found no evidence to support this belief.

OPTION   DEPOT PIPOTHIAZINE PALMITATE

One systematic review found limited evidence from two RCTs of no significant difference between depot pipothiazine palmitate and standard antipsychotic drugs.

Benefits: **Versus standard oral antipsychotic drugs:** We found one systematic review (search date 1999), which identified two RCTs, both conducted in the 1970s, comparing intramuscular pipothiazine palmitate versus normal treatment ("standard" oral antipsychotic drugs, chosen by physicians).[9] Neither found a significant difference between active treatment and control groups (first trial, 124 people: WMD in composite rating of psychotic symptoms at 18 months −3.1, 95% CI −7.3 to +1.2; second trial, 48 people: no quantified results available).

Harms: **Versus standard oral antipsychotic drugs:** One RCT (mean dose 90 mg a month) found that the number of people needing to take anticholinergic drugs for unspecified reasons was not significantly different between depot versus standard drugs (RR 0.9, 95% CI 0.7 to 1.1).[9] Meta-analysis combining both trials (mean dose 113 mg a month for 6 months) found no overall difference in the numbers of people leaving the trial early (25% in both groups, RR 1.0, 95% CI 0.5 to 1.9).

Comment: Several other depot preparations are commercially available in different countries, but we found even less evidence for their efficacy versus placebo or standard antipsychotic drugs.

OPTION   LOXAPINE

One systematic review of 22 small, brief RCTs comparing loxapine and standard antipsychotic drugs found no significant difference in benefits or harms.

Benefits: **Versus standard antipsychotic drugs:** We found one systematic review (search date 1999, 22 RCTs, 1073 people), which compared loxapine (dose range 25–250 mg daily) versus standard antipsychotic drugs, usually chlorpromazine.[10] It found no significant differences in global improvement (9 RCTs, 411 people; RR not improved 0.9, 95% CI 0.7 to 1.2).

Harms: The systematic review found no significant difference in adverse effects.[11]

Comment: All RCTs were conducted in the USA or India and none lasted longer than 12 weeks.

MOLINDONE

One systematic review of RCTs found no significant difference between molindone and standard antipsychotic drugs in benefits or harms, but the trials were short and of poor quality.

Benefits: **Versus standard antipsychotic drugs:** We found one systematic review of molindone versus standard antipsychotic drugs (search date 2000, 13 controlled trials, 469 people).[10] It found no significant differences in global efficacy between molindone and standard antipsychotic drugs (4 RCTs, 150 people; RR no improvement 1.1, 95% CI 0.7 to 1.8).

Harms: No significant differences were found between molindone and standard antipsychotic drugs in total numbers of adverse events. One trial found that the rate of confusion was higher in people taking molindone (RR 3.2, 95% CI 1.4 to 7.3). There were no significant differences in the rates of movement disorders between molindone and standard antipsychotic drugs. Weight loss was more frequent in those taking molindone (2 RCTs, 60 people; RR 2.8, 95% CI 1.1 to 7.0). Molindone was associated with less frequent weight gain than standard antipsychotic drugs (2 RCTs, 60 people; RR 0.4, 95% CI 0.1 to 1.0).

Comment: The RCTs in the review had methodological problems (in 4 trials it was unclear whether randomisation had been performed, 7 trials included people whose diagnosis was not operationally defined) and were brief (all lasted under 13 weeks). We found no reliable evidence comparing molindone with either placebo or new antipsychotic drugs.

PIMOZIDE

We found insufficient evidence from RCTs comparing pimozide versus placebo. One systematic review of 34 RCTs comparing pimozide versus standard antipsychotic drugs found no significant differences in benefits or harms.

Benefits: **Versus placebo:** We found one systematic review (search date 2000, 3 RCTs, 86 people) of pimozide versus placebo.[12] One RCT (20 people) found no significant difference in Clinical Global Impression at 3 months. Two further small RCTs (66 people) found greater improvement at 6 months with pimozide, the significance of which depend on the statistical method used. **Versus standard antipsychotic drugs:** We found one systematic review (search date 2000, 1155 people) of pimozide (mean dose 7.5 mg daily, range 1–75 mg daily) versus a variety of standard antipsychotic drugs.[12] It found no significant differences in clinical global impression rates (3 RCTs, 206 people; RR 0.9, 95% CI 0.8 to 1.1).

Harms: **Versus placebo:** One small short RCT found more electrocardiograph changes in the pimozide group (T wave changes, RR 5, 95% CI 0.3 to 93). Doses used were on a sliding scale up to 40 mg daily. **Versus standard antipsychotic drugs:** Pimozide caused less sedation than standard antipsychotic drugs alone (RR 0.4, 95% CI 0.2 to 0.7; NNT 6, 95% CI 4 to 16), but was more likely to cause tremor (RR 1.6, 95 CI 1.1 to 2.3; NNH 6, 95% CI 3 to 44). There was no overall difference in cardiovascular symptoms such as rise or fall in blood pressure and dizziness between pimozide and other drugs. There was little usable electrocardiogram (ECG) data. One RCT in the review found no difference in ECG changes (RR 0.67, 95 CI 0.1 to 3.7).

Comment: Sudden death has been reported in a number of people taking pimozide at doses over 20 mg daily, but we found no evidence that pimozide is more likely to cause sudden death than other antipsychotic drugs. The manufacturer recommends periodic ECG monitoring in all people taking more than 16 mg daily of pimozide and avoidance of other drugs known to prolong the QT interval on an ECG or cause electrolyte disturbances (other antipsychotics, antihistamines, antidepressants, and diuretics). The trials comparing pimozide versus placebo may be too small to detect a clinically significant difference.

OPTION   POLYUNSATURATED FATTY ACIDS

One systematic review found limited evidence from one small, brief RCT that polyunsaturated fatty acids compared with placebo reduced the subsequent use of antipsychotic medication.

Benefits: **Versus placebo:** We found one systematic review (search date 2000, 1 RCT, 30 people) of fatty acid supplementation versus placebo.[13] It found less need at 12 weeks for subsequent antipsychotic medication in those receiving fish oil compared with those receiving placebo (RR 0.6, 95% CI 0.4 to 0.9). The review also found a slight difference in average symptom severity scores favouring fish oil (26 people; WMD –13, 95% CI –22 to –3).

Harms: The RCT did not find significant adverse events.

Comment: The single relevant RCT cited in the systematic review is an unpublished conference proceeding. Other RCTs considered only augmentation of antipsychotic treatment, which may be covered in a later issue of *Clinical Evidence*.

OPTION   OLANZAPINE

Two systematic reviews of RCTs have found that olanzapine may be as effective as standard antipsychotic drugs and has fewer adverse effects. Three systematic reviews found no evidence that olanzapine is more effective than other new antipsychotic drugs.

Benefits: We found four systematic reviews.[14–17] **Versus standard antipsychotic drugs:** The first review (search date 1999, 15 RCTs, 3282 people) compared olanzapine with standard antipsychotic drugs, usually haloperidol.[14] It found olanzapine 2.5–25 mg daily compared with standard antipsychotic drugs did not significantly reduce psychotic symptoms over 6–8 weeks (2778 people; RR of no important response defined as a 40% reduction on any scale: 0.9, 95% CI 0.76 to 1.06). The second review (search date 1998, 4 RCTs, 2914 people) found that olanzapine was associated with slightly greater treatment success than haloperidol on a composite measure of positive and negative symptoms.[15] **Versus other new antipsychotic drugs:** The second review included one RCT (84 people) comparing olanzapine with risperidone.[15] It found no evidence of a difference in effectiveness (RR no important clinical response by 8 weeks 0.93, 95% CI 0.85 to 1.01). The third systematic review (search date 1999, 1 RCT, 180 people) comparing olanzapine versus clozapine found no significant difference in effectiveness (RR no important clinical response 0.7, 95% CI 0.5 to 1.1).[16] The fourth review (search date 2000) identified three RCTs comparing olanzapine versus risperidone.[17] It found that olanzapine was associated with a slightly greater reduction on a composite symptom severity scale in the medium but not the long term (392 people, 7.5 points on 210 point scale, 95% CI 2.9 to 12.0).

Harms: **Versus standard antipsychotic drugs:** Olanzapine versus standard antipsychotic drugs did not significantly reduce the number of people who withdrew from the trials at 6–8 weeks (36% v 49%; RR 0.9, 95% CI 0.7 to 1.1) or at 1 year (83% v 90%; OR 0.9, 95% CI 0.86 to 1.02).[14] Olanzapine versus standard antipsychotic drugs caused fewer extrapyramidal adverse effects (in heterogeneous data prone to bias), less nausea (2347 people; RR 0.7, 95% CI 0.6 to 0.9; NNT 25, 95% CI 14 to 85), vomiting (1996 people; RR 0.6, 95% CI 0.4 to 0.8; NNT 20, 95% CI 12 to 46), or drowsiness (2347 people; RR 0.8, 95% CI 0.7 to 0.9) than standard antipsychotic drugs.[14] Olanzapine was associated with a greater increase in appetite (1996 people; RR 1.7, 95% CI 1.4 to 2.0; NNH 10, 95% CI 7 to 15) and weight gain (heterogeneous data) than standard antipsychotic drugs.[14] **Versus other new antipsychotic drugs:** One RCT included in the first review (84 people) found that olanzapine compared with risperidone was associated with fewer extrapyramidal adverse effects (NNT 8), less parkinsonism (NNT 11), and less need for anticholinergic medication (NNT 8); but olanzapine caused more dry mouth (NNH 9) and greater weight gain (NNH 11).[14] The fourth review also found that risperidone was associated with more people leaving trials early than olanzapine (404 people, RR 1.3, 95% CI 1.1 to 1.6; ARR 0.13, 95% CI 0.03 to 0.22).[17] One RCT (180 people) found olanzapine versus clozapine was associated with less nausea (RR 0.1, 95% CI 0.01 to 0.8) and no significant difference in the number of people complaining of movement disorders (RR 0.4, 95% CI 0.1 to 1.4).[16]

Comment: The results of the reviews are dominated by one large multicentre RCT reported by drug company employees. Benefits seem to be maximal at a dose of 15 mg daily, and higher doses may be associated with more harms. The results depended on the precise statistical test used. Those presented in the benefits section are conservative estimates, which seem reasonable given the presence of heterogeneity and other possible biases. Some less conservative statistical methods indicate superior effectiveness for olanzapine compared with standard antipsychotic drugs.

OPTION QUETIAPINE

Two systematic reviews of RCTs comparing quetiapine with standard antipsychotic drugs found no significant differences in benefits, but significant reduction of some harms.

Benefits: **Versus standard antipsychotic drugs:** We found two systematic reviews.[15,18] The first review (search date 1998, 6 RCTs, 1414 people) identified two RCTs (809 people) comparing quetiapine with haloperidol and found no evidence of a difference in effectiveness on a composite measure of positive and negative symptoms.[15] The second review (search date 2000, 7 RCTs) of quetiapine (50–800 mg daily) versus standard antipsychotic drugs (usually haloperidol), found no significant differences in global improvement (1247 people; RR no important improvement in mental state 0.93, 95% CI 0.83 to 1.04).[18]

Harms: **Versus standard antipsychotic drugs:** The second review found quetiapine versus standard antipsychotic drugs was associated with less people leaving trials early (RR 0.87, 95% CI 0.76 to 0.99), less dystonia than standard antipsychotics (RR 0.14, 95% CI 0.04 to 0.49), less akathisia (RR 0.24, 95% CI 0.15 to 0.38), and parkinsonism (RR 0.22, 95% CI 0.15 to 0.33), but more dry mouth (RR 2.85, 95% CI 1.46 to 5.57).[17]

Comment: The evidence comes from a small number of short term trials that had substantial withdrawal rates and did not conduct intention to treat analyses.

OPTION RISPERIDONE

Two systematic reviews of RCTs comparing risperidone versus standard antipsychotic drugs (mainly haloperidol) found limited evidence that risperidone may be more effective than standard antipsychotic drugs and good evidence that at lower doses it has fewer adverse effects. Two systematic reviews found no significant difference between risperidone versus new antipsychotic drugs.

Benefits: **Versus standard antipsychotic drugs:** We found two systematic reviews and one additional RCT.[15,19,20] Both systematic reviews found that risperidone was more effective than haloperidol. The first review (search date 1997, 14 RCTs, 3401 people) found that, at 12 weeks, risperidone (mean daily dose range 6.1–12 mg) was more effective than standard antipsychotic drugs, usually haloperidol.[21] Outcome was "clinical improvement", variably defined but usually a 20% reduction in general symptoms (2171 people; 11 RCTs; RR no improvement 0.8, 95% CI 0.7 to 0.9; NNT 10, 95% CI 7 to 16). No benefit was observed for the outcome of global clinical impression. The second review (search date 1998, 9 RCTs, 2215 people) found that risperidone was associated with slightly greater success than haloperidol on a composite measure of positive and negative symptoms.[15] The additional RCT (99 people) comparing a range of doses of risperidone with haloperidol found no overall significant difference in global outcome.[20] **Versus other new antipsychotic drugs:** See olanzapine, p 700. We found two systematic reviews,[16,17] which found no significant difference between risperidone versus clozapine (5 RCTs) or versus amisulpiride (1 RCT) for outcomes including improvement in mental state, but the RCTs were small and short, with high withdrawal rates.

Harms: **Versus standard antipsychotic drugs:** The systematic review found that risperidone versus standard antipsychotic drugs caused no significant change in the number of people who withdrew from treatment (2166 people; RR 0.8, 95% CI 0.6 to 1.1). People taking risperidone developed fewer extrapyramidal effects (2279 people; RR 0.6, 95% CI 0.5 to 0.7; NNT 5, 95% CI 5 to 10), required less antiparkinsonian medication (2436 people; RR 0.6, 95% CI 0.5 to 0.7; NNT 7, 95% CI 5 to 10), and were less likely to develop daytime somnolence (2098 people; RR 0.9, 95% CI 0.7 to 0.99; NNT 22, 95% CI 11 to 500). Risperidone was associated with greater weight gain (1652 people; RR 1.4, 95% CI 1.1 to 1.7; NNH 13, 95% CI 8 to 36).[19] The additional RCT found no overall significant difference in the rate of adverse effects between risperidone and haloperidol.[20] **Versus other new antipsychotic drugs:** See olanzapine, p 713. We found two systematic reviews,[16,17] which found no significant difference between risperidone and clozapine. The second systematic review (search date 1999, 1 RCT, 228 people) found amisulpiride versus risperidone caused less agitation (RR 0.29, 95% CI 0.1 to 0.86) and less constipation (RR 0.13, 95% CI 0.2 to 1.0).

Comment: The reported benefits in the first review over standard antipsychotic drugs were marginal, and it found evidence of publication bias.[19] Sensitivity analyses found that benefits in clinical improvement and continuing treatment of risperidone compared with standard antipsychotic drugs were no longer significant if trials using more than 10 mg haloperidol daily were excluded.[19] This loss of significance could be because of loss of power when trials were excluded. Exclusion of the higher dosage trials did not remove the difference in rate of extrapyramidal adverse effects.[19]

OPTION ZIPRASIDONE

One systematic review of RCTs comparing ziprasidone with standard antipsychotic drugs found no significant difference in mental state improvement but did find a different profile of adverse effects.

Benefits: We found one systematic review (search date 2000, 7 RCTs, 824 people). **Versus standard antipsychotics:** It identified four RCTs of ziprasidone versus standard antipsychotic drugs.[21] It found no significant differences in mental state improvement in different trials (301 people; RR no important improvement in mental state 0.9, 95% CI 0.7 to 1.0).

Harms: **Versus standard antipsychotics:** The review found no clear difference in total adverse events between ziprasidone and haloperidol.[21] Ziprasidone was less likely to cause akathisia in the short term (438 people; RR 0.3, 95% CI 0.2 to 0.6; NNT 8, 95% CI 5 to 18) and in the long term (301 people; RR 0.3, 95% CI 0.1 to 0.7; NNT 9, 95% CI 5 to 21), and less likely to cause acute dystonia (438 people; RR 0.4, 95% CI 0.2 to 0.9; NNT 16, 95% CI 9 to 166). Ziprasidone was more likely to produce nausea and vomiting in both the short term (306 people; RR 3.6, 95% CI 1.8 to 7; NNT 5, 95% CI 4 to 8) and in the long term (301 people; RR 2.1, 95% CI 1 to 4; NNT 9, 95% CI 5 to 33). Intramuscular ziprasidone was significantly more likely to be associated with injection site pain than haloperidol (306 people; RR 5.3, 95% CI 1.3 to 22; NNT 12, 95% CI 7 to 27).

Comment: The duration of RCTs was less than 6 weeks. Most reported a withdrawal rate of over 20% and no RCT clearly described adequate precautions for the blinding of treatment allocation. We found no evidence comparing ziprasidone with other new antipsychotic drugs.

OPTION ZOTEPINE

One systematic review of small, brief RCTs, which compared zotepine with standard antipsychotic drugs, found weak evidence that zotepine reduced a standard symptom severity score and had fewer adverse effects. This finding was not robust as removal of a single RCT alters the conclusion. We found no evidence comparing zotepine with other new antipsychotic drugs.

Benefits: We found one systematic review (search date 1999, 10 RCTs, 537 people). **Versus standard antipsychotic drugs:** The systematic review included eight RCTs comparing zotepine (75–450 mg daily) versus a variety of standard antipsychotic drugs.[22] Zotepine was more likely than standard antipsychotic drugs to bring about "clinically important improvement" as defined by a pre-stated cut off point on the Brief Psychiatric Rating Scale (356 people; 4 RCTs; RR 1.25, 95% CI 1.1 to 1.4; NNT 7, 95% CI 4 to 22).

Harms: The review found zotepine caused less akathisia (396 people; RR 0.7, 95% CI 0.6 to 0.9; NNT 8, 95% CI 5 to 34), dystonia (70 people; RR 0.5, 95% CI 0.2 to 0.9; NNT 4, 95% CI 2 to 56), and rigidity (164 people; RR 0.6, 95% CI 0.4 to 0.9; NNT 7, 95% CI 4 to 360) than standard antipsychotic drugs.[22]

Comment: All but one trial were of 12 weeks or less duration and all were conducted in Europe. Only one RCT favoured zotepine over standard antipsychotic drugs, and removal of this RCT from the analysis changed the result from a significant to a non-significant effect. Two RCTs found abnormal ECG results in people taking zotepine, but few additional details were given. We found too few trials to compare zotepine reliably with other new antipsychotics.

OPTION CLOZAPINE

One systematic review of RCTs has found that clozapine is more effective than standard antipsychotic drugs. However, it is associated with potentially fatal blood dyscrasias. A second systematic review of RCTs found no strong evidence about the effectiveness or safety of clozapine compared with new antipsychotic drugs.

Benefits: We found three systematic reviews.[16,17,23] **Versus standard antipsychotics:** We found one systematic review (search date 1998, 31 RCTs, 2530 people, 73% men).[23] Clozapine versus standard antipsychotics, such as chlorpromazine and haloperidol, was associated with greater clinical improvement both in the short term (4–10 weeks, 14 RCTs, 1131 people; RR no important improvement 0.7, 95% CI 0.7 to 0.8; NNT 6, 95% CI 5 to 7) and the long term (heterogeneous data). **Versus new antipsychotics:** We found one systematic review (search date 2000, 8 RCTs), which compared clozapine versus new antipsychotics, including olanzapine and risperidone,[16] and a second, which included comparisons of clozapine versus risperidone (search date 2000, 5 RCTs).[17] Both reviews found no significant difference in efficacy, but the number of people studied was too small to rule out a clinically important difference.

Harms: **Versus standard antipsychotics:** Clozapine was more likely to cause hypersalivation (1419 people; RR 3.0, 95% CI 1.8 to 4.7; NNH 3), temperature increases (1147 people; RR 1.8, 95% CI 1.2 to 2.7; NNH 11), and sedation (1527 people; RR 1.2, 95% CI 1.1 to 1.4; NNH 10), but less likely to cause dry mouth (799 people; RR 0.4, 95% CI 0.3 to 0.6; NNT 6) and extrapyramidal adverse effects (1235 people; RR 0.7, 95% CI 0.5 to 0.9; NNT 6).[16] The review found blood problems occurred more frequently with clozapine than with standard antipsychotics (1293 people; AR 3.6% v 1.9%; NNH 58, 95% CI 31 to 111).[23] In a large observational case series, leucopenia was reported in 3% of 99 502 people over 5 years. However, it found monitoring white cell (neutrophil) counts was associated with a lower than expected rate of cases of agranulocytosis (382 v 995; AR 0.38% v 1%) and deaths (12 v 149).[24] Dyscrasias were more common in younger people in a single RCT included in the first systematic review (21 people; RR 5.4, 95% CI 10 to 162; NNH 2.5).[23,25] Despite the requirement for regular blood tests, fewer people withdrew from treatment with clozapine in the long term (1513 people; RR 0.8, 95% CI 0.6 to 0.9; NNH 3).[23] **Versus new antipsychotics:** Compared with new antipsychotic drugs (mainly risperidone), clozapine was less likely to cause extrapyramidal adverse effects (305 people; RR 0.3, 95% CI 0.1 to 0.6; NNT 6, 95% CI 4 to 9). Clozapine may also be less likely to cause dry mouth and more likely to cause fatigue, nausea, dizziness, hypersalivation, and hypersomnia, but these findings were from one or at most two trials.[16] Compared with new antipsychotics, people on clozapine tended to be more satisfied with their treatment, but also tended to withdraw from trials more easily.[16] Both reviews found no difference in rates of blood dyscrasias between clozapine and the new antipsychotics, but the number of people studied was too small (558) to rule out clinically important differences.[16,17]

Comment: Some of the benefits of clozapine were more apparent in the long term, depending on which drug was used for comparison in the trials.

OPTION   SULPIRIDE   New

One systematic review of 18 RCTs found no significant difference in benefits between sulpiride and other antipsychotic medication.

Benefits: We found one systematic review (search date 1998).[26] **Versus placebo:** The review (3 RCTs, 141 people) found that sulpiride was better than placebo for mental state but meta-analysis was not possible. **Versus standard antipsychotic drugs:** The review (13 RCTs, 97 people) found no significant differences in global improvement versus standard antipsychotic drugs (RR of not improved 0.96, 95% CI 0.90 to 1.02). Evidence on mental state was inadequate.[26]

Harms: **Versus placebo:** Limited adverse event data were reported.[26] No differences were found between sulpiride versus placebo for involuntary movements or hypersalivation. **Versus standard antipsychotic drugs:** The use of antiparkinson drugs was less frequent in the sulpiride group (RR 0.73, 95% CI 0.59 to 0.90).[26]

Comment: Trial quality was generally poor. Observational evidence and clinical experience suggest galactorrhoea may be a real problem, but trial data did not quantify the risk of occurrence.[27]

OPTION   THIORIDAZINE   New

One systematic review of 11 RCTs found limited evidence favouring thioridazine over placebo. It found no significant differences between thioridazine and standard antipsychotic medication, although thioridazine was less likely to cause symptoms of drug induced parkinsonism.

Benefits: We found one systematic review (search date 2000). **Versus placebo:** The review (11 RCTs, 560 people)[28] of short term RCTs (100 people) found no significant difference between thioridazine versus placebo in global mental state (RR 0.66, 95% CI 0.35 to 1.23). Two RCTs (65 people) found that thioridazine versus placebo improved global mental state at 6 months (RR 0.34, 95% CI 0.21 to 0.56; NNT 2, 95% CI 1 to 6). Three short term trials found no significant differences between thioridazine and placebo in global mental state improvement. **Versus standard antipsychotic drugs:** The review (26 RCTs, 2397 people) found no significant difference between thioridazine versus standard antipsychotic medication in the risk of "being better or no worse" on clinical global impression, or in mental state improvements.[28]

Harms: **Versus placebo:** The review found no significant differences in adverse events.[28] **Versus standard antipsychotic drugs:** The review found one RCT (74 people) comparing thioridazine versus chlorpromazine, which found that thioridazine caused more cardiovascular adverse events at 3 months (RR 3.2, 95% CI 1.4 to 7.0; NNH 3, 95% CI 2 to 7), although by 6 months the difference was not statistically significant. The review found that thioridazine caused less extrapyramidal adverse events (1082 people; RR 0.48, 95% CI 0.28 to 0.81), and parkinsonism (340 people; RR 0.29, 95% CI 0.12 to 0.70).[28]

Comment: We found limited data on retinopathy and RCTs were generally short.

| QUESTION | Which interventions reduce relapse rates? |

| OPTION | CONTINUED TREATMENT WITH ANTIPSYCHOTIC DRUGS |

One systematic review of follow up studies has found that continuing antipsychotic medication for at least 6 months after an acute episode significantly reduces relapse rates, and that some benefit of continuing treatment is apparent for up to 2 years. We found no evidence of a difference in relapse rates between standard antipsychotic drugs, but a systematic review of RCTs has found that relapse rates are lower with clozapine.

Benefits: **Versus no treatment or placebo:** We found two systematic reviews.[6,29] Both found evidence that continued treatment was beneficial for prevention of relapse. One review (search date not stated, 66 studies, 4365 people taking antipsychotic drugs, mean dose 630 mg chlorpromazine equivalents a day, mean follow up of 6.3 months) included 29 controlled trials with a mean follow up of 9.7 months.[29] It found significantly lower relapse in 1224 people maintained on treatment compared with 1224 withdrawn from treatment (16.2% v 51.5%; ARR 35%, 95% CI 33% to 38%; NNT 3, 95% CI 2.6 to 3.1). Over time, the relapse rate in people maintained on antipsychotic treatment approached that in those withdrawn from treatment, but was still lower in those on treatment at 2 years (ARR 22%; NNT 5). The other review (search date 1997) found that relapse rates over 6–24 months were significantly lower on chlorpromazine than placebo (3 heterogeneous RCTs; RR 0.7, 95% CI 0.5 to 0.9; NNT 3, 95% CI 2.5 to 4).[6] **Choice of drug:** We found eight systematic reviews, which found that the choice of drug or preparation did not seem to affect relapse rates. The first (search date 1995) identified six RCTs comparing oral with depot fluphenazine (see table 1, p 716).[30] A second (search date 1998) identified seven RCTs comparing haloperidol decanoate with other depot antipsychotics.[8] A third (search date 1999) identified eight RCTs comparing flupenthixol decanoate with other depot antipsychotics.[31] A fourth (search date 1999) identified seven RCTs comparing pipothiazine palmitate with other depots and two RCTs comparing pipothiazine palmitate with oral antipsychotics.[9] A fifth (search date 1999) identified one RCT comparing fluspirilene decanoate with oral chlorpromazine and three studies comparing fluspirilene decanoate with other depot preparations.[32] A sixth (search date 1999) found one RCT comparing perphenazine enanthate with clopenthixol decanoate.[33] The reviews comparing pimozide and olanzapine versus typical antipsychotic drugs also found no significant difference in relapse rates.[12,14] The number of people studied was too small to rule out clinically important differences. One systematic review comparing clozapine with standard antipsychotic drugs (search date 1999) found that relapse rates up to 12 weeks were significantly lower with clozapine (19 RCTs; RR 0.6, 95% CI 0.5 to 0.8; NNT 20).[23] Another systematic review found that significantly fewer people taking depot zuclopenthixol decanoate relapsed over 12 weeks to 1 year compared with people taking other depot preparations (3 RCTs, 296 people; RR 0.7, 95% CI 0.6 to 1.0; NNT 9, 95% CI 5 to 53).[34]

Harms: Mild transient nausea, malaise, sweating, vomiting, insomnia, and dyskinesia were reported in an unspecified number of people after sudden drug cessation, but were usually acceptable with gradual dose reduction.[35] Annual incidence of tardive dyskinesia was 5%.[34]

Comment: In the systematic review of continued versus withdrawal of treatment, meta-analysis of the 29 controlled trials gave similar results to those obtained when all 66 studies were included (ARR 37%, NNT 3).[34] The review was weakened because all RCT results were used rather than weighted comparisons, no length of time was given since the last acute episode, and no distinction was made between people experiencing a first episode and those with chronic illness.[34] Some clinicians use depot antipsychotic medication in selected people to ensure adherence to medication. We found no evidence from RCTs to support this practice.

OPTION   FAMILY INTERVENTIONS

One systematic review of RCTs has found that family intervention significantly reduces relapse rates compared with usual care.

Benefits: We found one systematic review (search date 1999, 13 RCTs) and one additional RCT comparing family interventions with usual care.[36,37] Family interventions consisted mainly of education about the illness and training in problem solving over at least six weekly sessions. Three of the trials included substantial proportions of people experiencing their first episode. Family interventions significantly reduced relapse rates at 12 and 24 months. At 12 months, the risk of relapse was reduced (6 RCTs, 516 people; RR 0.7, 95% CI 0.5 to 1.0), such that seven families would have to be treated to avoid one additional relapse (and likely hospitalisation) in the family member with schizophrenia (NNT 7, 95% CI 4 to 14).[38] We found one potentially relevant additional RCT of family interventions compared with psychoeducation.[39] It will be assessed in future issues of *Clinical Evidence*.

Harms: No harms were reported, although illness education could possibly have adverse consequences on morale and outlook.[38]

Comment: These results are likely to overestimate treatment effect because of the difficulty of blinding people and investigators and the likelihood of publication bias.[36] The trend over time is for results to tend to the null. The mechanism for the effects of family intervention remains unclear. It is thought to work by reducing "expressed emotion" (hostility and criticism) in relatives of people with schizophrenia, but may act through improved adherence to medication. The time consuming nature of this intervention, which must normally take place at evenings or weekends, can limit its availability. It cannot be applied to people who have little contact with home based carers.

OPTION   SOCIAL SKILLS TRAINING

Limited evidence from RCTs suggests that social skills training may reduce relapse rates.

Benefits: We found one non-systematic review and meta-analysis of 27 RCTs (search date not given) comparing social skills training with usual care.[40] The trials were mainly in men admitted to hospital, not all of whom had schizophrenia, using different techniques that generally included instruction in social interaction. Four studies provided quantitative information, of which three defined relapse as rehospitalisation. Social skills training significantly reduced relapse rates (WMD 0.47). However, sensitivity analysis indicated that five null results (in studies not identified by a search) would render the difference non-significant. One systematic review (search date 1988) identified 73 RCTs in people with a variety of psychiatric disorders and found similar results, but suggested that motivation was an important predictor of benefit from treatment.[41]

Harms: None reported.

Comment: Many of the trials simultaneously compared the effects of other interventions (medication, education), so the effects of individual interventions are difficult to assess. Overall, it remains uncertain whether people at different stages of illness and function require different approaches. Selected people may benefit even from interventions of short duration.

OPTION COGNITIVE BEHAVIOURAL THERAPY

Limited evidence from RCTs suggests that cognitive behavioural therapy may reduce relapse rates.

Benefits: We found one systematic review (search date 1998, 4 small RCTs) comparing cognitive behavioural therapy plus standard care with standard care alone.[42] All trials incorporated the challenging of key beliefs, problem solving, and enhancement of coping. Relapse rates were significantly reduced in the short, medium, and long term. In the long term (up to 18 months), cognitive behavioural therapy plus standard care reduced the risk of relapse (3 RCTs, 183 people; RR 0.7, 95% CI 0.5 to 0.9; NNT 6, 95% CI 3 to 30).

Harms: None reported.

Comment: None of the three trials contributing long term results were blinded, and each concentrated on different clinical issues — symptoms, adherence to treatment, or general rehabilitation. The fourth trial blinded outcome raters and included an additional supportive psychotherapy control group. It found non-significantly lower relapse rates with cognitive behavioural therapy (1 RCT, 59 people; RR 0.6, 95% CI 0.2 to 2.1).

OPTION PSYCHOEDUCATIONAL INTERVENTIONS New

One systematic review of RCTs has found that psychoeducation is effective for preventing relapse.

Benefits: **Versus usual treatment:** We found one systematic review (search date 2000, 10 RCTs, 1128 people, 53% male).[43] The systematic review included one RCT of a brief individual intervention (10 sessions or less), but no standard length individual psychoeducational interventions (11 sessions or more). It included six RCTs of brief group psychoeducational interventions, and four of standard length. Standard length interventions were significantly more effective than treatment as usual in preventing relapse during 9–18 months (6 RCTs, 720 people; RR 0.80, 95% CI 0.70 to 0.92; NNT 6, 95% CI 3 to 83). Brief group psychoeducational interventions were also more effective than treatment as usual in preventing relapse or re-admission by 1 year (RR 0.85, 95% CI 0.74 to 0.98; NNT 12 CI 6 to 83). When all trials were pooled, relapse rates at 9–18 months' follow up were significantly lower in the psychoeducation group than in the control intervention (6 RCTs; RR 0.80, 95% CI 0.70 to 0.92; NNT 9, 95% CI 6 to 22).

Harms: None reported.

Comment: The systematic review found few good RCTs. There was significant heterogeneity of both interventions and outcomes.

QUESTION   Which interventions are effective in people resistant to standard treatment?

One systematic review of RCTs has found that clozapine benefits people who are resistant to standard treatment.

Benefits: **Clozapine:** We found one systematic review (search 1998, 6 RCTs) comparing clozapine versus standard antipsychotic drugs in people who were resistant to standard treatment.[23] Clozapine achieved improvement both in the short term (6–12 weeks: 4 RCTs, 370 people; RR for no improvement compared with standard antipsychotic drugs 0.7, 95% CI 0.6 to 0.8; NNT 5) and in the longer term (12–24 months: 2 RCTs, 648 people; RR 0.8, 95% CI 0.6 to 1.0). There was no difference in relapse rates in the short term. **Other interventions:** We found no good evidence on the effects of other interventions in people resistant to standard treatment.

Harms: See harms of clozapine, p 705.

Comment: Trials are under way to clarify the mode of action of cognitive behavioural therapy and establish its effects in people who are resistant to standard treatments.

QUESTION   Which interventions improve adherence to antipsychotic medication?

OPTION   COMPLIANCE THERAPY

We found limited evidence from three RCTs that compliance therapy (see glossary, p 713) may increase adherence with antipsychotic medication.

Benefits: We found no systematic review. We found one RCT of compliance therapy versus supportive counselling, which included 47 people with acute psychoses, although the majority fulfilled criteria for schizophrenia or had been admitted with the first episode of a psychotic illness.[38,44] People treated with compliance therapy were significantly more likely to attain at least passive acceptance of antipsychotic medication versus people who received non-specific counselling, both immediately after the intervention (OR 6.3, 95% CI 1.6 to 24.6) and at 6 months follow up (OR 5.2, 95% CI 1.5 to 18.3). At 18 months (for an extended sample of 74 people), a significant improvement on a seven point scale of medication adherence was found for people treated with compliance therapy (mean difference 1.4, 95% CI 0.9 to 1.6).

Harms: None reported.

Comment: Other trials have examined the potential benefits of compliance therapy, but either did not employ a standardised measure of adherence, or adherence was not rated in a blind fashion. The RCT above requires independent replication. About a third of each group did not complete the trials, and missing data are estimated from the mean scores in each group. Calculation of NNTs was not possible because of missing data.

OPTION	FAMILY THERAPY

Limited evidence from three RCTs suggests that family therapy is an effective intervention for improving adherence with antipsychotic medication.

Benefits: We found one systematic review that will be assessed in a future issue of *Clinical Evidence*.[36] We found three RCTs of family therapy in schizophrenia, which directly assessed its impact on adherence to antipsychotic medication.[39,45,46] The first RCT, conducted in the UK, compared family therapy versus individual supportive therapy in 32 people recently discharged from hospital who all had at least one parent who exhibited high "expressed emotion".[39] People were followed up for 6 months. Individuals receiving family therapy were significantly more likely to take at least half of their prescribed antipsychotic dose than those receiving supportive therapy (ARI 0.54; NNT 2, 95% CI 2 to 5) as judged by tablet counts, reports from people with schizophrenia, their family, and blood levels. The second and third RCTs were conducted in China and used comparison with standard care only. The two trials may have included some or all of the same people. The first of these (63 people) measured adherence as "compliance with medication for at least 75% of the non-hospitalised follow up period".[45] The trial found no advantage of family therapy over standard care using the numbers of people in each group compliant with 50% of their medication dose, or when using the months of medication as an outcome measure. The third RCT (78 men with schizophrenia admitted to hospital for the first time) measured adherence as "people taking at least 33% of the dose prescribed at the time of the index discharge for at least 6 days per week". It found an increase in medicated adherence with family therapy versus standard care (ARI 0.23; NNT 5, 95% CI 3 to 34).

Harms: None reported.

Comment: The first trial was conducted in the UK and found that family therapy also improved attendance at clinic appointments. Both of the Chinese trials refer to the unique family structure in China. How adherence to medication was judged is unclear, but appears to have been rated blind to treatment allocation.

OPTION **PSYCHOEDUCATIONAL THERAPY**

One systematic review of RCTs has found limited evidence that psychoeducation improves adherence with antipyschotic medication.

Benefits: **Versus usual treatment:** We found one systematic review (search date 2000, 10 RCTs, 1128 people, 53% male).[43] The systematic review considered individual and group psychoeducation of either standard length (11 sessions or more) or brief interventional types (10 sessions or less). One trial (67 people with DSM-III-R schizophrenia) measured the effect of individual psychoeducation on compliance. It found no significant differences between the brief individual psychoeducation and treatment as usual on the compliance subscale of the Schedule for Assessment of Insight. Two RCTs compared brief group psychoeducational interventions versus control group. Both suggest psychoeducation to be more effective than the comparison treatment. The first trial (236 people) found a significant advantage group of psychoeducational intervention versus usual treatment on a continuous scale of medication concordance (WMD −0.4, 95% CI −0.6 to −0.2). The second trial (46 people) of a brief psychoeducational intervention versus usual treatment reported compliance episodes at 1 year follow up. Skewed data suggested an advantage of psychoeducational interventions (treatment group: 24 people, mean number of non-compliant episodes at 1 year 0.38; control group: 22 people, mean 1.14). One trial (82 people, 18 months duration) compared standard length group interventions versus treatment as usual and found no significant differences in compliance. **Versus behavioural therapy:** We found two RCTs.[47,48] One RCT (36 men) compared behavioural therapy versus psychoeducation versus usual treatment.[47] The behavioural training method comprised being told the importance of complying with antipsychotic medication and instructions on how to take medication. Each participant was given a self monitoring spiral calendar, which featured a dated slip of paper for each dose of antipsychotic. Adherence was estimated by pill counts. After 3 months, fewer people had high pill adherence after psychoeducation compared with behaviour therapy (3/11 v 8/11 had pill adherence scores of 80% measured by pill counts). The second RCT (39 people) compared a behavioural intervention given individually, a behavioural intervention involving the person with schizophrenia and their family, and a psychoeducational intervention.[48] The behavioural intervention consisted of specific written guidelines, and oral instructions, given to people to use a pill box consisting of 28 compartments for every medication occasion during a week. The behavioural intervention, when given to the individual and their family, also consisted of instructions for the family member to compliment the person with schizophrenia for taking their prescribed medication. The primary outcome measure was pill count at 2 months. Medication adherence was more likely with behavioural interventions than with psychoeducation (over 90% adherence at 2 months, 25/26 [96%] with behavioural methods v 6/13 [46%] with psychoeducation; ARR 0.5; RR 2.1; NNT 2 95% CI 2 to 5).

Harms: None reported.

Comment: There are few RCTs of psychoeducational interventions, and most do not measure medication adherence. Each psychoeducational intervention varied in the protocol used, and few employed the same outcome ratings.

OPTION | **BEHAVIOURAL THERAPY**

One RCT found that behavioural interventions improved adherence to antipsychotic medication compared with usual treatment. One RCT found that behavioural interventions improved adherence compared with psychoeducational therapy.

Benefits: We found no systematic review. **Versus usual treatment:** We found one RCT (36 men).[47] The behavioural training method comprised being told the importance of complying with antipsychotic medication and instructions on how to take medication. Each participant was given a self monitoring spiral calendar, which featured a dated slip of paper for each dose of antipsychotic. Adherence was estimated by pill counts. After 3 months fewer people had high pill adherence after usual treatment compared with behaviour therapy (figures not presented). **Versus psychoeducational therapy:** See option, p 709.

Harms: None reported.

Comment: See above.

GLOSSARY

Compliance therapy A treatment based on cognitive behavioural therapy and motivational interviewing techniques with a view to improving concordance to medication.

Negative symptoms This generally refers to qualities abnormal by their absence (e.g. loss of drive, motivation, and self care).

Positive symptoms This refers to symptoms that characterise the onset, or relapse of schizophrenia, usually hallucinations and delusions, but sometimes including thought disorder.

Substantive changes since last issue

Olanzapine New systematic review found medium but not long term reduction in symptom severity with olanzapine versus risperidone.[17]

Quetiapine New systematic review;[17] conclusions unchanged.

Clozapine New systematic review;[17] conclusions unchanged.

Psychoeducational therapy New systematic review found that psychoeducation improves adherence with antipsychotic medication.[43]

REFERENCES

1. Andreasen NC. Symptoms, signs and diagnosis of schizophrenia. *Lancet* 1995;346:477–481.

2. Cannon M, Jones P. Neuroepidemiology: schizophrenia. *J Neurol Neurosurg Psychiatry* 1996;61:604–613.

3. Jablensky A, Sartorius N, Ernberg G, et al. Schizophrenia: manifestations, incidence and course in different cultures. A World Health Organisation ten-country study. *Psychol Med* 1992;monograph supplement 20:1–97.

4. Hegarty JD, Baldessarini RJ, Tohen M, Waternaux C, Oepen G. One hundred years of schizophrenia: a meta-analysis of the outcome literature. *Am J Psychiatry* 1994;151:1409–1416.

5. Johnstone EC. Schizophrenia: problems in clinical practice. *Lancet* 1993; 341:536–538.

6. Thornley B, Adams C. Content and quality of 2000 controlled trials in schizophrenia over 50 years. *BMJ* 1998;317:1181–1184. Search date December 1997; primary sources hand searching of conference proceedings, Biological Abstracts, CINAHL, The Cochrane Library (issue 3, 1997), Embase, Lilacs, Psyclit, Pstndex, Medline, Sociofile.

7. Thornley B, Adams CE, Awad G. Chlorpromazine versus placebo for those with schizophrenia. In: The Cochrane Library, Issue 4, 2000. Oxford: Update Software. Search date 1999; primary sources Biological Abstracts; Embase; Medline; Psychlit; SciSearch; Cochrane Library; Cochrane Schizophrenia Groups register; hand searches of

reference lists; and personal contact with pharmaceutical companies and authors of trials.

8. Quraishi S, David A. Depot haloperidol decanoate for schizophrenia. In: The Cochrane Library, Issue 4, 2000. Oxford: Update Software. Search date 1998; primary sources Biological Abstracts; Embase; Medline; Psychlit; SciSearch; The Cochrane Library; reference lists; authors of studies; and pharmaceutical companies.

9. Quraishi S, David A. Depot pipothiazine palmitate and undeclynate for schizophrenia. In: The Cochrane Library, Issue 4, 2000. Oxford: Update Software. Search date 1998; primary sources Biological Abstracts; Cochrane Library; Cochrane Schizophrenia Group's Register; Embase; Medline; Psyclit; hand searches of reference lists; and personal communication with pharmaceutical companies.

10. Bagnall AM, Fenton M, Lewis R, Leitner ML, Kleijnen J. Molindone for schizophrenia and severe mental illness. In: The Cochrane Library, Issue 4, 2000. Oxford: Update Software. Search date 1999; primary sources Biological Abstracts; The Cochrane Library, The Cochrane Schizophrenia Group's Register, Cinahl; Embase; Psychlit; and pharmaceutical databases and hand searches of reference lists and personal contact with authors of trials.

11. Fenton M, Murphy B, Wood J, Bagnall AM, Schou P, Leitner M. Loxapine for schizophrenia. In: The Cochrane Library, Issue 4, 2000. Oxford: Update Software. Search date 1999; primary sources Biological Abstracts; The Cochrane Library; The Cochrane Schizophrenia Group's Register; Embase; Lilacs; Psyndex; Psychlit; and hand searches of reference lists.

12. Sultana A, McMonagle T. Pimozide for schizophrenia or related psychoses. In: The Cochrane Library, Issue 4, 2000. Oxford: Update Software. Search date 1999; primary sources Biological Abstracts; The Cochrane Schizophrenia Group's Register; Embase; Janssen-Cilag UK's register of studies; Medline; hand searches of reference lists; and personal contact with pharmaceutical companies.

13. Joy CB, Mumby-Croft R, Joy LA. Polyunsaturated fatty acid (fish or evening primrose oil) for schizophrenia. In: The Cochrane Library, Issue 4, 2000. Oxford: Update Software. Search date 2000; primary sources Biological Abstracts; Cinahl; The Cochrane Library; The Cochrane Schizophrenia Group's Register; Embase; Psychlit; hand searches of reference lists; and personal contact with the authors.

14. Duggan L, Fenton M, Dardennes RM, El-Dosoky A, Indran S. Olanzapine for schizophrenia. In: The Cochrane Library, Issue 4, 2000. Oxford: Update Software. Search date June 1998; primary sources Biological Abstracts; Embase; Medline; Psychlit; Cochrane Library; hand searches of reference lists and conference abstracts; and personal communication with authors of trials and pharmaceutical companies.

15. Leucht S, Pitschel-Walx G, Abraham D, Kissling W. Efficacy and extrapyramidal side-effects of the new antipsychotics olanzapine, quetiapine, risperidone and sertindole compared to conventional antipsychotics and placebo. A meta-analysis of randomised controlled trials. Schizophr Res 1999; 35:51–68. Search date 1999; primary sources Medline; Current Contents; hand searches of reference lists; and personal communication with pharmaceutical companies.

16. Tuunainen A, Gilbody SM. Newer atypical antipsychotic medication versus clozapine for schizophrenia. In: The Cochrane Library, Issue 4, 2000. Oxford: Update Software. Search date May 1998; primary sources Biological Abstracts; Cochrane Schizophrenia Group's Register; Cochrane Library; Embase; Lilacs; Medline; Psychlit; hand searches of reference lists; and personal contact with authors of trials and pharmaceutical companies.

17. Gilbody SM, Bagnall AM, Duggan L, Tuunainen A. Risperidone versus other atypical antipsychotic medication for schizophrenia. In: The Cochrane Library, Issue 4, 2000. Oxford: Update Software. Search date February 1999; primary sources Biological Abstracts 1980 to 1999; Cochrane Library Issue 1; Cochrane Schizophrenia Group's Register; Embase 1980 to 1999; Medline 1966 to 1999; Lilacs 1982 to 1999; Psyindex 1977 to 1999; Psychlit 1974 to 1999; pharmaceutical databases on the Dialog Corporation Datastar and Dialog services; hand search of reference lists; and contact with pharmaceutical companies and authors of trials.

18. Srisurapanont M, Disayavanish C, Taimkaew K. Quetiapine for schizophrenia. In: The Cochrane Library, Issue 4, 2000. Oxford: Update Software. Search date 1998; primary sources Biological Abstracts; Embase; Medline; Psychlit; The Cochrane Library; Cinahl; Sigle; Sociofile; hand searches of journals; and personal communication with authors of studies and pharmaceutical companies.

19. Kennedy E, Song F, Hunter R, Clarke Q, Gilbody S. Risperidone versus typical antipsychotic medication for schizophrenia. In: The Cochrane Library, Issue 4, 2000. Oxford: Update Software. Search date 1997; primary sources Biological Abstracts; The Cochrane Trials Register; Embase; Medline; Psychlit; hand searches of reference lists; and personal communication with pharmaceutical companies.

20. Lopez Ibor JJ, Ayuso JL, Gutierrez M, et al. Risperidone in the treatment of chronic schizophrenia: multicenter study comparative to haloperidol. Actas Luso Esp Neurol Psiquiatr Cienc Afines 1996;24:165–172.

21. Bagnall AM, Lewis RA, Leitner ML, Kleijnen J. Ziprasidone for schizophrenia and severe mental illness. In: The Cochrane Library, Issue 4, 2000. Oxford: Update Software. Search date 1999; primary sources Biological Abstracts; The Cochrane Library; The Cochrane Schizophrenia Group's Register; Embase; Lilacs; Psyndex; Psychlit; pharmaceutical databases; hand searches of reference lists; and personal contact with authors of trials.

22. Fenton M, Morris J, De Silva P, et al. Zotepine for schizophrenia. In: The Cochrane Library, Issue 4, 2000. Oxford: Update Software. Search date 1999; primary sources Biological Abstracts; The Cochrane Library; The Cochrane Schizophrenia Group's Register; Embase; Dialog Corporation Datastar service; Medline; Psychlit; hand searches of reference lists; and personal contact with authors of trials and pharmaceutical companies.

23. Wahlbeck K, Cheine M, Essali MA. Clozapine versus typical neuroleptic medication for schizophrenia. In: The Cochrane Library, Issue 4, 2000. Oxford: Update Software. Search date 1999; primary sources Biological Abstracts; Cochrane Schizophrenia Group's Register; Cochrane Library; Embase; Lilacs; Medline; Psychlit; SciSearch Science Citation Index; hand searches of reference lists; and personal communication with pharmaceutical companies.

24. Honigfeld G, Arellano F, Sethi J, Bianchini A, Schein J. Reducing clozapine-related morbidity and mortality: five years experience of the clozaril national registry. J Clin Psychiatry 1998;59(suppl 3):3–7.

25. Kumra S, Frazier JA, Jacobsen LK, et al. Childhood-onset schizophrenia. A double-blind clozapine-haloperidol comparison. Arch Gen Psychiatry 1996; 53:1090–1097.

26. Soares BGO, Fenton M, Chue P. Sulpiride for schizophrenia. In: The Cochrane Library, Issue 1, 2001. Oxford: Update Software. Search date 1998 primary sources Biological Abstracts; Cinahl; Cochrane Schizophrenia Group's Register; The Cochrane Library, Embase; Medline; Psyclit; Sigle; and Sociofile

27. Harnryd C, et al. Clinical evaluation of sulpiride in schizophrenic patients — a double-blind comparison with chlorpromazine. *Acta Psych Scand.* 1984;311: 7–30.

28. Sultana A, Reilly J, Fenton M. Thioridazine for schizophrenia. In: The Cochrane Library, Issue 1, 2001. Oxford: Update Software. Search date 1999; primary sources Biological Abstracts; Cinahl; The Cochrane Library; The Cochrane Schizophrenia Group's Register; Embase; Medline; Psyclit; Sociofile; reference lists; Pharmaceutical companies, and authors of trials.

29. Gilbert PL, Harris MJ, McAdams LA, Jeste DV. Neuroleptic withdrawal in schizophrenic people: a review of the literature. *Arch Gen Psychiatry* 1995; 52:173–188. Search date not given; primary source Medline.

30. Adams CE, Eisenbruch M. Depot fluphenazine versus oral fluphenazine for those with schizophrenia. In: The Cochrane Library, Issue 4, 2000. Oxford: Update Software. Search date May 1995; primary sources Biological Abstracts; The Cochrane Library; Cochrane Schizophrenia Group's Register; Embase; Medline; Psychlit; Science Citation Index; hand searches of reference lists; and personal communication with pharmaceutical companies.

31. Quraishi S, David A. Depot flupenthixol decanoate for schizophrenia or similar psychotic disorders. In: The Cochrane Library, Issue 4, 2000. Oxford: Update Software. Search date 1998; primary sources Biological Abstracts; The Cochrane Library; Cochrane Schizophrenia Group's Register; Embase; Medline; Psychlit; SciSearch; references, and personal communication with authors of trials and pharmaceutical companies.

32. Quraishi S, David A. Depot fluspirilene for schizophrenia. In: The Cochrane Library, Issue 4, 2000. Oxford: Update Software. Search date 1998; primary sources Biological Abstracts; The Cochrane Library; The Cochrane Schizophrenia Group's Register; Embase; Medline; Psychlit; and hand searches of reference lists.

33. Quraishi S, David A. Depot perphenazine decanoate and enanthate for schizophrenia. In: The Cochrane Library, Issue 4, 2000. Oxford: Update Software. Search date 1998; primary sources Biological Abstracts; The Cochrane Library; The Cochrane Schizophrenia Group's Register; Embase; Medline; Psychlit; hand searches of reference lists; and personal communication with the pharmaceutical companies.

34. Coutinho E, Fenton M, Quraishi S. Zuclopenthixol decanoate for schizophrenia and other serious mental illnesses. In: The Cochrane Library, Issue 4, 2000. Oxford: Update Software. Search date 1998; primary sources Biological Abstracts 1982 to 1998; Cinhal 1982 to 1998; The Cochrane Library Issue 2, 2000; The Cochrane Schizophrenia Group's Register April 1998' Embase 1980 to 1998; Medline 1966 to 1998; and Psychlit 1974 to 1998. References of all eligible studies were searched for further trials. The manufacturer of zuclopenthixol was contacted.

35. Jeste D, Gilbert P, McAdams L, Harris M. Considering neuroleptic maintenance and taper on a continuum: need for an individual rather than dogmatic approach. *Arch Gen Psychiatry* 1995;52:209–212.

36. Pharaoh FM, Mari JJ, Streiner D. Family intervention for schizophrenia. In: The Cochrane Library, Issue 4, 2000. Oxford: Update Software. Search date 1998; primary sources Medline; Embase; The Cochrane Library; Cochrane Schizophrenia Group's Register of Trials; and reference lists of articles.

37. McFarlane WR, Lukens E, Link B, et al. Multiple-family groups and psychoeducation in the treatment of schizophrenia. *Arch Gen Psychiatry* 1995;52: 679–687.

38. Kemp R, Kirov G, Everitt B, Hayward P, David A. Randomised controlled trial of compliance therapy. 18-month follow-up. *Br J Psychiatry* 1998;172: 413–419.

39. Strang JS, Falloon IRH, Moss HB, Razani J, Boyd JL. Drug treatment and family intervention during the aftercare treatment of schizophrenics. *Psychopharmacology Bull* 1981;17:87–88.

40. Benton MK, Schroeder HE. Social skills training with schizophrenics: a meta-analytic evaluation. *J Consult Clin Psychol* 1990;58:741–747. Search date not given.

41. Corrigan PW. Social skills training in adult psychiatric populations: a meta-analysis. *J Behav Ther Exp Psychiatry* 1991;22:203–210. Search date 1988; primary source Psychological Abstracts.

42. Jones C, Cormac I, Mota J, Campbell C. Cognitive behavioural therapy for schizophrenia. In: The Cochrane Library, Issue 4, 2000. Oxford: Update Software. Search date July 1998; primary sources Biological Abstracts; Cochrane Schizophrenia Group's Register of Trials; Cinahl; The Cochrane Library; Medline; Embase; Psychlit; Sigle; Sociofile; reference lists of articles; and personal communication with authors of trials.

43. Pekkala E, Merinder L. Psychoeducation for schizophrenia. In: The Cochrane Library, Issue 4, 2000. Oxford: Update Software. Search date 1999; primary sources Cinahl 1982 to 1999; The Cochrane Library Issue 1 1999; Cochrane Schizophrenia Group's Register January 1999; Embase 1980 to 1999; Medline 1966 to 1999; Psychlit 1974 to 1999; Sociofile 1974 to 1999; hand searched reference lists; and personal contact with authors.

44. Kemp R, Hayward P, Applewhaite G, Everitt B, David A. Compliance therapy in psychotic people: randomised controlled trial. *BMJ* 1996;312:345–349.

45. Xiong W, Phillips MR, Hu X, et al. Family-based intervention for schizophrenic people in China. A randomised controlled trial. *Br J Psychiatry* 1994; 165:239–247.

46. Zhang M, Wang M, Li J, Phillips MR. Randomised-control trial of family intervention for 78 first-episode male schizophrenic people. An 18-month study in Suzhou, Jiangsu. *Br J Psychiatry* 1994;165:96–102.

47. Boczkowski JA, Zeichner A, DeSanto N. Neuroleptic compliance among chronic schizophrenic outpeople: an intervention outcome report. *J Consult Clin Psychol* 1985;53:666–671.

48. Azrin NH, Teichner G. Evaluation of an instructional program for improving medication compliance for chronically mentally ill outpatients. *Behaviour Res Ther* 1998;36:849–861.

Andrew McIntosh
Lecturer in Psychiatry
Department of Psychiatry
University of Edinburgh
Edinburgh, UK

Stephen Lawrie
Senior Clinical Research Fellow and
Honorary Consultant Psychiatrist
University of Edinburgh
Edinburgh, UK

Competing interests: SL has been paid for speaking about critical appraisal and has had expenses to attend a conference reimbursed by the manufacturers of Risperidone, and has been paid for speaking about critical appraisal and chairing a symposium by the manufacturers of Olanzapine. AM, none declared.

TABLE 1 Continued treatment with antipsychotic drugs: choice of drugs (see text, p 707).

Review	Search Date	Number of RCTs	Comparisons	Main Conclusion
30	1995	6	Oral v depot fluphenazine	No significant difference
8	1998	7	Haloperidol decanoate v other depots	No significant difference
31	1998	8	Flupenthixol decanoate v other depots	No significant difference
9	1998	7	Pipothiazine palmitate v other depots	No significant difference
9	1998	2	Pipothiazine palmitate v oral antipsychotics	No significant difference
32	1998	1	Fluspirilene decanoate v oral chlorpromazine	No significant difference
32	1998	3	Fluspirilene decanoate v other depots	No significant difference
33	1998	1	Perphenazine enanthate v clopenthixol decanoate	No significant difference
12	1999	11	Pimozide v standard antipsychotics	No significant difference
14	1998	1	Olanzapine v standard antipsychotics	No significant difference
34	1998	3	Zuclopenthixol decanoate v other depots	People taking zuclopenthixol had lower relapse rates over 12 weeks to 1 year
23	1999	19	Clozapine v standard antipsychotics	Relapse rates up to 12 weeks were lower with clozapine

Search date August 2000: new for this issue

Shawn Marshall

Musculoskeletal disorders

Key Messages

- Two RCTs have found that oral corticosteroids relieve short term symptoms of carpal tunnel syndrome.

- We found no evidence that diuretics or non-steroidal anti-inflammatory drugs (NSAIDs) improve the clinical symptoms of carpal tunnel syndrome.

- Three RCTs found no benefit of pyridoxine versus placebo in the treatment of carpal tunnel syndrome.

- One systematic review has found that local corticosteroid injection for carpal tunnel syndrome relieves symptoms up to 1 month after injection.

- One RCT found no significant difference in clinical symptoms with full time versus night time only wearing of wrist splints.

- We found no evidence comparing wrist splints versus no treatment.

- We found no RCTs evaluating the effectiveness of nerve and tendon gliding exercises.

- One RCT found a benefit of therapeutic ultrasound versus placebo, but one smaller RCT found no significant difference.

- One systematic review and four additional RCTs found no evidence that endoscopic versus open carpal tunnel release influences ultimate clinical outcome. Some RCTs found earlier return to work but more surgical complications with endoscopic versus open carpal tunnel release.

- Three RCTs found no evidence of benefit for internal neurolysis in conjunction with open carpal tunnel release.

- Three RCTs found no benefit for wrist splinting after carpal tunnel release.

DEFINITION   Carpal tunnel syndrome is a neuropathy characterised by compression of the median nerve within the carpal tunnel.[1] Classical or probable symptoms of carpal tunnel syndrome include numbness, tingling, burning, or pain in at least two of digits 1, 2, or 3.[2] Diagnostic criteria vary: some include combinations of symptom characteristics and electrodiagnostic study findings to diagnose carpal tunnel syndrome and place less emphasis on physical examination.[2] The American Academy of Neurology has specified diagnostic criteria (see glossary, p 726) that rely more heavily on clinical symptoms and physical examination findings.[3]

INCIDENCE/ PREVALENCE   A general population survey in Rochester, Minnesota, found the age adjusted incidence of carpal tunnel syndrome to be 105 (95% CI 99 to 112) cases per 100 000 person years.[4,5] Age adjusted incidence rates were 52 (95% CI 45 to 59) for men and 149 (95% CI 138 to 159) for women per 100 000 person years. The study found incidence rates increased from 88 (95% CI 75 to 101) per 100 000 person years in 1961–1965; to 125 (95% CI 112 to 138) per 100 000 person years in 1976–1980. Incidence rates of carpal tunnel syndrome increased with age for men, whereas for women they peaked between the ages of 45–54 years. An industry wide survey in Washington State, USA, found a higher incidence of carpal tunnel syndrome for employed persons (1.74 claims per 1000 full time employees) compared with surveys in the general population.[6] A general population survey in the Netherlands found the prevalence to be 0.6% for men and 6.8% for women.[7] A more comprehensive study in southern Sweden found the general population prevalence for carpal tunnel syndrome (defined by clinical symptoms and electrophysiological studies) was 2.7% (95% CI 2.1 to 3.4%).[8] As in other studies, the overall prevalence in women was higher than for men (male to female ratio 1 : 1.4); however, among older people the prevalence in women was almost four times that for men (age group 65–74: men 1.3%, 95% CI 0.3 to 3.7; women 5.1%, 95% CI 2.8 to 8.1).

AETIOLOGY/ RISK FACTORS   Most cases of carpal tunnel syndrome have no easily identifiable cause (idiopathic). Non-specific tenosynovitis is believed to contribute to compression of the median nerve within the carpal tunnel.[4] Secondary causes of carpal tunnel syndrome include space occupying lesions such as tumours, hypertrophic synovial tissue, fracture callus, and osteophytes; metabolic and physiologic causes such as pregnancy, hypothyroidism, rheumatoid arthritis; infectious causes and neuropathies associated with diabetes mellitus, alcoholism, and familial disorders. Secondary causes are often excluded from RCTs of treatments for carpal tunnel syndrome. One case control study found that risk factors in the general population included repetitive activities requiring wrist extension or flexion, obesity, very rapid dieting, shorter height, hysterectomy without oopherectomy and recent menopause.[9] A general health survey found a strong association between carpal tunnel syndrome and obesity, as well as among manual versus sedentary workers, and for occupations involving excessive wrist flexion and extension.[8]

PROGNOSIS We found little good evidence. One natural history study (carpal tunnel syndrome defined by clinical symptoms and electrophysiologic studies) found that 34% of people with idiopathic carpal tunnel syndrome had complete resolution of symptoms, without treatment intervention, within 6 months of diagnosis.[10] Remission rates were higher for the younger age groups, for females, and for pregnant compared with non-pregnant women. Pregnant women had the highest rate of remission at 6 months (68%).

AIMS To improve the signs and symptoms of carpal tunnel syndrome; to prevent progression and loss of hand function secondary to carpal tunnel syndrome; to minimise loss of time from work.

OUTCOMES Clinical improvement in signs and symptoms; hand function; time to return to work. The global symptom score[11,12] is the sum of five common carpal tunnel syndrome symptoms (pain, numbness, paresthesia, weakness/clumsiness, and nocturnal wakening), which are each rated from 0 (no symptoms) to 10 (severe symptoms).

METHODS *Clinical Evidence* search and appraisal August 2000.

QUESTION What are the effects of drug treatment?

OPTION ORAL CORTICOSTEROIDS

RCTs have found that oral corticosteroids provide short term relief of carpal tunnel syndrome symptoms versus placebo, diuretic (trichlormethiazide), and an NSAID (tenoxicam). Lower dose prednisone did not provide benefit versus placebo beyond the time of administration. The effect of a higher dose is beneficial while administered, but the effect after 4 weeks is unknown.

Benefits: We found no systematic review. We found two RCTs of the short term use of oral prednisone in the treatment of carpal tunnel syndrome.[11,12] One small RCT found that a 2 week course of prednisone (6 people; 20 mg daily first week followed by 10 mg daily second week) versus placebo (9 people) significantly improved clinical symptoms, based on the Global Symptom Score, at 2 week follow up, but significance was not maintained at 4 and 8 weeks follow up, (results presented graphically, no P values provided).[11] The second RCT (4 weeks) compared oral prednisolone (23 people; prednisolone 20 mg daily for 2 weeks followed by 10 mg daily for another 2 weeks), versus placebo (16 people), versus a slow release NSAID (tenoxicam; 16 people), versus a diuretic (trichlormethiazide; 18 people).[12] Only prednisolone was significantly better than placebo on the Global Symptom Score at 2 and 4 weeks (mean difference 2 weeks: –6.6, 95% CI –10.8 to –2.4; and 4 weeks: –10.8, 95% CI –15.4 to –6.2).

Harms: In the first RCT, three people in each group reported adverse effects; however they did not discontinue treatment.[11] In the prednisone group, one person with diabetes reported mild hyperglycaemia; other reported symptoms included nausea/abdominal discomfort, constipation, and dysgeusia. Symptoms in the placebo group included nausea/abdominal discomfort, constipation, insomnia, headache, dysuria, and burning nostrils. The second RCT did not report adverse effects.[12] Common adverse reactions to oral corticosteroids include nausea, anxiety, acne, menstrual irregularities, insomnia, headaches, and mood swings. More serious adverse reactions include peptic ulcer, steroid psychosis, and adrenal insufficiency.[13]

Comment: The second RCT reported that five people "refused to continue participation", but did not comment on the reason for withdrawal.[11] A weakness of this RCT is the failure to report adverse effects of NSAIDs or oral steroids after 4 weeks.[12]

OPTION NON-STEROIDAL ANTI-INFLAMMATORY DRUGS

We found no evidence that NSAIDs improve clinical symptoms in carpal tunnel syndrome.

Benefits: We found no systematic reviews. We found one RCT comparing NSAIDs (16 people; slow release tenoxicam 20 mg daily) versus placebo (16 people) versus diuretics (trichlormethiazide; 18 people) versus oral steroids (prednisolone; 23 people).[12] It found no significant difference in clinical symptoms with the NSAID versus placebo. Another RCT (91 people, age 21–45 years) compared NSAIDs (ibuprofen 800 mg, 3 times daily for 1 week, then twice daily for 1 week, and then as needed for 7 weeks) plus nocturnal wrist splints, versus chiropractic manipulation, ultrasound treatments, and nocturnal wrist splints.[14] It found no significant difference in clinical improvement versus placebo at 2 or 4 weeks (mean difference at 2 weeks +3.1, 95% CI –2.1 to +8.3 and at 4 weeks +3.2, 95% CI –2.5 to +8.9).

Harms: The RCT using tenoxicam did not report adverse effects.[12] In the RCT of ibuprofen 10 of 46 (22%) people experienced intolerance of ibuprofen (acute gastrointestinal intolerance, headache, nausea, or both). Of these, five withdrew from the medication and five continued to take ibuprofen with a liquid antacid.

Comment: The first RCT reported that five people "refused to continue participation", but did not comment on the reason for withdrawal.[12] Other studies suggest adverse effects would be a concern with NSAIDs or oral steroid for 4 weeks (see harms of oral corticosteroids above, and harms of differences between available NSAIDs, p 800). the second RCT, the particular effect of ultrasound therapy in the treatment of carpal tunnel syndrome is difficult to determine because two interventions (manipulation and ultrasound) were compared with oral NSAID and each group also used nocturnal wrist splints.[13]

DIURETICS

We found no evidence that diuretics improve clinical symptoms in carpal tunnel syndrome.

Benefits: We found no systematic review. We found one RCT (73 people) comparing the effect of diuretic (trichlormethiazide 2 mg daily) versus NSAIDs (slow release tenoxicam) versus placebo versus oral steroids (prednisolone).[12] It found no significant difference in clinical symptoms between the diuretic versus placebo, at 2 or 4 weeks (Global Symptom Score, mean difference at 2 weeks +0.7, 95% CI –3.4 to +4.8, and at 4 weeks +0.8, –3.7 to +5.3, respectively).

Harms: This RCT did not report on adverse effects. Common adverse effects of hydrochlorothizide include hyperglycemia, hyperuricemia, dizziness, orthostatic hypotension, weakness, restlessness, muscle cramp, and rash.[13]

Comment: The first RCT reported that five people "refused to continue participation", but did not comment on the reason for withdrawal.[12] A weakness of this RCT is the failure to report adverse effects of diuretics after 4 weeks (see harms of oral corticosteroids, p 720, and harms of differences between available NSAIDs, p 800).

PYRIDOXINE (VITAMIN B6)

We found no evidence to support pyridoxine as an effective treatment for carpal tunnel syndrome.

Benefits: We found no systematic review. We found two small double blinded RCTs.[15,16] They found no significant difference in clinical symptoms between daily pyridoxine (vitamin B6 200 mg) versus placebo. The first small RCT (11 people) found fewer people improved at 10 weeks with pyridoxine but the difference was not significant (3/6 [50%] improved with pyridoxine v 4/5 [80%] with placebo; RR 1.6, 95% CI 0.6 to 4).[16] The second RCT (35 people) found a greater improvement in some symptom scores (swollen fingers, tingling, or discomfort after repetitive movement), but not for others (night discomfort, poor co-ordination) compared with baseline with pyridoxine versus placebo, but direct statistical comparisons were not provided.[15]

Harms: Adverse effects were not reported by either RCT. Common adverse reactions associated with pyridoxine include numbness, parathesiae, and unsteady gait.[13]

Comment: The first RCT simply reported people as improved, unchanged, or worsened.[16]

LOCAL CORTICOSTEROID INJECTION

One systematic review of RCTs has found that local corticosteroid injection significantly improves carpal tunnel syndrome symptoms up to 1 month after injection.

Benefits: We found one systematic review (search date 2000, 2 RCTs, 97 people) of local corticosteroid injection versus placebo injection.[17]

The first RCT found short term benefit for clinical symptoms up to 1 month after injection of local corticosteroid versus placebo injection.[18] The second RCT found a short term benefit at 1 month with local corticosteroid injection plus placebo injection into the deltoid muscle versus local placebo injection plus systemic corticosteroid injection into the deltoid muscle.[19] Meta-analysis found significant improvement in symptoms at 1 month (32/48 [AR 67%] with corticosteroid injection v 9/49 [AR 18%] with placebo injection; ARR 48%; RR 3.6, 95% CI 1.9 to 6.7; NNT 3, 95% 2 to 4).[17]

Harms: No adverse effects were reported in any of the RCTs. Known serious adverse effects of local corticosteroid injection into the carpal tunnel include tendon rupture and injection into the median nerve.[20]

Comment: One RCT was excluded from the analysis because only significance values from baseline comparisons were reported instead of direct comparisons between groups.[21]

QUESTION What are the effects of non-drug treatment?

OPTION WRIST SPLINTS

We found no RCTs comparing wrist splinting versus no treatment. One quasi-randomised trial found that neutral angle wrist splints provide more symptomatic relief than wrist splints set in extension. One RCT found that full time and night time wear provide similar clinical improvement.

Benefits: We found one systematic review (search date 1997) of splinting for treatment of carpal tunnel syndrome.[22] **Versus no treatment:** The review found no RCTs of splinting versus no treatment.[22] **Versus other treatments:** The review found no RCTs of splinting versus other treatments.[22] **Versus different splinting regimens:** The review found one quasi-randomised trial (59 people, 90 hands, alternate allocation by hands), which compared a neutral angle wrist splint versus a wrist splint in 20° extension. This found the neutral angle wrist splint group had better clinical improvement at 2 weeks follow up. One subsequent RCT (24 people) compared full time wear of neutral angle wrist splints versus night time only wear.[23] It found no clinical difference in symptoms between groups at 6 weeks' follow up (mean difference +0.1, 95% CI −0.3 to +0.5).[23]

Harms: No adverse effects were reported.[22,23]

Comment: In the RCT comparing full time versus night time wear only, night time wear was complete or nearly complete in 85% of people allocated to night time wear only, but 23% reported limited day time use, whereas complete or nearly complete day time wear was reported by only 27% of people allocated to full time wear.[23] Results from this trial may not be generalisable because it recruited more men than would be expected from the usual sex distribution of carpal tunnel syndrome.

NERVE AND TENDON GLIDING EXERCISES

We found no systematic reviews or RCTs of nerve gliding (see glossary, p 727) and tendon gliding exercises (see glossary, p 727).

Benefits: We found no systematic reviews or RCTs evaluating the effectiveness of nerve and tendon gliding exercises or range of motion exercises for the treatment of carpal tunnel syndrome.

Harms: None identified.

Comment: None.

OPTION THERAPEUTIC ULTRASOUND

One large RCT found a benefit of therapeutic ultrasound versus placebo, and one smaller RCT found no significant difference.

Benefits: We found no systematic review. We found three RCTs of therapeutic ultrasound.[14,24,25] The first RCT (45 people with bilateral carpal tunnel syndrome) compared 20 ultrasound treatments (5 times a week for 2 weeks followed by twice weekly for 5 weeks at intensity of 1.0 W/cm^2) lasting 15 minutes versus sham treatment.[24] The dominant wrist was randomly allocated to ultrasound or sham treatment and the contralateral wrist was allocated to the other group. Ultrasound was significantly superior on a visual analog scale from week 2 until the end of treatment (at 6 months follow up the mean change on a 10 cm Visual Analogue Scale for main complaints was 2.0 cm, 95% CI 0.9 to 3.0 cm). Good or excellent results occurred for more people with active ultrasound (26/34 [76%] of actively treated wrists v 11/34 [32%] for sham treated wrists; RR 2.4, 95% CI 1.4 to 4.0; NNT 3, 95% CI 2 to 5). The second RCT (30 wrists, 18 people) compared ultrasound at 1.5 W/cm^2 versus 0.8 W/cm^2 versus sham ultrasound.[24] Treatments were five times a week for 2 weeks and lasted 5 minutes. It found no significant difference in clinical symptoms at 2 week follow up. A third RCT (91 people) compared ultrasound (1.0 to 1.5 W/cm^2 for 5 minute treatment sessions) plus nocturnal wrist splints and chiropractic manipulation (3 sessions a week for 2 weeks, then 2 a week for 3 weeks, then 1 a week for 4 weeks) versus nocturnal wrist splints plus an NSAID.[14] It found no significant difference in clinical outcome (figures not available).

Harms: In the third RCT, adverse events were related to NSAID use and one sore neck occurred after chiropractic manipulation.[14]

Comment: The second RCT[24] with only 10 wrists per group (and less intense treatment than the first RCT[25]) may have been too small to detect a clinically important difference.[24] In the third RCT, the effect of ultrasound is difficult to disentangle because two interventions, manipulation and ultrasound, were compared with oral NSAIDs.[14]

QUESTION What are the effects of surgical treatment?

OPTION SURGERY

One non-systematic review has found that endoscopic carpal tunnel release and open carpal tunnel release provide similar clinical outcomes. Endoscopic release technique is associated with earlier return to work. Complications were more common using the endoscopic technique versus the open release technique.

Benefits: **Surgery versus placebo:** We found one non-systematic review (search date 1997).[26] It found no RCTs of surgery versus placebo or no treatment. **Endoscopic carpal tunnel release versus open carpal tunnel release:** We found one non-systematic review (search date 1997, 5 RCTs, plus prospective and retrospective cohort studies) of endoscopic treatment for carpal tunnel syndrome.[26] Meta-analysis was not appropriate because RCTs used different surgical techniques and outcome measures. We found four additional non-English language RCTs.[27-30] None of the RCTs in the review or additional RCTs found a significant difference in clinical symptom improvement for endoscopic versus open carpal tunnel release.[22,27-32] Three RCTs found grip strength and function was initially better in the endoscopic group, but significant differences did not last beyond 3 months.[31-33] Five RCTs found time to return to work after surgery was significantly less for the endoscopic carpal tunnel release group,[28,29,31-33] and two RCTs did not find a significant difference (see table 1, p 728).[27,34] Three RCTs found that endoscopic versus open carpal tunnel release resulted in less scar pain up to 84 days after operation.[31-33]

Harms: In a multicentre RCT (122 people), one person in the endoscopic group had incomplete release requiring open carpal tunnel release and two other people had transient ulnar neurapraxia (see glossary, p 727). In the open carpal tunnel release group one person had injury to the deep motor branch of the ulnar nerve, one person had bowstringing of the digital flexor tendons, and two people had wound dehiscence.[33] In another RCT (145 people), four complications occurred in the endoscopic release group (1 partial transection of the superficial palmar arch, 1 digital nerve contusion, 1 ulnar nerve neurapraxia, 1 wound hematoma).[32] Another RCT (29 people) found three people experienced transient numbness on the radial side of the ring finger after endoscopic release versus one person with prolonged weeping of the wound that resolved after antibiotic treatment.[34] In two other RCTs, complications occurred only in the endoscopic treatment groups. In the first RCT (39 people) four postoperative complications included ulnar nerve injury (2 people) and painful neuromas (2 people).[30] The second (178 people) found two complications.[27] One RCT (71 people) found no significant difference in complication rate with open versus endoscopic carpal tunnel release (7/52 [14%] v 2/53 [4%], RR 3.6, 95% CI 0.8 to 16).[33] In the open release group there were seven complications (5 scar hypertrophy, 1 wound tethering, 1 wound infection). In the endoscopic release group there were two complications (1 ulnar nerve paraesthesia, 1 symptom recurrence).

Comment: Endoscopic release techniques vary between RCTs, which may account for some of the variation in complication rates.[26] Another important factor is the increased technical demand for performing endoscopic versus open carpal tunnel release. One RCT found observational evidence of a "steep learning curve" for this technique before the surgeon becomes proficient.[31] This increased technical difficulty may account for the higher complication rates found in older studies comparing endoscopic and open carpal tunnel release.

OPTION	INTERNAL NEUROLYSIS IN CONJUNCTION WITH OPEN CARPAL TUNNEL RELEASE

Three RCTs have consistently found no difference in outcomes of open carpal tunnel release with or without internal neurolysis.

Benefits: We found no systematic review. We found three RCTs, which compared open carpal tunnel release with or without internal/interfascicular neurolysis.[35–37] They found no significant difference in clinical symptoms following carpal tunnel release with or without internal neurolysis (see glossary, p 727). The first RCT (79 people, 84 hands) found no significant difference in subjective improvement between simple decompression versus decompression with internal neurolysis (28/32 [88%] hands improved with simple decompression v 25/31 [81%] with decompression and internal neurolysis; P value not available, intention to treat analysis not reported). The second RCT (48 people) found no significant difference in improvement in paraesthesia at 6 months' follow up for decompression alone versus decompression and internal neurolysis (23/23 [100%] improved with decompression alone v 23/24 [96%] with internal neurolysis).[37] The third RCT (41 people, 47 hands) specifically examined severe carpal tunnel syndrome (thenar atrophy or markedly prolonged or absent distal sensory latency). It found no significant difference in symptoms between open carpal tunnel release with or without internal neurolysis (good or excellent outcome in 65% v 67%).[36]

Harms: In the RCT (47 hands) of internal neurolysis for severe carpal tunnel syndrome, complications were similar for the neurolysis and non-neurolysis groups.[36] The most common complication was persistent incisional pain (with neurolysis 4/24 [17%] of hands v with non-neurolysis 3/23 [13%] of hands). The neurolysis group had one case of hand swelling and one case of adhesive capsulitis versus one case of causalgia in the non-neurolysis group. The second RCT found no complications from internal neurolysis (48 people). The first RCT did not report complications.[35]

Comment: All three RCTs found no significant difference between groups, but the results do not exclude a clinically important difference.

QUESTION	What are the effects of postoperative treatment?

OPTION	WRIST SPLINTING AFTER CARPAL TUNNEL SYNDROME RELEASE

Three RCTs found no benefit from wrist splinting after carpal tunnel release. One RCT found earlier return to work for the non-splinted group. Another RCT found lower pain ratings for the non-splinted group after surgery.

Benefits:

Versus unrestricted range of motion: We found three RCTs of wrist splinting versus unrestricted range of motion following carpal tunnel release.[38-40] Two RCTs compared rigid splinting for 2 weeks versus no splinting.[39,40] A third RCT compared splinting for 4 weeks versus no splinting (74 people, 82 wrists).[38] The first RCT of postoperative splinting for 2 weeks (47 people, 51 wrists) found no significant differences in grip strength, lateral pinch strength, wrist range of motion, and subjective clinical improvement.[39] The second RCT (50 people, 50 wrists) of postoperative splinting for 2 weeks found that subjective rating of clinical improvement ($P = 0.001$), and grip strength ($P = 0.02$), were greater for the unsplinted group after 1 month, but there was no significant difference after 3 and 6 months (quantified results not available). The unsplinted group also had more rapid return to work (17 days unsplinted v 27 days splinted, $P = 0.005$).[40] The RCT (74 people, 82 wrists) of 4 weeks of postoperative splinting found no significant differences between the splinted versus unsplinted groups for grip strength (as a percentage of preoperative grip strength at 6 weeks: unsplinted 78%, 95% CI 70% to 86% v splinted 76%, 95% CI, 71% to 85%), pain symptoms based on visual analogue scale (unsplinted 2%, 95% CI 4 to 20 v splinted 6%, 95% CI 2 to 4), or time for return to work (unsplinted 6 weeks, 95% CI 5 to 6 weeks v splinted 6 weeks 95% CI 4 to 7 weeks) (confidence intervals for the differences not available).[40] **Versus bulky dressings:** We found one systematic review (search date 1997) of splinting versus bulky dressings after carpal tunnel decompression. It found no RCTs.[22]

Harms:

The second RCT reported complications for one person in the unsplinted group who had persistent symptoms and required reoperation.[39] The third RCT reported that pillar pain (see glossary, p 727) was increased at 1 month for the splinted group ($P = 0.02$) as was scar tenderness ($P = 0.04$).[40] The first RCT reported no adverse effects.

Comment:

The RCTs were too small to exclude the possibility of a clinically important increase in the risk of some complications (e.g. transient ulnar nerve injury) with splinting compared to no splinting.

GLOSSARY

Adhesive capsulitis A condition in which the joint capsule becomes contracted and thickened causing restriction in the range of movement.

American Academy of Neurology diagnostic criteria[3] The likelihood of carpal tunnel syndrome increases with the number of standard symptoms and provocative factors. **Symptoms** include dull aching discomfort in the hand, forearm or upper arm; paraesthesia in the hand; weakness or clumsiness of the hand; dry skin, swelling, or colour changes in the hand; or occurrence of any of these symptoms in the distribution of the median nerve. **Provocative factors** include sleep; sustained arm or hand positions; or repetitive actions of the hand or wrist. **Relieving factors** include changes in hand posture and shaking the hand. **Physical examination** may be normal; or symptoms may be elicited by tapping or direct pressure over the median nerve at the wrist or with forced flexion or extension of the wrist; or sensory loss in the median nerve distribution; or weakness or atrophy in the thenar muscles; or dry skin on thumb, index, or middle fingers. Electromyography and nerve conduction studies can confirm, but not exclude, the diagnosis of carpal tunnel syndrome.

Internal neurolysis Decompression within the nerve accomplished by performing an epineurotomy and then dividing the nerve into multiple fascicular groups.[36]

Nerve gliding exercises Exercise therapy directed at restoring and maximising excursion of the median nerve through the carpal tunnel.[41]

Pillar pain Pain at the radial or ulnar border of the carpal tunnel.

Tendon gliding exercises Exercise therapy directed at restoring and maximising excursion of the finger flexor tendons through the carpal tunnel.[41]

Ulnar neurapraxia Failure of nerve conduction of the ulnar nerve, usually reversible, due to metabolic or microstructural abnormalities without disruption of the axon.

REFERENCES

1. Rozmaryn LM. Carpal tunnel syndrome: a comprehensive review. Curr Opin Orthop 1997;8: 33–43.
2. Rempel D, Evanoff B, Amadio PC, et al. Consensus criteria for the classification of carpal tunnel syndrome in epidemiologic studies. Am J Public Health 1998;88:1447–1451.
3. Anonymous. Practice parameter for carpal tunnel syndrome (summary statement). Report of the Quality Standards Subcommittee of the American Academy of Neurology. Neurology 1993;43: 2406–2409.
4. von Schroeder H, Botte MJ. Carpal tunnel syndrome. Hand Clin 1996;12:643–655.
5. Stevens JC, Sun S, Beard CM, O'Fallon WM, Kurland LT. Carpal tunnel syndrome in Rochester, Minnesota, 1961 to 1980. Neurology 1988;38: 134–138.
6. Franklin GM, Haug J, Heyer N, Checkoway H, Peck N. Occupational carpal tunnel Syndrome in Washington state, 1984–1988. Am J Public Health 1991;81:741–746.
7. Dumitru D. Textbook of Electrodiagnostic Medicine. Hanley and Belfus, eds. Philadelphia: Mosby Publications, 1995.
8. Atroshi I, Gummesson C, Johnsson R, Ornstein E, Ranstam J, Rosen I. Prevalence of carpal tunnel syndrome in a general population. JAMA 1999; 282:153–158.
9. De Krom MCTF, Kester A, Knipschild P, Spaans F. Risk factors for carpal tunnel syndrome. Am J Epidemiol 1990;132:1102–1110.
10. Fatami T, Kobayashi A, Utika T, Endoh T, Fujita T. Carpal tunnel syndrome; its natural history. Hand Surgery 1997;2(2):129–130.
11. Herskovitz S, Berger AR, Lipton RB. Low-dose, short-term oral prednisone in the treatment of carpal tunnel syndrome. Neurology 1995;45: 1923–1925.
12. Chang MH, Chiang HT, Lee SS, Ger LP, Lo YK. Oral drug of choice in carpal tunnel syndrome. Neurology 1998;51:390–393.
13. Canadian Pharmacists Association. Compendium of pharmaceuticals and specialties 2000. Ottawa: Canadian Pharmacists Association, 2000.
14. Thomas P, James D, Hulbert R, Kassak KM, Meyer JJ. Comparative efficacy of conservative medical and chiropractic treatments for carpal tunnel syndrome: a randomized clinical trial. J Manipulative Physiol Ther 1998;21:317–326.
15. Spooner GR, Desai HB, Angel JF, Reeder BA, Donat JR. Using pyridoxine to treat carpal tunnel syndrome. Randomized control trial. Can Fam Physician 1993;39:2122–2127.
16. Stransky M, Rubin A, Lava NS, Lazaro RP. Treatment of carpal tunnel syndrome with vitamin B6: a double-blind study. South Med J 1989;82: 841–842.
17. Marshall S, Tardif G, Ashworth N. Local corticosteroid injection for carpal tunnel syndrome.

In: The Cochrane Library, Issue 4, 2000. Oxford: Update Software. Search date not stated; primary sources Cochrane Neuromuscular Disease Group Register, Medline, Embase, Cinahl. No company sponsorship supplied.
18. Dammers JW, Veering MM, Vermeulen M, Weinreb H. Injection with methyprednisolone proximal to the carpal tunnel: randomized double blind trial. BMJ 1999;319:884–886.
19. Ozdogan H, Yazici H. The efficacy of local steroid injections in idiopathic carpal tunnel syndrome: a double-blind study. Br J Rheumatol 1984;23: 272–275.
20. Babu SR, Britton JM. The role of steroid injection in the management of carpal tunnel syndrome. J Orthop Rheumatol 1994;7:59–60.
21. Girlanda P, Dattola R, Venuto C, Mangiapane R, Nicolosi C, Messina C. Local steroid treatment in idiopathic carpal tunnel syndrome: short and long-term efficacy. J Neurol 1993;240:187–190.
22. Feuerstein M, Burrell LM, Miller VI, Lincoln A, Huang GD, Berger R. Clinical management of carpal tunnel syndrome: a 12-year review of outcomes. Am J Ind Med 1999;35:232–245. Search date 1997; primary sources Medline, Cinahl, Psyclit, Nioshtic. No company sponsorship stated.
23. Walker WC, Metzler M, Cifu DX, Swartz Z. Neutral wrist splinting in carpal tunnel syndrome: a comparison of night-only versus full-time wear instructions. Arch Phys Med Rehabil 2000;81: 424–429.
24. Oztas O, Turan B, Bora I, Karakaya MK. Ultrasound therapy effect in carpal tunnel syndrome. Arch Phys Med Rehabil 1998;79:1540–1544.
25. Ebenbichler GR, Resch KL, Nicolakis P, et al. Ultrasound treatment for treating the carpal tunnel syndrome: randomised "sham" controlled trial. BMJ 1998;316:730–735.
26. Jimenez DF, Gibbs SR, Clapper AT. Endoscopic treatment of carpal tunnel syndrome: a critical review [see comments]. J Neurosurg 1998;88: 817–826. Search date 1997; primary sources not stated.
27. Hoefnagels WAJ, Van Kleef JGF, Mastenbroek GGA, De Blok JA, Breukelman AJ, De Krom MCTF. Surgical treatment of the carpal tunnel syndrome: Endoscopic or classical (open) surgery? A prospective randomised study. Ned Tijdschr Geneeskd 1997;141:878–882.
28. Benedetti RB, Sennwald G. Endoscopic decompression of the median nerve by the technique of Agee: A prospective study in comparison with the open decompression. Handchir Mikrochir Plast Chir 1996;28:151–155.
29. Stark B, Engkvist-Lofmark C. Carpal tunnel syndrome. Endoscopic release or conventional surgery. Handchir Mikrochir Plast Chir 1996;28: 128–132.

30. Herren DB. Complications after endoscopic carpal tunnel decompression. *Z Unfallchir Versicherungsmed* 1994;87:120–127.
31. Erdmann MWH. Endoscopic carpal tunnel decompression. *J Hand Surg* 1994;19:5–13.
32. Brown RA, Gelberman RH, Seiler III, Abrahamsson SO, Weiland AJ, Urbaniak JR, Schoenfeld DA, Furcolo D. Carpal tunnel release. A prospective, randomized assessment of open and endoscopic methods. *J Bone Joint Surg Am* 1993;75:1265–1275.
33. Agee JM, McCarroll J, Tortosa RD, et al. Endoscopic release of the carpal tunnel: a randomized prospective multicenter study. *J Hand Surg* 1992;17:987–995.
34. Jacobsen MB, Rahme H. A prospective, randomized study with an independent observer comparing open carpal tunnel release with endoscopic carpal tunnel release. *J Hand Surg* 1996;21:202–204.
35. Mackinnon SE, McCabe S, Murray JF, Szalai JP, Kelly L, Novak C, Kin B, Burke GM. Internal neurolysis fails to improve the results of primary carpal tunnel decompression. *J Hand Surg Am* 1991;16:211–218.

36. Lowry WE Jr, Follender AB. Interfascicular neurolysis in the severe carpal tunnel syndrome. A prospective, randomized, double-blind, controlled study. *Clin Orthop* 1988;227:251–254.
37. Holmgren-Larsson H, Leszniewski W, Linden U, Rabow L, Thorling J. Internal neurolysis or ligament division only in carpal tunnel syndrome — results of a randomized study. *Acta Neurochir* (Wien) 1985;74:118–121.
38. Finsen V, Andersen K, Russwurm H. No advantage from splinting the wrist after open carpal tunnel release. A randomized study of 82 wrists. *Acta Orthop Scand* 1999;70:288–292.
39. Bury TF, Akelman E, Weiss AP. Prospective, randomized trial of splinting after carpal tunnel release. *Ann Plastic Surg* 1995;35:19–22.
40. Cook AC, Szabo RM, Birkholz SW, King EF. Early mobilization following carpal tunnel release. A prospective randomized study. *J Hand Surg Br* 1995;20:228–230.
41. Rozmaryn LM, Dovelle S, Rothman ER, Gorman K, Olvey KM, Bartko JJ. Nerve and tendon gliding exercises and the conservative management of carpal tunnel syndrome. *J Hand Ther* 1998;11:171–179.

Shawn Marshall
Assistant Professor
University of Ottawa
Ottawa
Canada

Competing interests: None declared.

| TABLE 1 | Return to work times comparing open versus endoscopic carpal tunnel release (see text, p 724). | | | |

Reference	Mean return to work time (days)		P value	Difference (95% CI)
	Endoscopic	Open		
27	72	75	P > 0.05	3 days (−17.8 to +25.8)
28	24.5	41.9	P = 0.003	
34	17 (0–31)	19 (0–42)	P > 0.05	2 days (−3.3 to +7.1)
29	20 (8–34)	30 (8–64)	P < 0.01	
31	14	39	P < 0.05	
	Median return to work time (days)			
32	14	28	P < 0.05	
33	25	46.5	P < 0.01	

Search date May 2000

Steven Reid, Trudie Chalder, Anthony Cleare, Mattew Hotopf and Simon Wessely

Key Messages

- Limited data from four RCTs provide insufficient evidence to support the use of antidepressants in people with chronic fatigue syndrome (CFS).

- Limited data from three RCTs provide insufficient evidence to support the use of corticosteroids in people with CFS. Any benefit from low dose glucocorticoid treatment seems to be short lived, and higher doses are associated with adverse effects.

- One small RCT found limited benefit from oral nicotinamide adenine dinucleotide (NADH).

- Two RCTs found that a graded exercise programme produced substantial improvements in measures of fatigue and physical functioning in people with CFS.

- We found no evidence that prolonged rest is an effective treatment for CFS. We found indirect evidence suggesting that prolonged rest may be harmful.

- Limited data from three small RCTs provide no clear evidence of benefit from magnesium injections or oral evening primrose oil in people with CFS.

- Four small RCTs of Immunoglobulin G (IgG) in people with CFS found only limited benefit and adverse effects. RCTs of other forms of immunotherapy found no evidence of an advantage over placebo.

- A systematic review has found that cognitive behavioural therapy administered by highly skilled therapists in specialist centres is effective in people with CFS, with a number needed to treat of 2. This finding may be of limited relevance to less specialised settings.

DEFINITION Chronic fatigue syndrome (CFS) is characterised by severe, disabling fatigue and other symptoms, including musculoskeletal pain, sleep disturbance, impaired concentration and headaches. Two widely used definitions of CFS (see table 1, p 737) from the US Centers for Disease Control and Prevention [1] and Oxford, UK[2] were developed as operational criteria for research. There are two important differences between these definitions. The UK criteria insist upon the presence of mental fatigue, whereas the US criteria include a requirement for several physical symptoms, reflecting the belief that CFS has an underlying immunological or infective pathology.

INCIDENCE/ PREVALENCE Community and primary care based studies have reported the prevalence of CFS to be 0.2–2.6%, depending on the criteria used.[3,4] Systematic population surveys have found similar rates of CFS in people of different socioeconomic status, and in all ethnic groups.[4,5] Women are at higher risk than men (RR 1.3 to 1.7 depending on diagnostic criteria used).[6]

AETIOLOGY/ RISK FACTORS The cause of CFS is poorly understood.

PROGNOSIS Studies have focused on people attending specialist clinics. A systematic review of studies of prognosis (search date 1996) found that children with CFS had a notably better outcome than adults; 54–94% of children showed definite improvement (after up to 6 years' follow up) whereas 20–50% of adults showed some improvement in the medium term and only 6% returned to premorbid levels of functioning.[7] Despite the considerable burden of morbidity associated with CFS, we found no evidence of increased mortality. The systematic review found that outcome was influenced by the presence of psychiatric disorders and beliefs about causation and treatment.[7]

AIMS To reduce levels of fatigue and associated symptoms; to increase levels of activity; to improve quality of life.

OUTCOMES Severity of symptoms and their effects on physical function and quality of life. These outcomes are measured in several different ways: the medical outcomes survey short form general health survey (SF-36),[8] a rating scale measuring limitation of physical functioning caused by ill health; the Karnofsky scale,[9] a modified questionnaire originally developed for the rating of quality of life in people undergoing chemotherapy for malignancy; the Beck Depression Inventory;[10] the sickness impact profile,[11] a measure of the influence of symptoms on social and physical functioning; and self reported severity of symptoms and levels of activity.

METHODS *Clinical Evidence* search and appraisal May 2000.

QUESTION What are the effects of treatments?

OPTION ANTIDEPRESSANTS

Limited data from four RCTs provide insufficient evidence to support the use of antidepressants in people with CFS.

Benefits: We found no systematic reviews. We found three RCTs. One compared fluoxetine versus placebo in 96 people.[12] It found no significant benefit in terms of the Beck Depression Inventory and the sickness impact profile. Another RCT allocated 136 people to four groups: exercise plus fluoxetine; exercise plus placebo; appointments to review activity diary with physiotherapist plus fluoxetine; and appointments to review activity diary with physiotherapist plus placebo. It found no significant difference in outcome (level of fatigue), although there was a trend indicating some benefit and there were modest improvements in measures of depression.[13] A third RCT compared the monoamine oxidase inhibitor phenelzine versus placebo in 24 people with CFS, using a modified Karnofsky scale and other outcome measures.[14] This also found a non-significant trend towards improvement. We found one RCT comparing sertraline versus clomipramine in people with CFS. There was no placebo group, making it difficult to draw useful conclusions.[15]

Harms: Up to 15% of participants withdrew from active treatment because of adverse drug effects.[12-15]

Comment: To date, clinical trials have taken place in specialist clinics, which may actively select for people whose condition is more resistant to treatment. The first trial[12] used shorter treatment and studied people with a long duration of illness than the second trial.[13]

OPTION	CORTICOSTEROIDS

Limited data from three RCTs provide insufficient evidence about the effects of corticosteroids in people with CFS. Any benefit from low dose glucocorticoids seems to be short lived, and higher doses are associated with adverse effects.

Benefits: We found no systematic review. **Versus placebo:** We found three placebo controlled RCTs in people with CFS. One, a crossover RCT of fludrocortisone in 20 people, measured outcomes as change in symptom severity, on a visual analogue scale, and functional status (using the SF-36).[16] It found no significant difference between active treatment and placebo. The other two trials evaluated hydrocortisone. One compared hydrocortisone 25–35 mg daily versus placebo in 65 people and found a greater improvement in a self rated scale of "wellness" in the active treatment group. Other self rating scales did not show significant benefit.[17] The other trial used a lower dose of hydrocortisone (5 or 10 mg daily) in 32 people and found short term improvement in fatigue. Nine people (28%) taking hydrocortisone improved, as measured by a self report fatigue scale, compared with three (9%) taking placebo. The benefit rapidly attenuated when treatment was stopped.[18]

Harms: The trial using the higher doses of hydrocortisone found that 12 people (40%) on active treatment experienced adrenal suppression.[17] Minor adverse effects were reported in up to 10% of people in the other trials.[16,18]

Comment: The RCT of fludrocortisone may have had too few participants to detect a difference. The trials used different reasons for their choice of active treatment. The use of fludrocortisone, a mineralocorticoid, was based on the hypothesis that CFS is associated with neurally mediated hypotension.[19] The use of hydrocortisone in the other trials was based on evidence of underactivity of the hypothalamic-pituitary–adrenocortical axis in some people with CFS.[20]

| OPTION | ORAL NADH |

One small RCT found limited benefit from oral NADH.

Benefits: We found no systematic review. We found one randomised cross-over trial comparing NADH 10 mg per day) versus placebo for 4 weeks.[21] Of the 33 people with CFS who completed the trial, 26 were included in the analysis. Using a symptom rating scale, 8/26 attained a 10% improvement on active treatment compared with 2/26 on placebo.

Harms: Minor adverse effects (loss of appetite, dyspepsia, flatulence) were reported on active treatment but did not lead to cessation of treatment.

Comment: The rationale for this treatment is that NADH facilitates generation of adenosine triphosphate, which it is suggested may be depleted in CFS.[21] The authors are planning a larger trial.

| OPTION | EXERCISE |

Two RCTs found that a graded exercise programme substantially improved measures of fatigue and physical functioning in people with CFS.

Benefits: We found no systematic review. We found two RCTs. The first compared aerobic exercise versus flexibility training (control intervention) in 66 people.[22] The programmes involved individual weekly sessions over 12 weeks. The exercise group built up their level of activity to 30 minutes of exercise a day, with a maximum energy expenditure of 60% of maximum oxygen consumption (VO_2max). Using the self rated clinical global impression scales as an outcome measure, 55% of the aerobic exercise group reported feeling much better or very much better compared with 27% of the flexibility training group ($P = 0.05$). Significantly better outcomes were also reported as measured by physical fatigue and levels of physical functioning on SF-36. The flexibility training group crossed over to aerobic exercise at the end of the trial, and significant improvements from baseline were found. The second trial randomised 136 people with CFS to one of four groups: exercise plus fluoxetine; exercise plus placebo; appointments plus fluoxetine; and appointments plus placebo.[13] The exercise group undertook graded aerobic exercise for 20 minutes three times a week up to an energy expenditure of 75% of VO_2max. Exercise was associated with significant improvements in fatigue and functional work capacity. This trial was complicated by a high withdrawal rate, particularly in the exercise groups (37% v 22% in the appointment groups), but the differences remained significant after intention to treat analysis.

Harms: Neither trial reported data on adverse effects, and we found no evidence that exercise is harmful in people with CFS.

Comment: Experience suggests that symptoms of CFS may be exacerbated by over ambitious or over hasty attempts at exercise.

OPTION   PROLONGED REST

We found no evidence that prolonged rest is an effective treatment for CFS. We found considerable indirect evidence suggesting that prolonged rest may be harmful.

Benefits: We found no systematic reviews or RCTs of prolonged rest in people with CFS.

Harms: We found no direct evidence of harmful effects of rest in people with CFS. We found observational evidence suggesting that prolonged inactivity may perpetuate or worsen fatigue and its associated symptoms in both healthy volunteers[23] and in people recovering from viral illness.[24]

Comment: None.

OPTION   DIETARY SUPPLEMENTS

One small RCT found limited evidence of benefit from magnesium injections. Two small RCTs of oral evening primrose oil found mixed results.

Benefits: We found no systematic review. **Magnesium:** We found one RCT people comparing intramuscular injections of magnesium versus placebo in people with CFS over a 6 week period.[25] This trial found significant benefits with magnesium: 12/15 people on active treatment compared with 3/17 on placebo. **Evening primrose oil:** We found two RCTs comparing evening primrose oil versus placebo in people with a diagnosis of postviral fatigue syndrome or CFS. One RCT participants compared evening primrose oil (4 g orally per day) versus placebo in people with a diagnosis of postviral fatigue syndrome.[26] At 3 months, 85% of the people on active treatment had improved compared with 17% on placebo, a significant benefit. The other RCT 50 participants found no significant difference between evening primrose oil (4 g orally per day) and placebo, in people with CFS, at 3 months (using the Oxford, UK diagnostic criteria).[27]

Harms: These trials reported no adverse effects.

Comment: Subsequent studies have failed to find a deficiency of magnesium in people with CFS.[28–30] The difference in outcome for the studies of evening primrose oil may be partly explained by participant selection; the second study used currently accepted diagnostic criteria.[27] Also, whereas the first study used liquid paraffin as a placebo,[26] the second study used sunflower oil, which is better tolerated and less likely to affect the placebo response adversely.[27]

OPTION   IMMUNOTHERAPY

Four small RCTs of Immunoglobulin G (IgG) in people with CFS found only limited benefit and considerable adverse effects. RCTs of other forms of immunotherapy have found no evidence of a benefit over placebo.

Benefits: We found no systematic review. **IgG:** We found four RCTs comparing IgG versus placebo. In the first, 30 people were given either intravenous IgG 1 g/kg or albumin (placebo) every 30 days.[31] After 6 months no differences were found in measures of fatigue or physical and social functioning. A similar study randomised 49 people to three infusions of either intravenous IgG (2 g/kg) or placebo (a maltose solution).[32] Treatment was given monthly. Nearly half (10/23) of the immunoglobulin recipients improved in terms of a physician rated assessment of symptoms and disability, compared with 3/26 placebo recipients. A subsequent attempt by the same group to replicate the results was unsuccessful.[33] A further trial compared IgG 1 g/kg versus placebo in 71 adolescents aged 11–18 years.[34] Three infusions were given 1 month apart. There was a significant difference between the active treatment and control groups in mean functional outcome determined by taking the mean of clinician ratings from four areas of the participants' activities. Both groups showed significant improvements from baseline, however, continuing to the 6 month assessment after treatment. **Other immunotherapies:** We found one RCT comparing α interferon versus placebo 30 people.[35] In this study, treatment benefit was found only on subgroup analysis. Other RCTs found no significant advantage over controls from dialysable leucocyte extract (in a factorial design with cognitive behavioural therapy)[36] or terfenadine.[37]

Harms: Considerable adverse effects (gastrointestinal complaints, headaches, arthralgia, and worsening fatigue) were reported with IgG in up to 82% of trial participants.[31] Adverse effects were also notable with α interferon, and two of 13 participants on active treatment developed neutropenia.[35]

Comment: The first two studies differed in that the second used twice the dose of IgG, did not require that participants fulfil the operational criteria for CFS, and made no assessments of them during the study, waiting until 3 months after completion.[32] Terfenadine, particularly in increased blood concentrations, is associated with rare hazardous cardiac arrhythmias. Terfenadine has been withdrawn from sale in the US and UK.[38]

OPTION   **COGNITIVE BEHAVIOURAL THERAPY**

A systematic review has found that cognitive behavioural therapy administered by highly skilled therapists in specialist centres is effective in people with CFS, with a number needed to treat of 2. This finding may be of limited relevance to less specialised settings.

Benefits: We found one systematic review (updated August 1998, 13 RCTs) of cognitive behavioural therapy in people with CFS.[39] Three trials met the reviewers' inclusion criteria (all participants fulfilled diagnostic criteria for CFS, use of adequate randomisation, and use of controls).[30,36,40] The earliest trial 90 people used the Australian diagnostic criteria and evaluated cognitive behavioural therapy and immunotherapy using a factorial design.[36] The comparison group received standard medical care. Cognitive behavioural therapy was given every 2 weeks for six sessions lasting 30–60 minutes each. Treatment involved encouraging participants to exercise at home and feel less helpless. There was no significant difference in outcomes between cognitive behavioural therapy and standard care, using the Karnofsky scale and symptom report on a visual analogue scale. The second trial 60 people used the Oxford, UK diagnostic criteria and compared cognitive behavioural therapy versus normal general practice care in people attending a secondary care centre.[41] The active treatment consisted of a cognitive behavioural assessment, followed by 16 weekly sessions of behavioural experiments, problem solving activity, and re-evaluation of thoughts and beliefs inhibiting return to normal functioning. At 12 months, using the Karnofsky scale, 73% of those receiving cognitive behavioural therapy were improved compared with 27% receiving standard care. The relative benefit increase was 175% (95% CI 54% to 432%), with three people needing to be treated with cognitive behavioural therapy for one additional person to achieve normal functioning (NNT 3, 95% CI 2 to 5). The third trial 60 people was in people attending a different secondary care centre.[40] Cognitive behavioural therapy was given in 13 weekly sessions. The control group received relaxation therapy. Outcome was assessed using the medical outcomes survey short form. A good outcome was found in 63% of those treated with cognitive behavioural therapy compared with 17% receiving relaxation therapy. The relative benefit increase was 270% (95% CI 137% to 531%, NNT 3, 95% CI 1 to 7). In both the second and third trials, improvement continued over 6–12 months' follow up.[30,40]

Harms: No harmful effects were reported.

Comment: The negative results of the Australian trial[36] may have been because the therapy was less intense and no attempts at cognitive reappraisal were offered, and because routine care was itself reasonably effective. The conflict between the differing illness models for the two active treatments being evaluated, cognitive behavioural therapy and immunotherapy, may also have had an impact on effectiveness. The Australian diagnostic criteria are no longer widely used. The other two trials[40,41] took place in centres with highly skilled cognitive behavioural therapists. The applicability of their positive results to settings outside specialist centres remains uncertain. A large Dutch RCT (G Bleijenberg, personal communication, 1999) and a UK RCT based in primary care (L Ridsdale et al, personal communication, 1999) are due to report soon.

REFERENCES

1. Fukuda K, Straus S, Hickie I, et al. The chronic fatigue syndrome: a comprehensive approach to its definition and study. Ann Intern Med 1994; 121:953–959.

2. Sharpe M, Archard LC, Banatvala JE. A report - chronic fatigue syndrome: guidelines for research. J R Soc Med 1991;84:118–121.

3. Wessely S, Chalder T, Hirsch S, et al. The prevalence and morbidity of chronic fatigue and chronic fatigue syndrome: a prospective primary care study. Am J Public Health 1997;87:1449–1455.

4. Steele L, Dobbins JG, Fukuda K, et al. The epidemiology of chronic fatigue in San Francisco. Am J Med 1998;105(suppl 3A):83–90.

5. Lawrie SM, Pelosi AJ. Chronic fatigue syndrome in the community: prevalence and associations. Br J Psychiatry 1995;166:793–797.

6. Wessely S. The epidemiology of chronic fatigue syndrome. Epidemiol Rev 1995;17:139–151.

7. Joyce J, Hotopf M, Wessely S. The prognosis of chronic fatigue and chronic fatigue syndrome: a systematic review. QJM 1997;90:223–133. Search date March 1996; primary sources Medline; Embase; Current Contents; Psychlit.

8. Stewart AD, Hays RD, Ware JE. The MOS short-form general health survey. Med Care 1988;26: 724–732.

9. Karnofsky DA, Burchenal JH. MacLeod CM, eds. The clinical evaluation of chemotherapeutic agents in cancer. New York Academy of Medicine. New York: Columbia University Press, 1949:191–206.

10. Beck AT, Ward CH, Mendelson M, Mock JE, Erbaugh JK. An inventory for measuring depression. Arch Gen Psychiatry 1961;4:561–571.

11. Bergner M, Bobbit RA, Carter WB, et al. The sickness impact profile: development and final revision of a health status measure. *Med Care* 1981;19:787–805.

12. Vercoulen J, Swanink C, Zitman F. Randomised, double-blind, placebo-controlled study of fluoxetine in chronic fatigue syndrome. *Lancet* 1996;347:858–861.

13. Wearden AJ, Morriss RK, Mullis R, et al. Randomised, double-blind, placebo controlled treatment trial of fluoxetine and a graded exercise programme for chronic fatigue syndrome. *Br J Psychiatry* 1998;172:485–490.

14. Natelson BH, Cheu J, Pareja J, et al. Randomised, double blind, controlled placebo-phase in trial of low dose phenelzine in the chronic fatigue syndrome. *Psychopharmacology* 1996;124:226–230.

15. Behan PO, Hannifah H. 5-HT reuptake inhibitors in CFS. *J Immunol Immunopharmacol.* 1995;15:66–69.

16. Peterson PK, Pheley A, Schroeppel J, et al. A preliminary placebo-controlled crossover trial of fludrocortisone for chronic fatigue syndrome. *Arch Intern Med* 1998;158:908–914.

17. McKenzie R, O'Fallon A, Dale J, et al. Low-dose hydrocortisone for treatment of chronic fatigue syndrome. *JAMA* 1998;280:1061–1066.

18. Cleare AJ, Heap E, Malhi G, et al. Low-dose hydrocortisone in chronic fatigue syndrome: a randomised crossover trial. *Lancet* 1999;353:455–458.

19. Bou-Holaigah I, Rowe P, Kan J, et al. The relationship between neurally mediated hypotension and the chronic fatigue syndrome. *JAMA* 1995;274:961–967.

20. Demitrack M, Dale J, Straus S, et al. Evidence for impaired activation of the hypothalamic–pituitary–adrenal axis in patients with chronic fatigue syndrome. *J Clin Endocrinol Metab* 1991;73:1224–1234.

21. Forsyth LM, Preuss HG, MacDowell AL, et al. Therapeutic effects of oral NADH on the symptoms of patients with chronic fatigue syndrome. *Ann Allergy Asthma Immunol* 1999;82:185–191.

22. Fulcher KY, White PD. A randomised controlled trial of graded exercise therapy in patients with the chronic fatigue syndrome. *BMJ* 1997;314:1647–1652.

23. Sandler H, Vernikos J. *Inactivity: physiological effects.* London: Academic Press, 1986.

24. Dalrymple W. Infectious mononucleosis: 2. relation of bed rest and activity to prognosis. *Postgrad Med* 1961;35:345–349.

25. Cox IM, Campbell MJ, Dowson D. Red blood cell magnesium and chronic fatigue syndrome. *Lancet* 1991;337:757–760.

26. Behan PO, Behan WMH, Horrobin D. Effect of high doses of essential fatty acids on the postviral fatigue syndrome. *Acta Neurol Scand* 1990;82:209–216.

27. Warren G, McKendrick M, Peet M. The role of essential fatty acids in chronic fatigue syndrome. *Acta Neurol Scand* 1999;99:112–116.

28. Clague JE, Edwards RHT, Jackson MJ. Intravenous magnesium loading in chronic fatigue syndrome. *Lancet* 1992;340:124–125.

29. Hinds G, Bell NP, McMaster D, et al. Normal red cell magnesium concentrations and magnesium loading tests in patients with chronic fatigue syndrome. *Ann Clin Biochem* 1994;31:459–461.

30. Swanink CM, Vercoulen JH, Bleijenberg G, et al. Chronic fatigue syndrome: a clinical and laboratory study with a well matched control group. *J Intern Med* 1995;237:499–506.

31. Peterson PK, Shepard J, Macres M, et al. A controlled trial of intravenous immunoglobulin G in chronic fatigue syndrome. *Am J Med* 1990;89:554–560.

32. Lloyd A, Hickie I, Wakefield D, et al. A double-blind, placebo-controlled trial of intravenous immunoglobulin therapy in patients with chronic fatigue syndrome. *Am J Med* 1990;89:561–568.

33. Vollmer-Conna U, Hickie I, Hadzi-Pavlovic D, et al. Intravenous immunoglobulin is ineffective in the treatment of patients with chronic fatigue syndrome. *Am J Med* 1997;103:38–43.

34. Rowe KS. Double-blind randomized controlled trial to assess the efficacy of intravenous gammaglobulin for the management of chronic fatigue syndrome in adolescents. *J Psychiatr Res* 1997;31:133–47.

35. See DM, Tilles JG. Alpha interferon treatment of patients with chronic fatigue syndrome. *Immunol Invest* 1996;25:153–164.

36. Lloyd A, Hickie I, Boughton R, et al. Immunologic and psychological therapy for patients with chronic fatigue syndrome. *Am J Med* 1993;94:197–203.

37. Steinberg P, McNutt BE, Marshall P, et al. Double-blind placebo-controlled study of efficacy of oral terfenadine in the treatment of chronic fatigue syndrome. *J Allergy Clin Immunol* 1996;97:119–126.

38. British National Formulary 2000;40. London: British Medical Association and Royal Pharmaceutical Society of Great Britain.

39. Price JR, Couper, J. Cognitive behaviour therapy for CFS. In: The Cochrane Library, Issue 4, 1998. Oxford: Update Software. Search date May 1998; primary sources Medline; Embase; Biological Abstracts; SIGLE (System for Information on Grey Literature in Europe); Index to Theses of Great Britain and Ireland; Index to Scientific and Technical Proceedings; Science Citation Index; Trials Register of the Depression; Anxiety and Neurosis Group plus citation lists and personal contacts.

40. Deale A, Chalder T, Marks I, et al. Cognitive behaviour therapy for chronic fatigue syndrome: a randomized controlled trial. *Am J Psychiatry* 1997;154:408–414.

41. Sharpe M, Hawton K, Simkin S, et al. Cognitive behaviour therapy for chronic fatigue syndrome: a randomized controlled trial. *BMJ* 1996;312:22–26.

Steven Reid
Clinical Research Fellow

Trudie Chalder
Senior Lecturer

Anthony Cleare
Senior Lecturer

Matthew Hotopf
Senior Lecturer

Simon Wessely
Professor of Epidemiological and Liaison Psychiatry

Guys, Kings and St Thomas's School of Medicine and Institute of Psychiatry
London
UK

Competing interests: None declared.

TABLE 1	Diagnostic criteria for chronic fatigue syndrome (see text, p 730).

CDC 1994[1]

Clinically evaluated, medically unexplained fatigue of at least 6 months' duration that is:

- of new onset
- not a result of ongoing exertion
- not substantially alleviated by rest
- a substantial reduction in previous levels of activity

The occurrence of four or more of the following symptoms:

- subjective memory impairment
- tender lymph nodes
- muscle pain
- joint pain
- headache
- unrefreshing sleep
- postexertional malaise (> 24 hours)

Oxford, UK[2]

Severe, disabling fatigue of at least 6 months' duration that:

- affects both physical and mental functioning
- was present for more than 50% of the time

Other symptoms, particularly myalgia, sleep, and mood disturbance, may be present.

Exclusion criteria

- Active, unresolved, or suspected disease likely to cause fatigue
- Psychotic, melancholic, or bipolar depression (but not uncomplicated major depression)
- Psychotic disorders
- Dementia

- Anorexia or bulimia nervosa
- Alcohol or other substance misuse
- Severe obesity
- Same as US CDC, apart from substance misuse and obesity

Musculoskeletal disorders

Search date September 2000

Olivier Bruyere and Jean-Yves Reginster

INTERVENTIONS

Key Messages

Prevention

- Two RCTs have found that hormone replacement therapy (HRT) reduces the risk of vertebral fracture by 40–60% compared with placebo. Similar reductions have been found in observational studies.

- For hip fracture, two RCTs and several observational studies presented conflicting results.

DEFINITION	A fracture is a break or disruption of bone or cartilage. Symptoms may include immobility, pain, tenderness, numbness, bruising, joint deformity, joint swelling, and limb shortening.
INCIDENCE/ PREVALENCE	The lifetime risk of fracture in white women is 20% for the spine, 15% for the wrist, and 18% for the hip.
AETIOLOGY/ RISK FACTORS	Fractures usually arise from trauma. Risk factors include those associated with an increased tendency to fall (such as ataxia, drug and alcohol intake, loose carpets), age, osteoporosis, bony metastases, and other disorders of bone.
PROGNOSIS	Fractures may result in pain, short or long term disability, haemorrhage, shock, and death. Vertebral fractures are associated with pain, physical impairment, changes in body shape, loss of physical function, and lower quality of life. Around 20% of women die in the year after a hip fracture, representing an increase in mortality of 12–20% compared with women of similar age and no hip fracture. Half of elderly women who had been independent become partly dependent after hip fracture. One third become totally dependent.
AIMS	To prevent fractures with minimal adverse effects from treatment.
OUTCOMES	Incidence of hip, wrist, and vertebral fractures.
METHODS	*Clinical Evidence* update search and appraisal September 2000. We also hand searched journals of bone diseases and carried out manual searches using the bibliographies of review articles published after 1985. We considered all studies assessing the effects of HRT on fracture rates.

QUESTION   **What are the effects of treatment to prevent fractures in postmenopausal women?**

OPTION   **HORMONE REPLACEMENT THERAPY**

Two RCTs found fewer vertebral fractures after HRT than after placebo. For non-vertebral fractures, two RCTs and several observational studies found conflicting results. Reduced risk of hip fracture seems significant only in women who started HRT within 5 years of menopause and who have used it continuously.

Benefits: **Vertebral fractures:** We found no systematic review of RCTs. We found two RCTs. One RCT (75 postmenopausal women, 47–75 years of age with one or more vertebral fractures) evaluated transdermal HRT (17β estradiol and oral medroxyprogesterone acetate).[1] After 12 months it found fewer vertebral fractures with HRT than with placebo (8 fractures in 7 women with HRT v 20 fractures in 12 women with placebo; RR 0.39, 95% CI 0.16 to 0.95). The second RCT (100 postmenopausal women) found that, over a median of 9 years, oestrogen reduced total spine score, an indirect measurement of vertebral fracture rate (P < 0.01), but had no significant effect on the number of women with a vertebral crush fracture (1/57 with oestrogen, 5/42 with placebo; RR 0.15, 95% CI 0.02 to 1.15).[2] **Non-vertebral fractures:** We found two RCTs and several observational studies. One RCT (2763 postmenopausal women, age less than 80 years) compared HRT versus placebo for an average of 4.1 years in the secondary prevention of coronary artery disease; prevention of fracture was a secondary end point.[3] It found that oestrogen had no significant effect on the number of women with a hip fracture (0.9% with HRT, 0.8% with placebo; RR 1.09, 95% CI 0.48 to 2.46) or on the number with any fracture (9% with HRT, 10% with placebo; RR 0.94, 95% CI 0.75 to 1.18). The other RCT randomised 464 postmenopausal women to one of four groups: HRT alone (estradiol and cyproterone), vitamin D alone, HRT plus vitamin D, or placebo.[4] At a mean of 4.3 years follow up, 32 women had 39 non-vertebral fractures (HRT 4, vitamin D 10, HRT plus vitamin D 8, placebo 17). Women on HRT alone had fewer fractures but this did not quite reach significance on intention to treat analysis (RR 0.41, 95% CI 0.16 to 1.05). However, comparison of the two HRT groups versus the two groups not receiving HRT did find a significant reduction in the number of non-vertebral fractures (RR 0.44, 95% CI 0.21 to 0.93).

Harms: See HRT under secondary prevention of ischaemic cardiac events, p 95. In the second RCT of non-vertebral fractures, 96 women withdrew from the trial, 72 of whom were in groups receiving HRT. The most common reasons cited for withdrawal were menstrual disorders (19 women) and headache (14 women).[4]

Comment: In addition to these RCTs, we found many observational studies with conflicting results.[5–11] One non-systematic review of 11 observational studies found a reduced risk of hip fracture in women taking oestrogen compared with non-users (RR 0.75, 95% CI 0.68 to 0.84).[7] Other observational studies found no differences.[12,13] We found no observational studies that detected an increased risk of fracture with HRT. Several observational studies found that only 8–20% of women continued HRT for at least 3 years.[14,15]

REFERENCES

1. Lufkin E, Wahner H, O'Fallon W, et al. Treatment of postmenopausal osteoporosis with transdermal estrogen. Ann Intern Med 1992;117:1–9.

2. Lindsay R. Prevention of spinal osteoporosis in oophorectomised women. Lancet 1980;1:1152–1154.

3. Hulley S, Grady D, Bush T, et al. Randomized trial of estrogen plus progestin for secondary prevention of coronary heart disease in postmenopausal women. JAMA 1998;31:45–54.

4. Komulainen M, Kröger H, Tuppurainen M, et al. HRT and vitamin D in prevention of non-vertebral fractures in postmenopausal women; a 5 year randomized trial. Maturitas 1998;31:45–54.

5. Ettinger B, Genant H, Cann C. Long-term estrogen replacement therapy prevents bone loss and fractures. Ann Intern Med 1985;102:319–324.

6. Maxim P, Ettinger B, Spitalny M. Fracture protection provided by long-term estrogen treatment. Osteoporos Int 1995;5:23–29.

7. Grady D, Rubin S, Petitti D, et al. Hormone therapy to prevent disease and prolong life in postmenopausal women. Ann Intern Med 1992; 117:1016–1037.

8. Cauley J, Seeley D, Ensrud K, et al. Estrogen replacement therapy and fractures in older women. Ann Intern Med 1995;122:9–16.

9. Kanis J, Johnell O, Gullberg B, et al. Evidence for efficacy of drugs affecting bone metabolism in preventing hip fracture. BMJ 1992;305:1124–1128.

10. Michaélsson K, Varon J, Farahmand B, et al, on behalf of the Swedish Hip Fracture Study Group. Hormone replacement therapy and risk of hip fracture: population based case-control study. BMJ 1998;316:1858–1863.

11. Michaélsson K, Baron J, Johnell O, et al, for the Swedish Hip Fracture Study Group. Variation in the efficacy of hormone replacement therapy in the prevention of hip fracture. Osteoporos Int 1998;8:540–546.

12. Nguyen T, Jones G, Sambrook N, et al. Effects of estrogen exposure and reproductive factors on bone mineral density and osteoporotic fractures. J Clin Endocrin Metab 1995;80:2709–2714.

13. Kiel D, Baron J, Anderson J, et al. Smoking eliminates the protective effect of oral estrogens on the risk for hip fracture among women. Ann Intern Med 1992;116:716–721.

14. Ettinger B, Li D, Lein R. Continuation of postmenopausal hormone replacement therapy: comparison of cyclic versus continuous combined schedules. Menopause 1996;3:185–189.

15. Groeneveld F, Bareman F, Barentsen R, et al. Duration of hormonal replacement therapy in general practice: a follow up study. Maturitas 1998;29:125–131.

Olivier Bruyere
Research Fellow
WHO Collaborating Center
for Public Health Aspects
of Osteoarticular Diseases
Liege
Belgium

Jean-Yves Reginster
Professor of Epidemiology
and Public Health
Bone and Cartilage Metabolism Unit
University of Liege
Liege
Belgium

Musculoskeletal disorders

Competing interests: OB, none declared. JR has participated in several pre-clinical and clinical trials, reviewed and consulted scientific documentation, has been an author of publications, and has chaired and spoken at scientific meetings for the following companies: Asahi, Bayer, Boehringer Ingelheim, Chiesi, Eli Lilly, Hoechst-Marion-Roussel, Hologic, Hybritech, Igea, Johnson & Johnson, Merck Sharp & Dohme, Negma, Organon, Pfizer, Pharmascience, Procter & Gamble Pharmaceuticals, Rotta research, Sanofi, Servier, SmithKline Beecham, Teva, Therabel, Tosse, Byk, UCB, and Will Pharma.

Hallux valgus (bunions)

Search date January 2001

Jill Ferrari

INTERVENTIONS

Key Messages

- We found no strong evidence about optimal treatment for hallux valgus.
- We found few conservative treatments that have been evaluated by RCTs, and those that have show no clear benefit compared with placebo.
- One systematic review found little good evidence on the effects of Keller's arthroplasty versus other types of operation for hallux valgus.
- One systematic review of RCTs found limited evidence that chevron osteotomy (see glossary, p 748) was more likely to produce poor outcomes than comparable operations.
- Two RCTs comparing standard fixation using sutures or Kirschner wire with other methods of fixation following Mitchell's osteotomy have found no significant difference in clinical or radiological outcomes. One of the RCTs found that screw fixation with early mobilisation versus suture fixation with late mobilisation significantly accelerated return to activities.
- Three RCTs have found that new postoperative regimens (the use of crepe bandages, continuous passive motion, and allowing early weightbearing) are of similar effectiveness as older techniques (plaster slipper casts, routine physiotherapy, and delayed weightbearing).

DEFINITION **Hallux valgus** is a deformity of the great toe characterised by a lateral deviation (abduction) and valgus rotation of the toe with adduction and varus rotation of the first metatarsal.[1] Radiological criteria for hallux valgus vary, but a commonly accepted criterion is a metatarsal joint angle greater than 14.5°.[2] **Bunion** is the lay term used to describe a prominent and often inflamed metatarsal head and overlying bursa. Symptoms include pain, limitation in walking, and problems with wearing normal shoes.

INCIDENCE/ PREVALENCE The prevalence of hallux valgus varies in different populations. In a recent study of 6000 UK school children aged 9–10 years, 2.5% had clinical evidence of hallux valgus, and 2% met both clinical and radiological criteria for hallux valgus. An earlier study found hallux valgus in 48% of adults.[2] Different prevalences may result from different methods of measurement, varying age groups, or different diagnostic criteria (e.g. metatarsal joint angle $> 10°$ or $> 15°$).[3]

AETIOLOGY/ RISK FACTORS Nearly all population studies have found that hallux valgus is more common in women. Footwear may contribute to the deformity, but studies comparing people who wear shoes with those who do not have been contradictory. Hypermobility of the first ray (see glossary, p 748) and excessive foot pronation are associated with hallux valgus.[4]

PROGNOSIS We found no studies that looked at progression of hallux valgus. Progression of deformity and symptoms is rapid in some people, others remain asymptomatic. One study found that hallux valgus is often unilateral initially, but usually progresses to bilateral deformity.[2]

AIMS To reduce symptoms and deformity, with minimum adverse effects.

OUTCOMES Hallux abductus angle (the angle, usually measured from radiographs, between the shaft of the metatarsal and the hallux). The first intermetatarsal angle (the angle measured radiographically between the first and second metatarsal shafts). Range of motion of the first metatarsophalangeal joint (the total range of both dorsiflexion and plantarflexion). Incidence of complications such as infection; re-operation; non-union; avascular necrosis; pain; general satisfaction and satisfaction with appearance; requirement for specialist or extra-width footwear; proportion of people with mobility problems; time to healing; development of transfer lesions; and adverse effects of treatment.

METHODS *Clinical Evidence* update search and appraisal January 2001. An earlier search (October 1998) was also made using a strategy developed by the Cochrane Musculoskeletal Injuries Group. We also hand searched podiatry journals up to January 2001.

Hallux valgus (bunions)

QUESTION What are the effects of conservative treatments?

OPTION ORTHOSES

Two RCTs have evaluated the use of antipronatory orthoses (see glossary, p 748) in the treatment and prevention of hallux valgus. In children, deterioration of the deformity has been shown to occur regardless of orthotic intervention. In adult males with rheumatoid arthritis, orthoses have been shown to reduce the chance of developing hallux valgus.

Benefits: We found no systematic reviews. We found two RCTs. **In children:** One RCT screened 6000 British school children aged 9–10 years. On the basis of a clinical examination, 150 were selected for x-ray examination. Children (122, 13% boys) with metatarsophalangeal joint angles greater than 14.5° were randomised either to anti-pronatory orthoses for 3 years, or to no treatment.[2] For children with bilateral deformity (46 children), the hallux abductus angle increased for both treatment groups but the difference was not significant. For children with unilateral deformity (47 children), orthoses were associated with greater deterioration in joint position. **In adults:** We found no RCTs of orthoses in adults who already had hallux valgus. We found one RCT (102 men with rheumatoid arthritis), which compared the use of orthoses versus no treatment in preventing the development of hallux valgus.[5] None of the men had hallux valgus at inclusion. Hallux valgus was less frequent in those treated with orthoses compared with the control group, but the difference was not significant (AR 5/50 [10%] for adults with orthoses v 12/48 [25%] no treatment; RR 0.4, 95% CI 0.2 to 1.1). Orthoses did not improve pain, disability, or function.

Harms: The RCT of orthoses in children gave no information on complications.[2] A few men with rheumatoid arthritis experienced mild discomfort with orthoses.[5]

Comment: The use of this type of antipronatory orthoses in children is questionable because earlier studies have found that hallux valgus in children is not related to pronation but is because of positional changes in the first ray (see glossary, p 748).[6] Twenty nine children (mainly from the control group) were lost to follow up. The study in adults with rheumatoid arthritis only included men, although rheumatoid arthritis is more frequent in women. Generalisations from the results may be limited.

OPTION NIGHT SPLINTS

One RCT found no significant difference in deformity or pain with night splints compared with no treatment in people with hallux valgus.

Benefits: We found no systematic review. One RCT (28 people) compared the use of night splints versus no treatment, with follow up for 6 months.[6] It found no significant difference between groups in the hallux abductus angle or pain.

Harms: Eleven people (39%) failed to complete the trial; seven were from the treatment group.

Comment: None.

QUESTION What are the effects of surgical treatments?

OPTION KELLER'S ARTHROPLASTY

One systematic review found little good evidence on the effects of Keller's arthroplasty (see glossary, p 748) versus other types of operation for hallux valgus.

Benefits:
Versus no treatment: We found no RCTs. **Versus proximal osteotomy:** We found one systematic review (search date 1998, 3 RCTs)[7] that included one RCT (29 people) comparing Keller's arthroplasty with distal metatarsal osteotomy. The osteotomy gave better results for many outcomes but these were significant only for intermetatarsal angle (WMD −5.0°, 95% CI −1.1° to −8.9°), and for range of movement (WMD 13°, 95% CI 5.0° to 21.1°). **Versus arthrodesis:** The second RCT included in the review (81 people) compared Keller's arthroplasty with arthrodesis. It found no significant difference between procedures for any of the outcomes used except limitation in walking, where the Keller's arthroplasty was associated with significantly less reduction in mobility (AR 11/37 [30%] for arthrodesis v 4/44 [9%] for Keller's arthroplasty; RR 3.3, 95% CI 1.1 to 9.4; NNH 5, 95% CI 3 to 29). **Plus joint distraction:** The third RCT included in the review compared the use of a Kirschner wire to distract the joint during healing after Keller's arthroplasty. It found no significant difference in the hallux abductus angle or intermetatarsal angle, pain, or movement. However, a subjective assessment score for symptoms and activity was significantly better in the non-wire group (P < 0.05). A significant decrease in interphalangeal joint movement was noted when wire distraction was used (P < 0.05).

Harms:
No particular complications were described. Reduced toe function has been described after Keller's procedure.[7] The systematic review reported high levels of patient dissatisfaction (up to 33%) in most trials.[7]

Comment:
Most of the people having surgery were under 50 years old and were followed up for no more than 3 years. Longer term outcomes remain unclear. Many of the RCTs reported results for numbers of feet, and did not always report standard deviations of the results. The systematic review analysed the results by numbers of people.

OPTION CHEVRON OSTEOTOMY

One systematic review of RCTs found limited evidence that chevron osteotomy (see glossary, p 748) was more likely to produce poor outcomes than comparable operations.

Benefits:
Versus no treatment: We found no RCTs. **Versus proximal osteotomy:** We found one systematic review (search date 1998, 3 RCTs, 205 people).[7] The first RCT (75 people) compared proximal chevron osteotomy with proximal crescentic osteotomy (see glossary, p 749). In the 66 people assessed, it found no significant difference between the procedures for the hallux abductus angle, intermetatarsal angle, transfer lesions (see glossary, p 749), or

number of complications after 22 months. Chevron osteotomy was associated with significantly faster healing time (P < 0.001), and significantly less postoperative dorsiflexion at the healed site (P = 0.005). The second RCT (79 people) compared chevron osteotomy with proximal osteotomy (see glossary, p 749). After 2 years, it found that proximal osteostomy significantly improved the hallux abductus angle (WMD −5.0°, 95% CI −0.5° to −9.5°), and intermetatarsal angle (WMD −3.0°, 95% CI −1.0° to −5.0°). It found no significant difference between the procedures for pain, satisfaction, footwear, or limited walking. The third RCT (51 people) compared chevron versus Wilson osteotomy (see glossary, p 749). Forty six people were examined after 38 months. Wilson osteotomy significantly improved the hallux abductus angle (WMD −12.4°, 95% CI −17.5° to −7.5°). It found no significant differences in complications, footwear, or limited walking. **Plus adductor tenotomy:** One RCT in the review (84 people) compared the use of an additional adductor tenotomy plus chevron osteotomy versus chevron osteotomy alone. It found no significant differences in hallux abductus angle, range of motion, complications, pain, satisfaction, footwear, or limited walking.

Harms: Complications were found in most RCTs. Overcorrection and pin tract infections were reported in both groups of one trial. In the RCT of proximal osteotomy versus chevron osteotomy, there was one wound infection and two stress fractures in the chevron group, and 11 complications in the proximal osteotomy group, consisting mostly of pain in other areas of the forefoot (metatarsalgia). In the trial of Wilson osteotomy versus chevron osteotomy, complications were found in both groups. Transfer pain and lesions were recurring problems in both groups (18 v 17). Although Wilson osteotomy resulted in a significantly shortened metatarsal (P = 0.02) with metatarsal dorsiflexion in 20% of people, this change in position did not correlate with development of new lesions or pain. In the RCT of chevron osteostomy plus adductor tenotomy, about 25% of both groups remained dissatisfied during follow up. This may be related to greater postoperative reduction in the circumference of the ball of the foot; the ball circumference of dissatisfied people was greater than that of satisfied people (P > 0.005).[7]

Comment: No trial included long term follow up.

| OPTION | DIFFERENT METHODS OF BONE FIXATION |

Two RCTs comparing standard fixation using sutures or Kirschner wire (see glossary, p 748) with other methods of fixation following Mitchell's osteotomy (see glossary, p 748) found no significant difference in clinical or radiological outcomes. One of the RCTs found that screw fixation with early mobilisation versus suture fixation with late mobilisation significantly accelerated return to activities.

Benefits: We found no systematic review. We found two RCTs comparing methods of fixation following Mitchell's osteotomy.[8,9] The first RCT (28 people, 39 feet) compared a standard method of fixation with absorbable pin fixation.[8] The mean follow up was 11 months (2–24 months) and included radiological outcomes: hallux abductus angle, intermetatarsal angle and the ratio of the first to second metatarsal length; and clinical outcomes: range of movement, pain, metatarsalgia, walking ability, and cosmetic appearance. No significant differences were found between standard versus absorbable fixation. The second RCT (30 people) compared screw fixation followed by early weightbearing in a plaster shoe versus vicryl suture fixation followed by 6 weeks non-weightbearing in a plaster boot.[9] Follow up at 6 weeks, 3 months, 6 months, and 1 year included clinical and radiographic evaluation, range of motion assessment, patient satisfaction, and return to activity measures. Screw fixation versus sutures significantly accelerated return to social activities (mean 2.9 v 5.7 weeks, P < 0.001) and employment (mean 4.9 v 8.7 weeks, P < 0.001). At 3 and 6 months, metatarsophalangeal joint stiffness was the only outcome to be significantly worse in people with screw fixation. After 6 months, clinical and radiological outcomes were not significantly different.[9]

Harms: The first RCT reported more complications in people receiving standard fixation versus pin fixation (14/17 [82%] feet v 16/22 [73%] feet; P = 0.48). These included recurrence of deformity (3 v 2); problems primarily resulting in pain (5 v 6); and continued swelling (3 v 0). In the RCT of screw versus suture fixation, 2 of 15 people had the screw removed because of pain. Superficial infection occurred in three people overall (2 v 1).[9]

Comment: The first trial was limited because it used people as the unit of randomisation, and feet as the unit of analysis.

QUESTION What are the effects of postoperative care?

OPTION CONTINUOUS PASSIVE MOTION

One systematic review found no significant difference between continuous passive motion versus routine rehabilitation on joint range of motion or return to normal footwear, but was too small to rule out a clinically important effect.

Benefits: We found one systematic review (search date 1998, 1 small RCT).[7] For 3 months the RCT (39 people) compared continuous passive motion plus physiotherapy versus physiotherapy alone. It found no significant difference in the range of motion (WMD −6.7°, 95% CI −13.6° to +0.3°) or in the number of people who returned to normal footwear.

Harms: No complications were found in the trial.

Comment: None.

OPTION	EARLY WEIGHTBEARING

One systematic review has found that the incidence of non-union at the site of arthrodesis is similar after early compared with late weightbearing after surgery.

Benefits: We found one systematic review (search date 1998, 1 RCT).[7] The RCT (56 people) compared early with late weightbearing. One group (29 people) began to bear weight in a cast for 2–4 weeks after the operation, whereas 27 people did not bear weight until 4 weeks postoperatively. The only outcome assessed was non-union at the site of arthrodesis (see harms below).

Harms: The only complication considered was non-union at the site of arthrodesis. This occurred in one person allowed early weightbearing and in two from the late weightbearing group (OR 0.69, 95% CI 0.11 to 4.51). The RCT found no significant difference in the number of new complications.[7]

Comment: None.

OPTION	SLIPPER CAST

One RCT comparing crepe bandage with plaster cast slippers following a Wilson osteotomy found no significant difference in any outcome, but was too small to rule out a clinically important effect.

Benefits: We found no systematic review. We found one RCT (54 feet) comparing the use of plaster slipper cast (27 feet) with crepe bandage (27 feet) following a Wilson osteotomy.[10] Cast and dressings were changed 12 days after surgery and then kept on for a further 4 weeks. It found no significant difference between the groups for hallux valgus angle, pain, overall assessment, joint range of movement, or return to normal activities.

Harms: One failed union occurred in the crepe group versus none in the plaster group. Two people in the plaster group had a superficial wound infection.[10]

Comment: The RCT was small and could not exclude a clinically important difference between the groups.

GLOSSARY

Antipronatory orthoses Insoles designed to reduce the amount of in-roll or flattening of the foot during gait.

Chevron osteotomy A v-shaped wedge of bone is removed from the distal end of the metatarsal shaft allowing the metatarsal head to be realigned on the shaft.

First ray The first metatarsal and medial cuneiform function as a single unit called the first ray.

Keller's arthroplasty A procedure involving removal of the medial side of the metatarsal head and straight resection of the base of the proximal phalanx.

Kirschner wire A thin but rigid wire that is used to fix bone fragments. It is passed through drilled channels in the bone (sometimes called K-wire).

Mitchell's osteotomy A distal metatarsal osteotomy whereby an incomplete osteotomy is performed perpendicular to the long axis of the bone. The distal portion is moved laterally and fixed in position. This results in shortening of the bone.

Proximal chevron osteotomy Removal of a v-shaped wedge of bone from the base of the metatarsal shaft followed by displacement and fixation of the distal portion of bone.

Proximal crescentic osteotomy A curved cut is made across the base of the metatarsal shaft. The distal portion of bone is slid across the proximal end of bone and fixed in a corrected position.

Proximal osteotomy A similar procedure to the proximal chevron osteotomy.

Transfer lesions Areas of corns or callus that develop when the weightbearing forces are transferred from one area of the foot to another.

Wilson osteotomy A double oblique cut is made in the distal portion of the metatarsal shaft and the metatarsal head is slid into a corrected position.

Substantive changes since last issue

Different methods of bone fixation New RCT;[9] conclusion unchanged.

REFERENCES

1. Dykyj D. Pathological anatomy of hallux abducto valgus. *Clin Podiatr Med Surg* 1989;6:1–15.

2. Kilmartin TE, Barrington RL, Wallace WA. A controlled prospective trial of a foot orthosis for juvenile hallux valgus. *J Bone Joint Surg (Br)* 1994;76:210–214.

3. Morris JB, Brash LF, Hird MD. Chiropodial survey of Geriatric and Psychiatric hospital in-patients – Angus District. *Chiropodist* 1980;April:128–139.

4. LaPorta G, Melillo T, Olinsky D. X-ray evaluation of hallux abducto valgus deformity. *J Am Podiatr Med Assoc* 1974;64:544–566.

5. Budiman-Mak E, Conrad KJ, Roach KE, et al. Can orthoses prevent hallux valgus deformity in rheumatoid arthritis? A randomised clinical trial. *J Clin Rheumatol* 1995;1:313–321.

6. Juriansz AM. Conservative treatment of hallux valgus: a randomised controlled trial of a hallux valgus night splint. MSc Thesis 1996: Faculty of Science, Kings College, London University.

7. Ferrari J, Higgins JPT, William RL. Interventions for treating hallux valgus (abductovalgus) and bunions. In: The Cochrane Library, Issue 4, 2000. Oxford: Update Software. Search date 1998; primary sources Medline, Embase, Cinahl, Amed, Cochrane Controlled Trials Register, Cochrane Musculoskeletal Injuries Trials Register, bibliographies of identified trials, and hand searching of podiatry journals.

8. Prior TD, Grace DL, MacLean JB, et al. Correction of hallux abductovalgus by Mitchell's osteotomy: comparing standard fixation methods with absorbable polydioxanone pins. *Foot* 1997;7:121–125.

9. Calder JDF, Hollingdale JP, Pearse MF. Screw versus suture fixation of Mitchell's osteotomy. A prospective randomised study. *J Bone Joint Surg (Br)* 1999;81:621–624.

10. Meek RMD, Anderson EG. Plaster slipper versus crepe bandage after Wilson's osteotomy for hallux valgus. *Foot* 1999;9:138–141.

Jill Ferrari
Department of Podiatry
University College London
London
UK

Competing interests: None declared.

Musculoskeletal disorders

Hip fracture

Search date December 2000: expanded this issue

William Gillespie

QUESTIONS

INTERVENTIONS

Surgical treatment

- One systematic review of RCTs has found that regional anaesthesia compared with general anaesthesia may reduce short term mortality and deep venous thrombosis after hip fracture surgery.

- One systematic review has found that threaded screws are associated with fewer fracture healing complications than smooth pins. We found insufficient evidence on the effects of using one or more screws, or on the effects of side plate.

- Limited evidence from a systematic review of randomised and observational studies suggests that arthroplasty for displaced intracapsular fractures of the hip has no significant effect on mortality or morbidity compared with internal fixation.

- One systematic review of RCTs has found that leg deformity is more common after conservative treatment of extracapsular hip fractures. We found limited evidence of no significant difference between conservative and operative management in terms of medical complications, mortality, or long term pain.

- We found insufficient evidence from RCTs to determine whether replacement arthroplasty has any advantage over the sliding hip screw for extracapsular hip fractures.

- One systematic review of RCTs has found that sliding hip screws are associated with significantly fewer complications than fixed nail plates in the treatment of extracapsular hip fractures.

- One systematic review has found that, compared with cephalocondylic intramedullary devices, extramedullary fixation of hip fractures using sliding hip screw devices is associated with similar benefits and significantly fewer operative complications.

- One systematic review found that condylocephalic nails are less effective than extramedullary fixation for extracapsular hip fractures.

Preoperative medical treatment

- We found no evidence that routine preoperative traction causes any significant benefit or harm.

- One systematic review has found that nerve blocks for pain control reduce total analgesic intake.

- Systematic reviews of RCTs have found that multidose perioperative and single dose preoperative antibiotic prophylaxis is effective in reducing nosocomial infection following hip surgery.

- One systematic review of RCTs has found that prophylaxis with unfractionated heparin or low molecular weight heparin after hip fracture significantly reduces the incidence of deep venous thrombosis identified by imaging. We found insufficient evidence to confirm the effect on clinical outcomes (pulmonary thromboembolism or postphlebitic leg).

- One systematic review has found that aspirin is likely to be effective in reducing the risk of deep venous thrombosis and pulmonary embolism in patients undergoing hip fracture surgery when administered as preoperative prophylaxis.

- We found no RCT of thromboembolism stockings versus no stockings for hip fracture in elderly people. One systematic review of RCTs has found that graduated elastic compression versus no compression in elective total hip replacement reduces the risk of deep venous thrombosis by a third.

- One systematic review has found that cyclical compression devices (foot or calf pumps) reduce deep venous thrombosis in people with hip fracture. Problems with skin abrasion and compliance have been reported.

- One systematic review has found that high specification foam mattresses and pressure relieving mattresses on operating tables prevent pressure sores.

- One systematic review of poor quality RCTs has found weak evidence that nutritional supplementation (oral protein and energy feeds) reduces unfavourable outcomes after hip fracture surgery.

Rehabilitation programmes

- RCTs comparing geriatric orthopaedic rehabilitation units (GORU) versus conventional care found inconclusive results. Limited evidence from observational studies suggest that GORU may reduce the frequency of re-admission to hospital, improve the rate of return to previous residence, and provide improved function in mobility and activities of daily living.

- One systematic review of RCTs and observational studies, and a subsequent RCT, have found limited evidence that geriatric hip fracture programmes (GHFP) versus control programmes return more elderly people who have suffered hip fracture to their previous residence, and restore mobility and competence in activities of daily living. GHFP may be effective in reducing length of hospital stay and the incidence of hospital complications. We found no evidence of reduced mortality or re-admission to hospital.

- One systematic review has found that early supported discharge programmes (ESD) increase the number of people returning to their previous residence after hip fracture and reduce the length of hospital stay, but increase the number of people re-admitted to hospital.

DEFINITION	Hip fracture is a fracture of the femur above a point 5 cm below the distal part of the lesser trochanter.[1] **Intracapsular fractures** occur proximal to the point at which the hip joint capsule attaches to the femur, and can be subdivided into displaced and undisplaced fractures. Undisplaced fractures include impacted or adduction fractures. Displaced intracapsular fractures may be associated with disruption of the blood supply to the head of the femur. Numerous subdivisions and classification methods exist for these fractures. In the most distal part of the proximal femoral segment (below the lesser trochanter), the term "subtrochanteric" is used. **Extracapsular fractures** occur distal to the hip joint capsule.
INCIDENCE/ PREVALENCE	Hip fractures may occur at any age but are most common in elderly people. In industrialised societies, the lifetime risk of hip fracture is about 18% in women and 6% in men.[2] A recent study reported that prevalence increases from about three per 100 women aged 65–74 to 12.6 per 100 women aged 85 years and above.[3] The age stratified incidence has also increased in some societies during the past 25 years; not only are people living longer, but the incidence of fracture in each age group may have increased.[4]
AETIOLOGY/ RISK FACTORS	Hip fractures are usually sustained through a fall from standing height or less. The pattern of incidence is consistent with two main risk factors: increased risk of falling, and loss of skeletal strength from osteoporosis. Both are associated with aging.
PROGNOSIS	One in five people die in the first year after a hip fracture,[5] and one in four elderly people require a higher level of long term care after a

fracture.[5,6] Those who do return to live in the community after a hip fracture have greater difficulty with activities of daily living than age and sex matched controls.[3]

AIMS	To improve survival and quality of life; and to minimise complications and disability associated with hip fracture.
OUTCOMES	Incidence of preoperative, operative, and postoperative complications (infection, venous thromboembolism, refracture, fixation failure, pressure sores, medical complications); proportion of people returning to previous residential and mobility status; rates of re-admission to hospital and reoperation; measures of mobility and competence in activities of daily living; health related quality of life measures.
METHODS	*Clinical Evidence* search and appraisal December 2000. We searched for any systematic reviews and randomised or quasirandomised trials that evaluated a treatment or strategy relating to the prevention, management, or rehabilitation of proximal femoral fracture. This included any type of surgical or non-surgical intervention applied in the treatment of hip fracture, as well as any type of prophylactic treatment or dietary supplementation hypothesised to reduce the occurrence of complications of surgery or bed rest (e.g. antibiotic prophylaxis, prophylaxis against venous thromboembolism, dietary supplements, rehabilitation after acute treatment of hip fracture). The authors also searched the following databases: Current Contents to December 2000, Medline to December 2000, Embase to December 2000, Cinahl to December 2000, Cochrane Library to 2001, Issue 1, and Best Evidence to March 2000. We also scanned the bibliographies of included studies for additional references, and contacted known trialists for up to date information.

QUESTION   **What are the effects of specific surgical interventions in the treatment of hip fracture?**

OPTION   **GENERAL VERSUS REGIONAL ANAESTHESIA FOR HIP FRACTURE SURGERY**

One systematic review of RCTs has found that regional anaesthesia may reduce short term mortality after hip fracture surgery compared with general anaesthesia, and may be associated with a lower rate of deep venous thrombosis.

Benefits: We found one systematic review (search date 1999, 16 RCTs, 2191 participants).[7] Regional anaesthesia was associated with lower mortality at 1 month (53/781 with regional anaesthesia v 78/781 with general anaesthesia; RR 0.72, 95% CI 0.51 to 1.00; ARR 0.027; NNT 37). Too few people were seen at 1 year follow up to confirm any long term benefit. Regional anaesthesia was associated with reduced risk of deep venous thrombosis (39/129 v 61/130 with general anaesthesia; RR 0.64, 95% CI 0.48 to 0.86; ARR 0.169; NNT 6).

Harms: Regional anaesthesia was associated with marginally longer operation time (WMD 4.8 minutes, 95% CI 1.1 minutes to 8.6 minutes).

Comment: Although the pooled results indicated a significant reduction in risk of deep venous thrombosis, the three contributing trials had methodological limitations (probable selection and performance biases). Therefore, this association may be insecure.

OPTION **CHOICE OF IMPLANT FOR INTERNAL FIXATION OF INTRACAPSULAR HIP FRACTURES** New

One systematic review has found that threaded screws are associated with fewer fracture healing complications than smooth pins. We found insufficient evidence on the effects of using one or more screws, or the effects of a side plate.

Benefits: We found one systematic review (search date 1997, 25 RCTs, 4925 people).[8] Seven RCTs compared threaded with smooth devices. Fracture healing complications were significantly more frequent in patients treated with smooth devices (OR 1.63, 95% CI 1.22 to 2.18).

Harms: None identified.

Comment: The 25 RCTs reported 14 different comparisons; most had insufficient numbers to permit a confident conclusion on the performance of the individual devices.

OPTION **ARTHROPLASTY VERSUS INTERNAL FIXATION FOR INTRACAPSULAR HIP FRACTURES**

One systematic review of randomised and observational studies has found limited evidence that arthroplasty for displaced intracapsular fractures of the hip has no significant difference in mortality or morbidity compared with internal fixation.

Benefits: **Arthroplasty versus internal fixation:** We found one systematic review comparing arthroplasty versus internal fixation in people aged over 65 with a displaced intracapsular fracture (search date 1997, 1 RCT, 105 non-randomised studies).[9] Overall, the review found no significant differences between the two options in mortality, mobility, deep vein thrombosis, or pulmonary embolism. No health related quality of life results were available. Deep infection was slightly but significantly more common after arthroplasty than after internal fixation (no results provided). **Unipolar versus bipolar hemiarthroplasty:** We found no systematic review. We found two RCTs.[10,11] One RCT (250 people aged over 80 years, followed for 2 years) found that significantly more unipolar participants returned to preinjury status (numbers not given; OR 1.94, 95% CI 1.03 to 3.67).[10] The other RCT (48 people, mean age 77 years) found that at 6 months, performance in a 6 metre walk was better after bipolar hemiarthroplasty (unipolar 1.93 feet/second, range 1.16–3.30 v bipolar 2.67 feet/second, range 0.77–4.86).[11]

Harms: The need for reoperation was higher after internal fixation when assessed 12–15 months after surgery (3 studies, arthroplasty 36/285 [12.6%] v fixation 75/170 [44%]; RR 2.9, 95% CI 1.7 to 5.3) and 24 months after surgery (2 studies, arthroplasty 26/144 [18%] v fixation 61/194 [31%]; RR 2.6, 95% CI 1.4 to 4.6).[9]

Comment: The review included only one RCT. A Cochrane Review on this topic will be published in 2001, and will be included in the next issue of *Clinical Evidence*.

OPTION   CONSERVATIVE VERSUS OPERATIVE TREATMENT FOR EXTRACAPSULAR HIP FRACTURES

One systematic review of RCTs has found that leg deformity is more common after conservative treatment of extracapsular hip fractures. We found limited evidence of no significant difference between conservative and operative management in medical complications, mortality, or long term pain.

Benefits: We found one systematic review (search date 1999, 5 RCTs).[12] Only one RCT (106 people) used a fixation device with the dynamic features used in contemporary practice (sliding nail plate). Operative treatment was associated with shorter hospital stay, but no results were provided.

Harms: Conservative treatment was associated with leg shortening (conservative 29/39 v operative fixation 11/37; RR 2.5, 95% CI 1.47 to 4.24) and varus deformity (conservative 19/39 v operative fixation 3/35; RR 5.7, 95% CI 1.8 to 17.6).

Comment: Operative treatment was introduced in the 1950s with the expectation of improved functional outcome and reduced incidence of complications of immobilisation and prolonged bed rest. Although we found only limited evidence from RCTs about short term benefits of operation, the additional benefits of early mobilisation and early supported discharge (see option, p 764) can be realised only after surgery.

OPTION   ARTHROPLASTY VERSUS INTERNAL FIXATION FOR EXTRACAPSULAR FRACTURES

We found insufficient evidence from RCTs comparing replacement arthroplasty with a sliding hip screw for extracapsular hip fractures.

Benefits: We found one systematic review (search date 1999, 1 RCT, 90 people).[13] Participants with unstable extracapsular hip fractures were randomised to arthroplasty or a sliding hip screw. From the limited results available, there were no significant differences between the treatments for operating time, local wound complications, mortality at 12 months (RR 0.99, 95% CI 0.47 to 2.10; AR 23.4% for arthroplasty v 23.4% for sliding hip screw), or mobility of previously independent patients at discharge (RR 0.80, 95% CI 0.45 to 1.42; AR 40% v 50%).

Harms: More people received blood transfusion in the arthroplasty group (arthroplasty 34/43 v fixation 27/47; RR 1.38, 95% CI 1.03 to 1.84).

Comment: The RCT had limited methods (the method of randomisation was not specified, there was no blinding, analysis was not by intention to treat, and the outcome measures were not defined clearly).[13]

| OPTION | FIXED VERSUS DYNAMIC (SLIDING) EXTRAMEDULLARY FIXATION FOR EXTRACAPSULAR HIP FRACTURE |

One systematic review of RCTs has found that sliding hip screws are associated with significantly fewer complications than fixed nail plates in people with extracapsular hip fractures.

Benefits: We found one systematic review (search date 1999).[14] Three RCTs compared a fixed nail plate (Jewett or McLaughlin) versus a sliding hip screw. There were no significant differences in mortality or reported pain at follow up.

Harms: The use of fixed nail plates was associated with increased risk of fixation failure (2 trials, 38/62 v 12/83 with sliding hip screw; RR 4.3, 95% CI 2.4 to 7.5). Postoperative mobility was non-significantly poorer in participants whose fractures were fixed with fixed nail plates (1 trial, 15/36 v 11/42 with sliding hip screw; RR 1.6, 95% CI 0.8 to 3.0).

Comment: None.

| OPTION | CEPHALOCONDYLIC NAILS VERSUS EXTRAMEDULLARY FIXATION FOR EXTRACAPSULAR HIP FRACTURE |

One systematic review has found that, compared with cephalocondylic intramedullary devices, extramedullary fixation of hip fractures using sliding hip screw devices is associated with similar benefits and significantly fewer operative complications.

Benefits: We found one systematic review (search date 1999)[15] and one subsequent RCT.[16] **Intramedullary (Gamma nail) fixation versus extramedullary (sliding hip screw) fixation:** The review identified 14 RCTs (1977 people, follow up 3–12 months). The pooled results found no difference between cephalocondylic nails and sliding hip screws in mortality, incidence of wound infection, medical complications of surgery, blood transfusion, or functional outcomes at follow up. Radiological screening time, a measure of radiation exposure, was shorter in the Gamma nail group (Gamma nail 172 people, sliding hip screw 172 people; WMD –22.6 seconds, 95% CI –25.7 seconds to –19.5 seconds). **Intramedullary hip screw versus sliding hip screw:** The review identified two trials (231 people). Results for postoperative complications, mortality, and functional outcomes were similar in the two groups. The subsequent RCT (110 people) compared intramedullary hip screw with a sliding hip screw and found no difference between groups in fracture healing or functional outcomes.

Harms: The Gamma nail was associated with an increased risk of fracture of the femur during the operative procedure (RR 3.75, 95% CI 1.69 to 8.31) or later (RR 6.26, 95% CI 2.55 to 15.4) and an increased reoperation rate (RR 1.99, 95% CI 1.27 to 3.11). In the comparisons of intramedullary hip screw and sliding hip screw, more fracture fixation complications, including all of the intraoperative and later femur fractures, occurred in the intramedullary hip screw group, but the difference was not significant.

Comment: We found no evidence that the theoretical mechanical advantages of intramedullary cephalocondylic devices for operative fixation of extracapsular hip fractures have so far been confirmed or rejected. The designs tested have been associated with higher risk of fracture fixation complications than alternative devices. The evidence refers to extracapsular hip fractures in the trochanteric region and may not apply to people with subtrochanteric fractures.

OPTION **CONDYLOCEPHALIC NAILS OR EXTRAMEDULLARY FIXATION FOR EXTRACAPSULAR HIP FRACTURE**

One systematic review found that condylocephalic nails are less effective than extramedullary fixation for extracapsular hip fractures.

Benefits: We found one systematic review (search date 1997, 11 RCTs, 1667 people).[17] The advantages of condylocephalic nails were reduced deep wound sepsis (condylocephalic 5/554 v extramedullary 23/549; RR 0.26, 95% CI 0.11 to 0.62), shorter length of surgery (326 people; WMD −22.8 minutes, 95% CI −27.7 minutes to −17.8 minutes), and lower operative blood loss (326 people; WMD −208 ml, 95% CI −262 to −154 ml).

Harms: Use of condylocephalic nails was associated with several adverse outcomes: higher risk of reoperation for fixation failure (8 trials, condylocephalic 118/564 v extramedullary 31/566; RR 3.72, 95% CI 2.54 to 5.44), greater incidence of leg shortening (7 trials, condylocephalic 44/401 v extramedullary 19/442; RR 2.71, 95% CI 1.65 to 4.59), and higher incidence of external rotation deformity (5 trials, condylocephalic 86/345 v extramedullary 28/396; RR 3.73, 95% CI 2.47 to 5.64).

Comment: None.

QUESTION **What are the effects of perisurgical medical interventions on surgical outcome and prevention of complications?**

OPTION **TEMPORARY TRACTION BEFORE SURGERY FOR HIP FRACTURE**

We found no evidence that routine preoperative traction to the injured limb is associated with any significant benefit or harm.

Benefits: We found one systematic review (search date 2000, 6 RCTs, 938 people with recent hip fracture).[6] Traction had no effect on the number of people requiring analgesia in the 24 hours after admission (1 RCT, traction 54/101 v control 71/151; RR 1.14, 95% CI 0.89 to 1.46), or the difficulty of fracture reduction at time of surgery (1 RCT, traction 5/45 v control 7/64; RR 1.02, 95% CI 0.34 to 3.00). In one trial, which compared skeletal with skin traction, there was a small but significant reduction in the mean number of analgesic doses used by those treated with skeletal traction (1 RCT; skin traction 40 people, mean 2.5 doses, SD 1.6 v skeletal traction 38 people, mean 1.7, SD 1.4; WMD 0.80, 95% CI 0.13 to 1.46).

Harms: Two of the trials compared skeletal traction with skin traction. Although no important difference was identified between these two methods, initial skeletal traction was more painful.

Comment: We found no good evidence to support routine preoperative traction to the injured limb of people with hip fracture in hospital.

OPTION   NERVE BLOCKS FOR PAIN CONTROL BEFORE AND AFTER HIP FRACTURE

One systematic review has found that nerve blocks for pain control reduce total analgesic intake.

Benefits: We found one systematic review (search date 2000, 7 RCTs or case controlled trials, 269 people with recent hip fracture).[18] Two small trials studied the effects of nerve block at hospital admission, and the remaining five examined perioperative blocks. Nerve blocks were associated with reduced use of parenteral or oral analgesia to control pain from the fracture, operation, or during surgery. Reduced analgesic use was found with lateral cutaneous block (2 trials, block 19/26 v control 25/25; RR 0.73, 95% CI 0.58 to 0.92) and with triple block (1 trial, block 13/25 v control 22/24; RR 0.57, 95% CI 0.38 to 0.84). It is not clear whether this reduction in analgesia was associated with clinical benefit. Administration of a psoas block at hospital admission was associated with fewer complaints of unsatisfactory pain control, measured on a visual analogue scale both preoperatively (RR 0.25, 95% CI 0.08 to 0.75) and postoperatively (RR 0.10, 95% CI 0.01 to 0.71). A single small trial of femoral nerve block on admission found reduced incidence of respiratory infection (block 2/25 v control 11/25; RR 0.18, 95% CI 0.04 to 0.74).

Harms: None reported.

Comment: The trials were small, used different types of nerve blocks, and had varying times of insertion. It is unclear whether nerve blocks confer any benefit compared with other methods of analgesia in hip fracture. The possible reduction of respiratory infection is worthy of further study.

OPTION   PERIOPERATIVE ANTIBIOTICS

Systematic reviews of RCTs have found that multidose perioperative and single dose preoperative antibiotic prophylaxis are effective in reducing infection after hip surgery.

Benefits: **Multiple dose perioperative regimens:** We found one systematic review (search date 2000, 11 RCTs, 1896 people with recent hip fracture) of multiple dose regimens versus placebo or no prophylaxis.[19] The review found significant reduction in the incidence of deep wound infection (antibiotic 12/961 v control 40/935; RR 0.36, 95% CI 0.21 to 0.65; ARR 2.9%, 95% CI 1.3% to 4.4%), superficial wound infection (antibiotic 22/705 v control 38/661; RR 0.48, 95% CI 0.28 to 0.81), and urinary tract infection (antibiotic 31/259 v control 44/241; RR 0.66, 95% CI 0.43 to 1.00). The review found no significant reduction in the incidence of respiratory infection (antibiotic 14/259 v control 16/241; RR 0.81, 95% CI

0.41 to 1.63). **Single dose preoperative regimens:** We found one systematic review (search date 2000, 7 RCTs, 3500 people with recent hip fracture, including 2195 people from one multicentre trial).[19] Single dose prophylaxis, compared with placebo or no treatment, significantly reduced deep wound infection (antibiotic 20/1745 v control 51/1755; RR 0.41, 95% CI 0.25 to 0.65; ARR 1.8%, 95% CI 0.8% to 2.7%), superficial wound infection (antibiotic 59/1745 v control 87/1755; RR 0.69, 95% CI 0.50 to 0.95), urinary tract infection (antibiotic 131/1493 v control 212/1482; RR 0.63, 95% CI 0.53 to 0.76), and respiratory infection (antibiotic 41/1493 v control 92/1482; RR 0.46, 95% CI 0.33 to 0.65).

Harms: Adverse effects (allergy, rashes, gastrointestinal complaints) were rarely reported but were more common in people given multiple dose perioperative antibiotics (antibiotic 24/520 v control 12/362; RR 1.83, 95% CI 0.96 to 3.50).[19]

Comment: Many different antimicrobials were studied (all active against *Staphylococcus aureus*). The absolute risk reduction with single dose regimens was not significantly less than with multiple dose regimens.

OPTION	UNFRACTIONATED HEPARIN AND LOW MOLECULAR WEIGHT HEPARIN

One systematic review of RCTs has found that prophylaxis with unfractionated heparin or low molecular weight heparin (LMWH) after hip fracture significantly reduces the incidence of deep venous thrombosis identified by imaging. We found insufficient evidence to confirm the effect on clinical outcomes (pulmonary thromboembolism or postphlebitic leg).

Benefits: We found one systematic review (search date 2000, 22 RCTs in elderly people undergoing surgery for hip fracture).[20] Overall, trial quality was poor. **Heparin versus placebo or no treatment:** Ten trials evaluated unfractionated heparin and four trials evaluated LMWH. The trials found fewer lower limb deep vein thromboses (identified by imaging) with unfractionated heparin (103/407 [25.3%] with heparin v 166/409 [40.6%] with control; RR 0.59, 95% CI 0.49 to 0.72; ARR 17%; NNT 6) and with LMWH (18/104 with heparin v 37/110 with control; RR 0.55, 95% CI 0.34 to 0.88; ARR 0.15; NNT 7). **Unfractionated heparin versus LMWH:** Five trials compared unfractionated heparin versus LMWH. LMWH significantly reduced deep venous thrombosis identified by imaging (47/252 v 64/227 with unfractionated heparin; RR 0.67, 95% CI 0.48 to 0.94; ARR 0.09, 95% CI 0.02 to 0.16; NNT 11).

Harms: There was a non-significant increase in overall mortality after hip fracture in the group receiving heparin (heparin 46/420 [11%] v control 35/423 [8%]; RR 1.31, 95% CI 0.88 to 1.97).[20] One systematic review (search date not stated) summarised the risk of bleeding or transfusion in all RCTs of prophylactic subcutaneous unfractionated heparin in general, orthopaedic, and urological surgery.[21] Overall, excessive bleeding or need for transfusion was significantly increased with heparin (heparin 419/7027 v control

244/6504; OR 1.66). Another systematic review (search date 1991) included comparisons of unfractionated heparin and LMWH in general and orthopaedic surgery, and found insufficient evidence from published RCTs to confirm a difference in the rate of bleeding complications.[22]

Comment: We found no trials that reported the incidence of postphlebitic leg or wound complications.

OPTION ANTIPLATELET AGENTS

One systematic review and a large multicentre RCT have found that aspirin is likely to be effective in reducing the risk of deep venous thrombosis and pulmonary embolism in people undergoing hip fracture surgery when administered as preoperative prophylaxis.

Benefits: We found one systematic review (search date 1990, 898 people), which compared prophylaxis versus an antiplatelet agent versus placebo or no prophylaxis after fracture.[23] Most people in the review had a hip fracture. For this group of people, the reduction in deep venous thrombosis incidence was not significant (antiplatelet 163/454 v control 186/444; odds reduction 31%), but for pulmonary embolism it was significant (antiplatelet 14/504 v control 34/494, odds reduction 60%). We found one subsequent multicentre RCT (13 356 people having surgery for hip fracture), which compared aspirin with placebo started preoperatively and continued for 35 days.[24] It found that aspirin versus placebo significantly reduced the incidence of symptomatic deep vein thrombosis (69/6679 with aspirin v 97/6677 with placebo; RR 0.71, 95% CI 0.52 to 0.97), of venous thromboembolism (symptomatic deep vein thrombosis or non-fatal pulmonary embolism, 87/6679 with aspirin v 122/6677 with control; RR 0.71, 95% CI 0.54 to 0.94), and of fatal pulmonary embolism (18/6679 with aspirin v 43/6677 with control; RR 0.42, 95% CI 0.24 to 0.73).

Harms: The systematic review summarised the bleeding complications reported across all surgical procedures.[23] Fatal bleeds were rare (antiplatelet group 2/4441 v controls 0/4450). The need for transfusion was significantly more frequent in the antiplatelet group (28/2798 v controls 15/3808), as were other bleeding related complications (reoperation, haematoma, or infection because of a bleed) (antiplatelet agents 177/2269 v controls 129/2306). In the multicentre trial, fatal bleeds were also rare (aspirin 13/6679 v control 15/6677).[24] Non-fatal gastrointestinal bleeding was significantly more frequent in people given aspirin (aspirin 182/6679 v control 122/6677).

Comment: None.

OPTION GRADUATED ELASTIC COMPRESSION (THROMBOEMBOLISM STOCKINGS)

We found no RCT of thromboembolism stockings for hip fracture in elderly people. One systematic review of RCTs has found that graduated elastic compression in elective total hip replacement reduces the risk of deep venous thrombosis by a third compared with placebo.

Benefits: We found one systematic review (search date 1998), which found no RCTs in people with hip fracture.[25] It pooled data from four trials in people undergoing elective total hip replacement.[25] It found graduated elastic compression significantly reduced deep venous thrombosis (stockings 32/125 v control 61/111; RR 0.43, 95% CI 0.30 to 0.61; ARR 0.29; NNT 4). A second systematic review (search date 1999) included two of the three RCTs reported in the earlier review but did not present a separate analysis for lower limb surgery.[26]

Harms: The first systematic review reported that manufacturers of stockings advise against their use in people with an ankle : brachial pressure of less than 0.7. People with peripheral arterial disease or with diabetes and neuropathy were stated to be at higher risk of worsening ischaemia, but we found no evidence in RCTs to quantify this risk.

Comment: It is unclear whether extrapolation from elective hip replacement studies is appropriate for hip fracture.

OPTION **CYCLICAL COMPRESSION OF THE FOOT OR CALF**

One systematic review has found that cyclical compression devices (foot or calf pumps) reduce deep venous thrombosis in people with hip fracture. Problems with skin abrasion and compliance have been reported.

Benefits: We found one systematic review (search date 2000, 4 RCTs, 442 people) comparing mechanical pumping devices versus no intervention.[20] Cyclical compression devices reduced the risk of deep venous thrombosis (compression 12/202 v control 42/212; RR 0.30, 95% CI 0.17 to 0.53). We found no adequate evidence about any effect on the incidence of pulmonary embolism and overall mortality.

Harms: Problems with skin abrasion and compliance were reported in all four RCTs of cyclical compression devices.

Comment: None.

OPTION **BEDS, MATTRESSES, AND CUSHIONS FOR PREVENTING PRESSURE SORES**

One systematic review has found that high specification foam mattresses and pressure relieving mattresses on operating tables prevent pressure sores.

Benefits: We found one systematic review (search date 2000).[27] High specification foam mattresses compared with "standard hospital" foam mattresses significantly reduced pressure sores (4 RCTs; high specification 52/678 v standard 57/172; RR 0.29, 95% CI 0.19 to 0.43). Pressure relieving mattresses for high risk people in the operating theatre reduced postoperative pressure sores. Three RCTs evaluated different methods of pressure relief on the operating table. A viscoelastic polymer (gel) pad compared with a standard table reduced postoperative pressure sores (gel 22/205 v control 43/211; RR 0.53, 95% CI 0.33 to 0.85; ARR 9.6%; NNT 11). Two

RCTs compared an alternating system (applied during and after surgery) with a gel pad used during surgery plus standard mattress after surgery. Use of alternating pressure throughout significantly reduced pressure sores (alternation 3/188 v control 14/180; RR 0.21, 95% CI 0.06 to 0.7; ARR 6.2%; NNT 16).

Harms: None identified.

Comment: None.

OPTION   **NUTRITIONAL SUPPLEMENTATION AFTER HIP FRACTURE**

One systematic review has found that nutritional supplementation (oral protein and energy feeds) reduces unfavourable outcomes after surgery for hip fracture.

Benefits: We found one systematic review (search date 2000, 15 RCTs, 1054 people).[28] Six RCTs found that oral multinutrient feeds (providing non-protein energy, protein, some vitamins and minerals) reduced the overall incidence of death or complications by the end of the study (14/66 v 26/73; RR 0.52, 95% CI 0.32 to 0.84), but did not find an effect on mortality (12/91 v 14/97; RR 0.85, 95% CI 0.42 to 1.70). Three RCTs comparing nasogastric multinutrient feeding versus control found no evidence for an effect on mortality (RR 0.99, 95% CI 0.50 to 1.97), but the studies included people with differing characteristics. Three RCTs found that protein in an oral feed did not significantly reduce mortality, but significantly reduced unfavourable outcomes (complications or death combined) (66/113 with protein v 82/110 with no protein; RR 0.78, 95% CI 0.65 to 0.95). Two RCTs (one testing intravenous thiamine and other water soluble vitamins, the other testing alfacalcidiol), found no evidence of benefit for either vitamin supplement).

Harms: We found little evidence about harms. Nasogastric feeds were sometimes tolerated poorly. Complications, described in only one RCT, included bloating and anorexia. We found no reports of feed induced diarrhoea or aspiration pneumonia.

Comment: The quality of trials reported in the review was poor. Defects included inadequate size, method problems (inadequate allocation concealment, assessor blinding, and intention to treat analysis), and limited outcome assessment.

QUESTION   **What are the effects of rehabilitation programmes and treatment protocols after hip fracture?**

OPTION   **INPATIENT REHABILITATION IN A GERIATRIC ORTHOPAEDIC REHABILITATION UNIT**

The evidence from RCTs about the effectiveness of GORU is inconclusive. Limited evidence from observational studies suggests that GORU may reduce the frequency of re-admission for acute care, improve the rate of return to previous residence, and provide improved mobility and activities of daily living.

Benefits: We found one systematic review (search date 1998, 41 comparative studies, including 14 RCTs), which included seven studies (4 RCTs, 3 cohort studies) of GORU.[29] **Length of hospital stay:** Significant heterogeneity was present between RCT results.[29] The pooled results from RCTs (GORU 333 people v control 375; WMD 1.6 days, 95% CI −28.0 days to +31 days) were similar to those found in a cohort study. There was no evidence of a significant difference in total hospital stay between programmes with access to a GORU and those without. **Readmission for acute care:** The systematic review found a significant reduction in rate of readmission for acute care (GORU 36/182 v control 57/196; RR 0.68, 95% CI 0.47 to 0.97). **Return to previous residence after discharge:** There was a marginally significant improvement in the return to previous residence in the GORU group (4 RCTs, GORU 254/343 v control 255/380; RR 1.11, 95% CI 1.01 to 1.22). **Death:** The review found no reduction in death by follow up with rehabilitation in a GORU (GORU 79/383 v control 90/433; RR 0.98, 95% CI 0.75 to 1.28). **Hospital morbidity:** Two cohort studies found no significant difference in postoperative complications as a whole (1 study, 102 events from 521 admissions with GORU v 95 events from 202 admissions with control). **Mobility and activities of daily living:** One cohort study found that the proportion of participants independently mobile at 6 months was significantly higher with the orthopaedic unit (GORU 221/336 v control 104/127; RR 1.25, 95% CI 1.11 to 1.39). Rehabilitation in the GORU reduced loss of daily living ability score at 12 months (22/44 had loss of ability with GORU v 28/36 with control; RR 0.64, 95% CI 0.46 to 0.91). **Health related quality of life:** The systematic review included one RCT (108 people) and one cohort study (723 people) comparing health related quality of life scores for GORU versus control. They both found no significant difference.

Harms: Pressure sores were more common in GORU (1 study, GORU 17/142 v control 8/193; RR 2.89, 95% CI 1.28 to 6.50).

Comment: None.

OPTION **GERIATRIC HIP FRACTURE PROGRAMME WITHIN AN ACUTE ORTHOPAEDIC UNIT**

One systematic review of RCTs and observational studies, and a subsequent non-randomised controlled trial, found limited evidence that GHFP versus control programmes return more elderly people who have suffered hip fracture to their previous residence, and restore mobility and competence in activities of daily living. GHFP may reduce the length of hospital stay and the incidence of hospital complications. We found no evidence of reduced mortality or re-admission to hospital.

Benefits: We found one systematic review (search date 1998, 41 comparative studies, including 14 RCTs), which included five studies of GHFP versus control programmes.[29] **Length of hospital stay:** Introduction of GHFP was associated with a reduction in length of hospital stay in four of the five included studies. The crude average reduction from the published data was 9 days. **Re-admission for acute care:** One RCT found no significant effect on re-admission rate by 4 months (GHFP 16/127 v control 11/125; RR 1.43, 95% CI 0.69 to

2.96). **Return to previous residence after discharge:** GHFP reduced the risk of failing to return home (2 RCTs, GHFP 121/139 v control 100/131; RR 0.88, 95% CI 0.78 to 0.99). **Mortality:** Two RCTs found no significant reduction in mortality with GHFP (GHFP 27/165 v control 30/158; RR 0.87, 95% CI 0.54 to 1.39). **Morbidity:** The number of participants sustaining one or more complications in hospital was lower with GHFP (GHFP 162/431 v control 39/60; RR 0.58, 95% CI 0.46 to 0.72). **Mobility and activities of daily living:** One RCT found that GHFP did not significantly reduce the number of people failing to walk independently by discharge (1 RCT, GHFP 63/127 v control 51/125; RR 0.70, 95% CI 0.43 to 1.15). Another RCT found that performance of a 20 metre walk was quicker (1 RCT, GHFP mean 45 seconds v control 59 seconds, no SD provided). A third RCT found that the modified Barthel Index was higher in GHFP participants (1 RCT, GHFP mean 92.8, 95% CI 90.0 to 95.6 v control 85.6, 95% CI 81.3 to 89.8). **Health related quality of life:** The systematic review found no studies of this outcome. We found one subsequent RCT comparing GHFP with control programmes.[30] It found that GHFP significantly reduced hospital stay, but did not reduce complication or readmission rates.

Harms: We found no evidence of harms.

Comment: None.

| OPTION | EARLY SUPPORTED DISCHARGE PROGRAMMES |

One systematic review has found that ESD after hip fracture increases the number of people returning to their previous residence and reduces length of hospital stay, but increases the frequency of re-admission to hospital.

Benefits: We found one systematic review (search date 1998, 41 comparative studies, including 14 RCTs), which included six studies of ESD.[29] **Lengths of hospital stay:** Introduction of ESD was associated with reduced length of both acute hospital stay and total number of days in hospital. The crude average reduction (no standard deviations provided) was 6.9 days in acute hospital stay and 2 days in total duration of care. **Return to previous residence after discharge:** ESD was associated with a significantly increased rate of return to previous residence (3 cohort studies, ESD 203/247 v control 129/197; RR 1.25, 95% CI 1.11 to 1.41). **Mortality:** There was no evidence of benefit or disadvantage from introduction of ESD (1 RCT, ESD 12/160 v control 6/81; RR 1.01, 95% CI 0.39 to 2.60). **Morbidity:** One cohort study found no evidence of a significant difference in incidence of one or more hospital complications between ESD and control participants (ESD 17/63 v control 15/66; RR 1.19, 95% CI 0.65 to 2.17). **Mobility and activities of daily living:** One cohort study found no evidence of difference in Nottingham Health Profile mobility dimension mean score (ESD 48 v control 50, no SD provided). One RCT found no evidence of difference in improvement of Barthel Index over 3 months (ESD 160 people, mean change 1.9, SD 3.22 v control 81 people, mean change 1.7, SD 2.68). **Health related quality of life:** Two studies reported scores for this outcome. There was no evidence of difference in mean Nottingham Health Profile dimension score (1 cohort study, 110 people). One RCT found no evidence of difference in EUROQOL score at 3 months (mean difference −0.04, 95% CI −0.13 to +0.06).

Harms: ESD was associated with a significant increase in the frequency of readmission to hospital (3 cohort studies; 69/922 with ESD v 17/406 with control; RR 1.91, 95% CI 1.11 to 3.29).

Comment: None.

OPTION	SYSTEMATIC MULTICOMPONENT HOME REHABILITATION AFTER HIP FRACTURE

One RCT comparing a systematic home based rehabilitation programme with existing services found no important differences.

Benefits: We found no systematic review, but we found one RCT (304 people who had surgery for hip fracture and returned home within 100 days, follow up 12 months),[31] which compared systematic home based multicomponent rehabilitation addressing physical impairments and activities of daily living versus "usual care". It found no significant difference between groups in recovery to prefracture levels of self care, home management, social activity, balance, or lower extremity strength. The systematic programme was associated with slightly greater upper arm strength, and marginally better walking.

Harms: None reported.

Comment: The RCT examined whether systematising home assessment and treatment according to a protocol made a difference compared with "usual care". The failure of this trial to find a difference between the systematic programme and "usual care" may be contextual, indicating that "usual care" was already being delivered competently.

Substantive changes since last issue

Graduated elastic compression New systematic review;[26] conclusion unchanged.
Nutritional supplementation New RCT;[28] conclusion unchanged.
Geriatric hip fracture programme New RCT;[30] conclusion unchanged.

REFERENCES

1. Parker MJ, Pryor GA. *Hip fracture management*. Oxford: Blackwell Scientific Publications, 1993.
2. Meunier PJ. Prevention of hip fractures. *Am J Med* 1993;95(suppl):75–78.
3. Hochberg MC, Williamson J, Skinner EA, et al. The prevalence and impact of self-reported hip fracture in elderly community-dwelling women: The Women's Health and Aging Study. *Osteoporos Int* 1998;8:385–389.
4. Boyce WJ, Vessey MP. Rising incidence of fracture of the proximal femur. *Lancet* 1985;1:150–151.
5. Schurch M-A, Rizzoli R, Mermillod B, et al. A prospective study on the socio-economic aspects of fracture of the proximal femur. *J Bone Miner Res* 1996;11:1935–1942.
6. Parker MJ, Handoll HHG. Pre-operative traction for fractures of the proximal femur. In: The Cochrane Library, Issue 1, 2001. Oxford: Update Software.

Search date 2000; primary sources Cochrane Musculoskeletal Injuries Group Trials Register, Medline, and hand searches of reference bibliographies.
7. Parker MJ, Urwin SC, Handoll HHG, Griffiths R. General versus spinal/epidural anaesthesia for surgery for hip fractures in adults. In: The Cochrane Library, Issue 1, 2001. Oxford: Update Software. Search date 1999; primary sources Cochrane Musculoskeletal Injuries Group Trials Register, Medline, and hand searching of selected orthopaedic and anaesthetic journals, conference proceedings, and reference lists of relevant articles.
8. Lu-Yao GL, Keller RB, Littenberg B, Wenberg JE. Outcomes after displaced fractures of the femoral neck. A meta-analysis of one hundred and six published reports. *J Bone Joint Surg Am* 1994;76:

15–25. Search date 1990; primary sources Medline, and hand searches of reference lists.

9. Parker MJ, Blundell C. Choice of implant for internal fixation of femoral neck fractures: meta-analysis of 25 randomised trials including 4925 patients. *Acta Orthop Scand* 1998;69:138–143. Search date 1997; primary sources Cochrane, Medline, and hand searches of six orthopedic journals.

10. Calder SJ, Anderson GH, Jagger C, et al. Unipolar or bipolar prosthesis for displaced intracapsular hip fracture in octogenarians: a randomised prospective study. *J Bone Joint Surg Br* 1996;78: 391–394.

11. Cornell CN, Levine D, O'Doherty J, Lyden J. Unipolar versus bipolar arthroplasty for the treatment of femoral neck fractures in the elderly. *Clin Orthop* 1998;348;67–71.

12. Parker MJ, Handoll HHG. Conservative versus operative treatment for extracapsular hip fractures. In: The Cochrane Library, Issue 1, 2001. Oxford: Update Software. Search date 1999; primary sources Cochrane Musculoskeletal Injuries Group Trials Register, hand searches of reference bibliographies, and personal contact with trialists.

13. Parker MJ, Handoll HHG. Replacement arthroplasty versus internal fixation for extracapsular hip fractures. In: The Cochrane Library, Issue 1, 2001. Oxford: Update Software. Search date 1999; primary sources Cochrane Musculoskeletal Injuries Group Trials Register, hand searches of reference bibliographies, and personal contact with colleagues.

14. Parker MJ, Handoll HHG, Chinoy MA. Extramedullary fixation implants for extracapsular hip fractures. In: The Cochrane Library, Issue 1, 2001. Oxford: Update Software. Search date 1999; primary sources Cochrane Musculoskeletal Injuries Group trials register, and hand searches of reference lists of relevant articles.

15. Parker MJ, Handoll HHG. Gamma and other cephalocondylic intramedullary nails versus extramedullary implants for extracapsular hip fractures. In: The Cochrane Library, Issue 1, 2001. Oxford: Update Software. Search date 1999; primary sources Cochrane Musculoskeletal Injuries Group Trials Register, Medline, hand searching of selected orthopaedic journals, conference proceedings, reference lists of relevant articles, personal contact with trialists, colleagues, and implant manufacturers.

16. Hoffmann R, Schmidmaier G, Schulz R, Schutz M, Sudkamp NP. Classic nail versus DHS. A prospective randomised study of fixation of trochanteric femur fractures. *Unfallchirurg* 1999; 102:182–190.

17. Parker MJ, Handoll HHG, Bhonsle S, Gillespie WJ. Condylocephalic nails versus extramedullary implants for extracapsular hip fractures. In: The Cochrane Library, Issue 1, 2001. Oxford: Update Software. Search date 1997; primary sources Cochrane Musculoskeletal Injuries Group trials register, Medline, and hand searches of reference lists of relevant articles.

18. Parker MJ, Griffiths R, Appadu BN. Nerve blocks (subcostal, lateral cutaneous, femoral, triple, psoas) for hip fractures. In: The Cochrane Library, Issue 1, 2001. Oxford: Update Software. Search date 2000; primary sources Cochrane Musculoskeletal Injuries Group trials register, Medline, and hand searches of trial bibliographies.

19. Gillespie WJ, Walenkamp G. Antibiotic prophylaxis for surgery for proximal femoral and other closed long bone fractures. In: The Cochrane Library, Issue 1, 2001. Oxford: Update Software. Search date 2000; primary sources Medline, Embase,

Current Contents, Dissertation Abstracts, Index to UK theses, and hand searches of bibliographies of identified articles.

20. Handoll HHG, Farrar MJ, McBirnie J, et al. Heparin, low molecular weight heparin and physical methods for preventing deep vein thrombosis and pulmonary embolism following surgery for hip fractures. In: The Cochrane Library, Issue 1, 2001. Oxford: Update Software. Search date 2000; primary sources Cochrane Musculoskeletal Injuries Group Trials Register, Medline, Embase, hand searches of published papers and books, and personal contact with trialists and other workers in the field.

21. Collins R, Scrimgeour A, Yusuf S, Peto R. Reduction in fatal pulmonary embolism and venous thrombosis by perioperative administration of subcutaneous heparin. *N Engl J Med* 1988; 318:1162–1173. Search date not stated; primary sources Medline, hand searches of reference lists, and personal contact with colleagues, investigators, and manufacturers of heparin.

22. Jorgensen LN, Wille-Jorgensen P, Hauch O. Prophylaxis of postoperative thromboembolism with low molecular weight heparins. *Br J Surg* 1993;80:689–704. Search date 1991; primary sources Medline, Current Contents, hand searches of reference lists, and personal contact with authors of trials.

23. Antiplatelet Trialists' Collaboration. Collaborative review of randomized trials of antiplatelet therapy. III: Reduction in venous thrombosis and pulmonary embolism by antiplatelet prophylaxis among surgical and medical patients. *BMJ* 1994;308: 235–246. Search date 1990; primary sources Medline, Current Contents, hand searches of journals, reference lists, abstracts, conference proceedings, personal contact with the International Committee on Thrombosis and Haemostasis and colleagues and manufacturers.

24. Anonymous. Prevention of pulmonary embolism and deep vein thrombosis with low dose aspirin: Pulmonary Embolism Prevention (PEP) trial. *Lancet* 2000;355:1295–1302.

25. Agu O, Hamilton G, Baker D. Graduated compression stockings in the prevention of venous thromboembolism. *Br J Surg* 1999;86:992–1004. Search date 1998; primary sources Medline, Cochrane, and hand searches of reference lists.

26. Amarigiri SV, Lees TA. Elastic compression stockings for prevention of deep venous thrombosis. In: The Cochrane Library, Issue 1, 2001. Oxford: Update Software. Search date 1999; primary sources Cochrane Peripheral Vascular Disease Group trials register, Medline, Embase and hand searches of Index Medicus, and personal contact with manufacturers and trialists in ongoing trials.

27. Cullum N, Deeks J, Sheldon TA, Song F, Fletcher AW. Beds, mattresses and cushions for pressure sore prevention and treatment. In: The Cochrane Library, Issue 1, 2001. Oxford: Update Software. Search date 2000; primary sources Cochrane Wounds Group specialist trials register, hand searching of wound care journals, and relevant conference proceedings.

28. Avenell A, Handoll HHG. Nutritional supplementation for hip fracture aftercare in the elderly. In: The Cochrane Library, Issue 1, 2001. Oxford: Update Software. Search date 2000; primary sources Cochrane Musculoskeletal Injuries Group Trials Register, The Cochrane Controlled Trials Register, Medline, Nutrition Abstracts and Reviews, Healthstar, Embase, Biosis, Cinahl, hand searching of reference lists of selected nutrition journals.

29. Cameron I, Crotty M, Currie C, et al. Geriatric rehabilitation following fractures in older people: a systematic review. *Health Technol Assess* 2000;4. Search date 1998; primary sources Cochrane Musculoskeletal Injuries Group Trials Register, The Cochrane Controlled Trials Register, Medline, Cinahl, hand searches of reference lists.

30. Choong PFM, Langford AK, Dowsey MM, Santamaria NM. Clinical pathway for fractured neck of femur: a prospective, controlled study. *Med J Aust* 2000;172:423–426.

31. Tinetti ME, Baker DI, Gottschalk M, et al. Home-based multi-component rehabilitation program for older persons after hip fracture: a randomized trial. *Arch Phys Med Rehab* 1999;80:916–922.

William Gillespie

Professor

Dunedin School of Medicine

University of Otago

Dunedin

New Zealand

Competing interests: The author is coordinating editor of the Cochrane Musculo-skeletal Injuries Group, and has participated in several of the cited systematic reviews.

Leg cramps

Musculoskeletal disorders

Search date November 2000: new for this issue

Gavin Young

QUESTIONS

INTERVENTIONS

To be covered in future issues of
  Clinical Evidence
Leg cramps associated with
  pregnancy
Leg cramps associated with venous
  insufficiency
Leg cramps associated with dialysis

Covered elsewhere in this issue
Compression hosiery for venous
  ulcers, p 1365

See glossary, p 771

Key Messages

- We found no evidence on the effect of compression hosiery in idiopathic leg cramps.
- One systematic review has found that quinine significantly reduces the frequency of attacks of nocturnal leg cramps.
- We found limited evidence from one small RCT that quinine with theophylline versus quinine reduces the number of nights affected by leg cramps.
- We found limited evidence from one small RCT that vitamin E versus quinine sulphate or placebo produced no benefit in the frequency or severity of idiopathic leg cramps.
- We found no evidence on the effects of analgesics for the treatment of idiopathic leg cramps.
- We found no evidence on the effects of antiepileptic drugs for the treatment of idiopathic leg cramps.

Musculoskeletal disorders

DEFINITION	Leg cramps are painful spasms of the leg muscles. They occur most commonly at night. They can also occur after exercise.
INCIDENCE/ PREVALENCE	Leg cramps are common and increase with age. About half of the people attending a general medicine clinic have had leg cramps within 1 month of their visit, and over two thirds of people over 50 years of age have experienced leg cramps.[1]
AETIOLOGY/ RISK FACTORS	Very little is known about the cause of leg cramps. Risk factors include pregnancy, salt depletion, peripheral vascular disease (both venous and arterial), and myopathy.
PROGNOSIS	Leg cramps can cause severe pain and sleep disturbance, both of which are distressing.
AIMS	To reduce the number and the severity of attacks of cramp, with minimal adverse effects of treatment.
OUTCOMES	Number of attacks; severity of attacks; number of disturbed nights.
METHODS	*Clinical Evidence* search and appraisal November 2000.

QUESTION **What are the effects of treatments for idiopathic leg cramps?**

OPTION **COMPRESSION HOSIERY**

We found no evidence about the effects of compression hosiery on idiopathic leg cramps (see glossary, p 771).

Benefits: We found no systematic reviews or RCTs.

Harms: We found no systematic reviews or RCTs addressing harms related to the use of compression hosiery in idiopathic leg cramps (see compression under prevention and treatment of venous leg ulcers, p 1365).

Comment: None.

OPTION **QUININE**

One systematic review has found that quinine significantly reduces the frequency of attacks of leg cramp.

Benefits: We found one updated systematic review (4 published RCTs and 4 unpublished RCTs, 409 people).[2] Seven of the eight RCTs used a crossover design. The review found that quinine versus placebo significantly reduced the frequency of nocturnal leg cramps (frequency of cramps in a 4 week period reduced by 3.6, 95% CI 2.2 to 5.1; RRR 21%, 95% CI 12% to 30%).

Harms: Adverse effects of quinine include headache, digestive disorders, tinnitus, fever, blurred vision, dizziness, and pruritus.[2] Only tinnitus occurred with a marginally greater frequency in the quinine group compared with the placebo group. More people taking quinine versus placebo suffered tinnitus (18 v 7 people, significance not provided). Elevated quinine levels can cause cinchonism (see glossary, p 771), which includes nausea, vomiting, deafness, and tinnitus.[3]

Leg cramps

Comment: We found no evidence about the optimal dose or length of treatment.

OPTION   QUININE WITH THEOPHYLLINE

We found limited evidence from one RCT that addition of theophylline to quinine, compared with quinine alone, reduces the number of nights affected by leg cramp.

Benefits: We found no systematic review but found one double blinded RCT (164 people), which compared quinine sulphate for 2 weeks versus quinine with theophylline.[4] Baseline rates of leg cramp were measured during 1 week prior to randomisation, when all people received placebo (single blind). Pooled results for 126 people who completed at least 4 days' treatment in the 2 week period found quinine plus theophylline to be rated significantly more often as "good" or "very good" compared with quinine alone or placebo (87% with quinine and theophylline v 64% with quinine v 40% with placebo). The RCT did not specify criteria to categorise outcomes as "good" or "very good". After 2 weeks of treatment, theophylline plus quinine versus quinine alone significantly reduced the mean number of nights affected by cramp (from 4.7 to 1.1 with theophylline plus quinine v 4.8 to 2.2 with quinine alone, $P = 0.009$)

Harms: No evidence on specific harms was reported by the trial.

Comment: The results of the RCT should be treated with caution as it pooled results only of people who received treatment for at least 4 days out of 14, and did not use an intention to treat analysis.

OPTION   VITAMIN E

One small RCT found no significant difference in the number of nights disturbed by cramps with vitamin E versus placebo.

Benefits: We found no systematic reviews. We found one crossover RCT (27 men), which compared vitamin E versus quinine sulphate versus placebo.[5] It found that vitamin E versus placebo did not significantly reduce the median number of nights with leg cramps (15 v 13, $P > 0.05$).

Harms: Adverse effects were reported as similar in the vitamin E and placebo groups, but no details were provided.[5]

Comment: None.

OPTION   ANALGESICS

We found no evidence about the effects of analgesics for the treatment of idiopathic leg cramps.

Benefits: We found no systematic review or RCTs.

Harms: We found no evidence.

Comment: None.

OPTION	ANTIEPILEPTIC DRUGS

We found no evidence on the effects of antiepileptic drugs for the treatment of idiopathic leg cramps.

Benefits: We found no systematic review or RCTs.

Harms: We found no evidence on harms of antiepileptics on idiopathic leg cramps (see epilepsy, p 876).

Comment: None.

GLOSSARY

Cinchonism Adverse effects caused by quinine and other derivates of cinchona bark. It usually presents with nausea, vomiting, headache, tinnitus, deafness, vertigo, and visual disturbances.

Idiopathic leg cramps A phrase indicating that the underlying cause of the leg cramps is currently unknown, used in this review to distinguish the commonest type of leg cramps from leg cramps in people who are receiving dialysis, have venous insufficiency, or are pregnant.

REFERENCES

1. Hall AJ. Cramp and salt balance in ordinary life. *Lancet* 1947;3:231–233.
2. Man-Son-Hing M, Wells G, Lau A. Quinine for nocturnal leg cramps: a meta-analysis including unpublished data. *J Gen Intern Med* 1998;13: 600–606. Search date 1997; primary sources Medline, Embase, Current Contents, and contact with authorities.
3. McGee SR. Muscle cramps. *Arch Intern Med* 1990;150:511–518.
4. Gorlich HD, Gablez VE, Steinberg HW. Treatment of recurrent nocturnal leg cramps. A multicentric double blind, placebo controlled comparison between the combination of quinine and theophylline ethylene diamine and quinine *Arzneimittelforschung* 1991;41:167–175.
5. Connolly PS, Shirley EA, Wasson JH, Nierenberg DW. Treatment of nocturnal leg cramps: A crossover trial of quinine vs vitamin E. *Arch Intern Med* 1992;152:1877–1880.

Gavin Young
General Practitioner
Temple Sowerby Surgery
Penrith
UK

Competing interests: None declared.

Musculoskeletal disorders

Search date May 2000

Maurits van Tulder and Bart Koes

INTERVENTIONS

Key Messages

Acute low back pain

- Systematic reviews of RCTs have found:
  - That NSAIDs and muscle relaxants relieve pain more than placebo.
  - That advice to stay active speeds up symptomatic recovery and reduces chronic disability.
  - No evidence that bed rest, specific back exercises, or other interventions (traction or acupuncture) are effective.

Chronic low back pain

- Systematic reviews of RCTs have found:
  - That back exercises, back schools, behavioural therapy, and multidisciplinary pain treatment programmes are effective.
  - No evidence that other interventions (such as antidepressants, facet joint injections, and EMG biofeedback) are effective.

DEFINITION Low back pain is pain, muscle tension, or stiffness localised below the costal margin and above the inferior gluteal folds, with or without leg pain (sciatica).[1] It may be acute or chronic (persisting for 12 weeks or more).[2] Non-specific low back pain is low back pain not attributed to recognisable pathology (such as infection, tumour, osteoporosis, rheumatoid arthritis, fracture, or inflammation).[1] This review excludes low back pain or sciatica with symptoms or signs that suggest a specific underlying condition.

INCIDENCE/ Over 70% of people in developed countries will experience low back
PREVALENCE pain at some time in their lives.[3] Each year, 15–45% of adults suffer low backache, and one in 20 people present with a new episode. Low back pain is most common between the ages of 35 and 55.[3]

AETIOLOGY/ Symptoms, pathology, and radiological appearances are poorly
RISK FACTORS correlated. Pain is non-specific in about 85% of people. About 4% with low back pain in primary care have compression fractures, and about 1% have a neoplasm. Ankylosing spondylitis and spinal infections are rarer.[4] The prevalence of prolapsed intervertebral disc is about 1–3%.[3] Risk factors include heavy physical work, frequent bending, twisting, lifting, pulling and pushing, repetitive work, static postures, and vibrations. Psychosocial risk factors include anxiety, depression, job dissatisfaction, and mental stress at work.[3,5]

PROGNOSIS Acute low back pain is usually self limiting (90% recover within 6 weeks) but 2–7% develop chronic pain. One study found recurrent pain accounted for 75–85% of absenteeism.[6]

AIMS To relieve pain; to improve function; to learn to cope with pain, with minimal adverse effects from treatment.[2,7]

OUTCOMES Pain intensity (visual analogue or numerical rating scale); overall improvement (self reported or observed); back pain specific functional status (such as Roland Morris questionnaire, Oswestry questionnaire); impact on employment (days of sick leave, number of people returned to work); functional status (sickness impact profile); medication use; strength, mobility, fitness; intervention specific outcomes (such as coping and pain behaviour for behavioural treatment, strength and flexibility for exercise therapy, depression for antidepressants, and muscle spasm for muscle relaxants and EMG biofeedback).

METHODS

We searched Medline (1966 to December 1998), Embase drugs and pharmacology database (1980 to September 1998), and Psyclit (1984 to December 1998), using the search strategy recommended by the Cochrane Back Review Group.[8] *Clinical Evidence* search and appraisal May 2000. We examined the references in relevant publications and reviewed the titles and abstracts of identified articles to determine their relevance. In doubtful cases we read the article. We excluded abstracts and unpublished studies. We included all relevant systematic reviews and RCTs. Most RCTs of treatments for low back pain were small (< 50 people per intervention group, range 9–169), short term (mostly < 6 months' follow up), and of low overall quality. Problems included lack of power, no description of randomisation procedure, incomplete analysis with failure to describe dropouts, and lack of blinding.[9]

QUESTION   What are the effects of oral drug treatments?

OPTION   ANALGESICS (PARACETAMOL, OPIOIDS)

One placebo controlled trial of tramadol found decreased pain and improved function in people with chronic low back pain. Systematic reviews have found no clear difference between analgesics and non-steroidal anti-inflammatory drug (NSAIDs) in people with low back pain. Analgesics were less effective than electroacupuncture (see glossary, p 786) or ultrasound. There is considerable evidence from studies of other acute pain conditions that analgesics provide short term pain relief. One RCT found that analgesics were less effective than NSAIDs in people with chronic low back pain.

Benefits:

We found two systematic reviews (search date not given,[2] search date 1995;[9] no placebo controlled RCTs, seven comparative RCTs, no statistical pooling) and one subsequent RCT.[10] **Acute low back pain:** Of six RCTs identified in the reviews (329 people), three compared analgesics versus NSAIDs. Two of these (110 people) found no significant difference in the pain reduction from meptazinol, paracetamol, or diflunisal (an NSAID). The third trial found that mefenamic acid reduced pain more than paracetamol. One small trial (40 people) found that electroacupuncture reduced pain slightly more than paracetamol after 6 weeks. One RCT (73 people) found that ultrasound treatment substantially increased the proportion of people who were pain free after 4 weeks compared with (unspecified) analgesics. **Chronic low back pain:** One small RCT identified in the review (29 people, paracetamol versus diflunisal) found that more people treated with diflunisal rated the treatment as good or excellent. One subsequent RCT (254 people) found that tramadol decreased pain and increased functional status more than placebo.[10]

Harms:

The trials found adverse effects (constipation and drowsiness) with analgesics in about 50% of people. One systematic review comparing combinations of paracetamol and weak opioids versus paracetamol alone found that combination therapy increased the risk of adverse effects (single dose studies OR 1.1, 95% CI 0.8 to 1.5; multiple dose studies OR 2.5, 95% CI 1.5 to 4.2).[11]

Comment: None.

OPTION   ANTIDEPRESSANTS

We found insufficient evidence on the effects of antidepressants in acute low back pain. RCTs of antidepressants found conflicting results for relief of pain and depressive symptoms associated with chronic low back pain.

Benefits: We found four systematic reviews[2,7,9,12] and five additional RCTs (no statistical pooling of data).[13–18] **Acute low back pain:** We found no RCTs. **Chronic low back pain:** Overall, from four systematic reviews that did not pool data, and from additional RCTs, we identified seven placebo controlled RCTs (328 people) evaluating an antidepressant (imipramine, trazodone, nortriptyline, doxepin, or clomipramine) in people with chronic low back pain. Five trials reported on pain relief; three of these found no evidence that antidepressants reduced pain more than placebo, and two found that antidepressants were more effective. Six trials reported on antidepressant effects; five (one of which was not included in the systematic reviews[13]) found no evidence of benefit whereas one reported a significant reduction in depression with antidepressants compared with placebo.[14,15] We found three head to head RCTs. One (36 people) compared different antidepressants (doxepin v desipramine) and found no differences in pain relief or depression. The second RCT (67 people) also compared antidepressants and found better pain relief with maprotiline versus paroxetine.[18] The other (n = 39) compared antidepressants versus paracetamol in people with mild depression and chronic low back pain and found that antidepressants reduced pain more.[16]

Harms: Adverse effects of antidepressants included dry mouth, drowsiness, constipation, urinary retention, orthostatic hypotension, and mania.[2] One of the RCTs not included in the systematic reviews found that the prevalence of dry mouth, insomnia, sedation, and orthostatic symptoms was between 60–80% with tricyclic antidepressants; however, rates were only slightly lower in the placebo group and none of the differences was significant.[13]

Comment: None.

OPTION   COLCHICINE

We found insufficient evidence on the effects of colchicine in acute or chronic low back pain.

Benefits: We found one systematic review, which identified three RCTs (n = 135).[2] Two of the identified trials did not distinguish between acute and chronic low back pain. Of these, one (n = 48, intravenous colchicine v intravenous saline) found greater short term pain relief with colchicine. The other (n = 60, intravenous plus oral colchicine v placebo) found greater pain relief with colchicine. **Acute low back pain:** One identified trial (n = 27) compared oral colchicine with placebo and found no evidence of an effect; however, the trial was too small to rule out a clinically important difference.[2] **Chronic low back pain:** We found no RCTs.

Harms: The trials reported gastrointestinal irritation and skin problems in about 33% of people.[2] Other adverse effects included chemical cellulitis and agranulocytosis.[19]

Comment: None.

OPTION   MUSCLE RELAXANTS/BENZODIAZEPINES

Systematic reviews of RCTs have found that muscle relaxants reduce acute low back pain but have found no evidence to distinguish different muscle relaxants. One small RCT found that muscle relaxants reduced chronic low back pain in the short term.

Benefits: We found two systematic reviews (search date not given,[2] search date 1995;[9] 15 RCTs, no statistical pooling). **Acute low back pain:** Of 14 identified trials (total n = 1160), nine (n = 762) compared a muscle relaxant (tizanidine, cyclobenzaprine, dantrolene, carisoprodol, baclofen, orphenadrine, diazepam) versus placebo. Seven of these found that muscle relaxants reduced pain and muscle tension and increased mobility more than placebo between 1 and 2 weeks; two found no evidence of benefit. Three trials (total n = 236) compared different types of muscle relaxants. Two of these found that overall improvement was equivalent with cyclobenzaprine and with carisoprodol, both being better for overall improvement than diazepam. The trials found that all three treatments provided similar reductions in pain intensity. One RCT found no evidence of difference between methocarbamol and chlormezanone. **Chronic low back pain:** One trial in the reviews (n = 50, tetrazepam versus placebo) found that tetrazepam was associated with greater overall improvement (64% v 29% improved people) and reduced pain more than placebo after 10 days.

Harms: Adverse effects included drowsiness or dizziness in up to 70% of people and a risk of dependency even after 1 week of treatment.[2,9] Adverse effects were more common with muscle relaxants than placebo; 68% of people taking baclofen experienced one or more adverse reactions compared with 30% of those taking placebo. One RCT found more adverse effects (dyspepsia and drowsiness) with chlormezanone (14 of 52 people) than with methocarbamol (six of 55 people).[2,9]

Comment: None.

OPTION   NON-STEROIDAL ANTI-INFLAMMATORY DRUGS (NSAIDS)

RCTs in people with acute low back pain have found that NSAIDs are more effective than placebo for pain relief and overall improvement. They have found no evidence to distinguish different NSAIDs, no evidence that NSAIDs relieve radicular pain, and conflicting evidence for benefit compared with paracetamol, opioids, muscle relaxants, antidepressants, and non-drug treatments. Two RCTs in people with chronic low back pain found that NSAIDs were more effective than paracetamol for overall improvement and more effective than placebo for pain, and that NSAIDs plus vitamin B were more effective than NSAIDs alone.

Benefits: We found four systematic reviews and 25 additional RCTs (51 RCTs in total, statistical pooling only for NSAIDs versus placebo in acute low back pain).[2,9,20,21] (References for individual RCTs available on www.clinicalevidence.org). **Acute low back pain, NSAIDs versus placebo:** Nine RCTs (n = 1135) found that NSAIDs increased the number of people experiencing global improvement (pooled OR after 1 week 2.0, 95% CI 1.4 to 3.0) and reduced the number needing additional analgesics (pooled OR 0.64, 95% CI 0.45 to 0.91). Four RCTs (n = 313) found no evidence that NSAIDs relieved radicular pain. **Versus paracetamol:** Of three conflicting trials, two (n = 93) found no evidence of significant differences in recovery, and one (n = 60) found greater pain reduction with mefenamic acid than paracetamol. **Versus muscle relaxants and opioid analgesics:** Five out of six RCTs (n = 399 out of 459) found no evidence of significant differences in pain and overall improvement. One RCT (n = 60) found that mefenamic acid reduced pain more than dextropropoxyphene plus paracetamol. **Versus non-drug treatments:** We found three trials (n = 461). One (n = 110) found that NSAIDs improved range of movement more than bed rest and reduced the need for further treatment, although another trial (n = 241) found no evidence of an effect on these outcomes. Both this RCT and one further trial (total n = 354) found no evidence of benefit versus physiotherapy or spinal manipulation in terms of pain and mobility. **Versus each other:** 15 RCTs (n = 1490) found no evidence of significant differences in efficacy. **Versus NSAID plus adjuvant treatment:** Three RCTs (n = 232, NSAIDs v NSAIDs plus muscle relaxants) found no evidence of significant differences in efficacy between NSAID/muscle relaxant combinations versus NSAIDs alone. Two RCTs (n = 123) (one of which was not included in the systematic reviews[22]) comparing NSAIDs with NSAID/vitamin B combinations found no evidence of significant differences in pain, although one of these trials found that combination therapy was associated with a greater return to work within a week (78% of people with combination therapy v 35% with NSAIDs alone). **Chronic low back pain:** One RCT (n = 37) found that naproxen reduced pain more than placebo, but found no evidence that diflunisal was better than placebo for pain. One small RCT (n = 30) found more overall improvement with diflunisal compared with paracetamol. Three trials (n = 262) compared different NSAIDs and found no evidence of a significant difference. One RCT (n = 252, diclofenac versus diclofenac plus vitamins B1, B6, B12) found greater overall improvement for the NSAID/B complex combination.

Harms: Adverse effects (particularly at high doses and in elderly people) may be serious. Effects included gastritis and other gastrointestinal complaints (in 10% of people). Ibuprofen and diclofenac had the lowest gastrointestinal complication rate, mainly because of the low doses used in practice (pooled OR for adverse effects compared with placebo 1.3, 95% CI 0.91 to 1.8).[2,18,23] In two trials, adverse effects were more frequent with NSAID/muscle relaxant combinations.

Comment: None.

QUESTION **What are the effects of local injections for acute and chronic non-specific low back pain?**

OPTION **EPIDURAL STEROID INJECTIONS**

In people with acute low back pain, we found no evidence that epidural steroids are effective in the absence of sciatica. In chronic low back pain with sciatica, we found conflicting evidence on the effects of epidural steroids.

Benefits:
We found four systematic reviews.[2,9,24,25] **Acute low back pain:** We found two RCTs. One trial (n = 57, epidural steroids v subcutaneous lignocaine injections in people with acute pain and sciatica) found no differences after 1 month, but more people were pain free in the steroid group at 3 months. The second trial (n = 63, epidural steroids v epidural saline, bupivacaine, and dry needling) found no difference in the number of people improved or cured. **Chronic low back pain:** Seven trials were common to all four systematic reviews (n = 216, 3 RCTs of epidural steroids versus epidural saline, 4 RCTs of epidural steroids versus epidural bupivacaine, procaine, midazolam, or lignocaine and morphine). Three of the reviews (no statistical pooling) found insufficient evidence to draw conclusions. The fourth review found that steroids reduced pain in more people than the control interventions in the short term (pooled OR 2.60, 95% CI 1.9 to 3.8).[25]

Harms:
Adverse effects were infrequent and included headache, fever, subdural penetration, and more rarely epidural abscess and ventilatory depression.[2,24]

Comment:
Trials were small (range 22–73 participants) and included people with a variety of indications (chronic low back pain with and without sciatica, sciatica alone, lumbar radicular pain syndrome, postlaminectomy pain syndrome).

OPTION **FACET JOINT INJECTIONS**

One systematic review of RCTs has found no evidence that facet joint injections improve pain or function in people with chronic low back pain. We found insufficient evidence in people with acute low back pain.

Benefits:
We found one systematic review (search date not stated, published 1994, 5 RCTs, no statistical pooling).[2] Two trials did not distinguish between acute and chronic pain.[2] **Acute low back pain:** We found no RCTs. **Chronic low back pain:** Two trials (n = 206, intra-articular corticosteroid versus intra-articular saline) found no significant differences in pain, disability, and flexibility after 1, 3, and 6 months. One trial (n = 86) compared facet joint injections versus facet nerve block and found no significant difference in pain relief after 2 weeks, 1 month, and 3 months.

Harms:
Adverse effects included pain at injection site, infection, haemorrhage, neurological damage, and chemical meningitis.[2]

Comment:
None.

OPTION   TRIGGER POINT AND LIGAMENTOUS INJECTIONS

One systematic review of RCTs in chronic low back pain has found limited evidence that combined steroid and local anaesthetic injection of trigger points provides greater pain relief after 3 months than injection of local anaesthetic alone. It also found limited evidence that phenol injection of the lumbar interspinal ligament reduces disability compared with saline injection. We found insufficient evidence in acute low back pain.

Benefits: We found one systematic review (search date not given, published 1994, two RCTs, 138 people).[2] **Acute low back pain:** We found no RCTs. **Chronic low back pain:** One trial (n = 57) compared trigger point injection with methylprednisolone or triamcinolone plus lignocaine versus lignocaine alone. It found that combined lignocaine and steroid completely relieved pain in more people than lignocaine alone (60–80% v 20%). The other RCT (n = 81) compared injection of dextrose-glycerine-phenol into the lumbar interspinal ligament versus injection of saline. It found that phenol reduced pain and disability more than saline at 1, 3, and 6 months.

Harms: Potential harms included nerve or other tissue damage, infection, and haemorrhage.[2]

Comment: None.

QUESTION   What are the effects of non-drug treatments?

OPTION   ADVICE TO STAY ACTIVE

Systematic reviews of RCTs have found that, in people with acute low back pain, advice to stay active speeds symptomatic recovery, reduces chronic disability and results in less time off work compared with bed rest or usual care. We found insufficient evidence in people with chronic low back pain.

Benefits: We found two systematic reviews (search dates not given, no statistical pooling).[2,26] **Acute low back pain:** Two RCTs (n = 228) found faster rates of recovery, less pain, and less disability in people advised to stay active than in people receiving no advice. Five RCTs (n = 1500) found that advice to stay active led to less sick leave and less chronic disability compared with traditional medical treatment (analgesics as required, advice to rest and "let pain be your guide"). **Chronic low back pain:** We found no RCTs.

Harms: Harms were not addressed.

Comment: Limitations in methods preclude meaningful quantification of effect sizes. Advice to stay active was either provided as a single treatment or in combination with other interventions such as back schools, a graded activity programme, or behavioural counselling.

OPTION   BACK SCHOOLS

Systematic reviews of RCTs have found conflicting evidence on the effects of back schools in people with acute or chronic low back pain. In occupational settings, back schools have been shown to be more effective than no treatment in people with chronic low back pain.

Low back pain and sciatica

Benefits: We found one systematic review (16 RCTs, no statistical pooling),[27] and one subsequent RCT.[28] **Acute low back pain:** Two RCTs (n = 242) compared back schools versus McKenzie exercises (see glossary, p 786) and physical therapy. They found no evidence of improvements in pain, recovery rate, and rates of sick leave. One trial (n = 100, ongoing McKenzie exercises v one 45 minute session of back school) found that exercises improved pain and reduced sick leave more than back school up to 5 years. The other trial (n = 145) found that back schools speeded recovery and reduced sick leave in the short term compared with placebo (shortwave diathermy at lowest intensity). **Chronic low back pain:** Of 10 RCTs, five (861 people) compared back schools versus exercises, manipulation, NSAIDs, or physiotherapy. They found that back schools were better at reducing pain and disability up to 6 months, but found no evidence of an effect after 1 year. Of seven trials (529 people) comparing back schools versus no treatment, waiting list control, or detuned shortwave diathermy, four reported positive short term outcomes for the back school treatment, two found no short term differences, and two found no long term differences. Five RCTs (880 people) found that intensive back school programmes in an occupational setting improved pain and disability more than no treatment, but found no evidence that they were better than other treatments (physical therapy, calisthenics group training, usual care).

Harms: We found no evidence.

Comment: The risk of adverse effects is considered to be low.[2]

OPTION BED REST

Systematic reviews of RCTs have found no evidence that bed rest is better, and found evidence that it may be worse than back exercises, physiotherapy, spinal manipulation, NSAIDs, or no treatment in people with acute low back pain. We found insufficient evidence on the effects of bed rest in people with chronic low back pain.

Benefits: We found five systematic reviews (no statistical pooling).[2,7,9,26,29] **Acute low back pain:** Five RCTs (n = 921) compared bed rest versus other treatments (back exercises, physiotherapy, spinal manipulation, or NSAIDs). They found either no evidence of benefit or that bed rest was worse (using outcomes of pain, recovery rate, time to return to daily activities, and sick leave). Five RCTs (n = 663) found that bed rest was no different or worse than no treatment or placebo. Two RCTs (n = 254) found that 7 days of bed rest was no different from 2–4 of bed rest. **Chronic low back pain:** We found no RCTs.

Harms: Adverse effects of bed rest were joint stiffness, muscle wasting, loss of bone mineral density, pressure sores, and venous thromboembolism. Prolonged bed rest may lead to chronic disability and may impair rehabilitation.[26]

Comment: None.

| OPTION | BEHAVIOURAL THERAPY |

Two RCTs found that behavioural therapy reduced acute low back pain more than traditional care or EMG feedback. In people with chronic back pain, systematic reviews of RCTs have found that behavioural therapy has a moderate effect on pain and a mild effect on disability compared with no treatment. We found conflicting evidence comparing behavioural therapy with other treatments (usual care, back exercises), and found no evidence that one type of behavioural therapy is superior to another.

Benefits: We found five systematic reviews and additional RCTs (no statistical pooling).[2,7,9,30,31] (References for additional RCTs available on www.clinicalevidence.org) **Acute low back pain:** One RCT (n = 107) found that behavioural treatment reduced pain and perceived disability (at 9–12 months) more than traditional care (analgesics and back exercises until pain had subsided). A second RCT (50 people) found better pain relief in people with acute sciatica with risk factor based cognitive behavioural treatment (see glossary, p 786) than with EMG feedback.[32] **Chronic low back pain:** We found 9 RCTs that compared different types of behavioural therapy (cognitive behavioural treatment, operant behavioural treatmentsand respondent behavioural treatment, n = 308). They found no overall differences among the treatments (using functional status, pain, and behavioural outcomes, including anxiety, depression, pain behaviour, and coping). Eleven trials (n = 1223) found that behavioural treatment had a moderate effect on pain intensity and small effects on functional status and behavioural outcomes compared with no treatment, waiting list controls, or placebo. Of two RCTs (n = 202) comparing behavioural treatment versus other treatments, one found that a higher proportion of people returned to work within 12 weeks with operant behavioural treatment compared with traditional care (rest, analgesics, physical therapy). The other RCT found no evidence of differences in pain and depression after 6 and 12 months between operant behavioural treatment and back exercises. Six RCTs (n = 343) evaluated behavioural therapy in combination with other treatments (physiotherapy and back education, multidisciplinary treatment programmes, inpatient pain management programmes, and back exercises). These found that the addition of behavioural therapy had a small positive short term effect on functional status but no significant effect on pain or behavioural outcomes compared with the other treatments alone.

Harms: The trials did not assess harms.

Comment: None.

| OPTION | ELECTROMYOGRAPHIC (EMG) BIOFEEDBACK |

One small RCT found that EMG biofeedback (see glossary, p 786) produced less pain relief than cognitive behavioural treatment in acute low back pain. One systematic review found conflicting evidence in chronic low back pain.

Benefits: We found one systematic review (search date 1995, 5 RCTs, no statistical pooling)[9] and one subsequent RCT.[32] **Acute low back pain:** We found one small RCT (50 people) that found better pain relief in people with acute sciatica with risk factor based cognitive behavioural treatment than EMG biofeedback.[32] **Chronic low back pain:** The review found five small trials (total n = 168).[9] Three (n = 102) found no differences between EMG biofeedback and placebo or waiting list control (outcomes were pain and functional status). Two trials (n = 30) compared biofeedback versus progressive relaxation training and found conflicting effects on pain and functional status; one trial found EMG biofeedback better than relaxation training, and the other found the converse. One trial (n = 30) found no evidence of differences in pain and range of movement between rehabilitation programmes with and without biofeedback.

Harms: The trials did not address harms.

Comment: None.

| OPTION | BACK EXERCISES |

Systematic reviews of RCTs have found no evidence that specific back exercises (flexion, extension, aerobic, or strengthening exercises) are more effective than other conservative treatments in people with acute low back pain. RCTs have found that back exercises are more effective than other conservative measures in people with chronic low back pain.

Benefits: We found five systematic reviews and additional[2,7,9,33,34] RCTs (no statistical pooling). (References for additional RCTs available on www.clinicalevidence.org) Results for acute and chronic low back pain were not reported separately in three trials. **Acute low back pain:** Of 12 identified trials (n = 1894), eight compared specific back exercises (flexion, extension, aerobic or strengthening programmes, such as McKenzie exercises) versus other conservative treatments (usual care by the general practitioner, continuation of ordinary activities, bed rest, manipulation, NSAIDs, mini back school, or short wave diathermy). Seven of these found either no significant differences or that exercise mildly increased pain intensity and disability. The eighth trial found that exercise therapy improved pain and return to work compared with a mini back school. The four other trials (n = 1234) found no evidence that exercises had significant effects on pain, global improvement, or functional status compared with "inactive" treatment (bed rest, educational booklet, and placebo ultrasound). **Chronic low back pain:** We found four systematic reviews.[7,9,33,34] Three systematic reviews found 23 RCTs (2240 people) and found that overall, exercises improved pain, disability, and physical outcomes (e.g. strength and flexibility) in the short term, but the effects were small.[7,9,33] The fourth systematic review concluded that it is still unclear whether back exercises are more effective than inactive treatment for chronic low back pain.[34] Nine of the RCTs (1020 people) compared exercises versus conservative treatment. Three trials found no evidence that exercises had significant effects on pain, functional status, overall improvement, or return to work compared with conventional physiotherapy. Three trials found that exercises improved pain, functional status, and return to work compared with "usual care" by the general practitioner. The remaining three RCTs found that exercises improved pain and functional status more than back school education and early morning lumbar flexion control. Six trials (n = 587) compared exercises versus inactive treatments (hot packs and rest, semi hot packs and sham traction, waiting list controls, TENS, sham TENS, detuned ultrasound, or detuned shortwave diathermy). Three found better overall improvement or more pain reduction with exercises, whereas three found no evidence of significant differences. Three small trials (153 people) compared extension versus flexion exercises; two found no evidence of a significant difference in pain intensity and one found better global improvement with flexion exercises. One RCT (148 people) found no significant difference between active physiotherapy muscle reconditioning and low impact aerobics.[35]

Harms: Potential harms include increased stress on the spine.[2] Most trials did not assess harms.

Comment: None.

OPTION   LUMBAR SUPPORTS

We found insufficient evidence on the effects of lumbar supports in acute or chronic back pain.

Benefits: We found five systematic reviews and additional RCTs (six RCTs in total, no statistical pooling).[2,7,9,25,28–30,36] Five trials (1200 people) did not differentiate between acute and chronic pain. These compared lumbar supports for 3–6 weeks versus no treatment or versus treatments such as manipulation, physiotherapy, and analgesics.[2,7,37,38] Results for overall improvement, return to work, and functional status were conflicting. **Acute low back pain:** We found no RCTs specifically including people with acute low back pain. **Chronic low back pain:** One RCT (n = 19) evaluated a lumbar corset with or without a synthetic support. It found that the inclusion of a support improved symptom severity and functional disability, but found no evidence that it improved range of movement.

Harms: Adverse effects of prolonged lumbar support include decreased strength of the trunk musculature, a false sense of security, heat, skin irritation, and general discomfort.[2] The trials did not assess these.

Comment: None.

OPTION   MULTIDISCIPLINARY TREATMENT PROGRAMMES

One systematic review of two RCTs found limited evidence that multidisciplinary treatment (see glossary, p 787), which includes a workplace visit, leads to faster recovery from acute low back pain. A systematic review found that multidisciplinary treatment programmes improve pain, functional status, and return to work in people with chronic low back pain.

Benefits: **Acute low back pain:** We found one systematic review (search date 1998, 2 RCTs, 233 people).[39] It found that multidisciplinary treatment which includes a workplace visit leads to faster return to work and less sick leave than usual care. **Chronic low back pain:**

We found one systematic review and two additional RCTs (10 trials, n = 1691).[7,40-42] These found that, in people with severe chronic low back pain, multidisciplinary treatment programmes improved pain, functional status, and return to work moderately more than traditional inpatient rehabilitation (see glossary, p 787) or usual care, up to 1 year.

Harms: The trials gave no information on adverse effects.

Comment: None.

> **OPTION**   **PHYSICAL TREATMENTS (SHORT WAVE DIATHERMY, ULTRASOUND, ICE, HEAT, MASSAGE)**

We found insufficient evidence on the effects of physical treatments in acute and chronic low back pain.

Benefits: We found two systematic reviews, which found no RCTs.[2,43]

Harms: Insufficient information.

Comment: None.

> **OPTION**   **SPINAL MANIPULATION**

We found conflicting evidence on the effects of spinal manipulation in acute and chronic low back pain.

Benefits: We found five systematic reviews of 36 RCTs (no statistical pooling).[2,7,9,44,45] **Acute low back pain:** Of five placebo controlled trials (n = 383), two found slightly more pain relief with manipulation up to 3 weeks and two found no evidence of pain reduction compared with placebo. The remaining trial found slightly faster recovery in the manipulation group. The reviews identified 12 RCTs (n = 899) comparing manipulation versus short wave diathermy, massage, exercises, back school, or drug treatment. Four systematic reviews found that the results of these RCTs were conflicting.[2,7,9,44] The other review (7 RCTs, n = 731, manipulation versus other conservative treatments) found that manipulation increased recovery at 2–3 weeks (NNT 5, 95% CI 4 to 14).[45] **Chronic low back pain:** Four trials (n = 514) compared manipulation versus placebo. Eight trials (n = 545) compared manipulation versus other conservative treatments (such as usual care, short wave diathermy, massage, exercises, back schools, and drug treatment). Of four systematic reviews in chronic low back pain, three found that the results of these RCTs were conflicting.[7,44,45] One systematic review (no statistical pooling) found manipulation slightly more effective than placebo in five trials (n = 543).[9]

Harms: In the studies that used a trained therapist to select and manipulate people, the risk of serious complication was low (estimated risk: vertebrobasilar strokes 1 in 20 000 to 1 in 1 000 000; cauda equina syndrome < 1 in 1 000 000).

Comment: Current guidelines contraindicate manipulation in people with severe or progressive neurological deficit.[2,19]

OPTION	TRACTION

Systematic reviews of RCTs have found no evidence that traction is effective in either acute or chronic back pain.

Benefits: We found three systematic reviews[7,9,46] and two additional RCTs.[47–48] Of the 16 RCTs identified, 12 (n = 921) did not distinguish between acute and chronic low back pain. Ten of these trials found no significant differences between traction and placebo traction, exercises, hot packs, massage, interferential therapy or rest. Two found slightly better overall improvement after treatment. **Acute low back pain:** Two RCTs (total n = 225) compared traction versus bed rest plus corset, and traction versus infrared treatment. One study found more overall improvement after 1 and 3 weeks with traction, but the other found no significant difference in overall improvement after 2 weeks. **Chronic low back pain:** Two studies (total n = 176) compared traction versus placebo traction of maximum 25% of body weight. They found no significant differences in global improvement, pain or functional status after 5–9 weeks.[1,49]

Harms: The trials gave no information on harms. Potential adverse effects include debilitation, loss of muscle tone, bone demineralisation, and thrombophlebitis.[2]

Comment: None.

OPTION	TRANSCUTANEOUS ELECTRICAL NERVE STIMULATION (TENS)

We found insufficient evidence on the effects of TENS in either acute or chronic low back pain.

Benefits: We found three systematic reviews of five RCTs.[2,9,50] **Acute low back pain:** Of two identified RCTs, one (n = 58) compared rehabilitation programmes with and without TENS and found no difference in pain and functional status. The other (n = 40) found that TENS improved pain and mobility significantly more than paracetamol after 6 weeks of treatment. **Chronic low back pain:** Four identified RCTs (n = 253) compared TENS versus placebo. One trial (n = 42) found better pain relief with TENS after 1 week but not after 3 and 6 months, and one crossover trial (n = 33) found slightly better overall improvement with TENS. The other two trials (n = 178) found no differences in pain, functional status, or mobility. Two of the systematic reviews found that these RCTs conflicted (no statistical pooling performed).[2,9] The other review pooled the data and found that TENS did not significantly reduce the number of people with pain compared with placebo (OR no pain 1.62, 95% CI 0.90 to 2.68).[50]

Harms: The reviews gave no information on adverse effects.[2,9,50]

Comment: None.

Musculoskeletal disorders

| OPTION | ACUPUNCTURE |

We found no RCTs of acupuncture (see glossary, p 786) in people with acute low back pain. Two systematic reviews of RCTs found conflicting evidence of its effects in people with chronic low back pain.

Benefits: We found two systematic reviews (search dates 1996, 12 RCTs in total, of which six RCTs were unsuitable; see comment below),[51,52] and one subsequent RCT.[53] **Acute low back pain:** No RCTs. **Chronic low back pain:** Seven RCTs (380 people) compared acupuncture versus no treatment or waiting list or transcutaneous electrical nerve stimulation or placebo acupuncture in people with chronic low back pain. One systematic review (no statistical pooling) found that the overall quality of the RCTs was low, and found no evidence that acupuncture was more effective than placebo or no treatment.[52] The other review found that acupuncture was better than all other interventions analysed together (OR for overall improvement 2.3, 95% CI 1.3 to 4.1). It found no significant difference between acupuncture and placebo acupuncture (OR 1.4, 95% CI 0.84 to 2.3).[51] The subsequent RCT included 60 elderly people aged 60 or over found that acupuncture versus transcutaneous electrical nerve stimulation significantly reduced pain measured on a visual analogue scale (P < 0.001), pain measured on the pain subscale of the Nottingham Health Profile (P < 0.001) and the number of analgesic tablets consumed per week (P < 0.05).[53]

Harms: Acupuncture has been found to have fewer adverse effects than spinal manipulation.[51] One systematic review (search date 1996) found that serious, rare, adverse effects included infections (HIV, hepatitis, bacterial endocarditis) and trauma (pneumothorax, cardiac tamponade).[54]

Comment: Three of the identified RCTs combined acute and chronic low back pain and two did not specify the duration of symptoms. One RCT included people with back and neck pain.[51,52]

GLOSSARY

Acupuncture Needling of the skin at traditional "meridian" acupuncture points. Modern acupuncturists also use non-meridian points and trigger points (tender sites occurring in the most painful areas). The needles may be stimulated manually or electrically. Placebo acupuncture is needling of traditionally unimportant sites or non-stimulation of the needles once placed.

Cognitive behavioural treatment This aims to identify and modify patients' cognitions regarding their pain and disability using cognitive restructuring techniques (such as imagery and attention diversion) or by modifying maladaptive thoughts, feelings, and beliefs.

Electroacupuncture Non-penetrative electrical stimulation of classical acupuncture points with low amplitude, pulsed electrical current.

Electromyographic (EMG) biofeedback A person receives external feedback of their own electromyogram (using visual or auditory scales), and uses this to learn how to control the electromyogram, and hence the tension within their own muscles. Electromyogram biofeedback for low back pain aims to relax the paraspinal muscles.

McKenzie exercises Extension exercises that use self generated stresses and forces to centralise pain from the legs and buttocks to the lower back. This method emphasises self care.

Multidisciplinary treatment Intensive physical and psychosocial training by a team (e.g. a physician, physiotherapist, psychologist, social worker, and occupational therapist). Training is usually given in groups and does not involve passive physical therapy.

Operant behavioural treatments These include positive reinforcement of healthy behaviours and consequent withdrawal of attention from pain behaviours, time-contingent instead of pain-contingent pain management, and spouse involvement, while undergoing a programme aimed at increasing exercise tolerance towards a preset goal.

Respondent behavioural treatment This aims to modify physiological responses directly (e.g. reducing muscle tension by explaining the relation between tension and pain, and using relaxation techniques).

Traditional inpatient rehabilitation The components of inpatient rehabilitation may vary from country to country, and may include passive physical therapy (massage, ultrasound, electrotherapy, heat, traction), muscle training, relaxation exercises, pool exercises, back school education, and may last for about 3 weeks.

REFERENCES

1. Van der Heijden GJMG, Bouter LM, Terpstra-Lindeman E. De effectiviteit van tractie bij lage rugklachten. De resultaten van een pilotstudy. Ned T Fysiotherapie 1991;101:37–43.

2. Bigos S, Bowyer O, Braen G, et al. Acute low back problems in adults. Clinical Practice Guideline no.14. AHCPR Publication No. 95–0642. Rockville MD: Agency for Health Care Policy and Research, Public Health Service, US, Department of Health and Human Services. December 1994. Search date not given; primary sources The Quebec Task Force on Spinal Disorders Review to 1984; search carried out by National Library of Medicine from 1984; and references from expert panel.

3. Andersson GBJ. The epidemiology of spinal disorders. In: Frymoyer JW, ed. The adult spine: principles and practice. 2nd ed. New York: Raven Press, 1997:93–141.

4. Deyo RA, Rainville J, Kent DL. What can the history and physical examination tell us about low back pain? JAMA 1992;268:760–765.

5. Bongers PM, de Winter CR, Kompier MA, et al. Psychosocial factors at work and musculoskeletal disease. Scand J Work Environ Health 1993;19:297–312.

6. Frymoyer JW. Back pain and sciatica. N Engl J Med 1988;318:291–300.

7. Evans G, Richards S. Low back pain: an evaluation of therapeutic interventions. Bristol: Health Care Evaluation Unit, University of Bristol, 1996. Search date 1995; primary sources Medline; Embase; A-Med; Psyclit; and hand searched references.

8. Van Tulder MW, Assendelft WJJ, Koes BW, et al, and the Editorial Board of the Cochrane Collaboration Back Review Group. Method guidelines for systematic reviews in the Cochrane Collaboration back review group for spinal disorders. Spine 1997;22:2323–2330.

9. Van Tulder MW, Koes BW, Bouter LM. Conservative treatment of acute and chronic nonspecific low back pain: a systematic review of randomized controlled trials of the most common interventions. Spine 1997;22:2128–2156. Search date 1995; primary sources Medline; Embase; Psychlit; and hand searched references.

10. Schnitzer TJ, Gray WL, Paster RZ, et al. Efficacy of tramadol in treatment of chronic low back pain. J Rheumatol 2000;27:772–778.

11. De Craen AJM, Di Giulio G, Lampe-Schoenmaeckers AJEM, et al. Analgesic efficacy and safety of paracetamol–codeine combinations versus paracetamol alone: a systematic review. BMJ 1996;313:321–325. Search date 1995; primary sources Medline; Embase; International Pharmaceutical Abstracts; Biosis; contact with pharmaceutical companies; and hand searched references.

12. Turner JA, Denny MC. Do antidepressant medications relieve chronic low back pain? J Fam Pract 1993;37:545–553. Search date 1992; primary sources Medline; Psyclit; hand searches of bibliographies; and inquiries to researchers and drug companies.

13. Atkinson JH, Slater MA, Williams RA, et al. A placebo-controlled randomized clinical trial of nortriptyline for chronic low back pain. Pain 1998;76:287–296.

14. Hameroff SR, Cork RC, Scherer K, et al. Doxepin effects on chronic pain, depression and plasma opioids. J Clin Psychiatry 1982;43:22–27.

15. Hameroff SR, Weiss JL, Lerman JC, et al. Doxepin's effects on chronic pain and depression: a controlled study. J Clin Psychiatry 1984;45:47–52.

16. Stein D, Peri T, Edelstein E, et al. The efficacy of amitriptyline and acetaminophen in the management of acute low back pain. Psychosomatics 1996;37:63–70.

17. Treves R, Montane De La Roque P, Dumond JJ, et al. Prospective study of the analgesic action of clomipramine versus placebo in refractory low back pain and sciatica (68 cases). Rev Rhum 1991;58:549–552 (in French).

18. Atkinson JH, Slater MA, Wahlgren DR, et al. Effects of noradrenergic and serotonergic antidepressants on chronic low back pain intensity. Pain 1999;83:137–145.

19. Waddell G, Feder G, McIntosh A, et al. Low back pain evidence review. London: Royal College of General Practitioners, 1996. Search date 1996; primary sources Medline; Embase; Science Citation Index; Social Sciences Citation Index; correspondence with experts and researchers, and hand searched references.

20. Koes BW, Scholten RJPM, Mens JMA, et al. Efficacy of non-steroidal anti-inflammatory drugs for low back pain: a systematic review of

randomised clinical trials. *Ann Rheum Dis* 1997; 56:214–223. Search date 1994; primary sources Medline 1966 to 1994; Embase 1980 to 1994, and hand searched references.

21. Van Tulder MW, Scholten RJPM, Koes BW, et al. Non-steroidal anti-inflammatory drugs (NSAIDs) for non-specific low back pain. In: The Cochrane Library, Issue 3, 2000. Oxford: Update Software. Search date 1998; primary sources Medline; Embase; Cochrane Controlled Trials Register; and hand searched of reference lists.

22. Bruggemann G, Koehler CO, Koch EM. Results of a double-blind study of diclofenac + vitamin B1, B6, B12 versus diclofenac in patients with acute pain of the lumbar vertebrae: a multicenter study. *Klinische Wochenschrift* 1990;68:116–120.

23. Henry D, Lim LLY, Rodriguez LAG, et al. Variability in risk of gastrointestinal complications with individual non-steroidal anti-inflammatory drugs: results of a collaborative meta-analysis. *BMJ* 1996;312:1563–1566. Search date 1994; primary sources Medline, contact with study authors, and hand searched references.

24. Koes BW, Scholten RJPM, Mens JMA, et al. Efficacy of epidural steroid injections for low back pain and sciatica: a systematic review of randomized clinical trials. *Pain* 1995;63:279–288. Search date 1993; primary sources Medline 1966 to 1993, and hand searched references.

25. Watts RW, Silagy CA. A meta-analysis on the efficacy of epidural corticosteroids in the treatment of sciatica. *Anaesth Intensive Care* 1995;23:564–569.

26. Waddell G, Feder G, Lewis M. Systematic reviews of bed rest and advice to stay active for acute low back pain. *Br J Gen Pract* 1997;47:647–652. Search date not given; primary sources Medline; contacted recently published authors and pharmaceutical company; and hand searched references.

27. Van Tulder MW, Esmail R, Bombardier C, Koes BW. Back schools for non-specific low back pain. In: The Cochrane Library, Issue 3, 2000. Oxford: Update Software. Search date 1997; primary sources Medline, Embase, and hand searched references.

28. Dalichau S, Scheele K, Perrey RM, et al. Ultraschallgestützte Haltungs- und Bewegungsanalyse der Lendenwirbelsäule zum Nachweis der Wirksamkeit einer Rückenschule. *Zentralbl Arbeitsmed* 1999;49:148–156.

29. Koes BW, van den Hoogen HMM. Efficacy of bed rest and orthoses of low back pain. A review of randomized clinical trials. *Eur J Phys Med Rehabil* 1994;4:86–93. Search date not given; primary sources Medline 1966 to 1992, and hand searched references.

30. Turner JA. Educational and behavioral interventions for back pain in primary care. *Spine* 1996;21:2851–2859. Search date 1994; primary sources Medline; Psyclit; handsearches; and inquiries to pharmaceutical companies and expert researchers in the field.

31. Van Tulder MW, Ostelo R, Vlaeyen JWS, Linton SJ, Morley SJ, Assendelft WJJ. Behavioural treatment for chronic low back pain. In: The Cochrane Library, Issue 3, 2000. Oxford: Update Software. Search date 1999; primary sources Medline; Psyclit; Cochrane Controlled Trials Register; Embase; and hand searches of reference lists.

32. Hasenbring M, Ulrich HW, Hartmann M, et al. The efficacy of a risk factor-based cognitive behavioral intervention and electromyographic biofeedback in patients with acute sciatic pain: an attempt to prevent chronicity. *Spine* 1999;24:2525–2535.

33. Faas A. Exercises: which ones are worth trying, for which patients and when? *Spine* 1996;21:2874–

2879. Search date 1995; primary source Medline.

34. Van Tulder MW, Malmivaara A, Esmail R, Koes BW. Exercise therapy for non-specific low back pain. In: The Cochrane Library, Issue 3, 2000. Oxford: Update Software. Search date 1999; primary sources Medline; Psychlit; Cochrane Controlled Trials Register; Embase; and hand searches of reference lists.

35. Mannion AF, Müntener M, Taimela S, et al. A randomized clinical trial of three active therapies for chronic low back pain. *Spine* 1999;24:2435–2448.

36. Van Tulder MW, Jellema P, van Poppel MNM, et al. Lumbar supports for prevention and treatment of low back pain. In: The Cochrane Library, Issue 3, 2000. Oxford: Update Software. Search date 1999; primary sources Medline; Cinahl; Current Contents; Cochrane Controlled Trials Register; Embase; Science Citation Index; and hand searches of reference lists.

37. Penrose KW, Chook K, Stump JL. Acute and chronic effects of pneumatic lumbar support on muscular strength, flexibility, and functional impairment index. *Sports Train Med Rehab* 1991; 2:121–129.

38. Pope MH, Phillips RB, Haugh LD, et al. A prospective randomized three week trial of spinal manipulation, transcutaneous muscle stimulation, massage and corset in the treatment of subacute low back pain. *Spine* 1994;19:2571–2577.

39. Karjalainen K, Malmivaara A, van Tulder M, et al. Multidisciplinary biopsychosocial rehabilitation for subacute low back pain among working age adults. In: The Cochrane Library, Issue 3, 2000. Oxford: Update Software. Search date 1998; primary sources Medline; Embase; Psyclit; Cochrane Register of Controlled Clinical Trials; Science Citation Index; and hand searches of reference lists and personal contact with experts.

40. Bendix AF, Bendix T, Ostenfeld S, et al. Active treatment programs for patients with chronic low back pain: a prospective, randomized, observer-blinded study. *Eur Spine J* 1995;4:148–152.

41. Bendix AF, Bendix T, Vaegter K, et al. Multidisciplinary intensive treatment for chronic low back pain: a randomized, prospective study. *Cleve Clin J Med* 1996;63:62–69.

42. Bendix AF, Bendix T, Labriola M, et al. Functional restoration for chronic low back pain: two-year follow-up of two randomized clinical trials. *Spine* 1998;23:717–725.

43. Gam AN, Johannsen F. Ultrasound therapy in musculoskeletal disorders: a meta-analysis. *Pain* 1995;63:85–91. Search date 1992; primary sources Index Medicus, Medline, and hand searched references.

44. Koes BW, Assendelft WJJ, van der Heijden GJMG, et al. Spinal manipulation for low back pain. An updated systematic review of randomized clinical trials. *Spine* 1996;21:2860–2871. Search date 1995; primary sources Medline, and hand searched references.

45. Shekelle PG, Adams AH, Chassin MR, et al. Spinal manipulation for low back pain. *Ann Intern Med* 1992;117:590–598. Search date not given; primary sources Medline and Index Medicus from 1952; contacted experts; and hand searched references.

46. Van der Heijden GJMG, Beurskens AJHM, Koes BW, et al. The efficacy of traction for back and neck pain: a systematic, blinded review of randomized clinical trial methods. *Phys Ther* 1995;75:93–104. Search date 1992; primary sources Medline 1966 to 1992; Embase 1974 to 1992; Index to Chiropractic Literature 1980 to 1992; Physiotherapy Index 1986 to 1992; and

hand searched non-indexed journals.

47. Ljunggren E, Weber H, Larssen S. Autotraction versus manual traction in patients with prolapsed lumbar intervertebral discs. *Scand J Rehabil Med* 1984;16:117–124.

48. Werners R, Pynsent PB, Bulstrode CJK. Randomized trial comparing interferential therapy with motorized lumbar traction and massage in the management of low back pain in a primary care setting. *Spine* 1999;24:1579–1584.

49. Beurskens AJ, de Vet HCW, Köke AJ, et al. Efficacy of traction for non-specific low back pain: a randomised clinical trial. *Lancet* 1995;346:1596–1600.

50. Gadsby JG, Flowerdew MW. The effectiveness of transcutaneous electrical nerve stimulation (TENS) and acupuncture-like transcutaneous electrical nerve stimulation (ALTENS) in the treatment of patients with chronic low back pain. In: The Cochrane Library, Issue 3, 2000. Oxford: Update Software. Search date 1999; primary sources Medline; Embase; AMED; CISCOM; contacted investigators; hand searched references, conference proceedings and textbooks.

51. Ernst E, White AR. Acupuncture for back pain. A meta-analysis of randomized controlled trials. *Arch Intern Med* 1998;158:2235–2241. Search date 1996; primary sources Medline 1969 to 1996; Cochrane Controlled Trials Register; CISCOM November 1996; contacted authors and experts; and hand searched references.

52. Van Tulder MW, Cherkin DC, Berman B, et al. Acupuncture low back pain. In: The Cochrane Library, Issue 3, 2000. Oxford: Update Software. Search date 1996; primary sources Medline; Embase; Cochrane Complementary Medicine Field trials register; Cochrane Controlled Trials Register; Science Citation Index; and hand searched references.

53. Grant DJ, Bishop-Miller J, Winchester DM, et al. A randomized comparative trial of acupuncture versus transcutaneous electrical nerve stimulation for chronic back pain in the elderly. *Pain* 1999;82:9–13.

54. Ernst E, White A. Life-threatening adverse reactions after acupuncture? A systematic review. *Pain* 1997;71:123–126. Search date 1996; primary sources Medline; CISCOM; other specialised databases; contacted experts and hand searched references.

Maurits van Tulder

Institute for Research in Extramural
Medicine
Vrije Universiteit
Amsterdam
The Netherlands

Bart Koes

Department of General Practice
Eramus University
Rotterdam
Netherlands

Competing interests: None declared.

Search date January 2001: expanded this issue

Allan Binder

INTERVENTIONS

Key Messages

■ We found little good quality evidence, highlighting the need for prospective studies with standardised validation of diagnosis and good study design.

DEFINITION Neck pain can be divided into uncomplicated pain, whiplash, and pain with radiculopathy. Neck pain often occurs with limitation of movement and poorly defined neurological symptoms affecting the upper limbs. The pain can be severe and intractable, and can occur with radiculopathy or myelopathy.

INCIDENCE/ PREVALENCE About two thirds of people will experience neck pain at some time in their lives.[1,2] Prevalence is highest in middle age. In the UK about 15% of hospital based physiotherapy, and in Canada 30% of chiropractic referrals, are for neck pain.[3,4] In the Netherlands neck pain contributes up to 2% of general practitioner consultations.[5]

AETIOLOGY/ RISK FACTORS Most uncomplicated pain is associated with poor posture, anxiety and depression, neck strain, or occupational or sport injuries. With chronic pain, mechanical and degenerative factors, often referred to as cervical spondylosis, become more evident. Some neck pain results from soft tissue trauma, most typically seen in whiplash syndrome. Rarely disc prolapse and inflammatory, infective, or malignant conditions affect the cervical spine and present with neck pain with or without neurological features.

PROGNOSIS Neck pain usually resolves within days or weeks but can recur or become chronic. In some industries, neck related disorders account for as much time off work as low back pain (see low back pain and sciatica, p 772).[6] The percentage of people in whom neck pain becomes chronic depends on the cause but is thought to be about 10%,[1] similar to low back pain. It causes severe disability in 5% of affected people.[2] One systematic review of the clinical course and prognostic factors of non-specific neck pain identified six observational studies and 17 RCTs.[7] In people who had had pain for at least 6 months, a median of 46% (22–79%) improved with treatment. Whiplash injuries were more likely to cause disability; up to 40% of sufferers reported symptoms even after 15 years of follow up.[8] Factors associated with a poorer outcome after whiplash are not well defined.[9]

AIMS To recover from acute episode within 4 weeks; to maintain activities of daily living and reduce absenteeism from work; to prevent development of long term symptoms.

OUTCOMES Pain, range of movement, function, adverse effects of treatment, return to work, level of disability (Neck Disability Index).[10]

METHODS *Clinical Evidence* update search and appraisal January 2001. We also searched the following databases: Chirolars (now called Mantis) for English language articles from 1966 to November 1999; the Cochrane database;[11] Index Medicus (1966 to 1997); Bioethicsline (1973 to 1997); Cumulative Index to Nursing and Allied Health (Cinahl) (1982 to 1997); and Current Contents (1994 to 1997). Criteria for assessment of RCTs were based on a 100 point scale, including study population, interventions, effects, and data presentation and analysis.[12]

Musculoskeletal disorders

OPTION PHYSICAL TREATMENTS

We found insufficient evidence about the effects of most physical treatments — heat or cold, traction, biofeedback, spray and stretch, acupuncture, and laser — in people with uncomplicated neck pain without neurological deficit. Two RCTs found benefit from physiotherapy, and one RCT found limited evidence for benefit from pulsed electromagnetic field therapy.

Benefits:
We found five systematic reviews[11,13–16] and two subsequent RCTs.[17,18] Two of the systematic reviews[11,13] considered all physical modalities and the other three considered traction only[14] or acupuncture only.[15,16] The first systematic review (search date 1993) identified 13 RCTs (in 760 people with neck pain but without neurological deficit), which evaluated at least one form of physical treatment. It found no significant benefit from any of the following physical treatments: heat or cold, traction, electrotherapy (pulsing electromagnetic field or transcutaneous electrical nerve stimulation), biofeedback, spray and stretch, acupuncture, or laser.[11] The second general systematic review (search date 1995, 17 RCTs, 1202 people) found possible benefit for pulsed electromagnetic field therapy and active physiotherapy but not for traction, acupuncture, or other physical therapies.[13] One RCT (81 people with neck pain and radiographic evidence of cervical osteoarthritis and 86 people with osteoarthritis of the knee) included in the second systematic review compared true versus sham pulsed electromagnetic field therapy (given for at least 1 year).[19] In people with chronic neck pain, the RCT found that after 18 episodes of treatment there were significant reductions in pain ($P < 0.04$) and pain on passive motion ($P = 0.03$), but not in difficulty with activities of daily living, tenderness, self assessment of improvement, or physicians' global assessment. It found no significant differences between the effects in people with knee or neck problems. Data pooling found that more people had improved in at least three of six variables with active compared with sham therapy (ARs 57/82 [70%] v 37/82 [45%]; RR 1.54, 95% CI 1.21 to 1.80; NNT 4, 95% CI 3 to 11). This benefit was sustained up to 1 month (see comment below). The third systematic review (search date 1992, 3 RCTs, 639 people) comparing traction versus a range of alternative treatments, including heat, mobilisation, exercise, no treatment, collar, and analgesics. The RCTs found no consistent pain reduction from traction compared with any of the alternatives.[14] One RCT (47 people) included in both reviews found that active physiotherapy and exercise (for 60 minutes each visit, mean 13 visits) versus passive treatment (heat, massage, and light stretching for 20 minutes each visit, mean 10 visits) significantly reduced pain immediately after treatment ($P < 0.05$).[20] A subsequent single blind RCT (76 people with non-specific chronic neck pain) compared multimodal treatment emphasising proprioceptive training (active) versus supervised home exercises (home) versus a

recommendation to exercise (control).[18] It found that active and home treatments significantly reduced pain versus the control group at 3 months' follow up (active Visual Analogue Scale [VAS]– 29 mm v home VAS –28mm v control VAS –12 mm, P < 0.001), but at 12 months there was no significant difference. It also found no difference in mobility. Two further systematic reviews (search dates 1998) identified 13 RCTs comparing needle or laser acupuncture with a range of control procedures (sham therapies, diazepam, and physiotherapy) but found no consistent benefit for the acupuncture groups.[15,16] One subsequent RCT (103 women with work related neck pain) compared three exercise regimens (training strength v endurance v coordination) over 10 weeks versus stress management. It found exercise reduced pain significantly versus stress management (P < 0.05), but found no significant difference between any exercise programme.[17]

Harms: We found no good data on harms. The incidence of serious adverse events seems to be low for all physical treatments considered.

Comment: The RCT comparing true and sham pulsed electromagnetic field therapy was double blinded and used random numbers to allocate people to groups.[19] By chance, the baseline characteristics of treated and placebo groups were different: the people allocated to active treatment had higher pain scores, more tenderness, and more difficulty with the activities of daily living than the placebo group. The analysis in the RCT was based on changes from the baseline value, and it is not known how much of the observed effect was caused by bias introduced by the baseline differences.

OPTION	MANUAL TREATMENTS: MOBILISATION AND MANIPULATION

Four systematic reviews found evidence of benefit from manipulation and mobilisation that did not require instrumentation or anaesthesia. Rare but serious adverse effects have been reported following manipulation of the cervical spine.

Benefits: We found four systematic reviews (search dates 1990,[12] 1993,[21] 1995,[22] and 1995[13]), which evaluated mobilisation (defined as any manual treatment to improve joint function that does not involve high velocity movement, anaesthesia, or instrumentation) and manipulation (the use of short or long lever high velocity thrusts directed at one or more of the cervical spine joints that does not involve anaesthesia or instrumentation). **Mobilisation:** One RCT (included in all four systematic reviews; 30 people with acute pain) found no significant difference in pain reduction between mobilisation (10 people) versus transcutaneous nerve stimulation (10 people), versus control (10 people). All people were given a neck collar and allowed to take analgesics.[23] However, the trial was too small to rule out a beneficial effect. Two other RCTs included people with chronic neck pain and found modest benefit from mobilisation in the short term. The first (63 people) compared mobilisation plus analgesia versus less active physiotherapy plus analgesia.[24] It found significant pain reduction with mobilisation in the first month but not thereafter (83% of the mobilisation group improved v 60% of the physiotherapy group,

P < 0.05, 95% CIs not available). The second RCT (256 people with chronic neck and back pain, 64 having chronic neck pain alone) compared manual treatment (mobilisation, manipulation, or both) versus physical treatment (heat, electrotherapy, ultrasound, shortwave diathermy), placebo (detuned shortwave diathermy or ultrasound), or usual medical care (analgesics, advice, home exercise, and bed rest).[25] It found manual treatment was significantly better than all other treatments. This benefit was sustained for 12 months. However, it was not possible to compare directly the effects of the two manual treatments, and more people received manipulation. **Manipulation:** One of the reviews performed meta-analysis (3 RCTs in 155 people with chronic pain) of manipulation versus other treatments.[22] The RCTs compared manipulation versus diazepam,[26] anti-inflammatory drugs,[27] or usual medical care.[25] There was a non-significant greater improvement with manipulation versus the other treatments (–12.6 mm on a 100 mm VAS, 95% CI –0.15 to +25.5).[22] **Mobilisation versus manipulation:** We found one RCT (100 people with mainly chronic neck pain) comparing a single mobilisation treatment versus a single manipulation treatment.[28] It found no significant difference between groups (immediate improvement in pain found in 69% of people with mobilisation v 85% with manipulation, RR of improvement in pain with manipulation compared with mobilisation 1.23; P = 0.05, but corrected to P = 0.16 after adjusting for pretreatment differences between the groups). People in the manipulation group had improved range of movement, but the result was not significant. We found one subsequent RCT (119 people with chronic neck pain), which compared mobilisation physiotherapy versus manipulation versus intensive training.[29] There was no significant difference between groups at the end of treatment (P = 0.44) or at 12 months, but median pain on a 30 point scale improved from 12 to 6 with intensive training or mobilisation and from 13 to 6 with manipulation.

Harms: **Mobilisation:** We found occasional reports of increased pain, but no serious adverse effects or deaths. **Manipulation:** Rare but serious adverse effects have been reported, including death and serious disability caused by vertebrobasilar and other strokes, dissection of the vertebral arteries, disc herniation, and other serious neurological complications. The estimated risk from case reports of cerebrovascular accident is 1–3 per million manipulations,[30] and of all serious adverse effects is 5–10 per 10 million manipulations.[22] A non-systematic review of reported cases of injury attributable to manipulation of the cervical spine identified 116 articles published between 1925 and 1997 with 177 cases of injury. The most frequently reported injuries involved arterial dissection or spasm, lesions of the brain stem, and Wallenberg's syndrome (see glossary, p 798); death occurred in 32 (18%) of the cases. However, the method of data collection and analysis makes it impossible to assess the frequency of complications with this treatment.[31]

Comment: None.

OPTION	DRUG TREATMENTS FOR NECK PAIN	New

We found insufficient evidence on the effects of any drug treatments for neck pain, although they are widely used as a first line intervention.

Benefits: We found three systematic reviews (search dates 1993, 1993, and not stated).[9,21,32] **Simple analgesics (paracetamol, opioids) and oral non-steroidal anti-inflammatory drugs (NSAIDs):** The reviews found no RCTs. Several RCTs of other interventions include the use of analgesics or NSAIDs as adjunctive treatments but do not allow for subgroup analysis.[18,19,23–25,27,29] **Antidepressants:** The review found no RCTs. RCTs of antidepressants in chronic low back pain syndromes found conflicting results (see antidepressants under low back pain, p 772). **Muscle relaxants/benzodiazepines:** One systematic review identified two RCTs (159 people with chronic neck or back pain with acute spasm) comparing cyclobenzaprine versus diazepam or placebo.[21] The RCTs found significant benefit for the muscle relaxant at 2 weeks ($P < 0.05$), but quantified and follow up pain data could not be extracted.[33,34] One subsequent RCT (157 people with chronic neck pain) of eperisone versus placebo found significantly better pain control with eperisone at 6 weeks ($P < 0.05$).[35]

Harms: **Simple analgesics (paracetamol, opioids) and oral NSAIDs:** We found no reports of harm from simple analgesics. Adverse effects of NSAIDs are similar to other situations (See harms of NSAIDs, p 800). One systematic review calculated that the risk of a harm of NSAIDs was considerably greater than for manipulation, although no direct comparisons were made.[27] **Antidepressants:** The review found no RCTs (see harms of antidepressants under anxiety disorder, p 668). **Muscle relaxants/benzodiazepines:** The RCTs found minor adverse effects, including weakness, dizziness, drowsiness, and gastrointestinal problems occurring in 4% of people with muscle relaxants (see harms of benzodiazepines under generalised anxiety disorder, p 668).

Comment: Few RCTs have considered treatment for chronic whiplash, and many people with whiplash are included in general RCTs of chronic mechanical neck pain.

QUESTION	What are the effects of treatments for acute whiplash injury?

One systematic review of RCTs has found that, in people with acute whiplash injury, electrotherapy was more effective than placebo, early mobilisation physiotherapy was more effective than immobilisation, and return to normal activity was more effective than rest.

Benefits: We found one systematic review of treatment of whiplash injury (search date 1993), which highlighted the paucity of evidence on all treatment modalities.[9] **Physical treatments:** One RCT (40 people with acute whiplash) included in the review compared pulsing electromagnetic field therapy versus placebo pulsing electromagnetic field.[36] All participants received analgesia and collar. People in the active pulsing electromagnetic field group had significantly better pain relief after 4 weeks ($P < 0.05$) but not after

3 months. **Early mobilisation versus immobilisation or less active treatment:** The review (search date 1993, 2 RCTs, 165 people)[37,38] plus two subsequent RCTs[39,40] (total for 4 RCTs, 269 people) compared early mobilisation physiotherapy versus immobilisation, analgesics, rest, and education. The review found that people treated with mobilisation had significantly better pain relief and improved range of movement at 4 and 8 weeks (P < 0.01).[9] The first subsequent RCT found significantly quicker recovery with active therapy but no significant difference in outcome at 12 weeks.[39] The second subsequent RCT found that active mobilisation was significantly more effective than rest and a collar (P < 0.001), but only if started immediately after treatment. A 2 week delay resulted in no significant benefit at 6 months.[40] **Early resumption of normal activity versus immobilisation and rest:** We found one recent single blinded RCT (201 people presenting to an emergency department with acute whiplash), which compared an "act as usual" group (advice plus anti-inflammatory drugs) versus an immobilisation group (also given 14 days' sick leave).[41] The "act as usual" group did better for subjective symptoms, including pain during daily activities, neck stiffness, memory, concentration, and headache at 6 months, but with no benefit in objective variables such as neck range and length of sick leave. It found no significant difference in severe symptoms at 6 months (11% of the "act as usual" group v 15% of the immobilisation group; RR 0.75, 95% CI 0.08 to 1.42). The systematic review found no evidence of benefit from immobilisation, rest, traction, or other physical treatments in acute whiplash.[9] **Home exercise programmes:** We found one RCT (59 people with acute whiplash) comparing two home mobilisation regimes; a regular exercise treatment regimen versus instructions to perform an additional isometric exercise at least three times a day.[42] It found no significant difference between treatments at 3 or 6 months for self efficacy, disability, or pain intensity. **Drug treatments:** We found two additional systematic reviews (search dates 1993[21] and not stated[32]). The reviews found no RCTs. Simple analgesics and NSAIDs were adjuvant treatments in a variety of trials of acute whiplash.[38,39,41]

Harms: Adverse effects are not well documented, but early mobilisation physiotherapy is not always well tolerated (see harms of manual treatments, p 794).[43]

Comment: The management of acute whiplash injury remains controversial, and needs further investigation. In the first subsequent RCT comparing early mobilisation versus immobilisation, although early mobilisation led to early benefits in pain relief and movement, at 12 weeks follow up there was no difference compared with use of a collar.[39] In the second subsequent RCT, active mobilisation was only beneficial if started immediately after injury.[40] A 2 week delay resulted in no significant benefit at 6 months Only the 40% of people most severely affected by whiplash were included in the RCT comparing home exercise programs, which may have led to a poorer outcome.

QUESTION What are the effects of treatments for chronic whiplash injury?

We found little good quality information on the management of chronic whiplash injury, although one RCT found limited evidence that percutaneous radiofrequency neurotomy may be beneficial for zygapophyseal joint pain.

Benefits: We found one systematic review of treatment of whiplash injury (search date 1993), which highlighted the paucity of evidence on all treatment modalities.[9] It identified one RCT (24 people with chronic whiplash, 9 men; mean age 43 years) in whom the source of pain was confirmed by placebo controlled diagnostic blocks to be the zygapophyseal (excluding C2/3) joints.[44] **Percutaneous radiofrequency neurotomy versus sham procedure:** The median time taken for more than half of the pain to return was 263 days in the active group compared with 8 days in the control group (P = 0.04). At 27 weeks more people were free of pain in the active group then in the control group (AR 58% with active treatment v 8% with placebo; ARR 50%, 95% CI 3% to 85%; NNT 2, 95% CI 1 to 29).

Harms: Adverse effects are not well documented.

Comment: Few RCTs have considered treatment for chronic whiplash, and many people with whiplash are included in general RCTs of chronic mechanical neck pain.

QUESTION What are the effects of treatments for neck pain with radiculopathy?

OPTION SURGERY VERSUS CONSERVATIVE TREATMENT

We found insufficient evidence comparing the effects of conservative treatment and surgery in people with neck pain and radiculopathy.

Benefits: We found no systematic review. One non-blinded RCT (81 people with severe radicular symptoms) for at least 3 months (number with disc prolapse not stated) compared surgery versus physiotherapy or immobilisation in a collar.[45] Participants were reviewed at 12 months. Although the surgery group had more rapid pain reduction (P < 0.01), there was no difference between the groups at 1 year follow up. Between 3 and 12 months, people who did not improve were given additional treatments: one person in the physiotherapy group and five in the collar group underwent surgery; eight people in the surgery group underwent a second operation; and 12 people in the surgery group and 11 in the collar group received physiotherapy.

Harms: The RCT gave no information on adverse effects.

Comment: Conservative treatment needs further assessment, particularly in people considered to be poor risk candidates for surgery.

We found insufficient evidence on the effects of epidural steroid injection in people with neck pain and radiculopathy.

Benefits: **Periradicular, cervical epidural steroid injections, or both:** We found no systematic review or RCTs. One prospective study lacked a control group.[46] **Simple analgesics (paracetamol, opioids) and oral NSAIDs:** We found no systematic reviews or RCTs. **Antidepressants:** We found no systematic reviews or RCTs. **Muscle relaxants/benzodiazepines:** We found no systematic reviews or RCTs.

Harms: **Periradicular, cervical epidural steroid injections, or both:** Case reports have documented occasional complications, such as infection or bleeding after cervical epidural injection. The incidence of adverse events after different cervical injection techniques is unknown.

Comment: None.

GLOSSARY

Wallenberg's syndrome (lateral medullary syndrome) An infarction of the dorsolateral aspect of the medulla. Manifestations may include loss of pain and temperature sensation in the same side of the face and opposite side of the body.

Substantive changes since last issue

Physical treatments One new systematic review;[16] conclusion unchanged. One new RCT[18] found no difference between proprioceptive training and supervised home treatment at 12 months.

Acute whiplash Two new RCTs [39,40] found that early mobilisation improved pain relief and range of movement compared to immobilisation.

Acute whiplash One new RCT[42] compared two home exercise regimes and found that both led to improvement compared to baseline.

REFERENCES

1. Mäkelä M, Heliövaara M, Sievers K, Impivaara O, Knekt P, Aromaa A. Prevalence, determinants, and consequences of chronic neck pain in Finland. *Am J Epidemiol* 1991;134:1356–1367.

2. Cote P, Cassidy D, Carroll L. The Saskatchewan health and back pain survey: the prevalence of neck pain and related disability in Saskatchewan adults. *Spine* 1998;23:1689–1698.

3. Hackett GI, Hudson MF, Wylie JB, et al. Evaluation of the efficacy and acceptability to patients of a physiotherapist working in a health centre. *BMJ* 1987;294:24–26.

4. Waalen D, White P, Waalen J. Demographic and clinical characteristics of chiropractic patients: a 5-year study of patients treated at the Canadian Memorial Chiropractic College. *J Can Chiropract Assoc* 1994;38:75–82.

5. Lamberts H, Brouwer H, Groen AJM, Huisman H. Het transitiemodel in de huisartspraktijk. *Huisart Wet* 1987;30:105–113.

6. Kvarnstrom S. Occurrence of musculoskeletal disorders in a manufacturing industry with special attention to occupational shoulder disorders. *Scand J Rehabil Med* 1983(suppl 8):1–114.

7. Borghouts JA, Koes BW, Bouter LM. The clinical course and prognostic factors of non-specific neck pain: a systematic review. *Pain* 1998;77:1–13. Search date 1996; primary sources Medline, Embase.

8. Squires B, Gargan MF, Bannister GC. Soft-tissue injuries of the cervical spine: 15 year follow-up. *J*

   Bone Joint Surg Br 1996;78:955–957.

9. Spitzer WO, Skovron ML, Salmi LR, et al. Scientific monograph of the Quebec Task Force on whiplash-associated disorders: redefining "whiplash" and its management. *Spine* 1995;20(suppl 8):1–73. Search date 1993; primary sources Medline, TRIS, NTIS, plus personal contacts and Task Force reference lists.

10. Vernon H, Mior S. The neck disability index: a study of reliability and validity. *J Manipulative Physiol Ther* 1991;14:409–415.

11. Gross AR, Aker PD, Goldsmith CH, Peloso P. Physical medicine modalities for mechanical neck disorders. In: The Cochrane Library, Issue 2, 2000. Oxford: Update Software. Search date, 1985–1993; primary sources Medline; Embase; Chirolars; Index to Chiropractic Literature; Cinahl; and Science Citation Index

12. Koes BW, Assendelft WJ, Van der Heijden GJ, Bouter LM, Knipschild PG. Spinal manipulation and mobilisation for back and neck pain: a blinded review. *BMJ* 1991;303:1298–1303. (Comment in *BMJ* 1992;304:184; discussion 185, and *BMJ* 1992;304:184–185.) Search date 1990; primary sources Medline.

13. Kjellman GV, Skargren EI, Oberg BE. A critical analysis of randomised clinical trials on neck pain and treatment efficacy. A review of the literature. *Scand J Rehabil Med* 1999;31:139–152. Search date 1995; primary sources Medline, Cinahl, and hand searches of reference lists.

14. Van der Heijden GJ, Beurskens AJ, Koes BW, Assendelft WJ, de Vet HC, Bouter LM. The efficacy of traction for back and neck pain: a systematic, blinded review of randomized clinical trial methods. *Phys Ther* 1995;75:93–104. Search date 1992; primary sources Medline; Embase; Index to Chiropractic Literature; and Physiotherapy Index.

15. White AR, Ernst E. A systematic review of randomized controlled trials of acupuncture for neck pain. *Rheumatology* 1999;38:143–147. Search date 1998; primary sources Medline; Embase; Cochrane Library; and CISCOM (a database specialising in complementary medicine).

16. Smith LA, Oldman AD, McQuay HJ, Moore RA. Teasing apart quality and validity in systematic reviews: an example from acupuncture trials in chronic neck and back pain. *Pain* 2000;86:119–132. Search date 1998; Medline, Embase, CINAHL, Pychlit, PubMed, The Cochrane Library, Oxford Pain Relief Database, and hand searches of reference lists.

17. Waling K, Sundelin G, Ahlgren C, Jarvholm B. Perceived pain before and after three exercise programs–a controlled clinical trial of women with work-related trapezius myalgia. *Pain* 2000;85: 201–207.

18. Taimela S, Takala EP, Asklof T, Seppala K, Parviainen S. Active treatment of chronic neck pain: a prospective randomized intervention. *Spine* 2000;25:1021–1027.

19. Trock DH, Bollet AJ, Markoll R. The effect of pulsed electromagnetic fields in the treatment of osteoarthritis of the knee and cervical spine. Report of randomized double-blind placebo controlled trials. *J Rheumatol* 1994;21:1903–1911.

20. Levoska S, Keinänen-Kiukaanniemi S. Active or passive physiotherapy for occupational cervicobrachial disorders? A comparison of two treatment methods with a 1-year follow-up. *Arch Phys Med Rehabil* 1993;74:425–430.

21. Aker PD, Gross AR, Goldsmith CH, Peloso P. Conservative management of mechanical neck pain: systematic overview and meta-analysis. *BMJ* 1996;313:1291–1296. Search date 1985– 1993; primary sources Medlars, Embase, Cinahl, and Chirolars.

22. Hurwitz EL, Aker PD, Adams AH, Meeker WC, Shekelle PG. Manipulation and mobilization of the cervical spine: a systematic review of the literature. *Spine* 1996;21:1746–1760. Search dates 1966–1995; primary sources Medline, Embase, Chirolars, and Cinahl.

23. Nordemar R, Thörner C. Treatment of acute cervical pain: a comparative group study. *Pain* 1981;10:93–101.

24. Brodin H. Cervical pain and mobilization. *Manipulative Med* 1985;2:18–22.

25. Koes BW, Bouter LM, van Mameren H, et al. Randomised clinical trial of manipulative therapy and physiotherapy for persistent back and neck complaints: results of one year follow up. *BMJ* 1992;304:601–605.

26. Sloop PR, Smith DS, Goldenberg E, Dore C. Manipulation for chronic neck pain: a double-blind controlled study. *Spine* 1982;7:532–535.

27. Howe DH, Newcombe RG, Wade MT. Manipulation of the cervical spine: a pilot study. *J R Coll Gen Pract* 1983;33:574–579.

28. Cassidy JD, Lopes AA, Yong-Hing K. The immediate effect of manipulation versus mobilization on pain and range of motion in the cervical spine: a randomised controlled trial. *J Manipulative Physiol Ther* 1992;15:570–575.

29. Jordan A, Bendix T, Nielsen H, Hansen FR, Host D, Winkel A. Intensive training, physiotherapy, or manipulation for patients with chronic neck pain. A prospective, single-blinded, randomized clinical trial. *Spine* 1998;23:311–319.

30. Dabbs V, Lauretti WJ. A risk assessment of cervical manipulation vs NSAIDS for the treatment of neck pain. *J Manipulative Physiol Ther* 1995;18:530–536.

31. Di Fabio RP. Manipulation of the cervical spine: risks and benefits. *Phys Ther* 1999;79:50–65.

32. Bogduk N. Whiplash: why pay for what does not work? *J Musculoskel Pain* 2000;8:29–53. Search date and primary sources not stated.

33. Basmajian JV. Cyclobenzaprine hydrochloride effect on skeletal muscle spasm in the lumbar region and neck: two double-blind controlled clinical and laboratory studies. *Arch Phys Med Rehabil* 1978;59:58–63.

34. Bercel NA. Cyclobenzaprine in the treatment of skeletal muscle spasm in osteoarthritis of the cervical and lumbar spine. *Curr Ther Res* 1977; 22:462–468.

35. Bose K. The efficacy and safety of eperisone in patients with cervical spondylosis: results of a randomised double-blind placebo-controlled trial. *Meth Find Exp Clin Pharmacol* 1999;21:209–213.

36. Foley-Nolan D, Moore K, Codd M, Barry C, O'Connor P, Coughlun RJ. Low energy high frequency pulsed electromagnetic therapy for acute whiplash injuries. A double blind randomised controlled study. *Scand J Rehabil Med* 1992;24:51–59.

37. Mealy K, Brennan H, Fenelon GC. Early mobilization of acute whiplash injuries. *BMJ* 1986; 292:656–657.

38. McKinney LA, Dornan JO, Ryan M. The role of physiotherapy in the management of acute neck sprains following road-traffic accidents. *Arch Emerg Med* 1989;6:27–33.

39. Bonk AD, Ferrari R, Giebel GD, Edelmann M, Huser R. Prospective, randomized, controlled study of activity versus collar, and the natural history for whiplash injury, in Germany. *J Musculoskel Pain* 2000;8:123–132.

40. Rosenfeld M, Gunnarsson R, Borenstein P. Early intervention in whiplash–associated disorders: a comparison of two treatment protocols. *Spine* 2000;25:1782–1787.

41. Borchgrevink GE, Kaasa A, McDonagh D, Stiles TC, Haraldseth O, Lereim I. Acute treatment of whiplash neck sprain injuries: a randomised trial of treatment during the first 14 days after a car accident. *Spine* 1998;23:25–31.

42. Soderlund A, Olerud C, Lindberg P. Acute whiplash-associated disorders (WAD): the effects of early mobilization and prognostic factors in long-term symptomatology. *Clin Rehab* 2000;14:457–467.

43. Pennie BH, Agambar LJ. Whiplash injuries: a trial of early management. *J Bone Joint Surg Br* 1990; 72:277–279.

44. Lord SM, Barnsley L, Wallis BJ, McDonald GJ, Bogduk N. Percutaneous radio-frequency neurotomy for chronic cervical zygapophyseal-joint pain. *N Engl J Med*. 1996;335:1721–1726.

45. Persson LC, Carlsson CA, Carlsson JY. Long-lasting cervical radicular pain managed with surgery, physiotherapy, or a cervical collar: a prospective randomised study. *Spine* 1997;22:751–758.

46. Bush K, Hillier S. Outcome of cervical radiculopathy treated with periradicular/epidural corticosteroid injections: a prospective study with independent clinical review. *Eur Spine J* 1996;5:319–325.

Allan Binder

Consultant Rheumatologist, Lister Hospital, Stevenage, UK

Competing interests: None declared.

Musculoskeletal disorders

Search date September 2000

Peter C Gøtzsche

Key Messages

Differences between NSAIDs

- Systematic reviews have found no important differences in effect between different non-steroidal anti-inflammatory drugs (NSAIDs) or doses, but found differences in toxicity related to increased doses and to the nature of the NSAID itself.

- In acute musculoskeletal syndromes, we found no large double blind trial that compared an NSAID with paracetamol.

Preventing gastrointestinal adverse effects

- One large RCT has found that misoprostol slightly reduces the incidence of clinically significant gastrointestinal complications of oral NSAIDs.

- One large RCT has found that omeprazole 20 mg and 40 mg daily and misoprostol 800 µg daily produce similar reductions of endoscopically diagnosed ulceration. RCTs have found that misoprostol causes more adverse effects than placebo, omeprazole, and ranitidine (mostly diarrhoea and abdominal pain).

- RCTs have found H_2 blockers given in standard doses to be inferior to omeprazole and misoprostol at preventing adverse effects of NSAIDs.

© *Clinical Evidence* 2001;5:800–807.

Topical NSAIDs

- One systematic review has found that topical NSAIDs are effective compared with placebo in acute pain conditions (NNT 5 to obtain good pain relief) and chronic pain conditions (NNT 3).
- We found no high quality trials of topical NSAIDs versus oral forms of the same drug, or against paracetamol.

DEFINITION	NSAIDs have anti-inflammatory, analgesic, and antipyretic effects, and inhibit platelet aggregation. The drugs have no documented effect on the course of musculoskeletal diseases.
INCIDENCE/ PREVALENCE	NSAIDs are widely used. Almost 10% of people in the Netherlands used a non-aspirin NSAID in 1987, and the overall use was 11 defined daily doses (see glossary, p 806) per 1000 persons a day.[1] Australia in 1994, overall use was 35 defined daily doses per 1000 persons a day, with 36% of the people receiving NSAIDs for osteoarthritis, 42% for sprain and strain or low back pain, and 4% for rheumatoid arthritis; 35% were aged over 60 years.[2]
AIMS	To reduce symptoms in rheumatic disorders; to avoid severe gastrointestinal adverse effects.
OUTCOMES	**Primary outcomes:** pain intensity; person's preference for one drug over another; global efficacy; clinically significant gastrointestinal complications. **Secondary outcomes:** number of tender joints; perforation; gastrointestinal haemorrhage; dyspepsia; and ulcer detected by routine endoscopy.
METHODS	*Clinical Evidence* update search and appraisal September 2000. More than 100 systematic reviews and thousands of RCTs have compared various NSAIDs. Many trials are unpublished, or published in sources that are not indexed in publicly available databases. The quality of the trials is variable and bias is common, both in the design and analysis of the trials, to such an extent that a systematic review identified false significant findings favouring new drugs over control drugs in 6% of trials.[3] We included only large trials that provided clinically important information not already covered in the systematic reviews. We have favoured systematic reviews that have not been sponsored or authored by industry, as bias in such reviews has been repeatedly demonstrated, but may be difficult to detect.[4] For example, it is easy to seemingly follow the rules for systematic reviews and yet adopt inclusion and exclusion criteria that omit inconvenient studies. In fact, it is hard to find a systematic review sponsored by, or co-authored by, industry that concludes that the company's product is not better than those of its competitors.

QUESTION   **Are there any important differences between available NSAIDs?**

Systematic reviews found no important differences in effect between different NSAIDs or doses, but found differences in toxicity related to increased doses, and to the nature of the NSAID itself. In acute musculoskeletal syndromes, we found no large double blind trials comparing an NSAID with paracetamol. We found no evidence that NSAIDs are more effective than simple analgesics.

Benefits: **Rheumatoid arthritis:** We found two systematic reviews[5,6] and one subsequent RCT.[7] The first systematic review (search date 1985, 37 crossover trials, 1416 people) compared indomethacin with 10 newer NSAIDs in people treated for a median of 2 weeks with each drug.[5] Four of the trials included a placebo period and one trial compared four drugs. Only 5% more people (95% CI 0% to 10%) preferred the newer NSAID to indomethacin. The second systematic review (search date 1988, 88 trials comparing two NSAIDs, 27 trials comparing an NSAID with placebo, 6440 people), found no significant differences in the number of tender joints among 17 different NSAIDs.[6] The subsequent RCT (1149 people) compared three doses of the COX-2 inhibitor celecoxib versus naproxen 1 g.[7] It found a similar beneficial effect, with fewer endoscopically detected ulcers (5% v 26%; ARR 21%, 95% CI 13% to 29%). Only one of the ulcers was clinically significant and only seven (1%) of 692 people taking celecoxib and five (2%) of 225 people taking naproxen withdrew because of gastrointestinal adverse effects.[7] **Osteoarthritis:** Two systematic reviews (search dates 1994 and 1996) found no clear differences between various NSAIDs used to treat osteoarthritis of the hip (39 trials)[8] or the knee (16 trials).[9] One systematic review (search date 1990) of tenoxicam versus three other NSAIDs for osteoarthritis found superiority of tenoxicam over piroxicam both for global efficacy (10 trials, 834 people; RR 1.12, 95% CI 1.03 to 1.22), and for global tolerability (7 trials, 974 people; RR 1.06, 95% CI 1.00 to 1.12).[10] This result is at variance with a large RCT (1328 people with osteoarthritis or rheumatoid arthritis), which found no significant difference in global efficacy or tolerability between the two drugs. Improvement was noted for 55% of people taking tenoxicam versus 53% of people taking piroxicam (ARI +2%, 95% CI −5% to +9%) (see NSAIDs under osteoarthritis, p 808).[11] One review of eight RCTs (5435 people) of rofecoxib versus other NSAIDs found a cumulative incidence of clinically significant gastrointestinal adverse events of 1.3% versus 1.8% (CI not available; P = 0.46).[12] Fewer people taking rofecoxib withdrew because of gastrointestinal adverse effects (3.5% v 4.8%, ARR 1.3%; RR 0.73, 95% CI 0.55 to 0.97; NNT with rofecoxib versus other NSAIDs to avoid one additional withdrawal because of gastrointestinal adverse effects 78, 95% CI 46 to 790). **Acute musculoskeletal syndromes:** We found two systematic reviews, which identified generally poor quality RCTs.[13,14] The first systematic review (search date 1998) of 17 NSAID trials for shoulder pain was inconclusive (see NSAIDs under osteoarthritis, p 808).[14] Another systematic review (search date 1993, 84 trials, 32 025 people with soft tissue injuries of the ankle) was unable to pool data to perform a statistical analysis of the different forms of treatment.[13] We found no good evidence that NSAIDs are more effective than paracetamol in acute musculoskeletal syndromes. **Dose response relation:** One systematic review (search date 1989, 19 trials), in which participants were randomised to more than one dose of nine different NSAIDs found a dose response relation that saturated at high doses.[15] This and another systematic review (search date 1992) found that the recommended dosages were close to providing a ceiling effect.[15,16] The review of the 115 trials mentioned above found no significant differences between various doses of drugs;[6] 10 of 21 RCTs of ibuprofen had used a daily dosage of 1200 mg or less.[6]

Harms: **Versus placebo:** One systematic review (100 trials, 12 853 people) found a higher rate of gross haemorrhage (ARI for NSAID v placebo +0.7%, 95% CI –0.1% to +1.5%) and proven ulcer (ARI for NSAID v placebo +0.05%, 95% CI –0.01% to +0.11%) with NSAIDs compared with placebo. The differences did not quite reach significance. Mean treatment duration was short (2 months).[17] For 40 aspirin trials (22 234 people, mean treatment duration 1 year), the review found an increased risk of gross haemorrhage (ARI 0.6%, 95% CI 0.2% to 1.0%) and for proven ulcer (ARI 0.6%, 95% CI 0% to 1.2%).[17] The number needed to harm was in the range 100–1000. One systematic review (38 placebo controlled trials) found that NSAIDs raised mean blood pressure by 5.0 mm Hg (95% CI 1.2 mm Hg to 8.7 mm Hg).[18] **Versus other NSAIDs:** One meta-analysis of 11 case control studies and one cohort study found that ibuprofen was significantly less toxic than other NSAIDs. The 11 comparator drugs were associated with a 1.6–9.2 fold increase in risk of serious upper gastrointestinal complications.[19] COX-2 inhibitors were associated with less gastrointestinal toxicity than older NSAIDs, but the clinical significance is not clear (see above).[7,12] **Dose response relation:** Three systematic reviews found no ceiling effect for adverse effects; the incidence of adverse effects increased in an approximately linear fashion with dose.[16,19,20]

Comment: Important differences in adverse effects seem to exist between different NSAIDs. In contrast, the beneficial effects of NSAIDs seem similar. The only meta-analysis that found one drug to be more effective than another was funded by the manufacturer;[10] the studies it included were small and the result was not replicated in a large RCT. People's preferences for particular drugs have not been replicated and could therefore be because of chance or natural fluctuations in disease activity.[21,22] The evidence suggests that if the NSAID is unsatisfactory, switching to another NSAID will not solve the problem.[11] Likewise, doubling the dose of an NSAID leads to only a small increase in effect, which may not be clinically relevant. In acute musculoskeletal problems it is doubtful whether NSAIDs have any clinically relevant anti-inflammatory effect; we found no large double blind RCT comparing an NSAID with paracetamol. Paracetamol has been studied in osteoarthritis where it had much the same effect as ibuprofen or naproxen (see simple analgesics v NSAIDs under osteoarthritis, p 808).

QUESTION What are the effects of co-treatments to reduce the risk of gastrointestinal adverse effects of NSAIDs?

One systematic review found that misoprostol slightly reduced the incidence of clinically significant gastrointestinal complications of oral NSAIDs. One large RCT found that omeprazole 20 mg and 40 mg daily and misoprostol 800 µg daily had similar effects in reducing endoscopically diagnosed adverse effects. However, misoprostol caused more adverse effects (mostly diarrhoea and abdominal pain). The review found double doses, (see glossary, p 806) of H_2 blockers reduced the development of endoscopic ulcers compared with placebo. RCTs found H_2 blockers given in standard doses to be inferior to omeprazole and misoprostol, but the effect of H_2 blockers seems to increase with dose. The absolute risk of serious upper gastrointestinal complications is approximately doubled for people over 75 years old, and for those with a history of peptic ulcer, bleeding, or cardiovascular disease.

Benefits: We found one updated systematic review.[23] **Misoprostol versus placebo:** The systematic review (search date January 2000, 9 RCTs, 3329 people) included people who had received NSAIDs for at least 3 months and where ulcers were detected by routine endoscopy.[23] Misoprostol reduced the development of endoscopic ulcers compared with placebo (ARR 10%, 95% CI 9% to 12% for gastric ulcer and ARR 4%, 95% CI 2% to 5% for duodenal ulcer). Between trial comparisons suggested a dose response relationship (P = 0.006) for gastric ulcers in the dose range 400–800 µg. One additional 6 month RCT (8843 people with rheumatoid arthritis, mean age 68 years, all treated with NSAIDs) with clinically relevant outcomes compared misoprostol 800 µg daily versus placebo.[24] Serious upper gastrointestinal complications (such as perforation, gastric outlet obstruction, or bleeding detected by clinical symptoms or investigation) were reduced by misoprostol compared with placebo (AR 0.6% in misoprostol group v 1.0% in placebo group; ARR 0.4%, 95% CI 0% to 0.7%; NNT 263). The risk of serious upper gastrointestinal complications was approximately doubled for people above 75 years old, and for those with a history of peptic ulcer, bleeding, or cardiovascular disease. People with all four risk factors had an absolute risk of 9% for a major complication in 6 months, corresponding to a number needed to treat with misoprostol rather than placebo of 28 people. **H₂ blockers versus placebo:** The systematic review included seven RCTs with 1303 people who had received NSAIDs for at least 3 months.[23] Double doses reduced the development of endoscopic ulcers compared with placebo (ARR 14%, 95% CI 6% to 23% for gastric ulcer and ARR 10%, 95% CI 4% to 17% for duodenal ulcers). **Omeprazole versus placebo** The systematic review included three RCTs with 774 people who had received NSAIDs for at least 3 months.[23] Omeprazole compared with placebo reduced the development of endoscopic ulcers (ARR 13%, 95% CI 8% to 18% for gastric ulcer and ARR 9%, 95% CI 5% to 12% for duodenal ulcer). **Misoprostol versus omeprazole:** We found one RCT in 935 people treated with NSAIDs who had ulcers or more than 10 erosions at endoscopy. Treatment success was defined as fewer than five erosions at each site, no ulcers, and not more than mild dyspepsia.[25] At 8 weeks, treatment was successful in 76% of individuals given omeprazole 20 mg daily, 75% given omeprazole 40 mg daily, and 71% given misoprostol 800 µg daily. A total of 732 people in whom treatment was successful were re-randomised to maintenance treatment for 6 months. More people remained in remission with omeprazole 20 mg than with misoprostol 400 µg (61% v 48%), and with either drug than with placebo (27% with placebo; ARR for omeprazole v placebo 34%, 95% CI 25% to 43%; NNT 3; ARR for misoprostol v placebo 21%, 95% CI 12% to 30%; NNT 5). **Omeprazole versus H₂ blockers:** In a similarly designed RCT (541 people), treatment was successful in 80% given omeprazole 20 mg, 79% given omeprazole 40 mg, and 63% of people given ranitidine 300 mg daily.[26] The estimated proportions in remission after 6 months were 72% with omeprazole 20 mg and 59% with ranitidine 300 mg (ARR for omeprazole v ranitidine 13%, 95% CI 4% to 22%; NNT 8). **Misoprostol versus H₂ blockers:** One 8 week RCT (538 people with NSAID related upper gastrointestinal pain without endoscopic evidence of ulcers) compared misoprostol 800 µg versus ranitidine 300 mg daily.[27] A third were excluded from analysis because of problems with adherence and missing endoscopic examinations. Gastric ulcers at least 3 mm in diameter were found in 1% of people taking misoprostol and in 6% of people taking ranitidine (ARR for misoprostol v ranitidine 5%, 95% CI 2% to 9%; NNT 20). Duodenal ulcer rate was 1% with both drugs.

Harms: In one of the large trials, significantly more people receiving misoprostol than placebo withdrew from the study because of adverse events, primarily diarrhoea, and abdominal pain (27% v 20%, P > 0.001).[23] There were 17 deaths in the misoprostol group versus 21 deaths in the placebo group. One person on placebo died as a direct result of gastrointestinal toxicity. Few adverse events were reported in the trial comparing omeprazole with ranitidine. Treatment discontinuations (all causes) occurred in 10% of people taking omeprazole 20 mg, 10% omeprazole taking 40 mg, and 14% taking ranitidine.[26] In the trial comparing misoprostol with ranitidine, adverse events (mostly gastrointestinal) occurred in 77% of people taking misoprostol and 66% taking ranitidine, with withdrawal rates of 13% on misoprostol and 7% on ranitidine (ARR for ranitidine v misoprostol 6%, 95% CI 1% to 11%; NNT 17).[27]

Comment: The clinical relevance of these findings is doubtful. The only trial that used clinically relevant outcomes found little difference between active drug and placebo, except for people at high risk.[24] The rate of ulcers was more than 10 times higher in the studies where the investigators looked for them with regular endoscopy than in earlier trials of NSAIDs.[18] These ulcers were sometimes defined as endoscopic lesions with a size of only 3 mm, sometimes as any lesion of an unequivocal depth, and sometimes no definition was provided at all.

QUESTION   What are the effects of topical NSAIDs?

One systematic review has found that topical NSAIDs are effective compared with placebo in acute pain conditions (NNT 5 to obtain good pain relief) and chronic pain conditions (NNT 3). We found no high quality trials of topical versus oral formulations of the same drug, and found no direct comparisons of topical NSAIDs versus paracetamol. It is therefore uncertain whether topical treatment is advantageous over these alternatives.

Benefits: **Versus placebo:** We found one systematic review (86 RCTs, search date 1996) in 10 160 people, which primarily compared a topical NSAID with placebo.[28] The review was partly sponsored by two manufacturers. Many trials of acute pain conditions (soft tissue trauma, strains, and sprains) were small; in 37 trials, the average number of actively treated people was 32, and the effect declined significantly with sample size. In seven trials with more than 80 people per group, the number of people that would need to be treated for one extra good outcome was five (RR 1.6, 95% CI 1.3 to

1.9; NNT 5, 95% CI 4 to 6). In 12 RCTs in chronic pain conditions (osteoarthritis, tendinitis) the number of people that would need to be treated for one extra good outcome was three (RR 2.0, 95% CI 1.5 to 2.7; NNT 3, 95% CI 3 to 4). In one trial, additional to the review (116 people with osteoarthritis of the hip or knee) copper salicylate gel or placebo was applied to the forearm.[29] It found no significant difference in effect (22% v 21% of participants reported good effect). **Versus oral NSAIDs:** Five trials in the systematic review compared topical versus oral NSAIDs, but they all had inadequate design and power.[28] No high quality trial compared the same NSAID given orally and topically (see effects of topical agents under osteoarthritis, p 808). **Versus paracetamol:** We found no RCTs.

Harms: In the systematic review, local adverse effects occurred in 3% of people in both groups and systemic adverse events in 1%.[28] In the trial of copper salicylate gel, more people receiving treatment reported adverse reactions, most commonly skin reactions (83% v 52%), and more people withdrew from the trial because of these reactions (17% v 2%).[29]

Comment: Sample size bias hampers the interpretation of the available trials. We found no high quality trials comparing topical versus systemic administration of the same NSAID, and no trials comparing a topical NSAID with paracetamol.

GLOSSARY
Defined daily dose The assumed average daily dose for the main indication of a specified drug. The defined daily dose per 1000 population per day is an estimate of the proportion of that population receiving treatment with that drug.
Double doses Twice the daily defined dose.

Substantive changes since last issue
Misoprostol versus placebo Updated systematic review;[23] conclusions unchanged.
H$_2$ blockers versus placebo Updated systematic review[23] found double doses reduced the development of gastric and duodenal ulcers compared with placebo, whereas normal doses only significantly reduced the development of duodenal ulcers.

REFERENCES

1. Leufkens HG, Ameling CB, Hekster YA, Bakker A. Utilization patterns of non-steroidal anti-inflammatory drugs in an open Dutch population. Pharm Weekbl Sci 1990;12:97–103.
2. McManus P, Primrose JG, Henry DA, et al. Pattern of non-steroidal anti-inflammatory drug use in Australia 1990–1994. A report from the drug utilization sub-committee of the pharmaceutical benefits advisory committee. Med J Aust 1996; 164:589–592.
3. Gøtzsche PC. Methodology and overt and hidden bias in reports of 196 double-blind trials of nonsteroidal anti-inflammatory drugs in rheumatoid arthritis (published erratum appears in Control Clin Trials 1989;10:356). Control Clin Trials 1989;10:31–56. Search date May 1985; primary source Medline.
4. Smith GD, Egger Matthias. Meta-analysis: unresolved issues and future developments. BMJ 1998;316:221–225.
5. Gøtzsche PC. Patients' preference in indomethacin trials: an overview. Lancet 1989;i:88–91. Search

date 1985; primary sources Medline, personal contact with companies that marketed proprietary products, and hand searching of reference lists of collected articles.
6. Gøtzsche PC. Meta-analysis of NSAIDs: contribution of drugs, doses, trial designs, and meta-analytic techniques. Scand J Rheumatol 1993;22:255–260. Search dates May 1985 and September 1988; primary source Medline.
7. Simon LS, Weaver AL, Graham DY, et al. Anti-inflammatory and upper gastrointestinal effects of celecoxib in rheumatoid arthritis. JAMA 1999;282: 1921–1928.
8. Towheed T, Shea B, Wells G, Hochberg M. Analgesia and non-aspirin, non-steroidal anti-inflammatory drugs in osteoarthritis of the hip. In: The Cochrane Library, Issue 3, 2000. Oxford: Update Software. Search date 1994; primary sources Cochrane Controlled Trials Register; Medline; and hand searched references.
9. Watson MC, Brookes ST, Kirwan JR, Faulkner A. Non-aspirin, non-steroidal anti-inflammatory drugs

for treating osteoarthritis of the knee. In: The Cochrane Library, Issue 3, 2000. Oxford: Update Software. Search date November 1996; primary sources Medline; and Embase.

10. Riedemann PJ, Bersinic S, Cuddy J, Torrance GW, Tugwell PX. A study to determine the efficacy and safety of tenoxicam versus piroxicam, diclofenac and indomethacin in patients with osteoarthritis: a meta-analysis. J Rheumatol 1993;20:2095–2103. Search date 1990; primary source Medline.

11. Simpson J, Golding DN, Freeman AM, et al. A large multicentre, parallel group, double-blind study comparing tenoxicam and piroxicam in the treatment of osteoarthritis and rheumatoid arthritis. Br J Clin Pract 1989;43:328–333.

12. Langman MJ, Jensen DM, Watson DG, et al. Adverse upper gastrointestinal effects of rofecoxib compared with NSAIDs. JAMA 1999;282:1929–1933.

13. Ogilvie Harris DJ, Gilbart M. Treatment modalities for soft tissue injuries of the ankle: a critical review. Clin J Sport Med 1995;5:175–186. Search date 1993; primary sources Medline and Embase.

14. Green S, Buchbinder R, Glazier R, Forbes A. Interventions for shoulder pain. In: The Cochrane Library, Issue 3, 2000. Oxford: Update Software. Search date May 1998; primary sources Cochrane Musculoskeletal Group Trials Register; Cochrane Controlled Trials Register; Medline; Embase; Cinahl; and Science Citation Index.

15. Gøtzsche PC. Review of dose-response studies of NSAIDs in rheumatoid arthritis. Dan Med Bull 1989;36:395–399. Search date May 1985; primary sources Medline and hand searches of reference lists and contact with companies marketing proproctary preparations.

16. Eisenberg E, Berkey CS, Carr DB, Mosteller F, Chalmers TC. Efficacy and safety of nonsteroidal antiinflammatory drugs as a meta-analysis. J Clin Oncol 1994;12:2756–2765. Search date up to 1992; primary source Medline.

17. Chalmers TC, Berrier J, Hewitt P, et al. Meta-analysis of randomized controlled trials as a method of estimating rare complications of non-steroidal anti-inflammatory drug therapy. Aliment Pharmacol Ther 1988;2(suppl 1):9–26. Search date not available; primary source Medline.

18. Johnson AG, Nguyen TV, Day RO. Do nonsteroidal anti-inflammatory drugs affect blood pressure? A meta-analysis. Ann Intern Med 1994;121:289–300. Search date 1990; primary sources Medline, Embase, Biosis, Diagenes, Science Citation Abstracts, International Pharmaceutical Abstracts, IOWA Drug Information Service, Combined Health Informatics Database, and hand searches of bibliographies, text books, and reference lists

19. Henry D, Lim LL, Garcia Rodriguez LA, et al. Variability in risk of gastrointestinal complications with individual non-steroidal anti-inflammatory drugs: results of a collaborative meta-analysis.

BMJ 1996;312:1563–1566. Search date up to 1994; primary source Medline.

20. Cappelleri JC, Lau J, Kupelnick B, Chalmers TC. Efficacy and safety of different aspirin dosages on vascular diseases in high-risk patients. A meta-regression analysis. Online J Curr Clin Trials 1995; Doc No 174. Search date up to 1992; primary sources Medline, and Current Contents.

21. Huskisson EC, Woolf DL, Balme HW, Scott J, Franklin S. Four new anti-inflammatory drugs: responses and variations. BMJ 1976;i:1048–1049.

22. Cooperating Clinics Committee of the American Rheumatism Association. A seven-day variability study of 499 patients with peripheral rheumatoid arthritis. Arthritis Rheum 1965;8:302–334.

23. Rostom A, Wells G, Tugwell P, Welch V, Dube C, McGowan J. Prevention of chronic NSAID induced upper gastrointestinal toxicity. In: The Cochrane Library, Issue 3, 2000. Oxford: Update Software. Search date 2000, primary sources Medline, Current Contents, Embase, Cochrane Controlled Trials Register, hand searches of conference proceedings, and personal contact with experts and companies.

24. Silverstein FE, Graham DY, Senior JR, et al. Misoprostol reduces serious gastrointestinal complications in patients with rheumatoid arthritis receiving nonsteroidal anti-inflammatory drugs. A randomized, double-blind, placebo-controlled trial. Ann Intern Med 1995;123:241–249.

25. Hawkey CJ, Karrasch JA, Szczepanski L, et al. Omeprazole compared with misoprostol for ulcers associated with nonsteroidal antiinflammatory drugs. Omeprazole versus misoprostol for NSAID-induced ulcer management (OMNIUM) study group. N Engl J Med 1998;338:727–734.

26. Yeomans ND, Tulassay Z, Juhasz L, et al. A comparison of omeprazole with ranitidine for ulcers associated with nonsteroidal antiinflammatory drugs. Acid suppression trial: ranitidine versus omeprazole for NSAID associated ulcer treatment (ASTRONAUT) study group. N Engl J Med 1998;338:719–726.

27. Raskin JB, White RH, Jaszewski R, Korsten MA, Schubert TT, Fort JG. Misoprostol and ranitidine in the prevention of NSAID-induced ulcers: a prospective, double-blind, multicenter study. Am J Gastroenterol 1996;91:223–227.

28. Moore RA, Tramer MR, Carroll D, Wiffen PJ, McQuay HJ. Quantitative systematic review of topically applied non-steroidal anti-inflammatory drugs. BMJ 1998;316:333–338. Search date 1996; primary sources Medline; Embase; Oxford Pain Relief Database 1950 to 1994; contact with pharmaceutical companies, and hand searched references.

29. Shackel NA, Day RO, Kellett B, Brooks PM. Copper-salicylate gel for pain relief in osteoarthritis: a randomised controlled trial. Med J Aust 1997;167:134–136.

Peter C Gøtzsche
Director
The Nordic Cochrane Centre
Copenhagen
Denmark

Competing interests: None declared.

Musculoskeletal disorders

Search date November 2000

Paul Dieppe, Jiri Chard, Alex Faulkner and Stefan Lohmander

INTERVENTIONS

Key Messages

Non-surgical treatments

- Systematic reviews have found that non-steroidal anti-inflammatory drugs (NSAIDs) and simple analgesics, such as paracetamol (acetaminophen), reduce the pain of osteoarthritis. We found no good evidence that NSAIDs are superior to simple analgesics, such as paracetamol (acetaminophen), or that any one of the many NSAIDs is more effective than the others in relieving the pain of osteoarthritis.

- One systematic review has found that topical agents relieve pain in people with osteoarthritis and have fewer adverse effects than systemic treatments. However, we found no evidence that prescribed agents are superior to cheaper non-prescription alternatives or to other local treatments, such as heat or cold packs.

- Systematic reviews and subsequent RCTs have found that both exercise and education may help reduce the burden of pain and disability in people with hip or knee osteoarthritis.

- Systematic reviews have found no clear evidence of benefit from intra-articular injection of various drugs over placebo injection in people with osteoarthritis of the knee.

Surgical treatments

- Systematic reviews have found that hip and knee replacements are effective in relieving pain and improving function in a wide range of people. One RCT found limited evidence that unicompartmental knee operations are more effective than tricompartmental replacement. We found limited evidence that unicompartmental knee operations are more effective than bicompartmental operations.

- We found limited evidence suggesting that hip replacement is less effective in younger people.

- We found conflicting evidence from observational studies about the effects of old age and obesity on the balance of benefits and harms from knee surgery.

DEFINITION	Osteoarthritis is a heterogeneous condition for which the prevalence, risk factors, clinical manifestations, and prognosis vary according to the joints affected. It most commonly affects hands, knees, hips, and spinal apophyseal joints. It is usually defined by pathological or radiological criteria rather than clinical features, and is characterised by focal areas of damage to the cartilage surfaces of synovial joints, associated with remodelling of the underlying bone and mild synovitis. When severe, there is characteristic joint space narrowing and osteophyte formation, with visible subchondral bone changes on radiography.
INCIDENCE/ PREVALENCE	Osteoarthritis is common and an important cause of pain and disability in older adults.[1,2] Radiographic features are practically universal in at least some joints in people aged over 60 years, but significant clinical disease probably affects 10–20% of people. Knee disease is about twice as prevalent as hip disease in people aged over 60 (about 10% v 5%).[3,4]
AETIOLOGY/ RISK FACTORS	The main initiating factors are abnormalities in joint shape or injury.

PROGNOSIS	The natural history of osteoarthritis is poorly understood. Only a minority of people with clinical disease of the hip or knee joint progress to surgery.
AIMS	To reduce pain, stiffness, and disability; to limit the risk of progressive joint damage; to improve quality of life, with minimal adverse effects.
OUTCOMES	Frequency and severity of joint pain (particularly activity related pain and night pain); stiffness; functional impairment and disability; quality of life; perioperative complications (infection, bleeding, venous thromboembolism, and death); prosthesis survival and the need for revision surgery. A global knee rating scale that includes measures of pain, function, and range of movement. A modified Knee Society score: this instrument combines three different domains (pain, function, and joint status) into a single score (patient function [i.e. walking ability and stair climbing] accounts for about 50% of the total score, with pain and joint status [i.e. stability and deformity] each accounting for about 25%).[5] The Western Ontario and McMaster osteoarthritis index (WOMAC) is a validated instrument for assessing lower limb (hip and knee) osteoarthritis and is sensitive to change. It is a self assessment questionnaire and includes questions on pain, stiffness, and physical function (such as walking ability). WOMAC is disease specific, but not intervention specific; it can be used to assess any intervention in osteoarthritis.[6–8]
METHODS	*Clinical Evidence* update search and appraisal November 2000.

QUESTION **What are the effects of exercise and physical therapy?**

Evidence from systematic reviews and subsequent RCTs suggests that exercise and physical therapy reduces pain and disability in people with hip or knee osteoarthritis.

Benefits: We found three systematic reviews, one subsequent non-systematic review, and two subsequent RCTs of exercise in people with osteoarthritis of the knee or hip. The first review (search date 1997, 11 RCTs) concluded that exercise regimens were beneficial but that more evidence was needed (see table 1, p 822).[9] The second systematic review (search date 1993) of non-medicinal and non-invasive treatments for hip and knee osteoarthritis concluded that, of seven modalities reviewed, exercise had the strongest evidence of benefit.[10] The third systematic review (search date 1994) of aerobic exercises for osteoarthritis of the knee found only three admissible RCTs.[11] The review concluded that, despite a favourable impression, the evidence currently available was inadequate. The non-systematic review identified 13 RCTs.[12] The review found that there was small to moderate beneficial effects for pain and function from use of strength, aerobic exercise interventions, or both. The first subsequent RCT (24 obese people with osteoarthritis, body mass index $\geq 28\,kg/m^2$) compared an exercise plus weight loss diet versus an exercise programme alone. It found no significant differences in 6 month pain or function scores (no figures reported).[13] The second subsequent RCT (179 older people with osteoarthritis, average age 74 years) found that exercise was significantly better than control for pain (WOMAC pain subscale, $P = 0.003$), physical activity (WOMAC physical activity subscale, $P = 0.006$), and pain at rest (Visual Analogue Scale [VAS]: $P = 0.02$), and pain when walking (VAS: $P = 0.002$).[14]

Harms: We found no evidence of harm.

Comment: The trials are limited by methodological and reporting issues.

QUESTION   What are the effects of education and behavioural change?

Evidence from one systematic review and three RCTs suggests that education reduces pain and disability in people with hip or knee osteoarthritis.

Benefits: We found one systematic review and three subsequent RCTs. The systematic review (search date 1993) included 10 controlled trials of education over 2–48 weeks.[15] One trial, which found benefit from a combination of exercise and education, was excluded from the main analysis (see comment below). Effect sizes associated with education were not significant for pain (0.16, 95% CI −0.69 to +1.02) and disability (0.0, 95% CI −0.61 to +0.61). The first subsequent RCT (211 people with osteoarthritis of the knee) compared self care education (see glossary, p 819) versus attention only education (see glossary, p 819) over 1 year. The self care education group derived greater benefit for both pain and disability.[16] At both 4 and 12 months, there was a significant difference between self care education versus attention only for function and pain. The second subsequent RCT (252 people) assessed methods to improve adherence to treatment plans. The trial compared a targeted education programme versus an information pack, both delivered through a computer over 8 weeks, and found no significant difference in quality of life, pain, or disability between groups. The targeted education programme was associated with significant improvement in stiffness compared with controls (effect size −0.63, 95% CI −0.81 to −0.45 v −0.39, 95% CI −0.53 to −0.25).[17] The third subsequent RCT (113 people) compared an isokinetic exercise regime versus generic information lectures given by health professionals over 12 weeks. It found no significant difference in leg strength, pain, or function between the groups; both improved from baseline.[18]

Harms: No harms were reported.

Comment: We found few well designed RCTs, and the participants in many trials were not representative of those in the general population. Individual patient education studies in the systematic review also included biofeedback, exercises, and social support.[15] One trial that found a very large improvement for pain and disability was excluded from the analysis because its results were so different from the others. It also included exercise in the intervention. The remaining nine trials showed no evidence of heterogeneity of effects.

QUESTION   What are the effects of physical aids?

We found limited evidence on the effectiveness of physical aids. Physical aids refer to shoe wedges/insole, walking aids, joint braces, and taping of the joint.

Benefits: We found no systematic reviews. We found two RCTs on the use of physical aids. One RCT (119 people) compared two forms of valgus knee bracing (neoprene sleeve and unloader-brace) against a control group. It found that both the knee brace groups versus the control group significantly improved disease specific quality of life (P = 0.001) and function (P < 0.001). No significant difference was found between WOMAC scores for the two braces (P = 0.062).[19] The second small RCT (14 people) found that taping of the knee versus control was associated with a reduction in pain (difference in pain score on 10 cm VAS between neutral versus medical taping 15.5, 95% CI 2.4 to 28.6, differences in pain score between neutral and lateral taping −8, 95% CI −22.5 to +6.5, figures as presented in original paper, units not clear).[20]

Harms: We found no evidence of adverse effects from using physical aids.

Comment: In addition to the two RCTs identified, we found several observational studies, which all found positive effects from using physical aids.

QUESTION What are the effects of oral drug treatments?

OPTION ANALGESICS

Two systematic reviews found that simple analgesics such as paracetamol (acetaminophen) control short term pain associated with osteoarthritis.

Benefits: We found one systematic review evaluating analgesics in osteoarthritis of the hip (search date 1994, 3 RCTs)[21] and one systematic review in osteoarthritis of the knee (search date 1994).[22] The reviews found limited evidence that simple analgesics versus placebo were effective in controlling pain associated with osteoarthritis. A small RCT included in the review (44 people with osteoarthritis of the knee)[22] found that paracetamol (acetaminophen) was superior to placebo for short term pain relief (improvement in pain at rest in 73% of knees with paracetamol v 5% of knees with control) and global responses (improved global response 18/22 [82%] with paracetamol v 1/22 [5%] with control; ARI 77%; RR 18, 95% CI 6.9 to 22; NNT 1, 95% CI 1 to 4).[23]

Harms: Liver damage results from overdose of paracetamol, or at lower doses in people with existing liver damage.[24]

Comment: None.

OPTION NON-STEROIDAL ANTI-INFLAMMATORY DRUGS

Three systematic reviews have found that NSAIDs reduce short term pain in osteoarthritis (see NSAIDs, p 800).

Benefits: We found three systematic reviews of analgesic and anti-inflammatory treatment in osteoarthritis of the hip (search date 1994, 14 RCTs)[21] and knee (search dates 1996, 16 RCTs,[25] and search date 1994, 45 RCTs[22]). The reviews found that NSAIDs were effective at reducing short term pain. We identified hundreds of

RCTs comparing NSAIDs with other NSAIDs or placebo for treatment of osteoarthritis. Most of these trials found benefit from using NSAIDs to treat osteoarthritis. **Oral versus topical NSAIDs:** See topical agents, p 814.

Harms: Indomethacin (and possibly other NSAIDs) may accelerate joint damage in osteoarthritis, and there is a risk of gastrointestinal or renal damage in older people with osteoarthritis, particularly those with intercurrent disease.[26] Case control studies of several thousand people suggest that the odds ratio of gastrointestinal haemorrhage when taking any NSAID is about 4–5, the risk increasing with certain drugs and with increased doses.[27,28] A meta-analysis (search date 1994) ranked the risk from different drugs and found it to be dose dependent (see table 2, p 822).[29] We found insufficient evidence about the gastrointestinal effects of COX-2 inhibitors versus traditional NSAIDs to calculate the comparative risk for more recently introduced NSAIDs (see COX-2 option under NSAIDs, p 800).

Comment: Despite the many studies of NSAIDs use in osteoarthritis, the evidence we found on efficacy remains poor and difficult to generalise. Most RCTs suffer from weak methods, including short duration; exclusion of older people, those with intercurrent disease, or those at risk of gastrointestinal and other drug complications; variable outcome measures; comparison of one drug versus another rather than versus placebo; and funding bias.[30,31] In the absence of clear evidence of the superiority of one type of treatment or product, other considerations, such as safety (particularly the risk of gastrointestinal bleeding with NSAIDs) and cost should determine the choice of drug (see NSAIDs, p 800).

OPTION	ANALGESICS VERSUS NON-STEROIDAL ANTI-INFLAMMATORY DRUGS

Two systematic reviews have found that simple analgesics and NSAIDs produce short term pain relief in osteoarthritis. However, we found no good evidence that NSAIDs are superior to simple analgesics such as paracetamol (acetaminophen) (see NSAIDs, p 800).

Benefits: We found two systematic reviews (17 RCTs in one review of which one is a comparison of NSAIDs versus other analgesics;[21] 48 RCTs in the other review[22] of which five[32–36] compared NSAIDs and analgesics). The systematic reviews found no evidence for the superiority of NSAIDs over simple analgesics. One RCT (178 people with knee osteoarthritis) compared naproxen versus paracetamol (acetaminophen) over 2 years. The trial found no significant difference in effects.[32] Another RCT (184 people with osteoarthritis) compared two doses of ibuprofen versus paracetamol. The trial concluded that there were no differences in the three groups.[33] Twenty crossover trials of one person each ("n of 1" trials) compared paracetamol (acetaminophen) versus diclofenac and concluded that, although some people's pain was adequately controlled by paracetamol (acetaminophen) alone, others responded better to an NSAID.[37]

Harms: See above.

Comment: None.

| QUESTION | What are the effects of topical agents? |

We found limited evidence that topical agents provide some pain relief for people with osteoarthritis and that they are less toxic than systemic drug treatments. We found no evidence comparing different topical agents or comparing topical agents with other local treatments such as heat or cold packs.

Benefits:
Topical NSAIDs versus placebo: See NSAIDs, p 800. We found one recent systematic review (search date 1996, 86 trials) comparing topically applied agents containing NSAIDs versus placebo.[38] It found that these agents reduced pain compared with placebo (RR for relief of chronic musculoskeletal pain due to osteoarthritis and tendinitis 2.0, 95% CI 1.5 to 2.7). One subsequent RCT (119 people with osteoarthritis) found better pain relief with a topical NSAID (diclofenac-hyaluronan gel) versus placebo gel, but the difference was not significant (P = 0.057).[39] One further RCT (70 people with mild knee osteoarthritis) showed a significant improvement (measured by WOMAC) in the treatment group receiving diclofenac gel compared with the control group receiving vehicle gel (P = 0.05).[40] **Topical NSAIDs versus oral NSAIDs:** We found no RCT comparing the same NSAID given orally and topically. One good quality RCT (included in the review) in 235 people with mild osteoarthritis of the knee compared topical piroxicam gel versus oral ibuprofen 1200 mg daily and found no significant difference in pain relief between the two groups (good or excellent relief in 60% v 64%, P = 0.56).[41] **Capsaicin:** One nonsystematic meta-analysis of three RCTs of topically applied capsaicin found that capsaicin cream reduced pain compared with placebo (OR 4.4, 95% CI 2.8 to 6.9).[42] One RCT (70 people with osteoarthritis) compared 0.025% capsaicin cream versus nonmedicated cream. Active treatment resulted in significantly greater pain reduction than placebo (no quantified estimates of benefit available).[43] **Versus other local treatments:** We found no systematic review or RCTs comparing agents containing NSAIDs or capsaicin with simple rubefacients (see glossary, p 819), or local applications such as hot packs.

Harms:
The main adverse effect of topical treatment is local skin irritation; systemic adverse effects were no more common than with placebo.[38] We found no reports of gastric or renal problems.

Comment:
The evidence is poor, most studies being short term, including a mixture of patient groups, and comparing different agents with no placebo control. The RCT comparing topical versus oral NSAIDs did not use the same drug so it is difficult to disentangle the effects of this and the different routes of administration.

| QUESTION | What are the effects of intra-articular injection of the knee? |

Systematic reviews have found no clear evidence of benefit from intra-articular injection of various drugs over placebo injection in people with osteoarthritis of the knee.

Benefits: **Glucocorticoids:** We found one systematic review (published in 1997, 10 RCTs)[44] and one subsequent RCT.[45] The systematic review found that intra-articular injection of glucocorticoids into the knee (one trial used four injections, the rest used single injections) provided little additional pain relief compared with placebo. Pain reduction lasted from 1 week to 1 month.[44] The subsequent RCT (89 people randomised to 4 groups) evaluated a single injection with 24 weeks' follow up.[45] The trial found a short term benefit (1–4 weeks) of the steroid injection compared with placebo for both pain and for a functional index.[44] **Hyaluronan:** We found one systematic review (search date not stated)[44] and four subsequent RCTs.[46–49] The review identified 10 trials of hyaluronan in the knee joint.[44] Treatment consisted of several injections of high molecular weight hyaluronan complexes over several weeks. The review found slightly greater benefit with the injections versus placebo at 1–6 months after treatment. Three of the four subsequent RCTs of hyaluronan injections versus placebo found no significant difference at 2–5 months' follow up, but both active and placebo groups improved compared with baseline.[46–48] One of the trials (240 people) included a subgroup analysis of people aged over 60 years with moderate to severe symptoms; these benefited more with active treatment than placebo.[46] The fourth subsequent RCT (100 people) found significant benefit on the Lequense index with hyaluronan versus placebo, both at 5 weeks ($P = 0.03$) and 4 months ($P = 0.04$).[49] **Other intra-articular treatments:** Several other intra-articular treatments exist, but we found only limited evidence on their effects. Treatments include radioactive isotopes, glycosaminoglycan polysulfuric acid, orgotein, and morphine.[4,50,51]

Harms: We found no reports of serious adverse effects. Localised discomfort after injection is common. A theoretical risk of infection exists, but we found no evidence of this.

Comment: There seems to be little benefit from intra-articular injection beyond any placebo effect. Placebo injection seems to have a substantial beneficial effect. Whether simple aspiration of the knee would be as beneficial as injection remains to be established. We found two non-systematic reviews. Both found no good evidence in favour of hyaluronan.[52,53]

| QUESTION | What are the effects of joint replacement surgery? |

| OPTION | TOTAL HIP REPLACEMENT |

One systematic review and observational studies have found that hip replacement is effective for at least 10 years. Many uncontrolled, observational studies suggest that even better results can be obtained over longer time periods.

Benefits: We found one systematic review (search date 1995, 17 RCTs, 61 observational studies of hip replacements).[54] Mean ages of people in the trials ranged from 43–71 years. The review found that at least 70% of people without prosthetic failure were rated "good/excellent" for pain and function at 10 year follow up (see comment, p 816).

Harms: **Death:** We found one recent systematic review (search date 1995). It pooled data from 130 000 people who had undergone hip replacement and had not received thromboprophylaxis, and found that the rate of fatal pulmonary embolism was 0.1–0.2%, and overall mortality was 0.3–0.4%.[55] One retrospective cohort study (11 607 hip replacements) found mortality to be higher in the first 3 months after surgery than in the subsequent 9 months.[56]

Revision and infection: Two good observational studies found that the risk of a revision operation was about 1% per annum, ranging from 0.2–2.0%.[54,57] Most studies found that revisions were not required until at least 10 years after implantation. One large study, of a patient register in Sweden, found that the proportion of revised hip replacements that were caused by deep infection fell to less than 0.5% between 1978 and 1990. It also found that after the immediate postoperative period aseptic loosening accounted for about 80% of all requirements for replacement or revision surgery.[58] Observational studies found that the initial results of revision surgery were only slightly worse than primary surgery. However, the prostheses deteriorated more quickly.[59–61] One prospective cohort study (39 543 people) on the Norwegian Hip Replacement register found a lower standardised mortality ratio (0.81) for people who had undergone total hip replacement, at mean follow up of 5.2 years (range 0 to 10.4 years).[62]

Comment: A second systematic review (search date 1995) identified 11 RCTs and 180 observational studies comparing different prostheses.[63] It found wide variations in outcome with primary evidence too weak to make valid comparisons. We also found a weak narrative review of 20 mainly small uncontrolled studies evaluating self assessed quality of life (at least two out of the following factors: physical, social, emotional, economic, and overall satisfaction).[64] It found that improvement in non-physical measures occurred most often within 3 months. Benefit was sustained for up to 5 years after surgery. We found no longer term evidence. Most studies did not distinguish between hip replacement for osteoarthritis, and hip replacement for other reasons, which may confound data for osteoarthritis. Outcome of hip replacement for osteoarthritis differs significantly from that for other conditions (e.g. hip fracture in the very elderly and frail, or replacement for rheumatoid arthritis). Additionally, hundreds of observational studies are available. These studies generally find that hip replacement is effective and beneficial. One recent observational study using the Swedish National Total Hip Arthoplasty register (1056 randomly selected people who had not had revision surgery) found that 10 years after surgery people usually had good health (based on SF-36 measures).[65]

OPTION	KNEE REPLACEMENT

One systematic review of RCTs has found that tricompartmental knee joint replacement is effective. One systematic review of observational studies has found better outcomes with unicompartmental versus bicompartmental operations. One subsequent RCT has found that unicompartmental knee replacement is more effective than tricompartmental knee replacement at 5 years follow up. Most studies concentrated on prosthesis survival rather than clinical outcomes.

Benefits: We found one systematic review (search date 1992).[58] **Tricompartmental prostheses:** The review identified 154 studies (4 RCTs, 130 cohort studies, 20 others) of 37 different tricompartmental prostheses in 9879 people (63% with osteoarthritis, mean follow up 4.1 years).[57] Good or excellent outcomes were reported in 89% of people (improved function 5 years after surgery; pain relief after 5 years; mortality rate at 30 days and at 1 year; thromboembolism by 30 days after surgery; no failure of knee prosthesis).[66] **Bicompartmental prostheses:** The review identified no RCTs but found 18 cohort studies (884 people).[58] The review found that bicompartmental prostheses was effective (based on a global knee rating scale that includes pain, function, and range of movement). **Unicompartmental prostheses:** The review identified no RCTs but found 46 cohort studies (2391 people).[58] We found one subsequent RCT.[67] The review found that both procedures were effective (based on a global knee rating scale that includes measures of pain, function, and range of movement), with better outcomes from unicompartmental operations, particularly since 1987.[68] The subsequent RCT (112 people) found that unicompartmental knee replacement is more effective than tricompartmental knee replacement at 5 years follow up. Pain relief was good in both groups, but the number of knees able to flex 120° or more was significantly higher in people treated with unicompartmental replacement (P < 0.001) and there were more excellent results in this group (34/45 v 26/46).[67] **Quality of life:** Two observational studies published since the review found improvement in quality of life after all forms of knee replacement. The first found that knee replacement improved function (measured by WOMAC, from 58.2 before surgery to 18.4 at time of survey).[69] The second, a cross sectional community survey, found that more people had moderate to severe pain (assessed using a modified Knee Society score) before surgery (361/487 people [74%]), than 1 or more years afterwards (100/487 [21%]).[70]

Harms: **Death:** In one 6 year cohort of 338 736 US Medicare patients, the death rate within 30 days of hospital admission for total knee replacement was 2147 (0.63%).[71] The same study reported a mean mortality of 1.5% per annum (no comparative data available).[66] One observational study (208 people) found no significant increase in the risk of death after knee arthoplasty for women (standardized mortality ratio: 1.03, 95% CI 0.76 to 1.37) or men (standardized mortality ratio 1.14, 95% CI 0.68 to 1.80), after a mean follow up of 6 years (range 0 to 20 years).[72] **Thrombosis:** We found one RCT[73] and one prospective cohort study,[63] which reported rates of venous thrombosis: about 24% of people who had a total knee replacement developed a deep vein thrombosis.[74] **Revision and infection:** This is the main long term risk. The first review, mentioned above, found a revision rate of 3.8% during 4.1 years of follow up after tricompartmental replacements.[66] The second review found a revision rate of 9.2% over 4.6 years for unicompartmental prostheses and 7.2% over 3.6 years for bicompartmental prostheses.[68] Large patient register based studies in Sweden found that the cumulative 10 year risk for revision surgery due to infection had fallen to less than 1%. Most implant revision surgery was because of aseptic loosening. For unicompartmental osteoarthritis, unicompartmental knee replacement was an effective alternative to total knee replacement.[75,76]

Postoperative pain: This was rarely recorded, but seemed to be absent or mild in most people. **Wound infection:** We found no good evidence on the frequency of wound infections. One large retrospective cohort study found lower complication rates in centres with a higher volume of procedures.[77]

Comment: We found hundreds of observational studies that reported the time to prosthesis failure or revision surgery, but less evidence on patient related outcomes. The evidence suggests that benefits and harms of knee replacement now appear to be comparable to that of hip replacement.

QUESTION   Which people are most likely to benefit from hip replacement?

Observational studies have found younger age (under 45 years), old age (over 75 years), and obesity to be associated with worse outcomes from hip replacement, in terms of self assessed satisfaction and failure rates.

Benefits: We found no RCTs. One systematic review (published in 1998) identified 40 observational studies (number of people not stated) relating individual characteristics to outcome after hip replacement.[78] It found that the following factors predicted better outcomes in terms of pain relief and function: age 45–75 years; weight less than 70 kg; good social support; higher educational level; and less preoperative morbidity. **Obesity:** One prospective cohort study (176 people) found no difference in the quality of life after a primary hip replacement between the non-obese and moderately obese either at 1 or 3 years, but the study reported results in people with body mass index greater than 40 kg/m^2.[79] **Age:** We found a few large observational studies. They found conflicting evidence, which suggested that older people had good self reported outcomes in terms of pain and function, but spent longer in hospital, needed more rehabilitation, and experienced more perioperative complications.[64,80–85]

Harms: **Revision and infection:** One Swedish cohort study found that younger people and those doing heavy physical work were at greater risk of revision.[58] Another study found lower rates of long term survival of the implant in obese people.[60]

Comment: Consensus groups have reported from Sweden, USA, Canada, and New Zealand.[86–89] Constant pain, particularly night or rest pain, with or without substantial functional impairment, were the generally agreed criteria for joint replacement (see table 3, p 822). In practice, most surgeons prefer to have radiographic evidence of joint damage as well.

QUESTION   Which people are most likely to benefit from knee replacement?

We found limited and conflicting evidence from observational studies.

Benefits: **Obesity:** We found limited and conflicting evidence from observational studies on the effects of obesity on outcome of knee replacement.[90–93] **Age:** We found limited evidence from observational studies suggesting that knee replacement is effective in elderly people.[94,95]

Harms: None found.

Comment: None.

GLOSSARY

Attention only education Information about arthritis but no guidance on self treatment.

Rubefacient An agent that produces mild irritation and redness of the skin.

Self care education Individualised arthritis self care instruction based on patients needs assessment.

Substantive changes since last issue

Exercise New non-systematic review and two subsequent RCTs;[12–14] conclusions unchanged.

Hip replacement New prospective cohort study;[62] conclusions unchanged.

Knee replacement New RCT and new observational study;[72] conclusions unchanged.

REFERENCES

1. Petersson IF. Occurrence of osteoarthritis of the peripheral joints in European populations. *Ann Rheum Dis* 1996;55:659–661.
2. Felson DT. Epidemiology of hip and knee osteoarthritis. *Epidemiol Rev* 1988;10:1–28.
3. Gaffney KL. Intra-articular triamcinolone hexacetonide in knee osteoarthritis: factors influencing the clinical response. *Ann Rheum Dis* 1995;54:379–381.
4. Pavelka JKS. Glycosaminoglycan polysulfuric acid (GAGPS) in osteoarthritis of the knee. *Osteoarthritis Cartilage* 1995;3:15–23.
5. Insall JN, Dorr LD, Scott RD, Scott WN. Rationale of the Knee Society clinical rating system. *Clin Orthopaed Rel Res* 1988;248:13–14.
6. Bellamy N, Buchanan WW, Goldsmith CH, et al. Validation study of WOMAC: A health status instrument for measuring clinically important patient relevant outcomes to antirheumatic drug therapy in patients with osteoarthritis of the hip or knee. *J Rheumatol* 1988;15:1833–1840.
7. Dougados M, Devogelaer JP, Annefeldt M, et al. Recommendations for the registration of drugs used in the treatment of osteoarthritis. *Ann Rheum Dis* 1996;55:552–557.
8. Altman R, Brandt K, Hochberg M, et al. Design and conduct of clinical trials in patients with osteoarthritis: recommendations from a task force of the Osteoarthritis Research Society. *Osteoarthritis Cartilage* 1996;4:217–243.
9. Van Baar ME, Assendelft WJ, Dekker J, et al. Effectiveness of exercise therapy in patients with osteoarthritis of the hip or knee: a systematic review of randomized clinical trials. *Arthritis Rheum* 1999;42:1361–1369. Search date September 1997; primary sources Medline; Embase; Cinahl; and Cochrane Controlled Trials Register.
10. Puett DW, Griffin MR. Published trials of non-medicinal and non-invasive therapies for hip and knee osteoarthritis. *Ann Intern Med* 1994;121:133–140. Search date 1993; primary source Medline.
11. La Mantia K, Marks R. The efficacy of aerobic exercises for treating osteoarthritis of the knee. *NZ J Physiother* 1995;23:23–30. Search date 1994; primary sources Medline; Cinahl; hand searched references; and personal contacts.
12. Baker K, McAlindon TE. Exercise for knee osteoarthritis. *Curr Opin Rheumatol* 2000;12:456–463.
13. Messier SP, Loeser RF, Mitchell MN, et al. Exercise and weight loss in obese older adults with knee osteoarthritis: a preliminary study. *J Am Geriat Soc* 2000;48:1062–1072.
14. Petrella RJ, Bartha C. Home based exercise therapy for older patients with knee osteoarthritis: A randomized clinical trial. *J Rheumatol* 2000;27:2215–2221.
15. Superio-Cabuslay E, Ward MM, Lorig KR. Patient education interventions in osteoarthritis and rheumatoid arthritis: a meta-analytic comparison with non-steroidal anti-inflammatory drug treatment. *Arthritis Care Res* 1996;9:292–301. Search date 1993; primary sources Medline and hand searched references.
16. Mazzuca SA, Brandt KD, Katz BP, et al. Effects of self-care education on the health status of inner-city patients with osteoarthritis of the knee. *Arthritis Rheum* 1997;40:1466–1474.
17. Edworthy SM, Devins GM. Improving medication adherence through patient education distinguishing between appropriate and inappropriate utilization. Patient Education Study Group. *J Rheumatol* 1999;26:793–1801.
18. Maurer BT, Stern AG, Kinossian B, et al. Osteoarthritis of the knee: Isokinetic quadriceps exercise versus and educational intervention. *Arch Phys Med Rehab* 1999;80:1293–1299.
19. Kirkley A, Websterbogaert S, Litchfield R, et al. The effect of bracing on varus gonarthrosis. *J Bone Joint Surg* 1999;81:539–548.
20. Cushnaghan J, McCarthy C, Dieppe P. Taping the patella medially: a new treatment for osteoarthritis of the knee-joint. *BMJ* 1994;308:753–755.
21. Towheed T, Shea B, Wells G, Hochberg M. Analgesia and non-aspirin, non-steroidal anti-inflammatory drugs for osteoarthritis of the hip. In: The Cochrane Library, Issue 3, 2000. Search date 1994; primary sources Medline; Cochrane Library; and Controlled Clinical Trials Register.
22. Towheed TE, Hochberg MC. A systematic review of randomized controlled trials of pharmacological therapy in osteoarthritis of the knee, with an emphasis on trial methodology. *Semin Arthritis Rheum* 1997;26:755–770. Search date August 1994; primary sources Medline and hand searched references.
23. Amadio P, Cummings DM. Evaluation of acetaminophen in the management of osteoarthritis of the knee. *Curr Ther Res Clin Exp* 1983;34:59–66.

24. Hawton K, Ware C, Mistry H, et al. Why patients choose paracetamol for self poisoning and their knowledge of its dangers. BMJ 1995;310:164.

25. Watson MC, Brookes ST, Kirwan JR, Faulkner A. Osteoarthritis: the comparative efficacy of non-aspirin non-steroidal anti-inflammatory drugs for the management of osteoarthritis of the knee. In The Cochrane Library, Issue 4, 1999. Search dates and primary sources Medline January 1980 to December 1995; BIDS 1996; Embase 1995.

26. Huskisson EC, Berry H, Gishen P, et al. Effects of anti-inflammatory drugs on the progression of osteoarthritis of the knee. J Rheumatol 1995;22: 1941–1946.

27. Langman MJ. Non-steroidal anti-inflammatory drugs and peptic ulcer. Hepatogastroenterology 1992;39(suppl 1):37–39.

28. Garcia Rodriguez LA, Williams R, Derby LE, et al. Acute liver injury associated with non-steroidal anti-inflammatory drugs and the role of risk factors. Arch Intern Med 1994;154:311–316.

29. Henry D, Lim LL, Garcia Rodriguez LA, et al. Variability in risk of gastrointestinal complications with individual non-steroidal anti-inflammatory drugs: results of a collaborative meta-analysis. BMJ 1996;312:1563–1566.

30. Brandt KD. Nonsurgical management of osteoarthritis, with an emphasis on nonpharmacologic measures. Arch Fam Med 1995;4:1057–1064.

31. Wollheim FA. Current pharmacological treatment of osteoarthritis. Drugs 1996;52(suppl 3):27–38.

32. Williams HJ, Ward JR, Egger MJ, et al. Comparison of naproxen and acetaminophen in a 2-year study of treatment of osteoarthritis of the knee. Arthritis Rheum 1993;36:1196–1206.

33. Bradley JD, Brandt KD, Katz BP, et al. Comparison of an anti-inflammatory dose of ibuprofen, an analgesic dose of ibuprofen, and acetaminophen in the treatment of patients with osteoarthritis of the knee. N Engl J Med 1991;325:87–91.

34. Solomon I, Abrams G. Orudis in the management of osteoarthritis of the knee. S Afr Med J 1974; 48:1526–1529.

35. Muller F, Gosling J, Erdman G. A comparisonof tolemetin with aspirin in the treatment of osteoarthritis of the knee. S Afr Med J 1977;51: 794–796.

36. Valtonen EJ. Clinical comparison of fenbufen and aspirin in osteoarthritis. Scand J Rheumatol 1979; 27:3–7.

37. March L, Irwig L, Schwarz J, et al. N of 1 trials comparing non-steroidal anti-inflammatory drug with paracetamol in osteoarthritis. BMJ 1993; 309:1041–1046.

38. Moore RA, Tramer MR, Carroll D, et al. Quantitative systematic review of topically applied non-steroidal anti-inflammatory drugs. BMJ 1998; 316:333–338. Search date September 1996; primary sources Embase; Medline; Oxford Pain Relief Database; hand searched references; and librarians and medical directors of 12 pharmaceutical companies asked for reports of their products.

39. Roth SH. A controlled clinical investigation of 3% diclofenac/2.5% sodium hyaluronate topical gel in the treatment of uncontrolled pain in chronic oral NSAID users with osteoarthritis. Int J Tissue React 1995;17:129–132.

40. Grace D, Rogers J, Skeith K, et al. Topical diclofenac versus placebo: a double blind, randomized clinical trial in patients with osteoarthritis of the knee. J Rheumatol 1999;26: 2659–2663.

41. Dickson DJ. A double-blind evaluation of topical piroxicam gel with oral ibuprofen in osteoarthritis of the knee. Curr Ther Res Clin Exp 1991;49: 199–207.

42. Zhang WY, Po ALW. The effectiveness of topically applied capsaicin: a meta-analysis. Eur J Clin Pharmacol 1994;46:517–522. Search date 1994; primary sources BIDS 1980 to 1994; Medline 1980 to 1994, and hand searches of relevant published references.

43. Deal CL, Schnitzer TJ, Lipstein E, et al. Treatment of arthritis with topical capsaicin: a double-blind trial. Clin Ther 1991;13:383–395.

44. Kirwan JRR. Intra-articular therapy in osteoarthritis. Baillieres Clin Rheumatol 1997;11: 769–794. Search date not stated. RCTs cited from 1958 to 1996; primary sources Medline, Embase.

45. Ravaud P, Moulinier L, Giraudeau B, et al. Effects of joint lavage and steroid injection in patients with osteoarthritis of the knee: results of a multicenter, randomized, controlled trial. Arthritis Rheum 1999;42:475–482.

46. Lohmander LSD. Intra-articular hyaluronan injections in the treatment of osteoarthritis of the knee: a randomised, double blind, placebo controlled multicentre trial. Ann Rheum Dis 1996; 55:424–431.

47. Corrado EM, Peluso GF, Gigliotti S. The effects of intra-articular administration of hyaluronic acid on osteoarthritis of the knee: a clinical study with immunological and biochemical evaluations. Eur J Rheumatol Inflamm 1995;15:47–56.

48. Formiguera SSE. Intra-articular hyaluronic acid in the treatment osteoarthritis of the knee: a short term study. Eur J Rheumatol Inflamm 1995;15: 33–38.

49. Huskisson EC, Donnelly S. Hyaluronic acid in the treatment of osteoarthritis of the knee. Rheumatology 1999;38:602–607.

50. McIlwain HSJ. Intra-articular orgotein in osteoarthritis of the knee: a placebo-controlled efficacy, safety, and dosage comparison. Am J Med 1989;87:295–300.

51. Likar RS. Intraarticular morphine analgesia in chronic pain patients with osteoarthritis. Anesth Analg 1997;84:1313–1317.

52. Brandt KD, Smith GN Jr, Simon LS. Intraarticular injection of hyaluronan as treatment for knee osteoarthritis: what is the evidence? Arthritis Rheum 2000;43:1192–203.

53. Adams ME, Lussier AJ, Peyron JG. A risk-benefit assessment of injections of hyaluronan and its derivatives in the treatment of osteoarthritis of the knee. Drug Safety 2000;23:115–130.

54. Faulkner A, Kennedy LG, Baxter K, et al. Effectiveness of hip prostheses in primary total hip replacement: a critical review of evidence and an economic model. Health Technol Assess 1998;2: 1–33. Search date 1995; primary sources Embase, Medline, in-house database on epidemiology and service provision for total hip replacement; additional search on Embase 1990–1996.

55. Murray DW, Britton AR, Bulstrode CJ. Thromboprophylaxis and death after total hip replacement. J Bone Joint Surg Br 1996;78:863–870. Search date 1995; primary source Medline.

56. Seagroatt V, Soon Tan H, Goldacre M, et al. Elective total hip replacement: incidence, emergency readmission rate, and postoperative mortality. BMJ 1991;303:1431–1435.

57. Chang RW, Pellissier JM, Hazen GB. A cost-effectiveness analysis of total hip arthroplasty for osteoarthritis of the hip. JAMA 1996;275:858–865.

58. Malchau H, Herberts P, Ahnfelt L. Prognosis of total hip replacement in Sweden. Follow up of 92 675 operations performed 1978–1990. Acta

Orthop Scand 1993;64:497–506.

59. Robinson AH, Palmer CR, Villar RN. Is revision as good as primary hip replacement? A comparison of quality of life. *J Bone Joint Surg Br* 1999;81: 42–45.

60. Espehaug B, Havelin LI, Engesaeter LB, et al. Patient-related risk-factors for early revision of total hip replacements. A population register-based case-control study of 674 revised hips. *Acta Orthop Scand* 1997;68:207–215.

61. Johnsson R, Franzen H, Nilsson LT. Combined survivorship and multivariate analyses of revisions in 799 hip prostheses. A 10 to 20-year review of mechanical loosening. *J Bone Joint Surg Br* 1994; 76:439–443.

62. Lie SA, Engesaeter LB, Havelin LI, Gjessing HK, Vollset SE. Mortality after total hip replacement: 0–10-year follow-up of 39 543 patients in the Norwegian Arthroplasty Register. *Acta Orthop Scand* 2000;71:19–27.

63. Fitzpatrick R, Shortall E, Sculpher M, et al. Primary total hip replacement surgery: a systematic review of outcomes and modelling of cost-effectiveness associated with different prostheses. *Health Technol Assess* 1998;2:1–64. Search date 1995; primary sources Medline and hand searched references.

64. Towheed TE, Hochberg MC. Health-related quality of life after total hip replacement. *Semin Arthritis Rheum* 1996;26:483–491.

65. Soderman P, Malchau H, Herberts P. Outcome after total hip arthroplasty. Part I. General health evaluation in relation to definition of failure in the Swedish National Total Hip Arthroplasty register. *Acta Ortho Scand* 2000;71:354–359.

66. Callahan CM, Drake BG, Heck DA, et al. Patient outcomes following tricompartmental total knee replacement: a meta-analysis. *JAMA* 1994;271: 1349–1357. Search date 1992; primary sources Medlars and hand searched references.

67. Newman JH, Ackroyd CE, Shah NA. Unicompartmental or total knee replacement? Five-year results of a prospective, randomised trial of 102 osteoarthritic knees with unicompartmental arthritis. *J Bone Joint Surg* 1998;80:862–865.

68. Callahan CM, Drake BG, Heck DA, et al. Patient outcomes following unicompartmental or bicompartmental knee arthroplasty: a meta-analysis. *J Arthroplasty* 1995;10:141–150. Search date 1992; primary sources Medlars and hand searched references.

69. Kiebzak GM, Vain PA, Gregory AM, et al. SF-36 general health status survey to determine patient satisfaction at short-term follow up after total hip and knee arthroplasty. *J South Orthop Assoc* 1997;6:169–172.

70. Hawker G, Wright J, Coyte P, et al. Health related quality of life after knee replacement. *J Bone Joint Surg* 1998;80:163–173.

71. Freund DA. *Assessing and improving outcomes: total knee replacement: patient outcomes research team (PORT): final report.* Maryland, Agency for Health Care Policy and Research, 1997.

72. Bohm P, Holy T, Pietsch-Breitfeld B, Meisner C. Mortality after total knee arthroplasty in patients with osteoarthrosis and rheumatoid arthritis. *Arch Ortho Trauma Surg* 2000;120:75–78.

73. Kim YH. The incidence of deep vein thrombosis after cementless and cemented knee replacement. *J Bone Joint Surg* 1990;72:779–783.

74. Fauno P, Suomalained O, Rehnberg V, et al. Prophylaxis for the prevention of venous thromboembolism after total knee arthroplasty. *J Bone Joint Surg Am* 1994;76:1814–1818.

75. Knutson K, Lewold S, Robertsson O, Lidgren L. The Swedish knee arthroplasty register. A nation-wide study of 30 003 knees. *Acta Orthop Scand* 1994;65:375–386.

76. Robertsson O, Borgquist L, Knutson K, et al. Use of unicompartmental instead of tricompartmental prostheses for unicompartmental arthrosis of the knee is a cost-effective alternative. 15 437 primary tricompartmental prostheses were compared with 10 624 primary medical or lateral unicompartmental prostheses. *Acta Orthop Scand* 1999;70:170–175.

77. Norton EC, Garfinkel SA, McQuay LJ, et al. The effect of hospital volume on the in-hospital complication rate in knee replacement patients. *Health Serv Res* 1998;33:1191–1210.

78. Young NL, Cheah D, Waddell JP, et al. Patient characteristics that affect the outcome of total hip arthroplasty: a review. *Can J Surg* 1998;41:188–195. Search date not stated; primary sources Medline and hand search of references.

79. Chan CL, Villar RN. Obesity and quality of life after primary hip arthroplasty. *J Bone Joint Surg Br* 1996;78:78–81.

80. Espehaug B, Havelin LI, Engesaeter LB, et al. Patient satisfaction and function after primary and revision total hip replacement. *Clin Orthop* 1998; 351:135–148.

81. Garellick G, Malchau H, Herberts P, et al. Life expectancy and cost utility after total hip replacement. *Clin Orthop* 1998;346:141–151.

82. Brander VA, Malhotra S, Jet J, et al. Outcome of hip and knee arthroplasty in persons aged 80 years and older. *Clin Orthop* 1997;345:67–78.

83. Levy RN, Levy CM, Snyder J, et al. Outcome and long-term results following total hip replacement in elderly patients. *Clin Orthop* 1995;316:25–30.

84. Boettcher WG. Total hip arthroplasties in the elderly – morbidity, mortality, and cost-effectiveness. *Clin Orthop* 1992;274:30–34.

85. Braeken AM, Lochaas-Gerlach JA, et al. Determinants of 6–12 month postoperative functional status and pain after elective total hip replacement. *Int J Qual Health Care* 1997;9:413–418.

86. Swedish web site: http://www.sos.se/ sosmenye.htm. Last accessed 27.03.01.

87. National Institutes of Health. Total hip replacement. NIH consensus development panel on total hip replacement. *JAMA* 1995;273:1950–1956.

88. Naylor CD, Williams JI. Primary hip and knee replacement surgery: Ontario criteria for case selection and surgical priority. *Qual Health Care* 1996;5:20–30.

89. Hardorn DC, Holmes AC. The New Zealand priority criteria project. *BMJ* 1997;314:131–134.

90. Donnell ST, Neyret P, Dejour H, et al. The effect of age on the quality of life after knee replacement. *Knee* 1998;5:125–112.

91. De Leeuw JM, Villar RN. Obesity and quality of life after primary total knee replacement. *Knee* 1998; 5:119–23.

92. Lubitz R, Dittus R, Robinson R, et al. Effects of severe obesity on health status 2 years after knee replacement. *J Gen Intern Med* 1996;11:145.

93. Winiarsky R, Barth P, Lotke P. Total knee arthroplasty in morbidly obese patients. *J Bone J Surg Am* 1998;80;1770–1774.

94. Ettinger WH Jr, Burns R, Messier SP, et al. A randomized trial comparing aerobic exercise and resistance exercise with a health education program in older adults with knee osteoarthritis. The fitness arthritis and seniors trial (FAST). *JAMA* 1997;277:25–31.

95. Laskin, RS. Total knee replacement in patients older than 85 years. *Clin Orthop* 1999;367:43–49.

Paul Dieppe
Director

Jiri Chard
Research Associate

MRC Health Services
Research Collaboration
University of Bristol
Bristol
UK

Alex Faulkner
Research Fellow
University of Wales
Cardiff, UK

Stefan Lohmander
Professor
Department of Orthopaedics
Lund University
Lund, Sweden
Competing interests: None declared.

TABLE 1	Estimated relative risk of gastrointestinal adverse effects with the use of individual NSAIDs (pooled data from 12 studies) (see text, p 810).[29]

Drug	Pooled RR	95% CI for pooled RR
Ibuprofen (low dose)*	1.0	–
Fenoprofen	1.6	1.0 to 2.5
Aspirin	1.6	1.3 to 2.0
Diclofenac	1.8	1.4 to 2.3
Sulindac	2.1	1.6 to 2.7
Diflunisal	2.2	1.2 to 4.1
Naproxen	2.2	1.7 to 2.9
Indomethacin	2.4	1.9 to 3.1
Tometin	3.0	1.8 to 4.9
Piroxicam	3.8	2.7 to 5.2
Ketoprofen	4.2	2.7 to 6.4
Azapropazone	9.2	4.0 to 21.0

*Comparative data used low dose ibuprofen as the reference control for calculating the relative risk of other drugs.

TABLE 2	Effect sizes (95% CI) of exercise in osteoarthritis of the knee and hip: results of the best three RCTs identified in a systematic review (see text, p 813).[9]

RCT	Pain	Observed disability
1	0.31 (0.28 to 0.34)	0.31 (0.28 to 0.34)
2	0.47 (0.44 to 0.50)	0.89 (0.85 to 0.93)
3	0.58 (0.54 to 0.62)	0.28 (0.24 to 0.32)

TABLE 3	Summary of New Zealand priority criteria for joint replacement (see text, p 818).[89]

Severity is scored out of a possible 100 on the basis of:
Pain: severity 0–20; duration 0–20
Function: walking difficulty 0–10; other 0–10
Joint damage: pain on passive movement 0–10; other/X-ray 0–10
Other: other joints 0–10; work, care giving, independence 0–10

Plantar heel pain (including plantar fasciitis)

Search date January 2001

Fay Crawford

QUESTIONS

Effects of treatments for plantar heel pain. 825

INTERVENTIONS

Unknown effectiveness

Steroid injections alone or plus local anaesthetic injection versus placebo (short term) 825

Casted orthoses (custom made insoles). 827

Heel pads. 828

Pain medication 828

Extracorporeal shock wave therapy (ESWT) 829

Surgery 830

Lasers 830

Ultrasound 830

Night splints 831

Trade off between benefits and harms

Steroid plus local anaesthetic injection versus local anaesthetic injections alone or plus pads (short term). 825

Likely to be ineffective or harmful

Steroid injections alone versus placebo (medium to long term) 825

Steroid plus local anaesthetic injection versus pads (medium to long term) 825

Steroid plus local anaesthetic injection versus local anaesthetic alone (medium to long term) 829

To be covered in future issues of *Clinical Evidence*

Prevention of heel pain

Oral analgesics

See glossary, p 831

Key Messages

■ RCTs have found that symptoms resolve spontaneously in most people allocated to placebo.

■ One RCT found limited evidence of short term improvement in pain for steroid injections plus lignocaine versus rignocaine alone. This small clinical effect was not found in the group receiving lignocaine plus local anaesthetic plus nerve block, and no evidence of medium to long term benefit was found.

■ Observational studies have found a high rate of plantar fascia rupture and other complications associated with steroid injections, which may lead to chronic disability in some people.

■ We found conflicting evidence on the effect of steroid plus local anaesthetic injections versus pads. One RCT found limited evidence of effectiveness for short term improvement in pain for steroid plus lignocaine injections versus pads. A second RCT using a different type of pad and different outcomes found no significant difference. Neither RCT found medium to long term benefit from steroid plus lignocaine injections.

■ We found no evidence from systematic reviews or RCTs of medium to long term benefit for steroid injections with or without local anaesthetics versus placebo or other treatments.

Plantar heel pain (including plantar fasciitis)

- We found conflicting evidence about the benefit of orthoses versus heel pads. Trials involved different regimens.
- One systematic review of one weak RCT found limited evidence of a benefit with extracorporeal shock wave therapy (ESWT) versus placebo.
- We found no RCTs of surgery.
- One systematic review found no significant benefit from laser, ultrasound, or night splints versus placebo or no treatment.

DEFINITION Plantar heel pain is soreness or tenderness of the heel. It often radiates from the central part of the heel pad or the medial tubercle of the calcaneum, but may extend along the plantar fascia into the medial longitudinal arch of the foot. Severity may range from an irritation at the origin of the plantar fascia, noticeable on rising after rest, to an incapacitating pain. This review excludes clinically evident underlying disorders, for example, infection, calcaneal fracture, and calcaneal nerve entrapment, which can be distinguished by their characteristic history and signs. (A calcaneal fracture may present after trauma, whereas calcaneal nerve entrapment gives rise to shooting pains and feelings of "pins and needles" on the medial aspect of the heel.)

INCIDENCE/ PREVALENCE The incidence and prevalence of plantar heel pain is uncertain. Plantar heel pain primarily affects those in mid to late life.[1]

AETIOLOGY/ RISK FACTORS Unknown.

PROGNOSIS One systematic review (search date 1998) found that almost all the included trials reported an improvement in discomfort regardless of the intervention received (including placebo).[1] A telephone survey of 100 people treated conservatively (average follow up 47 months) found that 82 people had resolution of symptoms, 15 had continued symptoms but no limitations of activity or work, and three had continued symptoms that limited activity or changed work status.[2] Thirty one people said that they would have seriously considered surgical treatment at the time medical attention was sought. The three people still with limitation had bilateral symptoms but no other clear risk factors.

AIMS To reduce pain and immobility, with minimal adverse effects.

OUTCOMES Pain reduction (using visual analogue scales [VAS]); walking distance.

METHODS *Clinical Evidence* search and appraisal January 2001.

What are the effects of treatments for plantar heel pain?

STEROID INJECTIONS

One systematic review of one small RCT found no significant reduction in pain with steroid injection versus placebo. One systematic review of one small RCT found no significant difference in pain relief with steroid injection versus heel pads (see glossary, p 831).

Benefits: We found one systematic review (search date 1998).[1] **Versus placebo or no treatment:** The review found one small RCT of steroid (hydrocortisone acetate 25 mg) versus saline injection in 19 people with recalcitrant heel pain but not arthritis.[1] It found no significant difference in pain relief (RR 0.52, 95% CI 0.15 to 1.79). **Versus orthoses:** The review found no RCTs. **Versus pads:** The review found one small RCT (17 people) of steroid (20 mg triamcinolone 2%) versus a prefabricated silicone type heel pad. Although more people improved after treatment with the heel pad (66% v 33% at 12 weeks) the difference was not significant at 1, 2, or 12 weeks. **Versus pain medication alone:** The review found no RCTs.

Harms: Steroid injections can be painful. In one study of 106 people, all heels were injected through the medial aspect of the heel pad. Half of the participants were given a tibial nerve block to reduce discomfort during the injection, but there was no significant difference in pain at time of injection between those who received the nerve block and those who did not. Local steroid injection may lead to infection, subcutaneous fat atrophy, skin pigmentation changes, fascial rupture, infection, peripheral nerve injury, or muscle damage.[3] Observational studies have reported rupture of the plantar fascia in people receiving steroid injections.[4,5] One study reported a 10% incidence of rupture out of 122 injected heels,[4] and a second study reported ruptures in 33% of 37 people given injections.[5] The original heel pain may be relieved after rupture, but arch and midfoot strain, lateral plantar nerve dysfunction, stress fracture, deformity, and swelling may result from plantar fascia rupture, and may persist.

Comment: All trials were small. Heterogeneity of interventions prevented data pooling. The evidence from observational studies makes it difficult to define the clinical importance of rupture of the plantar fascia, and may incorporate confounding factors.

STEROID INJECTIONS PLUS LOCAL ANAESTHESIA

One systematic review and a subsequent RCT found no evidence of a significant long term benefit from steroid plus local anaesthetic injections versus alternative treatments, and only limited evidence of a short term benefit.

Benefits: We found one systematic review (search date 1998), which included RCTs of injected steroid plus local anaesthetic versus various other treatments.[1] **Versus placebo or no treatment:** The review found no RCTs. **Versus heel pads:** See glossary, p 831. The

Plantar heel pain (including plantar fasciitis)

review[1] found one RCT, and we found one subsequent RCT.[6] The first RCT included people with pain on the plantar aspect of the heel but excluded people on anti-inflammatory medication, people who had a steroid injection in the last 6 months, people with rheumatoid arthritis, and people with pain that radiated along the plantar fascia more distally. It compared three arms, a heel pad alone versus an injection alone (triamcinolone hexacteonide + 2% lignocaine) versus injection plus pad. Analysis was not by intention to treat, and four people (5%) were lost to follow up. After 1 month, the greatest improvement in pain was in people who received the injection alone (22 people), with the least improvement in people who had the pad alone (26 people) (100 mm VAS scale, injection alone v pad alone WMD −45 mm, 95% CI −59 to −31). At 24 weeks, there was greater pain reduction with the injection alone versus the pad alone, but the difference was not significant (85% v 75%). The subsequent RCT included 103 people with plantar heel tenderness, a history of pain upon rising in the morning (first step pain), and no history of trauma in the previous 3 months.[6] Analysis was not intention to treat and 18 people were lost to follow up. It compared three arms: non-steroidal anti-inflammatory drugs (NSAIDs) plus three steroid plus local anaesthetic injections into the heel (anti-inflammatory, 35 people) versus heel pads plus paracetamol (acetaminophen) as required (accommodative, 33 people) versus a heel pad prior to fitting of custom made orthoses (see glossary, p 831) (mechanical, people). The anti-inflammatory regimen consisted of 2 x 300 mg capsules of etodolac and 0.5 ml dexamethasone sodium phosphate 4 mg/ml plus 0.55 bupivacaine hydrochloride without epinephrine. If there was no response then 0.2 ml of dexamethasone acetate 16 mg/ml injection was added cumulatively to the second (2 weeks) and third (4 weeks) injections. The RCT found slightly greater pain relief among people treated by the anti-inflammatory regimen compared with the accommodative regimen at 3 months, but the difference was not significant (10 cm VAS, WMD −1.2 cm, 95% CI −2.8 to +0.4). **Versus heel pad and orthoses:** The review found no RCTs. We found no RCTs versus orthoses alone. We found one subsequent RCT comparing an anti-inflammatory regimen versus mechanical regimen.[6] At 3 months, people treated with a heel pad and orthoses had improved more, but the difference was not significant (WMD −1, 95% CI −2.5 to +0.5). **Versus local anaesthetic alone:** The review found no RCTs. We found one subsequent RCT (106 people).[7] It compared a single injection of 1 ml 25 mg/ml prednisolone acetate plus 1 ml 2% lignocaine hydrochloride versus 2 ml 2% lignocaine hydrochloride alone. It found a small benefit with the combined injection at 1 month, the clinical relevance of which is considered small (10 cm VAS, WMD −0.8, 95% CI −1.5 to −0.2), but no significant difference in pain thereafter (3 months, WMD 0.1, 95% CI −1.2 to +1.3 and 6 months, 0.5, 95% CI −0.8 to +1.7). **Versus steroid alone:** The review found no RCTs. **Versus steroid plus local anaesthetic plus pad:** The review[1] found one RCT in 76 people, which found significantly worse results at 1 month after treatment with the heel pad plus injection versus steroid injection plus local anaesthetic (100 mm VAS, WMD −16 mm, 95% CI −31 to −1). However, at 24 weeks, people treated with pad plus injection versus injection alone had less pain, but this was not significant (94% v 85%). **Steroid plus local anaesthetic plus pad versus pad alone:** The review[1] found one RCT in 76 people. It found a significantly better response with injection plus pad versus pad alone at 4 weeks and 12 weeks, but not at 24 weeks (100 mm VAS; at 4 weeks figures not available; at 24 weeks WMD −10.7 mm, 95% CI −25.5 to +4.1, 94% v 75% pain reduction).

Harms: No trials reported on harms.

Comment: All trials were small. Heterogeneity of interventions prevented data pooling. A recent survey of UK rheumatologists found that corticosteroid injections are the most common treatment of heel pain and are used by 98% of UK rheumatologists (F Crawford, personal communication, 2000), confirming the results of similar surveys.[3] We found no placebo controlled RCTs of steroid injections plus local anaesthesia, and no evidence of medium to long term efficacy in RCTs comparing this treatment with other options. We found evidence from two observational studies of high rates of moderate harms from this treatment (see harms of steroid injections, p 825). This is also consistent with evidence about harms of steroid injections in other areas.[3] These harms are particularly relevant because the evidence of benefit is poor, and spontaneous resolution of symptoms is common. The RCTs have many flaws (lack of intention to treat analysis, high withdrawal rates, and lack of placebo control). Limitations of the available evidence make the use of steroid injections in heel pain difficult to categorise.

OPTION	CUSTOM MADE ORTHOSES

A systematic review found no evidence about the benefit of orthoses versus placebo or no treatment for heel pain. A few RCTs found limited evidence about the benefit of orthoses versus other treatments for heel pain.

Benefits: We found one systematic review (search date 1998).[1] **Versus placebo or no treatment:** The review found no RCTs. **Orthoses plus heel pad versus steroid plus pain medication:** The review[1] found no RCTs. We found one subsequent RCT, which found no significant difference in pain improvement.[6] **Orthoses plus heel pad versus heel pads plus pain medication:** The review found one RCT of a heel pad applied for 4 weeks prior to fitting of custom made orthoses heel pad (28 people) versus a viscoelastic heel pad plus paracetamol (acetaminophen) as required (26 people). It found significantly better pain reduction with pad plus orthoses (10 cm VAS; WMD −2.2 mm, 95% CI −3.8 to −0.5). **Orthoses plus stretching versus heel pad plus stretching:** The review found no RCTs. We found one subsequent RCT (236 people, 5 groups) in people with maximal tenderness over the medial calcaneal tuberosity for which they had received no previous treatment.[8] People with systemic disease, sciatica, or local nerve entrapment were excluded. The RCT compared customised orthoses plus stretching exercises versus prefabricated shoe inserts made from three different materials (silicone, felt, and rubber) plus stretching exercises (achilles and plantar fascial stretching for 10 minutes twice daily). It found significantly less pain at 8 weeks in people who were assigned to prefabricated inserts (results combined) versus orthoses (P = 0.007). **Orthoses plus stretching versus stretching alone:** The review found no RCTs. We found one subsequent RCT of custom made orthoses plus stretching exercises versus stretching exercises alone. It found no significant difference in pain improvement at 8 weeks (100 mm VAS; WMD −3.2 mm, 95% CI −17.4 to +11.0).

Harms: No trials reported on harms.

Comment: Subgroup analysis in the RCT comparing orthoses versus heel pads found that, among people who stood for more than 8 hours daily, a greater reduction in pain was achieved with stretching alone than with customised insoles.[8] It found no significant difference in people who stood for less than 8 hours a day. This hypothesis requires testing as the primary outcome in an RCT. Only half the participants in this subgroup analysis responded to the pain questionnaire.

OPTION   **HEEL PADS AND HEEL CUPS**

One systematic review found no evidence about heel pads and heel cups (see glossary, p 831) versus placebo or no treatment for heel pain. A few small RCTs of heel pads and heel cups versus other treatments for heel pain provided no strong evidence.

Benefits: We found one systematic review (search date 1998),[1] which included RCTs of heel pads and heel cups versus various treatments. **Versus placebo or no treatment:** The review found no RCTs.[1] **Versus steroid:** The review found one small RCT, which found no significant difference in pain improvement (see benefits of steroids versus heel pads, p 825 and benefits of steroids plus pain mediation versus heel pads, p 825). **Versus steroid plus pain medication:** The review found one RCT, which found better short term outcomes with steroid plus lignocaine injections.[1] One subsequent RCT found no significant difference in pain improvement between steroid injection plus NSAIDs versus pads plus paracetamol (see benefits under steroids plus local anaesthesia, p 825).[6] **Versus customised orthoses:** The review found one RCT[1] and we found one subsequent RCT.[6] They found conflicting evidence on improvement in pain (see benefits under customised orthoses, p 827). **Heel pad plus steroid plus local anaesthetic versus steroid plus local anaesthetic:** The review found one RCT.[1] It found a short term benefit with the steroid plus local anaesthetic injection alone (see benefits under steroids plus local anaesthesia, p 825).

Harms: None of the trials reported harms.

Comment: Heel cups and heel pads can be made from several different materials, but rubber, viscoelastic, and silicone can be bought as prefabricated shoe inserts. Podiatrists or orthotists sometimes use felt and foam to construct heel pads.

OPTION   **LOCAL ANAESTHETIC INJECTION**

One systematic review found no evidence about the benefit of local anaesthesia versus placebo or no treatment for heel pain. A few small RCTs found limited evidence about the benefit of local anaesthesia versus other treatments.

Benefits: We found one systematic review (search date 1998).[1] **Local anaesthetic versus placebo or no treatment:** The review found no RCTs.[1] **Local anaesthetic versus steroids plus local anaesthetic:** The review found one RCT (see benefits of steroids plus local anaesthesia, p 825), which found a short term benefit with combined treatment.[1] **Local anaesthetic plus steroid versus orthoses:** The review found one RCT of NSAIDs plus up to three steroid injections versus orthoses (see benefits under customised orthoses, p 827, or heel pads, p 828).[1] It found no advantage with NSAIDs. **Local anaesthetic plus steroid versus local anaesthetic plus steroid plus pad:** The review identified one RCT, which found a better result at 1 month without the pad (see benefits under steroids plus local anaesthesia, p 825).[1] **Local anaesthetic plus steroid plus pad versus pad alone:** The review found one RCT, which found a better result at 1 month with lignocaine plus pads versus pads alone (see benefits under steroids plus local anaesthesia, p 825).[1]

Harms: None of the trials reported on harms.

Comment: Adrenaline is not recommended in local anaesthetics for procedures involving the appendages because of the risk of ischaemic necrosis.[9]

| OPTION | EXTRACORPOREAL SHOCK WAVE THERAPY |

One systematic review of one poor quality RCT found limited evidence of a benefit with ESWT versus sham. One subsequent RCT found a small, non-significant reduction of pain with ESWT versus sham ESWT. Two RCTs found limited evidence of a greater improvement with high dose versus low dose ESWT.

Benefits: **Versus placebo:** We found one systematic review (search date 1998)[1] and one subsequent RCT of ESWT (see glossary, p 831).[10] The review found one single blind RCT in 36 people with recalcitrant heel pain, which compared 1000 impulses ($0.06 \, mJ/mm^2$) versus placebo (sham ESWT) three times at weekly intervals. It found that pain on manual pressure and pain free walking ability were significantly improved at 6 weeks ($P < 0.005$). Six people withdrew from the trial and analysis was not intention to treat. The small subsequent RCT in people with recalcitrant heel pain found no significant difference between ESWT at 1500 pulses at 3 Hz versus sham treatment (37 people, 100 mm VAS; WMD −15 mm, 95% CI −45 to +15).[10] **Different doses:** The review identified one non-blinded RCT[1] and one additional RCT.[11] The RCT in the review (119 people) compared 1000 impulses versus 10 impulses of $0.08 \, mJ/mm^2$ in people with recalcitrant heel pain. All treatments were given three times at weekly intervals. It found greater improvements in pressure pain between weeks 0–12 with the higher dose (100 mm VAS, WMD −47 mm, 95% CI −54 to −40). The additional RCT (50 people) compared 3×500 impulses of ESWT versus 3×100 impulses (both at intensity $0.08 \, mJ/mm^2$) in people with recalcitrant heel pain.[11] It found no significant difference in pain on pressure at 6 weeks (10 cm VAS: WMD −0.4, 95% CI −2.0 to +1.2) or at 12 weeks (WMD −1.4, 95% CI −3.0 to 0.2). There was also no significant difference in walking pain at 6 weeks (WMD −0.8, 95% CI −2.4 to +0.7) or at 12 weeks (WMD −0.9, 95% CI −2.5 to +0.7). Self reported walking pain at 12 months suggested a marginal long term benefit from higher doses of ESWT (10 cm VAS: WMD −2.0 cm, 95% CI −3.7 to −0.2).

Harms: ESWT without local anaesthetic can be painful.

Comment: All trial participants had recalcitrant heel pain. Availability of ESWT is limited. RCTs and reviews are mainly from German speaking countries. Pain associated with ESWT and differences in procedures mean the single blinding in the first placebo controlled RCT was probably not maintained.[1]

OPTION   SURGERY

One systematic review found no RCTs of surgery for heel pain.

Benefits: We found one systematic review (search date 1998).[1] It identified no RCTs of surgery for heel pain.

Harms: We found no evidence.

Comment: One systematic review (search date 1998) identified many observational studies of surgery for chronically painful heels.[1] One of the largest observational studies (76 people) compared postoperative complication rates after endoscopic fasciotomy versus traditional plantar fasciotomy.[12] It found that serious complications were more common in people treated with endoscopic fasciotomy (35% v 17%).

OPTION   LASERS

One systematic review of one small RCT found no evidence of benefit with lasers versus placebo.

Benefits: One systematic review (search date 1998) identified one small RCT of laser therapy versus placebo (treatment with a disabled laser) in 32 people with pain of at least 1 months' duration, tenderness to pressure at the origin of the plantar fascia, on the mid-anterior inferior border of the calcaneus, and sharp shooting, and/or localised inferior foot pain made worse with activity or on rising in the morning.[1] It found no evidence of a significant effect.

Harms: The RCT[1] reported that 96% of people had no adverse effects, and the rest (4%) reported a mild sensation during or after treatment.

Comment: None.

OPTION   ULTRASOUND

One systematic review of one small RCT found no evidence of a significant effect.

Benefits: One systematic review (search date 1998) included one small RCT in 19 people (7 with bilateral heel pain) of eight treatments of true ultrasound versus the same number of applications of placebo (sham ultrasound).[1] Inclusion criteria were pain radiating from the medial tubercle of the calcaneum in response to both pressure and weight bearing first thing in the morning. The trial found no significant effect (WMD 0.1, 95% CI −1.8 to +2.1).

Harms: The trial did not look for harms.

Comment: None.

OPTION	NIGHT SPLINTS

One RCT found no evidence of an effect from wearing night splints.

Benefits: One systematic review found no good quality trials.[1] We found one additional RCT in 116 people with recalcitrant heel pain (people with bilateral presentations of heel pain were excluded).[13] All participants received ankle dorsiflexion exercises and piroxicam 20 mg daily for 30 days, with (54 people) or without (59 people) a night splint which dorsiflexed the ankle joint by 5°. The night splint was worn for 3 months. The trial found no evidence of an effect on pain (RR 1.0, 95% CI 0.8 to 1.3).

Harms: The trial did not look for harms.

Comment: The trial excluded people with bilateral disease because of potential inconvenience and poor compliance from wearing two night splints simultaneously.

GLOSSARY

Custom made orthoses Made from polyurethene or similar material to a negative cast of a person's foot.

Extracorporeal shock wave therapy (ESWT) Shock waves are pulsed acoustic waves that dissipate mechanical energy at the interface of two substances with different acoustic impedance.

Heel cups Prefabricated rubber heel cups (firmer than viscoelastic heel pads) that extend up the sides of the heel and enclose the fibro fatty heel pad.

Heel pads Prefabricated viscoelastic heel pads made of malleable material.

REFERENCES

1. Atkins D, Crawford F, Edwards J, et al. A systematic review of treatments for the painful heel. *Rheumatology* 1999;38:968–973. Search date 1998; BIDS database, and hand searches of *The Chiropodist, The Journal of British Podiatric Medicine,* and *The Foot* and personal contact with experts.
2. Wolgin M, Cook C, Graham C, et al. Conservative treatment of plantar heel pain: long term follow up. *Foot Ankle Int* 1994;15:97–102.
3. Fadale PD, Wiggins MD. Corticosteroid Injections: their use and abuse. *J Am Acad Orthop Surg* 1994;2:133–140.
4. Acevedo JI, Beskin JL. Complications of plantar fascial rupture associated with steroid injection. *Foot Ankle Int* 1998;19:91–97.
5. Sellman JR. Plantar fascial rupture associated with corticosteroid injection. *Foot Ankle Int* 1994;15: 376–381.
6. Lynch DM, Goforth WP, Martin JE, et al. Conservative treatment of plantar fasciitis. A prospective study. *J Am Podiatr Assoc* 1998;88: 377–380.
7. Crawford F, Atkins D, Young P, et al. Steroid injection for heel pain: evidence of short term effectiveness. A randomised controlled trial. *Rheumatology* 1999;38:974–977.
8. Pfeffer G, Bacchetti P, Deland J, et al. Comparison of custom and prefabricated orthoses in the initial treatment of proximal plantar fasciitis. *Foot Ankle Int* 1999;20:214–221.
9. McCauley WA, Gerace RV, Scilley C. Treatment of accidental digital injection of epinephrine. *Ann Emerg Med* 1991;6:665–668.
10. Speed CA, Nichols DW, Burnett SP, et al Extracorporeal shock wave therapy (ESWT) in plantar fasciitis. A pilot double blind randomised placebo controlled study [abstract]. *Rheumatology* 2000;39(suppl 123):230.
11. Krischeck O, Rompe JD, Herbsthrofer B, et al. Symptomatic low-energy shockwave therapy in heel pain and radiologically detected plantar heel spur [in German]. *Z Orthop Ihre Grenzgeb* 1998; 136:169–174.
12. Kinley S, Frascone S, Calderone D, et al. Endoscopic plantar fasciotomy versus traditional heel spur surgery: a prospective study. *J Foot Ankle Surg* 1993;32:595–603.
13. Probe RA, Baca M, Adams R, et al. Night splint treatment for plantar fasciitis. *Clin Orthop* 1999; 368:191–195.

Fay Crawford
MRC Fellow, University of York, York, UK

Competing interests: None declared.

Rheumatoid arthritis

Musculoskeletal disorders

Search date February 2001

Maria Suarez-Almazor and Wednesday Foster

QUESTIONS

INTERVENTIONS

Key Messages

- Systematic reviews of RCTs have found that early intervention with a disease modifying antirheumatic drug (DMARD) improves outcome at 1 year.

- Most DMARDs have been shown to be more effective than placebo in reducing disease activity and joint inflammation, but the effect of prolonged treatment with DMARDs (for more than a year) has not been adequately evaluated in RCTs.

- Systematic reviews of RCTs found no evidence of a difference in effectiveness between most DMARDs, although auranofin seems to be the least effective.

- One systematic review and five subsequent RCTs have found that some combinations of two or more DMARDs might be beneficial. The long term effects of these combined therapies have not been established.

- Systematic reviews of RCTs have found that low dose oral steroids relieve symptoms and may slow radiological progression. However, long term use carries the risk of serious adverse effects.
- Five RCTs have found that tumour necrosis factor antagonists reduce disease activity and joint inflammation. Short term toxicity was low, but the long term risk is unknown. Optimal dosages and duration of treatment have not been clearly established.

DEFINITION　　Rheumatoid arthritis is a chronic inflammatory disorder. It is characterised by a chronic polyarthritis affecting primarily the peripheral joints and related periarticular tissues. It usually starts as an insidious symmetric polyarthritis, often with non-specific systemic symptoms. Diagnostic criteria include arthritis lasting longer than 6 weeks, positive rheumatoid factor, and radiological damage.[1]

INCIDENCE/　Prevalence ranges from 0.5 to 1.5% of the population in industria-
PREVALENCE　lised countries.[2,3] Rheumatoid arthritis occurs more frequently in women than men (ratio 2.5 to 1).[2,3] The annual incidence in women was recently estimated at 36/100 000 and in men 14/100 000.[3]

AETIOLOGY/　The evidence suggests that the cause is multifactorial in people with
RISK FACTORS genetic susceptibility.[4]

PROGNOSIS　The course of rheumatoid arthritis is variable and unpredictable. Some people experience flares and remissions, and others a progressive course. Over the years, structural damage may occur, often leading to articular deformities and functional impairment. About half of people will be disabled or unable to work within 10 years.[5] Rheumatoid arthritis shortens life expectancy.[6]

AIMS　　　To relieve symptoms; and to reduce mortality and disability, with minimum adverse effects.

OUTCOMES　Number of swollen or tender joints; pain score; acute phase reactants such as erythrocyte sedimentation rate (ESR); functional status; patient and physician global assessments; radiological progression; and rates of withdrawal from treatment. Many of the RCTs in rheumatoid arthritis use, as some of their primary outcomes, proxy measures such as acute phase reactants and radiological progression. These measures are normally not clinically relevant to people with rheumatoid arthritis. Many meta-analyses also report outcomes as effect sizes, which are difficult to interpret clinically. In future editions, *Clinical Evidence* will attempt to include more quality of life measures, measures of function, and report results in the most clinically relevant form possible. The American College of Rheumatology has established criteria for improvement to be used in clinical trials. ACR20 criteria specify a 20% reduction in swollen and tender joints and 20% improvement in at least three of the following: pain, function, patient and physician global assessments, and acute phase reactants. ACR50 and ACR70 use a 50% or 70% improvement in the same parameters. RCTs of many new treatments, such as biological agents, use these aggregate indices as primary end points.[7] Radiological progression is assessed in many RCTs by reference to standard films. The Larsen score, for instance, provides six grades of severity ranging from normal (Larsen Grade 0) to mutilating abnor-

Musculoskeletal disorders

mality (Larsen Grade V). However, the question of what constitutes a clinically important change remains unresolved.

METHODS   *Clinical Evidence* update search and appraisal February 2001.

QUESTION   What are the effects of disease modifying antirheumatic drugs?

OPTION   METHOTREXATE

One systematic review of short term RCTs has found that methotrexate is more effective than placebo in reducing joint inflammation and radiological progression, and improving functional status in people with rheumatoid arthritis. Four systematic reviews of RCTs have found no consistent differences between methotrexate and other DMARDs, but observational studies have found that people are more likely to continue therapy with methotrexate than with other DMARDs.

Benefits: **Versus placebo:** We found one systematic review (search date 1997, 5 RCTs, 161 people) of low dose methotrexate for 12–18 weeks (usually < 20 mg per week) versus placebo.[8] It found a significant improvement in the number of swollen and tender joints, pain score, physician and patient global assessment, and functional status. There was no significant difference in ESR. **Versus other DMARDs:** We found four systematic reviews of comparative RCTs (search dates 1989,[9] 1990,[10] 1988,[11] not specified[12]). They found no consistent differences between methotrexate and other DMARDs. RCTs, found methotrexate versus placebo reduced radiological progression, but was not significantly different from leflunomide (see benefits of leflunomide, p 840).[13]

Harms: One systematic review (search date 1997, 5 RCTs, 161 people)[8] of methotrexate versus placebo found more people on methotrexate withdrew because of adverse effects (22% v 7%). The adverse effects were mainly liver enzyme abnormalities (AR for liver abnormalities: 11% on methotrexate v 2.6% on placebo; ARI 9%; RR 4.5, 95% CI 1.6 to 11.0; NNH 11, 95% CI 4 to 65).[8] Other common adverse effects were mucocutaneous, gastrointestinal, or haematological. Pulmonary toxicity, hepatic fibrosis, and infections occur occasionally, even at the low dosages usually used in rheumatoid arthritis. Another systematic review found that concurrent administration of folic acid decreased the risk of gastrointestinal and mucocutaneous adverse effects (AR 51% with folic acid v 83% without folic acid; ARR 33%, 95% CI 14% to 51%; NNT 3, 95% CI 2 to 7) with no adverse impact on the efficacy of methotrexate.[14] Although some studies reported an increased risk of tumours, results have not been consistent.[15]

Comment: Observational studies (3 prospective, 1 retrospective) have found that people with rheumatoid arthritis are more likely to continue methotrexate than any other DMARD.[16–19] One systematic review of observational studies comparing methotrexate versus other DMARDs on radiological progression found a significant benefit from methotrexate only when compared with azathioprine (P = 0.049).[20] It found no significant difference between methotrexate and parenteral gold (results not quantified).

OPTION | **ANTIMALARIALS**

One systematic review of RCTs has found that hydroxychloroquine versus placebo reduces disease activity and joint inflammation in people with rheumatoid arthritis. Older, poorer quality RCTs also found benefit from chloroquine versus placebo. Two RCTs found no evidence of a benefit on functional status and radiological progression. Systematic reviews of RCTs found no significant difference in effectiveness between antimalarials and other DMARDs.

Benefits: **Versus placebo:** We found one systematic review (search date 1997, 4 RCTs of hydroxychloroquine given for 6–12 months, 371 people).[21] The review reported a significant improvement in the number of swollen and tender joints, pain score, physician and patient global assessment, and ESR. One RCT found no significant difference in functional status (119 people), and another RCT (91 people) found no significant difference in radiological progression. **Versus other DMARDs:** We found four systematic reviews of RCTs (search dates 1989,[9] 1990,[10] 1988,[11] not specified[12]). They found no significant differences between antimalarials and other DMARDs. Individual RCTs found no consistent advantage for any one drug, although some found better results with penicillamine and sulfasalazine than with antimalarials. **Hydroxychloroquine versus chloroquine:** We found no RCTs adequately comparing chloroquine versus hydroxychloroquine; one older RCT included both drugs but did not report a direct comparison.[22]

Harms: The systematic review (search date 1997, 4 placebo controlled RCTs) found no significant difference in the number of withdrawals because of adverse effects.[21] **Ocular toxicity:** No participants discontinued treatment because of ocular adverse effects, and mild toxicity was reported in only one person.[21] One long term retrospective observational study (97 people) found that more people receiving chloroquine alone versus hydroxychloroquine developed retinopathy (6/31 [19.4%] v 0/66 [0%]).[23] We found no good evidence on the optimal frequency for eye examinations; expert opinion ranges from every 6 months to 2 years. **Non-ocular adverse effects:** The most common are gastrointestinal disturbances, occurring in about 25% of people.[24] Skin reactions and renal abnormalities occasionally occur. Mild neurological abnormalities include non-specific symptoms such as vertigo and blurred vision. Cardiomyopathy and severe neurological disease are extremely rare.

Comment: Older RCTs of chloroquine versus placebo (not included in the systematic review because of weak methods) found a beneficial effect. Observational studies (2 prospective, 1 retrospective) found that people with rheumatoid arthritis were more likely to continue on other DMARDs than on antimalarials.[16–18] Most people discontinued treatment because of lack of efficacy. Typical median duration of courses was about 20 months for hydroxychloroquine, 25 months for parenteral gold, and 60 months for methotrexate.[17] One recent RCT found that dose loading for 6 weeks at a higher dose than that usually recommended when initiating treatment with hydroxychloroquine increased the clinical response.[25]

OPTION   SULFASALAZINE

One systematic review of RCTs has found that sulfasalazine is more effective than placebo in reducing disease activity and joint inflammation. We found inadequate evidence on radiological progression and functional status. Six systematic reviews found no consistent evidence of a difference between sulfasalazine and other DMARDs.

Benefits: **Versus placebo:** We found two systematic reviews and one subsequent RCT.[26–28] The first review (search date 1997, 6 RCTs, 252 people) of sulfasalazine given for 6 months found improvement in the number of tender and swollen joints, pain score, and ESR.[23] Only two RCTs (155 people) included global assessments and they found no significant effect. None evaluated functional status. The second review (search date 1998, 8 RCTs, 903 people) of sulfasalazine versus placebo found better results with sulfasalazine on all outcome measures (decrease in number of swollen joints: 51% in the sulfasalazine group v 26% in the placebo group, P < 0.0001).[27] The subsequent RCT found that sulfasalazine (133 people) versus placebo (92 people) significantly improved patient and physician global assessment (P< < 0.001).[28] **Versus other DMARDs:** We found five systematic reviews (search dates 1989, 1990, 1988, not specified, and 1998)[9–12,27] of sulfasalazine versus other DMARDs. The most recent review (search date 1998) identified nine RCTs in 785 people. All reviews found no significant differences between sulfasalazine and other DMARDs.[9–12,27] One RCT (60 people) comparing sulfasalazine versus hydroxychloroquine found that sulfasalazine was significantly better in controlling radiological damage, although progression occurred with both drugs (median erosion scores at week 48: hydroxychloroquine 16, sulphasalazine 5, P < 0.02). However, hydroxychloroquine was given at a lower dose than is usually recommended.[29] One RCT found no significant difference between sulfasalazine versus leflunomide.[28] One RCT (200 people) comparing sulfasalazine versus penicillamine found significantly better functional status with sulfasalazine after 12 years.[30] However, differences were small and many people had changed treatment or died during the 12 years.

Harms: Common adverse effects included gastrointestinal discomfort, rash, and liver enzyme abnormalities.[26] More serious haematological or hepatic toxicity was uncommon. Reversible leucopenia or agranulocytosis was occasionally observed. Treatment was discontinued for adverse effects less often than with other DMARDs, with the exception of antimalarials.

Comment: Observational studies have reported lower long term efficacy of sulfasalazine versus other DMARDs, such as methotrexate or parenteral gold, with most people who withdrew from treatment doing so because of lack of efficacy.[19]

Systematic reviews of RCTs have found that parenteral gold versus placebo reduces disease activity, joint inflammation, and slows radiological progression in people with rheumatoid arthritis. We found no evidence on long term functional status. Systematic reviews found no significant difference between parenteral gold and other DMARDs.

Benefits: **Versus placebo:** We found one systematic review (search date 1997, 4 RCTs, 309 people) of parenteral gold for 6 months versus placebo.[31] The review found significant improvement in the number of swollen joints, patient and physician global assessments, and ESR. Functional status was not evaluated. One overview (9 RCTs and 1 observational study) that included radiological assessment found that parenteral gold decreased radiological progression.[32] **Versus other DMARDs:** We found four systematic reviews of RCTs.[9–12] They found no consistent differences between parenteral gold and other DMARDs. Some RCTs found that parenteral gold was more effective, but also more toxic, than its oral counterpart, auranofin. A few RCTs comparing parenteral gold versus methotrexate found no difference in short term efficacy.

Harms: The systematic review (search date 1997, 4 RCTs, 309 people) of parenteral gold versus placebo found that more people receiving gold discontinued treatment because of adverse effects, including dermatitis, stomatitis, proteinuria, and haematological changes (withdrawals because of adverse events with parenteral gold 66/223 [30%] v with placebo 29/192 [15%], RR 1.9, 95% CI 1.3 to 2.8).[31] Life threatening reactions such as aplastic anaemia or nephrotic syndrome are rare.

Comment: Use of parenteral gold is limited mainly by toxicity.

Systematic reviews of RCTs have found that auranofin (oral gold) versus placebo reduces disease activity and joint inflammation. We found no evidence on radiological progression or long term functional status. We found limited evidence from RCTs that auranofin is less effective than other DMARDs.

Benefits: **Versus placebo:** We found three systematic reviews (search dates 1989, 1990, and 1999), which identified several RCTs.[9,10,33] They consistently found that auranofin was superior to placebo.[9,10] The most recent review (9 RCTs, 1049 people) found significantly better results with auranofin for tender joints (effect size 0.39; small to moderate difference), swollen joint scores (effect size 0.08; small difference), pain (4.68, scale 0 to 100), and ESR (fell by 9.9 mm). **Versus other DMARDs:** RCTs comparing auranofin versus other DMARDs such as antimalarials found no consistent differences. However, one systematic review (search date 1990) of RCTs concluded that auranofin was significantly less effective than other DMARDs.[10] Data pooling found auranofin to be less effective than parenteral gold in controlling disease activity.[34] One RCT (200 people) of auranofin versus sulfasalazine found that people were more than twice as likely to continue with sulfasalazine than auranofin (people continuing treatment over 5 years: sulfasalazine 31% *v* auranofin 15%; P < 0.05).[35]

Harms: The major adverse effects of auranofin were diarrhoea and gastrointestinal discomfort.[9,10] A review of adverse effects found that serious adverse effects, such as those associated with parenteral gold, were rare with auranofin (number of participants developing serious organ specific toxicity was < 0.5%; blood 0.2%, renal 0.1%, lung 0.1%, and hepatic 0.4%).[36]

Comment: None.

OPTION   MINOCYCLINE

Three RCTs have found that minocycline versus placebo improves control of disease activity in people with rheumatoid arthritis. We found no evidence on radiological progression or functional status. We found no RCTs versus other DMARDs.

Benefits: **Versus placebo:** We found no systematic review. We found three RCTs of minocycline versus placebo.[37–39] They found that minocycline improved control of disease activity. The RCTs reported different outcomes: a typical result was that minocycline versus placebo at least halved the proportion of people who did not improve (AR 3/23 [13%] with minocycline, 11/20 [55%] with placebo; ARR 42%, 95% CI 15% to 52%; RRR 76%, 95% CI 27% to 94%; NNT 2, 95% CI 2 to 7).[39] **Versus other DMARDs:** We found no RCTs.

Harms: Adverse reactions included nausea (AR at 26 weeks 50% with minocycline, 13% with placebo), dyspepsia, dizziness (AR 40% with minocycline, 15% with placebo), and skin pigmentation.[37] Other important but less frequent reactions include hepatitis and drug induced systemic lupus erythematosus.

Comment: The magnitude of the beneficial effects of minocycline seems moderate, similar to that observed with antimalarials or sulfasalazine. However, we found no direct comparisons with other DMARDs.

OPTION   PENICILLAMINE

One systematic review of RCTs has found that penicillamine versus placebo reduces disease activity and joint inflammation. We found no evidence of its effect on radiological progression or long term functional status. Systematic reviews of RCTs found no significant difference versus other DMARDs. Common and potentially serious adverse effects limit its usefulness.

Benefits: **Versus placebo:** We found one systematic review (search date 1998, 6 RCTs of penicillamine versus placebo, 683 people).[40] The review found significant improvement in the number of swollen joints and ESR. Only some of the RCTs evaluated global assessment and functional status, and results were inconclusive. **Versus other DMARDs:** We found one systematic review (search date 1990, 79 RCTs, 6518 people, 22 treatment arms using penicillamine, 583 people completing the trial).[10] It found no consistent differences between penicillamine and other drugs, although some trials found penicillamine to be superior to antimalarials.[10]

Harms: Adverse effects were common and sometimes serious. Reactions included mucocutaneous reactions, altered taste, gastrointestinal reactions, proteinuria, haematological effects, myositis, and autoimmune induced disease.

Comment: The use of penicillamine is limited by the frequency of serious adverse effects. Observational studies found that most people discontinued the drug within the first 2 years of treatment.[16–19]

OPTION **AZATHIOPRINE**

One systematic review of three small RCTs has found that azathioprine versus placebo reduces disease activity. We found no evidence on radiological progression or long term functional status. We found no evidence that it is superior to other DMARDs. Toxicity limits its usefulness.

Benefits: **Versus placebo:** We found one systematic review (published in 1999, 3 RCTs of azathioprine versus placebo, 81 people).[41] The review found a significant benefit in the tender joint score from azathioprine versus placebo. However, not all trials reported all outcomes, and benefits were observed in only one trial. **Versus other DMARDs:** One RCT found azathioprine to be less effective than methotrexate. No other consistent differences between azathioprine and other DMARDs have been reported.

Harms: Nausea and abnormal liver enzymes were commonly reported adverse effects. Serious haematological adverse reactions included leucopenia, thrombocytopenia, and anaemia. Azathioprine is an immunosuppressive drug and its use has been associated with increased risk of infection and tumours.

Comment: Because of its toxicity profile, azathioprine tends to be reserved for people who have not responded to other DMARDs.

OPTION **CYCLOPHOSPHAMIDE**

One systematic review of three small RCTs has found that cyclophosphamide is more effective than placebo in reducing disease activity and joint inflammation in people with rheumatoid arthritis. It may also reduce the rate of radiological progression, but the evidence we found was limited. We found no evidence of its effect on long term functional status. We found no evidence that it is more effective than other DMARDs. Severe toxicity limits its usefulness.

Benefits: **Versus placebo:** We found one systematic review (search date 1997, 3 placebo controlled RCTs of cyclophosphamide given for 6 months).[42] Pooled data from 70 people found significant reduction in number of tender and swollen joints. One trial reported radiological progression, which appeared to be delayed in the cyclophosphamide group. **Versus other DMARDs:** We found two RCTs of cyclophosphamide versus other DMARDs.[9,10] They found no significant difference between groups.

Harms: Adverse effects included nausea or vomiting (58%), alopecia (26%), dysuria (26%), and amenorrhoea.[42] Severe reactions include leucopenia, thrombocytopenia, anaemia, and haemorrhagic cystitis.

People on cyclophosphamide were at increased risk of infections such as herpes zoster. Prolonged use has been associated with increased risk of cancer, in particular bladder cancer.[43]

Comment: Because of its cytotoxic effects, cyclophosphamide is usually reserved for people who have not responded to other DMARDs. Another related drug, chlorambucil, has also been used in people with severe rheumatoid arthritis that is unresponsive to other DMARDs.

OPTION | CYCLOSPORIN

One systematic review of three RCTs has found that, compared with methotrexate, cyclosporin reduces disease activity and joint inflammation, improves functional status, and may decrease the rate of radiological progression. Severe toxicity limits its usefulness.

Benefits: **Versus placebo:** We found one systematic review (search date 1997, 3 RCTs of cyclosporin given for a minimum of 4 months, 318 people).[44] The review found significant improvement in the number of tender and swollen joints and in functional status. Radiological progression was also reduced. **Versus other DMARDs:** Only a few trials compared cyclosporin with other DMARDs such as methotrexate, antimalarials, and gold, with no clear evidence of a difference.[45]

Harms: **Renal toxicity:** People given cyclosporin may develop nephropathy, which can be irreversible, and hypertension. **Other adverse reactions:** These included nausea and dyspepsia, hypertrichosis, gingival hyperplasia, and hepatotoxicity. Cyclosporin has been associated with increased risk of infections and tumours.

Comment: Cyclosporin is usually reserved for people with severe disease or those who do not respond to other less toxic DMARDs.

OPTION | LEFLUNOMIDE

One RCT has found that, in people with rheumatoid arthritis, leflunomide versus placebo reduces disease activity and joint inflammation, improves functional status and health related quality of life, and decreases radiological progression.

Benefits: **Versus placebo:** We found one systematic review (search date 1999, 3 RCTs, 1242 people)[46] of leflunomide versus placebo. The RCTs consistently found that leflunomide improved quality of life and radiological progression. The first RCT (402 people with active rheumatoid disease) compared leflunomide (two dosages) versus placebo.[47] Leflunomide (10 or 25 mg) was significantly more effective than placebo in reducing the number of swollen joints (−20 with leflunomide v −13 with placebo, P < 0.05). The second RCT (358 people) compared leflunomide versus placebo versus sulfasalazine.[28] The RCT found a significant reduction in the number of swollen joints with leflunomide (44%) versus placebo (21%) (P < 0.0001). The third RCT (482 people) compared leflunomide versus methotrexate versus placebo over 12 months.[13] Twenty per cent improvement (ACR20 criteria) was achieved by 52% with leflunomide, 46% with methotrexate, and 26% with placebo. ACR50 response criteria were achieved by 34% with leflunomide, 23% with methotrexate, and 8% with placebo (P ≤ 0.001). Radiological progression was reduced in people receiving leflunomide compared with placebo. It found significant improvements in the quality of life with leflunomide.[48] **Versus other DMARDs:** We found three RCTs. Two RCTs found no evidence of significant differences between leflunomide and sulfasalazine or methotrexate in controlling disease activity or radiological progression.[13,28] The third RCT (999 people) comparing methotrexate versus leflunomide found that at 1 year, methotrexate reduced the number of tender joints (reduction 9.7 v 8.3), swollen joints (reduction 9.0 v 6.8), and ESR (reduction 28.2 v 14.4), and improved patient and physician global assessments (P < 0.05 for all outcomes).[49] At 2 years, radiological disease progression was significantly less with methotrexate but there was no significant difference in tender joint count and patient global assessment.

Harms: In one of the trials, adverse effects included diarrhoea (17% with leflunomide v 5% with placebo), nausea (10% v 7%), rash (10% v 4%), alopecia (8% v 2%), and liver enzyme abnormalities (2% v 0%).[28] Adverse reactions were observed more frequently in the study comparing leflunomide with methotrexate, but the rate of serious adverse events was similar for all three groups (methotrexate, leflunomide, and placebo).[13] We found no evidence on long term adverse effects.

Comment: Leflunomide is a new drug, which seems to be as effective as other DMARDs in the short term. Studies of longer duration are required to adequately evaluate the efficacy of leflunomide against that of other drugs.

QUESTION   Which DMARD is the treatment of choice?

We found no good evidence to suggest that one DMARD is more effective than another for initial treatment of rheumatoid arthritis, although auranofin seems to be the least effective. Penicillamine, azathioprine, cyclophosphamide, and cyclosporin are considered too toxic for first line treatment.

Benefits: We found two systematic reviews evaluating placebo controlled RCTs of various different DMARDs. The first review (search date 1988, 33 RCTs, 3409 people) found the efficacy of most drugs to be modest, with overall risk of discontinuing treatment greater for active drug than for placebo.[11] The second review (search date not given, published 1998) found no significant differences between most DMARDs compared with placebo; only methotrexate seemed slightly better for some outcomes such as joint inflammation.[12] We found two systematic reviews comparing the efficacy and toxicity of various DMARDs (search dates 1989[9], 1990[10]; 66 trials with 117 treatment groups). When results were pooled, auranofin was significantly less effective than other drugs, but more effective than placebo. The differences between methotrexate, penicillamine, parenteral gold, and sulfasalazine were not significant. One subsequent RCT (541 people) compared hydroxychloroquine, parenteral gold, penicillamine, and auranofin over 5 years.[50] No major differences were observed between these drugs. In observational studies, more participants are likely to continue with methotrexate compared to other DMARDs.[16–19,51]

Harms: Two systematic reviews found that parenteral gold had the highest withdrawal rate because of toxicity, and auranofin had the lowest withdrawal rate.[9,10] Methotrexate had more adverse effects than antimalarials or sulfasalazine.

Comment: The method of analysis used in the two systematic reviews of comparative RCTs removed the benefit of randomisation, and the summary results cannot truly be considered as summary measures of RCTs.[9,10] The approach recommended by the Cochrane Collaboration is to conduct various meta-analyses, one for each specific group of comparisons, and to evaluate the effects of each drug within each group. The various interventions can then be compared by examining the magnitude of the effect sizes. Observational studies found that the DMARDs most frequently prescribed as initial treatment were methotrexate, sulfasalazine, and antimalarials.[16–19]

QUESTION What are the effects of combining DMARDs?

One systematic review of RCTs has found that combining certain DMARDs is more effective than using individual drugs alone. However, the evidence remains conflicting, and the balance between benefits and harms varies between combinations.

Benefits: We found one systematic review[52] and five subsequent RCTs.[53–57] The review (search date 1997, 20 RCTs, 1956 people) concluded that many combinations of DMARDs may be useful. Nine of the RCTs (1240 people) compared methotrexate plus another DMARD versus methotrexate or the other DMARD alone. A wide range of other DMARDs were included. The review found that methotrexate combined with most other DMARDs was more beneficial than treatment with a single drug.[51] Five subsequent RCTs have found that combinations of different agents (antimalarials, sulfasalazine, methotrexate, cyclosporin, and steroids) have a greater beneficial effect than monotherapy.[53–57] Some RCTs included in the systematic review have not found significant differences between combinations of different agents and monotherapy.[52]

Harms: Toxicity of combination treatments depends on the drugs used. Potential synergistic interactions should also be considered. Combination treatments may be worse than using a single drug because of interactions between drugs.

Comment: An additional meta-analysis (search date 1992) pooled data from RCTs comparing single versus combination drug treatment.[58] However, the analysis did not provide adequate data on specific combinations. We found no evidence that any one or more DMARD combination therapies are more effective than any one of the other combination therapies.

We found limited evidence from RCTs suggesting that people with active rheumatoid arthritis should start treatment with DMARDs early in the course of their disease.

Benefits: We found no systematic review but found four RCTs. One RCT (238 people with recently diagnosed rheumatoid arthritis) compared early treatment with DMARDs (within 1 year of symptom onset) versus delayed treatment.[59] People who received early treatment had significantly better outcomes at 12 months, including improved measures of disability, pain, joint inflammation, and ESR. It found no difference in radiological progression between the early and delayed treatment. A second RCT compared early treatment with auranofin versus placebo for 2 years followed by open treatment with DMARDs for a further 3 years. Five year follow up found better outcomes with auranofin. However, this analysis included only 75 of the original 137 people.[60] A third prospective 3 year follow up of an RCT (119 people with early disease) of hydroxychloroquine versus placebo, found that a 9 month delay in instituting DMARD treatment had a significant detrimental effect on pain intensity and patient global well being.[61] A fourth RCT (38 people with disease for < 1 year) compared minocycline versus placebo.[62] All participants were given DMARDs at the end of the 3 month study. After 4 years of follow up, eight people who originally received minocycline were in remission compared with one in the placebo group (P = 0.02). The need for DMARDs at 4 years was also reduced in the minocycline group.

Harms: We found no evidence comparing the harms of early versus delayed DMARDs.

Comment: About 10% of people with rheumatoid arthritis experience a short illness that resolves and remains largely quiescent. Early treatment may expose them to adverse effects unnecessarily.

We found no good evidence about optimum duration of treatment with DMARDs. Few trials have followed people for more than a year, and most people discontinue treatment with an individual drug within a few years because of toxicity or lack of effectiveness.

Benefits: We found one review of 122 studies of DMARDs (including 57 single or double blinded RCTs, 35 open label RCTs, and 19 observational studies) in 16 071 people. The review found that 90% of participants had been followed for 1 year or less.[63] Short term clinical trials in people with rheumatoid arthritis found beneficial effects for most DMARDs, but in the longer term effectiveness of these drugs seemed to decline. Observational studies have found that after a few years most people discontinued the prescribed DMARD, either because of toxicity or lack of effectiveness. We found limited evidence suggesting that discontinuing DMARDs, even for people in remission, may result in disease exacerbation or flare. These effects may vary according to the DMARD being discontinued. One RCT comparing gold and methotrexate found that people discontinuing methotrexate because of adverse effects were more likely to relapse than people discontinuing gold (joint counts as % of baseline: gold 30% v methotrexate 70%, P < 0.05).[64] One additional RCT (51 people with early disease and in remission, 24 weeks follow up) found no significant difference between weekly versus every second week low dose methotrexate (7.5 mg).[65]

Harms: Adverse effects requiring discontinuation are common, limiting long term usefulness of DMARDs.[16]

Comment: Trials of longer duration may not be feasible because many people will eventually receive a different or additional DMARD, contaminating the original groups.

QUESTION What are the effects of low dose oral corticosteroids?

Three systematic reviews of RCTs have found benefit from both short and longer term treatment (more than 3 months) with low dose oral corticosteroids. Short term treatment reduces disease activity and joint inflammation. Longer term treatment may reduce radiological progression while treatment continues. However, long term use is associated with considerable adverse effects.

Benefits: **Versus placebo or non-steroidal anti-inflammatory drugs (NSAIDs):** We found two systematic reviews. The first review (search date 1997, 10 RCTs, 402 people) compared short term treatment with low dose prednisolone (15 mg/day for several weeks) versus placebo or NSAIDs.[66] The review found that, in the short term, prednisolone had a greater effect than placebo or NSAIDs in controlling disease activity. Prednisolone versus placebo improved pain, grip strength, and joint tenderness (WMD for the number of tender joints −12, 95% CI −18 to −6). The second review (search date 1998, 7 RCTs, 508 people)[6] evaluated longer term treatment with corticosteroids (for at least 3 months). The review found that moderate term treatment with prednisolone was superior to placebo (WMD for tender joints −0.37, 95% CI −0.59 to −0.14; swollen joints −0.41, 95% CI −0.67 to −0.16; pain −0.43, 95% CI −0.74 to −0.12; and functional status −0.57, 95% CI −0.92 to −0.22). The review also found that prednisolone was comparable to aspirin or chloroquine.[67] One RCT (128 people) included in the review evaluated radiological damage. It found a significant decrease in the rate of progression in people treated with prednisolone 7.5 mg daily versus placebo over 2 years.[68] One follow up study of people in this RCT found that joint destruction resumed after discontinuing prednisolone.[69] **Versus chloroquine:** One systematic review (search date 1998, 1 RCT, 56 people) found no significant difference between oral prednisolone and chloroquine in improving disease activity.[67]

Harms: Serious long term adverse effects of corticosteroids include hypertension, diabetes, osteoporosis, infections, gastrointestinal ulcers, obesity, and hirsutism. Observational studies of people with rheumatoid arthritis have suggested that mortality may be increased by long term treatment with steroids.[70] However, many of these studies included people receiving dosages over 7.5 mg, which were higher than those currently recommended. One systematic review found that bone loss was limited when lower dosages were prescribed.[71]

Comment: The decision to give oral corticosteroids should balance the potential for increased comorbidity, which is affected by individual risk factors, and the potential improvement in disease activity.

QUESTION What are the effects of biological agents?

OPTION TUMOUR NECROSIS FACTOR ANTAGONISTS

Five RCTs have found that tumour necrosis factor antagonists (etanercept and infliximab) reduce disease activity and joint inflammation. Short term toxicity is low, but long term safety is unknown. Optimal dosages and duration of treatment have not been clearly established.

Benefits: **Etanercept:** We found no systematic review. We found two 6 month placebo controlled RCTs. One RCT (234 people who had failed to respond to other DMARDs) compared two doses of etanercept (25 mg and 10 mg) versus placebo.[72] More people improved by at least 20% (ACR20 criteria) with etanercept 25 mg than with the lower dose or with placebo (59% v 51% v 11%: 10 mg v placebo, P < 0.001; 25 mg v placebo, P < 0.001; 25 mg v 10 mg, P = 0.2). Improvement by at least 50% (ACR50 criteria) was found in 40% of people with high dose etanercept, 24% with low dose etanercept, and 5% with placebo (10 mg v placebo, P < 0.001; 25 mg v placebo, P < 0.001; 25 mg v 10 mg, P = 0.032). The RCT also found that etanercept improved functional status (disability index; 25 mg v placebo, P < 0.05) and quality of life (general health status; 25 mg v placebo, P < 0.05). The second RCT (89 people with inadequate response to methotrexate) compared etanercept (25 mg) versus placebo.[73] People were allowed to continue methotrexate. More people achieved ACR20 criteria with etanercept (71%) than with placebo (27%) (P < 0.001). **Infliximab:** We found three placebo controlled RCTs. The first RCT (73 people) compared infliximab 1 mg/kg, versus infliximab 10 mg/kg, versus placebo over 4 weeks.[74] More people experienced at least 20% improvement in the 10 mg group (79%) than in the 1 mg group (44%) or in the placebo group (8%) (placebo v 1 mg/kg, P = 0.0083; placebo v 10 mg/kg, P < 0.0001). A second RCT (1010 people) compared 1, 3, or 10 mg/kg of infliximab with or without methotrexate versus placebo (ACR 20 improvement; 60% in people taking 3 or 10 mg/kg infliximab v 15% in people taking placebo).[75] A third large multicentre RCT (428 people with active disease not responsive to methotrexate) compared five groups over 7 months: placebo versus infliximab at 3 mg or 10 mg/kg, administered every 4 or 8 weeks.[76] All continued to receive methotrexate. ACR20 criteria were reached by 50–58% receiving infliximab/methotrexate and 20% with the methotrexate/placebo group. ACR50 was attained by 26–31% of the people receiving infliximab and 5% in the placebo group (P < 0.001).

Harms: **Etanercept:** The most common adverse effect was mild injection site reaction: 42–49% in the treated group versus 7–13% in the placebo group. Other adverse effects included upper respiratory symptoms or infections, headache, and diarrhoea. Auto-antibodies to double stranded DNA developed in 5–9% of the treated group. Less than 1% of people developed malignancies or infections within the 6 months of the trials. We found no long term studies. **Infliximab:** In the RCTs, common adverse reactions were upper respiratory infections, headache, diarrhoea, and abdominal pain. Reactions during or immediately after the injection (headache, nausea, and urticaria) were also observed in the placebo groups, but were more frequent with infliximab. Antibodies to double stranded DNA were found in about 16% of people taking infliximab. The rates of serious adverse effects in treated and placebo groups were not significantly different, but there was insufficient power to detect clinically important differences.

Comment: Etanercept and infliximab were administered by injection (twice weekly subcutaneously only for etanercept and intravenously every 4 or 8 weeks for infliximab). The effects on disease activity occurred within weeks, unlike other DMARDs that may take several months to act. The optimal dosage and duration of treatment are unclear. We found insufficient evidence to estimate the rates and severity of adverse reactions.

Substantive changes since last issue

Sulfasalazine versus placebo One subsequent RCT;[28] conclusions unchanged.
Sulfasalazine versus other DMARDs Long term RCT;[30] found long term treatment was more effective with sulfasalazine.
Auranofin versus placebo New systematic review;[33] conclusions unchanged.
Leflunomide versus placebo New systematic review;[46] conclusions unchanged.
Leflunomide versus other DMARDs New RCT;[49] it found that methotrexate versus leflunomide significantly reduced the number of tender and swollen joints, and ESR score.

REFERENCES

1. Arnett FC, Edworthy SM, Bloch DA, et al. The American Rheumatism Association 1987 revised criteria for the classification of rheumatoid arthritis. *Arthritis Rheum* 1987;31:315–324.
2. Lawrence RC, Helmick CG, Arnett FC, et al. Estimates of the prevalence of arthritis and selected musculoskeletal disorders in the United States. *Arthritis Rheum* 1998;41:778–781.
3. Symmons DP, Barrett EM, Bankhead CR, Scott DG, Silman AJ. The incidence of rheumatoid arthritis in the United Kingdom: results from the Norfolk Arthritis Register. *Br J Rheumatol* 1994; 33:735–739.
4. Winchester R, Dwyer E, Rose S. The genetic basis of rheumatoid arthritis: the shared epitope hypothesis. *Rheum Dis Clin North Am* 1992;18: 761–783.
5. Yelin E, Henke C, Epstein W. The work dynamics of the person with rheumatoid arthritis. *Arthritis Rheum* 1987;30:507–512.
6. Mutru O, Laakso M, Isomäki H, Koota K. Ten year mortality and causes of death in patients with rheumatoid arthritis. *BMJ* 1985;290:1811–1813.
7. Felson DT, Anderson JJ, Boers M, et al. American College of Rheumatology preliminary definition of improvement in rheumatoid arthritis. *Arthritis Rheum* 1995;38:727–735.
8. Suarez-Almazor ME, Belseck E, Shea B, Wells G, Tugwell P. Methotrexate for rheumatoid arthritis. In: The Cochrane Library, Issue 3, 2000. Oxford:

Update Software. Search date 1997; primary sources Medline; Embase; Cochrane Controlled Trials Register; and hand search of reference lists.
9. Felson DT, Anderson JJ, Meenan RF. The comparative efficacy and toxicity of second-line drugs in rheumatoid arthritis: results of two meta-analyses. *Arthritis Rheum* 1990;33:1449–1461. Search date 1989; primary sources Medline 1966 to August 1989; hand search of two key journals and reference lists.
10. Felson DT, Anderson JJ, Meenan RF. Use of short-term efficacy/toxicity trade-offs to select second-line drugs in rheumatoid arthritis: a meta-analysis of published clinical trials. *Arthritis Rheum* 1992; 35:1117–1125. Search date 1990; primary sources Medline 1966 to December 1990; hand search of two key journals and reference lists.
11. Gotzsche PC, Podenphant J, Olesen M, Halberg P. Meta-analysis of second-line antirheumatic drugs: sample size bias and uncertain benefit. *J Clin Epidemiol* 1992;45:587–594. Search date 1988; primary source Medline September 1966 to 1988; hand searching of reference lists, and drug companies contacted for unpublished trials.
12. Suarez-Almazor ME, Belseck E, Wells G, Shea B, Tugwell P. Meta-analyses of placebo controlled trials of disease-modifying antirheumatic drugs (DMARD) for the treatment of rheumatoid arthritis (RA). *Arthritis Rheum* 1998;41:S153. Search date

not specified; primary sources Medline and Embase.

13. Strand V, Cohen S, Schiff M, et al. Treatment of active rheumatoid arthritis with leflunomide compared with placebo or methotrexate. *Arch Intern Med* 1999;159:2542–2550.

14. Ortiz Z, Shea B, Suarez-Almazor ME, Moher D, Wells GA, Tugwell P. The efficacy of folic acid and folinic acid in reducing methotrexate gastrointestinal toxicity in rheumatoid arthritis: a meta-analysis of randomised controlled clinical trials. *J Rheumatol* 1998;25;36–43. Search date 1996; primary sources Medline 1966 to December 1996; hand search bibliographic references; Current Contents June 1996 to December 1996; and abstracts selected from rheumatology meetings and journals.

15. Beauparlant P, Papp K, Haroui B. The incidence of cancer associated with the treatment of rheumatoid arthritis. *Semin Arthritis Rheum* 1999; 29:145–148.

16. Wolfe F, Hawley DJ, Cathey MA. Termination of slow acting anti-rheumatic therapy in rheumatoid arthritis: a 14 year prospective evaluation of 1017 starts. *J Rheumatol* 1990;17:994–1002.

17. Pincus T, Marcum SB, Callahan LF. Long-term drug therapy for rheumatoid arthritis in seven rheumatology private practices: II. second line drugs and prednisone. *J Rheumatol* 1992;19: 1885–1894.

18. Fries JF, Williams CA, Ramey D, Bloch DA. The relative toxicity of disease-modifying antirheumatic drugs. *Arthritis Rheum* 1993;36:297–306.

19. Suarez-Almazor ME, Soskolne CL, Saunders LD, Russell AS. Use of second-line drugs in the treatment of rheumatoid arthritis in Edmonton, Alberta: patterns of prescription and long-term effectiveness. *J Rheumatol* 1995;22:836–843.

20. Alarcon GS, Lopez-Mendez A, Walter J, et al. Radiographic evidence of disease progression in methotrexate treated and nonmethotrexate disease modifying antirheumatic drug treated rheumatoid arthritis patients: a meta-analysis. *J Rheumatol* 1992;19:1868–1873. Search date 1991; primary sources Medline 1970 to May 1991. Handsearch of bibliographies and meetings abstract of the American College of Rheumatology 1988–1991.

21. Suarez-Almazor ME, Belseck E, Shea B, Homik J, Wells G, Tugwell P. Antimalarials for rheumatoid arthritis. In: The Cochrane Library, Issue 1, 2000. Oxford: Update Software. Search date 1997; primary sources Medline; Embase; Cochrane Controlled Trials Register; and hand search of reference lists.

22. Scull E. Chloroquine and hydroxychloroquine therapy in rheumatoid arthritis. *Arthritis Rheum* 1962;5:30–36.

23. Finbloom DS, Silver K, Newsome DA, Gunke R. Comparison of hydroxychloroquine and chloroquine use and the development of retinal toxicity. *J Rheumatol* 1985;12:692–694.

24. The Hera Study Group. A randomised trial of hydroxychloroquine in early rheumatoid arthritis: the Hera study. *Am J Med* 1995;156–158.

25. Furst DE, Lindsley H, Baethge B, et al. Dose-loading with hydroxychloroquine improves the rate of response in early, active rheumatoid arthritis: A randomized, double-blind six-week trial with eighteen-week extension. *Arthritis Rheum* 1999; 42:357–365.

26. Suarez-Almazor ME, Belseck E, Shea B, Wells G, Tugwell P. Sulfasalazine for rheumatoid arthritis. In: The Cochrane Library, Issue 1, 2000. Oxford: Update Software. Search date 1997; primary sources Medline; Embase; Cochrane Controlled Trials Register; and hand search of reference lists.

27. Weinblatt ME, Reda D, Henderson W, et al. Sulfasalazine treatment for rheumatoid arthritis: a metaanalysis of 15 randomized trials. *J Rheumatol* 1999;26:2123–2130. Search date 1998; primary sources Medline 1966 to 1998; Excerpta Medica 1974 to 1998; and Derwent Drug File 1964 to 1998.

28. Smolen JS, Kalden JR, Scott, DL, et al. Efficacy and safety of leflunomide compared with placebo and sulphasalazine in active rheumatoid arthritis: A double-blind, randomised, multicentre. Trial. *Lancet* 1999;353:259–266.

29. Van der Heijde DM, van Riel PL, Nuver-Zwart IH, Gribnau FW, van de Putte LB. Effects of hydroxychloroquine and sulphasalazine on progression of joint damage in rheumatoid arthritis. *Lancet* 1989;1:1036–1038.

30. Capell HA, Maiden N, Madhok R, Hampson R, Thomson EA. Intention-to-treat analysis of 200 patients with rheumatoid arthritis 12 years after random allocation to either sulfasalazine or penicillamine. *J Rheumatol* 1998;25:1880–1886.

31. Clark P, Tugwell P, Bennet K, et al. Injectable gold for rheumatoid arthritis. In: The Cochrane Library, Issue 1, 2000. Oxford: Update Software. Search date 1997; primary sources Medline and hand search of reference lists and bibliographies in selected textbooks.

32. Rau R. Does parenteral gold retard radiological progression in rheumatoid arthritis? *Z Rheumatol* 1996;55:307–318.

33. Suarez-Almazor ME, Spooner CH, Belseck E, Shea B. Auranofin versus placebo in rheumatoid arthritis. In: The Cochrane Library, Issue 4, 2000. Oxford: Update Software. Search date December 1998; primary sources Medline; Embase; Cochrane Controlled Trials Register; and hand searches of reference lists of retrieved articles.

34. Berkey CS, Anderson JJ, Hoaglin DC. Multiple outcome meta-analysis of clinical trials. *Stat Med* 1996;15:537–557.

35. McEntegart A, Porter D, Capell HA, Thomson EA. Sulfasalazine has a better efficacy/toxicity profile than auranofin — evidence from a 5 year prospective randomized trial. *J Rheumatol* 1996; 23:1887–1890.

36. Singh G, Fieis JF, Williams CA, et al. Toxicity profiles of disease modifying antirheumatic drugs in rheumatoid arthritis. *J Rheumatol* 1991;18: 188–194.

37. Kloppenburg M, Breedveld FC, Terwiel JP, Mallee C, Dijkmans BA. Minocycline in active rheumatoid arthritis: a double-blind, placebo-controlled trial. *Arthritis Rheum* 1994;37:629–636.

38. Tilley BC, Alarcon GS, Heyse SP, et al. Minocycline in rheumatoid arthritis: a 48-week, double-blind, placebo-controlled trial. MIRA trial group. *Ann Intern Med* 1995;122:81–89.

39. O'Dell JR, Haire CE, Palmer W, et al. Treatment of early rheumatoid arthritis with minocycline or placebo: results of a randomized, double-blind, placebo-controlled trial. *Arthritis Rheum* 1997;40: 842–848.

40. Suarez-Almazor ME, Spooner C, Belseck E. Penicillamine for rheumatoid arthritis. In: The Cochrane Library, Issue 1, 2000. Oxford: Update Software. Search date 1998; primary sources Cochrane Musculoskeletal Group's Trials Register; Cochrane Controlled Trials Register; Medline; Embase; and hand searching of reference lists of trials retrieved.

41. Suarez-Almazor ME, Spooner C, Bekseck E. Azathioprine for rheumatoid arthritis. In: The Cochrane Library, Issue 1, 2000. Oxford: Update Software. Search date 1998; primary sources Cochrane Musculoskeletal Group's Trials Register; Cochrane Controlled Trials Register; Medline;

Embase; and hand searching of reference lists of trials retrieved.

42. Suarez-Almazor ME, Belseck E, Shea B, Wells G, Tugwell P. Cyclophosphamide for rheumatoid arthritis. In: The Cochrane Library, Issue 1, 2000. Oxford: Update Software. Search date 1997; primary sources Medline; Embase; and hand search of reference lists.

43. Radis CD, Kahl LE, Baker GL, et al. Effects of cyclophosphamide on the development of malignancy and on long-term survival of patients with rheumatoid arthritis. A 20-year follow up study. Arthritis Rheum 1995;38:1120–1127.

44. Wells G, Haguenauer D, Shea B, Suarez-Almazor ME, Welch VA, Tugwell P. Cyclosporin for rheumatoid arthritis. In: The Cochrane Library, Issue 1, 2000. Oxford: Update Software. Search date 1997; primary sources Medline; hand search of reference lists; consultation with experts.

45. Drosos AA, Voulgari PV, Papadopoulos IA, Politi EN, Georgiou PE. Cyclosporin A in the treatment of early rheumatoid arthritis. A prospective, randomized 24-month study. Clin Exp Rheumatol 1998;16:695–701.

46. Hewitson PJ, DeBroe S, McBride A, Milne R. Leflunomide and rheumatoid arthritis: a systematic review of effectiveness, safety and cost implications. J Clin Pharm Ther 2000;25:295–302. Search date: 1999, Primary sources: Medline, Embase, the Cochrane Library, Econlit, HMIC (Dhdata), HMIC (Helmis), HMIC (King's Fund Database) and Best Evidence3.

47. Mladenovic V, Domljan Z, Rozman B, et al. Safety and effectiveness of leflunomide in the treatment of patients with active rheumatoid arthritis. Arthritis Rheum 1995;38:1595–1603.

48. Strand V, Tugwell P, Bombardier C, et al. Function and health-related quality of life: results from a randomized controlled trial of leflunomide versus methotrexate or placebo in patients with active rheumatoid arthritis. Arthritis Rheum 1999;42:1870–1878.

49. Emery P, Breedveld FC, Lemmel EM, et al. A comparison of the efficacy and safety of leflunomide and methotrexate for the treatment of rheumatoid arthritis. Rheumatology 2000;39:655–665.

50. Jessop JD, O'Sullivan MM, Lewis PA, et al. A long-term five-year randomized controlled trial of hydroxychloroquine, sodium aurothiomalate, auranofin and penicillamine in the treatment of patients with rheumatoid arthritis. Br J Rheumatol 1998;37:992–1002.

51. Maetzel A, Wong A, Strand V, Tugwell P, Wells G, Bombardier C. Meta-analysis of treatment termination rates among rheumatoid arthritis patients receiving disease-modifying anti-rheumatic drugs. Rheumatology 2000;39:975–981.

52. Verhoeven AC, Boers M, Tugwell P. Combination therapy in rheumatoid arthritis: updated systematic review. Br J Rheumatol 1998;37:612–619. Search date 1997; primary source Medline, and hand searches of article bibliographies.

53. Van den Borne BE, Landewe RB, Goei HS, et al. Combination therapy in recent onset rheumatoid arthritis: a randomized double blind trial of the addition of low dose cyclosporin to patients treated with low dose chloroquine. J Rheumatol 1998;25:1493–1498.

54. Boers M, Verhoeven AC, Markusse HM, et al. Randomised comparison of combined step-down prednisolone, methotrexate and sulphasalazine with sulphasalazine alone in early rheumatoid arthritis. Lancet 1997;350:309–318.

55. Mottonen T, Hannonen P, Leirisalo-Repo M, et al. Comparison of combination therapy with single-drug therapy in early rheumatoid arthritis: a randomised trial. FIN-RACo trial group. Lancet 1999;353:1568–1573.

56. Calguneri M, Pay S, Caliskaner Z, et al. Combination therapy versus monotherapy for the treatment of patients with rheumatoid arthritis. Clin Exp Rheumatol 1999;17:699–704.

57. O'Dell JR, Haire CE, Erikson N, et al. Treatment of rheumatoid arthritis with methotrexate alone, sulfasalazine and hydroxychloroquine, or a combination of all three medications. N Engl J Med 1996; 334:1287–1291.

58. Felson DT, Anderson JJ, Meenan RF. The efficacy and toxicity of combination therapy in rheumatoid arthritis: a meta-analysis. Arthritis Rheum 1994; 37:1487–1491. Search date 1992; primary sources: Medline; hand searches of five international rheumatology journals; abstracts of rheumatology society meetings.

59. Van Der Heide A, Jacobs JWG, Bijlsma JWJ, et al. The effectiveness of early treatment with 'second-line' antirheumatic drugs: a randomized, controlled trial. Ann Intern Med 1996;124:699–707.

60. Egsmose C, Lund B, Borg G, et al. Patients with rheumatoid arthritis benefit from early second line therapy: 5 year follow up of a prospective double blind placebo controlled study. J Rheumatol 1995; 22:2208–2213.

61. Tsakonas E, Fitzgerald AA, Fitzcharles MA, et al. Consequences of delayed therapy with second line agents in rheumatoid arthritis: a 3 year follow up on the hydroxychloroquine in early rheumatoid arthritis (HERA) study. J Rheumatol 2000;27:623–629.

62. O'Dell JR, Paulsen G, Haire CE, et al. Treatment of early seropositive rheumatoid arthritis with minocycline: four-year follow up of a double blind, placebo-controlled trial. Arthritis Rheum 1999;42:1691–1695.

63. Hawley DJ, Wolfe F. Are the results of controlled clinical trials and observational studies of second line therapy in rheumatoid arthritis valid and generalizeable as measures of rheumatoid arthritis outcomes? An analysis of 122 studies. J Rheumatol 1991;18:1008–1014.

64. Sander O, Herborn G, Bock E, Rau R. Prospective six year follow up of patients withdrawn from a randomised study comparing parenteral gold salt and methotrexate. Ann Rheum Dis 1999;58:281–287.

65. Luis M, Pacheco-Tena C, Cazarin-Barrientos J, et al. Comparison of two schedules for administering oral low-dose methotrexate (weekly versus every-other-week) in patients with rheumatoid arthritis in remission: a twenty-four week, single blind, randomized study. Arthritis Rheum 1999;42:2160–2165.

66. Gotzsche PC, Johansen HK. Meta-analysis of short term low dose prednisolone versus placebo and non-steroidal anti-inflammatory drugs in rheumatoid arthritis. BMJ 1998;316:811–818. Search date 1997; primary sources Medline 1966 to Sept 1997; Cochrane Controlled Trials Register searched up to September 1997; and hand search of reference lists.

67. Criswell LA, Saag KG, Sems KM, et al. Moderate-term low dose corticosteroids for rheumatoid arthritis. In: The Cochrane Library, Issue 1, 2000. Oxford: Update Software. Search date 1998; primary sources Medline; and hand search of selected journals.

68. Kirwan JR. Arthritis and Rheumatism Council low dose glucocorticoid study group: the effect of glucocorticoids on joint destruction in rheumatoid arthritis. N Engl J Med 1995;333:142–146.

69. Hickling P, Jacoby RK, Kirwan JR, et al. Joint destruction after glucocorticoids are withdrawn in early rheumatoid arthritis. *Br J Rheumatol* 1998; 37:930–936.

70. Wolfe F, Mitchell DM, Sibley JT, et al. The mortality of rheumatoid arthritis. *Arthritis Rheum* 1994;37: 481–494.

71. Verhoeven AC, Boers M. Limited bone loss due to corticosteroids: a systematic review of prospective studies in rheumatoid arthritis and other diseases. *J Rheumatol* 1997;24:1495–1503. Search date 1995; primary source Medline.

72. Moreland LW, Schiff MH, Baumgartner SW, et al. Etanercept therapy in rheumatoid arthritis. A randomized, controlled trial. *Ann Intern Med* 1999;130:478–486.

73. Weinblatt ME, Kremer JM, Bankhurst AD, et al. A trial of etanercept, a recombinant tumor necrosis factor receptor: Fc fusion protein, in patients with rheumatoid arthritis receiving methotrexate. *N Engl J Med* 1999;340:253–259.

74. Elliott MJ, Maini RN, Feldmann M, et al. Randomised double-blind comparison of chimeric monoclonal antibody to tumour necrosis factor alpha (cA2) versus placebo in rheumatoid arthritis. *Lancet* 1994;344:1105–1110.

75. Maini RN, Breedveld FC, Kalden JR, et al. Therapeutic efficacy of multiple intravenous infusions of anti-tumor necrosis factor α monoclonal antibody combined with low-dose weekly methotrexate in rheumatoid arthritis. *Arthritis Rheum* 1998;41:1552–1563.

76. Maini RN, St Clair EW, Breedweld F, et al. Infliximab (chimeric anti-tumour necrosis factor α monoclonal antibody) versus placebo in rheumatoid arthritis patients receiving concomitant methotrexate: a randomized phase III trial. ATTRACT study group. *Lancet* 1999;354: 1932–1939.

Maria Suarez-Almazor
Associate Professor of Medicine
Baylor College of Medicine
Houston, Texas
USA

Wednesday Foster
Research Health Science Specialist
Veterans Affairs Medical Center and
Baylor College of Medicine
Houston, Texas
USA

Competing interests: The author has been reimbursed by Sanofi-Winthrop, manufacturer of hydroxychloroquine, for attending conferences and as a consultant, and has received research funds from Connetics, manufacturer of auranofin.

Search date September 2000: expanded this issue

Cathy Speed and Brian Hazelman

QUESTIONS

INTERVENTIONS

Key Messages

- Systematic reviews have emphasised a lack of uniformity of RCTs, poor methods, and pronounced heterogeneity of study populations and outcome measures.

- Shoulder pain is not a diagnosis. Well designed, double blind RCTs of specific interventions in specific shoulder disorders are needed.

- We found insufficient evidence on the effects of most interventions in people with non-specific shoulder pain.

- We found no evidence about the effect of analgesics specifically for shoulder disorders.

- Two systematic reviews found weak evidence for short term benefits with oral non-steroidal anti-inflammatory drugs (NSAIDs) in shoulder pain.

- We found insufficient evidence about the effects of topical and intra-articular NSAIDs specifically in shoulder pain.

- One systematic review of two small RCTs, and one additional small RCT, have found that subacromial corticosteroid injections improve range of movement but found no evidence of an effect on pain compared with placebo.

- One small RCT has found that, in people with frozen shoulder, distending the glenohumeral joint, in addition to intra-articular corticosteroid injection, may increase range of movement and reduce severity of symptoms.

- We found no evidence that ultrasound for shoulder pain improved pain or quality of life compared with sham treatment.

- One small RCT found limited evidence that extracorporeal shock wave therapy might improve function in calcifying tendinitis.

- Four small RCTs found conflicting evidence on effects of laser treatment in people with shoulder pain.

- One small RCT found limited evidence that intra-articular guanethidine reduced pain more than placebo 8 weeks after treatment.

- One small RCT found limited evidence that high intensity transcutaneous nerve stimulation (TNS) during distension arthrography reduced pain of the procedure compared with low intensity treatment or placebo in people with frozen shoulder.

- We found no evidence on most surgical interventions in shoulder pain. We found limited evidence from one small RCT that forced manipulation and intra-articular corticosteroid injection reduced the number of people with disability due to frozen shoulder at 3 months' follow up compared with intra-articular corticosteroid injection alone.

- One systematic review found no good evidence that multidisciplinary biopsychosocial rehabilitation is effective in people with shoulder pain.

DEFINITION	Shoulder pain arises in or around the shoulder from the glenohumeral, acromioclavicular, sternoclavicular, "subacromial", and scapulothoracic articulations and surrounding soft tissues. Regardless of the disorder, pain is the reason for most consultations. In adhesive capsulitis (frozen shoulder), pain is associated with pronounced restriction of movement. For most shoulder disorders, diagnosis is based on clinical features, with imaging studies playing a role in some. Non-articular shoulder disorders are the most common, involving rotator cuff, subacromial bursa, joint capsule, glenoid labrum, or ligaments within the shoulder complex.
INCIDENCE/ PREVALENCE	Each year in primary care in the UK, about 1% of adults aged over 45 years present with a new episode of shoulder pain.[1] Prevalence is uncertain, with estimates from 4–20%.[2-6] One survey reported a 1 month prevalence of shoulder pain of 34% in a general community sample of 392 people.[7] The age distribution of specific shoulder disorders in the community is unknown. A second community survey (644 elderly people aged over 70 years) reported a point prevalence of 21%.[8] It was more common in women than men (25% v 17%). Seventy per cent of cases involved the rotator cuff. One survey of 134 people in a community based rheumatology clinic found that 65% of cases were rotator cuff lesions; 11% were caused by localised tenderness in the pericapsular musculature; 10% acromioclavicular joint pain; 3% glenohumeral joint arthritis; and 5% were referred pain from the neck.[9] One survey found that in adults the annual incidence of frozen shoulder was about 2%, with those aged 40–70 years most commonly affected.[10]
AETIOLOGY/ RISK FACTORS	Rotator cuff disorders are associated with excessive overloading; instability of the glenohumeral and acromioclavicular joints; muscle imbalance; adverse anatomical features, such as a narrow

coracoacromial arch and a hooked acromion; cuff degeneration with aging; ischaemia; and musculoskeletal diseases that result in attrition of the cuff.[11–14] Risk factors for frozen shoulder include female sex, older age, shoulder trauma, and surgery.[10,15] It is associated with diabetes, cardiorespiratory disorders, cerebrovascular events, thyroid disease, and hemiplegia.[10,16] Arthritis of the glenohumeral joint can occur in numerous forms, including primary and secondary osteoarthritis, rheumatoid arthritis, and crystal arthritides.[11]

PROGNOSIS   One survey in an elderly community found that most people with shoulder pain were still affected 3 years after the initial survey.[17] One prospective cohort study of 122 people in primary care found that a quarter of people with shoulder pain reported previous episodes, and 49% reported full recovery at 18 months' follow up.[18]

AIMS   To reduce pain and to improve range of movement and function, with minimal adverse effects.

OUTCOMES   Pain scores (overall score, on activity, at night, at rest, during the day, analgesia count); range of movement measures; assessment of overall severity (self assessed or by blinded assessor); functional score; global improvement scores (self assessed or by blinded assessor); tenderness; strength; stiffness; and adverse effects of treatment. The shoulder pain and disability index (SPADI) is a validated, shoulder related pain and disability questionnaire.[19–24] Other validated patient rated disability scores have been developed.[20]

METHODS   *Clinical Evidence* update search and appraisal September 2000.

QUESTION   What are the effects of treatments?

OPTION   SIMPLE ANALGESICS (PARACETAMOL OR OPIATES)

We found no evidence about the effect of analgesics specifically for shoulder disorders.

Benefits: We found no systematic reviews or RCTs of analgesics in shoulder pain.

Harms: We found no evidence.

Comment: None.

OPTION   ORAL NON-STEROIDAL ANTI-INFLAMMATORY DRUGS (NSAIDS)

Two systematic reviews found weak evidence for short term benefits with oral NSAIDs in shoulder pain (see acute musculoskeletal syndromes under NSAIDs topic, p 800).

Benefits: **NSAIDs versus placebo:** We found two systematic reviews of NSAIDs in shoulder pain.[25,26] One of the reviews (search date 1995, 4 RCTs, 151 people) compared oral NSAIDs versus placebo in shoulder pain lasting more than 72 hours.[25] Data pooling from two small RCTs (90 people with rotator cuff tendinitis) found no significant effect at 4 weeks for pain measured using a visual analogue scale (WMD +3%, 95% CI −19% to +25%, positive values represent deterioration) and no significant effect on abduction (WMD +26, 95% CI −9 to +61, positive values represent improvement).[27,28] The third RCT found a small improvement in pain and no change in abduction; the final RCT did not allow assessment of pain or abduction. The other systematic review (search date 1993) identified three RCTs, including two trials pooled in the first review.[26] The third RCT (69 people) compared oral NSAIDs versus placebo for 14 days in acute shoulder pain of less than 96 hours' duration. NSAIDs were associated with a higher rate of effective pain relief as judged by the investigator (86% of people v 56% with placebo; ARR 30%, 95% CI 10% to 50%).[29]

Harms: One systematic review of NSAIDs in shoulder pain (search date 1993, 5 RCTs, 14 comparative studies) found adverse events reported in 10 studies that involved NSAIDs in shoulder pain. The review noted a wide range in the incidence of adverse events across studies (8–76%). Adverse events were generally mild to moderate. Withdrawal because of adverse events was less than 10% in most comparative studies. However, RCTs reported that withdrawal because of adverse events was up to 20%. Adverse events were mostly gastrointestinal, skin rash, headache, or dizziness.[26] The review found no evidence that agents differed with respect to the incidence or nature of adverse effects. One RCT (not included in either review, 224 adults with musculoskeletal sprains or tendinitis) compared two NSAIDs and found adverse events in 12–18%, causing 5–7% of people to withdraw.[30] We found no systematic review of the adverse effects of cyclo-oxygenase type II selective agents (see differences between NSAIDs under NSAIDs topic, p 800).

Comment: The quality of research on the effects of NSAIDs in shoulder disorders is limited by the lack of standardised approaches to research in this field: diverse disorders are considered under the universal term shoulder pain, different types of NSAIDs are used, and outcome measures and follow up periods vary.

OPTION   TOPICAL NSAIDS

We found insufficient evidence about the effects of topical NSAIDs specifically in shoulder pain (see topical NSAIDs under NSAIDs topic, p 800).

Benefits: We found no systematic review or RCTs of topical NSAIDs specifically in shoulder disorders.

Harms: We found no systematic review or RCTs of the harms of topical NSAIDs specifically in shoulder disorders.

Comment: None.

OPTION   INTRA-ARTICULAR NSAIDS

We found insufficient evidence on the beneficial effects on pain of intra-articular injection of NSAIDs in people with shoulder pain.

Benefits: We found no systematic review. One RCT (80 people with acute or subacute rotator cuff tendinitis) found that local injection of NSAIDs was more effective than placebo for pain control, and found no significant difference in active abduction.[3] At 4 weeks, active treatment was associated with greater improvement than placebo in mean pain at rest (visual analogue scale, range not stated, from 4.7 [95% CI 3.8 to 5.6] to 1.7 [95% CI 0.95 to 2.5] v from 4.8 [95% CI 4.1 to 5.6] to 3.2 [95% CI 2.3 to 4.1]; WMD and 95% CI not available); greater improvement in mean pain during active movement (from 7.4 [95% CI 6.9 to 7.8] to 2.4 [95% CI 1.5 to 3.2] v from 7.0 [95% CI 6.5 to 7.5] to 5.0 [95% CI 4.1 to 5.9]); and greater improvement in mean active abduction (from 111° [95% CI 98° to 124°] to 142° [95% CI 130° to 153°] v from 116° [95% CI 105° to 128°] to 129° [95% CI 116° to 142°]). Participants were offered further injections at weekly intervals if the assessor felt this was indicated. There were no differences in the total number of injections per group.

Harms: The RCT reported episodes of a vagal reaction (2/80 people [2%]) and one episode of nausea in the treatment group, and single separate episodes of nausea, hotness, gastric pain, and flu-like symptoms in the placebo group after injection (time interval not stated). There were no withdrawals from the RCT as a result.[31]

Comment: Eight people did not complete the RCT (3 in the treatment group, 5 on placebo) and follow up was limited to 4 weeks after the initial injection. The clinical importance of the benefits found in the trial is uncertain.

OPTION   SUBACROMIAL CORTICOSTEROID INJECTIONS

One systematic review found limited evidence of improved range of abduction but no evidence of an effect on pain. One additional RCT found no evidence of an effect on pain or abduction.

Benefits: **Versus placebo:** We found one systematic review (search date 1995), which identified two placebo controlled RCTs of corticosteroid injections for shoulder pain with 4 weeks' follow up.[25] One RCT (50 people with rotator cuff tendinitis) was of subacromial bursa injection (triamcinolone 40 mg) and the other (40 people with rotator cuff tendinitis) was of subacromial and intra-articular injection (2 ml of 0.5% lignocaine plus 1 ml of triamcinolone).[27,28] The review found that abduction improved at 4 weeks (WMD 35°, 95% CI 14° to 55°) but there was no evidence of an effect on pain (WMD +7%, 95% CI –33% to +47%). We found one additional RCT (55 people with rotator cuff tendinitis), which compared subacromial methylprednisolone plus lignocaine versus lignocaine alone. It found no evidence of a significant effect on pain or abduction at 12 weeks (median pain improved by 8 with active treatment v 8 with placebo, visual analogue scale 0–30). Range of abduction did not change from baseline with either active treatment or placebo.[32]

Harms: One RCT (20 people with rotator cuff tendinitis receiving subacromial corticosteroid injections) reported no adverse effects apart from mild postinjection discomfort.[27] In another RCT (25 people with rotator cuff tendinitis) of subacromial corticosteroid injection and placebo tablets, one person developed mild gastrointestinal upset, one developed pityriasis rosea 2 days after the injection, and one experienced increased frequency of urination. This compared with adverse effects in three of 25 people in the placebo group (subcromial lignocaine and placebo tablets). One person had mild gastrointestinal upset, one had diarrhoea, and one had a vasovagal reaction after the injection.

Comment: Range of movement is not a satisfactory surrogate measure of function.

OPTION   **INTRA-ARTICULAR CORTICOSTEROID INJECTIONS**

Two systematic reviews found no evidence of beneficial effects. We found limited evidence from one small RCT in people with frozen shoulder that distending the glenohumeral joint, in addition to intra-articular steroid injection, may increase range of movement and reduce severity of symptoms.

Benefits: **Versus placebo:** We found two systematic reviews (search dates 1995[25] and 1993[26]), which identified the same two RCTs.[33,34] Neither the first RCT (24 people with shoulder pain, 4 week follow up) nor the second RCT (30 people with adhesive capsulitis, 24 week follow up) found a benefit in either pain or range of movement. In the first RCT, mean pain scores, assessed on a 100 mm visual analogue scale, improved from 39 mm at baseline to 27 mm at week 4 with active treatment, compared with 52 mm at baseline and 22 mm at week 4 with placebo; mean range of shoulder abduction was 86° at baseline and 101° at week 4 with active treatment, compared with 92° and 121° with placebo (no CI available).[33] The second RCT (30 people) assessed pain using a 6 point rating system, on which 0 was no pain and 5 was extreme pain. Mean pain improved from 3.9 at baseline to 3.2 at 24 weeks with active treatment, compared with 4.1 at baseline to 3.0 at 24 weeks with placebo.[34] Mean total degrees of shoulder movement improved from 303° at baseline to 351° at 24 weeks with active treatment compared with 300° at baseline to 347° at 24 weeks with placebo (no CI available). **Different doses:** One RCT compared low dose versus higher dose triamcinolone injections in people with adhesive capsulitis (10 mg, 32 people; 40 mg, 25 people). It found the higher dose more effective for relieving pain, movement restriction, and functional impairment.[35] Pain scores improved over 6 weeks (100 mm visual analogue scale) by 31 mm (low dose) compared with 49 mm (high dose); movement restriction improved by 0.7 versus 1.1; and self rated functional impairment was reduced by 0.7 versus 1.3 (4 point ordinal scale; no CI available). The RCT found no significant difference in sleep disturbance between treatment and control groups (4 point ordinal scale, both improved from baseline).[36] **Combined intra-articular and subacromial corticosteroid injections versus placebo:** Two systematic reviews (search dates 1995 and 1993) of interventions in shoulder pain[25,26] identified two RCTs (42 people with adhesive capsulitis and 101 people with shoulder pain) of combined intra-articular and subacromial corticosteroid.[35,37] Data could not be pooled because of diversity in study designs. Both found no significant benefit from injections at 6 weeks' follow up (figures not available). **Hydrodistension with corticosteroid versus corticosteroid alone:** We found no systematic review. We found one small RCT in people with frozen shoulder comparing intra-articular corticosteroid alone (8 people) or in combination with hydrodistension (12 people) given weekly for 6 weeks or until symptoms resolved.[38] Hydrodistension involved injection of 19 ml of 0.5% lignocaine. Distension of the glenohumeral joint was confirmed by ultrasound. At 12 weeks, distension of the joint was associated with a significant increase in the number of people with a range of external rotation in the affected shoulder of at least 75% of that in the opposite shoulder (10/12 with distension, 1/8 with steroid alone; RR for improvement 7, 95% CI 1 to 42). There were also significant improvements in physicians' impression of severity of symptoms (number with light or no symptoms 12/12 [100%] with distension v 3/8 [37.5%] with steroid alone; NNT 2, 95% CI 2 to 9), and in the use of analgesics. No significant improvement was found in visual analogue scores of function or pain at rest.

Harms: Intra-articular injections were associated with infection in up to one in 14 000–50 000 injections.[39,40] An acute self limited synovitis was reported in up to 2%. Prevalence of tendon rupture, including rupture of the bicipital tendon and rotator cuff, has been reported at less than 1% after local injection.[39] Prevalence of subcutaneous fat necrosis or skin atrophy was estimated at less than 1%. There are reports of corticosteroid arthropathy and osteonecrosis, which are rare (< 0.8%) and seem to affect mostly weight bearing joints.[27] One RCT of corticosteroid injection versus physiotherapy in painful stiff shoulders reported more facial flushing (9/52 [17%] people treated with corticosteroid injections v 1/56 [2%] treated with physiotherapy), and more new menstrual irregularities (6/52 [12%] people treated with local corticosteroid injections v none after physiotherapy).[41] Two of the 12 people treated with intra-articular corticosteroid and hydrodistension complained of unacceptable pain after the injection.[38]

Comment: The systematic reviews of interventions in shoulder pain emphasise the lack of adequately designed RCTs on the subject. One case control study found that clinical outcome correlated with accuracy of injection.[42] Another case control study found that only 10% of intra-articular injections were placed correctly even with experienced operators.[43] Confirmation of injection accuracy can be obtained through fluoroscopy or ultrasound. We found no evidence on the accuracy of placement of subacromial injections. The RCT of hydrodistension included only 20 people with frozen shoulder, but it used specific inclusion criteria (only 26 people with frozen shoulder were recruited out of 120 referred). They were recruited from a hospital rheumatology clinic and may not be representative of people with frozen shoulder in the community. Twenty two people were randomised, but one dropped out of each group. The reported results were not analysed on an intention to treat basis, but they remain significant even when re-analysed in that way. There was no placebo group, and it is not clear whether any effect of distension was dependent on the intra-articular steroid injection.[38] We found no other RCTs of hydrodistension. The possibility of publication and other biases cannot be assessed until the results have been replicated in other studies.

ORAL CORTICOSTEROIDS

Two small RCTs found no evidence of an effect from oral corticosteroids.

Benefits: **Versus placebo:** We found no systematic review. One placebo controlled RCT of oral corticosteroids (32 people with frozen shoulder) found no evidence of an effect.[44] Active treatment was associated with a mean pain improvement from 1.4 at baseline to 0.5 at 18 weeks, compared with 1.4 to 0.6 with placebo (4 point rating scale, 0 is no pain and 3 is severe), and an improvement in mean range of abduction from 75° at baseline to 154° at 18 weeks, compared with 82° to 153° with placebo (no CI available). Another RCT (40 people with frozen shoulder) of 4 weeks' oral corticosteroid treatment versus no treatment found no benefit at 8 months' follow up in pain and range of motion (no figures available).[45]

Harms: The adverse effect of corticosteroids are well documented (see rheumatoid arthritis, p 832, and asthma, p 1011). One RCT (40 people with adhesive capsulitis) reported mild indigestion in two people in the oral corticosteroid group that settled on reducing the dose from 10 mg.[45] No other adverse events were reported. The other RCT did not report adverse events.[44]

Comment: None.

PHYSIOTHERAPY (MANUAL THERAPY AND EXERCISES)

Systematic reviews of one small RCT found no evidence of an effect for manual therapy and exercises in shoulder pain.

Benefits: We found two systematic reviews (search dates 1995 and 1993), which identified one small RCT (19 people) of manual therapy and exercises in frozen shoulder.[25,26,35] The RCT compared a particular type of physiotherapy (Maitland mobilisations) versus no treatment. It found no significant difference in shoulder pain between the groups at 3 months (no figures available).

Harms: One RCT of corticosteroid injection versus physiotherapy in people with painful stiff shoulders found adverse events in 56% of the 57 people treated with physiotherapy. These effects lasted longer than 2 days in 13%.[41] Fever during treatment was found in 1% and local skin irritation in 2%; 4% reported tingling, radiation of pain down the arm, or slight swelling after treatment.

Comment: The quality of research on the effects of physiotherapy in shoulder disorders is limited by the lack of standardised approaches to research in this field: diverse disorders are considered under the universal term shoulder pain, widely diverse forms of physiotherapy are evaluated, and outcome measures and follow up periods vary.

ULTRASOUND

One systematic review and two subsequent RCTs found no evidence of an effect for ultrasound.

Benefits: We found one systematic review and two subsequent RCTs. The systematic review (search date 1997, 5 RCTs, 136 people) compared ultrasound versus placebo treatment for shoulder disorders.[46] Follow up was 4–6 weeks. Clinical heterogeneity and insufficient data on outcome measures precluded pooling of results, but none of the individual trials found evidence of a clinically important effect of ultrasound versus placebo. The subsequent RCT involved 180 people with shoulder disorders who had failed to respond to six sessions of exercise therapy.[47] It compared pulsed ultrasound versus dummy ultrasound and bipolar interferential electrotherapy versus dummy electrotherapy in a blinded two by two factorial design. It also included an additional control group that received no active or dummy treatments (39 people received only pulsed ultrasound and 68 received no active treatment, either no treatment or two dummy treatments). After 6 weeks, ultrasound was not significantly associated with improvement on a 7 point Likert scale (improvement occurred in 7/35 [20%] with no treatment v 19/73 [26%] with active ultrasound v 14/72 [19%] with dummy ultrasound; ARR for failure to improve with ultrasound v control treatments +6%, 95% CI −5% to +22%). Follow up at 12 months found no significant effect of ultrasound versus control treatments on proportion reporting substantial improvement in functional status, pain, or range of movement. One additional double blind RCT (63 people, 70 shoulders) found no evidence that ultrasound for shoulder pain improved pain or quality of life scores at 9 months compared with sham treatment. Shoulders, not individuals, were randomised to pulsed ultrasound (frequency 0.89 MHz; intensity 2.5 W/cm^2; pulsed mode 1 : 4) or an indistinguishable sham treatment over the area of calcification. The first 15 treatments were given daily (5 times per week) and the remainder three times weekly for 3 weeks. The treating therapist was blinded. Sixty one shoulders completed the RCT. At 6 weeks, ultrasound versus sham treatment significantly improved pain, quality of life, and function (pain: mean change in 15 point pain score 6.4, 95% CI 5.1 to 7.7 [ultrasound] v 1.6, 95% CI 0.01 to 3.1 [sham]; P < 0.001; quality of life: mean change in 10 cm quality of life visual analogue scale 2.6, 95% CI 1.7 to 3.6 [ultrasound] v 0.4, 95% CI 0.6 to 1.4 [sham]; P = 0.002; function: mean change in total Constant score — a functional shoulder score 17.8, 95% CI 12.0 to 23.8 [ultrasound] v +3.7, 95% CI −3.3 to +10.7 [sham]; P = 0.002). At 9 months, there were no significant differences between groups for pain, quality of life, or function (pain: 5.7, 95% CI 4.0 to 7.3 [ultrasound] v 4.0, 95% CI 1.8 to 6.2 [sham]; P = 0.23; quality of life: 2.4, 95% CI 1.2 to 3.5 [ultrasound] v 1.9, 95% CI 0.8 to 2.9; P = 0.52; function: 15.7, 95% CI 8.5 to 22.9 [ultrasound] v 12.4, 95% CI 4.8 to 19.9 [sham]; P = 0.52). Nine people (nine shoulders) did not complete the treatment: three in the ultrasound group and six in the sham group, two in the latter owing to pain.[48]

Harms: We found no systematic review and no RCTs specifically addressing adverse effects. The trials described above gave no information on adverse events.

Comment: In most RCTs, with the exception of the most recent,[48] there was considerable heterogeneity of the groups, interventions, and follow up duration among the RCTs. It is not clear that ultrasound machines were always adequately calibrated before use.

OPTION	LASER TREATMENT

We found conflicting evidence from four small RCTs.

Benefits: We found no systematic review. We found four placebo controlled RCTs. One RCT (35 people) found no significant effect of laser treatment at 8 weeks. With active treatment, pain score on a 10 cm visual analogue scale improved by 3.6 cm compared with 1.2 cm with placebo (P = 0.34), and range of movement improved by 36° compared with 29° with placebo (P = 0.23).[49] The second trial (91 people) found that more people recovered at 1 month follow up with laser treatment than with placebo (42/47 [89%] v 18/44 [41%]; mean difference 48%, 95% CI 31% to 65%).[50] The third RCT (20 people with rotator cuff tendinitis) of low level laser treatment versus placebo found less pain at 2 weeks with treatment (mean score difference of 2.5%) (95% CI 2% to 3%).[51] The fourth RCT (24 people with supraspinatus tendinitis) of low level laser treatment versus placebo found no significant difference in shoulder pain at 12 weeks' follow up (no figures available).[52]

Harms: We found no evidence on harms.

Comment: As with other interventions, the quality of research on the effects of laser treatment in shoulder disorders is limited by the lack of standardised approaches to research in this field.

OPTION	ELECTROTHERAPY

We found no evidence of a significant effect.

Benefits: We found no systematic review. **Pulsed electromagnetic field treatment versus placebo:** One RCT (29 people with rotator cuff tendinitis) of pulsed electromagnetic field treatment (5–9 hours daily for 4 weeks) versus placebo found no difference in the number recovered at 4 weeks (figures not available).[53] **Bipolar interferential electrotherapy versus ultrasound:** One RCT (see ultrasound, p 857) involved 180 people with shoulder disorders who had failed to respond to six sessions of exercise therapy.[48] It compared pulsed ultrasound versus dummy ultrasound and bipolar interferential electrotherapy versus dummy electrotherapy in a blinded two by two factorial design. At 6 weeks, there was no difference between the groups with respect to the percentage reporting large improvements (20% without electrotherapy or ultrasound, 23% and 22% with active and dummy electrotherapy, 26% and 19% with active and dummy ultrasound).

Harms: We found no evidence on harms.

Comment: As with other interventions, the quality of research on the effects of pulsed electromagnetic field treatment in shoulder disorders is limited by the lack of standardised approaches to research in this field.

OPTION   ICE

We found insufficient evidence on the effects of ice.

Benefits: We found no systematic review or RCTs.

Harms: We found no evidence.

Comment: None.

OPTION   INTRA-ARTICULAR GUANETHIDINE

One small RCT of intra-articular guanethidine found significant pain benefit 8 weeks after treatment, but no evidence of an effect on range of abduction.

Benefits: We found no systematic review. We found one RCT (18 people with resistant shoulder pain) of intra-articular sympathetic block with guanethidine versus placebo. It found greater improvement in pain over time with guanethidine, reaching significance at 8 weeks ($P < 0.05$; mean reduction in pain 10 cm on a vertical visual analogue scale: 9% v 7 % at week 1, 15% v 6% at week 4, 36% v 16% at week 8).[54] No significant change in range of movement was found. Mean range of abduction was 53° at baseline and 52° at 8 weeks with active treatment, compared with 57° and 56° with placebo (no CI available).

Harms: Not reported.

Comment: This single RCT involved a heterogeneous population, including people with osteoarthritis, frozen shoulder, and rotator cuff tendinitis. The effects of treatment in individual disorders remain uncertain.

OPTION   TRANSDERMAL GLYCERYL TRINITRATE

We found insufficient evidence that transdermal glyceryl trinitrate is superior to placebo for pain relief in people with supraspinatus tendinitis.

Benefits: We found no systematic review. We found one RCT (20 people with supraspinatus tendinitis) of local transdermal glyceryl trinitrate versus placebo. It found significant decreases in pain scores at 24 hours.[55] Mean pain intensities with active treatment (measured on a 0 to 10 analogue scale) were 7.1 at baseline compared with 4.5 at 24 hours ($P < 0.001$) and 2.0 at 48 hours ($P < 0.001$). The RCT reported no changes in the placebo group (data not given). Relief was maintained at 15 days' follow up (values not reported). Mean duration of pain was also significantly reduced with active treatment (figures not available). Mean mobility (assessor rated 4 point scale) significantly improved with active treatment (2.0 at baseline v 0.1 at 5 days; $P < 0.0001$), but not with placebo (1.2 at baseline v 1.2 at 15 days).

Harms: Headaches were reported in 20% of the treatment group 24 hours after the treatment was started (no comparative figures available).[55]

Comment: The significance figures quoted are not direct comparisons. Significance figures for treatment versus placebo are not stated.

TRANSCUTANEOUS NERVE STIMULATION

One RCT of TNS during distension arthrography found improved pain relief with high intensity TNS compared with low intensity treatment or placebo.

Benefits: We found no systematic review. One RCT of TNS (60 people with frozen shoulder) compared high intensity TNS versus low intensity treatment or placebo.[56] Pain of the procedure (distension arthrography) was measured using a 0 to 100 mm visual analogue scale. No baseline measures were taken. Mean pain scores after the procedure were 19 (high intensity), 23.5 (low intensity), and 37.5 (placebo); no CI available. Difference from the control groups was significant ($P < 0.001$ for high intensity and $P < 0.05$ for low intensity TNS). No further data were available.

Harms: We found no adverse events reported in RCTs.

Comment: None.

PHONOPHORESIS

One small RCT found no evidence of an effect of phonophoresis (see glossary, p 863).

Benefits: We found no systematic review. We found one RCT (24 people: 13 with rotator cuff tendinitis, 1 with tendinitis of the biceps, 1 triceps, and 9 with a knee tendinitis) comparing phonophoresis using a coupling medium of dexamethasone, lignocaine, and aqueous gel (5 sessions of treatment lasting 5–10 days) versus placebo.[57] It found no significant difference for perceived pain (measured on 10 cm visual perception scale from 0 no pain to 10 extreme pain). Between sessions one and five, active treatment was associated with a reduction in pain from 2.4 (95% CI 1.5 to 3.3) to 1.3 (95% CI 0.7 to 1.9), compared with placebo (2.6, 95% CI 1.4 to 3.8) to 1.5 (95% CI 0.77 to 2.3). No significant effect was found in punctate tenderness (degree of force in ounces before pain elicited). With active treatment, this rose from 7.0 (95% CI 5.8 to 8.3) at session one to 7.2 (95% CI 6.0 to 8.4) at session five, compared with 6.9 (95% CI 5.4 to 8.3) to 8.8 (95% CI 7.8 to 9.7) with placebo.

Harms: Adverse effects were not reported.

Comment: None.

EXTRACORPOREAL SHOCK WAVE THERAPY

Limited evidence from one RCT suggests that extracorporeal shock wave therapy (ESWT) may improve function in calcifying tendinitis.

Benefits: We found no systematic review. We found one RCT with two parts.[58] The first compared three different ESWT regimens (low energy treatment in a single session, a single high energy session, and 2 high energy sessions 1 week apart) versus placebo in 80 people with calcifying tendinitis. It found that more people experienced subjective improvement of pain after high energy treatment than after less intense treatment (0/20 [0%] with placebo, 6/21 [29%] with low energy treatment, 12/20 [60%] with 1 high energy session, 14/20 [70%] with 2 high energy sessions; NNT 2 for high energy treatment compared with placebo, 95% CI 1 to 21 for single session and 1 to 14 for 2 session treatment). A combined measure of pain and function in activities of daily living (the Constant score) found significant improvement for both high energy groups versus the placebo group (P < 0.0001). The second part compared one versus two high energy sessions in 115 people with calcifying tendinitis (91 followed for 6 months). More people experienced relief of pain with two sessions than with a single session, but the result was not significant (19/42 [45%] with 1 session v 26/49 [53%] with 2 sessions; RR of continued pain 0.85, 95% CI 0.50 to 1.23). The difference in Constant scores after 6 months was also not significant.

Harms: High intensity ESWT may be painful during treatment. Small haematomas were reported in the RCT, but the incidence was not stated and they may have been related to subcutaneous infiltration of local anaesthetic before treatment.[58]

Comment: The mechanism of action of ESWT remains unclear. There was radiological disappearance or disintegration of calcium deposits in a significantly greater proportion of people who received high energy treatment than control treatment: 77% of those receiving two sessions of treatment had radiological disappearance or disintegration of calcium deposits after 6 months, compared with 47% who had one session (P = 0.05).

OPTION   SURGERY

We found no evidence on most surgical interventions in shoulder pain. One small RCT found that forced manipulation was more effective in the short term management of frozen shoulder (3 months) than intra-articular injection of corticosteroid, although we found no placebo controlled trials.

Benefits: We found one RCT (30 people with frozen shoulder, 15 in each group).[59] It compared forced manipulation and intra-articular hydrocortisone injection versus intra-articular hydrocortisone injection alone. Manipulation and injection versus injection alone increased the number of people who completely recovered (no disability) at 3 months (7/15 [47%] v 2/15 [13%]; ARI 33%, 95% CI 1% to 65%).[59]

Harms: Adverse effects were not reported.

Comment: There is a need for RCTs of specific surgical interventions in people with specific shoulder disorders.

OPTION   MULTIDISCIPLINARY BIOPSYCHOSOCIAL REHABILITATION   New

One systematic review found no evidence that multidisciplinary biopsychosocial rehabilitation was effective.

Benefits: We found one systematic review (search date 1998, 1 RCT and 1 controlled trial) of multidisciplinary biopsychosocial rehabilitation for neck and shoulder pain among working age adults.[60] Neither trial found a significant difference from usual treatment.

Harms: No systematic review and no RCTs were found that specifically addressed this issue.

Comment: The review found that both trials had weak methods. The rehabilitation combined physical therapy with psychological, behavioural and educational interventions.

GLOSSARY

Phonophoresis This is the application of topical medication followed by ultrasound to the same area; the theory being that the ultrasound energy drives the medication through the skin.

REFERENCES

1. Royal College of General Practitioners; Office of Populations, Censuses and Surveys. Third National Morbidity Survey in General Practice, 1980–1981; Department of Health and Social Security, series MB5 No 1. London: HMSO.

2. Bergnnud H, Lindgarde F, Nilsson B, Petersson CJ. Shoulder pain in middle age. Clin Orthop 1988;231:234–238.

3. McCormack RR, Inman RD, Wells A, Bernsten C, Imbus HR. Prevalence of tendinitis and related disorders of the upper extremity in a manufacturing workforce. J Rheumatol 1990;17: 958–964.

4. Allander E. Prevalence, incidence and remission rates of some common rheumatic diseases or syndromes. Scand J Rheumatol 1974;3:145–153.

5. Badley EM, Tennant A. Changing profile of joint disorders with age: findings from a postal survey of the population of Calderdale, West Yorkshire, UK. Ann Rheum Dis 1992;51:366–371.

6. Andersson HI, Ejlertsson G, Leden I, Rosenberg C. Chronic pain in a geographically defined general population: studies of differences in age, gender, social class and pain localisation. Clin J Pain 1993;9:174–182.

7. Pope DP, Croft PR, Pritchard CM, Macfarlane GJ, Silman AJ. The frequency of restricted range of movement in individuals with self-reported shoulder pain: results from a population-based survey. Br J Rheumatol 1996;35;1137–1141.

8. Chard M, Hazleman R, Hazleman BL, King RH, Reiss BB. Shoulder disorders in the elderly: a community survey. Arthritis Rheum 1991;34:766–769.

9. Vecchio-P, Kavanagh R, Hazleman BL, King RH. Shoulder pain in a community-based rheumatology clinic. Br J Rheumatol 1995;34: 440–442.

10. Lundberg B. The frozen shoulder. Acta Orthop Scand 1969: suppl 119.

11. Riordan J, Dieppe PA. Arthritis of the glenohumeral joint. In: The shoulder joint. Baillieres Clin Rheumatol 1989;3:607–626.

12. Bonutti PM, Hawkins RJ. Rotator cuff disorders. Baillieres Clin Rheumatol 1989;3:535–550.

13. Jobe FW, Kvitne RS. Shoulder pain in the overhand or throwing athlete: the relationship of anterior instability and rotator cuff impingement. Orthop Rev 1989;18:963–975.

14. Soslowsky LJ, An CH, Johnston SP, Carpenter JE. Geometric and mechanical properties of the coracoacromial ligament and their relationship to rotator cuff disease. Clin Orthop 1994;304:10–17.

15. Nash P, Hazleman BL. Frozen shoulder. Baillieres Clin Rheumatol 1989;3:551–566.

16. Wohlgethan JR. Frozen shoulder in hyperthyroidism. Arthritis Rheum 1987;30:936–939.

17. Vecchio PC, Kavanagh RT, Hazleman BL, King RH. Community survey of shoulder disorders in the elderly to assess the natural history and effects of treatment. Ann Rheumatol Dis 1995;54:152–154.

18. Croft P, Pope D, Silman A. The clinical course of shoulder pain: prospective cohort study in primary care. BMJ 1996;313:601–602.

19. Roach KE, Budiman-Mak E, Songsiridej N, Lertratanakul Y. Development of a shoulder pain and disability index. Arthritis Care Res 1991;4: 143–149.

20. Croft P, Pope D, Zonca M, O'Neill T, Silman A. Measurement of shoulder related disability: results of a validation study. Ann Rheum Dis 1994;53: 525–528.

21. Beaton DE, Richards RR. Measuring function of the shoulder. A cross-sectional comparison of five questionnaires. J Bone Joint Surg Am 1996;78; 882–890.

22. Gerber C. Integrated scoring systems for the functional assessment of the shoulder. In: Matsen III FA, Fu EH, Hawkins RJ, eds. The shoulder: a balance of mobility and stability. Rosemont, Illinois: The American Academy of Orthopaedic Surgeons, 1993:531–550.

23. Richards RR, An KN, Bigliani LU, et al. A standardised method for the assessment of shoulder function. J Shoulder Elbow Surg 1994;3:347–352.

24. L'Insalata JC, Warren RF, Cohen SF, et al. A self-administered questionnaire for assessment of symptoms and function of the shoulder. J Bone Joint Surg 1997;79:738–748.

25. Green S, Buchbinder R, Glazier R, Forbes A. Systematic review of randomised controlled trials of interventions for painful shoulder: selection criteria, outcome assessment and efficacy. BMJ 1998;316:354–360. Search date 1995; primary sources Medline, Embase, Cinahl, hand searched references, and conference proceedings.

26. Van der Windt DAWM, Van der Heijden GJMG, Scholten RJPM, Koes BW, Bouter, LM. The efficacy of non-steroidal anti-inflammatory drugs (NSAIDs) for shoulder complaints. A systematic review. J Clin Epidemiol 1995;48:691–704. Search date 1993; primary sources Medline and hand searched references.

27. Adejabo AO, Nash P, Hazleman BL. A prospective blind dummy placebo controlled study comparing triamcinolone hexacetonide injection with oral diclofenac 50 mg tds in patients with rotator cuff tendinitis. J Rheumatol 1990;17:1207–1210.

28. Petri M, Dobrow R, Neiman R, Whiting-O'Keefe Q, Seaman WE. Randomised double blind, placebo controlled study of the treatment of the painful shoulder. Arthritis Rheum 1987;30:1040–1045.

29. Mena HR, Lomen PL, Turner LF, et al. Treatment of acute shoulder syndrome with flurbiprofen. Am J Med 1986;80:141–144.

30. Auvinet B, Crielaard JM, Manteuffel GE, Muller P. A double-blind comparison of piroxicam fast-dissolving dosage form and diclofenac enteric-coated tablets in the treatment of patients with acute musculoskeletal disorders. Curr Ther Res Clin Exp 1995;56:1142–1153.

31. Itzkowitch D, Ginsberg F, Leon M, Bernard V, Appelboom T. Peri-articular injection of tenoxicam for painful shoulders: a double-blind, placebo controlled trial. *Clin Rheumatol* 1996;15:604–609.

32. Vecchio PC, Hazleman BL, King RH. A double-blind trial comparing subacromial methylprednisolone and lignocaine in acute rotator cuff tendinitis. *Br J Rheumatol* 1993;32:743–745.

33. Berry H, Fernandes L, Bloom B, Clarke R, Hamilton E. Clinical study comparing acupuncture, physiotherapy, injection and oral anti-inflammatory therapy in the shoulder. *Curr Med Res Opin* 1980; 7:121–126.

34. Rizk T, Pinals R, Talaiver A. Corticosteroid injections in adhesive capsulitis: investigation of their value and site. *Arch Phys Med* 1991;72:20–22.

35. Bulgen D, Binder A, Hazleman B, Dutton J, Roberts S. Frozen shoulder: prospective clinical study with an evaluation of three treatment regimes. *Ann Rheum Dis* 1984;43:353–360.

36. De Jong BA, Dahmen R, Hogeweg JA, Marti RK. Intra-articular triamcinolone acetonide injection in patients with capsulitis of the shoulder: a comparative study of two dose regimens. *Clin Rehabil* 1998;12:211–215.

37. Richardson AT. The painful shoulder. *Proc R Soc Med* 1975;68:11–16.

38. Gam AN, Schydlowsky P, Rossel I, Remvig L, Jensen EM. Treatment of "frozen shoulder" with distension and glucocorticoid compared with glucocorticoid alone. *Scand J Rheumatol* 1998; 27:425–430.

39. Gray RG, Gottlieb NL. Intra-articular corticosteroids. An updated assessment. *Clin Orth* 1983;177:235–263.

40. Hollander JL. The use of intra-articular hydrocortisone, its analogues, and its higher esters in arthritis. *Md Med J* 1970;61:511.

41. Van der Windt DA, Koes BW, Deville W, Boeke AJP, de Jong BA, Bouter LM. Effectiveness of corticosteroid injections versus physiotherapy for treatment of painful stiff shoulder in primary care: randomised trial. *BMJ* 1998;317:1292–1296.

42. Eustace JA, Brophy DP, Gibney RP, Bresnihan B, FitzGerald O. Comparison of the accuracy of steroid placement with clinical outcome in patients with shoulder symptoms. *Ann Rheum Dis* 1997;56:59–63.

43. Jones A, Regan M, Ledingham J, Patrick M, Manhire A, Doherty M. Importance of placement of intra-articular steroid injections. *BMJ* 1993; 307:1329–1330.

44. Blockey N, Wright J. Oral cortisone therapy in periarthritis of the shoulder. *BMJ* 1954;i:1455–1457.

45. Binder A, Hazleman BL, Parr G, Roberts S. A controlled study of oral prednisolone in frozen shoulder. *Br J Rheum* 1986;25:288–292.

46. Van der Windt DAWM, Van der Heijden GJMG, Van der Berg SGM, ter Riet G, de Winter AF, Bouter LM. Ultrasound therapy for musculoskeletal disorders: a systematic review. *Pain* 1999;81: 257–271. Search date July 1997; primary sources Medline, Embase, Cochrane Database of Randomised Clinical Trials.

47. Van der Heijden GJMG, Leffers P, Wolters PJMC, et al. No effect of bipolar interferential electrotherapy and pulsed ultrasound for soft tissue shoulder disorders: a randomised controlled trial. *Ann Rheum Dis* 1999;58:530–540.

48. Ebenbichler GR, Erdogmus CB, Resch KL, et al. Ultrasound treatment for calcific tendinitis of the shoulder. *N Engl J Med* 1999;340:1533–1588.

49. Vecchio P, Cave C, King V, et al. A double blind study of the effectiveness of low energy laser treatment of rotator cuff tendinitis. *Br J Rheumatol* 1993;32:740–742.

50. Gudmundssen J, Vikne J. Laser treatment for epicondylitis humeri and rotator cuff syndrome. *Nord Tidskr Idrettsmed* 1987;2:6–15.

51. England S, Farrell A, Coppock J, Struthers G, Bacon P. Low laser therapy of shoulder tendonitis. *Scand J Rheumatol* 1989;18:427–443.

52. Saunders L. The efficacy of low level laser therapy in supraspinatus tendinitis. *Clin Rehabil* 1995;9: 126–134.

53. Binder A, Parr G, Hazleman B. Pulsed electromagnetic field therapy of persistent rotator cuff tendonitis. *Lancet* 1984;1:695–698.

54. Gado I, Emery P. Intra-articular guanethidine injection for resistant shoulder pain: a preliminary double blind study of a novel approach. *Ann Rheum Dis* 1996;55:199–201.

55. Berrazueta JR, Losada A, Poveda J, et al. Successful treatment of shoulder pain syndrome due to supraspinatus tendinitis with transdermal nitroglycerin. A double blind study. *Pain* 1996;66: 63–67.

56. Nash TP, Williams JD, Machin D. TENS: does the type of stimulus really matter? *Pain Clinic* 1990;3: 161–168.

57. Penderghest CE, Kimura IF, Gulick DT. Double-blind clinical efficacy study of pulsed phonophoresis on perceived pain associated with symptomatic tendinitis. *J Sport Rehab* 1998;7:9–19.

58. Loew M, Daecke W, Kusnierczak D, Rahmanzadeh M, Ewerbeck V. Shock-wave therapy is effective for chronic calcifying tendinitis of the shoulder. *J Bone Joint Surg Br* 1999;81:863–867.

59. Thomas D, Williams R, Smith D. The frozen shoulder. A review of manipulative treatment. *Rheumatol Rehab* 1980;19:173–179.

60. Karjalainen K, Malmivaara A, van Tulder M, et al. Multidisciplinary biopsychosocial rehabilitation for neck and shoulder pain among working age adults. In: The Cochrane Library, Issue 3, 2000. Oxford: Update Software. Search date 1998; primary sources Medline, Embase, Cochrane Library, Medic (Finnish medical database), Science Citation Index, and hand searches of reference lists and contact with 24 experts in the field of rehabilitation.

Cathy Speed

Rheumatologist/Director of Sports and Exercise Medicine Unit

Brian Hazelman

Senior Consultant Addenbrooke's Hospital Cambridge UK

Competing interests: None declared.

Search date November 2000: expanded this issue

Rodrigo Salinas

QUESTIONS

Effects of medical treatments in adults and children. 866

INTERVENTIONS

Unknown effectiveness

Steroids 866
Antiviral treatment. 867
Surgery New 868

See glossary, p 868

Key Messages

- Two systematic reviews of RCTs and one subsequent RCT found no good evidence that steroids provide long term benefit compared with placebo.
- One RCT found limited evidence that prednisone is more effective than aciclovir in improving recovery of facial motor function.
- One RCT found limited evidence that aciclovir is more effective than placebo in people receiving prednisone.
- We found insufficient evidence about the effects of surgery for Bell's palsy.

Bell's palsy

DEFINITION Bell's palsy is an acute, unilateral paresis or paralysis of the face in a pattern consistent with peripheral nerve dysfunction, without detectable causes.[1] Additional symptoms may include pain in or behind the ear, numbness in the affected side of the face, hyperacusis, and disturbed taste on the ipsilateral anterior part of the tongue.[2-5]

INCIDENCE/ PREVALENCE The incidence is about 23 of 100 000 people a year, or about one in 60–70 people in a lifetime.[6] Bell's palsy affects men and women more or less equally, with a peak incidence between the ages of 10 and 40 years. It occurs with equal frequency on the right and left sides of the face.[7]

AETIOLOGY/ RISK FACTORS The cause is unclear. Viral infection, vascular ischaemia, autoimmune inflammatory disorders, and heredity have been proposed as the underlying causes.[2,8,9] A viral cause has gained popularity since the isolation of the herpes simplex virus-1 genome from facial nerve endoneurial fluid in people with Bell's palsy.[10]

PROGNOSIS More than two thirds of people with Bell's palsy achieve full spontaneous recovery. The largest series of people with Bell's palsy who received no specific treatment (1011 people) found the first signs of improvement within 3 weeks of onset in 85% of people.[11] For the other 15%, some improvement occurred 3–6 months later. The same series found that 71% of people recovered normal function of the face, 13% had insignificant sequelae, and the remaining 16% had permanently diminished function, with contracture and synkinesis (see glossary, p 868). These figures are roughly similar to those of other series of people receiving no specific treatment for Bell's palsy.[7,8,12]

AIMS To maximise recovery of facial function and to reduce the risk of complications, with minimum adverse effects.

OUTCOMES Grade of recovery of motor function of the face; presence of sequelae (motor synkinesis, autonomic dysfunction, hemifacial spasm); time to full recovery.

METHODS *Clinical Evidence* update search and appraisal November 2000. All identified trials were reviewed. Trials used different scoring systems for reporting outcomes.

QUESTION What are the effects of treatments in adults and children?

OPTION CORTICOSTEROIDS

Two systematic reviews of RCTs found no significant difference between steroids and placebo either in the proportion of people achieving good recovery of facial motor function, or in the proportion left with permanent complications. One poor quality RCT found that steroids decreased the frequency of motor synkinesis and autonomic dysfunction.

Benefits: **Versus placebo or no specific treatment:** We found two systematic reviews. One review[13] (search date 1998, 2 trials, 206 people; 113 given steroid v 93 controls) included two trials in the analysis, one of them was not randomised.[14] The other systematic review[15] (search date 1995, 4 RCTs, 390 people; 180 given steroids v 210 controls) included two good quality trials. We found one subsequent RCT of sufficient quality.[16] Both reviews found that steroids significantly improved the recovery of facial motor function. However, this conclusion was affected by the inclusion of an RCT (in both reviews), in which 29% of participants were lost to follow up,[17] and the inclusion (in one of them) of a non-randomised clinical trial.[14] If this RCT[17] was excluded, the result was no longer significant. Pooled results of the two high quality RCTs (75 people, both double blind), and one subsequent trial of sufficient quality[16] (42 people, not blind), found recovery of facial motor function in 46 of 59 people taking steroids and 46 of 58 controls (RR 0.97, 95% CI 0.71 to 1.34). They found no significant difference in the time to recovery. **Versus aciclovir:** See antiviral treatment below.

Harms: No serious adverse effects were reported in these trials.

Comment: None.

| OPTION | ANTIVIRAL TREATMENT |

One RCT has found that aciclovir in combination with prednisone is better than placebo in improving recovery of facial motor function.

Benefits: We found no systematic review. **Versus placebo:** We found two RCTs.[18,19] The first enrolled 119 participants, of which 20 people (16%) were lost to follow up, 53 people received aciclovir (400 mg 5 times daily for 10 days), and 46 people received placebo. All participants received prednisone. The proportion of people with good recovery of facial motor function was significantly higher in those receiving the aciclovir and prednisone combination (good recovery AR 49/53 [93%] with aciclovir plus prednisone v 35/46 [76%] with prednisone alone; RR 1.22, 95% CI 1.02 to 1.45; ARR 16%; NNT 6, 95% CI 3 to 50). There was no significant difference in the incidence of sequelae (AR 7/53 [13%] receiving aciclovir plus prednisone v 13/46 [28%] with prednisone alone; RR 0.47, 95% CI 0.20 to 1.07).[18] The second trial enrolled 30 people, of whom 14 received prednisone and aciclovir (200 mg 5 times daily for 10 days) and 16 received prednisone alone. All achieved good recovery of facial motor function.[19] **Versus prednisone:** We found one RCT.[20] The trial was not blinded or placebo controlled, and the randomisation technique was not stated. Of the 113 people enrolled, 12 (11%) were lost to follow up, 54 (48%) received aciclovir, and 47 (41%) received prednisone. Prednisone was associated with a significantly higher rate of good facial motor recovery (AR 44/47 [94%] good recovery with prednisone v 42/54 [78%] with aciclovir; RR 1.2, 95% CI 1.03 to 1.41; NNT 6, 95% CI 3 to 56).

Harms: No serious adverse effects were reported in these trials.

Comment: The final trial comparing aciclovir versus prednisone was of poor quality and should be interpreted cautiously.[20]

Neurological disorders

We found insufficient evidence on the effects of surgical treatment in people suffering from Bell's palsy.

Benefits: We found no systematic review and no RCTs.

Harms: None reported.

Comment: None.

GLOSSARY

Synkinesis Involuntary movement accompanying a voluntary movement.

Substantive changes since last issue

Corticosteroids One additional systematic review identified and included;[13] conclusion unchanged.

REFERENCES

1. Niparko JK, Mattox DE. Bell's palsy and herpes zoster oticus. In: Johnson RT, Griffin JW, eds. *Current therapy in neurologic disease.* St Louis: Mosby, 1993:355–361.
2. Burgess LPA, Capt MC, Yim DWS, Lepore ML. Bell's palsy: the steroid controversy revisited. *Laryngoscope* 1984;94:1472–1476.
3. Knox GW. Treatment controversy in Bell's palsy. *Arch Otolaryngol Head Neck Surg* 1998;124:821–824.
4. May M, Klein SR, Taylor FH. Idiopathic (Bell's) facial palsy: natural history defies steroid or surgical treatment. *Laryngoscope* 1985;95:406–409.
5. Rowland LP. Treatment of Bell's palsy. *N Engl J Med* 1972;287:1298–1299.
6. Victor M, Martin J. Disorders of the cranial nerves. In: Isselbacher KJ, et al, eds. *Harrison's principles of internal medicine* 13th ed. New York: McGraw-Hill, 1994:2347–2352.
7. Prescott CAJ. Idiopathic facial nerve palsy. *J Laryngol Otol* 1988;102:403–407.
8. Adour KK. Diagnosis and management of facial paralysis. *N Engl J Med* 1982;307:348–351.
9. Lorber B. Are all diseases infectious? *Ann Intern Med* 1996;125:844–851.
10. Murakami S, Mizobuchi M, Nakashiro Y, et al. Bell palsy and herpes simplex virus: identification of viral DNA in endoneurial fluid and muscle. *Ann Intern Med* 1996;124:27–30.
11. Peitersen E. The natural history of Bell's palsy. *Am J Otol* 1982;4:107–111.
12. Brown JS. Bell's palsy: a 5 year review of 174 consecutive cases: an attempted double blind study. *Laryngoscope* 1982;92:1369–1373.
13. Ramsay MJ, DerSimonian R, Holtel MR, Burgess LPA. Corticosteroid treatment for idiopathic facial nerve paralysis: a meta-analysis. *Laryngoscope* 2000;110:335–341. Search date January 1998;

primary sources Medline and handsearches of Current Contents and bibliographies.
14. Shafshak TS, Essa AY, Bakey FA. The possible contributing factors for the success of steroid therapy in Bell's palsy: a clinical and electrophysiological study. *J Laryngol Otol* 1994; 108:940–943.
15. Williamson IG, Whelan TR. The clinical problem of Bell's Palsy: is treatment with steroids effective? *Br J Gen Pract* 1996;46:743–747. Search date 1995; primary sources Medline, BIDS, Science Citation Index, and communication with manufacturers and specialists.
16. Unuvar E, Oguz F, Sidal M, Kilic A. Corticosteroid treatment of childhood Bell's palsy. *Pediatr Neurol* 1999;21:814–816.
17. Austin JR, Peskind SP, Austin S, Rice DH. Idiopathic facial nerve paralysis: a randomized double blind controlled study of placebo versus prednisone. *Laryngoscope* 1993;103:1326–1333.
18. Adour KK, Ruboyianes JM, Von Doersten PG, et al. Bell's palsy treatment with acyclovir and prednisone alone: a double blind, randomized, controlled trial. *Ann Otol Rhinol Laryngol* 1996; 105:371–378.
19. Ramos-Macias A, De Miguel Martinez I, Martin Sanchez AM, Gomez Gonzalez JI, Martin Galan A. The incorporation of acyclovir into the treatment of peripheral paralysis. A study of 45 cases [in Spanish]. *Acta Otorrinolaringol Esp* 1992;43:117–120.
20. De Diego JI, Prim MP, De Sarriá MJ, Madero R, Gavilán J. Idiopathic facial paralysis: a randomized, prospective, and controlled study using single-dose prednisone versus acyclovir three times daily. *Laryngoscope* 1998;108:573–575.

Rodrigo Salinas
Ministry of Health
Santiago
Chile

Competing interests: None declared.

Search date August 2000

Anish Bahra and Peter Goadsby

QUESTIONS

Effects of treatments for chronic tension-type headache. 870

INTERVENTIONS

Beneficial
Amitriptyline (only short term
  evidence) 870

Likely to be beneficial
Relaxation therapy and
  electromyographic biofeedback
  therapy 872

Unknown effectiveness
Other tricyclic antidepressants .870
Serotonin reuptake inhibitors . .871
Cognitive behavioural therapy. .873

Likely to be ineffective or harmful
Regular acute relief
  medication 871

Benzodiazepines 871

To be covered in future issues of
  Clinical Evidence
Other non-pharmacological
  treatments, including
  acupuncture
Other pharmacological treatments,
  including botulinum toxin and
  antiepileptic drugs
Treatment in children and
  adolescents

See glossary, p 873

Key Messages

- We found only limited evidence about the treatment of chronic tension-type headache (CTTH).
- Systematic reviews of limited evidence from small, brief RCTs have found that amitriptyline may improve CTTH. It is difficult to interpret older studies that were carried out without standard patient inclusion criteria (International Headache Society criteria).
- We found insufficient evidence about other tricyclic antidepressants and serotonin reuptake inhibitors.
- We found insufficient evidence about any benefits of benzodiazepines to outweigh the harms associated with their regular use.
- A systematic review of observational studies has suggested that regular analgesic medication may lead to a daily headache and reduce the effectiveness of prophylactic medication.
- Small, earlier, mainly poor quality RCTs have found modest improvement with relaxation and electromyographic (EMG) biofeedback therapy in a selective group of patients.
- We found insufficient evidence about the use of cognitive behavioural therapy for CTTH.

DEFINITION The 1988 International Headache Society criteria for CTTH are headaches on 15 or more days per month (180 days per year) for at least 6 months; pain that is bilateral, pressing or tightening in quality, of mild or moderate intensity, that does not prohibit activities, and that is not aggravated by routine physical activity; presence of no more than one additional clinical feature (nausea, photophobia, or phonophobia); and no vomiting.[1] CTTH is distinguished from the other causes of chronic daily headache (e.g. migraine, analgesic related headache).[2] In contrast to CTTH, episodic tension-type headache can last for 30 minutes to 7 days and occurs for fewer than 180 days per year. Terms based on assumed mechanisms (muscle contraction headache, tension headache) are not operationally defined, and old studies that used these terms may have included people with many different types of headache.

INCIDENCE/ PREVALENCE The prevalence of chronic daily headache from a survey of the general population in the USA was 4.1%. Half of sufferers met the criteria for CTTH.[3] In a survey of 2500 undergraduate students in the USA, the prevalence of CTTH was 2%.[4] The prevalence of CTTH was 2.5% in a Danish population based survey of 975 individuals.[5]

AETIOLOGY/ RISK FACTORS Tension-type headache is more prevalent in women.[6] Symptoms begin before the age of 10 years in 15% of people with CTTH. The prevalence declines with age.[7] There is a family history of some form of headache in 40% of people with tension-type headache.[8]

PROGNOSIS The prevalence of CTTH declines with age.[7]

AIMS To reduce frequency, severity, and duration of headache, with minimal adverse effects from treatment.

OUTCOMES Headache frequency, intensity and duration.

METHODS We searched the Cochrane Library, Medline, and Embase from 1966 to August 2000, and performed a hand search of the references in recent books on headache. We reviewed all systematic reviews and RCTs. Unless stated otherwise, we selected studies that used a definition of headache consistent with current International Headache Society criteria,[1] and which excluded patients with concomitant analgesic or other drug misuse. One systematic review of chronic daily headache (a term that includes, but is not limited to, CTTH) was not included.[9]

| QUESTION | What are the effects of treatments for chronic tension-type headache? |

| OPTION | PHARMACOLOGICAL TREATMENTS |

Small, short duration RCTs have found benefit from amitriptyline compared with placebo for the treatment of CTTH. We found insufficient evidence on the effects of other types of tricyclic antidepressants, serotonin reuptake inhibitors, or benzodiazepines.

Benefits: **Tricyclic antidepressants versus placebo:** We found one systematic review[10] (search date 1994, 2 RCTs), a non-systematic review (published in 1997, 4 further RCTs),[11] and two additional RCTs.[12,13] Six of the eight RCTs looked at amitriptyline specifically.

All six had methodological flaws (see additional table on clinicalevi-dence.org web site).[13–18] Treatment duration ranged from 4 to 32 weeks. Doses of amitriptyline ranged from 10 mg to 150 mg daily. Outcomes used in the trials varied considerably. The two RCTs of highest quality[12,19] found significant improvement in headache duration and frequency with amitriptyline (see table 1, p 875). The other four RCTs showed variable results. All RCTs had methodological problems. **Serotonin reuptake inhibitors versus tricyclic antidepressants or placebo:** We found one RCT, which found no significant benefit from citalopram versus placebo in headache duration, frequency; or severity.[12] It also found amitriptyline improved headache duration, frequency, and severity more than citalopram (see table 1, p 875). **Regular analgesics:** We found no RCTs (see comment below). **Benzodiazepines:** We found no systematic reviews and two RCTs.[20,21] One small RCT (16 people) found that diazepam versus placebo produced modest improvement over 12 weeks.[20] The dose of diazepam was not stated, and International Headache Society criteria were not used. The other RCT (crossover design) compared alprazolam 250 µg three times daily versus placebo over 16 weeks.[21] The trial also found a modest short term improvement.

Harms: **Tricyclic antidepressants:** One RCT found increased rates of dry mouth (54% with amitriptyline 75 mg daily v 17% with placebo, $P < 0.05$), drowsiness (62% v 27%, $P < 0.05$), and weight gain (16% v 0%, NS).[19] Similar results have been found for amitriptyline[12] and other tricyclic antidepressants.[15,22] **Serotonin reuptake inhibitors:** Four of eight people taking fluvoxamine in a cohort study had transient nausea, two complained of anorexia, and three complained of irritability.[22] **Regular analgesics:** We found no RCTs but found one systematic review of 29 observational studies (2612 people).[23] Maintained frequent analgesic use (2–3 times a week) in people with episodic headache was associated with chronic headache and reduced effectiveness of prophylactic treatment. Many, but not all, people improved following withdrawal of the acute relief medication. **Benzodiazepines:** Harms of benzo-diazepines found in studies for other indications include increased risk of motor vehicle accidents, falls and fractures, fatal poisonings, depression, dependency, decline in functional status, cognitive decline, confusion, bizarre behaviour, and amnesia.[24]

Comment: Most RCTs were small, short term, and used different outcome measures. Not all studies excluded people taking regular analgesics. The quality of the studies often did not conform to current International Headache Society guidelines. Observational studies are also difficult to interpret. One cohort study found significant benefit from fluvoxamine, but the people recruited were not randomised, and those responding to placebo were excluded before the trial.[22] The available evidence supports the view that prophylactic treatment with amitriptyline is likely to be superior to the habitual use of short term analgesics. It is not clear whether benzodiazepines alone might contribute to the development of a daily headache, but the modest benefit found in the two small RCTs is unlikely to outweigh the risk of dependence with prolonged use.

Neurological disorders

| OPTION | RELAXATION THERAPY AND ELECTROMYOGRAPHIC BIOFEEDBACK THERAPY |

Small, mainly poor quality RCTs have found modest improvement with relaxation and electromyographic (EMG) biofeedback therapy (see glossary, p 873). People most likely to benefit seem to be younger individuals, women, and those who volunteer for treatment.

Benefits:

We found two systematic reviews (published in 1986[25] and 1994[10]) and one subsequent RCT.[4] **Adults:** The first systematic review evaluated 37 small, short term, prospective studies of relaxation and EMG biofeedback therapy in people with CTTH.[25] The review found results from 66 treatment groups. Only a third reported criteria used for diagnosing "tension headache". Three treatments were used: EMG biofeedback training (26 treatment groups), relaxation training (15 groups), and combined EMG biofeedback and relaxation training (9 groups). Two control conditions were used: non-contingent biofeedback (see glossary, p 873) training (6 groups), and headache monitoring (see glossary, p 873) (10 groups). Pooling the results from many studies found that improvement in headache frequency, intensity, and duration varied between the interventions (46% with EMG biofeedback, 45% with relaxation, 57% with both EMG biofeedback and relaxation, 15% with non-contingent biofeedback and −4% with headache monitoring or other control treatments). However, the apparent difference in effectiveness of the different interventions was explained best by differences in the people recruited to the studies rather than by differences in the effectiveness of the interventions or study designs. Outcomes were better in groups with mean age below 35 years, a greater proportion of women, small size, lower withdrawal rates, and when people were asked to enter the study rather than being referred. Half the studies reported follow up data; greater improvement was reported at follow up than immediately after treatment for at least 3–6 months. The second review included 29 EMG biofeedback treatment groups, 38 treated with relaxation therapy (see glossary, p 873), 11 with both, 17 control groups (no treatment), and 28 sham treatment or placebo groups from many small studies. The review found that EMG biofeedback and relaxation therapy alone or in combination were better than no treatment, sham treatments, or placebo. Retrospective analysis found greater improvements in younger people with short duration of headache but no greater improvement with gender, method of recruitment, quality of the study, sample size, diagnostic criteria, or withdrawal rate. The review selected studies that used specified diagnostic criteria, but did not differentiate between episodic tension-type headache or CTTH. Treatment outcome measures were variable. Concomitant analgesic use was not considered. Smaller benefits of treatment were reported in the most recent studies. The subsequent RCT compared six sessions of relaxation plus EMG biofeedback therapy versus three sessions of assessment only in 44 paid undergraduate college students (mean age 19 years, 86% women in both groups, all with International Headache Society defined CTTH).[4] Of the 30 people in the treatment group, 52% had at least a 50% reduction in headache activity (based on headache intensity and indirectly on frequency) compared with

15% of the controls. EMG biofeedback versus control treatment significantly increased the number of headache free days ($P < 0.05$) and non-significantly reduced analgesic consumption ($P = 0.065$).

Harms: We found no reported adverse effects of EMG biofeedback or relaxation therapy.

Comment: Relaxation and biofeedback require additional trained staff and are time consuming. The finding of smaller benefits in recently published studies may reflect publication bias (earlier studies with negative results failing to be published) or possibly because recent studies are less prone to systematic bias.

<table><tr><td>OPTION</td><td>COGNITIVE BEHAVIOURAL THERAPY</td></tr></table>

One systematic review found limited evidence from three small RCTs that cognitive therapy versus no treatment is effective for the treatment of CTTH.

Benefits: **Versus placebo:** We found one systematic review (published in 1994, 3 small RCTs), which found greater improvement with cognitive therapy compared with no treatment, sham treatment, or placebo groups.[10] **Versus another treatment:** Nine additional comparative studies of relaxation and/or EMG biofeedback therapy compared with either cognitive therapy alone (2 studies) or in combination with relaxation or EMG biofeedback therapy (7 studies) found inconclusive results.

Harms: We found no reported adverse effects of cognitive behavioural therapy.

Comment: The studies were small and had as few as five people in a group. The evidence is too limited to define the role of cognitive therapy in CTTH.

GLOSSARY

Electromyographic (EMG) biofeedback Feedback of the amplified EMG signal from forehead and neck muscles through earphones or a loudspeaker to enable people to reduce the amount of muscle contraction.

Headache monitoring People in a study who make daily recordings of headache symptoms without additional therapeutic intervention.

Non-contingent biofeedback Sounds uncorrelated with muscle activity are played to the person.

Relaxation therapy Includes Jacobson's progressive relaxation exercises, meditation, passive relaxation, and autogenic training.[25]

REFERENCES

1. Headache Classification Committee of the International Headache Society. Classification and diagnostic criteria for headache disorders, cranial neuralgias and facial pain. *Cephalalgia* 1988;8:1–96.

2. Silberstein SD, Lipton RB, Sliwinski M. Classification of daily and near-daily headaches: field trial of revised IHS criteria. *Neurology* 1996; 47:871–875.

3. Schwartz BS, Stewart WF, Simon D, Lipton RB. Epidemiology of tension-type headache. *JAMA* 1998;279:381–383.

4. Rokicki LA, Holroyd KA, France CR, et al. Change mechanisms associated with combined relaxation/ EMG biofeedback training and chronic tension-type headache. *Appl Psychophysiol Biofeedback* 1997;22:21–187.

5. Rasmussen BK, Jensen R, Olesen J. A population-based analysis of the diagnostic criteria of the International Headache Society. *Cephalalgia* 1991;11:129–134.

6. Friedman AP, von Storch TJC, Merritt HH. Migraine and tension headaches: a clinical study of two thousand cases. *Neurology* 1954;4:773–788.

Neurological disorders

7. Lance JW, Curran DA, Anthony M. Investigations into the mechanism and treatment of chronic headache. Med J Aust 1965;2:909–914.

8. Russell MB, Ostergaard S, Bendtsen L, Olesen J. Familial occurrence of chronic tension-type headache. Cephalalgia 1999;19:207–210.

9. Redillas C, Solomon S. Prophylactic treatment of chronic daily headache. Headache 2000;40:83–102. Search date not given; primary sources Medline 1988 to search date for open studies; Medline 1966 to date for double-blind studies.

10. Bogaards MC, Moniek M, ter Kuile M. Treatment of recurrent tension-type headache: A meta-analytic review. Clin J Pain 1994;10:174–190. Search date 1994; primary sources Compact Cambridge, Psychlit and reference lists of relevant articles.

11. Schoenen J, Wang W. Tension-type headache. In: Goadsby PJ, Silberstein SD, eds. Headache. 1st ed. Newton: Butterworth-Heinemann, 1997:177–200.

12. Bendtsen L, Jensen R, Olesen J. A non-selective (amitriptyline), but not a selective (citalopram), serotonin reuptake inhibitor is effective in the prophylactic treatment of chronic tension-type headache. J Neurol Neurosurg Psychiatry 1996; 61:285–290.

13. Holroyd KA, O'Donnell FJ, Lipchik GL, Cordingley GE, Carlson B. Management of chronic tension-type headache with (tricyclic) antidepressant medication, stress-management therapy and their combination: a randomized controlled trial [abstract]. Cephalalgia 2000;20 (in press).

14. Diamond S, Baltes BJ. Chronic tension headache treated with amitriptyline: A double-blind study. Headache 1971;11:110–116.

15. Fogelholm R, Murros K. Maprotiline in chronic tension headache: a double-blind cross-over study. Headache 1985;25:273–275.

16. Langemark M, Loldrup D, Bech P, Oleson J. Clompramine and mianserin in the treatment of chronic tension headache. A double-blind, controlled study. Headache 1990;30:118–21.

17. Pfaffenrath V, Essen D, Islet H, et al. Amitriptyline versus amitriptyline-N-oxide versus placebo in the treatment of chronic tension-type headache : A multi-centre randomised parallel-group double-blind study. Cephalalgia 1991;11(suppl).

18. Lance JW. Mechanism and Management of Headache. London: Butterworth, 1973.

19. Gobel H, Hamouz V, Hansen C, et al. Chronic tension-type headache: amitriptyline reduces clinical headache-duration and experimental pain sensitivity but does not alter pericranial muscle activity readings. Pain 1994;59:241–249.

20. Paiva T, Nunes JS, Moreira A, et al. Effects of frontalis EMG biofeedback and diazepam in the treatment of tension headache. Headache 1982; 22:216–220.

21. Shukla R, Nag D, Ahuja RC. Alprazolam in chronic tension-type headache. J Assoc Physician India 1996;44:641–644.

22. Manna V, Bolino F, Di Cicco L. Chronic tension-type headache, mood depression and serotonin: therapeutic effects of fluvoxamine and mianserin. Headache 1994;34:44–49.

23. Diener H-C, Tfelt-Hansen P. Headache associated with chronic use of substances. In: Oleson J, Tfelt-Hansen P, Welch KMA, eds. The Headaches. New York: Raven, 1993:721–727.

24. Holbrook AM, Crowther R, Lotter A, et al. The diagnosis and management of insomnia in clinical practice: a practical evidence-based approach. CMAJ 2000;162:216–220.

25. Holroyd KA, Penzien DB. Client variables and the behavioural treatment of recurrent tension headache: A meta-analytic review. J Behav Med 1986;9:515. Search date not stated; primary sources Eric, Medlars, Psycinfo, Psycalert, and hand searches of key journals, book reviews and conference proceedings.

Anish Bahra
Research Fellow

Peter Goadsby
Professor of Clinical Neurology

Institute of Neurology
London
UK

Competing interests: None declared.

TABLE 1 RCTs of tricyclic antidepressants versus placebo for the treatment of chronic tension-type headache, including a comparative study with serotonin reuptake inhibitor (see text, p 871).

RCT	Treatment	Number of people	CTTH definition	Analgesic overuse excluded?	Total duration and type of study	Outcome	Effect of drug compared with placebo
19	Amitriptyline 75 mg, placebo	2429	*IHS[1]	Yes	6 weeks Parallel group	Mean daily headache duration	At 6 weeks, pain reduced by 3.2 hours per day with amitriptyline v 0.28 hours per day with placebo (P < 0.01)
12	Amitriptyline 75 mg, citalopram 20 mg, placebo	34	*IHS[1]	Yes	32 weeks total Cross-over	Headache duration and intensity, analgesic intake	Reduced analgesic intake (P = 0.01), and headache duration and frequency (P = 0.002) with amitriptyline; no significant difference in headache intensity. No significant difference in headache duration, frequency, and severity with citalopram.

CTTH, chronic tension-type headache; *IHS, International Headache Society criteria.

Epilepsy

Search date November 2000

Anthony Marson

QUESTIONS

INTERVENTIONS

Beneficial
Antiepileptic monotherapy in partial
  epilepsy* 878
Antiepileptic monotherapy in
  generalised epilepsy* 879
Addition of second line drugs for
  drug resistant partial
  epilepsy 880

**Trade off between benefits and
harms**
Antiepileptic drugs after a single
  seizure 877

**To be covered in future issues of
*Clinical Evidence***
Treatment of infantile spasms
Treatment of drug resistant
  generalised epilepsy
Temporal lobe surgery and vagus
  nerve stimulation for drug
  resistant epilepsy

* We found no placebo controlled
  RCTs. However, widespread
  consensus holds that these
  drugs are effective.

Key Messages

- RCTs have found that treatment of single seizures reduces the risk of further seizures by about half. However, we found no evidence that treatment alters long term prognosis. Long term antiepileptic drug treatment is potentially harmful.

- We found no placebo controlled trials of the main antiepileptic drugs (carbamazepine, lamotrigine, phenobarbitone, phenytoin, primidone, valproate) in people with newly diagnosed partial or generalised epilepsy. We found no good evidence on which to base a choice between drugs in terms of efficacy. RCTs have found that phenobarbitone and primidone are less well tolerated than other drugs.

- Four systematic reviews of RCTs have found that the addition of second line drugs significantly reduces the seizure frequency in people with partial epilepsy who have not responded to usual treatment. Each additional drug increases the frequency of adverse effects, the need for withdrawal of additional treatment, or both. We found no good evidence from RCTs on which to base a choice between drugs.

- One systematic review of observational studies and one RCT have found that antiepileptic drug withdrawal for people in remission is associated with a higher risk of seizure recurrence than continued treatment. Clinical predictors of relapse after drug withdrawal include age, seizure type, number of antiepileptic drugs being taken, whether seizures have occurred since antiepileptic drugs were started, and the period of remission before drug withdrawal.

DEFINITION	Epilepsy is a group of disorders rather than a single disease. Seizures can be classified by type as partial (categorised as simple partial, complex partial, and secondary generalised tonic clonic seizures), or generalised (categorised as generalised tonic clonic, absence, myoclonic, tonic, and atonic seizures).[1] See glossary, p 881.
INCIDENCE/ PREVALENCE	Epilepsy is common, with an estimated prevalence in the developed world of 5–10 per 1000 and an annual incidence of 50 per 100 000 people.[2] About 3% of people will be given a diagnosis of epilepsy at some time in their lives.[3]
AETIOLOGY/ RISK FACTORS	Epilepsy can also be classified by cause.[1] Idiopathic generalised epilepsies (such as juvenile myoclonic epilepsy or childhood absence epilepsy) are largely genetic. Symptomatic epilepsies result from a known cerebral abnormality — for example, temporal lobe epilepsy may result from a congenital defect, mesial temporal sclerosis, or a tumour. Cryptogenic epilepsies are those that cannot be classified as idiopathic or symptomatic and in which no causative factor has been identified, but is suspected.
PROGNOSIS	For most people with epilepsy the prognosis is good. About 70% go into remission, defined as being seizure free for 5 years on or off treatment. This leaves 20–30% who develop chronic epilepsy, often treated with multiple antiepileptic drugs.[4] About 60% of untreated people suffer no further seizures in the 2 years after their first seizure.[5]
AIMS	To reduce the risk of subsequent seizures and to improve the prognosis of the seizure disorder; in people in remission, to withdraw antiepileptic drugs without causing seizure recurrence; and to minimise adverse effects of treatment.
OUTCOMES	For treatment after a single seizure: time to subsequent seizures, time to achieve remission, proportion achieving remission. For treatment of newly diagnosed epilepsy: retention on allocated treatment or time to withdrawal of allocated treatment, time to remission, time to first seizure after treatment. For treatment of drug resistant epilepsy: percentage reduction in seizure frequency, proportion of responders (response defined as ≥ 50% in reduction in seizure frequency). For drug withdrawal: time to seizure recurrence.
METHODS	*Clinical Evidence* update search and appraisal November 2000.

QUESTION Should single seizures be treated?

RCTs have found that treatment with antiepileptic drugs reduces the risk of further seizures by about half. However, we found no evidence that treatment alters long term prognosis. Long term antiepileptic drug treatment is potentially harmful.

Benefits: We found no systematic review. We found three RCTs, the largest of which compared immediate with no treatment in 419 people (42% women, 28% aged 16 years or under, 65% aged 16–65 years, 6% aged 60 years or over).[6,7] Participants were randomised within 7 days of their first tonic clonic seizure and were followed for a minimum of 3 years. At 2 years, there were half as many second seizures in the treatment group compared with the control group (HR 0.36, 95% CI 0.24 to 0.53). However, there was no significant difference in the proportion of people achieving a 2 year remission (AR 60% v 68%; RR 0.82, 95% CI 0.64 to 1.03; RR 0.96, 95% CI 0.77 to 1.22).

Harms: The largest RCT gave no information on adverse effects.[6,7] However, these are well known and include idiosyncratic reactions, teratogenesis, and cognitive effects.

Comment: One systematic review of prospective observational studies (search date not stated, about 2500 people, 30% receiving treatment) concluded that, at 2 years from their first seizure, 40% (95% CI 37% to 43%) of people will have had further seizures.[5] The largest RCT was too small to rule out the possibility that treating a first seizure alters the long term prognosis of epilepsy.[6,7]

QUESTION   **What are the effects of monotherapy in newly diagnosed partial epilepsy?**

We found no placebo controlled RCTs of the main antiepileptic drugs (carbamazepine, lamotrigine, phenobarbitone, phenytoin, primidone, valproate) used as monotherapy in people with partial epilepsy. Trials comparing one drug with another have found that phenobarbitone and primidone are less well tolerated than other drugs. With respect to effect on seizures, we found no evidence on which to base a choice between drugs in partial epilepsy.

Benefits: **Versus placebo:** We found no systematic reviews or RCTs. **Versus each other:** We found one systematic review (search date 1999, 5 RCTs of valproate versus carbamazepine, 1265 people of which 830 had partial epilepsy, and 395 had generalised epilepsy, age 3–83 years, follow up < 5 years).[8] The systematic review included a meta-analysis of the subgroup of people with partial epilepsy (with results expressed as hazard ratios [HR]; HR > 1 for an event that is more likely with valproate). It found no significant difference for time to treatment withdrawal (HR 1.00, 95% CI 0.79 to 1.26), an advantage with carbamazepine for time to 12 month remission (HR 0.82, 95% CI 0.67 to 1.00), and a significant advantage with carbamazepine for time to first seizure (HR 1.22, 95% CI 1.04 to 1.44). A test for statistical interaction was performed to test the robustness of these subgroup analyses. This was significant for time to first seizure but not for time to 12 month remission, and so these subgroup analyses must be treated with caution. The largest RCT that was not included in the meta-analysis (622 people, mean age 41 years, 87% men) compared carbamazepine versus phenobarbitone versus phenytoin versus primidone. At 36 months, people allocated to primidone were less likely to be still taking the allocated treatment (P < 0.001). In people with predominantly simple and/or complex partial seizures, those allocated to phenobarbitone or primidone were less likely to be taking allocated treatment (P < 0.02). At 3 years, 39% of participants remained seizure free, and no significant difference was found between groups. In people with predominantly tonic clonic seizures, the proportion remaining seizure free was not significantly different between treatment groups (43–48%; no P value given). In people with predominantly complex partial seizures, the proportion of people who remained seizure free was significantly higher with carbamazepine (43%) than with phenobarbitone (16%) or primidone (15%) (P < 0.03).

Harms: See benefits above.

Comment: Placebo controlled trials of these drugs would now be considered unethical. People recruited into the two largest comparative trials were predominantly male veterans and were therefore more likely to have epilepsy as a consequence of brain trauma, which may result in a more resistant form of partial epilepsy. The meta-analysis provides weak evidence in support of the consensus view to use carbamazepine as the drug of choice in people with partial epilepsy.

QUESTION **What are the effects of monotherapy in newly diagnosed generalised epilepsy (generalised tonic clonic seizures with or without other generalised seizure types)?**

We found no placebo controlled trials of the main antiepileptic drugs (carbamazepine, lamotrigine, phenobarbitone, phenytoin, valproate) used as monotherapy in people with generalised epilepsy. Trials comparing one drug with another have failed to find consistent differences between drugs.

Benefits: **Versus placebo:** We found no systematic reviews or RCTs. **Versus each other:** We found one systematic review (search date 1999, 5 RCTs of carbamazepine versus valproate, 4 of the RCTs included 395 people with generalised epilepsy, age 3–79 years, follow up < 5 years).[8] People were recruited into the RCTs if they had generalised tonic clonic seizures with or without other types of generalised seizure (e.g. absence or myoclonus). Only generalised tonic clonic seizures were documented during follow up. A meta-analysis of the generalised epilepsy subgroup found no significant differences between valproate and carbamazepine for time to treatment withdrawal (HR 0.89, 95% CI 0.62 to 1.29), time to 12 month remission (HR 0.96, 95% CI 0.75 to 1.24), and time to first seizure (HR 0.86, 95% CI 0.68 to 1.67) (see comment below).

Harms: Two RCTs found similar prevalence of adverse effects with carbamazepine and valproate.[9,10] Rashes occurred more often in people on carbamazepine than on valproate (11% v 1.7%, P < 0.05; 6.3% v 3.4%, NS).[9,10] More people on carbamazepine reported weight gain (12% v 1.1%, P < 0.05; 10% v 3.9%, NS),[9,10] usually after at least 3 months of treatment. Other adverse events with carbamazepine were dizziness (6.7% v 2.9%, NS; 6.3% v 0.8%, P < 0.05),[9,10] headaches (6.1% v 3.4%), ataxia (2.2% v 0%), somnolence (20% v 9.3%, P < 0.05), fatigue (10% v 5.1%, NS), diplopia (3.9% v 0%, NS), and insomnia (3.9% v 0%, NS).[9,10] Other drug related adverse events with valproate were tremor (5.2% v 1.7%, NS), alopecia (2.9% v 0.6%, NS; 4.2% v 1.6%, NS), and appetite increase (2.3% v 0%, NS; 9.3% v 0%, P < 0.01).[9,10] Treatment was withdrawn because of adverse events in 9% of people on valproate compared with 18% on carbamazepine (18 v 15 people).[9,10]

Comment: Although no difference was found by the meta-analysis between valproate and carbamazepine, the confidence intervals are wide and these results do not establish equivalence of valproate and carbamazepine. Also, the age distribution of people classified as having generalised epilepsy suggests significant errors in the classification of epilepsy type. Failure of the RCTs to document generalised seizures other than tonic clonic seizures is a significant limitation. The meta-analysis does not provide evidence to support or refute the use of valproate for people with generalised tonic clonic seizures as part of generalised epilepsy.

QUESTION Does the addition of second line drugs benefit people with drug resistant partial epilepsy?

Four systematic reviews have found that the addition of second line drugs significantly reduces the seizure frequency in people with partial epilepsy who have not responded to usual treatment. Each additional drug increases the frequency of adverse effects, the need for withdrawal of additional treatment, or both. We found no good evidence from RCTs on which to base a choice between these drugs.

Benefits: We found four systematic reviews (search dates 1995, 1998, 1999, and 1999). For gabapentin the systematic reviews identified four RCTs (750 people with drug resistant partial epilepsy), for lamotrigine 10 RCTs (1044 people), for tiagabine three RCTs (769 people), for topiramate six RCTs (743 people), for vigabatrin four RCTs (495 people), and for zonisamide three RCTs (499 people).[11–14] These reviews found that the addition of each drug to usual treatment significantly reduced seizure frequency versus placebo (see table 1, p 883).

Harms: Adverse effects were more frequent with additional treatment versus placebo (see table 1, p 883).[12,13] Lamotrigine is associated with a rash, which may be avoided by slower titration of the drug. Vigabatrin causes concentric visual field abnormalities in about 40% of people, which are probably irreversible.[15]

Comment: Few RCTs have compared these drugs directly with each other. Consensus about the irreversibility of the visual field abnormalities with vigabatrin have meant that few neurologists recommend this drug.

QUESTION Which people are at risk of relapse on withdrawal of drug treatment?

Observational studies have found that nearly a third of people will relapse within 2 years if antiepileptic drugs are withdrawn. Clinical predictors of relapse after drug withdrawal include age, seizure type, number of antiepileptic drugs being taken, whether seizures have occurred since antiepileptic drugs were started, and the period of remission before drug withdrawal.

Benefits: We found no systematic review of RCTs. The largest single RCT (1013 people who had been seizure free for at least 2 years) compared continued antiepileptic treatment with slow antiepileptic drug withdrawal.[16,17] At 2 years, 78% of people who continued treatment remained seizure free, compared with 59% in the with-drawal group. Risk reductions with 95% confidence intervals for the main factors predicting recurrence of seizures are given in table 2 (see table 2, p 884). One systematic review of observational studies (search date not stated) found that, at 2 years, 29% (95% CI 24% to 34%) of people in remission from all types of epilepsy would relapse if antiepileptic drugs were withdrawn.[18]

Harms: Sixteen people died during the trial, 10 in the continued treatment group and six in the withdrawal group.[16,17] Only two deaths were attributed to epilepsy, and both of these occurred in people ran-domised to continued treatment.

Comment: There were no significant differences in psychosocial outcomes between groups. People with a seizure recurrence were less likely to be in paid employment at 2 years.[16,17]

GLOSSARY

Absence seizure Previously known as "petit mal", brief episodes of unconscious-ness with vacant staring, sometimes with fluttering of the eyelids, as if "daydream-ing". No falling to the ground. Rapid recovery. Rare in adults.

Atonic seizure Momentary loss of limb muscle tone causing sudden falling to the ground or drooping of the head.

Complex partial seizure Consciousness is impaired, memory of the episode is distorted but the person may not collapse. The subject may exhibit automatic behaviours ("automatisms" such as chewing, scratching the head, undressing). They can spread to the rest of the brain to become a secondary generalised tonic clonic seizure. The electrical abnormality commonly starts in the temporal lobes.

Myoclonic seizure Sudden, symmetrical, shock like limb movements with or without loss of consciousness.

Simple partial seizure Electrical activity confined to one localised part of the brain causing symptoms and signs that depends on the part of the brain affected. The person remains conscious and fully aware.

Tonic clonic seizure Also known as a convulsion or "grand mal" attack. The person will become stiff (tonic) and collapse and have generalised jerking (clonic) move-ments. Breathing might stop and the bladder might empty. Generalised jerking movements lasting typically for a few minutes are followed by relaxation and deep unconsciousness, before slowly coming round. People are often tired, confused, and may remember nothing. Tonic clonic seizures may follow simple partial or complex partial seizures, where they are classified as secondary generalised tonic clonic seizures. Tonic clonic seizures occurring without warning and in the context of a generalised epilepsy are classified as generalised tonic clonic seizures.

Tonic seizure Stiffening of the whole body with or without loss of consciousness.

Substantive changes since last issue

Monotherapy for partial seizures One new systematic review;[8] conclusions unchanged.

Monotherapy for generalised seizures One new systematic review;[8] conclu-sions unchanged.

REFERENCES

1. Commission on classification and terminology of the international league against epilepsy. Proposal for revised classification of epilepsies and epileptic syndromes. *Epilepsia* 1989;30:389–399.
2. Hauser AW, Annegers JF, Kurland LT. Incidence of epilepsy and unprovoked seizures in Rochester, Minnesota 1935–84. *Epilepsia* 1993;34:453–468.
3. Hauser WA, Kurland LT. The epidemiology of epilepsy in Rochester, Minnesota, 1935 through 1967. *Epilepsia* 1975;16:1–66.
4. Cockerell OC, Johnson AL, Sander JW, Hart YM, Shorvon SD. Remission of epilepsy: results from the national general practice study of epilepsy. *Lancet* 1995;346:140–144.
5. Berg AT, Shinnar S. The risk of seizure recurrence following a first unprovoked seizure: a quantitative review. *Neurology* 1991;41:965–972. Search date not given; primary sources Cumulated Index Medicus, and bibliographies of relevant papers.
6. First Seizure Trial Group (FIRST Group). Randomized clinical trial on the efficacy of antiepileptic drugs in reducing the risk of relapse after a first unprovoked tonic clonic seizure. *Neurology* 1993;43:478–483.
7. Musicco M, Beghi E, Solari A, Viani F, for the FIRST group. Treatment of first tonic clonic seizure does not improve the prognosis of epilepsy. *Neurology* 1997;49:991–998.
8. Marson AG, Williamson PR, Hutton JL, Clough HE, Chadwick DW, on behalf of the epilepsy monotherapy trialists. Carbamazepine versus valproate monotherapy for epilepsy. In: The Cochrane Library, Issue 3, 2000. Oxford: Update Software. Search date 1999; primary sources Medline, Cochrane Library, manufacturers, investigators.
9. Richens A, Davidson DL, Cartlidge NE, Easter DJ. A multicentre comparative trial of sodium valproate and carbamazepine in adult onset epilepsy: adult EPITEG collaborative group. *J Neurol Neurosurg Psychiatry* 1994;57:682–687.
10. Verity CM, Hosking G, Easter DJ. A multicentre comparative trial of sodium valproate and carbamazepine in paediatric epilepsy: the paediatric EPITEG collaborative group. *Dev Med Child Neurol* 1995;37:97–108.
11. Marson AG, Kadir ZA, Hutton JL, Chadwick DW. The new antiepileptic drugs: a systematic review of their efficacy and tolerability. *Epilepsia* 1997;38: 859–880. Search date 1995, primary sources Medline 1966 to December 1995, hand search of key journals, and contacting pharmaceutical companies.
12. Marson AG, Kadir ZA, Hutton JL, Chadwick DW. Gabapentin for drug-resistant partial epilepsy. In: The Cochrane Library, Issue 2, 2000. Oxford: Update Software. Search date 1999; primary sources Cochrane Controlled Trials Register, Cochrane Epilepsy Group Trials Register, and personal contact with Johnson and Johnson, manufacturer of topiramate, and experts in the field.
13. Jette NJ, Marson AG, Kadir ZA, Hutton JL. Topiramate in drug-resistant partial epilepsy. In: The Cochrane Library, Issue 3, 2000. Oxford: Update Software. Search date 1998; primary sources Cochrane Epilepsy Group Trial Register, Cochrane Controlled Trials Register, and personal contact with Parke Davis, manufacturer of gabapentin, and experts in the field.
14. Chadwick DW, Marson AG. Zonisamide for drug-resistant partial epilepsy. In: The Cochrane Library, Issue 3, 2000. Oxford: Update Software. Search date 1999; primary sources Cochrane Controlled Trials Register, Cochrane Epilepsy Group Trials Register, and personal contact with Dainippon and Elan Pharma, manufacturers of zonisamide, and experts in the field.
15. Kalviainen R, Nousiainen I, Mantyjarvi M, et al. Vigabatrin, a gabaergic antiepileptic drug, causes concentric visual field defects. *Neurology* 1999; 53:922–926.
16. Medical Research Council Antiepileptic Drug Withdrawal Study Group. Prognostic index for recurrence of seizures after remission of epilepsy. *BMJ* 1993;306:1374–1378.
17. Medical Research Council Antiepileptic Drug Withdrawal Study Group. Randomised study of antiepileptic drug withdrawal in patients in remission. *Lancet* 1991;337:1175–1180.
18. Berg AT, Shinnar S. Relapse following discontinuation of antiepileptic drugs. *Neurology* 1994;44:601–608. Search date not given; primary sources Index Medicus and bibliographies of relevant papers.

Anthony Marson
Lecturer in Neurology
University of Liverpool
Liverpool
UK

Competing interests: AM has been paid for speaking at meetings by Johnson and Johnson, manufacturers of topiramate, and by Janssen Cilag, Sanofi, and Glaxo Wellcome for attending conferences.

TABLE 1 Effects of additional drug treatment in people not responding to usual treatment: results of four systematic reviews (see text, p 880).[11], [12-14]

Drug added to usual treatment	Daily dose (mg)	Percentage responding (95% CI) (≥ 50% reduction in seizure frequency)‡	OR treatment withdrawal (95% CI)‡	OR adverse effects (95% CI)	Comment
Gabapentin	Placebo	9.9 (7.2 to 13.5)	1.4 (0.8 to 2.5)	Dizziness 2.25 (1.3 to 4) Fatigue 2.25 (1.1 to 4.6) Somnolence 2.04 (1.2 to 3.4)	4 RCTs. Efficacy increased with increasing dose. No plateauing of therapeutic effect, so doses tested may not have been optimal
	600	14.4 (12.0 to 17.3)			
	900	17.3 (14.6 to 20.3)			
	1200	20.6 (17.1 to 24.6)			
	1800	28.5 (21.5 to 36.7)			
Lamotrigine†	200–500	OR versus placebo 2.32 (1.5 to 3.7)	1.2 (0.8 to 1.8)	Ataxia 3.0 (1.86 to 4.8) Diplopia 3.4 (2.1 to 5.6) Dizziness 2.4 (1.6 to 3.5) Nausea 1.7 (1.1 to 2.7)	10 RCTs
Tiagabine	Placebo	6.2 (3.9 to 9.7)	1.8 (1.2 to 2.7)	Dizziness 1.9 (1.2 to 3) Tremor 3.2 (1.2 to 8.8)	3 RCTs
	16	9.8 (4.5 to 20.1)			
	30–32	21.6 (17.7 to 26.0)			
	56	29.8 (19.4 to 42.8)			
Topiramate	Placebo	11.6 (8.0 to 16.6)	2.6 (1.6 to 4.0)	Dizziness 1.99 (1.20 to 3.28) Fatigue 2.52 (1.47 to 4.31) Somnolence 2.86 (1.71 to 4.79) Difficulty thinking 3.95 (1.86 to 8.39)	6 RCTs. Clear plateauing of therapeutic effect. No better with doses >400 mg.
	200	26.7 (15.8 to 41.3)			
	400–1000	45.7 (41.3 to 50.1)			
Vigabatrin	Placebo	13.8 (9.7 to 19.2)	2.58 (1.3 to 5.3)	With vigabatrin, no adverse effects significantly more frequent but 40% develop concentric visual field abnormalities.[15]	4 RCTs
	1000 or 2000	22.8 (14.5 to 34.0)			
	3000 or 6000	45.9 (39.5 to 52.5)			
Zonisamide	400	OR versus placebo 2.72 (1.7 to 4.3)	1.74 (1.0 to 3.0)	Ataxia 4.0 (1.23 to 12.6) Somnolence 2.1 (1.1 to 4) Agitation 2.4 (1.0 to 5.7) Anorexia 3 (1.3 to 6.4)	3 RCTs

*Results were generated from regression models rather than from multiple subgroup analyses.
†Lamotrigine has been evaluated in several crossover trials and one parallel group trial. As a result we were unable to investigate the effects of different lamotrigine doses in regression models.
‡OR of overall treatment withdrawal of usual treatment plus active drug versus usual treatment plus placebo.

TABLE 2 Relative risks of seizure recurrence within 2 years of treatment withdrawal, according to prognostic variable (see text, p 881).[16,17]

Prognostic variable	RR (95% CI) of seizure recurrence within 2 years
Age < 16 years	1.8 (1.3 to 2.4)
Tonic clonic seizures	1.6 (1.1 to 2.2)
Myoclonus	1.8 (1.1 to 3.0)
Treatment with more than one antiepileptic drug	1.9 (1.4 to 2.4)
Seizures since antiepileptic drugs were started	1.6 (1.2 to 2.1)
Any electroencephalographic abnormality	1.3 (1.0 to 1.8)

Risk of recurrence also declined as the seizure free period increased, but in a complex manner.

Search date July 2000: new for this issue

Cristina Sampaio and Joaquim Ferreira

INTERVENTIONS

Key Messages

- We found no RCTs that reported the long term effects of treatments for essential tremor.

- Several small RCTs have found that propranolol (60–240 mg) versus placebo for 1 month improves short term clinical scores, tremor amplitude, and self-evaluation of severity. We found no RCTs of the long term effects of propranolol in essential tremor.

- Four small, brief RCTs found weak evidence that sotalol and atenolol are beneficial for treatment of essential hand tremor. We found no adequate evidence comparing propranolol with other β blockers.

- Two small and brief RCTs have found that primidone versus placebo improves clinical scores. One small brief RCT has found that phenobarbitone versus placebo improves clinical scores. We found no long term RCTs.

- We found no reliable RCTs of the effects of benzodiazepines in people with essential tremor.

- One RCT found no evidence of benefit with methazolamide compared with placebo.

- RCTs found conflicting evidence about the benefit of dihydropyridine calcium channel blockers versus placebo in essential hand tremor.

© Clinical Evidence 2001;5:885–893.

Essential tremor

- One small RCT found weak evidence that flunarizine compared with placebo may reduce the symptoms of essential hand tremor.
- Single RCTs found no evidence of benefit from clonidine or isoniazid on the symptoms of essential tremor.
- Two brief RCTs found conflicting evidence about the effects of gabapentin in essential hand tremor.
- One small RCT of botulinum A toxin-haemagglutinin complex versus placebo in essential hand tremor found short term improvement of clinical scores. We found no RCTs addressing long term benefits or harms.

DEFINITION	Tremor is a rhythmic, mechanical oscillation of at least one body region. The term essential tremor is used when there is either a persistent bilateral tremor of hands and forearms, or an isolated tremor of the head without abnormal posturing, and when there is no evidence that the tremor arises from another identifiable or separately named cause. The diagnosis is not made if there are abnormal neurological signs, known causes of enhanced physiological tremor, a history or signs of psychogenic tremor, sudden change in severity, primary orthostatic tremor, isolated voice tremor, isolated position specific or task specific tremors, and isolated tongue, chin or leg tremor.[1]
INCIDENCE/ PREVALENCE	Essential tremor is one of the most common movement disorders throughout the world, with a prevalence of 0.4–3.9% in the general population.[2]
AETIOLOGY/ RISK FACTORS	Essential tremor is sometimes inherited with an autosomal dominant pattern. About 40% of people with essential tremor have no family history. Alcohol ingestion provides symptomatic benefit in 50–70% of people.[3]
PROGNOSIS	Essential tremor is a persistent and progressive condition. It usually begins during young adulthood and the severity of the tremor increases slowly. Only a small proportion of people with essential tremor seek medical advice, but the proportion in different surveys varies from 0.5–11%.[2] Most people with essential tremor are only mildly affected. However, most of the people who seek medical care are disabled to some extent, and most are socially handicapped by the tremor.[4] A quarter of people receiving medical care for the tremor change jobs or retire because of essential tremor induced disability.[3,5]
AIMS	To reduce tremor; to minimise disability and social embarrassment; to improve quality of life, with minimal adverse effects from treatment.
OUTCOMES	Severity of symptoms and disability measured by clinical rating scales or patient self evaluation. Clinical rating scales are often composite scores that grade tremor amplitude in each body segment in specific postures or tasks. Few scales have been formally validated. Tremorgraphic recordings are reported in many trials but they are proxy outcomes that have been included in this review only when clinical outcomes were not available.
METHODS	*Clinical Evidence* search and appraisal July 2000. We excluded single dose studies and RCTs lasting under 1 week.

OPTION PROPRANOLOL

Several small RCTs have found that propranolol (60–240 mg) versus placebo for 1 month improves short term clinical scores, tremor amplitude, and self evaluation of severity. We found no RCTs of the long term effects of propranolol in essential tremor.

Benefits: **Propranolol versus placebo:** We found no systematic review but found nine[6–14] small (10–24 people) and brief (up to 6 weeks) RCTs, many of which had a crossover design. One RCT[11] compared propranolol versus metoprolol versus placebo (see β blockers other than propranolol below). Seven of the nine RCTs evaluated clinical outcomes, including self evaluations of severity.[6–8,11–14] Propranolol (60–160 mg/day) versus placebo significantly increased the number of people categorised as "responders". The precise definition of responder varied among the RCTs, but the results were similar (22/23 [96%] with propranolol v 5/23 [22%] with placebo; ARR 69%, 95% CI 49% to 89%, NNT 2;[6] ARR 80%, 95% CI 69% to 91%, NNT 2;[7] ARR 64%, 95% CI 33% to 95%, NNT 2, 95% CI 2 to 4;[8] ARs 10/16 [63%] with propranolol v 5/16 [31%] with placebo, ARR 32%, 95% CI 17% to 47%, NNT 4, 95% CI 2 to 6.[14]). Six RCTs found that propranolol versus placebo significantly improved symptom scores (P < 0.05 in each RCT).[7,8,11–14]

Harms: Withdrawals (mainly because of fatigue and bradycardia) were rare (e.g. 1/10 people in 1 RCT).[8] Depression, diarrhoea, breathlessness, sedation, blurred vision, and sexual problems were each reported in less than 5% of people taking propranolol.

Comment: We found no RCTs on the long term effects of propranolol in essential tremor. All trials were analysed as "on treatment" rather than by intention to treat, and this may have biased results. Accelerometry (see glossary, p 892) is a proxy outcome that was reported in five of the RCTs. All five accelerometry results were favourable to propranolol, but there is an inconsistent relationship between accelerometry and clinical measures of effectiveness. People with congestive heart failure, second degree heart block, asthma, severe allergy, and insulin dependent diabetes were generally excluded from the RCTs. All the studies were small. The possibility of publication bias has not been excluded.

OPTION β BLOCKERS OTHER THAN PROPRANOLOL

Four small, brief RCTs found weak evidence that sotalol and atenolol are beneficial for treatment of essential hand tremor. We found no adequate evidence comparing propranolol with other β blockers.

Benefits: **β blockers other than propranolol versus placebo:** We found no systematic review, but found four small (9–24 people) and brief (1–4 weeks) RCTs of different β blockers (sotalol, atenolol, metoprolol, nadolol) versus placebo.[12,15–17] Two RCTs selected participants known to be responders or non-responders to propranolol.[12,16] The RCTs found limited evidence that both sotalol and atenolol versus placebo reduce symptom scores (P < 0.02),[12] and that sotalol versus placebo improves self evaluated measures of tremor (P < 0.05).[17] A small RCT of nadolol versus placebo found significant results only with a subgroup analysis.[16] The fourth crossover RCT (24 people) compared propranolol versus atenolol versus placebo. It found atenolol versus placebo improved accelerometer readings.[15] **β blockers other than propranolol versus propranolol:** We found no systematic review but found two small (14–24 participants) crossover, double blind RCTs.[11,15] The first RCT compared propranolol (120–240 mg/day) versus metoprolol (150–300 mg/day) versus placebo.[11] The RCT reported three outcomes: a composite clinical score, self evaluation, and accelerometer records. Propranolol 120 mg versus metoprolol 150 mg significantly improved clinical scores (P < 0.05) and self assessment (P < 0.01). Propranolol 240 mg versus metoprolol 300 mg significantly improved self assessment (P < 0.05). Propranolol was statistically superior to placebo (P < 0.05), but metoprolol was not. The second RCT compared propranolol versus atenolol versus placebo. It found no significant difference between propranolol and atenolol in accelerometer readings, but more people preferred propranolol to atenolol (12/24 v 1/24).[15]

Harms: See harms of propranolol, p 887.

Comment: We found no long term RCTs. People with congestive heart failure, second degree heart block, asthma, severe allergy, and insulin dependent diabetes were usually excluded from the RCTs. All the studies were small. Publication bias has not been excluded. The weak evidence suggests but does not confirm that β blockers other than propranolol improve essential hand tremor compared with placebo.

| OPTION | BARBITURATES |

Two small and brief RCTs have found that primidone versus placebo improves clinical scores. One small brief RCT has found that phenobarbitone versus placebo improves clinical scores. We found no long term RCTs.

Benefits: We found no systematic reviews. **Primidone versus placebo:** We found two crossover RCTs.[18,19] Both were small (8–22 people) and brief (2–5 weeks). The first RCT[18] compared primidone (up to 750 mg/day) versus phenobarbitone (up to 150 mg/day) versus placebo. Primidone versus placebo significantly improved a clinical score and self evaluation of tremor (P < 0.05). In the second RCT (22 people), primidone (up to 750 mg/day) versus placebo significantly improved clinical scores (P < 0.02), functional tests (P < 0.01), and self evaluation (P < 0.01). Only 16 of 22 people completed the trial.[19] **Phenobarbitone versus placebo:** We found three RCTs.[13,18,20] One crossover RCT (12 people, 5 weeks duration) found that phenobarbitone (120 mg/day) versus placebo significantly improved accelerometer recordings (P < 0.01), symptom rating scale (P < 0.05), but found no significant differences for handwriting tests or self evaluation of tremor.[20] More people responded (decrease in tremor score ≥ 15%) to phenobarbitone than to placebo (11/11 [100%] with phenobarbitone v 6/11 [55%] with placebo; ARR 45%, 95% CI 15% to 75%; NNT 3, 95% CI 2 to 7). The second RCT (double blind, 17 people, only 12 completed the study) compared propranolol (1.7 mg/kg/day) versus phenobarbitone (1.25 mg/kg/day) versus placebo.[13] Phenobarbitone versus placebo produced no significant differences in a clinical tremor score or functional tests.[13] The third small RCT (8 people) found no significant difference between phenobarbitone and placebo.[18]

Harms: **Primidone:** In one RCT[19] five of 12 people taking primidone withdrew because of adverse effects (first dose acute toxic reaction, sedation, daytime sleepiness, tiredness, and depression). **Other barbiturates:** Both primidone (metabolised to phenobarbitone) and phenobarbitone are associated with depression and cognitive and behavioural effects (particularly in children, elderly people, and people with neuropsychiatric problems). See epilepsy, p 876.

Comment: The RCTs were short term, small, and many randomised people did not complete the trials. We found no controlled long term RCTs. Publication bias has not been excluded.

OPTION BENZODIAZEPINES

Two brief RCTs found weak evidence that benzodiazepines versus placebo have no significant clinical benefits in essential hand tremor.

Benefits: We found no systematic reviews. We found two RCTs.[21,22] **Clonazepam versus placebo:** We found one RCT (15 people), which found no significant differences for any outcome.[21] However, nine people withdrew during an open run in period with clonazepam, so only six entered the double blind phase. Potential selection bias makes it difficult to interpret the results of this RCT. **Alprazolam versus placebo:** We found one double blind RCT (24 people), which found alprazolam (up to 3 mg/day) versus placebo improved investigator global impression, but produced no significant difference in clinical scores, functional tests, or self evaluation of tremor.[22]

Harms: We found no data addressing harms of benzodiazepines specifically in populations with essential tremor. Adverse effects with benzodiazepines, including sedation and cognitive and behavioural effects, have been well described for other conditions.

Comment: None.

OPTION METHAZOLAMIDE

One RCT found no evidence of benefit with methazolamide compared with placebo.

Benefits: We found no systematic review. **Versus placebo:** We found one double blind, crossover RCT (25 people with essential tremor), which found methazolamide (up to 300 mg/day) versus placebo produced no significant differences in clinical score, functional tasks, or self evaluation (7/18 [39%] improved with methazolamide v 4/18 [22%] with placebo; ARR +16%, 95% CI −15% to +45%).[23]

Harms: The RCT did not look for adverse effects. Paraesthesias, drowsiness, and headaches are associated with methazolamide.

Comment: Methazolamide is a carbonic anhydrase inhibitor. The RCT was small, and limited by being a crossover study. The results were analysed on treatment rather than by intention to treat, but seven people withdrew from the trial.

OPTION DIHYDROPYRIDINE CALCIUM CHANNEL BLOCKERS

Three RCTs, with weak methods, compared calcium channel blockers with placebo and found conflicting results.

Benefits: We found no systematic review. **Nicardipine versus placebo:** We found two RCTs.[24,25] One double blind, crossover RCT (11 people) found that nicardipine versus placebo produced no significant differences in accelerometer recordings after 1 month.[24] No clinical outcomes were assessed. Another crossover RCT (14 people) compared nicardipine (1 mg/kg/day) for 1 month versus propranolol (160 mg/day) for 1 month versus placebo.[26] Both nicardipine and propranolol versus placebo improved a symptom score. **Nimodipine versus placebo:** We found one double blind, crossover RCT (15 people), which found that nimodipine (90 mg/day) versus placebo produced no difference in clinical scores after 2 weeks of treatment (ARR +20%, 95% CI −15% to +55%).[25]

Harms: Nicardipine and nimodipine can provoke or aggravate heart failure. They are associated with dizziness, flushing, peripheral oedema, lethargy, headache, and fatigue. Adverse gastrointestinal effects (nausea/vomiting, loss of appetite, constipation, weight gain, thirst, indigestion, or altered taste) are reported by 1–3% of people. Abnormalities of laboratory tests (liver function tests) have been observed, usually within 1–8 weeks after starting treatment.

Comment: The RCTs were small, brief, and used crossover design. Publication bias has not been excluded. The evidence is too weak to assess the role of calcium channel blockers in essential hand tremor.

OPTION FLUNARIZINE

One small RCT found weak evidence that flunarizine compared with placebo may reduce the symptoms of essential hand tremor.

Benefits: We found no systematic review. **Flunarizine versus placebo:** We found one double blind, crossover RCT (17 people), which found that flunarizine (10 mg/day) versus placebo significantly improved clinical scores and tremor amplitude after 1 month of treatment (P = 0.0006).[27] Most of the people who completed the study were considered improved with flunarizine (13/15), but the number improving with placebo was not reported.[9]

Harms: Flunarizine is associated with adverse neuropsychiatric effects, and with the development of parkinsonism and other movement disorders.[28–31]

Comment: The RCT was small and brief. The evidence is inconclusive.

<table>
<tr><td>OPTION</td><td>CLONIDINE</td></tr>
</table>

One RCT found no improvement of essential hand tremor with clonidine versus placebo.

Benefits:	**Versus placebo:** We found no systematic review. One small (10 people), brief crossover RCT of clonidine (up to 0.6 mg/day) versus placebo found no significant difference in the number of people who improved (1/10 [10%] with clonidine v 1/10 [10%] with placebo).[32]
Harms:	The RCT did not look for adverse effects. Clonidine has been associated in other studies with sedation, lethargy, drowsiness, constipation, dry mouth, headache, dizziness, fatigue, and weakness.
Comment:	None.

<table>
<tr><td>OPTION</td><td>ISONIAZID</td></tr>
</table>

One RCT found no benefit with isoniazid versus placebo in essential hand tremor.

Benefits:	We found no systematic review. **Versus placebo:** We found one small (15 people, 11 with essential tremor), brief, crossover RCT of isoniazid (up to 1200 mg/day) versus placebo.[33] No significant differences were found in clinical scores or in accelerometer recordings.
Harms:	Isoniazid has been associated in other studies with hepatotoxicity and peripheral neuropathy.
Comment:	None.

<table>
<tr><td>OPTION</td><td>GABAPENTIN</td></tr>
</table>

Two brief RCTs found conflicting evidence about the effects of gabapentin in essential hand tremor.

Benefits:	We found no systematic review. **Versus placebo:** We found two small crossover RCTs (16–20 people).[14,34] The first RCT of gabapentin (1800 mg/day) versus placebo found no difference in clinical scores, activities of daily living, or self evaluation.[35] The second RCT compared gabapentin (up to 1200 mg/day) versus propranolol (up to 120 mg/day) versus placebo. Compared with placebo, gabapentin improved the number of people who responded (10/16 [63%] with gabapentin v 5/16 [31%] with placebo; ARR 32%, 95% CI 17% to 47%; NNT 4, 95% CI 2 to 6), clinical scores ($P < 0.05$), disability ($P < 0.01$), self evaluation ($P < 0.006$), and accelerometer recordings ($P < 0.05$).[14]
Harms:	The RCTs reported fatigue, nausea, and dizziness in people taking gabapentin.[14,34] See epilepsy, p 876.
Comment:	The results of the two RCTs are contradictory. It is unclear whether the difference arose by chance or whether confounding variables, such as prior use of antitremor medications and different baseline severity, explain the difference.

Neurological disorders

| OPTION | BOTULINUM A TOXIN-HAEMAGGLUTININ COMPLEX |

One small RCT of botulinum A toxin-haemagglutinin complex versus placebo in essential hand tremor found short term improvement of clinical scores. We found no RCTs addressing long term benefits or harms.

Benefits: We found no systematic review. We found one RCT (25 people with essential hand tremor unresponsive to medical therapy),[35] which compared placebo versus botulinum A toxin-haemagglutinin complex. The botulinum toxin (50 U) was injected in forearm muscles and repeated if necessary after 1 month (100 U). A successful response to the first injection was more likely with the botulinum toxin than with placebo (12/13 [92%] with botulinum toxin v 1/12 [8%] with placebo). After 4 weeks, mild to moderate improvement was more likely with botulinum toxin (75% with botulinum toxin v 27% with placebo; ARR 48%, 95% CI 30% to 66%; NNT 3, 95% CI 2 to 4). Clinical scores were significantly improved by botulinum toxin versus placebo (P < 0.05), but functional tests and accelerometer measurements were not significantly different.

Harms: The main adverse effect of botulinum A toxin-haemagglutinin complex is transient local weakness.

Comment: None.

GLOSSARY

Accelerometer recording Recording of the movements from a body segment to allow measurement of frequency and amplitude of a tremor.

REFERENCES

1. Deuschl G, Bain P, Brin M, and an Ad Hoc Scientific Committee. Consensus statement of the Movement Disorder Society on Tremor. *Mov Disord* 1998;13(suppl 3):2–23.
2. Louis ED, Ottman R, Hauser WA. How common is the most common adult movement disorder? Estimates the prevalence of essential tremor throughout the world. *Mov Disord* 1988;13:803–808.
3. Koller WC, Busenbark K, Miner K. The relationship of essential tremor to other movement disorders: report on 678 patients. Essential Tremor Study Group. *Ann Neurol* 1994;35:717–723.
4. Auff E, Doppelbauer A, Fertl E. Essential tremor: functional disability vs. subjective impairment. *J Neural Transm Suppl* 1991;33:105–110.
5. Bain PG, Findley LJ, Thompson PD, et al. A study of hereditary essential tremor. *Brain* 1994;117:805–824.
6. Winkler GF, Young RR. Efficacy of chronic propranolol therapy in action tremors of the familial, senile or essential varieties. *N Engl J Med* 1974;290:984–988.
7. Tolosa ES, Loewenson RB. Essential tremor: treatment with propranolol. *Neurology* 1975;25:1041–1044.
8. Morgan MH, Hewer RL, Cooper R. Effect of the beta adrenergic blocking agent propranolol on essential tremor. *J Neurol Neurosurg Psychiatry* 1973;36:618–624.
9. Calzetti S, Findley LJ, Perucca E, Richens A. The response of essential tremor to propranolol evaluation of clinical variables governing its

efficacy on prolonged administration. *J Neurol Neurosurg Psychiatry* 1983;46:393–398.
10. Cleeves L, Findley LJ. Propranolol and propranolol-LA in essential tremor: a double blind comparative study. *J Neurol Neurosurg Psychiatry* 1988;51:379–384.
11. Calzetti S, Findley LJ, Perucca E, et al. Controlled study of metoprolol and propranolol during prolonged administration in people with essential tremor. *J Neurol Neurosurg Psychiatry* 1982;45:893–897.
12. Jefferson D, Jenner P, Marsden CD. Beta-adrenoreceptor antagonists in essential tremor *J Neurol Neurosurg Psychiatry* 1979;42:904–909.
13. Baruzzi A, Procaccianti G, Martinelli P, et al. Phenobarbitone and propranolol in essential tremor: a double-blind controlled clinical trial. *Neurology* 1983;33:296–300.
14. Gironell A, Kulisevsky J, Barbanoj M, et al. A randomised placebo-controlled comparative trial of gabapentin and propranolol in essential tremor. *Arch Neurol* 1999;56:475–480.
15. Larsen TA, Teravainen H, Calne DB. Atenolol vs. propranolol in essential tremor. A controlled, quantitative study. *Acta Neurol Scand* 1982;66:547–554.
16. Koller WC. Nadolol in essential tremor. *Neurology* 1983;33:1076–1077.
17. Leigh PN, Jefferson D, Twomey A, at al. Beta-adrenoreceptor mechanisms in essential tremor; a double-blind placebo controlled trial of metoprolol, sotalol and atenolol. *J Neurol Neurosurg Psychiatry* 1983;46:710–715.

18. Sasso E, Perucca E, Calzetti S. Double-blind comparison of primidone and phenobarbitone in essential tremor. *Neurology* 1988;38:808–810.

19. Findley LJ, Cleeves L, Calzetti S. Primidone in essential tremor of the hands and head: a double-blind controlled clinical study. *J Neurol Neurosurg Psychiatry* 1985;48:911–915.

20. Findley LJ, Cleeves L. Phenobarbitone in essential tremor. *Neurology* 1985;35:1784–1787.

21. Thompson C, Lang A, Parkes JD, et al. A double-blind trial of clonazepam in benign essential tremor. *Clin Neuropharmacol* 1984;7:83–88.

22. Huber SJ, Paulson GW. Efficacy of alprazolam for essential tremor. *Neurology* 1988;38:241–243.

23. Busenbark K, Pahwa R, Hubble J, Hopfensberg K, Koller W. Double-blind controlled study of methazolamide in treatment of essential tremor. *Neurology* 1993;43:1045–1047.

24. Garcia-Ruiz PJ, Garcia-de-Yebenes-Prous J, Jimenez-Jimenez J. Effect of nicardipine on essential tremor: brief report. *Clin Neuropharmacol* 1993;16:456–459.

25. Biary N, Bahou Y, Sofi MA, et al. The effect of nimodipine on essential tremor. *Neurology* 1995;45:1523–1525.

26. Jimenez-Jimenez FJ, Garcia-Ruiz PJ, Cabrera-Valdivia F. Nicardipine versus propranolol in essential tremor. *Acta Neurol (Napoli)* 1994;16:184–188.

27. Biary N, Deeb S, Langenberg P. The effect of flunarizine in essential tremor. *Neurology* 1991;41:311–312.

28. Micheli FE, Pardal MM, Giannaula R, Gatto M, et al. Movement disorders and depression due to flunarizine and cinnarizine. *Mov Disord* 1989;4:139–146.

29. Capella D, Laporte JR, Castel JM, Tristan C, Cos A, Morales-Olivas FJ. Parkinsonism, tremor, and depression induced by cinnarizine and flunarizine. *BMJ* 1988;297:722–723.

30. Chouza C, Caamano JL, Alijanabi R, et al. Parkinsonism tardive dyskinesia, akathisia and depression induced by flunarizine, *Lancet* 1986;i:1303–1304.

31. Micheli F, Pardal MF, Gatto M. Flunarizine and cinnarizine induced extrapyramidal reactions. *Neurology* 1987;37:881–884.

32. Koller W, Herbster G, Cone S. Clonidine in the treatment of essential tremor. *Mov Disord* 1986;4:235–237.

33. Hallett M, Ravitis J, Dubinsky RM, et al. A double-blind trial of isoniazid for essential tremor and other action tremors. *Mov Disord* 1991;6:253–256.

34. Pahwa R, Lyons K, Hubble JP, et al. Double-blind controlled trial of gabapentin in essential tremor. *Mov Disord* 1988;13:465–467.

35. Jankovic J, Schwartz K, Clemence W, et al. A randomised, double-blind, placebo-controlled study to evaluate botulinum toxin type A in essential hand tremor. *Mov Disord* 1996;11:250–256.

Cristina Sampaio
Assistant Professor

Joaquim Ferreira
Neurologist

Instituto de Farmacologia e Terapêutica
Geral
Lisbon School of Medicine
University of Lisbon
Lisbon
Portugal

Competing interests: CS has accepted reimbursement for attending symposium, fees for speaking, fees for organising education and funds for a member of staff from Allergan (Botox) and IPSEN (Dysport). JF, none declared.

Neurological disorders

Search date May 2000

Helen Ford and Mike Boggild

Key Messages

Relapse rates and disability

- We found no evidence that any treatment alters long term outcome in multiple sclerosis (MS).
- Large RCTs in people with active relapsing and remitting MS have found that interferon beta-1a/b reduces relapse rates by a third and may delay development of neurological disability.
- One RCT in people with secondary progressive MS found that interferon beta-1b delayed development of disability by 9–12 months.
- One systematic review of RCTs has found that azathioprine has a modest effect on relapse rates.
- Evidence from single RCTs suggests modest benefit from glatiramer acetate, intravenous immunoglobulin (Ig), and methotrexate.
- Limited evidence from small RCTs suggests that pulsed intravenous mitoxantrone improves outcome in people with very active MS, in whom the risk of severe neurological disability may outweigh the risks of cytotoxic treatment.

- We found insufficient evidence about the effects of plasma exchange on neurological disability.

- We found no evidence about the effects of corticosteroids on long term outcome.

Fatigue

- One short term RCT found that amantadine modestly reduced MS related fatigue. It found no evidence of a benefit from pemoline.

- We found insufficient evidence on the effects of behavioural modification therapy or exercise in people with MS related fatigue.

Spasticity

- Two RCTs have found that tizanidine reduces spasticity in people with MS.

- We found insufficient evidence on the effects of other oral drug treatments or of physical therapy in people with MS related spasticity.

- One small RCT found benefit from intrathecal baclofen in non-ambulant patients with symptomatic spasticity resistant to oral drug treatment.

Multidisciplinary care

- Limited evidence from two RCTs suggests that 3–4 weeks of inpatient rehabilitation results in short term improvements in disability, despite no evidence of an effect on neurological impairment. The duration of this effect is uncertain.

- One small RCT found that prolonged outpatient rehabilitation reduced MS symptom frequency and fatigue.

DEFINITION	MS is a chronic inflammatory disease of the central nervous system. Diagnosis requires evidence of lesions that are separated in both time and space and the exclusion of other inflammatory, structural, or hereditary conditions that might give a similar clinical picture. The disease takes three main forms: relapsing and remitting MS, characterised by episodes of neurological dysfunction interspersed with periods of stability; primary progressive MS, where progressive neurological disability occurs from the outset; and secondary progressive MS, where progressive neurological disability occurs later in the course of the disease.
INCIDENCE/ PREVALENCE	Prevalence varies with geography and racial group; it is highest in white populations in temperate regions.[1] In Europe and North America, prevalence is 1 in 800 people, with an annual incidence of 2–10 per 100 000, making MS the most common cause of neurological disability in young adults. Age of onset is broad, peaking between 20 and 40 years.[2]
AETIOLOGY/ RISK FACTORS	The cause remains unclear, although current evidence suggests that MS is an autoimmune disorder of the central nervous system resulting from an environmental stimulus in genetically susceptible individuals. MS is currently regarded as a single disorder with clinical variants, but there is some evidence that it may comprise several related disorders with distinct immunological, pathological, and genetic features.[1,3]
PROGNOSIS	In 90% of people, early disease is relapsing and remitting. Although some people follow a relatively benign course over many years, most develop secondary progressive disease, usually 6–10 years after onset. In 10% of people, initial disease is primary progressive.

Apart from a minority of people with "aggressive" MS, life expectancy is not greatly affected, and the disease course is often of more than 30 years' duration.

| AIMS | To prevent or delay disability; to improve function; to alleviate symptoms of spasticity; to prevent complications (contractures, pressure sores); to optimise quality of life. |

AIMS To prevent or delay disability; to improve function; to alleviate symptoms of spasticity; to prevent complications (contractures, pressure sores); to optimise quality of life.

OUTCOMES Neurological disability, spasticity, fatigue, general health, relapse rate, quality of life. **Neurological disability:** In clinical trials, disability in MS is usually measured using the disease specific expanded disability status scale (EDSS), which ranges from 0 (no disability) to 10 (death from MS) in half point increments.[4] Lower scores (0–4) reflect specific neurological impairments and disability; higher scores reflect reducing levels of mobility (4–7) and upper limb and bulbar function (7–9.5). The scale is non-linear and has been criticised for indicating change poorly, for emphasising neurological examination and mobility, and for failing to reflect other disabilities (such as fatigue and sexual disability). Some timed outcomes include ambulation (time taken to walk a specified short distance), the nine-hole peg test (time taken to place some pegs into holes in a block), and the box and block test (time taken to transfer blocks between boxes). **Sustained disease progression:** This is reported when an increase in disability from either disease progression or incomplete recovery from relapse is sustained for 3 or 6 months. A relapse that resolves within this time period constitutes non-sustained progression. **Spasticity:** A variety of clinical measures are used, the most common being the Ashworth scale, which scores muscle tone on a scale of 0–4 with 0 representing normal tone and 4 severe spasticity. Other measures include examination findings, neurophysiological techniques, and patient/physician ratings. **General health:** Attempts have been made to customise generic health status scales, but these scales have not been widely used.[5]

METHODS *Clinical Evidence* search and appraisal May 2000. We included only trials focusing on clinical outcomes (disability, relapses, and symptoms) and commonly used drug treatments.

QUESTION What are the effects of treatments aimed at reducing relapse rates and disability?

OPTION INTERFERON BETA-1A/B

We found three large RCTs in people with active relapsing and remitting MS have found that interferon beta-1a/b reduces relapse rates by a third and may delay development of neurological disability. Limited evidence from one RCT in people with secondary progressive disease suggests that interferon beta-1b delays development of disability by 9–12 months. The effect of interferon beta on long term outcome and quality of life is unknown.

Benefits: We found no systematic review. **Relapsing and remitting MS:** We found three large placebo controlled RCTs with 2–3 years' follow up in people with active relapsing and remitting MS.[6–8] One RCT (560 people, disability range EDSS 0–5) compared interferon beta-1a

(22 µg and 44 µg given subcutaneously on alternate days) versus placebo.[6] The trial found significant reductions in relapse rate with both doses over 2 years (22 µg ARR 27%, 95% CI 14% to 39%; 44 µg ARR 33%, 95% CI 21% to 44%) and delayed time to sustained progression of disability (1 or more steps in the EDSS, sustained for at least 3 months). The average time to progression with placebo was 11.9 months versus 18.5 months with 22 µg (P < 0.05, RR progression within 6 months 0.68, 95% CI 0.48 to 0.98) and 21.4 months with 44 µg (P 0.05, RR progression within 6 months 0.62, 95% CI 0.43 to 0.91). A second RCT (372 people, EDSS 0–5.5) compared interferon beta-1b 1.6 MIU and 8 MIU given subcutaneously on alternate days versus placebo.[7] The trial found no significant effect of the lower dose compared with placebo. With the higher dose, the exacerbation rate was significantly reduced (RRR 33%, average number of exacerbations per year 0.84 v 1.27) on placebo, and at 2 years more people were relapse free (OR 2.38, 95% CI 1.25 to 4.25). A third RCT (301 people, EDSS 1–3.5) compared interferon beta-1a 6 MIU given intramuscularly every week versus placebo.[8] At 2 years' follow up (172 people), the trial found a significant reduction in the exacerbation rate (RRR 32%, average number of exacerbations per year 0.61 v 0.9 on placebo) and fewer people had sustained progression of disability (21.9% v 34.9% on placebo, OR not reported). **Secondary progressive MS:** We found one large RCT comparing interferon beta-1b (8 MIU on alternate days) versus placebo in 718 people with secondary progressive MS (EDSS 3–6.5).[9] The average length of follow up was 30 months. It found that average time to sustained progression of disability (as measured by EDSS) was longer with active treatment by 9–12 months (OR 0.65, 95% CI 0.52 to 0.83). To prevent one additional person becoming wheelchair bound, 13 people need to be treated over 30 months (NNT 13, 95% CI 8 to 49). The treatment effect was apparent in people of all levels of baseline disability. There were a large number of withdrawals from both groups (27% placebo and 25% interferon), and no data on quality of life were reported.

Harms: The trials did not report any major adverse effects.[6–9] Mild to moderate effects included early flu-like symptoms (50% of people) and, rarely, leucopenia and asymptomatic elevation of transaminases. Injection site reactions occurred with subcutaneous administration in 80% of people.

Comment: None.

| OPTION | GLATIRAMER ACETATE |

One RCT found a modest effect on relapse rate over 2 years, but found no evidence of an effect on disability.

Benefits: We found no systematic review. **Relapsing and remitting MS:** We found one placebo controlled RCT in 251 people (EDSS 0–5.0).[10] At 2 years, the trial found significantly reduced relapse rates with glatiramer acetate 20 mg daily (ARR 29%, P = 0.007). No significant effect on disability was found. **Secondary progressive MS:** We found no good large RCTs.

Harms: Glatiramer acetate seems to be well tolerated. A self limiting allergic type reaction (flushing, chest tightness, and anxiety) lasting up to 30 minutes was reported by 15% of people on active treatment on at least one occasion (maximum 7 reactions).[10]

Comment: None.

OPTION   INTRAVENOUS IMMUNOGLOBULIN

We found limited evidence from one RCT in people with relapsing and remitting MS suggesting that monthly intravenous immunoglobulin (Ig) reduced disability compared with placebo.

Benefits: We found no systematic review. **Relapsing and remitting MS:** We found one RCT comparing intravenous Ig 0.2 g/kg per month versus placebo in 150 people with relapsing and remitting MS.[11] Treatment was for a maximum of 2 years, but average duration was 21 months. The level of disability decreased in the experimental group (change in EDSS −0.23, 95% CI −0.43 to −0.03) compared with no significant change in the placebo group (change in EDSS 0.12, 95% CI −0.13 to +0.37). The trial did not report data on the time to development of sustained progression of disability. **Secondary progressive MS:** We found no good large RCTs.

Harms: No significant adverse effects were reported.[11] However, higher dosages of intravenous Ig have been associated with aseptic meningitis and several other systemic reactions.[12]

Comment: None.

OPTION   AZATHIOPRINE

One systematic review of RCTs has found a modest reduction in relapse rates but no evidence of a significant effect on disability over 2–3 years.

Benefits: We found one systematic review of azathioprine (search date 1989, 7 RCTs, 793 people with both relapsing remitting MS and progressive MS).[13] At 2 years, the trial found that azathioprine reduced the relapse rate compared with placebo or no treatment (OR 2.04, 95% CI 1.42 to 2.93) and just failed to reduce disability significantly (EDSS mean score difference −0.22, 95% CI −0.43 to +0.003).

Harms: About 10% of people were unable to tolerate therapeutic doses of azathioprine. Well documented adverse effects include hepatotoxicity and bone marrow suppression.[13] There are concerns about long term cancer risk.[14] In one large RCT, 21% of people on azathioprine withdrew after 1 year compared with 12% on placebo.[15]

Comment: The methods used in MS trials have improved over the past 10 years, making it hard to compare older and more recent studies. Trials in the review included people with different categories of MS and used different definitions of relapse.[13]

OPTION   METHOTREXATE

We found weak evidence from one small RCT suggesting that low dose, weekly methotrexate may delay disease progression marginally in people with secondary progressive disease.

Benefits: We found no systematic review. We found one RCT comparing low dose methotrexate (7.5 mg) versus placebo in 60 people with primary or secondary progressive disease.[16] The trial found that methotrexate reduced the risk of progression (ARR 31%, P = 0.01), defined by a composite outcome measure, including EDSS, ambulation, nine-hole peg test, and box and block test.

Harms: No major toxicity was reported in the RCT, but marrow suppression and hepatotoxicity can occur with low dose methotrexate; regular monitoring is advised.[16]

Comment: The trial's findings mainly reflected changes in upper limb function.[16] Studies of other drugs have not used composite outcome measures, which makes comparisons difficult. Relative risks for treatment failure were not reported.

OPTION   MITOXANTRONE

Limited evidence from small RCTs suggests that pulsed intravenous mitoxantrone reduces disease activity in people with very active MS, in whom the risk of severe neurological disability may outweigh the risks of cytotoxic treatment.

Benefits: We found no systematic review. Several small RCTs have evaluated this cytotoxic antibiotic in people with MS, finding a positive or neutral effect. One non-blinded RCT in 42 people with very active disease compared 6 months of treatment with monthly intravenous mitoxantrone 20 mg plus methylprednisolone 1 g versus methylprednisolone alone.[17] The trial found mitoxantrone plus methylprednisolone significantly reduced disease activity (as assessed by appearance on magnetic resonance imaging) and lower annual clinical relapse rates (0.7 v 3.0, P < 0.01) compared with methylprednisolone alone.

Harms: The major risk is dose related cardiotoxicity, but this is rare at the doses used in trials in people with MS. Leucopenia, nausea, and amenorrhoea are commonly reported.[18]

Comment: A larger blinded RCT has recently been completed and results are awaited.

QUESTION   What are the effects of treatments for acute relapse?

OPTION   CORTICOSTEROIDS

We found evidence from a large RCT in people with acute optic neuritis, and several small RCTs in people with acute MS relapse, that pulsed intravenous methylprednisolone improves recovery at 4 weeks. We found no evidence that steroids affect long term outcome. None of the available studies of steroids include quantitative data on the effects of treatment.

Benefits: We found no systematic review. **Oral steroids versus placebo:** We found one RCT comparing oral methylprednisolone (500 mg daily for 5 days with 10 day taper) versus placebo in 51 people with acute MS relapse.[19] The trial found that oral steroid treatment improved outcome at 3 and 8 weeks, as measured by EDSS, Scripps neurological rating scale (derived from the neurological examination), and visual analogue scores. **Intravenous steroids versus placebo:** Two small RCTs (45 people) compared intravenous methylprednisolone (500 mg for 5 days or 15 mg/kg per day) versus placebo for acute relapses.[20,21]In both trials, methylprednisolone improved the chance of recovery (no OR or RR given). One large RCT in 457 people with acute optic neuritis compared intravenous methylprednisolone (151 people, 1 g daily for 3 days followed by an oral steroid taper 11 days) versus oral prednisolone (156 people, 1 mg/kg per day for 14 days) versus placebo (150 people). Compared with placebo, intravenous methylprednisolone significantly improved the visual fields at 4 weeks (P = 0.0001) but not at 6 months. **Oral versus intravenous steroids:** We found two small RCTs comparing intravenous versus oral methylprednisolone.[23,24] These trials found no significant differences between the effects of each treatment on functional or disability scores, as measured by the EDSS. The first RCT (35 people with acute relapse) compared identical doses of methylprednisolone (500 mg/day for 5 days).[23] At 4 weeks' follow up, there was no significant difference in disability scores between the groups. The second RCT (n = 80) compared high dose intravenous methylprednisolone (1 g for 3 days) versus intermediate dose oral methylprednisolone.[24] The trial found no significant difference between treatments in terms of EDSS at predetermined time points after relapse.

Harms:
In the trial in people with acute optic neuritis, oral steroids were associated with an increased risk of recurrence of optic neuritis at 2 years (RR of a "new episode" of optic neuritis in either eye with oral steroids versus placebo 1.79, 95% CI 1.08 to 2.95).[22] This effect was no longer evident at 3 years. Occasional serious complications of intravenous methylprednisolone include acute psychosis, avascular necrosis of the femoral head, and sudden death caused by cardiac arrhythmia. A retrospective analysis of 350 treatment courses in people with MS found one episode of psychotic depression and one case of severe duodenitis, but no cardiac events or avascular necrosis.[25]

Comment:
In one RCT, minor adverse effects from steroid treatment were common and may have compromised blinding.[19]

OPTION   PLASMA EXCHANGE

We found insufficient evidence on the effectiveness of plasma exchange in people with acute demyelinating episodes who had previously failed to respond to intravenous steroids.

Benefits:
We found no systematic review. We found one randomised, double blinded crossover trial of plasma exchange versus a sham control in people with acute relapses of MS (n = 12) or other demyelinating disease (n = 10) who had previously failed to respond to intravenous steroids.[26] The trial found moderate or greater improvement in neurological disability in people receiving plasma exchange compared with sham treatment (8/19 [42%] v 1/17 [6%]; ARI 36%, 95% CI 1% to 81%; RR 7.2, 95% CI 1.2 to 15; NNT 3, 95% CI 1 to 68).

Harms: The trial reported no major complications.[26]

Comment: At the time of randomisation, all patients had failed to respond to standard doses of intravenous corticosteroids, and were within 3 months of onset of the acute deficit. This is a small study in a difficult area and further data are needed.

QUESTION What are the effects of treatments for fatigue in multiple sclerosis?

OPTION DRUG TREATMENT: AMANTADINE AND PEMOLINE

One short term RCT found that amantadine modestly reduced MS related fatigue. This trial, and a small crossover RCT, found no evidence of benefit from pemoline.

Benefits: We found no systematic review but found two RCTs.[27,28] One RCT (119 people) compared amantadine and pemoline versus placebo.[27] Amantadine significantly reduced fatigue, measured by the MS specific fatigue scale ($P = 0.04$), but there was no significant difference in the effects of pemoline and placebo. After a 2 week washout period, the proportions of people who reported feeling better on than off the study medication were 79% (15/19) with amantadine, 32% (7/22) with pemoline, and 52% with placebo. Neither amantadine nor pemoline affected the secondary outcome measures of sleep or depression. A crossover RCT in 46 people found no significant benefit of pemoline over placebo.[28]

Harms: Two people taking amantadine withdrew from the trial because of rash or anxiety. Other reported adverse effects of amantadine included sleep disturbance (2 people) and palpitations (1 person).[27]

Comment: None.

OPTION BEHAVIOURAL MODIFICATION THERAPY

We found insufficient evidence on the effects of behavioural modification therapy in people with MS related fatigue.

Benefits: We found no systematic review and no RCTs.

Harms: None reported.

Comment: None.

OPTION EXERCISE

We found insufficient evidence on the effects of exercise in people with MS related fatigue.

Benefits: We found no systematic review. We found one RCT (46 people, EDSS 0–6.0), which compared 15 weeks of aerobic training versus no exercise.[29] Using a scale that measures mental and physical fatigue, there was a significant reduction in fatigue at 10 weeks but not after completion of the exercise programme. A different scale that measured only physical fatigue remained unchanged in both groups of people. The trial found improvements in emotional behaviour and quality of life.

Harms: None reported.

Comment: People with moderate disability or severe fatigue may have difficulty adhering to an aerobic exercise programme.

QUESTION **What are the effects of treatments for spasticity?**

OPTION **PHYSICAL THERAPY**

One small RCT of inpatient physiotherapy found no evidence of benefit in terms of mobility or activities of daily living.

Benefits: We found no systematic review. One non-blinded RCT compared early versus delayed physiotherapy (9 weeks of inpatient treatment) in 45 people with progressive MS.[30] The trial found no evidence of an effect of treatment on measures of mobility (timed walk, Rivermead mobility index) or activities of daily living. Treated people reported reduced mobility related stress (P < 0.001).

Harms: None reported.

Comment: The study lacked the power to detect a small effect of treatment on mobility.

OPTION **ORAL DRUG TREATMENT**

Two RCTs have found that tizanidine reduces spasticity in people with MS, but with no evidence of a beneficial effect on mobility. We found insufficient evidence to assess other oral drug treatments.

Benefits: **Versus placebo:** We found no systematic review. We found two large RCTs comparing tizanidine versus placebo in people with MS related spasticity.[31,32] One RCT (220 people, tizanidine 2–36 mg daily) found no significant difference in Ashworth scores (see Outcomes, p 896) but found that tizanidine reduced self reported clonus and spasm.[31] The other RCT (187 people, tizanidine 24–36 mg daily) found that tizanidine significantly reduced muscle tone (P < 0.05), although the trial found no impact of tizanidine on mobility related activities of daily living.[32] **Versus each other:** We found one systematic review (published 1998, 10 European RCTs, 70 people with both cerebrovascular disease and MS) comparing tizanidine versus baclofen (7 RCTs) or diazepam (3 RCTs). The review found no difference between the three drugs in their effects on muscle tone.[33] The trials were too small to rule out clinically important differences.

Harms: Comparative studies of baclofen and tizanidine found similar levels of adverse effects (including muscle weakness, sedation, and dry mouth), but tizanidine may be less likely than baclofen to cause muscle weakness.[33]

Comment: Increased muscle tone is not always detrimental or disabling; mild or moderate spasticity may aid standing or transfers.

INTRATHECAL BACLOFEN

Limited evidence from one small RCT suggests benefit in non-ambulant people with symptomatic spasticity resistant to oral drug treatment.

Benefits: We found no systematic review. We found one small RCT comparing intrathecal baclofen versus intrathecal saline in 20 (19 non-ambulant) people with spasticity resistant to oral baclofen.[34] Participants suffered from MS or spinal cord injury. Baclofen significantly reduced spasticity and spasm frequency. Average Ashworth scores (see outcomes, p 896) fell from 4.0 to 1.2 (P < 0.0001), with scores for all participants improving from baseline.

Harms: Potential problems include pump failure, infection, and, rarely, baclofen overdose.

Comment: We found no evidence on the role of intrathecal baclofen in ambulant patients.

What are the effects of a multidisciplinary approach to patient management?

INPATIENT REHABILITATION

Two RCTs found that 3–4 weeks of inpatient rehabilitation resulted in short term improvements in disability, despite no evidence of an effect on levels of neurological impairment. The duration of this effect is uncertain.

Benefits: We found no systematic review but found two RCTs.[35,36] The first trial compared a short period of inpatient rehabilitation (average 25 days) versus remaining on the waiting list (non-treatment control group) in 66 people with progressive MS who were selected as "good candidates" for rehabilitation.[35] Rehabilitation significantly improved disability, assessed by the functional independence measure and the London handicap scale, despite unchanged levels of neurological impairment (EDSS). Follow up of these people found that benefit persisted for up to 9 months. The second RCT compared 3 weeks of inpatient rehabilitation versus exercises at home in 50 (ambulant) people. The trial found improvements in disability, as measured by the functional independence measure (P < 0.004), which persisted at 9 but not at 15 weeks' follow up.[36]

Harms: None reported.

Comment: Many centres lack appropriate rehabilitation facilities.

OUTPATIENT REHABILITATION

One small RCT found that prolonged outpatient rehabilitation reduced MS symptom frequency and fatigue.

Benefits: We found no systematic review. We found one RCT comparing outpatient rehabilitation (5 hours per week for 1 year) versus remaining on the waiting list (non-treatment control group) in 46 people with progressive MS. Rehabilitation reduced the frequency

Multiple sclerosis

of fatigue (effect size −0.27) and MS symptoms (effect size −0.32), despite no evidence of a change in neurological impairment in either group.[37]

Harms: None reported.

Comment: Future trials need to record effects on disability and quality of life as well as impairment.

REFERENCES

1. Compston A. Genetic epidemiology of multiple sclerosis. *J Neurol Neurosurg Psychiatry* 1997;62: 553–561.

2. Weinshenker BG, Bass B, Rice GPA, et al. The natural history of multiple sclerosis: a geographically based study. 1. Clinical course and disability. *Brain* 1989;112:133–146.

3. Lucchinetti CF, Bruck W, Rodriguez M, Lassmann H. Distinct patterns of multiple sclerosis pathology indicates heterogeneity in pathogenesis. *Brain Pathol* 1996;6:259–274.

4. Kurtzke JF. Rating neurological impairment in multiple sclerosis: an expanded disability status scale (EDSS). *Neurology* 1983;33:1444–1452.

5. Vickrey BG, Hays RD, Genovese BJ, Myers LW, Ellison GW. Comparison of a generic to disease-targeted health-related quality-of-life measures for multiple sclerosis. *J Clin Epidemiol* 1997;50:557–569.

6. PRISMS Study Group. Randomised double-blind placebo-controlled study of interferon beta-1a in relapsing/remitting multiple sclerosis. *Lancet* 1998;352:1498–1504.

7. The IFNB Multiple Sclerosis Study Group. Interferon beta-1b is effective in relapsing-remitting multiple sclerosis. Clinical results of a multicenter, randomised, double-blind, placebo-controlled trial. *Neurology* 1993;43:655–661.

8. Jacobs LD, Cookfair DL, Rudick RA, et al. Intramuscular interferon beta-1a for disease progression in relapsing multiple sclerosis. *Ann Neurol* 1996;39:285–294.

9. European Study Group on Interferon Beta-1b in Secondary Progressive MS. Placebo-controlled multicentre randomised trial of interferon beta-1b in treatment of secondary progressive multiple sclerosis. *Lancet* 1998;352:1491–1497.

10. Johnson KP, Brooks BR, Cohen JA, et al. Copolymer-1 reduces relapse rate and improves disability in relapsing-remitting multiple sclerosis: results of a phase III multicenter, double-blind, placebo-controlled trial. *Neurology* 1995;45: 1268–1276.

11. Fazekas F, Deisenhammer F, Strasser-Fuchs S, Naylor G, Mamoli M, for the Austrian Immunoglobulin in Multiple Sclerosis Study Group. Randomised placebo-controlled trial of monthly intravenous immunoglobulin therapy in relapsing-remitting multiple sclerosis. *Lancet* 1997;349: 589–593.

12. Stangel M, Hartung HP, Marx P, Gold R. Side-effects of high-dose intravenous immunoglobulins. *Clin Neuropharmacol* 1997;20:385–393.

13. Yudkin PL, Ellison GW, Ghezzi A, et al. Overview of azathioprine treatment in multiple sclerosis. *Lancet* 1991;338:1051–1055. Search date 1989; primary sources Medline 1966 to 1989; and hand searched references.

14. Confavreux C, Saddier P, Grimaud J, et al. Risk of cancer from azathioprine therapy in multiple sclerosis: a case-control study. *Neurology* 1996; 46:1607–1612.

15. British and Dutch Multiple Sclerosis Azathioprine Trial Group. Double masked trial of azathioprine in multiple sclerosis. *Lancet* 1988;2:179–183.

16. Goodkin DE, Rudick RA, VanderBrug Medendorp S, et al. Low-dose (7.5 mg) oral methotrexate reduces the rate of progression in chronic progressive multiple sclerosis. *Ann Neurol* 1995; 37:30–40.

17. Edan G, Miller D, Clanet M, et al. Therapeutic effect of mitoxantrone combined with methylprednisolone in multiple sclerosis: a randomised multicentre study of active disease using MRI and clinical criteria. *J Neurol Neurosurg Psychiatry* 1997;62:112–118.

18. MacDonald M, Posner LE, Dukart G, et al. A review of the acute and chronic toxicity of mitoxantrone. *Future Trends Chemother* 1985;6: 443–450.

19. Sellebjerg F, Frederiksen JL, Nielsen PM, Olesen J. Double-blind, randomised, placebo-controlled study of oral, high-dose methylprednisolone in attacks of MS. *Neurology* 1998;51:529–534.

20. Milligan NM, Newcombe R, Compston DAS. A double-blind controlled trial of high dose methylprednisolone in patients with multiple sclerosis: 1. Clinical effects. *J Neurol Neurosurg Psychiatry* 1987;50:511–516.

21. Durelli L, Cocito D, Riccio A, et al. High-dose intravenous methylprednisolone in the treatment of multiple sclerosis. *Neurology* 1986;36:238–243.

22. Beck RW, Cleary PA, Anderson MM, et al. A randomised controlled trial of corticosteroids in the treatment of acute optic neuritis. *N Engl J Med* 1992;326:581–588.

23. Alam SM, Kyriakides T, Lawden M, Newman PK. Methylprednisolone in multiple sclerosis: a comparison of oral with intravenous therapy at equivalent high dose. *J Neurol Neurosurg Psychiatry* 1993;56:1219–1220.

24. Barnes D, Hughes RAC, Morris RW, et al. Randomised trial of oral and intravenous methylprednisolone in acute relapses of multiple sclerosis. *Lancet* 1997;349:902–906.

25. Lyons PR, Newman PK, Saunders M. Methylprednisolone therapy in multiple sclerosis; a profile of adverse events. *J Neurol Neurosurg Psychiatry* 1988;51:285–287.

26. Weinshenker BG, O'Brien PC, Petterson TM, et al. A randomised trial of plasma exchange in acute central nervous system inflammatory demyelinating disease. *Neurology* 1999;46:878–886.

27. Fuller KJ, Dawson K, Wiles CM. Physiotherapy in chronic multiple sclerosis: a controlled trial. *Clin Rehabil* 1996;10:195–204.

28. Krubb LB, Coyle PK, Doscher C, et al. Fatigue therapy in multiple sclerosis: results of a double-blind, randomised parallel trial of amantadine, pemoline and placebo. *Neurology* 1995;45: 1956–1961.

29. Weinshenker BG, Penman M, Bass B. A double-blind, randomised, crossover trial of pemoline in fatigue associated with multiple sclerosis.

Neurology 1992;42:1468–1471.

30. Petajan JH, Gappmaier E, White AT, et al. Impact of aerobic training on fitness and quality of life in multiple sclerosis. _Ann Neurol_ 1996;39:432–441.

31. Smith C, Birnbaum G, Carter JL, Greenstein J, Lublin FD. Tizanidine treatment of spasticity caused by multiple sclerosis: results of a double-blind, placebo-controlled trial. US tizanidine study group. _Neurology_ 1994;44(suppl):34–42.

32. UK Tizanidine Trial Group. A double-blind, placebo-controlled trial of tizanidine in the treatment of spasticity caused by multiple sclerosis. _Neurology_ 1994;44:S70–S78.

33. Groves L, Shellenberger MK, Davis CS. Tizanidine treatment of spasticity: a meta-analysis of controlled, double-blind, comparative studies with baclofen and diazepam. _Adv Ther_ 1998;15:241–251. Search date not given; primary sources

records of Sandoz (now Novartis).

34. Penn RD, Savoy SM, Corcos D, et al. Intrathecal baclofen for severe spinal spasticity. _N Engl J Med_ 1989;320:1517–1521.

35. Freeman JA, Langdon DW, Hobart JC, Thompson AJ. The impact of inpatient rehabilitation on progressive multiple sclerosis. _Ann Neurol_ 1997; 42:236–244.

36. Solari A, Fillipini G, Gasco P, et al. Physical rehabilitation has a positive effect on disability in multiple sclerosis patients. _Neurology_ 1999;52: 57–62.

37. Di Fabio RP, Soderberg J, Choi T, Hanson CR, Schapiro RT. Extended outpatient rehabilitation: its influence on symptom frequency, fatigue and functional status for persons with progressive multiple sclerosis. _Arch Phys Med Rehabil_ 1998; 79:141–146.

Helen Ford
Consultant Neurologist
St James's Hospital
Leeds
UK

Mike Boggild
Consultant Neurologist
The Walton Centre for Neurology and
Neurosurgery
Liverpool
UK

Competing interests: HF has been paid by Schering and Biogen for speaking at meetings, and by Serono Pharmaceuticals and Biogen for attending conferences; MB has received financial support for attending scientific meetings from Biogen, Serono Pharmaceuticals, and Teva Pharmaceuticals, and has organised educational sessions for Serono.

Parkinson's disease

Search date December 2000

A Peter Moore and Carl Clarke

INTERVENTIONS

Key Messages

- We found no good evidence that any drug delays the progression of Parkinson's disease.

- Five RCTs have found that selegiline delays the need for levodopa, but one of these RCTs found increased mortality in people treated with selegiline.

- Two RCTs found no evidence of a difference in long term motor complications with controlled release or immediate release levodopa monotherapy in people with early Parkinson's disease.

- One systematic review and six long term RCTs have found that dopamine agonist monotherapy reduces the incidence of motor complications. However, levodopa monotherapy is slightly more effective in treating motor impairments and disability. The strategy of starting people with early disease on dopamine agonists to defer the need for levodopa needs further evaluation.

- Six systematic reviews have found that, when used in later stage disease, adjuvant dopamine agonists reduce "off" time (see glossary, p 913), improve motor impairments and activities of daily living, and reduce levodopa dose, but increase dopaminergic adverse effects and dyskinesia (see glossary, p 913).

- Two systematic reviews found limited evidence that pallidotomy (see glossary, p 913) may be effective for the control of tremor, rigidity and dyskinesia, although serious complications of surgery can occur.

DEFINITION   Idiopathic Parkinson's disease is an age related neurodegenerative disorder and the most common cause of the parkinsonian syndrome: a combination of asymmetric bradykinesia, hypokinesia, and rigidity, sometimes combined with rest tremor and postural changes. Clinical diagnostic criteria have a sensitivity of 80% and specificity of 30% compared with the gold standard of diagnosis at autopsy.[1] The primary pathology is progressive loss of dopaminergic cells from the substantia nigra in the brainstem. Treatment aims to replace or compensate for the lost dopamine. A good response to treatment supports, but does not confirm, the diagnosis. Several other catecholaminergic neurotransmitter systems are also deranged in Parkinson's disease.

INCIDENCE/ PREVALENCE   Parkinson's disease occurs worldwide with equal incidence in both sexes. In 5–10% of people who develop Parkinson's disease it appears before the age of 40 years (young onset), with a mean age of onset of about 65 years. Overall age adjusted prevalence is 1% worldwide and 1.6% in Europe, rising from 0.6% at age 60–64 years to 3.5% at age 85–89 years.[2,3] First degree relatives of affected people may have twice the risk of developing Parkinson's disease (17% chance of developing the condition in their lifetime) compared with people in the general population.[4–6]

AETIOLOGY/ RISK FACTORS   The cause is unknown. Parkinson's disease may represent different conditions with a final common pathway. People may be affected differently by a combination of genetic and environmental factors (viruses, toxins, 1-methyl-4-phenyl-1,2,3,6-tetrahydropyridine [MPTP], well water, vitamin E, and smoking).[7–10] Purely genetic varieties probably comprise a small minority of people with Parkinson's disease.[11,12]

PROGNOSIS   Parkinson's disease is currently incurable. Disability is progressive and associated with increased mortality (RR death compared with the general population ranges from 1.6 to 3).[13] Treatment may reduce symptoms and slow progression but rarely achieves complete control. The question of whether treatment reduces mortality remains controversial.[14] Levodopa seemed to reduce mortality in the UK for 5 years after its introduction, before a "catch up" effect was noted and overall mortality rose towards previous levels. This suggested a limited prolongation of life.[15] An Australian cohort study followed 130 people treated for 10 years. The standardised mortality ratio was 1.58 (P < 0.001). At 10 years, 25% had been admitted to a nursing home and only four were still employed. The mean duration of disease until death was 9.1 years.[16] In a similar Italian cohort study[17] over 8 years, RR death for affected people versus healthy controls was 2.3 (95% CI 1.60 to 3.39). Age at initial census date was the main predictor of outcome: for age under 75 years, RR death was 1.80 (95% CI 1.04 to 3.11); for age over 75 years, RR death was 5.61 (95% CI 2.13 to 14.8).

AIMS   To improve symptoms and quality of life; to slow disease progression; to limit short and long term adverse effects of treatment, such as motor fluctuations (see glossary, p 913).

OUTCOMES Disease severity; severity of drug induced symptoms or signs; rate of progression of symptoms; need for levodopa or other treatment; adverse effects of treatment; withdrawals from treatment; and quality of life measures. There are no universal scales, but commonly used scales are the Hoehn and Yahr scale, Webster scale, the Unified Parkinson's Disease Rating Scale (UPDRS), the Core Assessment Programme for Intracerebral Transplantation (CAPIT),[18,19] the Parkinson's Disease Quality of Life questionnaire (PDQL),[20] and the UK Parkinson's Disease Quality of Life questionnaire 39 (PDQ-39).[21]

METHODS *Clinical Evidence* update search and appraisal December 2000. Unless stated otherwise, we have used the term "levodopa" to refer to a combination of levodopa and a peripheral decarboxylase inhibitor.

QUESTION What are the effects of drug treatments in people with early Parkinson's disease?

OPTION SELEGILINE

Five large RCTs have found that selegiline delays the need for levodopa, but one of these trials found increased mortality in people treated with selegiline.

Benefits: We found no systematic review. We found five large placebo controlled RCTs in people with early Parkinson's disease.[22–26] The first RCT (800 people) found that selegiline delayed the need for levodopa for 9 months (HR 0.50 for requiring levodopa in each time period, 95% CI 0.41 to 0.62; P < 0.001).[22] The second RCT (101 people newly diagnosed with Parkinson's disease) found that after 12 months of treatment and 2 months of washout there was a significantly smaller deterioration in total UPDRS score with selegiline versus placebo.[23] The third RCT (782 people) found no evidence of a clinically important difference after 4 years of selegiline.[24] The fourth RCT (116 people) found that significantly fewer people randomised to selegiline required a 50% or greater increase in their levodopa dose after 5 years (50% on selegiline v 74% on placebo; P = 0.027).[25] The fifth RCT (163 people) found significantly better motor function in those treated with selegiline for 5 years.[26] The absence of any deterioration on selegiline withdrawal argues against any symptomatic effect after 5 years of treatment. Other studies of early selegiline treatment were either too small or too short to reach a conclusion.[27]

Harms: One large RCT and one non-systematic review (see comment below) found no evidence of a difference in mortality between selegiline and placebo.[27,28] Another RCT found (at interim analysis after 5.6 years of follow up) higher mortality in those treated with selegiline (HR 1.57, 95% CI 1.07 to 2.31); the selegiline arm of the trial was terminated early.[24] Updated analysis (including blinded assessment of cause specific mortality) found that the increase in mortality did not quite reach significance (HR 1.30, 95% CI 0.99 to 1.72), perhaps because the study was stopped when, by chance, mortality was high.[29,30] One retrospective observational study in

12 621 people who had taken an antiparkinsonian drug (excluding those also taking antipsychotic drugs) found increased mortality in people prescribed selegiline, but the CI included zero (ARI 11%, 95% CI 0% to 23%).[31]

Comment: The review[27] claimed to be systematic but omitted at least one relevant study. A systematic review is under way, and a large RCT is planned.

OPTION **MODIFIED RELEASE LEVODOPA**

Two RCTs found no evidence that modified release levodopa reduced motor complications or improved disease control at 5 years versus immediate release levodopa in people with early Parkinson's disease.

Benefits: We found no systematic review. Two long term RCTs (134 and 618 people with early Parkinson's disease) compared modified versus immediate release levodopa preparations (co-beneldopa and co-careldopa).[32,33] At 5 years, the trials found no significant differences in the incidence of dyskinesia (41% with modified release v 34% with immediate release co-beneldopa), motor fluctuations (59% v 57%), motor impairment, or activities of daily living.

Harms: The RCT of co-careldopa found that nausea was more common with the immediate release preparation.[33]

Comment: In both trials, levodopa was combined with a peripheral decarboxylase inhibitor.[32,33]

OPTION **DOPAMINE AGONIST VERSUS LEVODOPA IN EARLY DISEASE**

Widespread experience suggests dyskinesias and fluctuations in motor response are related to long term levodopa treatment and are irreversible. One systematic review and six long term RCTs have found that dopamine agonist monotherapy reduces the incidence of these motor complications. However, levodopa monotherapy is slightly more effective in treating motor impairments and disability.

Benefits: We found two systematic reviews of bromocriptine monotherapy. The first review (search date not stated) identified six RCTs comparing bromocriptine versus levodopa and found that bromocriptine delayed motor complications and dyskinesias.[34] The second review (search date not stated) identified eight RCTs comparing bromocriptine plus levodopa versus levodopa alone, and found a trend towards reduced dyskinesia with combination treatment but no difference in duration of "off" time.[35] Neither review reported effects on disability or motor impairment. We found six additional long term RCTs. The first (268 people) compared ropinirole plus rescue levodopa if needed versus levodopa alone, and found that at 5 years dyskinesias were more common with levodopa alone (OR 3.8, 95% CI 2.1 to 6.9).[36] The trial found no difference in disability at 5 years (UPDRS activities of daily living scale) and a small increase in motor impairments with ropinirole. The second RCT (301 people) compared pramipexole plus rescue levodopa with levodopa alone. It found that pramipexole plus rescue levodopa versus levodopa significantly reduced all motor complications at

2 years (motor complications 28% with pramipexole v 51% with levodopa alone; HR 0.45, 95% CI 0.30 to 0.66).[37] Improvements in UPDRS motor and ADL scores were greater in the levodopa group. The third RCT (419 people), published as an abstract, compared cabergoline plus rescue levodopa versus levodopa alone. It found that cabergoline versus levodopa significantly reduced motor complications at 5 years (motor complications with cabergoline 22% v 34% with levodopa group; P < 0.05).[38] However, activities of daily living scores were worse with cabergoline. The fourth RCT (294 people), published in preliminary form, compared pergolide alone (without rescue levodopa) versus levodopa. The trial found that pergolide versus levodopa significantly reduced motor complications at 3 years (one or more motor complications with pergolide 16% v 33% with levodopa; P < 0.004).[39] The fifth RCT (90 people) was unblinded, and compared lisuride (plus rescue levodopa) versus levodopa alone; it found fewer motor complications in the lisuride group at 4 years, although motor function was worse in those treated with lisuride.[40] The sixth RCT (82 people) was partially blinded, and compared lisuride plus levodopa versus levodopa alone; it found no significant difference in complications rates between the two arms of the study at 5 years.[41]

Harms:
Adverse events were similar in all treatment groups, except hallucinations, which were more frequent with ropinirole,[36] and somnolence with pramipexole.[37] The RCT comparing pergolide versus levodopa found that motor UPRDS scores were worse in people taking pergolide, and significantly more people in the pergolide group withdrew from treatment (18% with pergolide v 10% with levodopa; P < 0.05).[39]

Comment:
The subsequent 5 year RCTs had withdrawal rates of about 50%.[36,38,41] The doses of levodopa and lisuride were low in this trial and paradoxically the UPDRS motor and ADL scores were better in the combined therapy group. We found no direct comparisons of individual dopamine agonists. A large, UK based RCT is examining quality of life and health economic outcomes of agonist monotherapy in people likely to develop motor complications. A multicentre North American study is investigating the effect of levodopa on dopaminergic cell death.[42]

QUESTION | **What are the effects of adding a dopamine agonist in people with a fluctuating response to levodopa?**

Systematic reviews have found that certain dopamine agonists reduce "off" time, improve motor impairment and activities of daily living, and reduce requirement for levodopa, but increase dopaminergic adverse effects and dyskinesia.

Benefits:
Versus placebo: We found six systematic reviews of placebo controlled RCTs.[43-48] The first (search date 1998, 7 RCTs, 396 people with later Parkinson's disease) compared adjuvant bromocriptine versus placebo.[43] Heterogeneity in trial design and outcomes made it impossible to draw conclusions. The second review (search date 1998) identified no trials comparing lisuride versus placebo.[44] The third review (search date 1999) identified one RCT (376 people) comparing pergolide versus placebo.[45] It

found that pergolide reduced daily "off" time (mean difference 1.6 hours, P < 0.001), reduced daily levodopa dose (mean 184 mg, P < 0.001), and improved activities of daily living scores. The fourth review (search date 1999) identified four trials comparing pramipexole versus placebo in a total of 669 people.[48] Pramipexole reduced daily "off" time (WMD 1.8 hours, 95% CI 1.2 hours to 2.3 hours), reduced levodopa dose (WMD 115 mg, 95% CI 87 mg to 143 mg), and improved activities of daily living scores. The fifth systematic review (search date 2000, 149 people) compared ropinirole versus placebo, and identified one RCT using sufficient dosage of the agonist.[46] It found that ropinirole did not significantly reduce "off" time, but did reduce the required dose of levodopa (WMD 180 mg, 95% CI 106 mg to 253 mg). Incomplete information was available on motor impairments and disability. The sixth systematic review (search date 2000, 3 RCTs, 268 people)[47] compared cabergoline versus placebo. It found that cabergoline did not significantly reduce "off" time but did reduce the required dose of levodopa "off" time (WMD 1.1 hours, 95% CI 0.06 hours to 2.33 hours; levodopa dose WMD 150 mg, 95% CI 94 mg to 205 mg). Small but significant benefits in UPDRS, ADL, and motor scores were seen with cabergoline in one study only. **Versus each other:** We found five systematic reviews.[44,49–53] One review (search date 1999, 3 RCTs) comparing pergolide versus bromocriptine found that pergolide slightly improved motor impairment compared with bromocriptine; however, this small advantage may not be clinically important.[50] Another systematic review (search date 1998) found insufficient evidence on the effect of lisuride versus bromocriptine.[49] We found three systematic reviews comparing pramipexole (search date 1999, 1 RCT, 163 people), ropinirole (search date 2000, 3 RCTs, 482 people), and cabergoline (search date 2000, 5 RCTs, 1071 people) with bromocriptine.[51–53] The newer agonists versus bromocriptine showed trends toward a reduction in "off" time but there was no significant difference in the reduction of levodopa dose. Motor impairments and activities of daily living were improved to a similar degree by the newer agonists and bromocriptine.

Harms: **Versus placebo:** The systematic reviews found increased rates of dopaminergic adverse effects with agonist therapy. In particular, dyskinesia was increased significantly with pergolide (OR 4.6, 95% CI 3.1 to 7.0), pramipexole (OR 2.1, 95% CI 1.5 to 2.9), and ropinirole (OR 2.9, 95% CI 1.4 to 6.2).[45,46,48] However, rates of withdrawal from treatment were significantly lower with pramipexole compared with placebo (OR 0.64, 95% CI 0.44 to 0.93) but not with pergolide, ropinirole, or cabergoline.[45–47] **Versus each other:** Systematic reviews found no difference in adverse events between pergolide, pramipexole, and cabergoline versus bromocriptine,[50–52] but nausea was significantly less frequent with ropinirole (OR 0.50, 95% CI 0.29 to 0.84).[53]

Comment: We found no studies that directly compared the newer dopamine agonists.

Parkinson's disease

QUESTION	What are the effects of surgery in people with later Parkinson's disease?

OPTION	PALLIDOTOMY

Two systematic reviews, including two RCTs, found limited evidence that pallidotomy reduces contralateral tremor and rigidity during "off" time, and dyskinesia during "on" time (see glossary, p 913), but with significant risk of morbidity and mortality. Bilateral surgery is associated with a variety of axial effects (see glossary, p 913), including mutism.

Benefits:
Versus medical treatment: We found two systematic reviews (search dates 1998 and 1999),[54,55] which between them included evidence from two short term RCTs (64 people)[56,57] and 15 uncontrolled trials (551 people), evaluating mainly unilateral posteroventral pallidotomy in people with advanced Parkinson's disease. We found one recent systematic review of mainly observational studies (search date 1999, 1959 people) that did not include the two RCTs.[58] The first short term RCT, published only as an abstract, compared medical treatment versus pallidotomy with 6 months' follow up.[56] Pallidotomy achieved greater improvements in tremor, bradykinesia, rigidity, gait, postural stability, and "off" time. It found no evidence that pallidotomy reduced the need for medical treatment. The second RCT (37 people with advanced Parkinson's disease) compared unilateral pallidotomy versus best medical treatment over 6 months' follow up.[57] It found that pallidotomy was associated with improved "off" phase median motor score (UPDRS part 3) from 47 to 32.5 compared with a deterioration from 52.5 to 56.6 in those receiving medical treatment only ($P < 0.001$); improved contralateral dyskinesia, which decreased in duration by 50%, compared with no change on medical treatment; improved duration of independence, which increased by 2.2 hours a day compared with a decrease of 0.4 hours a day with medical treatment (difference 2.6 hours/day, 95% CI 0.0 hours/day to 5.3 hours/day, $P < 0.05$); and improved quality of life (PDQL) ($P < 0.004$). Unilateral pallidotomy had no cognitive or behavioural effects, except that left sided pallidotomy reduced verbal fluency.[59] One recent non-systematic review and consensus statement (evaluating one RCT[60] plus 13 uncontrolled studies) suggested that gait, balance disorders, and hypophonia were less responsive to surgery.[61] **Versus stimulation of the posteroventral pallidum:** One small RCT (13 people) found no significant difference over 3 months with lesioning versus deep brain stimulation (see glossary, p 913) but was probably too small to exclude a clinically important difference.[62] **Versus stimulation of the subthalamic nucleus:** We found one small RCT (28 people) of pallidal stimulation versus subthalamic nucleus stimulation.[63] It found that, at 6–8 months after surgery, pallidal stimulation reduced motor scores during "off times" (reduction 57% v 29%) and dyskinesias during "on times" (reduction 36% v 25%). However, there was no untreated control group, and the differences between the two treatment groups were ascribed to baseline differences in preoperative symptoms.

Harms: The incidence of permanent adverse effects of pallidotomy was 4–46%, with a risk of a serious complication (including death) of 3–10%.[54] Complication rates decline with experience.[61] Bilateral procedures may worsen axial effects, including dysarthria, dysphonia, and gait disturbances.

Comment: The studies cited in the reviews followed different protocols.[54] Transplants or implants of dopaminergic tissue remain experimental. Most reports of stereotactic lesioning (see glossary below) or stimulation are uncontrolled. A US RCT of pallidotomy versus delayed pallidotomy is currently under way.[60]

GLOSSARY

Axial effects Changes affecting axial body sections, such as head and trunk, rather than the limbs.

Deep brain stimulation Prolonged focal electrical brain stimulation through a stereotactically implanted wire.

Dopaminergic adverse effects Include dyskinesia, hallucinations, and psychosis.

Dyskinesia Abnormal or involuntary writhing or jerky movements distinct from tremor.

Motor fluctuations Fluctuations in motor symptoms, such as bradykinesia, rigidity, and tremor during a day. Response fluctuations are fluctuations in a person's overall response to treatment during a day.

"Off" time Periods when treatment is not working.

"On" time Periods when treatment is working.

Pallidotomy Making a permanent surgical lesion, usually thermally or electrically, in the globus pallidum.

Stereotactic lesioning Placing a lesion using stereotactic techniques; a kind of three-dimensional triangulation.

Substantive changes since last issue

L-dopa v dopaminergics New RCT;[37] conclusion unchanged.

L-dopa v dopaminergics New RCT;[39] conclusion unchanged.

L-dopa v dopaminergics New RCT;[41] conclusion unchanged.

L-dopa + dopaminergics New systematic review comparing ropinirole with placebo;[46] conclusion unchanged.

L-dopa + dopaminergics New systematic review comparing cabergoline versus placebo;[47] conclusion unchanged.

L-dopa + dopaminergics Three new systematic reviews comparing newer dopamine agonists versus bromocriptine;[51–53] conclusion unchanged.

Pallidotomy New systematic review;[58] conclusion unchanged.

Pallidotomy New RCT comparing pallidal versus subthalamic stimulation;[63] conclusion unchanged.

REFERENCES

1. Hughes AJ, Daniel SE, Blankson S, Lees AJ. A clinico-pathologic study of 100 cases of Parkinson's disease. *Arch Neurol* 1993;50:140–148.

2. Zhang Z, Roman G. Worldwide occurrence of Parkinson's disease: an updated review. *Neuroepidemiology* 1993;12:195–208.

3. De Rijk MC, Tzourio C, Breteler MMB, et al. Prevalence of parkinsonism and Parkinson's disease in Europe: the EUROPARKINSON collaborative study. *J Neurol Neurosurg Psychiatry* 1997;62:10–15.

4. Marder K, Tang M, Mejia H, et al. Risk of Parkinson's disease among first degree relatives: a community based study. *Neurology* 1996;47:155–160.

5. Jarman P, Wood N. Parkinson's disease genetics comes of age. *BMJ* 1999;318:1641–1642.

6. Lazzarini A, Myers R, Zimmerman T, et al. A clinical genetic study of Parkinson's disease: evidence for dominant transmission. *Neurology* 1994;44:499–506.

7. Ben-Shlomo Y. How far are we in understanding the cause of Parkinson's disease? *J Neurol Neurosurg Psychiatry* 1996;61:4–16.

8. De Rijk M, Breteler M, den Breeilnen J, et al. Dietary antioxidants and Parkinson's disease: the Rotterdam study. *Arch Neurol* 1997;54:762–765.

9. Hellenbrand W, Seidler A, Robra B, et al. Smoking and Parkinson's disease: a case-control study in Germany. Int J Epidemiol 1997;26:328–339.

10. Tzourio C, Rocca W, Breteler M, et al. Smoking and Parkinson's disease: an age-dependent risk effect? Neurology 1997;49:1267–1272.

11. Gasser T, Müller-Myhsok B, Wszolek Z, et al. A susceptibility locus for Parkinson's disease maps to chromosome 2p13. Nat Genet 1998;18:262–265.

12. Tanner C, Ottman R, Goldman S, et al. Parkinson's disease in twins. An etiologic study. JAMA 1999;281:341–346.

13. Parkinson Study Group. Mortality in DATATOP: a multicenter trial in early Parkinson's disease. Ann Neurol 1998;43:318–325.

14. Rajput A, Uitti J, Offord K. Timely levodopa (LD) administration prolongs survival in Parkinson's disease. Parkinson Relat Disord 1997;3:159–165.

15. Clarke CE. Does levodopa therapy delay death in Parkinson's disease? A review of the evidence. Mov Disord 1995;10:250–256.

16. Hely MA, Morris JGL, Traficante R, et al. The Sydney multicentre study of Parkinson's disease: progression and mortality at 10 years. J Neurol Neurosurg Psychiatry 1999;67:300–307.

17. Morgante L, Salemi G, Meneghini F, et al. Parkinson disease survival. A population-based study. Arch Neurol 2000;57:507–512.

18. Fahn S, Elton L, for the UPDRS Development Committee. Unified Parkinson's disease rating scale. In: Fahn S, Marsden C, Calne D, et al, eds. Recent Developments in Parkinson's Disease, Vol. 2. Florham Park: Macmillan Healthcare Information, 1987:153–163.

19. Langston JW, Widner H, Goetz CG, et al. Core Assessment Program for Intracerebral Transplantations (CAPIT). Mov Disord 1992;7:2–13.

20. De Boer A, Wijker W, Speelman J, de Haes JCJM. Quality of life in people with Parkinson's disease: development of a questionnaire. J Neurol Neurosurg Psychiatry 1996;61:70–74.

21. Peto V, Jenkinson C, Fitzpatrick R, Greenhall R. The development and validation of a short measure of functioning and well being for individuals with Parkinson's disease. Qual Life Res 1995;4:241–248.

22. The Parkinson's Disease Study Group. Effects of tocopherol and deprenyl on the progression of disability in early Parkinson's disease. N Engl J Med 1993;328:176–183.

23. Olanow CW, Hauser RA, Gauger L, et al. The effect of deprenyl and levodopa on the progression of Parkinson's disease. Ann Neurol 1995;38:771–777.

24. Lees AJ, for the Parkinson's Disease Research Group of the United Kingdom. Comparison of therapeutic effects and mortality data of levodopa and levodopa combined with selegiline in people with early, mild Parkinson's disease. BMJ 1995;311:1602–1607.

25. Przuntek H, Conrad B, Dichgans J, et al. SELEDO: a 5-year long-term trial on the effect of selegiline in early Parkinsonian people treated with levodopa. Eur J Neurol 1999;6:141–150.

26. Larson JP, Boas J, Erdal JE, et al. Does selegiline modify the progression of early Parkinson's disease? Results from a five-year study. Eur J Neurol 1999;6:539–547.

27. Olanow CW, Mylla V, Sotaniemi K, et al. Effect of selegiline on mortality in people with Parkinson's disease. Neurology 1998;51:825–830.

28. Penny J, for the Parkinson Study Group. Impact of deprenyl and tocopherol treatment for Parkinson's disease in DATATOP people requiring levodopa.

29. Ben-Shlomo Y, Churchyard A, Head J, et al. Investigation by Parkinson's Disease Research Group of United Kingdom into excess mortality seen with combined levodopa and selegiline treatment in people with early, mild Parkinson's disease: further results of randomised trial and confidential inquiry. BMJ 1998;316:1191–1196.

30. Counsell C. Effect of adding selegiline to levodopa in early, mild Parkinson's disease. BMJ 1998;17:1586.

31. Thorogood M, Armstrong B, Nichols T, et al. Mortality in people taking selegiline: observational study. BMJ 1998;317:252–254.

32. Dupont E, Andersen A, Boas J, et al. Sustained-release Madopar HBS compared with standard Madopar in the long-term treatment of de novo Parkinsonian people. Acta Neurol Scand 1996;93:14–20.

33. Block G, Liss C, Reines S, Irr J, Nibbelink D, for the CR First Study Group. Comparison of immediate release and controlled release carbidopa/levodopa in Parkinson's disease. Eur Neurol 1997;37:23–47.

34. Ramaker C, van Hilten J. Bromocriptine versus levodopa in early Parkinson's disease. In: The Cochrane Library, Issue 1, 2001. Oxford: Update Software. Search date January 1999; primary sources Cochrane Movement Disorders Group Specialised Register, Cochrane Controlled Trials Register, Medline, Embase, pharmaceutical companies, experts for unpublished studies, and hand searched references and selected neurology journals.

35. Ramaker C, van Hilten J. Bromocriptine/levodopa versus levodopa in early Parkinson's disease. Parkinson Relat Disord 1999;5(suppl):82.

36. Rascol O, Brooks D, Korczyn A, De Deyn P, Clarke C, Lang A. A five-year study of the incidence of dyskinesia in people with early Parkinson's disease who were treated with ropinirole or levodopa. N Engl J Med 2000;342:1484–1491.

37. Parkinson Study Group. Pramipexole versus levodopa as initial treatment for Parkinson's disease. JAMA 2000;284:1931–1938.

38. Rinne U. A 5-year double-blind study with cabergoline versus levodopa in the treatment of early Parkinson's disease. Parkinsonism & Related Disorders 1999;5(suppl):84.

39. Oertel WH. Pergolide versus levodopa monotherapy (PELMOPET). Mov Disord 2000;15(suppl 3):4.

40. Rinne U. Lisuride, a dopamine agonist in the treatment of early Parkinson's disease. Neurology 1989;39:336–339.

41. Allain H, Destee A, Petit H, et al. Five-year follow-up of early lisuride and levodopa combination therapy versus levodopa monotherapy in de novo Parkinson's disease. Eur Neurol 2000;44:22–30.

42. Fahn S. Parkinson's disease, the effect of levodopa and the ELLDOPA trial. Arch Neurol 1999;56:529–535.

43. Van Hilten J, Beek W, Finken M. Bromocriptine for levodopa-induced motor complications in Parkinson's disease. In: The Cochrane Library, Issue 1, 2001. Oxford: Update Software. Search date January 1998; primary sources Cochrane Controlled Trials Register, Medline, Scisearch, pharmaceutical companies, experts for unpublished studies, and hand searched references.

44. Clarke C, Speller J. Lisuride for levodopa-induced complications in Parkinson's disease. In: The Cochrane Library, Issue 1, 2001. Oxford: Update Software. Search date November 1998; primary sources Medline, Embase, Cochrane Controlled

Trials Register, pharmaceutical companies, and hand searched references.

45. Clarke C, Speller J. Pergolide for levodopa-induced complications in Parkinson's disease. In: The Cochrane Library, Issue 1, 2001. Oxford: Update Software. Search date January 1999; primary sources Medline, Embase, Cochrane Controlled Trials Register, pharmaceutical companies, and hand searched references.

46. Clarke C, Deane K. Ropinirole for levodopa-induced complications in Parkinson's disease. In: The Cochrane Library, Issue 1, 2001. Oxford: Update Software. Search date not stated; primary sources Cochrane Movement Disorders Group Specialised Register, Cochrane Controlled Trials Register, Medline, Embase, pharmaceutical companies, experts for unpublished studies, and hand searched references and selected neurology journals.

47. Clarke C, Deane K. Cabergoline for levodopa-induced complications in Parkinson's disease. In: The Cochrane Library, Issue 1, 2001. Oxford: Update Software. Search date not stated; primary sources Medline, Embase, Cochrane Controlled Trials Register, hand searches of reference lists and selected neurology journals, and contact with Pharmacia Upjohn Ltd.

48. Clarke C, Speller J, Clarke J. Pramipexole for levodopa-induced complications in Parkinson's disease. In: The Cochrane Library, Issue 1, 2001. Oxford: Update Software. Search date not stated; primary sources Cochrane Movement Disorders Group Specialised Register, Cochrane Controlled Trials Register, Medline, Embase, pharmaceutical companies, experts for unpublished studies, and hand searched references and selected neurology journals.

49. Clarke CE, Speller JM. Lisuride versus bromocriptine for levodopa-induced complications in Parkinson's disease. In: The Cochrane Library, Issue 1, 2001. Oxford: Update Software. Search date not stated; primary sources Medline, Embase, Cochrane Controlled Trials Register, hand searches of the neurology literature, reference lists of identified studies, and contact with pharmaceutical companies.

50. Clarke C, Speller J. Pergolide versus bromocriptine for levodopa-induced motor complications in Parkinson's disease. In: The Cochrane Library, Issue 1, 2001. Oxford: Update Software. Search date 1998; primary sources Medline, Embase, Cochrane Controlled Trials Register, pharmaceuticals companies, and hand searched references.

51. Clarke C, Speller J, Clarke J. Pramipexole versus bromocriptine for levodopa-induced complications in Parkinson's disease. In: The Cochrane Library, Issue 1, 2001. Oxford: Update Software. Search date not stated; primary sources Cochrane Movement Disorders Group Specialised Register; Cochrane Controlled Trials Register, Medline, Embase, pharmaceutical companies, experts for unpublished studies, and hand searched references and selected neurology journals.

52. Clarke C, Deane K. Cabergoline versus bromocriptine for levodopa-induced complications in Parkinson's disease. In: The Cochrane Library, Issue 1, 2001. Oxford: Update Software. Search date not stated; primary sources Cochrane Movement Disorders Group Specialised Register; Cochrane Controlled Trials Register, Medline, Embase, pharmaceutical companies, experts for unpublished studies, and hand searched references and selected neurology journals.

53. Clarke C, Deane K. Ropinirole versus bromocriptine for levodopa-induced complications in Parkinson's disease. In: The Cochrane Library, Issue 1, 2001. Oxford: Update Software. Search date not stated; primary sources Cochrane Movement Disorders Group Specialised Register; Cochrane Controlled Trials Register, Medline, Embase, pharmaceutical companies, experts for unpublished studies, and hand searched references and selected neurology journals.

54. Gregory R. Posteroventral pallidotomy for advanced Parkinson's disease: a systematic review. *Neurol Rev Int* 1999;3:8–12. Search date 1998; primary sources not stated.

55. Development and Evaluation Committee. Report 105. *Pallidotomy, Thalotomy and Deep Brain Stimulation for Severe Parkinson's Disease.* Southampton: Wessex Institute for Health Research and Development, 1999. Search date September 1999; primary sources Cochrane Library; Health Technology Assessment database; Medline; Science Citation Index; BIOSIS; Embase; Index to Scientific and Technical Proceedings; Inspec; Best Evidence.

56. Vitek J, Bakay R, Freeman A, et al. Randomised clinical trial of pallidotomy for Parkinson's disease. *Neurology* 1998; 50(suppl 4):A80.

57. De Bie R, de Haan R, Nijssen P, et al. Unilateral pallidotomy in Parkinson's disease: a randomised, single-blind, multicentre trial. *Lancet* 1999;354: 1665–1669.

58. Alkhani A, Lozano A. Pallidotomy for Parkinson's disease: a review of contemporary literature. *J Neurosurg* 2001;94:43–49. Search date 1999; primary source Medline.

59. Schmand B, de Bie R, Koning-Haanstra M, et al. Unilateral pallidotomy in PD. A controlled study of cognitive and behavioural effects. *Neurology* 2000;54:1058–1064.

60. Vitek J, Bakay R, Freeman A, et al. Randomised clinical trial of pallidotomy versus medical therapy for Parkinson's disease [abstract]. *Mov Disord* 1998;13(suppl 2):266.

61. Bronstein JM, DeSalles A, DeLong MR. Sterotactic pallidotomy in the treatment of Parkinson's disease. *Arch Neurol* 1999;56:1064–1069.

62. Merello M, Nouzeilles MI, Kuzis G, et al. Unilateral radiofrequency lesion versus electrostimulation of posteroventral pallidum: a prospective randomized comparison. *Mov Disord* 1999;14:50–56.

63. Katayama Y, Kasai M, Oshima H, Fukaya C, Yamamoto T, Mizutani T. Double-blinded evaluation of the effect of pallidal and subthalamic nucleus stimulation on daytime activity in advance Parkinson's disease. *Parkinson Relat Disord* 2000; 7:35–40.

A Peter Moore
Senior Lecturer in Neurology
University of Liverpool
Liverpool
UK

Carl Clarke
Reader in Clinical Neurology
University of Birmingham
Birmingham
UK

Competing interests: APM, none declared. CC has been paid by various manufacturers of the drugs dealt with above for speaking at meetings and attending conferences.

Trigeminal neuralgia

Search date July 2000: new for this issue

Joanna Zakrzewska

Neurological disorders

QUESTIONS

INTERVENTIONS

Key Messages

- Three crossover RCTs have found that carbamazepine versus placebo increases the number of people who have pain relief in the short term (1 in 3 people respond), but one in three people have adverse effects.
- One small RCT found weak evidence about the effects of tizanidine.
- Small, poorly randomised trials found limited evidence for the effectiveness of baclofen.
- One RCT found that pimozide was more effective than carbamazepine, but caused adverse effects in the majority of people.
- One crossover RCT found weak evidence of benefit with tocainide versus carbamazepine. The use of tocainide is limited by considerable harms.
- One small crossover RCT found limited evidence about the effects of lamotrigine versus placebo as an additional therapy to other anticonvulsants for trigeminal neuralgia.
- One RCT found no evidence of benefit from a single application of anaesthetic agent to the ipsilateral eye.

DEFINITION	Trigeminal neuralgia is a characteristic pain in the distribution of one or more branches of the fifth cranial nerve. The diagnosis is made on the history alone, based on characteristic features of the pain. It occurs in paroxysms that last a few seconds to 2 minutes. The frequency of paroxysms is highly variable: from hundreds of attacks a day to long periods of remission that can last years. The pain is severe and described as intense, sharp, superficial, stabbing, burning, or like an electric shock. In any individual, the pain has the same character in different attacks. It is often triggered by touch in a specific area or by eating, talking, washing the face, or cleaning the teeth. Between paroxysms the person is asymptomatic. Other causes of facial pain may need to be excluded.[1] In trigeminal neuralgia the neurological examination is usually normal.[2,3]
INCIDENCE/ PREVALENCE	Most evidence about the incidence and prevalence of trigeminal neuralgia is from the USA.[4] The annual incidence, when age adjusted to 1980 age distribution of the USA, is 5.9 of 100 000 women and 3.4 of 100 000 men. The incidence tends to be slightly higher in women at all ages. The incidence rises with age. In men aged over 80 years the incidence is 45.2 of 100 000.[5] Other published surveys are small: one questionnaire survey of neurological disease in a single French village found one person with trigeminal neuralgia among 993 people.[6]
AETIOLOGY/ RISK FACTORS	The cause of trigeminal neuralgia remains unclear.[7] It is more common in people with multiple sclerosis (RR 20, 95% CI 4.1 to 59).[5] Hypertension is a risk factor in women (RR 2.1, 95% CI 1.2 to 3.4) but the evidence is less clear for men (RR 1.53, 95% CI 0.3 to 4.5). A study in the USA found that people with trigeminal neuralgia smoked less, consumed less alcohol, had fewer tonsillectomies, and were less likely than matched controls to be Jewish or an immigrant.[8]
PROGNOSIS	One study found no reduction of 10 year survival with trigeminal neuralgia.[9] We found no evidence about the natural history of trigeminal neuralgia. Many people have periods of remission with no pain for months or years.[3] Anecdotal reports suggest that in many people it becomes more severe and less responsive to treatment with time.[10] Most people with trigeminal neuralgia are initially managed medically, and a proportion eventually have a surgical procedure.[1] We found no good evidence about the proportion of people who require surgical treatment for pain control.
AIMS	To relieve pain with minimal adverse effects.
OUTCOMES	Pain frequency and severity scores; measures of psychological distress; ability to perform normal activities; side effects.
METHODS	*Clinical Evidence* search and appraisal July 2000. The author also searched her own extensive bibliography accumulated over 15 years.

Trigeminal neuralgia

QUESTION	What are the effects of medical treatments on trigeminal neuralgia?

OPTION	CARBAMAZEPINE

Three crossover RCTs have found that carbamazepine versus placebo increases the number of people who have pain relief (1 in 3 people respond) but causes adverse effects (1 in 3 people).

Benefits: **Versus placebo:** We found two systematic reviews[11,12] (see table 1, p 923). The first systematic review (search date 1999, 3 crossover RCTs,[13,14,17] 161 people with trigeminal neuralgia)[11] found that treatment with carbamazepine versus placebo (for 5 days to 2 weeks) significantly increased the number of people having a good or excellent response (57% with carbamazepine v 18% with placebo; OR 4.8, 95% CI 3.4 to 6.9; NNT 3, 95% CI 2 to 4). The second systematic review (search date 1999, 2 RCTs, 107 people with trigeminal neuralgia) found similar results.[12]

Harms: The review found significantly more minor adverse effects (drowsiness, dizziness, constipation, and ataxia) with carbamazepine than with placebo (NNH 3, 95% CI 2 to 7).[11] In the RCTs major side effects were more likely with carbamazepine than with placebo and more people withdrew from the RCTs because of adverse effects (NNH for withdrawal 24, CI 14 to 112).[22] Major adverse effects described in observational studies include rashes, leucopenia, and abnormal liver function tests.

Comment: The RCTs used crossover design, and one RCT[13] used multiple crossovers so that each individual was counted more than once when calculating the estimates of effectiveness in the systematic review.[11,22] The RCTs included in the systematic review were small and short term. All the RCTs used simple measures for pain outcomes and no quality of life measures. Diagnostic criteria were not clearly stated. Previous therapy and duration of pain varied considerably. Longer term effects of carbamazepine have been assessed only in open trials. We found one report (143 people followed for up to 16 years) on the long term effects of carbamazepine.[23] Initially carbamazepine was successful in 69% of participants, but by 5–16 years only 31 people (22%) were still finding carbamazepine effective and 44% required additional or alternative treatment.

OPTION	TIZANIDINE

We found inadequate evidence from one small RCT about the effects of tizanidine.

Benefits: **Versus placebo:** We found no RCTs. **Versus carbamazepine:** We found one systematic review (search date 1999, 1 double blind RCT,[15] 12 people).[11] It found that tizanidine (up to 18 mg/day) versus carbamazepine (up to 900 mg/day) reduced the number of people with relief of pain after treatment for 3 weeks, but the result was not significant (4/6 [67%] with carbamazepine v 1/6 [17%] with tizanidine; P = 0.08) (see table 1, p 923).

Harms: No adverse effects were reported but one person withdrew because of inadequate pain control.

Comment: The RCT was too small to establish or exclude clinically important effects.

OPTION **PIMOZIDE**

One RCT found pimozide versus carbamazepine reduced pain but caused more adverse effects.

Benefits: **Versus placebo:** We found no RCTs. **Versus carbamazepine:** We found one systematic review (search date 1999, 1 double blind, crossover RCT,[16] 48 people with trigeminal neuralgia who were refractory to medical treatment)[11] of pimozide versus carbamazepine. It found (using pre-crossover results) that significantly more people achieved a large reduction in pain with 8 weeks of pimozide treatment (48/48 [100%] with pimozide v 28/48 [56%] with carbamazepine; NNT 3, 95% CI 2 to 4) (see table 1, p 923).

Harms: The RCT found that more people experienced adverse effects with pimozide than with carbamazepine (40/48 [83%] with pimozide v 22/48 [46%] with carbamazepine; NNH 3, 95% CI 2 to 6; OR 7.8, 95% CI 3.7 to 20). Adverse effects included physical and mental retardation, hand tremors, memory impairment, and involuntary movements.

Comment: This was a well conducted multicentre trial using a variety of outcome measures. The crossover design limits interpretation of the results, because untested assumptions are required to perform the statistical analyses.

OPTION **TOCAINIDE**

We found limited evidence of benefit with tocainide versus carbamazepine. The use of tocainide is limited by harms.

Benefits: **Versus placebo:** We found no RCTs. **Versus carbamazepine:** We found one systematic review (search date 1999, 1 RCT,[24] 12 people with trigeminal neuralgia).[11] The double blind, crossover RCT had weak methods. It found that tocainide versus carbamazepine had no significant effect on the number of people who improved after 2 weeks of treatment (8/12 [67%] with tocainide v 9/12 [75%] with carbamazepine; ARR +8.3%, 95% CI −28% to +45%).

Harms: The RCT found severe adverse effects (1 person withdrew because of a skin rash and 3 others had adverse effects). The postscript to the paper reported a death attributed to haematological effects of tocainide.

Comment: The available evidence is poor, but provides no support for the use of tocainide in trigeminal neuralgia.

Trigeminal neuralgia

LAMOTRIGINE

We found limited evidence that lamotrigine versus placebo (added to other anticonvulsants) improves short term pain in trigeminal neuralgia.

Benefits:	**Versus placebo:** We found two systematic reviews (both search dates 1999),[11,12] which identified one RCT.[18] The RCT (double blind, crossover, 14 people with refractory trigeminal neuralgia using either carbamazepine or phenytoin) found that lamotrigine (400 mg) versus placebo in addition to the current medication increased the number of people who improved after 4 weeks of treatment (10/13 [77%] with lamotrigine v 8/14 [57%] with placebo; ARR +20%, 95% CI –16% to +55%) (see table 1, p 923). Although these results show no significant differences, a composite efficacy score based on total pain scores, global evaluations, and use of escape medication was higher with lamotrigine than with placebo (P = 0.01).
Harms:	In the RCT, adverse effects with lamotrigine included dizziness, constipation, nausea, and drowsiness. The total number of people reporting adverse effects was the same as with placebo (7/14 [50%] with lamotrigine v 7/14 [50%] with placebo).
Comment:	This RCT was a small study and lamotrigine was used in addition to existing treatment. The crossover design and short period of treatment limits interpretation. It is not clear which of the outcomes and analyses were defined a priori as the primary outcomes and analyses. The available evidence suggests, but does not establish, that lamotrigine is effective in the short term treatment of trigeminal neuralgia.

BACLOFEN

We found inadequate evidence of beneficial effects of baclofen compared with placebo.

Benefits:	**Versus placebo:** We found one systematic review,[12] which included one controlled RCT.[19] The RCT (double blind, crossover, 10 people, 4 using carbamazepine or phenytoin) found that baclofen versus placebo in addition to pre-existing treatment increased the number of people with relief of pain after treatment for 2 weeks (7/10 [70%] with baclofen v 1/10 [10%] with placebo; NNT 2, 95% CI 1 to 6).[19] It is not clear that randomisation was used to allocate people to baclofen or placebo before the crossover. **Versus other active drugs:** We found one trial (double blind, crossover, 15 people, not clearly randomised) compared racemic baclofen versus L-baclofen over 2 weeks.[20] It found no significant difference in response (9/15 [60%] with L-baclofen v 6/15 [40%] with racemic baclofen; ARI +20%, 95% CI –16% to +56%).
Harms:	In the first RCT[19] drowsiness was reported in one of 10 people on baclofen. In the second RCT more people with racemic baclofen versus L-baclofen reported dizziness, confusion, or lethargy (6/15 [40%] v 1/15 [7%]; ARI 33%, 95% CI 3.1% to 64%).
Comment:	Both RCTs were small and it is not clear that randomisation occurred. In four people the baclofen was used as add on therapy to

other anticonvulsants. In others it was used as monotherapy, making evaluations difficult. Standard baclofen is a racemic mixture. The first RCT,[19] after the initial 2 week period, became an open label trial during which 28 of 60 people using baclofen were pain free over 1–5 years, although many needed additional phenytoin or carbamazepine. Another small, brief trial of carbamazepine plus baclofen had a low quality score, with six of 30 withdrawals unexplained. The evidence does not provide adequate evidence about the effectiveness of baclofen for trigeminal neuralgia.

| OPTION | PROPARACAINE HYDROCHLORIDE DROPS |

One RCT found no evidence of benefit from a single application of anaesthetic eye drops to the ipsilateral eye.

Benefits: **Versus placebo:** We found no systematic review but found one RCT (double blind, 47 people with trigeminal neuralgia) of proparacaine hydrochloride versus placebo instilled for 20 minutes on the same side as the trigeminal neuralgia on one occasion only.[21] It found no significant reduction of pain after 3, 10, and 30 days (at 30 days: 6/25 [24%] improved with proparacaine v 5/22 [23%] with placebo; ARI +1.3%, 95% CI −23% to +26%).

Harms: None reported.

Comment: This study found no evidence of benefit from the single application of topical eye drops.

REFERENCES

1. Anonymous. *Classification of chronic pain. Descriptors of chronic pain syndromes and definitions of pain terms.* Seattle: IASP Press, 1994.
2. Katusic S, Williams DB, Beard CM, Bergstralh EJ, Kurland LT. Epidemiology and clinical features of idiopathic trigeminal neuralgia and glossopharyngeal neuralgia: similarities and differences, Rochester, Minnesota, 1945–1984. *Neuroepidemiology* 1991;10:276–281.
3. Zakrzewska JM. *Trigeminal Neuralgia.* London: WB. Saunders,1995.
4. Zakrzewska JM, Hamlyn PJ. Facial pain. In: Crombie IKCPR, Linton SJ, LeResche L, Von Korff M, eds. *Epidemiology of Pain.* Seattle: IASP,1999: 171–202.
5. Katusic S, Beard CM, Bergstralh E, Kurland LT. Incidence and clinical features of trigeminal neuralgia, Rochester, Minnesota, 1945–1984. *Ann Neurol* 1990;27:89–95.
6. Munoz M, Dumas M, Boutros-Toni F, et al. A neuro-epidemiologic survey in a Limousin town. *Rev Neurol (Paris)* 1988;144:266–271.
7. Burchiel KJ. Pain in neurology and neurosurgery: tic douloureux (trigeminal neuralgia). In: Campbell JN ed. *Pain 1996 – an updated review.* Seattle: IASP Press, 1996:41–60.
8. Rothman KJ, Monson RR. Epidemiology of trigeminal neuralgia. *J Chronic Dis* 1973;26:3–12.
9. Rothman KJ, Monson RR. Survival in trigeminal neuralgia. *J Chronic Dis* 1973;26:303–309.
10. Burchiel KJ, Slavin KV. On the natural history of trigeminal neuralgia. *Neurosurgery* 2000;46:152–155.
11. Wiffen P, Collins S, McQuay H, Carroll D, Jadad A, Moore A. Anticonvulsant drugs for acute and chronic pain. In: The Cochrane Library, Issue 4, 2000. Oxford: Update Software. Search date 1999; primary sources Medline; Embase; SIGLE; Cochrane Controlled Trials Register; handsearch of 40 medical journals and authors of published reports.
12. Sindrup SH, Jensen TS. Efficacy of pharmacological treatments of neuropathic pain: an update and effect related to mechanisms of drug action. *Pain* 1999 83:389–400. Search date not stated but trials included up to 1999; primary sources not stated.
13. Campbell FG, Graham JG, Zilkha KJ. Clinical trial of carbazepine (tegretol) in trigeminal neuralgia. *J Neurol Neurosurg Psychiatry* 1966;29:265–267.
14. Killian JM, Fromm GH. Carbamazepine in the treatment of neuralgia. Use of side effects. *Arch Neurol* 1968;19:129–136.
15. Vilming ST, Lyberg T, Latase X. Tizanidine in the management of trigeminal neuralgia. *Cephalalgia* 1986;6:181–182.
16. Lechin F, van der Dijs B, Lechin ME, et al. Pimozide therapy for trigeminal neuralgia. *Arch Neurol* 1989;46:960–963.
17. Nicol CF. A four year double blind study of tegretol in facial pain. *Headache* 1969;9:54–57.
18. Zakrzewska JM, Chaudhry Z, Patton DW, Mullens EL. Lamotrigine in refractory trigeminal neuralgia: results from a double-blind placebo controlled crossover study. *Pain* 1997;73:223–230.
19. Fromm GH, Terrence CF, Chattha AS. Baclofen in the treatment of trigeminal neuralgia: double-blind study and long-term follow-up. *Ann Neurol* 1984; 15:240–244.
20. Fromm GH, Terrence CF. Comparison of L-baclofen and racemic baclofen in trigeminal neuralgia. *Neurology* 1987;37:1725–1728.
21. Kondziolka D, Lemley T, Kestle JR, et al. The effect of single-application topical ophthalmic anesthesia in patients with trigeminal neuralgia. A randomized

Trigeminal neuralgia

double-blind placebo-controlled trial. *J Neurosurg* 1994;80:993–997.

22. McQuay H, Carroll D, Jadad AR, Wiffen P, Moore A. Anticonvulsant drugs for management of pain: a systematic review. *BMJ* 1995;311:1047–1052. Search date 1994; primary sources Medline; handsearch of 40 medical journals and reference lists; authors of published reports.

23. Taylor JC, Brauer S, Espir MLE. Long-term treatment of trigeminal neuralgia. *Postgrad Med J* 1981;57:16–8.

24. Lindstrom P, Lindblom V. The analgesic effect of tocainide in trigeminal neuralgia. *Pain* 1987;28:45–50.

Joanna Zakrzewska
Barts and the London School of
Medicine and Dentistry
London
UK

Competing interests: The author has been reimbursed by Glaxo Wellcome (manufacturer of lamotrigine) for attending a conference and for conducting the lamotrigine RCT.

TABLE 1 RCTs of drugs used in the management of trigeminal neuralgia (see text, p 918).

Ref	Interventions (daily dosage)* Active arm	Comparison	Duration	Design	Diagnostic criteria	Number of people randomised (analysed)	NNT (95% CI)	NNH (95% CI)
13	Carbamazepine (400–800 mg)	Placebo	8 weeks	Crossover	–	77 (70)	2.8 (2.3 to 3.7)	4.3 (2.6 to 11.7)
14	Carbamazepine (400 mg–1 g)	Placebo	2 weeks to 36 months	Crossover	–	30 (27)	1.4 (1.14 to 1.88)	1.6 (1.3 to 2.1)
15	Tizanidine (900 mg)	Carbamazepine	3 weeks	Parallel	–	12 (11)	NS	–
16	Pimozide (4–12 mg)	Carbamazepine (300 mg–1.2 g)	24 weeks	Crossover	–	48 (48)	1 (2 to 3)	2.9 (2 to 4)
17	Carbamazepine (100 mg–2.4 g)	Placebo	46 months	Partial crossover	–	54 (44)	NS	3.7 (2.4 to 7.9)
18	Lamotrigine† (400 mg)	Placebo	4 weeks	Crossover	IHS	14 (14)	2.1 (1.3 to 6.1)	NS
19	Baclofen‡ (40–80 mg)	Placebo	2 weeks	Crossover	IHS	10 (10)	1.4 (1 to 2.6)	NS
20	L-Baclofen (6–12 mg)	Racemic baclofen(60 mg)	2 weeks	Crossover	IHS	15 (15)	2 (1 to 4)	2 (1 to 4)
21	Proparacaine (0.5% for 20 min)	Placebo	30 days	Parallel	IHS	47 (47)	NS	–

*All daily doses were given as divided doses. IHS, International Headache Society criteria; NS, non-significant.
†Added to pre-existing therapy; ‡used as add on to other anticonvulsant in 4 of 10 people.

Aphthous ulcers: recurrent

Search date December 2000

Stephen Porter and Crispian Scully

QUESTIONS

INTERVENTIONS

Likely to be beneficial
Chlorhexidine (but no effect on
   recurrence rates) 926

Unknown effectiveness
Topical corticosteroids 925

Unlikely to be beneficial
Hexidine. 926

To be covered in future issues of
   Clinical Evidence
Other drug treatments
Low intensity ultrasound
Novel toothpastes
Barrier techniques
Laser

Key Messages

- Nine small RCTs found no consistent effect of topical corticosteroids on the incidence of new ulcers, compared with control preparations. They found weak evidence that topical corticosteroids may reduce duration of ulcers and hasten pain relief without causing notable local or systemic adverse effects.

- RCTs have found that chlorhexidine gluconate mouth rinses may reduce the duration and severity of each episode of ulceration, but do not effect the incidence of recurrent ulceration.

- Single RCTs provide no evidence of benefit from hexidine mouthwash or from a proprietary antiseptic mouthwash compared with control mouthwashes.

| DEFINITION | Recurrent aphthous ulcers are superficial and rounded, with painful mouth ulcers usually occurring in recurrent bouts at intervals of a few days to a few months.[1] |

| INCIDENCE/ PREVALENCE | The point prevalence of recurrent aphthous ulcers in Swedish adults has been reported as 2%.[1] Prevalence may be 5–10% of some groups of children. Up to 66% of young adults give a history consistent with recurrent aphthous ulceration.[1] |

| AETIOLOGY/ RISK FACTORS | The causes of aphthous ulcers remain unknown. Associations with haematinic deficiency, infections, gluten sensitive enteropathy, food sensitivities, and psychological stress have rarely been confirmed. Similar ulcers are seen in Behçet's syndrome. |

| PROGNOSIS | About 80% of people with recurrent aphthous ulcers develop a few ulcers smaller than 1 cm in diameter that heal within 5–14 days without scarring (the pattern known as minor aphthous ulceration). The episodes recur typically after an interval of 1–4 months. One in 10 sufferers has a more severe form (major aphthous ulceration) with lesions larger than 1 cm that may recur after a shorter interval and can cause scarring. Likewise perhaps 1 in 10 people with such recurrent ulceration may have multiple minute ulcers (herpetiform ulceration). |

| AIMS | To reduce pain, frequency, and duration of ulceration, with minimal adverse effects. |

| OUTCOMES | Number of new ulcers appearing within a specified period, usually 4–8 weeks; ulcer day index (the sum of the number of ulcers each day over a period, usually 4–8 weeks, which indicates the severity of the episode and reflects the mean prevalence and duration of ulcers); symptom score based on subjective pain severity recorded in categories on a questionnaire (e.g. from 0 to 3, ranging from no pain to severe pain) or on a 10 cm visual analogue scale; mean duration of individual ulcers (difficult to determine because of uncertainty in detecting the point of complete resolution); number of ulcer free days during a specified period; preference of people for one treatment over another. Diameter of lesions is a proxy measure of these clinical outcomes. |

| METHODS | *Clinical Evidence* update search and appraisal December 2000. |

QUESTION What are the effects of treatments for recurrent aphthous ulcers?

OPTION TOPICAL CORTICOSTEROIDS

Nine small RCTs found no consistent effect of topical corticosteroids on the incidence of new ulcers compared with control preparations. They found weak evidence that topical corticosteroids may reduce duration of ulcers and hasten pain relief without causing notable local or systemic adverse effects.

Benefits: We found no systematic review but found nine RCTs of corticosteroids versus placebo that reported relevant clinical outcomes in the management of recurrent aphthous ulcers.[2-9] Overall, one RCT found larger effect sizes than the others.[2] **Incidence of new ulcers:** Five randomised crossover trials (102 people) found inconsistent effects on the incidence of new ulcers (see table 1, p 929). **Ulcer duration:** Six RCTs reported data on ulcer duration, but the data were not presented in comparable forms.[3,4,6-9] Four RCTs reported the mean duration of ulcers, and no consistent effect was seen (see table 1, p 929). One RCT found topical steroids reduced mean ulcer duration below 6 days (ulcer duration ≤6 days, AR 25/33 [76%] people receiving topical steroid v 14/30 [47%] with control preparations; ARI 29%, 95% CI 5% to 43%; RR 1.62, 95% CI 1.06 to 2.49; NNT 3, 95% CI 2 to 20).[6] One crossover trial found that 13 of 15 people had shorter mean duration with topical steroid versus the control preparation.[8] **Ulcer days index:** Four trials found that topical steroids reduced the number of ulcer days compared with control; the reduction was significant in two of the trials[2,4,5,7] (see table 1, p 929). **Symptom scores:** Four trials reported symptom scores with topical steroids versus control, but all four presented their results in different ways.[6-9] One found that more people using steroids had symptom relief compared with those using a control preparation (29/33 v 18/30; ARI 27%, 95% CI 5% to 43%; RRI 46%, 95% CI 19% to 91%; NNT 4, 95% CI 2 to 20).[6] One crossover trial found that symptom scores were lower with topical steroids than the control preparation (2.77 v 3.54), but the results were not significantly different.[7] Another crossover trial found that 11 of 15 people using topical steroid versus the control preparation had lower pain scores.[8] One further crossover trial found that the pain score fell with time whether using topical steroids or control applications, but that the rate of fall was significantly faster when using topical steroids.[9] **User preference:** Two crossover trials found that more users preferred topical steroids than control preparations (20/26 in one study[4] and 10/17 in the other[6]).

Harms: The nine trials reported no serious adverse effects. Long term use of corticosteroid mouth rinses was occasionally associated with oral candidiasis (rate not specified). Limited studies of adrenal function found no evidence that 0.05% fluocinonide in adhesive paste and betamethasone-17-valerate mouth rinse caused adrenal suppression.[8,10] One RCT reported adrenal suppression in one man using betamethasone disodium phosphate.[5]

Comment: The trials differed in many ways: selection of people, type of topical corticosteroid and formulation used, control preparation used (although this was usually a base without topical steroid), duration of treatment, reported outcomes, and design (double or single blind, parallel group or crossover, use of washout period or not). Withdrawal rates were high. Most people in the trials had more severe ulceration than the average person with recurrent aphthous ulceration.

OPTION   CHLORHEXIDINE AND SIMILAR AGENTS

RCTs have found that chlorhexidine gluconate mouth rinses may reduce the duration and severity of each episode of ulceration, but do not effect the incidence of recurrent ulceration. Single RCTs found no significant benefit from hexidine mouthwash or a proprietary antiseptic mouthwash compared with control mouthwashes.

Benefits: We found no systematic review but found five RCTs (203 people with recurrent aphthous ulceration) of chlorhexidine gluconate or similar preparations versus assumed inactive control preparations.[11–15] Four of the RCTs used a crossover design with randomised sequence comparing a control preparation versus 1% chlorhexidine gel,[11] 0.2% chlorhexidine gel,[12] 0.2% chlorhexidine mouthwash,[13] or 0.1% hexetidine mouthwash.[14] One trial was a parallel group RCT of a proprietary antiseptic rinse versus a hydroalcoholic control.[15] **Incidence of ulceration:** All trials reported the number of ulcers as either the total number of ulcers or the number of new ulcers with each treatment (see table 1, p 929). Only one of the five RCTs found significantly fewer ulcers with active treatment.[13] Three RCTs noted that the number of ulcers fell during the course of the study, irrespective of the treatment received.[13–15] The crossover trial that found a significant difference in numbers of ulcers did not overtly account for this effect: data were available from only 12 of 26 people who were recruited, and it is not clear if there was a balanced sequencing of active and placebo treatments among these people. **Duration of ulceration:** The mean duration of individual ulcers was reported in four of the RCTs (see table 1, p 929). The mean duration of individual ulcers was reduced by active treatment in all four trials, but the difference was significant in only one trial and the mean difference was less than 1 day in the others. **Ulcer days index:** Three RCTs reported the ulcer days index. Both studies of chlorhexidine versus control found significant reduction in the ulcer day index. One RCT found that chlorhexidine significantly increased the number of ulcer free days compared with an inert preparation, from a mean of 17.5 to 22.9 over 6 weeks — an extra 5.4 ulcer free days per 6 weeks of treatment.[13] Another RCT found that hexidine had no significant effect.[14] **Severity of pain:** All five RCTs reported severity scores (see table 1, p 929). Two RCTs found that chlorhexidine significantly reduced the mean severity of pain compared with an inert preparation.[11] One RCT of a proprietary antiseptic mouthwash versus the alcohol containing control preparation found no difference between the treatment groups, but found a large improvement in clinical outcomes in both groups compared with baseline levels.[15] The evidence relating to other antibacterial agents such as triclosan will be reviewed in future issues of *Clinical Evidence*.

Harms: The RCTs reported few adverse events. Chlorhexidine had a bitter taste and was associated with brown staining of teeth and tongue, and with nausea.[12]

Comment: Four of the RCTs used a crossover design. A consistent observation was that outcomes improved during the course of the trials irrespective of the treatment received. One of the studies did not make clear if the effect of sequencing had been allowed for.[12] The withdrawal rates in the crossover trials were high. The parallel group trial had fewer withdrawals; 106 people with recurrent aphthous ulceration were recruited and 96 completed the study. Analysis was not by intention to treat and the method of randomisation was not specified.[15] People recruited to the trials might not be typical of the average person with recurrent aphthous ulceration.

Aphthous ulcers: recurrent

REFERENCES

1. Porter SR, Scully C, Pedersen A. Recurrent aphthous stomatitis. *Crit Rev Oral Biol Med* 1998; 9:306–321.
2. Cooke BED, Armitage P. Recurrent Mikulicz's aphthae treatment with topical hydrocortisone hemisuccinate sodium. *BMJ* 1960;1:764–766.
3. Walter T, McFall JR. Effect of flurandrenolone on oral aphthae. *J Periodontol* 1968;39:364–365.
4. Browne RM, Fox EC, Anderson RJ. Topical triamcinolone acetonide in recurrent aphthous stomatitis. *Lancet* 1968;1:565–567.
5. MacPhee IT, Sircus W, Farmer ED, Harkness RA, Cowley GC. Use of steroids in treatment of aphthous ulceration. *BMJ* 1968;2:147–149.
6. Merchant HW, Gangarosa LP, Glassman AB, Sobel RE. Betamethasone-17-benzoate in the treatment of recurrent aphthous ulcers. *Oral Surg Oral Med Oral Pathol* 1978;45:870–875.
7. Pimlott SJ, Walker DM. A controlled clinical trial efficacy of topically applied fluocinonide in the treatment of recurrent aphthous ulceration. *Br Dent J* 1983;154:174–177.
8. Thompson AC, Nolan A, Lamey P-J. Minor aphthous oral ulceration: a double-blind cross-over study of beclomethasone dipropionate aerosol spray. *Scot Med J* 1989;34:531–532.
9. Miles DA, Bricker SL, Razmus TF, Potter RH. Triamcinolone acetonide versus chlorhexidine for treatment of recurrent stomatitis. *Oral Surg Oral Med Oral Pathol* 1993;75:397–402.
10. Lehner T, Lyne C. Adrenal function during topical oral corticosteroid treatment. *BMJ* 1969;4:138–141.
11. Addy M, Carpenter R, Roberts WR. Management of recurrent aphthous ulceration – a trial of chlorhexidine gluconate gel. *Br Dent J* 1976;141:118–120.
12. Addy M. Hibitane in the treatment of recurrent aphthous ulceration. *J Clin Periodontol* 1977;4:108–116.
13. Hunter L, Addy M. Chlorhexidine gluconate mouthwash in the management of minor aphthous stomatitis. *Br Dent J* 1987;162:106–110.
14. Chadwick B, Addy M, Walker DM. Hexetidine mouthrinse in the management of minor aphthous ulceration and as an adjunct to oral hygiene. *Br Dent J* 1991;171:83.
15. Meiller TF, Kutcher MJ, Overholser CD, Niehaus C, DePaola LG, Siegel MA. Effect of an antimicrobial mouthrinse on recurrent aphthous ulcerations. *Oral Surg Oral Med Oral Pathol* 1991;72:425–429.

Stephen Porter
Professor of Oral Medicine

Crispian Scully
Professor of Special Needs Dentistry

Eastman Dental Institute for Oral Health
Care Sciences
University College London
London
UK

Competing interests: None declared.

TABLE 1 Effects of treatments on different outcomes: results of RCTs (see text, p 926, p 927).

Intervention	Study	Number	Treatment duration (weeks)	Outcomes Treatment	Outcomes Control	Effect (%)* (significance)
Incidence new ulcers (ulcers per week): topical corticosteroids versus inert preparations	2	17	8	0.51	1.15	−55% (P < 0.05)
	4	26	8	0.84	0.94	−11% (NS)
	5 pilot	8	4	2.07	1.85	+12% (NS)
	5 main	31†	4	0.73	0.82	−11% (NS)
	5	20	6	1.27	1.92	+6% (NS)
Mean ulcer duration (days): topical corticosteroids versus inert preparations	3	50	Until complete healing	6	6	0% (NS)
	4	26	8	8.07	8.94	−10% (NS)
	7	20	6	4.93	7.83	−37% (P < 0.001)
	9	19	12	5.93	5.92	0% (NS)
Ulcer days index: topical corticosteroids versus inert preparations	2	17	8	26.3	65.9	−60% (P < 0.01)
	4	26	8	58.3	71.3	−18% (NS)
	5 main	25	4	24.0	30.7	−22% (NS)
	7	20	6	48.3	70.6	−32% (P < 0.05)

TABLE 1 continued

Number of ulcers (ulcers/person/week): topical antibacterial versus presumed inert preparations					
11	20	5	1.04	1.40	NS
12	12	5	0.6	1.02	P < 0.05
13	38	6	1.26	1.38	NS
14	37	6	1.48	1.39	NS
15	96	26	0.09	0.13	NS
Mean duration of ulcers (days): topical antibacterial versus inert preparation					
11	20	5	4.8	7.8	P < 0.01
13	38	6	5.02	5.78	NS
14	37	6	6.64	6.80	NS
15	96	26	Median fall in ulcer duration from start of trial 2.42 days	Median fall in ulcer duration from start of trial 1.58 days	NS
Ulcer days index: topical antibacterial versus inert preparations					
12	12	5	9.5	17	P < 0.05
13	38	6	42.8	52.3	P < 0.05
14	37	6	79.7	65.7	NS

*Defined as difference between outcome measures for control and treatment, expressed as a fraction of the control.

†Each participant received one treatment for 4 weeks, a blank month, then another treatment with another drug. The trial compared an inert base, two local steroids and two other preparations. The figures given here are those during treatment with local steroids, and with the inert base; NS, not significant.

Search date October 2000

John Buchanan and Joanna Zakrzewska

QUESTIONS

INTERVENTIONS

Key Messages

- We found insufficient evidence about the effects of any treatment for people with burning mouth syndrome.
- One small RCT found that cognitive behavioural therapy reduced symptom intensity.

DEFINITION Burning mouth syndrome is a psychogenic or idiopathic burning discomfort or pain affecting people with clinically normal oral mucosa in whom a medical or dental cause has been excluded.[1-3] Terms previously used to describe what is now called burning mouth syndrome include glossodynia, glossopyrosis, stomatodynia, stomatopyrosis, sore tongue, and oral dysaesthesia.[4] A survey of 669 men and 758 women randomly selected from 48 500 people aged between 20 and 69 years found that people with burning mouth also have subjective dryness (66%), take some form of medication (64%), report other systemic illnesses (57%), and have altered taste (11%).[5] Many studies of people with symptoms of burning mouth do not distinguish those with burning mouth syndrome (i.e. idiopathic disease) from those with other conditions (such as vitamin B deficiency), making results unreliable.

INCIDENCE/ PREVALENCE Burning mouth syndrome mainly affects women,[6-8] particularly after the menopause, when its prevalence may be 18-33%.[9] One recent study in Sweden found a prevalence of 3.7% for the symptom of burning mouth without clinical abnormality of the oral mucosa (11/669 [1.6%] men, mean age 59 years; 42/758 [5.5%] women, mean age 57 years), with the highest prevalence (12%) in women aged 60-69 years.[5] Reported prevalence in general populations varies from 0.7%[10] to 15%.[6] Incidence and prevalence vary according to diagnostic criteria,[4] and many studies included people with the symptom of burning mouth rather than with burning mouth syndrome as defined above.

AETIOLOGY/ RISK FACTORS The cause is unknown, and we found no good aetiological studies. Hormonal disturbances associated with the menopause[7-9] and psychogenic factors (including anxiety, depression, stress, life events, personality disorders, and phobia of cancer) are possible causal factors.[11-13] Local and systemic factors (such as infections, allergies, ill fitting dentures,[12] hypersensitivity reactions,[14] and hormone and vitamin deficiencies[15-17]) may cause the symptom of burning mouth and should be excluded before diagnosing burning mouth syndrome.

PROGNOSIS We found no prospective cohort studies or other reliable evidence describing the natural history of burning mouth syndrome.[18] We found anecdotal reports of at least partial spontaneous remission in about half of people with burning mouth syndrome within 6-7 years.[12]

AIMS To alleviate symptoms, with minimal adverse effects.

OUTCOMES Self reported relief of symptoms (burning mouth, altered taste, dry mouth); incidence and severity of anxiety and depression; quality of life using a validated ordinal scale.

METHODS *Clinical Evidence* update search and appraisal October 2000, using the following terms: burning mouth, burning mouth syndrome, dysaesthesia or dysesthesia, stomatodynia or glossopyrosis, sore tongue, glossodynia or glossalgia.

QUESTION   What are the effects of treatments?

OPTION   COGNITIVE BEHAVIOURAL THERAPY

One small RCT found that cognitive behavioural therapy relieved symptoms.

Benefits: We found no systematic review. We found one small RCT in 30
             people with resistant burning mouth syndrome.[19] It found that
             12–15 sessions of cognitive behavioural therapy for 1 hour a week
             significantly reduced the intensity of symptoms (measured on a
             visual analogue scale) compared with the control group who
             received similar attention but without the cognitive therapy ses-
             sions. The difference remained at 6 month follow up (mean pre-
             treatment score 5.0 v 4.3 on placebo; mean score 6 months after
             treatment 1.4 v 4.7 on placebo, P < 0.001; 4/15 v 0/15 people
             symptom free 6 months after treatment).

Harms: The trial gave no information on adverse effects.[19]

Comment: The trial was small and individual characteristics of the two groups
             were not described, so the groups may not have been comparable.
             The visual analogue scale for assessing oral burning was not
             validated.[19]

OPTION   HORMONE REPLACEMENT THERAPY IN
             POSTMENOPAUSAL WOMEN

**We found insufficient evidence on the effects of hormone replacement
therapy in postmenopausal women with burning mouth syndrome.**

Benefits: We found no systematic review and no RCTs of sufficient quality.

Harms: Adverse effects of hormone replacement therapy are well docu-
             mented (see oestrogen under menopausal symptoms, p 1303).

Comment: We found three non-randomised intervention studies with no clear
             diagnostic criteria or outcome measures.[20–22]

OPTION   VITAMIN B REPLACEMENT OR SUPPLEMENTATION

**We found no reliable evidence about the effects of vitamin B
supplementation in people with burning mouth with or without vitamin B
deficiency.**

Benefits: We found no systematic reviews or RCTs, either in people with
             burning mouth syndrome, or in people with vitamin B deficiency and
             symptoms of burning mouth (see comment below).

Harms: We found no reliable evidence.

Comment: People with vitamin B group deficiencies and symptoms of burning
             mouth should no longer be classified as having burning mouth
             syndrome (see definition, p 932). One case control study in 70
             people found that those with symptoms of burning mouth were

more likely to have vitamin B deficiency (28/70 v 6/80).[16] One study of 16 people with vitamin deficiencies given vitamins or placebo found no improvement.[17]

OPTION   ANTIDEPRESSANTS

We found insufficient evidence on the effects of antidepressants in people with burning mouth syndrome.

Benefits: We found no systematic review. **Clomipramine and mianserin:** We found one short term RCT (253 people with chronic idiopathic pain syndrome, including 77 people with burning mouth syndrome) comparing clomipramine versus mianserin versus placebo for 6 weeks.[23] After 6 weeks there was no significant improvement in either group. **Trazodone:** One double blind RCT (37 women with burning mouth syndrome) compared trazodone (200 mg/day) versus placebo.[24] After 8 weeks there was no significant difference in pain or related symptoms between groups: mean pain on a visual analogue scale decreased in both groups at 8 weeks (from 59 to 45 with trazodone, and from 47 to 34 with placebo).

Harms: The first RCT did not report on adverse effects.[23] Adverse effects caused seven of 18 people taking trazodone to withdraw from the trial compared with two of 19 taking placebo. Adverse effects reported with trazodone were dizziness (11 people) and drowsiness (9 people).[24] Adverse effects of clomipramine, mianserin, and other antidepressants are documented elsewhere (see depressive disorders, p 652).

Comment: The trial of clomipramine and mianserin versus placebo was too small to exclude an effect of treatment, did not use adequate diagnostic criteria, was of short duration, and had limited follow up.[23] It therefore does not provide sufficient evidence to determine the role of antidepressants in treating burning mouth syndrome. Although the trial of trazodone versus placebo was well conducted and used several pertinent outcome measures, including psychological ones, it was too small and short term to detect clinically important effects.[24] The widespread use of antidepressants in burning mouth syndrome may be because of their effects on neuropathic pain[25] and the association of burning mouth syndrome with generalised anxiety disorder, depression, and adverse life events.[26]

OPTION   BENZYDAMINE HYPOCHLORIDE

We found insufficient evidence on the effects of benzydamine hypochloride in burning mouth syndrome.

Benefits: We found no systematic review. We found one small RCT (30 people with burning mouth syndrome), which compared benzydamine hypochloride (15 ml of 0.15%, for 1 minute 3 times daily for 4 weeks) versus placebo versus no treatment.[27] It found no significant difference among groups for symptoms (using a visual analogue scale), but the trial was too small to exclude a clinically important difference.

Harms: No adverse effects were reported.

Comment: Inclusion criteria were well defined. The trial was incompletely blinded, because the third group received no treatment.

REFERENCES

1. Fox H. Burning tongue glossodynia. *N Y State J Med* 1935;35:881–884.
2. Zakrzewska JM. The burning mouth syndrome remains an enigma. *Pain* 1995;62:253–257.
3. van der Waal I. *The burning mouth syndrome*. 1st ed. Copenhagen: Munksgaard, 1990.
4. Merksey H, Bogduk N, eds. *Classification of chronic pain*. 2nd ed. Seattle: International Association for the Study of Pain Press, 1994.
5. Bergdahl M, Bergdahl J. Burning mouth syndrome: prevalence and associated factors. *J Oral Pathol Med* 1999;28:350–354.
6. Tammiala-Salonen T, Hiidenkarii T, Parvinen T. Burning mouth in a Finnish adult population. *Community Dent Oral Epidemiol* 1993;21:67–71.
7. Basker RM, Sturdee DW, Davenport JC. Patients with burning mouths. A clinical investigation of causative factors, including the climacteric and diabetes. *Br Dent J* 1978;145:9–16.
8. Grushka M. Clinical features of burning mouth syndrome. *Oral Surg Oral Med Oral Pathol Oral Radiol Endod* 1987;63:30–36.
9. Wardrop RW, Hailes J, Burger H, Reade PC. Oral discomfort at the menopause. *Oral Surg Oral Med Oral Pathol Oral Radiol Endod* 1989;67:535–540.
10. Lipton JA, Ship JA, Larach-Robinson D. Estimated prevalence and distribution of reported orofacial pain in the United States. *J Am Dent Assoc* 1993; 124:115–121.
11. Rojo L, Silvestre FJ, Bagan JV, De Vicente T. Psychiatric morbidity in burning mouth syndrome. Psychiatric interview versus depression and anxiety scales. *Oral Surg Oral Med Oral Pathol Oral Radiol Endod* 1993;75:308–311.
12. Grushka M, Sessle BJ. Burning mouth syndrome. *Dent Clin North Am* 1991;35:171–184.
13. Lamey PJ, Lamb AB. The usefulness of the HAD scale in assessing anxiety in patients with burning mouth syndrome. *Oral Surg Oral Med Oral Pathol* 1989;67:390–392.
14. Bergdahl J, Anneroth G, Anneroth I. Clinical study of patients with burning mouth. *Scad J Dent Res* 1994;102:299–305.
15. Maragou P, Ivanyi L. Serum zinc levels in patients with burning mouth syndrome. *Oral Surg Oral Med Oral Pathol* 1991;71:447–450.
16. Lamey PJ, Allam BF. Vitamin status of patients with burning mouth syndrome and the response

to replacement therapy. *Br Dent J* 1986;168:81–84.
17. Hugoson A, Thorstensson B. Vitamin B status and response to replacement therapy in patients with burning mouth syndrome. *Acta Odontol Scand* 1991;49:367–375.
18. Zakrzewska JM, Hamlyn PJ. Facial pain. In: Crombie IK, Croft PR, Linton SJ, Le Resche L, Von Korff M, eds. *Epidemiology of pain*. Seattle: International Association for the Study of Pain Press, 1999:177–202.
19. Bergdahl J, Anneroth G, Perris H. Cognitive therapy in the treatment of patients with burning mouth syndrome: a controlled study. *J Oral Pathol Med* 1995;24:213–215.
20. Pisanty S, Rafaely B, Polshuk WZ. The effects of steroid hormones on buccal mucosa of menopausal women. *Oral Surg Oral Med Oral Pathol Oral Radiol Endod* 1975;40:346–353.
21. Ferguson MM, Boyle P, Hart D McK, Lindsay R. Oral complaints related to climacteric symptoms in oophorectomized women. *J R Soc Med* 1981;74: 492–497.
22. Forabosco A, Crisculo M, Coukos G, et al. Efficacy of hormone replacement therapy in postmenopausal women with oral discomfort. *Oral Surg Oral Med Oral Pathol Oral Radiol Endod* 1992;73:570–574.
23. Loldrup D, Langemark M, Hansen HJ, Olesen J, Bech P. Clomipramine and mianserin in chronic idiopathic pain syndrome. A placebo controlled study. *Psychopharmacology* 1989;99:1–7.
24. Tammiala-Salonen T, Forssell H. Trazodone in burning mouth pain: placebo-controlled, double-blind study. *J Orofac Pain* 1999;13:83–88.
25. McQuay HJ, Tramer M, Nye BA, Carroll D, Wiffen PJ, Moore RA. A systematic review of antidepressants in neuropathic pain. *Pain* 1996; 68:217–227.
26. Bogetto F, Maina G, Ferro G, Carbone M, Gandolfo S. Psychiatric comorbidity in patients with burning mouth syndrome. *Psychosom Med* 1998;60:378–385.
27. Sardella A, Uglietti D, Demarosi F, Lodi G, Bez C, Carrassi A. Benzydamine hypochloride oral rinses in management of burning mouth syndrome. A clinical trial. *Oral Surg Oral Med Oral Pathol Oral Radiol Endod* 1999;88:683–686.

John Buchanan
Clinical Lecturer in Oral Medicine

Joanna Zakrzewska
Senior Lecturer/Honorary Consultant in Oral Medicine

St Bartholomew's and The Royal London School of Medicine and Dentistry London UK

Competing interests: None declared.

Impacted wisdom teeth

Search date May 2000

Stephen Worrall

QUESTIONS
Effects of removing impacted wisdom teeth prophylactically 937

INTERVENTIONS

Likely to be ineffective or harmful
Prophylactic removal of
   asymptomatic impacted wisdom
   teeth 937

Key Messages

- We found limited evidence suggesting that harms of removing asymptomatic impacted wisdom teeth outweigh the benefits.

DEFINITION	Wisdom teeth are third molars that develop in almost all adults by about the age of 20. In some people, the teeth become partially or completely impacted below the gumline because of lack of space, obstruction, or abnormal position. Impacted wisdom teeth may be diagnosed because of pain and swelling, or incidentally by routine dental radiography.
INCIDENCE/ PREVALENCE	Third molar impaction is common. Over 72% of Swedish people aged 20–30 have at least one impacted lower third molar.[1] The surgical removal of impacted third molars (symptomatic and asymptomatic) is the most common procedure performed by oral and maxillofacial surgeons. It is performed on about 4/1000 people per year in England and Wales, making it one of the top ten inpatient and day case procedures.[2–4] Up to 90% of people on oral and maxillofacial surgery hospital waiting lists in the UK are awaiting removal of wisdom teeth.[3]
AETIOLOGY/ RISK FACTORS	Impacted wisdom teeth are partly a result of improved oral hygiene and changes in diet. Less gum disease and dental caries, and less wear and tear on teeth because of more refined diet, have increased the likelihood of retaining teeth into adult life, leaving less room for wisdom teeth.
PROGNOSIS	Impacted wisdom teeth can cause pain, swelling, and infection, as well as destroying adjacent teeth and bone. The removal of diseased and symptomatic wisdom teeth alleviates pain and improves oral health and function. We found no good data on what happens without treatment in people with asymptomatic impacted wisdom teeth.
AIMS	To reduce morbidity associated with impacted wisdom teeth with minimal adverse effects of treatments.
OUTCOMES	Pain; rates of infection; oral health and function.
METHODS	*Clinical Evidence* search and appraisal May 2000.

QUESTION   Effects of prophylactic removal of impacted wisdom teeth

We found no RCTs on the effects of prophylactic removal of asymptomatic impacted wisdom teeth. Non-randomised studies provide no evidence of benefit. Removal of lower wisdom teeth causes permanent numbness of the lower lip or tongue in about one in 200 people.

Benefits:	We found one systematic review (published in 1997), which identified 12 published reviews concerning the surgical removal of third molars.[5] No RCTs were found. There was no good evidence of benefit from the removal of impacted third molars that were free from disease. Two formal decision analyses also concluded that non-intervention was the optimal treatment for disease free, asymptomatic third molars.[6,7]
Harms:	Pain and swelling are almost universal after removing impacted wisdom teeth.[8,9] Removing lower wisdom teeth carries the risk of damage to the inferior alveolar nerve (injured in 1.3–7.8% of people,[10,11] permanently injured in 0.5–1%[12]), and to the lingual

nerve (permanently injured in up to 0.8% of people[13]). The risks appear to be greater with greater depth of impaction. The risks are the same whether the wisdom tooth is symptomatic or asymptomatic.

Comment: All studies identified in the review were of poor quality. It is likely to require an RCT with 10 years follow up to reliably answer the question. Anecdotal accounts and evidence from developing countries suggest that the answer would not be in favour of surgery.[5] Surgical morbidity following third molar removal increases with age. Where there are compelling reasons to remove them, it is prudent to do so in early adulthood.[14] Surgical morbidity is operator and technique sensitive.[15] A recently reported 20 year follow up including more than 2000 procedures reported no cases of permanent sensory lingual nerve disturbance.[15,16]

REFERENCES

1. Hugoson A, Kugelberg CF. The prevalence of third molars in a Swedish population. An epidemiological study. *Community Dent Health* 1988;5:121–138.
2. Mercier P, Precious D. Risks and benefits of removal of impacted third molars. *Int J Oral Maxillofac Surg* 1992;21:17–27.
3. Shepherd JP, Brickley M. Surgical removal of third molars. *BMJ* 1994;309:620–621.
4. Worrall SF, Riden K, Corrigan AM. UK National Third Molar project: the initial report. *Br J Oral Maxillofac Surg* 1998;36:14–18.
5. Song F, Landes DP, Glenny A-M, et al. Prophylactic removal of impacted third molars: an assessment of published reviews. *Br Dent J* 1997;182:339–346.
6. Tulloch JFC, Antczak AA, Wilkes JW. The application of decision analysis to evaluate the need for extraction of asymptomatic third molars. *J Oral Maxillofac Surg* 1987;45:855–863.
7. Brickley M, Kay E, Shepherd JP, et al. Decision analysis for lower third molar surgery. *Med Decis Making* 1995;15:143–151.
8. Bramley P. Sense about wisdoms? *J R Soc Med* 1981;74:867–868.
9. Capuzzi P, Montebugnoli L, Vaccaro MA. Extraction of impacted third molars. *Oral Surg Oral* 1994;77:341–343.
10. Schultze-Mosgau S, Reich RH. Assessment of inferior alveolar and lingual nerve disturbances after dentoalveolar surgery, and recovery of sensitivity. *Int J Oral Maxillofac Surg* 1993;22:214–217.
11. Rood JP. Permanent damage to inferior alveolar nerves during the removal of impacted mandibular third molars: comparison of two methods of bone removal. *Br Dent J* 1992;172:108–110.
12. Blackburn CW, Bramley PA. Lingual nerve damage associated with removal of lower third molars. *Br Dent J* 1989;167:103–107.
13. Robinson PP, Smith KG. Lingual nerve damage during lower third molar removal: a comparison of two surgical methods. *Br Dent J* 1996;180:456–461.
14. Bruce RA, Frederickson GC, Small GS. Age of patients and morbidity with mandibular third molar surgery. *J Am Dent Assoc* 1980;101:240–245.
15. Sisk AL, Hammer WB, Shelton DW, et al. Complications following removal of impacted third molars: the role of the experience of the surgeon. *J Oral Maxillofac Surg* 1986;44:855–859.
16. Moss CE, Wake MJC. Lingual access for third molar surgery: a 20-year retrospective audit. *Br J Oral Maxillofac Surg* 1999;37:255–258.

Stephen Worrall
Consultant Surgeon
St Luke's Hospital
Bedford
UK

Competing interests: None declared.

Search date January 2001

Caroline Pankhurst

QUESTIONS

INTERVENTIONS

PREVENTION

Beneficial

Likely to be beneficial

Unknown effectiveness

TREATMENT

Beneficial

Likely to be beneficial

Unknown effectiveness

**To be covered in future issues of
  *Clinical Evidence***

Treatment of systemic candidiasis
Prevention in people with dentures
Prevention and treatment in
  neonates

Key Messages

In people receiving chemotherapy or radiotherapy

- Two systematic reviews have found that antifungal drugs prevent oropharyngeal candidiasis in people with neutropenia and in people with cancer. RCTs have found that fluconazole is more effective than topical oral polyenes. Two RCTs found conflicting evidence of the preventive value of chlorhexidine versus placebo.

- Limited evidence from one small RCT suggests that fluconazole is more effective than amphotericin B lozenges for treatment of oropharyngeal candidiasis in people undergoing treatment for cancer.

In infants and children

- One RCT has found that fluconazole is more effective than oral polyenes in prevention of oropharyngeal candidiasis in immunocompromised infants and children.

- Two RCTs have found that in immunocompetent infants, miconazole gel is superior to nystatin suspension in the speed and effectiveness of treating oropharyngeal candidiasis. One RCT has found that fluconazole is more effective than oral polyenes in the treatment of oropharyngeal candidiasis in immunocompromised infants and children.

In people with diabetes mellitus

- We found no systematic reviews or RCTs on the prevention or treatment of oropharyngeal candidiasis in people with diabetes.

In people with denture stomatitis

- One small RCT found weak evidence that oral polyenes (nystatin, amphotericin B) were more effective than placebo at curing denture stomatitis. One RCT found no good evidence that miconazole dental lacquer benefits denture stomatitis. Trial methods included professional cleaning of the dentures at the start of the study, combined with advice on denture hygiene and advice not to wear the dentures while asleep at night. This cleaning and advice may explain the high clinical cure rate in the placebo groups.

In people with HIV infection

- RCTs have found that daily or weekly antifungal prophylaxis with fluconazole or nystatin reduces the incidence of oropharyngeal candidiasis. Most absolute benefit was found in people with AIDS who had low CD4 cell counts ($\leq 200/mm^3$) and a history of recurrent oropharyngeal candidiasis.

- RCTs have found that topical preparations of itraconazole, fluconazole, and clotrimazole effectively treat oropharyngeal candidiasis in people with HIV infection. One RCT has found that topical nystatin was inferior to fluconazole.

- RCTs have found that daily or weekly antifungal prophylaxis with fluconazole, itraconazole, and nystatin reduces the incidence of oropharyngeal candidiasis.

Reducing risk of antifungal resistance

- One RCT in people with HIV infection and acute episodes of oropharyngeal candidiasis found no significant difference between continuous prophylaxis and intermittent treatment in terms of the emergence of antifungal resistance.

DEFINITION Oropharyngeal candidiasis is an opportunistic mucosal infection, caused in over 85% of cases by *Candida albicans*. The four main types of oropharyngeal candidiasis are: (1) pseudomembranous (thrush), comprising white discrete plaques on an erythematous background, located on the buccal mucosa, throat, tongue, or gingivae; (2) erythematous, comprising smooth red patches on the hard or soft palate, dorsum of tongue, or buccal mucosa; (3) hyperplastic, comprising white, firmly adherent patches or plaques, usually bilateral on the buccal mucosa; (4) denture induced stomatitis, presenting as either a smooth or granular erythema confined to the denture-bearing area of the hard palate. Symptoms vary, ranging from none to a sore, painful mouth with a burning tongue and altered taste, which can impair speech, nutritional intake, and quality of life.

INCIDENCE/ Candida species are commensals in the gastrointestinal tract.
PREVALENCE Transmission occurs directly between infected people or on fomites. Candida is found in the mouth of 31–60% of healthy people.[1] Denture stomatitis associated with candida is prevalent in 65% of denture wearers.[1] Oropharyngeal candidiasis affects 15–60% of people with haematological or oncological malignancies during periods of immunosuppression.[2] Oropharyngeal candidiasis occurs in 7–48% of people with HIV infection and in over 90% of those with advanced disease. In severely immunosuppressed people, relapse rates are high (30–50%) and usually occur within 14 days of treatment cessation.[3]

AETIOLOGY/ Risk factors associated with symptomatic oropharyngeal candidi-
RISK FACTORS asis include local or systemic immunosuppression, haematological disorders, broad spectrum antibiotic use, inhaled or systemic steroids, xerostomia, diabetes, and wearing dentures, obturators, or orthodontic appliances. The same strain may persist for months or years in the absence of infection. In people with HIV infection, there is no direct correlation between the number of organisms and the presence of clinical disease. Symptomatic oropharyngeal candidiasis associated with *in vitro* resistance to fluconazole occurs in 5% of people with advanced HIV disease.[4] Resistance to azole antifungals is associated with severe immunosuppression (≤ 50 CD4 cells/mm^3), more episodes treated with antifungal drugs, and longer median duration of systemic azole treatment.[5]

PROGNOSIS Untreated candidiasis persists for months or years unless associated risk factors are treated or eliminated. In neonates, spontaneous cure of oropharyngeal candidiasis usually occurs after 3–8 weeks.

AIMS To resolve signs and symptoms of oropharyngeal candidiasis; to prevent or delay relapse in immunocompromised people; and to minimise drug induced resistance, with minimum adverse effects.

OUTCOMES Resolution of signs and symptoms; rate of recurrence on the basis of scoring of signs and symptoms. Many RCTs report the results of mycological culture but, whenever possible, this review has not used these intermediate outcomes because the relation between the clinical and mycological culture findings is uncertain.

METHODS   *Clinical Evidence* update search and appraisal January 2001, supplemented by a literature search of Medline and the author's library, selecting publications in English, from 1975 to 1999. We included only systematic reviews and RCTs that specified oropharyngeal candidiasis in the protocol design and outcome measurements; those dealing with oesophagitis and invasive, systemic candidal infections were excluded.

QUESTION   **What are the effects of interventions to prevent and treat oropharyngeal candidiasis in people receiving chemotherapy or radiotherapy?**

OPTION   **ANTIFUNGAL PROPHYLAXIS**

Two systematic reviews of RCTs have found that antifungal drugs prevent oropharyngeal candidiasis in neutropenic adults and cancer patients undergoing treatment. RCTs have found that fluconazole is more effective than topical oral polyenes. Two RCTs found conflicting evidence of the value of chlorhexidine oral rinse.

Benefits: We found two systematic reviews.[6,7] The earlier review (search date 1991, 9 RCTs, 710 people) compared systemic or topical anti-fungal agents with placebo in the prevention of oropharyngeal candidiasis in people with cancer and neutropenia.[6] Participants were immunosuppressed. They were not selected according to their fungal colonisation status before initiation of treatment. Treatments included amphotericin B, clotrimazole, miconazole, ketoconazole, fluconazole, and itraconazole. The duration of the prophylaxis was not stated. No eligible RCTs of nystatin were identified. Continuing colonisation of the throat after starting treatment was found to be a risk factor for development of oropharyngeal candidiasis (OR 3.66, 95% CI 1.74 to 5.18). Compared with placebo, antifungal drugs reduced the number of episodes of oropharyngeal candidiasis (AR 17/372 [5%] with antifungal v 109/338 [32%] with placebo; ARR 26%, 95% CI 23% to 28%; OR 0.15, 95% CI 0.10 to 0.22; NNT 4, 95% CI 4 to 5). Subgroup analysis for clotrimazole or fluconazole versus placebo was consistent with the global result. The second review (search date 1999, 15 RCTs, 1164 people) compared 3–10 weeks of oral and topical prophylaxis versus placebo or no treatment in people of all ages with cancer (excluding people with head and neck cancer) who were receiving chemotherapy. The review found significant reduction of oral candidiasis compared with placebo or no treatment for drugs that were partially absorbed from the gastrointestinal tract (miconazole, clotrimazole: RR 0.13, 95% CI 0.06 to 0.27; NNT 3, 95% CI 3 to 5), and for fully absorbed drugs (fluconazole, itraconazole, metoconazole: RR 0.36, 95% CI 0.19 to 0.69), but not for unabsorbed drugs (nystatin, amphotericin B, natamycin, chlorhexidine: RR 0.81, 95% CI 0.58 to 1.12).[7] One subsequent RCT (210 people with neutropenia) compared itraconazole (100 mg twice daily) with placebo as antifungal prophylaxis for superficial and systemic infections.[8] The RCT found no significant difference in oral candidiasis (AR 1/104 [0.96%] with itraconazole v 5/106 [4.7%] with placebo; RR 0.20, 95% 0.02 to 1.72), but fewer cases occurred with itraconazole. **Azoles versus polyenes:** We found no systematic review, but found three RCTs (see table 1, p 952).[9-11] One multicentre RCT (536 people with cancer and neutropenia associated with chemotherapy, radiotherapy or bone marrow transplant) compared prophylaxis for 30 days versus fluconazole 50 mg daily versus the oral polyenes amphotericin B (2 g daily), nystatin (4 x 106 units/day), or both, for the prevention of oropharyngeal candidiasis and invasive fungal infection.[9] Oropharyngeal candidiasis was less likely in people treated with fluconazole. Two smaller RCTs in people with liver transplant compared the prevention of oropharyngeal candidiasis by azoles with prevention by polyenes.[10,11] The first multicentre RCT (143 people given prophylaxis for 28 days after liver transplantation) of fluconazole versus nystatin found a lower incidence of oropharyngeal candidiasis with fluconazole, but the result was not significant.[10] The other RCT found no significant difference between nystatin and clotrimazole for prophylaxis during hospital stay after transplantation.[11] However, the two smaller RCTs had insufficient power individually to show a clinically important difference. We found no systematic review, but the results of the three RCTs were consistent with each other and the pooled results suggest that use of azoles instead of polyenes reduces the risk of oropharyngeal candidiasis by at least 40%. **Chlorhexidine oral rinse:** We found two RCTs in people who had received bone marrow transplants.[12,13] One RCT (51 people) compared prophylaxis for 60 days with chlorhexidine oral rinse versus a placebo rinse. All participants received oral nystatin suspension 100 000 units. Compared with placebo, chlorhexidine reduced oropharyngeal candidiasis (2/24 [8%] with chlorhexidine v 15/27 [56%] with control; ARR 47%, 95% CI 24% to 54%; RR 15%, 95% CI 3% to 57%; NNT 2, 95% CI 2 to 4) and mucositis.[12] The other RCT found no significant difference in the development of oropharyngeal candidiasis in 86 adults with leukaemia and bone marrow transplant randomly assigned to rinses containing saline alone, chlorhexidine alone, nystatin alone, or nystatin with chlorhexidine (no statistical analysis available).[13]

Harms: In one RCT with no placebo arm, the rates of adverse reactions over 30 days were 5.6% with fluconazole and 5.2% with oral polyenes.[9] The most common adverse events were abdominal pain, nausea and vomiting, and rash. There was no increased hepatotoxicity, cyclosporin interaction, or emergence of clinically relevant resistant strains reported in people receiving antifungal prophylaxis after liver transplantation.[10]

Comment: We found no RCTs comparing nystatin versus placebo. The RCTs of chlorhexidine found conflicting results about its effect on oropharyngeal candidiasis and mucositis,[12,13] but the second RCT had four parallel arms and was not powered to detect a clinically important difference.[13]

OPTION	ANTIFUNGAL TREATMENT

Inadequate evidence from one small RCT suggests that fluconazole is more effective than amphotericin B lozenges for treating oropharyngeal candidiasis in people undergoing treatment for cancer.

Benefits: We found no systematic reviews. We found one RCT (73 people), which compared fluconazole 50 mg tablets daily for 1 week with

Oropharyngeal candidiasis

amphotericin B 10 mg lozenges four times daily for 2 weeks in people with oropharyngeal candidiasis undergoing radiotherapy for head and neck cancer.[14] Clinical cure was more likely with fluconazole (34/37 [92%] v 26/36 [72%] with amphotericin; RR of cure 1.27, 95% CI 1.02 to 1.35; NNT with fluconazole rather than amphotericin to cure one additional person 5, 95% CI 4 to 60). For both treatments, cure rate was lower in denture wearers than in people who did not wear dentures.

Harms: The trial did not give details of adverse effects.

Comment: None.

QUESTION   What are the effects of interventions to prevent and treat oropharyngeal candidiasis in infants and children?

OPTION   ANTIFUNGAL PREVENTION IN IMMUNOCOMPROMISED INFANTS AND CHILDREN

One RCT has found that fluconazole is more effective than oral polyenes in prevention of oropharyngeal candidiasis in immunocompromised infants and children.

Benefits: We found no systematic reviews. We found one large, unblinded, multicentre RCT (502 people) comparing fluconazole 3 mg/kg versus oral polyenes (nystatin 50 000 units/kg 4 times daily, oral amphotericin B 25 mg/kg 4 times daily, or both) for the prevention of fungal infections, including oropharyngeal candidiasis. Participants were immunocompromised infants and children aged 6 months to 17 years, admitted to hospital and scheduled within the next 48 hours to undergo initial or repeat courses of chemotherapy or radiotherapy for haematological or oncological malignancies.[2] The mean duration of prophylaxis was 28 days. Fluconazole was associated with reduced incidence of oropharyngeal candidiasis (3/236 [1.3%] for fluconazole v 15/249 [6.0%] for oral polyenes; RR 0.21, 95% CI 0.06 to 0.72; NNT 21, 95% CI 18 to 58).[2] Subsequently 18 of the children from the multicentre RCT[2] were enrolled in a second RCT (25 children in each arm), which compared fluconazole 3 mg/kg once daily versus oral nystatin 50 000 units/kg four times daily in the prevention of oropharyngeal candidiasis.[15] The RCT found no significant difference in the incidence of oral candidiasis between the two arms (AR 2/25 [8%] with fluconazole v 3/25 [12%] with nystatin; P = 0.63).

Harms: Eight of 245 children on fluconazole and three of 257 on an oral polyene were withdrawn from the RCT because of adverse events.[2] In the second RCT, no children were withdrawn from the study, but three treated with fluconazole reported nausea and abdominal discomfort and one reported pruritus.[15]

Comment: None.

OPTION **ANTIFUNGAL TREATMENT IN CHILDREN**

Two RCTs have found that in immunocompetent infants, miconazole gel is superior to nystatin suspension in the speed and effectiveness of treating oropharyngeal candidiasis. One RCT has found that fluconazole is more effective than oral polyenes in the treatment of oropharyngeal candidiasis occurring in immunocompromised infants and children.

Benefits: We found no systematic review. **Immunocompetent infants and children:** We found no placebo controlled RCTs. We found two RCTs in immunocompetent infants, which compared miconazole with nystatin for treatment of oropharyngeal candidiasis.[16,17] In both RCTs, miconazole resulted in higher rates of clinical cure. In the larger RCT (183 people), quicker clinical cure was obtained with miconazole (at day 5: cure rate 83/98 [85%] for miconazole gel 25 mg 4 times daily v 18/85 [21%] for nystatin suspension 100 000 units 4 times daily; at day 12: 97/98 [99%] for miconazole v 46/85 [54%] for nystatin).[16] The clinical cure rates were not influenced significantly by the presence or absence of nappy rash. **Immunocompromised infants and children:** We found no placebo controlled RCTs. We found one multicentre RCT (32 centres, 182 immunocompromised infants and children aged 6 months to 17 years), which compared fluconazole suspension 3 mg/kg versus nystatin 400 000 units four times daily for 14 days for the treatment of oropharyngeal candidiasis. Participants were immunocompromised for different reasons: 64 were infected with HIV, 92 had a malignancy, and 26 were receiving immunosuppressive treatment.[18] Fluconazole was associated with a higher clinical cure rate than nystatin (78/86 [91%] with fluconazole v 37/73 [51%] with nystatin; RR of cure 1.8, 95% CI 1.6 to 1.9; NNT 2, 95% CI 2 to 3). In subgroup analyses, clinical cure with fluconazole was superior to nystatin for children with HIV infection (28/35 [80%] with fluconazole v 6/29 [21%] for nystatin) and for people with malignancy (49/50 [98%] for fluconazole v 30/42 [71%] for nystatin). Clinical relapse rates after 2 weeks were similar (18% for fluconazole v 24% for nystatin).

Harms: The most common adverse events with both miconazole and nystatin were vomiting and, more rarely, diarrhoea, affecting less than 4.5% of immunocompetent infants.[16,17] Two of 94 immunocompromised children were withdrawn from the fluconazole group and none of the 88 children from the nystatin group as a result of adverse events.[17]

Comment: **Immunocompetent infants and children:** The RCTs were not blinded or placebo controlled.[16,17] There is potential for observer bias, but the clinical results were corroborated by the mycological findings, which were blinded.[16] The larger RCT was carried out in 26 general practices,[16] so it is representative of the context in which most otherwise healthy infants with oropharyngeal candidiasis would be treated, especially regarding compliance and cure rate. **Immunocompromised infants and children:** The RCT showed the benefit of fluconazole for infants and children presenting with a wide range of different haematological malignancies, solid tumours, or HIV infection with no apparent differential effect dependant on age, sex, or race.[18]

QUESTION   What are the effects of interventions to prevent and treat oropharyngeal candidiasis in people with diabetes?

OPTION   ANTIFUNGAL DRUGS

We found insufficient evidence on prevention or treatment of oropharyngeal candidiasis in people with diabetes.

Benefits: We found no systematic reviews or RCTs.

Harms: Insufficient data available.

Comment: None.

QUESTION   What are the effects of treatments for oropharyngeal candidiasis in people with dentures?

One small RCT found weak evidence that oral polyenes (nystatin, amphotericin B) were more effective than placebo at curing denture stomatitis. One RCT found no good evidence that miconazole dental lacquer benefits denture stomatitis. Trial methods included professional cleaning of the dentures at the start of the study, combined with advice on denture hygiene and advice not to wear the dentures while asleep at night, which may explain the high clinical cure rate in the placebo groups.

Benefits: We found no systematic reviews, but we found several RCTs. **Versus placebo:** Four RCTs compared topical oral antifungals with placebo for the treatment of denture stomatitis.[19–22] One RCT (46 people) found that topical oral polyenes (nystatin, amphotericin B) were associated with a significant improvement in the clinical cure of denture stomatitis.[21] The second RCT (22 people) found no significant difference between polyenes and placebo in the clinical appearance of denture stomatitis.[20] The third RCT (49 people) compared amphotericin B with and without a hydrogen peroxide denture cleanser versus placebo. No combination was better than placebo for clinical cure.[19] The fourth RCT (36 people) compared miconazole dental lacquer applied to the fit surface of an upper denture as a single application versus a placebo lacquer, but found no significant difference in the resolution of palatal symptoms by day 14 (symptom resolution in 54% with placebo; RR 2.4, 95% CI 0.89 to 3.8).[22] **Different antifungal treatments:** We found three small RCTs. One RCT compared miconazole dental lacquer versus 2% miconazole gel applied to the denture four times a day and found no significant difference in palatal erythema after 14 days of treatment (13/20 [65%] with lacquer v 16/21 [76%] with gel; RR of erythema with lacquer v gel 0.85, 95% CI 0.42 to 1.2).[23] The second RCT (19 elderly, chronically ill, institutionalised adults) compared nystatin denture soaking solution (10 000 units/ml) versus tap water as a soaking solution; both groups were given nystatin pastilles (10 000 units/g 3 times daily).[24] The RCT found no additional advantage from the use of nystatin as a soaking agent: all participants in both groups were clinically cured at 7 days.[24] The third RCT (29 people) compared fluconazole 50 mg daily for 14 days versus amphotericin B lozenges plus denture cream for 28 days.[25] At 28 days there was no significant difference in the clinical cure rate (84% for fluconazole v 90% for amphotericin B). Clinical relapse was common in both groups at 12 weeks. We found one large multicentre RCT (305 elderly people from 56 investigational sites; 176 wore dentures). The RCT compared daily administration of fluconazole (50 mg) suspension versus amphotericin B (0.5 g) oral suspension three times daily for 2 weeks. It found no significant difference between fluconazole and amphotericin for either clinical or mycological cure. Wearing dentures did not affect the response to antifungal therapy (clinical cure rate 151/176 [86%] of denture wearers v 102/124 [82%] of non-denture wearers).[26]

Harms: None of the trials exclusively enrolling people with dentures were large enough to report accurately on the incidence of adverse effects. In the large RCT of elderly people,[26] six of 150 (4%) in the fluconazole arm and none of the 155 (0%) in the amphotericin arm experienced adverse events, including diarrhoea, buccal bitterness, aggravation of pre-existing renal dysfunction (1, withdrawn from RCT), and increased liver transaminases (1, not withdrawn).

Comment: Trial methods included professional cleaning of the dentures at the start of the study, combined with advice on denture hygiene and advice not to wear the dentures while asleep at night. Because the fit surface of the denture acts as a reservoir of primary and recurrent infection, this cleaning and advice may explain the high clinical cure rate in the placebo groups. There was poor correlation between clinical cure and mycological cure. The RCTs comparing different antifungals were not sufficiently powerful to detect clinically important differences.

QUESTION What are the effects of interventions to prevent and treat oropharyngeal candidiasis in people with HIV infection?

OPTION CONTINUOUS ANTIFUNGAL PROPHYLAXIS

RCTs have found that daily or weekly antifungal prophylaxis with fluconazole, itraconazole, or nystatin reduces the incidence of oropharyngeal candidiasis in people with HIV infection. Most absolute benefit was found in people with AIDS who had low CD4 cell counts ($\leq$ 200 cells/mm^3) and a history of recurrent oropharyngeal candidiasis.

Benefits: We found no systematic reviews. We found eight RCTs using different prophylaxis protocols with follow up from 3 to 29 months.[27–34] All RCTs enrolled people with AIDS, AIDS related complex, or CD4 cell counts $\leq$ 300 cells/mm^3. **Fluconazole versus placebo:** Five RCTs using daily or weekly regimens found significant reduction in oropharyngeal candidiasis with fluconazole.[27,28,30–32] Three of these RCTs compared weekly fluconazole versus placebo. Clinical relapse during 6 months' prophylaxis was reduced by fluconazole 150 mg weekly (relapse: 4/9 with fluconazole v 5/5 with placebo;[27] and 13/31 with fluconazole v 25/26 with placebo;[30] pooled AR 43% with fluconazole v 97% with placebo; RR 0.4, 95% CI 0.1 to 0.9; NNT 2). The third RCT (323 women infected with HIV) compared fluconazole 200 mg weekly versus placebo and found similar results: fluconazole reduced the risk of recurrent oropharyngeal candidiasis over 29 months (RR 0.50, 95% CI 0.33 to 0.74).[28] For people with a history of oropharyngeal candidiasis, the absolute benefit of treatment with weekly fluconazole was higher than in those with no history of infection (ARR 25.6/100 person years for those with previous infection v 11.2/100 person years for those with no history of infection).[28] In one RCT, the median time to relapse was 168 days with fluconazole versus 37 days with placebo ($P \leq 0.0001$).[30] We found no RCTs comparing weekly versus daily regimens. No significant difference was found between 50 mg or 100 mg daily doses (oropharyngeal candidiasis: 2/18 [11%] with 50 mg v 4/19 [21%] with 100 mg; RR 0.53, 95% CI 0.09 to 2.09).[31] **Itraconazole versus placebo:** One placebo controlled RCT found that daily prophylaxis with 200 mg of itraconazole for 24 weeks reduced the number of people who relapsed (5/24 [21%] with itraconazole v 14/20 [70%] with placebo; ARR 49%, 95% CI 19% to 64%; NNT 2, 95% CI 2 to 5) and increased the time interval before relapse occurred (median time to relapse 8.0 with placebo v 10.4 weeks with itraconazole; $P = 0.001$).[34] **Nystatin versus placebo:** One RCT found that, compared with placebo, prophylaxis with nystatin 200 000 unit pastille once daily over 20 weeks delayed the onset of oropharyngeal candidiasis (HR 0.56, no 95% CI given).[29] **Fluconazole versus clotrimazole:** One large RCT (428 people from 29 sites) compared fluconazole 200 mg daily versus clotrimazole 10 mg five times daily over 35 months, and found that fluconazole was associated with reduced recurrent oropharyngeal candidiasis (fluconazole 5.7 episodes/100 person years v clotrimazole 38.1 episodes/100 person years, $P \leq 0.001$).[33]

Harms:

The most commonly reported adverse events were gastrointestinal symptoms, rash, and headache, but data on adverse effects were incomplete and were not presented in all RCTs. No participants withdrew owing to adverse changes in liver function or haematological variables. Concomitant medication and severe underlying disease may have confounded attribution of adverse events.

Comment:

Many of the RCTs were small and not blinded, and most did not adjust for confounding factors such as anti-retroviral treatment and other established risk factors for oropharyngeal candidiasis. No RCTs used quality of life scores. The optimal dosage schedule and frequency of administration of preventive treatment have not been established.

OPTION TOPICAL TREATMENT

RCTs have found that topical preparations of itraconazole, fluconazole, and clotrimazole effectively treat oropharyngeal candidiasis in people with HIV infection. One RCT found that topical nystatin was inferior to fluconazole.

Benefits:

We found no systematic review. We found four RCTs comparing topical (suspensions or pastilles) versus orally absorbed antifungals for treatment of oropharyngeal candidiasis in people with HIV infection. Three RCTs found itraconazole oral solution 100 mg or

200 mg used in a swish and swallow mode was as effective as fluconazole 100 mg once daily for 14 days or clotrimazole 10 mg five times a day. All three RCTs achieved clinical response rates over 90%.[35–37] The fourth RCT found that complete resolution of signs and symptoms of oropharyngeal candidiasis was more common with fluconazole 100 mg daily than with nystatin liquid for 14 days (fluconazole 60/69 [87%] v 36/69 [52%] for nystatin liquid; ARI 35%, 95% CI 22% to 42%; RR 1.67, 95% CI 1.42 to 1.80; NNT 3, 95% CI 2 to 5).[38]

Harms: No consistent changes in results of haematology tests or blood or urine biochemistry tests were noted in any of the RCTs. The most frequently reported adverse effects were gastrointestinal symptoms (nausea, diarrhoea, vomiting). Altered taste, dry mouth, headache, and rashes were also recorded. On the basis of data from the six RCTs (861 people), in which adverse events were considered to be drug induced and resulted in withdrawal from the study, adverse events were reported with fluconazole (4 people), itraconazole (14 people), clotrimazole (12 people), and nystatin (1 person).[29,33,35–38]

Comment: Once daily dosing is associated with good adherence to treatment. Non-adherence because of the inconvenience of taking multiple doses was documented with clotrimazole.

QUESTION **Which treatments reduce the risk of acquiring resistance to antifungal drugs?**

OPTION **CONTINUOUS ANTIFUNGAL PROPHYLAXIS VERSUS INTERMITTENT ANTIFUNGAL TREATMENT**

One RCT in people with HIV infection and acute episodes of oropharyngeal candidiasis found no significant difference between continuous antifungal prophylaxis and intermittent antifungal treatment in terms of the emergence of antifungal resistance.

Benefits: We found no systematic review. We found one RCT comparing the effects of different treatment regimens on the development of acquired resistance in people with HIV infection over a mean follow up of 11 months.[39] Antifungal sensitivity testing followed the National Committee for Clinical Laboratory Standards guidelines.[40] Continuous prophylaxis compared with intermittent treatment with fluconazole 200 mg a day reduced median annual relapse rates (0 episodes/year for continuous prophylaxis v 4.1 episodes/year for intermittent treatment, P ≤ 0.001). Antifungal resistance developed in more people on continuous prophylaxis than on intermittent treatment, but the difference was not significant (9/16 [56%] for continuous v 13/28 [46%] for intermittent, P = 0.75).

Harms: No adverse reactions were reported.

Comment: Optimal treatment regimens to reduce the risk of acquiring resistance have not been evaluated adequately. In a prospective observational study of protease inhibitor treatment, 93 people with HIV and with a history of recurrent oropharyngeal candidiasis were followed up for 1 year. Oropharyngeal candidiasis was diagnosed in two of 30 people (7%) given protease inhibitors and 23 of 63 (37%) given other treatment (P ≤ 0.001, no 95% CI given).[41] Immuno-modulating anti-retroviral treatments (e.g. highly active anti-retroviral therapy), by reducing the number of recurrences of oropharyngeal candidiasis, are acting indirectly as antifungal sparing agents, thereby reducing exposure to antifungals and the potential risk of resistance.

Substantive changes since last issue

Antifungal prophylaxis New RCT;[8] conclusion unchanged.
Antifungal prevention in immunocompromised infants and children New RCT;[15] conclusion unchanged.

REFERENCES

1. Webb BC, Thomas CJ, Willcox MD, et al. Candida-associated denture stomatitis. Aetiology and management: a review. Part 3. Treatment of oral candidosis. Aust Dent J 1998;43:244–249.
2. Ninane JA. Multicentre study of fluconazole versus oral polyenes in the prevention of fungal infection in children with hematological or oncological malignancies. Multicentre study group. Eur J Clin Microbiol Infect Dis 1994;13:330–337.
3. Philips P, Zemcov J, Mahmood W, et al. Itraconazole cyclodextrin solution for fluconazole-refractory oropharyngeal candidiasis in AIDS: correlation of clinical response with in vitro susceptibility. AIDS 1996;10:1369–1376.
4. Rex JH, Rinald MG, Pfaler MA. Resistance of candida species to fluconazole. Antimicrob Agents Chemother 1995;39:1–8.
5. Maenza JR, Keruly JC, Moore RD, et al. Risk factors for fluconazole-resistant candidiasis in human immuno-deficiency virus-infected patients. J Infect Dis 1996;173:219–225.
6. Meunier F, Paesmans M, Autier P. Value of antifungal prophylaxis with antifungal drugs against oropharyngeal candidiasis in cancer patients. Eur J Cancer B Oral Oncol 1994;30:196–199. Search date 1991; primary sources English language papers from Medline and author's library.
7. Clarkson JE, Worthington HV, Eden OB. Prevention of oral mucositis or oral candidiasis for patients with cancer receiving chemotherapy (excluding head and neck cancer). In: The Cochrane Library, Issue 4, 2000. Oxford: Update Software. Search date July 1999; primary sources Medline, Embase, CINAHL, Cancerlit, the Cochrane Controlled Trials Register, and the Cochrane Oral Health Group Specialist Register.
8. Nucci M, Biasoli I, Akiti T, et al. A double-blind, randomized, placebo-controlled trial of itraconazole capsules as antifungal prophylaxis for neutropenic patients. Clin Infect Dis 2000;31:300–305.
9. Philpott-Howard JN, Wade JJ, Mufti GJ, et al. Randomized comparison of oral fluconazole versus oral polyenes for the prevention of fungal infection in patients at risk of neutropenia. Multicentre study group. J Antimicrob Chemother 1993;31:973–984.
10. Lumbreras C, Cuervas-Mons V, Jara P, et al. Randomized trial of fluconazole versus nystatin for the prophylaxis of candida infection following liver transplantation. J Infect Dis 1996;174:583–588.
11. Ruskin JD, Wood RP, Bailey MR, et al. Comparative trial of oral clotrimazole and nystatin for oropharyngeal candidiasis prophylaxis in orthotopic liver transplant patients. Oral Surg Oral Med Oral Pathol Oral Radiol Endod 1992;74:567–571.
12. Ferretti GA, Ash RC, Brown AT, Parr MD, Romond EH, Lillich TT. Control of oral mucositis and candidiasis in marrow transplantation: a prospective, double-blind trial of chlorhexidine digluconate oral rinse. Bone Marrow Transplant 1988;3:483–493.
13. Epstein JB, Vickars L, Spinelli J, Reece D. Efficacy of chlorhexidine and nystatin rinses in prevention of oral complications in leukemia and bone marrow transplantation. Oral Surg Oral Med Oral Pathol Oral Radiol Endod 1992;73:682–689.
14. Finlay PM, Richardson MD, Robertson AG. A comparative study of the efficacy of fluconazole and amphotericin B in the treatment of oropharyngeal candidosis in patients undergoing radiotherapy for head and neck tumours. Br J Oral Maxillofac Surg 1996;34:23–25.
15. Groll AH, Just-Nuebling G, Kurz M, et al. Fluconazole versus nystatin in the prevention of candida infections in children and adolescents undergoing remission induction or consolidation chemotherapy for cancer. J Antimicrob Chemother 1997;40:855–862.
16. Hoppe J, Burr R, Ebeling H, et al. Treatment of oropharyngeal candidiasis in immunocompetent infants: a randomized multicenter study of miconazole gel vs. nystatin suspension. Pediatr Infect Dis J 1997;16:288–293.
17. Hoppe JE, Hahn H. Randomized comparison of two nystatin oral gels with miconazole oral gel for treatment of oral thrush in infants. Antimycotics study group. Infection 1996;24:136–139.
18. Flynn PM, Cunningham CK, Kerkering T, et al. Oropharyngeal candidiasis in immunocompromised children: a randomized, multicenter study of orally administered fluconazole suspension versus nystatin. The multicenter fluconazole study group. J Pediatr 1995;127:322–328.
19. Walker DM, Stafford GD, Huggett R, et al. The treatment of denture stomatitis: evaluation of two agents. Br Dent J 1981;151:416–419.
20. Naim RI. Nystatin and amphotericin B in the treatment of denture-related candidiasis. Oral Surg Oral Med Oral Pathol Oral Radiol Endod 1975;40:68–75.
21. Johnson GH, Taylor TD, Heid DW. Clinical evaluation of a nystatin pastille for treatment of denture-related oral candidiasis. J Prosthet Dent 1989;61:699–703.
22. Konsberg R, Axell T. Treatment of candida-infected denture stomatitis with a miconazole lacquer. Oral Surg Oral Med Oral Pathol Oral Radiol Endod 1994;78:306–311.

23. Budtz-Jorgensen E, Carlino P. A miconazole lacquer in the treatment of candida-associated denture stomatitis. *Mycoses* 1994;37:131–135.

24. Banting DW, Greenhorn PA, McMinn JG. Effectiveness of a topical antifungal regimen for the treatment of oral candidiasis in older, chronically ill, institutionalized adults. *J Can Dent Assoc* 1995;61:199–195.

25. Bissell V, Felix DH, Wray D. Comparative trial of fluconazole and amphotericin B in the treatment of denture stomatitis. *Oral Surg Oral Med Oral Path Oral Radiol Endod* 1993;76:35–39.

26. Taillandier J, Esnault Y, Alemanni M, and the multicentre study group. A comparison of fluconazole oral suspension and amphotericin B oral suspension in older patients with oropharyngeal candidosis. *Age Ageing* 2000;29: 117–123.

27. Leen CLS, Dunbar EM, Ellis ME, et al. Once-weekly fluconazole to prevent recurrence of oropharyngeal candidiasis in patients with AIDS and AIDS-related complex: a double-blind placebo controlled study. *J Infect* 1990;21:55–60.

28. Schuman P, Capps L, Peng G, et al. Weekly fluconazole for the prevention of mucosal candidiasis in women with HIV infection. A randomized, double-blind, placebo-controlled trial. Terry Beirn community programs for clinical research on AIDS. *Ann Intern Med* 1997;126: 689–696.

29. MacPhail LA, Hilton JF, Dodd CL, et al. Prophylaxis with nystatin pastilles for HIV-associated oral candidiasis. *J Acquir Immune Defic Syndr* 1996; 12:470–476.

30. Marriott DJE, Jones PD, Hoy JF, et al. Fluconazole once a week as secondary prophylaxis against oropharyngeal candidiasis in HIV-infected patients. A double-blind placebo-controlled study. *Med J Aust* 1993;158:312–316.

31. Just-Nubling G, Gentschew G, Meissner K, et al. Fluconazole prophylaxis of recurrent oral candidiasis in HIV-positive patients. *Eur J Clin Microbiol Infect Dis* 1991;10:917–921.

32. Stevens DA, Greene SI, Lang OS. Thrush can be prevented in patients with acquired immunodeficiency syndrome and the acquired immunodeficiency syndrome-related complex. Randomized, double-blind, placebo-controlled study of 100 mg oral fluconazole daily. *Arch Intern Med* 1991;151:2458–2464.

33. Powderly WG, Finklestein DM, Feinberg J, et al. A randomised trial comparing fluconazole with clotrimazole troches for the prevention of fungal infection in patients with advanced human immunodeficiency virus infection. *N Engl J Med* 1995;332:700 705.

34. Smith D, Midgley J, Gazzard B. A randomised, double-blind study of itraconazole versus placebo in the treatment and prevention of oral or oesophageal candidosis in patients with HIV infection. *Int J Clin Pract* 1999;53:349–352.

35. Graybill JR, Vazquez J, Darouiche RO, et al. Randomized trial of itraconazole oral solution for oropharyngeal candidiasis in HIV/AIDS patients. *Am J Med* 1998;104:33–39.

36. Phillips P, De Beule K, Frechette G, et al. A double-blind comparison of itraconazole oral solution and fluconazole capsules for the treatment of oropharyngeal candidiasis in patients with AIDS. *Clin Infect Dis* 1998;26:1368–1373.

37. Murray PA, Koletar SL, Mallegol I, et al. Itraconazole oral solution versus clotrimazole troches for the treatment of oropharyngeal candidiasis in immunocompromised patients. *Clin Ther* 1997;19:471–480.

38. Pons V, Greenspan D, Lozada-Nur F, et al. Oropharyngeal candidiasis in patients with AIDS: randomized comparison of fluconazole versus nystatin oral suspensions. *Clin Infect Dis* 1997; 24:1204–1207.

39. Revankar SG, Kirkpatrick WR, McAtee RK, et al. A randomized trial of continuous or intermittent therapy with fluconazole for oropharyngeal candidiasis in HIV-infected patients: clinical outcomes and development of fluconazole resistance. *Am J Med* 1998;105:7–11.

40. National Committee for Clinical Laboratory Standards. *Reference Method for Broth Dilution Antifungal Susceptibility Testing of Yeasts: Approved Standard*. Wayne, Penn: NCCLS, 1997 (document M27-A).

41. Cauda R, Tacconelli E, Tumbarello M, et al. Role of protease inhibitors in preventing recurrent oral candidiasis in patients with HIV infections: a prospective case control study. *J Acquir Immune Defic Syndr* 1999;21:20–25.

Caroline Pankhurst
Guy's, King's College, and
St Thomas's Dental Institute
London
UK

Competing interests: The author has been reimbursed for a conference registration fee in 1994 by Pfizer, the manufacturer of fluconazole.

TABLE 1 RCTs of azoles versus polyenes in prevention of oropharyngeal candidiasis in people with impaired immunity (see text, p 943).

RCT	AR with azole	AR with nystatin	ARR	RR	NNT
Fluconazole v amphotericin and/or nystatin[9]	4/256 (1.6 %)	22/255 (8.6%)	7% (4.2% to 8.1%)	0.18 (0.06 to 0.52)	14 (12 to 24)
Fluconazole v nystatin[10]	7/76 (9%)	14/67 (21%)	12%	0.44 (0.18 to 1.01)	–
Clotrimazole v nystatin[11]	1/17 (6%)	1/17 (6%)	0%	1.00 (0.06 to 8.86)	–
Pooled results	**12/349 (3%)**	**37/339 (11%)**	**7.5% (4.4% to 9.1%)**	**0.32 (0.16 to 0.59)**	**13 (11 to 23)**

Search date November 2000

Michael Eddleston and Nick Buckley

QUESTIONS

INTERVENTIONS

Key Messages

- We found no good evidence on the effectiveness of ipecacuanha, gastric lavage, or activated charcoal in paracetamol poisoning.
- One small RCT found that acetylcysteine reduced mortality in people with established paracetamol induced liver failure. One observational study found that people given early treatment with acetylcysteine were less likely to develop liver damage than untreated historical controls.
- One small RCT found that the risk of hepatotoxicity was lower with methionine than with supportive care.

Paracetamol (acetaminophen) poisoning

DEFINITION	Paracetamol poisoning occurs as a result of either accidental or intentional overdose with paracetamol (acetaminophen).
INCIDENCE/ PREVALENCE	Paracetamol is the commonest drug used for self poisoning in the UK.[1] It is also a common means of self poisoning in Europe, North America, and Australasia. An estimated 41 200 cases of poisoning with products containing paracetamol occurred in 1989–1990 in England and Wales, with a case fatality rate of 0.4% (95% CI 0.38% to 0.46%). Overdoses due to paracetamol alone result in an estimated 150–200 deaths and 15–20 liver transplants each year in England and Wales.
AETIOLOGY/ RISK FACTORS	Most cases in the UK are impulsive acts of self harm in young people.[1,2] In one study of 80 people, 42 had obtained the tablets for the specific purpose of taking an overdose, and 33 had obtained them less than 1 hour before the act.[2]
PROGNOSIS	People with blood paracetamol concentrations above the standard treatment line (defined in the UK as a line joining 200 mg/l at 4 hours and 30 mg/l at 15 hours on a semilogarithmic plot) have a poor prognosis without treatment (see figure 1, p 959).[3,4] In one study of 57 untreated people with blood concentrations above this line, 33 developed severe liver damage and three died.[3] People with a history of chronic alcohol misuse, use of enzyme inducing drugs, eating disorders, or multiple paracetamol overdoses may be at risk of liver damage with blood concentrations below this line.[5] In the USA, a lower line is used as an indication for treatment, but we found no data relating this line to prognostic outcomes.[6] **Dose effect:** The dose ingested also indicates the risk of hepatotoxicity. People ingesting less than 125 mg/kg had no significant hepatotoxicity with a sharp dose dependent rise for higher doses.[7] The threshold for toxicity after acute ingestion may be higher in children, where a single dose of less than 200 mg/kg has not been reported to lead to death and rarely causes hepatotoxicity.[8]
AIMS	To prevent liver failure; liver transplantation; or death, with minimal adverse effects.
OUTCOMES	Rates of death, liver failure, liver transplantation, or hepatotoxicity (most commonly defined by the objective criterion of an aspartate aminotransferase of > 1000 U/l).
METHODS	*Clinical Evidence* search and appraisal November 2000. We also contacted experts in the field to identify unpublished studies. We evaluated only interventions that are currently in common use (not for example mercaptamine [cysteamine], cimetidine, or dimercaprol).

What are the effects of treatments for acute paracetamol poisoning?

OPTION   **IPECACUANHA**

We found no evidence of the effectiveness of ipecacuanha in paracetamol poisoning.

Benefits: We found no systematic review and no RCTs that reported clinical end points.

Harms: We found no large study of complications in paracetamol poisoned people receiving ipecacuanha. Specific complications of ipecacuanha may include aspiration, diarrhoea, ileus, arrhythmia during vomiting, dystonia from treatment for vomiting, and haematemesis from vomiting.[9]

Comment: Human simulated overdose studies suggest that ipecacuanha given within 1 hour could reduce paracetamol absorption, but no studies have shown a change in clinical outcome.[10] One non-systematic review of ipecacuanha in all forms of poisoning found no evidence that ipecacuanha improved outcome in poisoned people.[10] Administration of ipecacuanha may delay the administration of activated charcoal and oral antidotes.

OPTION   **GASTRIC LAVAGE**

We found no evidence of the effectiveness of gastric lavage in paracetamol poisoning.

Benefits: We found no systematic review and no RCTs that reported clinical outcomes.

Harms: We found no large study of complications in paracetamol poisoned people receiving gastric lavage. Harms may include aspiration of stomach contents, hypoxia, and oesophageal perforation.[9]

Comment: Studies of simulated overdose in human volunteers suggest that gastric lavage carried out within 1 hour removes a variable number of paracetamol tablets and that the number diminishes with time.[11] One cohort study in 450 consecutive people who took at least 10 g or more of paracetamol found that those given activated charcoal were significantly less likely to have high risk blood paracetamol concentrations (OR 0.36, 95% CI 0.23 to 0.58).[12] However, the addition of gastric lavage did not further decrease the risk (OR 1.12, 95% CI 0.57 to 2.20). One non-systematic review of gastric lavage in all forms of poisoning found no evidence that gastric lavage improved outcome in poisoned people.[11]

OPTION   **ACTIVATED CHARCOAL (SINGLE OR MULTIPLE DOSE)**

We found no evidence of the effectiveness of activated charcoal, whether in single or multiple dose regimens, in paracetamol poisoning.

Benefits: We found no systematic review and no RCTs that reported clinical outcomes.

Paracetamol (acetaminophen) poisoning

Harms: We found no large study of complications in paracetamol poisoned people receiving single doses of activated charcoal. We found no large, high quality RCT comparing activated charcoal with placebo in any form of poisoning that might have allowed calculation of the incidence of complications. Harms may include aspiration pneumonia, vomiting, diarrhoea, constipation, ileus, and interference with regular medications.

Comment: **Single dose regimens:** Studies of simulated overdose in human volunteers suggest that activated charcoal given within 2 hours decreases paracetamol absorption by a variable amount and that this amount diminishes with time.[13,14] One cohort study in 450 consecutive people who had taken 10 g or more of paracetamol found that those who had been given activated charcoal were significantly less likely to have high risk blood paracetamol concentrations (OR 0.36, 95% CI 0.23 to 0.58).[12] The effect was seen only in those treated within 2 hours, and the study was not large enough to assess the effect of numerous potential confounders.[12] One non-systematic review of activated charcoal in all forms of poisoning found no evidence that activated charcoal improved outcome in poisoned people.[13] **Multiple dose regimens:** We found no studies of simulated overdose that evaluated multiple dose regimens in paracetamol poisoning. A non-systematic review of multiple dose regimens in all forms of poisoning found no evidence that multiple dose regimens improve outcomes in poisoned people.[15] The rapid absorption and short half life of paracetamol suggest a beneficial effect is unlikely.

OPTION   ACETYLCYSTEINE

One small RCT found that acetylcysteine reduced mortality in people with established paracetamol induced liver failure. One observational study found that people given early treatment with acetylcysteine were less likely to develop liver damage than untreated historical controls.

Benefits: We found no systematic review. We found one RCT (50 people with established paracetamol induced liver failure), which compared intravenous acetylcysteine (150 mg/kg over 15 minutes, 50 mg/kg over 4 hours, and then 100 mg/kg over 16 hours, continued until death or recovery) versus a placebo infusion of 5% dextrose.[16] It found that significantly more people survived in the treated group compared with controls (48% v 20%; ARR 28%, 95% CI 3% to 53%).

Harms: The RCT did not specifically assess adverse outcomes and none were noted. Four case series suggested that the incidence of adverse effects from intravenous acetylcysteine is 5–15%.[17–20] These were predominantly rash, urticaria, and occasionally more serious anaphylactoid reactions occurring with the initial "loading" dose. In most or all cases, adverse effects responded to temporary cessation of infusions and symptomatic treatment, and did not recur when treatment was recommenced. Two deaths have been reported due to a tenfold miscalculation of the dose, although only half of the loading dose was given in one case.[20] Vomiting is common after oral acetylcysteine and occurred in 63% of people in one series despite prior administration of metoclopramide.[21] Oral acetylcysteine can also cause hypersensitivity and anaphylactoid reactions.[22]

Comment: In the RCT, allocation was concealed but treatment was not blinded. There were differences between the groups in prognostic variables (prothrombin time, coma grade) and other treatments, but a possible confounding effect could not be adequately assessed because of the small size of the study.[16] One observational study evaluated the use of intravenous acetylcysteine in people presenting early to hospital. It found that people treated within 10 hours of ingestion were less likely to develop liver damage than untreated historical controls (1.6% in treated group v 57.9% of controls; ARR 56%, 95% CI 47% to 58%; RRR 97%, 95% CI 81% to 99.6%; NNT 2, 95% CI 2 to 3).[3] As a result, subsequent RCTs were considered unethical. A systematic review of numerous case series found evidence that acetylcysteine is beneficial in paracetamol poisoning.[17] For both oral and intravenous acetylcysteine, the overall rate of hepatotoxicity was worse if treatment was delayed beyond 8 to 10 hours (1% in those treated within 8 hours v 46% in those treated after 16 hours).[3,17] We found no RCTs of different regimens and no evidence of a difference between oral and intravenous routes of administration.[17] The optimal dose, route, and duration of treatment is unknown. Two recent observational studies comparing different protocols for intravenous[23] and oral[24] acetylcysteine did not find marked differences in outcomes.

OPTION   METHIONINE

One RCT was too small to detect a clinically important effect of methionine on the death rate in people with blood paracetamol concentrations above the UK standard treatment line. The RCT found a lower risk of hepatotoxicity with methionine than supportive care.

Benefits: We found no systematic review. One RCT (40 people) compared methionine (2.5 g 4 hourly for 4 doses), mercaptamine, and supportive care in people with blood paracetamol concentrations above the UK standard treatment line.[25] There was no significant effect on death (0 deaths in the methionine group v 1 in the supportive care group). Only 27 people had a liver biopsy. Fewer people suffered grade III hepatic necrosis (0/9 v 6/10 after supportive care), or had peak aspartate aminotransferase greater than 1000 U (1/13 [7%] v 8/13 [62%] with supportive care; ARR 54%, 95% CI 16% to 61%; RRR 88%, 95% CI 25% to 99%; NNT 2, 95% CI 2 to 6).

Harms: No serious adverse effects associated with treatment were reported in the RCT, but vomiting after administration of methionine occurred in eight of 13 people. The incidence of adverse effects in the control group was not reported.

Comment: Interpretation of liver biopsy results from the RCT was difficult as not all people were tested and an intention to treat analysis was not possible. We found one case series in people treated with methionine in early and late paracetamol poisoning, but there was no comparison group.[26]

REFERENCES

1. Gunnell D, Hawton K, Murray V, et al. Use of paracetamol for suicide and non-fatal poisoning in the UK and France: are restrictions on availability justified? *J Epidemiol Community Health* 1997; 51:175–179.

2. Hawton K, Ware C, Mistry H, et al. Paracetamol self-poisoning. Characteristics, prevention and harm reduction. *Br J Psychiatry* 1996;168:43–48.

3. Prescott LF, Illingworth RN, Critchley JAJH, Stewart MJ, Adam RD, Proudfoot AT. Intravenous N-acetylcysteine: the treatment of choice for paracetamol poisoning. *BMJ* 1979;2:1097–1100.

4. Rumack BH, Matthew H. Acetaminophen poisoning and toxicity. *Pediatrics* 1975;55:871–876.

5. Vale JA, Proudfoot AT. Paracetamol (acetaminophen) poisoning. *Lancet* 1995;346: 547–552.

6. Smilkstein MJ, Knapp GL, Kulig KW, Rumack B. Efficacy of oral N-acetylcysteine in the treatment of acetaminophen overdose. Analysis of the National Multicentre Study (1976–1985). *N Engl J Med* 1988;319:1557–1562.

7. Prescott LF. Paracetamol overdosage. Pharmacological considerations and clinical management. *Drugs* 1983;25:290–314.

8. Caravati EM. Unintentional acetaminophen ingestion in children and the potential for hepatotoxicity. *J Toxicol Clin Toxicol* 2000;38:291–296.

9. Pond SM, Lewis-Driver DJ, Williams GM, Green AC, Stevenson NW. Gastric emptying in acute overdose: a prospective randomised controlled trial. *Med J Aust* 1995;163:345–349.

10. Krenzelok EP, McGuigan M, Lheur P. Position statement: ipecac syrup. American Academy of Clinical Toxicology and European Association of Poisons Centres and Clinical Toxicologists. *J Toxicol Clin Toxicol* 1997;35:699–709.

11. Vale JA. Position statement: gastric lavage. American Academy of Clinical Toxicology and European Association of Poisons Centres and Clinical Toxicologists. *J Toxicol Clin Toxicol* 1997; 35:711–719.

12. Buckley NA, Whyte IM, O'Connell DL, Dawson AH. Activated charcoal reduces the need for N-acetylcysteine treatment after acetaminophen (paracetamol) overdose. *J Toxicol Clin Toxicol* 1999;37:753–757.

13. Chyka PA, Seger D. Position statement: single-dose activated charcoal. American Academy of Clinical Toxicology; European Association of Poisons Centres and Clinical Toxicologists. *J Toxicol Clin Toxicol* 1997;35:721–741.

14. Rose SR, Gorman RL, Oderda GM, Klein-Schwartz W, Watson WA. Simulated acetaminophen overdose: pharmacokinetics and effectiveness of activated charcoal. *Ann Emerg Med* 1991;20: 1064–1068.

15. American Academy of Clinical Toxicology, European Association of Poison Centres and Clinical Toxicologists. Position statement and practice guidelines on the use of multi-dose activated charcoal in the treatment of acute poisoning. *J Toxicol Clin Toxicol* 1999;37:731–751.

16. Keays R, Harrison PM, Wendon JA, et al. Intravenous acetylcysteine in paracetamol induced fulminant hepatic failure: a prospective controlled trial. *BMJ* 1991;303:1026–1029.

17. Buckley NA, Whyte IM, O'Connell DL, Dawson AH. Oral or intravenous N-acetylcysteine: which is the treatment of choice for acetaminophen (paracetamol) poisoning? *J Toxicol Clin Toxicol* 1999;37:759–767.

18. Chan TY, Critchley JA. Adverse reactions to intravenous N-acetylcysteine in Chinese patients with paracetamol (acetaminophen) poisoning. *Hum Exp Toxicol* 1994;13:542–544.

19. Schmidt LE, Dalhoff KP. Side-effects of N-acetylcysteine treatment in patients with paracetamol poisoning [in Danish]. *Ugeskri Laeger* 1999;161:2669–2672.

20. Wright RO, Anderson AC, Lesko SL, Woolf AD, Linakis JG, Lewander WJ. Effect of metoclopramide dose on preventing emesis after oral administration of N-acetylcysteine for acetaminophen overdose. *J Toxicol Clin Toxicol* 1999;37:35–42.

21. Perry HE, Shannon MW. Efficacy of oral versus intravenous N-acetylcysteine in acetaminophen overdose: results of an open-label, clinical trial. *J Pediatr* 1998;132:149–152.

22. Mant TG, Tempowski JH, Volans GN, Talbot JC. Adverse reactions to acetylcysteine and effects of overdose. *BMJ* 1984;289:217–219.

23. Dougherty T, Greene T, Roberts JR. Acetaminophen overdose: comparison between continuous and intermittent intravenous N-acetylcysteine 48-hour protocols. *Ann Emerg Med* 2000;36:S83

24. Woo OF, Mueller PD, Olson KR, Anderson IB, Kim SY. Shorter duration of oral N-acetylcysteine therapy for acute acetaminophen overdose. *Ann Emerg Med* 2000;35:363–368.

25. Hamlyn AN, Lesna M, Record CO, et al. Methionine and cysteamine in paracetamol (acetaminophen) overdose; prospective controlled trial of early therapy. *J Int Med Res* 1981;9:226–231.

26. Vale JA, Meredith TJ, Goulding R. Treatment of acetaminophen poisoning. The use of oral methionine. *Arch Intern Med* 1981;141:394–396.

Michael Eddleston
Research Fellow
Centre for Tropical Medicine
University of Oxford
Oxford
UK

Nick Buckley
Consultant Clinical Pharmacologist
and Toxicologist
Royal Adelaide Hospital
Adelaide
Australia
Competing interests: None declared.

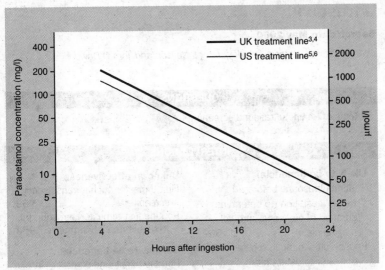

FIGURE 1 Nomograms used to determine acetylcysteine or methionine treatment, based on the blood concentrations between 4 and 24 hours after ingestion of paracetamol. Published with permission (see text, p 954).[12]

Antenatal care of low risk pregnancies: ultrasound

Search date May 2000

Leanne Bricker, Patricia Crowley, James Neilson and Tom O'Dowd

INTERVENTIONS

Key Messages

- A systematic review of RCTs has found that routine ultrasound screening before 24 weeks' gestation leads to earlier diagnosis of multiple pregnancies but has not been shown to have an important positive impact on the outcome of multiple pregnancies.

- A systematic review of RCTs has found that routine ultrasound screening before 24 weeks' gestation is associated with fewer inductions of labour for "post-term" pregnancy.

- One large RCT found that routine ultrasound screening before 24 weeks' gestation reduced perinatal mortality if detection of fetal malformation was an important objective, there was a high level of diagnostic expertise, and termination of pregnancy for fetal abnormality was widely accepted in the population screened.

- Routine ultrasound screening in the first trimester for increased nuchal translucency, fetal abnormalities, or both has not yet been evaluated in controlled trials.

- A systematic review of RCTs and primary observational studies has found that detection rates of fetal abnormality by screening ultrasound examinations vary with the organ system affected, with generally high rates of detection of abnormalities of the central nervous system, and low rates for skeletal and cardiac abnormalities. Similar variations are seen at both second and third trimester examinations.

© Clinical Evidence 2001;5:960–971.

Antenatal care of low risk pregnancies: ultrasound

- A systematic review of RCTs has found no evidence that routine ultrasound after 24 weeks confers clear benefit to mother or baby, except that assessment of placental appearances may, as an adjunct to fetal measurement, help reduce perinatal mortality.
- In a systematic review of RCTs, Doppler ultrasound in pregnancy has not been shown to be of benefit, and may even increase the risk of adverse outcome.

DEFINITION	A low risk pregnancy is one in which a rate of perinatal and maternal mortality and morbidity lower than that in the overall population can be achieved without a high rate of obstetric or paediatric intervention.
INCIDENCE/ PREVALENCE	In England, Wales, and Northern Ireland in 1995 the stillbirth rate was 5.48 per 1000 deliveries and the neonatal death rate was 4.04 per 1000 deliveries.[1] In the UK during the same period, the maternal death rate was 12.2 per 100 000,[2] the caesarean section rate was 17%,[3] and the rate of induction of labour was 27%.[3]
AETIOLOGY/ RISK FACTORS	Obstetric factors associated with an increased risk of perinatal morbidity or mortality include pre-eclampsia, prematurity, antepartum and postpartum haemorrhage, and intrauterine growth retardation. Perinatal morbidity and mortality are higher if the fetus is congenitally abnormal. Obstetric factors associated with maternal mortality and morbidity are pre-eclampsia, haemorrhage, and venous thromboembolism.
AIMS	To prevent avoidable maternal and perinatal mortality and morbidity; to enhance satisfaction with pregnancy, childbirth, and parenting; to avoid unnecessary intervention; and to improve convenience of care.
OUTCOMES	Perinatal death; maternal death; incidence and detection of fetal malformation; incidence of termination of pregnancy for medical reasons; rates of normal and uncomplicated birth; quality of experience of pregnancy and childbirth including feeling worried or not feeling relaxed about the pregnancy. Some intermediate outcomes (such as incidence of undiagnosed multiple pregnancy at 26 weeks, low birth weight, and rates of induction of labour for post-term pregnancy) have also been used.
METHODS	We searched the Cochrane Controlled Trials Register and the Cochrane Pregnancy and Childbirth Group's Register in May 2000. We included only randomised and quasi-randomised trials (e.g. those using allocation by date of birth). Primary studies assessing the detection of fetal anomalies by routine ultrasound before 1995 were taken from Chitty;[4] for subsequent primary studies we searched Medline from 1995 to May 2000 using the terms: pregnancy, ultrasound, prenatal and abnormalities. Predefined quality criteria were: population based study of unselected or low risk population; clearly stated study aim, setting, participants and time period; ultrasound intervention fully described, including gestation at the time of ultrasound, diagnostic approach, quality control, operators and skills, equipment used, anomalies sought, method of postnatal ascertainment (including description of false positives and false negatives), anomalies detected reported per fetus or per system. A few other good quality studies are quoted in the text to demonstrate particular issues.

Pregnancy and childbirth

Leanne Bricker, James P Neilson

OPTION   ROUTINE ULTRASOUND SCREENING BEFORE 24 WEEKS'
GESTATION TO ESTABLISH GESTATIONAL AGE, DETECT
FETAL HEART ACTIVITY AND MULTIPLE PREGNANCY, AND
DETERMINE CHORIONICITY (IF APPROPRIATE)

One systematic review of RCTs has found better gestational age
assessment and earlier detection of multiple pregnancy with routine than
with selective early ultrasound screening (before 24 weeks' gestation).
The effects on substantive clinical outcomes are unclear.

Benefits: We found one systematic review of routine versus selective ultrasound in pregnancy before 24 weeks (search date 1998, 9 RCTs,
34 245 pregnancies),[5] and one subsequent RCT.[6] Routine ultrasound examination before 24 weeks' gestation was associated with
earlier detection of multiple pregnancies (twins undiagnosed at 26
weeks 2/116 [1.7%] of screened group v 41/104 [39%] of control
group; OR 0.08, 95% CI 0.04 to 0.16; three twin pregnancies need
scanning in early pregnancy to diagnose one additional twin pregnancy), but with no demonstrable improvement in perinatal outcome of twin pregnancies (perinatal mortality of twins: 12/228
[5.2%] for screened group v 13/262 [5.0%] for controls; pooled RRI
6%, 95% CI –51% to +123%), and reduced rates of induction of
labour for post-term pregnancy (220/12 149 [1.8%] for screened
group v 357/12 046 [3.0%] for controls; OR 0.61, 95% CI 0.52 to
0.72; 87 women would need ultrasound screening in early pregnancy to prevent one induction for post-term pregnancy, 95% CI 70
to 121), presumably because of more accurate gestational dating.
There were no differences detected for substantive clinical outcomes, such as perinatal mortality (111/17 192 [0.65%] for
screened group v 127/17 053 [0.74%] for controls; OR 0.86, 95%
CI 0.67 to 1.12). The subsequent RCT (648 women) assessed the
efficacy of an ultrasound assessment of gestational age at the first
antenatal visit (≤ 17 weeks' gestation) as an adjunct to the routine
second trimester anomaly scan (18–20 weeks' gestation).[6] Fewer
women needed adjustment of their expected date of delivery at their
second trimester anomaly scan (9% v 18%; RR 0.52, 95% CI 0.34
to 0.79). The number of women who had a repeat blood sample
taken for maternal serum screening was similar in the ultrasound
and control groups (AR 6% v 6%). Fewer women in the ultrasound
group reported feeling worried (AR 32% v 40%; RR 0.80, 95% CI
0.65 to 0.99) or not feeling relaxed about their pregnancy compared with the control group (AR 22% v 30%; RR 0.73, 95% CI 0.56
to 0.96). The pregnancy outcomes were similar in the two groups,
including rates of induction of labour, but the numbers are too small
to draw conclusions about effects on substantive outcomes relating
to maternal and perinatal morbidity and mortality.

Harms: At present there is no clear evidence that ultrasound examination
during pregnancy is harmful. Long term follow up of children in
Norway who, as fetuses, were entered into the Alesund and Trond-
heim trials found no adverse influence on school performance or

screening was to be introduced it may need to be supplemented with a further scan in the second trimester.[12]

OPTION **ULTRASOUND SCREENING FOR FETAL ANOMALIES IN THE SECOND TRIMESTER**

Leanne Bricker, James P Neilson

We found that no easily generaliseable conclusions could be drawn from the available evidence. One RCT found that second trimester ultrasound screening performed specifically to detect fetal abnormality was associated with increased rates of planned termination of pregnancy and fewer perinatal deaths. Another RCT found conflicting results.

Benefits:
We found no systematic review of RCTs, but found two large RCTs.[13,14] We also found one unpublished systematic review (L Bricker et al, unpublished data, 2000) mainly of observational studies (see comment below). The two RCTs compared screening for fetal abnormalities by routine ultrasound before 24 weeks versus selective ultrasound in 24 017 pregnancies.[13,14] The findings of these trials were conflicting. In one RCT,[13] in which detection of fetal abnormality was a specific aim of ultrasound screening, the number of planned terminations of pregnancy increased (11/4353 [0.25%] for the screened group, 0/4309 for the control group; for every 415 women screened there was one additional termination of pregnancy, 95% CI 24 to 30 508 women) and there were fewer perinatal deaths (20/4389 [0.46%] for the screened group v 39/4347 [0.90%] for controls; OR 0.51, 95% CI 0.30 to 0.87; NNT 227, 95% CI 158 to 853). There were large differences in the detection rates between the two hospitals involved in this study (36% v 77% of babies with fetal abnormalities). In the other RCT,[14] only 17% of babies with abnormalities were identified in the ultrasound screened group before 24 weeks of pregnancy, and there was minimal impact on perinatal mortality (52/7685 [0.68%] for the screened group v 41/7596 [0.54%] for controls; OR 1.25, 95% CI 0.83 to 1.88). We found no RCTs that addressed the psychological impact or long term maternal and childhood outcomes associated with prenatal detection of fetal abnormalities. We found no RCTs evaluating the overall long term effect of fetal abnormality detection. However, prior knowledge of the presence of some abnormalities associated with possible survival and long term handicap may alter the management of the pregnancy, with regard to mode of delivery or place of delivery, in an attempt to improve outcome. We found several studies suggesting that the outcome of conditions such as gastroschisis[15] and cardiac abnormalities[16] may be improved by prenatal detection.

Harms:
There is a risk of pregnancy loss from invasive procedures to investigate positive ultrasound results, and a risk of psychological sequelae. Available evidence does not allow quantification of the risk of increased intervention and hence the risk of maternal morbidity in pregnancies where abnormalities are diagnosed prenatally, or of any subsequent improvement in long term outcome. One non-randomised study found that prenatal diagnosis of congenital diaphragmatic hernia, abdominal wall defects, meningomyelocele, or bladder exstrophy resulted in all diagnosed fetuses being

delivered by caesarean section in a hospital attached to a neonatal surgical unit, but it found no obvious difference in neonatal outcome between fetuses diagnosed and fetuses not diagnosed prenatally.[17] The gestational age at birth was significantly lower in the prenatally diagnosed group. The absence of randomisation makes comparison difficult because diagnosed cases may have been more severe or serious.

Comment: Many factors affect detection rates for fetal abnormalities: technical difficulties such as maternal obesity and fetal position at the time of scanning; the fact that sonographic signs for some anomalies are subtle or absent at the particular gestation of scanning; the anatomical system affected; and the equipment used. There was a difference in detection rates between different centres and between the two RCTs. The findings of studies may not generalise. One explanation is that experience and skill in performing ultrasonography affects detection rates. The detection rate of major fetal malformation was low in the RCT[14] undertaken in 109 centres where staff may have had different levels of skill. The limit of less than 24 weeks' gestation for legal termination of pregnancy in this trial may have contributed to the lack of impact on perinatal outcomes. Some studies report number of anomalies and not number of anomalous fetuses, thus overestimating sensitivity, as a fetus with multiple anomalies would be included more than once. Some exclude minor anomalies, or anomalies not detectable by ultrasound scan, or both. We found one unpublished systematic review (L Bricker et al, unpublished data, 2000) of 11 primary studies[18-28] that included one RCT, four prospective observational studies and six retrospective studies. The review assessed in 96 633 pregnancies the overall detection of fetal abnormalities by routine ultrasound (L Bricker et al, unpublished data, 2000). Overall the sensitivity for detection of fetal anomalies was 45% (range 15–85%). Detection rates by routine second trimester ultrasound for different anatomical systems were: central nervous system 76%, urinary tract 67%, pulmonary 50%, gastrointestinal 42%, skeletal 24%, and cardiac 17%. Overall detection rates for chromosomal abnormalities was 19%. Only one termination of pregnancy occurred as a result of false positive diagnosis (L Bricker et al, unpublished data, 2000). All studies reviewed had high specificity, confirming that normal ultrasound examinations may be reassuring. Only one study in the review addressed the role of ultrasonographic soft markers in improving detection of chromosomal abnormalities; it found that for a 4% increase in the detection rate of congenital abnormalities (from 51% to 55%) there was a 12-fold increase in false positives.[26]

OPTION   ROUTINE ULTRASOUND AFTER 24 WEEKS' GESTATION

One systematic review of routine late pregnancy ultrasound (> 24 weeks' gestation) in low risk or unselected populations found no significant benefit for mother or baby. We found no evidence about the psychological effects of routine ultrasound in late pregnancy, or about the effects on neonatal and childhood outcomes. One RCT found that placental grading in the third trimester may be beneficial.

Benefits:
We found one systematic review (search date 1999, seven RCTs, 25 036 unselected or low risk pregnancies) comparing routine ultrasound after 24 weeks' gestation versus concealed or selective ultrasound after 24 weeks gestation.[29] One of the seven trials combined repeated ultrasound scan for fetal biometry and amniotic fluid assessment with Doppler ultrasound, and its data were analysed separately. **Routine ultrasound after 24 weeks:** Meta-analysis of the results of six trials comprising 22 202 unselected or low risk pregnancies found no difference between the screened and control groups in the following outcomes: antenatal admissions or other tests of fetal wellbeing; obstetric interventions such as induction of labour, instrumental delivery and caesarean section; preterm delivery rates and birthweight; neonatal interventions such as resuscitation, ventilation, admission to special care; and neonatal morbidity such as Apgar score at 5 minutes. One RCT found no difference between screened and unscreened groups in the rates of moderate and severe neonatal morbidity. Overall, there was no difference between the groups in perinatal mortality, including congenital abnormalities (77/11199 [0.69%] v 74/11079 [0.67%]; OR 1.03, 95% CI 0.75 to 1.42) or in perinatal mortality excluding congenital abnormalities (50/9924 [0.50%] v 44/9812 [0.45%]; OR 1.12, 95% CI 0.75 to 1.68). There was also no difference in perinatal mortality of twins (6/168 [3.6%] v 8/146 [5.5%] for controls; OR 0.60, 95% CI 0.20 to 1.76). One of the RCTs found reduced stillbirth rate when placental grading was incorporated into routine third trimester ultrasound scan (1/1014 [0.10%] with placental assessment v 12/1011 [1.2%] for controls; OR 0.13, 95% CI 0.04 to 0.50; NNT 92 to prevent one additional stillbirth, 95% CI 85 to 231). Psychological and other maternal outcomes were not reported in any of the studies. **Intensive ultrasound screening including Doppler:** The review identified one RCT (2834 unselected pregnancies) comparing the combination of repeated ultrasound scanning for fetal biometry, amniotic fluid assessment plus Doppler ultrasound (intensive screening) with selective ultrasound. It found no significant difference between the two groups in other tests of fetal wellbeing, obstetric interventions, neonatal interventions, or perinatal mortality. **Routine ultrasound after 24 weeks to detect fetal abnormalities:** We found one systematic review (11 primary studies, 96 633 pregnancies) assessing the differential performance associated with different anatomical systems. Four of these primary studies (35 834 screened fetuses) included a routine third trimester ultrasound scan.[19,22,23,25] One of these studies was an RCT, two were prospective studies, and one was a retrospective study. However, all included second trimester scans and some anomalies were detected before routine scans in the third trimester. At routine third trimester ultrasound, the overall detection rate for fetal abnormalities was 19% (range 16–40%).

Harms:
The trial of intensive ultrasound screening unexpectedly found significantly more babies in the intensive screening group had birthweight under the 10th centile (179/1415 [12.7%] v 132/1419 [9.3%]; OR 1.41, 95% CI 1.11 to 1.78; NNH 30, 95% CI 16 to 106), and under the third centile (58/1415 [4.1%] v 35/1419 [2.5%]; OR 1.67, 95% CI 1.11 to 2.53; NNH 61, 95% CI 27 to

402).[30] This may have arisen by chance or frequent exposure to ultrasound may reduce fetal growth. There was no association with increased perinatal morbidity or mortality (perinatal mortality: 13/1415 [0.92%] v 22/1419 [1.55%] for controls; OR 0.60, 95% CI 0.31 to 1.17). Follow up of 2222 (81%) of these children at 1 year of age found no difference between those given intensive as opposed to selective screening (J Newnham, Australian Perinatal Society in conjunction with the New Zealand Perinatal Society, 1996).

Comment: Routine ultrasound in late pregnancy (after 24 weeks' gestation) is aimed at assessing some of the following: fetal size, amniotic fluid volume, placental site, placental grading, fetal structural abnormality, or fetal presentation. The trials used different ultrasound examination options and evaluated different outcomes. Some offered the control group no routine scans at any time in pregnancy. Some offered routine scans to all participants earlier in pregnancy (that is, before 24 weeks' gestation), whereas others offered routine scan at all stages of the trial, but only revealed results of late pregnancy ultrasound (after 24 weeks' gestation) for the study groups. It is unclear whether the specific nature of the ultrasound regimens affected the outcome measures.

OPTION   **ROUTINE DOPPLER ULTRASOUND OF THE UMBILICAL OR UTERINE ARTERIES IN UNSELECTED OR LOW RISK PREGNANCIES**

One systematic review of RCTs has found that routine Doppler ultrasound in low risk or unselected pregnancies benefits neither mother nor baby, and may be harmful. One systematic review of primary observational diagnostic studies has found that routine Doppler ultrasound of the uterine artery has limited diagnostic accuracy in predicting pre-eclampsia, intrauterine growth retardation, and perinatal death. We found no evidence to assess the effect on long term outcomes such as childhood neurological development and maternal outcomes, particularly psychological effects.

Benefits: We found two systematic reviews.[31,32] The first systematic review (search date 1999; 5 RCTs, 14 338 unselected or low risk pregnancies) compared routine Doppler ultrasound of the umbilical artery or a combination of the umbilical and uterine arteries versus control (no, concealed, or selective Doppler ultrasound).[31] Meta-analysis found no difference between groups in antenatal admissions, obstetric interventions, neonatal interventions, or overall perinatal mortality (perinatal mortality: 27/5853 [0.46%] v 29/5522 [0.53%] for controls; OR 0.88, 95% CI 0.52 to 1.48). In one trial, the screened group was more likely to have further Doppler ultrasound examinations (296/1950 [15.2%] v 198/1948 [10.2%] for controls; OR 1.57, 95% CI 1.30 to 1.90). Another trial found increased perinatal mortality among congenitally normal fetuses/neonates in the screened group (16/1246 [1.3%] v 4/1229 [0.3%]; OR 3.31, 95% CI 1.37 to 7.97; NNH 104, 95% CI 29 to 941) (see harms below). The second systematic review (search date not clearly specified, last included reference published 1998; 27 primary observational diagnostic studies comprising 12 994 women in low and high risk populations) evaluated Doppler ultrasound of the uterine artery in the prediction of pre-eclampsia, intrauterine growth retardation and perinatal death.[32] The predictive value of this test in low risk populations (9806 people) was poor with pooled likelihood ratios for both positive and negative tests all falling below 5.0 (see table 1, p 971). **Intensive screening including Doppler:** See benefits of routine ultrasound after 24 weeks' gestation, p 967.

Harms: The higher perinatal mortality among normal fetuses or neonates in the screened group in one trial raised fears that routine Doppler ultrasound in unselected pregnancies may do more harm than good. However, this was an unexpected finding that may have occurred by chance. The trial was not powered to test the ability of routine Doppler ultrasound examinations to reduce perinatal mortality. In the systematic review,[31] meta-analysis of perinatal outcome in normal fetuses included data from 9359 pregnancies, and no such effect was found (perinatal mortality of normal fetuses: 21/4838 [0.43%] v 18/4521 [0.40%]; OR 1.10, 95% CI 0.59 to 2.07) (See also harms under routine ultrasound after 24 weeks' gestation, p 967).

Comment: The five RCTs included in the first systematic review had different designs. Two trials studied unselected populations and three studied low risk populations. No trials included a standardised management protocol for abnormal Doppler results. The type of Doppler ultrasound differed; two trials evaluated umbilical and uterine artery Doppler and three trials evaluated umbilical artery Doppler alone.

REFERENCES

1. Maternal and Child Health Consortium. *Confidential enquiry into stillbirths and deaths in infancy, 4th annual report.* London: Maternal and Child Health Consortium, 1997:8.
2. Department of Health. Why mothers die. *Report on confidential enquiries into maternal deaths in the United Kingdom 1994–1996.* London: The Stationery Office, 1998.
3. Audit Commission. *First class delivery. Improving maternity services in England and Wales.* London: Audit Commission, 1997.
4. Chitty LS. Ultrasound screening for fetal abnormalities. *Prenat Diagn* 1995;15:1241–1257.
5. Neilson JP. Ultrasound for fetal assessment in early pregnancy. In: The Cochrane Library, Issue 4, 1999. Oxford: Update Software. Search date July 1998; primary sources Cochrane Pregnancy and Childbirth Groups Trials Register, and the Cochrane Controlled Trials Register.
6. Crowther CA, Kornman L, O'Callaghan S, George K, Furness M, Willson K. Is an ultrasound assessment of gestational age at the first antenatal visit of value? A randomised clinical trial. *Br J Obstet Gynaecol* 1999;106:1273–1279.
7. Royal College of Obstetricians and Gynaecologists. *Ultrasound screening for fetal abnormalities: report of the RCOG Working Party.* London: RCOG, 1997.
8. Chitty LS, Pandya PP. Ultrasound screening for fetal abnormalities in the first trimester. *Prenat Diagn* 1997;17:1269–1281.
9. Snijders RJM, Noble P, Sebire N, Souka A, Nicolaides KN. UK multicentre project on assessment of risk of trisomy 21 by maternal age and fetal nuchal-translucency thickness at 10–14 weeks of gestation. *Lancet* 1998;351:343–346.
10. Alfirevic Z, Gosden C, Neilson JP. Chorion villus sampling versus amniocentesis for prenatal diagnosis. In: The Cochrane Library, Issue 4, 1999. Oxford: Update Software. Search date 1996; primary sources Cochrane Pregnancy and Childbirth Groups Trials Register and the Cochrane Controlled Trials Register.
11. Alfirevic Z. Early amniocentesis versus transabdominal chorion villus sampling for prenatal diagnosis. In: The Cochrane Library, Issue 4, 1999. Oxford: Update Software. Search date October 1998; primary sources Cochrane Pregnancy and Childbirth Groups Trials Register and the Cochrane Controlled Trials Register.
12. Economides DL, Whitlow BJ, Braithwaite JM. Ultrasonography in the detection of fetal anomalies in early pregnancy. *Br J Obstet Gynaecol* 1999;106:516–523.
13. Saari-Kemppainen A, Karjalainen O, Ylostalo P, Heinonen OP. Fetal anomalies in a controlled one-stage ultrasound screening trial. A report from the Helsinki ultrasound group. *J Perinat Med* 1994; 22:279–289.
14. Ewigman BG, Crane JP, Frigoletto FD, LeFevre ML, Bain RP, McNellis D, and the RADIUS study group. Effect of prenatal ultrasound screening on perinatal outcome. *N Engl J Med* 1993;329:821–827.
15. Roberts JP, Burge DM. Antenatal diagnosis of abdominal wall defects: a missed opportunity? *Arch Dis Child* 1990;65(7 Spec No):687–689.
16. Cohen DM. Surgical management of congenital heart disease in the 1990s. *Am J Dis Child* 1992; 146:1447–1452.

17. Skari H, Bjornland K, Bjornstad Ostensen A, Haugen G, Emblem R. Consequences of prenatal ultrasound diagnosis: a preliminary report on neonates with congenital malformations. Acta Obstet Gynecol Scand 1998;77:635–642.

18. Chitty LS, Hunt GH, Moore J, Lobb MO. Effectiveness of routine ultrasonography in detecting fetal structural abnormalities in a low risk population. BMJ 1991;303:1165–1169.

19. Levi S, Hyjazi Y, Schaaps JP, Defoort P, Coulon R, Buekens P. Sensitivity and specificity of routine antenatal screening for congenital anomalies by ultrasound: the Belgian multicentric study. Ultrasound Obstet Gynecol 1991;1:366–371.

20. Shirley IM, Bottomley F, Robinson VP. Routine radiographer screening for fetal abnormalities by ultrasound in an unselected low risk population. Br J Radiol 1992;65:564–569.

21. Luck CA. Value of routine ultrasound scanning at 19 weeks: a four year study of 8849 deliveries. BMJ 1992;304:1474–1478.

22. Crane JP, LeFevre ML, Winborn RC, et al. A randomized trial of prenatal ultrasonographic screening: impact on the detection, management, and outcome of anomalous fetuses. Am J Obstet Gynecol 1994;171:392–399.

23. Levi S, Schaaps JP, De Havay P, Coulon R, Defoort P. End-result of routine ultrasound screening for congenital anomalies: the Belgian multicentric study 1984–92. Ultrasound Obstet Gynecol 1995; 5:366–371.

24. Skupski DW, Newman S, Edersheim T, et al. The impact of routine obstetric ultrasonographic screening in a low-risk population. Am J Obstet Gynecol 1996;175:1142–1145.

25. Lee K, Kim SY, Choi SM, et al. Effectiveness of prenatal ultrasonography in detecting fetal anomalies and perinatal outcome of anomalous fetuses. Yonsei Med J 1998;39:372–382.

26. Boyd P, Chamberlain P, Hicks N. Six-year experience of prenatal diagnosis in an unselected population in Oxford, UK. Lancet 1998;352: 1577–1581.

27. Van Dorsten JP, Hulsey TC, Newman RB, Menard MK. Fetal anomaly detection by second-trimester ultrasonography in a tertiary center. Am J Obstet Gynecol 1998;178:742–749.

28. Magriples U, Copel JA. Accurate detection of anomalies by routine ultrasonography in an indigent clinic population. Am J Obstet Gynecol 1998;179:978–981.

29. Bricker L, Neilson JP. Routine ultrasound in late pregnancy (> 24 weeks gestation). In: The Cochrane Library, Issue 1, 2000. Oxford: Update Software. Search date 1999; primary sources Cochrane Pregnancy and Childbirth Groups Trials Register, and the Cochrane Controlled Trials Register.

30. Newnham JP, Evans SF, Michael CA, Stanley FJ, Landau LI. Effects of frequent ultrasound during pregnancy: a randomised controlled trial. Lancet 1993; 342: 887–891.

31. Bricker L, Neilson JP. Routine Doppler ultrasound in pregnancy. In: The Cochrane Library, Issue 2, 2000. Search date 1999; primary sources Cochrane Pregnancy and Childbirth Groups Trials Register, and the Cochrane Controlled Trials Register.

32. Chien PF, Arnott N, Gordon A, Owen P, Khan KS. How useful is uterine artery Doppler flow velocimetry in the prediction of pre-eclampsia, intrauterine growth retardation and perinatal death? An overview. Br J Obstet Gynaecol 2000; 107:196–208. Search date 1997; primary sources Medline, hand searches of bibliographies and known unpublished studies

Leanne Bricker

Clinical Lecturer in Obstetrics
University Department of Obstetrics
and Gynaecology
Liverpool Women's Hospital
Liverpool
UK

James Neilson

Professor of Obstetrics and
Gynaecology
University of Liverpool
Liverpool
UK

Patricia Crowley

Consultant Obstetrician and
Gynaecologist
Coombe Women's Hospital
Dublin
Ireland

Tom O'Dowd

Professor of General Practice
Trinity College
Dublin
Ireland

Competing interests: None declared.

TABLE 1 Operative characteristics of Doppler ultrasound of the uterine artery in the prediction of three outcomes (see benefits of Doppler ultrasound, p 969).[32]

Predicted outcome	Abnormal test result (true positive/all positive)	Normal test result (false negative/all negative)	Sensitivity (95% CI)*	Specificity (95% CI)*	LR+ (95% CI)*	LR− (95% CI)*
Pre-eclampsia	150/891	117/6724	56% (50% to 62%)	90% (89% to 91%)	5.57 (4.9 to 6.3)	0.49 (0.43 to 0.56)
Intrauterine growth retardation	303/1076	665/8730	31% (29% to 34%)	91% (91% to 92%)	3.58 (3.19 to 4.02)	0.75 (0.72 to 0.79)
Perinatal death	12/607	43/3795	22% (13% to 34%)	86% (85% to 87%)	1.59 (0.96 to 2.60)	0.91 (0.79 to 1.04)

LR+ is the positive likelihood ratio (see main glossary); LR− is the negative likelihood ratio (see main glossary). Sensitivity and specificity are defined in the main glossary.

Pregnancy and childbirth

Search date October 2000

Chris Kettle

INTERVENTIONS

Beneficial

Restrictive use of episiotomy (reduces risk of posterior trauma). 975

"Hands on" versus "hands poised" method of delivery (reduces short term pain). 979

Absorbable synthetic material for perineal repair of first and second degree tears and episiotomies (reduces short term pain). 980

Continuous subcutaneous technique of perineal skin closure of first and second degree tears and episiotomies (reduces short term pain) . . .980

Likely to be beneficial

Vacuum extractor (less perineal trauma than with forceps). . .976

Continuous support during labour (reduces instrumental delivery) 977

Non-suturing of perineal skin in first and second degree tears and episiotomies (reduces dyspareunia) 980

Unknown effectiveness

Sustained breath holding (Valsalva) method of pushing. 979

Non-suturing of perineal muscle in second degree tears and episiotomies 981

Different methods and materials for repair of third and fourth degree tears. 981

Trade off between benefits and harms

Upright versus recumbent position during delivery 978

Unlikely to be beneficial

"Hands poised" versus "hands on" method of delivery (no significant difference in rate of perineal trauma). 979

Likely to be ineffective or harmful

Midline episiotomy incision (associated with higher risk of third/fourth degree tears compared with mediolateral incision) 975

Epidural anaesthesia (increases instrumental delivery). 976

To be covered in future issues of *Clinical Evidence*

Third trimester perineal massage

Postnatal interventions to reduce morbidity associated with perineal trauma

Key Messages

Intrapartum surgical interventions

- One systematic review of RCTs has found that restricting episiotomy to specific fetal and maternal indications reduces rates of posterior perineal trauma but slightly increases the rates of anterior vaginal and labial trauma.

- We found no evidence that midline episiotomy incision improves outcome compared with mediolateral incision. Limited evidence suggests that midline incision may increase the risk of third and fourth degree tears.

- One systematic review of RCTs found no direct evidence about the effect of epidural anaesthesia on rates of perineal trauma. However, epidural anaesthesia was associated with an increased risk of instrumental delivery, which in turn is associated with an increased risk of perineal trauma.

- One systematic review of RCTs has found that the use of the vacuum extractor versus forceps delivery reduces the rate of perineal trauma, but increases the incidence of neonatal cephalhaematoma and retinal haemorrhage.

Intrapartum non-surgical interventions

- One systematic review of RCTs has found that providing continuous support for women during childbirth versus usual care reduces the rate of instrumental delivery. Two RCTs found no significant difference in the risk of perineal trauma but were too small to rule out a clinically important difference.

- One systematic review of RCTs comparing an upright versus a recumbent position during delivery found no significant difference in overall rates of perineal trauma, but an increase in labial tears. A subsequent RCT found a reduced episiotomy rate in women who delivered in an upright position.

- One systematic review of controlled trials found no significant difference in the extent or rate of perineal trauma when sustained breath holding (Valsalva) versus spontaneous exhalatory methods of pushing are used during the second stage of labour.

- One RCT found that the "hands poised" method (not touching the baby's head or supporting the mother's perineum) versus the conventional "hands on" method (applying pressure to the baby's head during delivery and supporting the mother's perineum) increased short term perineal pain. However, it found no evidence of an effect on the risk of perineal trauma or third/fourth degree tears.

Methods and materials for primary repair

- Two systematic reviews of RCTs have found that use of absorbable synthetic suture materials with a continuous subcuticular stitch to appose the skin reduces short term pain compared with catgut sutures. The effects on long term pain and other complications remain uncertain.

- One large RCT found no evidence that leaving the perineal skin unsutured altered short term pain compared with conventional care that included skin sutures, but dyspareunia was reduced at 3 months postpartum.

- We found no good evidence on the best method or material for repairing third and fourth degree tears and major vaginal lacerations.

DEFINITION   Perineal trauma is any damage to the genitalia during childbirth that occurs spontaneously or intentionally by surgical incision (episiotomy). Anterior perineal trauma is injury to the labia, anterior vagina, urethra, or clitoris, and is usually associated with little morbidity. Posterior perineal trauma is any injury to the posterior vaginal wall, perineal muscles, or anal sphincter. Depending on severity, posterior perineal trauma is associated with increased morbidity. First degree spontaneous tears involve only skin; second degree involve perineal muscles; third degree partially or completely disrupt the anal sphincter; and fourth degree tears completely disrupt the external and internal anal sphincter and epithelium.[1]

INCIDENCE/   Over 85% of women having a vaginal birth sustain some form of
PREVALENCE   perineal trauma,[2] and 60–70% receive stitches — equivalent to 400 000 women per year in the UK in 1997.[2,3] There are wide variations in rates of episiotomy: 8% in the Netherlands, 26–67% in the UK, 50% in the USA, and 99% in east European countries.[4–8] Sutured spontaneous tears are reported in about a third of women in the USA[4] and the UK,[6] but this is probably an underestimate because of inconsistency of reporting and classification of perineal trauma. The incidence of anal sphincter tears varies between 0.5% in the UK, 2.5% in Denmark, and 7% in Canada.[9]

AETIOLOGY/   Perineal trauma occurs during spontaneous or assisted vaginal
RISK FACTORS delivery and is usually more extensive after the first vaginal delivery.[1] Associated risk factors include parity, size of baby, mode of delivery, malpresentation, and malposition of the fetus. Other maternal factors that may contribute to the extent and degree of trauma are ethnicity, age, tissue type, and nutritional state.[10] Clinicians' practices or preferences in terms of intrapartum interventions may influence the severity and rate of perineal trauma.

PROGNOSIS   Perineal trauma affects womens' physical, psychological, and social wellbeing in the immediate postnatal period as well as the long term. It can also disrupt breast feeding, family life, and sexual relations. In the UK, about 23–42% of women will continue to have pain and discomfort for 10–12 days postpartum, and 7–10% of women will continue to have long term pain (3–18 months after delivery);[2,3,11] 23% of women will experience superficial dyspareunia at 3 months; 3–10% will report faecal incontinence,[12,13] and up to 24% will have urinary problems.[2,3] Complications depend on severity of perineal trauma and on effectiveness of treatment.

AIMS   To reduce the rate and severity of trauma; to improve the short and long term maternal morbidity associated with perineal injury and repair.

OUTCOMES   Quality of life, incidence and severity of perineal trauma, psychological trauma, short and long term perineal pain, blood loss, infection, wound dehiscence, superficial dyspareunia, stress incontinence, faecal incontinence, adverse effects of treatment.

METHODS   *Clinical Evidence* update search and appraisal October 2000, supplemented by a detailed hand search of relevant journals.

QUESTION   What effects do intrapartum surgical interventions have on the risk of perineal trauma?

OPTION   RESTRICTIVE VERSUS ROUTINE USE OF EPISIOTOMY

One systematic review of RCTs has found that restricting the use of episiotomy to specific fetal and maternal indications reduces rates of posterior perineal trauma, need for suturing, and healing complications. Rates of anterior vaginal and labial trauma are slightly increased.

Benefits: We found one systematic review (search date not stated, 6 RCTs, 4850 women) comparing restricted versus routine episiotomy.[14] In the routine episiotomy group, 1752 of 2409 women (73%) had an episiotomy compared with 673 of 2441 women (28%) in the restricted group. Restricted use of episiotomy was associated with lower risk of posterior perineal trauma (AR 72% for restricted v 82% for routine; ARR 10%, 95% CI 6% to 14%; RRR 12%, 95% CI 7% to 18%; NNT 10, 95% CI 7 to 17); less perineal pain at discharge from hospital (AR 31% for restricted v 42% for routine; ARR 12%, 95% CI 8% to 15%; RRR 27%, 95% CI 19% to 36%; NNT 9, 95% CI 7 to 12); less suturing (AR 64% v 86%; ARR 22%, 95% CI 19% to 26%; RRR 26%, 95% CI 22% to 30%; NNT 4, 95% CI 4 to 5); and fewer healing complications (AR 21% v 30%; ARR 9%, 95% CI 4% to 13%; RRR 31%, 95% CI 15% to 45%; NNT 11, 95% CI 7 to 23). There were no significant differences in the two groups in overall rates of severe vaginal or perineal trauma (AR 4% v 4%; ARI 0%, 95% CI −1% to +2%; RRI 11%, 95% CI % −11% to +50%); dyspareunia (AR 52% v 51%; ARI 1%, 95% CI −6% to +7%; RRI 2%, 95% CI −11% to +15%); and urinary incontinence (AR 18% v 19%; ARR 1%, 95% CI −4% to +4%; RRR 2%, 95% CI −20% to +21%).

Harms: We found no reports of serious harms associated with restricted use of episiotomy apart from higher rates of anterior perineal trauma, which carries minimal morbidity (AR 20% for restricted v 11% for routine; ARI 9%, 95% CI 6% to 12%; RRI 79%, 95% CI 56% to 105%; NNH 11, 95% CI 9 to 16).[14]

Comment: The six RCTs included in the review varied in quality. The method of randomisation was not clear in one trial. All trials performed intention to treat analysis. The trials took place in the UK, Canada, and Argentina. The types of episiotomy performed were mediolateral in five of the trials and midline in the sixth.

OPTION   TYPE OF EPISIOTOMY INCISION

We found no evidence that midline episiotomy incision improves outcome compared with mediolateral incision. Limited evidence suggests that midline incision may increase the risk of third and fourth degree tears.

Benefits: We found no systematic review comparing mediolateral versus midline episiotomy incisions. However, stratified analysis of data from the systematic review of routine versus restricted episiotomy[14] found no difference in the overall results between midline and mediolateral episiotomies. We found two published RCTs comparing midline versus mediolateral episiotomies. These were of poor quality and found no evidence of a difference in perineal pain or wound dehiscence.[15,16] Women who had a midline episiotomy experienced significantly less perineal bruising and resumed intercourse earlier.

Harms: One of the RCTs found that midline episiotomies increased the risk of third or fourth degree tears (RRI 126%, 95% CI 64% to 330%).[15] Two retrospective cohort studies, including 5376 primiparous and 341 multiparous women, also found that midline episiotomies were associated with a fourfold increased risk of third and fourth degree tears after allowing for multiple confounders (CI not available).[17,18]

Comment: It has been claimed that midline incision causes less blood loss, easier repair, better healing, less pain, and earlier resumption of sexual intercourse, but at an increased risk of anal sphincter trauma. We found no good evidence to support these claims. One of the trials had an increased risk of selection bias owing to a quasi random method of treatment allocation and because analysis was not by intention to treat.[15] The other trial did not describe the method of treatment allocation.[16]

OPTION   EPIDURAL ANAESTHESIA

One systematic review of RCTs found no direct evidence about the effect of epidural anaesthesia on rates of perineal trauma. However, epidural anaesthesia is associated with an increased risk of instrumental delivery, which in turn is associated with an increased risk of perineal trauma.

Benefits: We found one systematic review (search date not stated, 11 RCTs comparing epidural anaesthesia versus other forms of analgesia, 3157 women).[19] The RCTs did not report the incidence of perineal trauma. Six trials (1252 women) provided data on rates of instrumental delivery when the epidural block was maintained beyond the first stage of labour. The women who had epidurals had increased risk of instrumental delivery (AR 27% for epidural v 16% for no epidural; ARI 10%, 95% CI 5% to 16%; RRI 64%, 95% CI 33% to 99%; NNH 10, 95% CI 6 to 19).

Harms: Analysis of observational evidence found that epidural block was associated with an increased incidence of chronic backache, chronic headache, bladder problems, tingling and numbness, and "sensory confusion".[20]

Comment: The quality of the trials was variable.

OPTION   VACUUM EXTRACTOR VERSUS FORCEPS

One systematic review of RCTs has found that the use of a vacuum extractor versus forceps delivery reduces the rate of perineal trauma, but increases the incidence of neonatal cephalhaematoma and retinal haemorrhage. One additional case of severe perineal trauma was prevented for every nine occasions that vacuum extraction was used instead of forceps.

Benefits: We found one systematic review (search date 1999, 10 RCTs comparing vacuum extraction v forceps, 2885 women).[21] Women allocated to vacuum extraction sustained significantly less perineal trauma (AR 9.8% for vacuum extraction v 20.3% for forceps; ARR 11%, 95% CI 8% to 12%; RRR 52%, 95% CI 41% to 61%; NNT to prevent one case of severe perineal trauma 10, 95% CI 8 to 12), and suffered less short term pain (AR 9% for vacuum extraction, 15% for forceps; ARR 6%, 95% CI 0.8% to 10%; RRR 43%, 95% CI 6% to 67%; NNT 16, 95% CI 10 to 119).

Harms: The systematic review found that babies delivered by vacuum extraction were at higher risk of cephalhaematoma (AR 10% v 4%; ARI 6%, 95% CI 3% to 10%; RRI 139%, 95% CI 69% to 234%; NNH 17, 95% CI 10 to 35) and retinal haemorrhage (AR 49% v 33%; ARI 15%, 95% CI 6% to 25%; RRI 45%, 95% CI 17% to 74%; NNH 7, 95% CI 4 to 17).[21]

Comment: The trials in the review varied in quality, some using quasi random methods of treatment allocation. None of the trials attempted to "blind" the allocated intervention during the postnatal assessments. The trials took place in different countries (UK, USA, South Africa, Denmark, Sweden, and Greece), and the procedures in the studies were comparable to everyday practice when an assisted delivery is required. Although some studies were performed in teaching hospitals, they were pragmatic, with wide inclusion criteria. The evidence is likely to be generaliseable.[21]

QUESTION **What effect do intrapartum non-surgical interventions have on the risk of perineal trauma?**

OPTION CONTINUOUS SUPPORT DURING LABOUR

One systematic review of RCTs has found that providing continuous support for women during childbirth versus usual care reduces the rate of instrumental delivery. Two small RCTs found no significant difference in the risk of perineal trauma but could not rule out a clinically important difference.

Benefits: We found one systematic review (search date 2000, 14 RCTs, ≥ 5000 women) comparing usual care versus continuous support from a professional nurse, midwife, or lay person.[22] Women given continuous support versus usual care were less likely to have instrumental delivery (AR 14% v 17%; ARR 2%, 95% CI 0.4% to 4%; RRR 14%, 95% CI 3% to 25%; NNT 41, 95% CI 24 to 239), or episiotomy (1 RCT; AR 42% v 62%; ARR 21%, 95% CI 5% to 36%; RRR 34%, 95% CI 8% to 57%; NNT 5, 95% CI 3 to 21), but there was no overall reduction in the risk of perineal trauma (2 RCTs; AR 224/281 [80%] for continuous care v 233/277 [84%] for usual care; ARR 4%, 95% CI −2% to +12%; RRR 5%, 95% CI −2% to +15%).

Harms: We found no evidence of harmful effects. The trials in the review examined a wide range of outcomes, but none revealed harmful effects.[22]

Comment: The trials were of reasonable quality, with 11 using sequentially numbered sealed opaque envelopes for treatment allocation. Only one trial "blinded" the participants to the experimental intervention before randomisation and maintained this throughout the study. Although the experimental intervention was always described as

Pregnancy and childbirth

one to one support, the timing and duration varied between trials. The pragmatic trials took place in a wide variety of settings (Europe, Scandinavia, South Africa, and the USA) and found similar results, which suggests that the results are generaliseable.[22]

OPTION **POSITION DURING DELIVERY**

One systematic review comparing upright versus recumbent positions during delivery found no significant difference in overall rates of perineal trauma, but an increase in labial trauma. One subsequent RCT found a reduction in episiotomies in the upright group, but this was offset by an increase in second degree tears.

Benefits:
We found one systematic review (search date not stated, 16 RCTs) comparing upright position for delivery (birthing chairs, cushions, and squatting) versus conventional recumbent position,[23] and one subsequent South African RCT.[24,25] Only eight of the trials from the review and the subsequent RCT (total 3627 women) provided data regarding perineal trauma. Analysis of the combined data[23,24] found no significant difference between groups in the number of women with perineal trauma requiring suturing (AR 61% for upright v 64% for recumbent; ARR 3%, 95% CI −0.2% to +6%; RRR 5%, 95% CI −0.3% to +95%). There were only eight third degree tears, and there was no significant difference in rate between groups (AR 0.2% for upright v 1.5% for recumbent; ARR 1.3%, 95% CI −0.2% to +1.5%; RRR 86%, 95% CI −15% to +98%). The subsequent RCT found that delivery in an upright (squatting) position versus a recumbent position significantly reduced the episiotomy rate (AR 17% v 25%; ARR 8%, 95% CI 1% to 14%; RRR 33%, 95% CI 6% to 54%; NNT 12, 95% CI 7 to 73), but significantly increased second degree tears (AR 8.9% v 3.4%; ARR 5.5%; OR 2.74, 95% CI 1.24 to 6.05).[24,25]

Harms:
Women in the upright group suffered more labial tears, which are thought to be associated with minimal long term morbidity (AR 37% v 28%; ARI 9%, 95% CI 2% to 17%; RRI 33%, 95% CI 7% to 61%; NNH 11, 95% CI 6 to 52).[23] The combined data suggest an increased risk in rate of postpartum haemorrhage (blood loss estimated as ≥ 500 ml) with upright delivery, mainly in women delivering on the birthing chair (RRI 78%, 95% CI 35% to 136%). However, this was not supported by the more objective measurement of haemoglobin (RRI for haemoglobin < 11 g/dl 7%, 95% CI −13% to +31%) or the small number of women requiring blood transfusions (RRI 93%, 95% CI −17% to +349%).

Comment:
We found a more recent version of the systematic review,[26] but it was not used to update this section because it used a different format to determine outcomes, and does not alter the data presented. The RCTs included in the earlier systematic review varied in quality.[23] It is difficult to interpret the results of some of the RCTs because of non-compliance and diversity of the treatment interventions (squatting, kneeling, Gardosi cushion, birthing chair). The South African RCT was of high quality, including full compliance with the allocated intervention.[24] The original publication[24] contained incorrect data regarding the total number of episiotomies in each intervention group; the corrected data have been published and are included here.[25]

OPTION   ALTERNATIVE METHODS OF BEARING DOWN (PUSHING)

A systematic review comparing sustained breath holding (Valsalva) with spontaneous exhalatory methods of pushing during the second stage of labour found no significant difference in the extent or rate of perineal trauma.

Benefits: We found one systematic review (search date 1993, 5 trials, 471 women) comparing bearing down by sustained breath holding (Valsalva) versus exhalatory or spontaneous pushing.[27] Only two of the trials provided data on perineal trauma requiring suturing, and they found no significant difference between the two interventions (AR 33% for Valsalva method v 40% for exhalatory method; ARR 7%, 95% CI −4% to +16%; RRR 16%, 95% CI −10% to +40%).

Harms: It is unclear whether the rate of adverse perineal outcomes is affected by different types of bearing down during the second stage of labour.

Comment: The review included published and unpublished trials. Three of the trials were small and of very poor quality. Two of these trials found reduced rates of perineal trauma in the spontaneous bearing down group but this was not supported by data from the two subsequent, more robust controlled trials.[27]

OPTION   "HANDS POISED" VERSUS "HANDS ON"

One RCT found that the "hands poised" method (not touching the baby's head or supporting the mother's perineum) versus the conventional "hands on" method (applying pressure to the baby's head during delivery and supporting the mother's perineum) increased short term perineal pain. It found no evidence of an effect on the risk of perineal trauma or third/fourth degree tears.

Benefits: We found no systematic review. We found one multicentre RCT (5471 women), which compared the "hands poised" to the "hands on" method of delivery.[2] There was no significant difference between groups in the risk of perineal trauma requiring suture (AR 60% for "hands poised" v 59% for "hands on"; ARI 1%, 95% CI −1.7% to +3.5%; RRI 1.6%, 95% CI −3% to +6%) or third/fourth degree tears (AR 1% in each group; ARI 0.3%, 95% CI −0.2% to +1.2%; RRI 28%, 95% CI −19% to +104%). In the "hands poised" group, the episiotomy rate was significantly reduced (AR 10% v 13%; ARR 3%, 95% CI 1% to 4%; RRR 20%, 95% CI 8% to 32%; NNT 38, 95% CI 25% to 100%), and perineal pain at day 10 was increased (AR 34% v 31%; ARI 3%, 95% CI 0.5% to 6%; RRI 10%, 95% CI 1.5% to 18%; NNH 33, 95% CI 18 to 212).

Harms: There was a significant increase in manual removal of placenta in the "hands poised" group (AR 2.6% v 1.5%; ARI 1.1%, 95% CI 0.2% to 2.2%; RRI 69%, 95% CI 16% to 145%; NNH 95, 95% CI 45 to 417).[2]

Comment: This was the only identified trial comparing "hands poised" with "hands on". It was a large, robust multicentred pragmatic trial, and the results are likely to be generaliseable.

Pregnancy and childbirth

OPTION   IN FIRST AND SECOND DEGREE TEARS AND EPISIOTOMIES

Two systematic reviews have found that use of absorbable synthetic suture materials with a continuous subcuticular stitch to appose the skin reduces short term pain compared with catgut sutures. The effects on long term pain and other complications remain uncertain. One large RCT found no evidence that leaving the perineal skin unsutured altered short term pain compared with conventional care that included skin sutures, but dyspareunia was reduced at 3 months postpartum.

Benefits: We found two systematic reviews (search dates 1999, 12 RCTs conducted in Europe and the USA, 5506 primiparous and multiparous women). They compared absorbable synthetic versus catgut suture material for repair of episiotomies and second degree tears,[28] and continuous subcuticular versus interrupted sutures to appose the perineal skin.[29] **Absorbable synthetic versus catgut sutures:** Absorbable synthetic material was associated with less analgesia use within 7 days (AR 38% v 49% with catgut; ARR 11%, 95% CI 5% to 17%; RRR 22%, 95% CI 10% to 34%; NNT 9, 95% CI 6 to 20) and less suture dehiscence, resuturing, and short term pain. There was no clear difference in long term pain with different materials (2 RCTs; AR perineal pain at 3 months 92/1061 [8.7%] with absorbable synthetic sutures, 112/1068 [10.5%] with catgut). **Continuous subcutaneous versus interrupted transcutaneous suture:** Short term pain was also reduced when a continuous subcutaneous suture was used compared with the interrupted, transcutaneous method of repairing perineal skin (AR 20% with continuous, 27% with interrupted; ARR 7%, 95% CI 3% to 11%; RRR 26%, 95% CI 11% to 39%; NNT 14, 95% CI 10 to 34), but there was no clear difference in long term pain (1 RCT; AR of pain at 3 months 58/465 [12.5%] with continuous, 51/451 [11.3%] with interrupted; ARI 1.2%, 95% CI −3% to +6%; RRI 10%, 95% CI −23% to +55%). Sutures were removed less frequently (up to 3 months postpartum) in the continuous subcuticular group compared with the interrupted group (AR 26% v 37%; ARR 11%, 95% CI 5% to 16%; RRR 29%, 95% CI 14% to 43%; NNT 9, 95% CI 6 to 20), probably as a result of them being less accessible. **Non-suturing of perineal skin:** We found no systematic review. We found one RCT carried out in a single centre in the UK in 1780 primiparous and multiparous women who sustained perineal trauma (first and second degree tears or episiotomies) after spontaneous or assisted vaginal delivery.[30] It compared a two stage method of repair (the vagina and perineal muscle was sutured, leaving the perineal skin unsutured but apposed) versus a conventional three stage method (the vagina, perineal muscle, and skin were sutured). It found no significant difference between the two and three stage groups in terms of pain at 10 days post partum (AR 25% v 28%; RR 0.90, 95% CI 0.77 to 1.06), but at 3 months fewer women reported dyspareunia in the two stage group (AR 15% v 19%; RR 0.80, 95% CI 0.65 to 0.99; NNT to avoid one additional woman developing dyspareunia 25). **Non-suturing of perineal muscle:** We found one small RCT (78 primiparous women in Sweden) comparing non-suturing to suturing of first and second degree tears. Outcomes were assessed after 2 to 3 days and 8 weeks.[31] It found that the type of pain was different between the two groups (burning sensation 9/40 v 1/38; soreness 3/40 v 1/38), but there was no significant difference in healing.[31]

Harms: Up to 3 months postpartum, suture removal was more common in the absorbable synthetic group than in the catgut group (AR 191/1061 [18%] v 108/1068 [10%] for catgut; RRI 78%, 95% CI 43% to 122%).[28] We found no reliable evidence that qualifies the harms of leaving perineal muscle unsutured.

Comment: The trials varied in quality and in operator skills and training. It was not possible to "blind" outcome assessment because of the obvious differences in method and materials used. Most of the trials used "intention to treat" as the method of analysis. One RCT (1542 women), comparing an interrupted method of perineal repair versus a loose continuous technique using two types of absorbable synthetic suture materials, is in progress (C Kettle, personal communication, 2001). Another RCT (pilot study) comparing two different methods for repair of third and fourth degree anal sphincter tears following childbirth is also in progress (R Fernando, personal communication, 2001). The RCT comparing "non-suturing of perineal skin to suturing of perineal skin" was a pragmatic study, and the results are likely to be generaliseable.[30] An RCT is in progress evaluating short term outcomes of non-suturing and suturing in 300 women (V Fleming, personal communication, 2000). We found no reliable evidence to support a policy of leaving minor perineal trauma unsutured (first or second degree tears). The findings of the small RCT on non-suturing of perineal muscle are difficult to interpret: published data are inconsistent with reported conclusions.[31]

OPTION **IN THIRD AND FOURTH DEGREE TEARS**

We found no good evidence on the effects of different methods and materials for repair of third and fourth degree tears.

Benefits: We found no systematic review or RCTs.

Harms: Insufficient data.

Comment: None.

Substantive changes since last issue

Upright versus recumbent position during delivery Recategorised following reappraisal of the evidence.

REFERENCES

1. Sultan AH, Kamm MA, Bartram CI, Hudson CN. Perineal damage at delivery. *Contemp Rev Obstet Gynaecol* 1994;6:18–24.
2. McCandlish R, Bowler U, van Asten H, et al. A randomised controlled trial of care of the perineum during second stage of normal labour. *Br J Obstet Gynaecol* 1998;105:1262–1272.
3. Sleep J, Grant A, Garcia J, et al. West Berkshire perineal management trial. *BMJ* 1984;298:587–690.
4. Graves EJ. 1993 summary: National hospital discharge survey. *Advance Data* 1995;264:1–11.
5. Graham ID, Graham DF. Episiotomy counts: trends and prevalence in Canada, 1981/1982 to 1993/1994. *Birth* 1997;24:141–147.
6. Audit Commission. First class delivery: improving maternity services in England and Wales. London: Audit Commission Publications, 1997.
7. Wagner M. *Pursuing the birth machine: the search for appropriate technology.* Camperdown: ACE Graphics, 1994;165–174.
8. Williams FL, Florey C du V, Mires GJ, Ogston SA. Episiotomy and perineal tears in low-risk UK primigravidae. *J Pub Health Med* 1998;20;422–427.
9. Sultan AH, Monga AK, Kumar D, et al. Primary repair of anal sphincter using the overlap technique. *Br J Obstet Gynaecol* 1999;106:318–323.
10. Renfrew MJ, Hannah W, Albers L, et al. Practices that minimize trauma to the genital tract in childbirth: a systematic review of the literature. *Birth* 1998;25:143–160. Search date May 1997; primary sources Cochrane Database of Systematic Reviews, Medline, Cinahl, Miriad, Midirs, Index Medicus, plus hand searches of current textbooks of obstetrics, midwifery, and nursing.
11. Glazener CMA, Abdalla M, Stroud P, et al. Postnatal maternal morbidity: extent, causes, prevention and treatment. *Br J Obstet Gynaecol* 1995;102:286–287.
12. Sleep J, Grant A. Pelvic floor exercises in postnatal care. *Br J Midwifery* 1987;3:158–164.
13. Sultan AH, Kamm MA, Hudson CN. Anal sphincter disruption during vaginal delivery. *N Engl J Med* 1993;329:1905–1911.
14. Carroli G, Belizan J, Stamp G. Episiotomy for vaginal births. In: The Cochrane Library, Issue 4, 2000. Oxford: Update Software. Search date not stated; primary sources Cochrane Pregnancy and Childbirth Group Trials Register.
15. Coats PM, Chan KK, Wilkins M, et al. A comparison between midline and mediolateral episiotomies. *Br J Obstet Gynaecol* 1989;87:408–412.
16. Werner CH, Schuler W, Meskendahl I. Midline episiotomy versus mediolateral episiotomy: a randomised prospective study. *Int J Gynaecol Obstet.* Proceedings of 13th World Congress of Gynaecology and Obstetrics (FIGO), Singapore 1991; Book 1:33.
17. Shiono P, Klebanof MD, Carey JC. Midline episiotomies: more harm than good? *Obstet Gynecol* 1990;75:756–770.
18. Klein MC, Gauthier MD, Robbins JM, et al. Relationship of episiotomy to perineal trauma and morbidity, sexual function, and pelvic floor relaxation. *Am J Obstet Gynecol* 1994;17:591–598.
19. Howell CJ. Epidural versus non-epidural analgesia for pain relief in labour. In: The Cochrane Library, Issue 4, 2000. Oxford: Update Software. Search date not stated; primary source Cochrane Pregnancy and Childbirth Group Trials Register.
20. Howell CJ, Chalmers I. A review of prospectively controlled comparisons of epidural with non-epidural forms of pain relief during labour. *Int J Obstet Anaesth* 1992;1:93–110.
21. Johanson RB, Menon VJ. Vacuum extraction versus forceps delivery for assisted vaginal delivery. In: The Cochrane Library, Issue 4, 2000. Oxford: Update Software. Search date February 1999; primary source Cochrane Pregnancy and Childbirth Group Trials Register.
22. Hodnett ED. Caregiver support for women during childbirth. In: The Cochrane Library, Issue 4, 2000. Oxford: Update software. Search date April 2000; primary sources Cochrane Pregnancy and Childbirth Group Trials Register; Cochrane Controlled Trials Register.
23. Nikodem VC. Upright vs recumbent position during the second stage of labour. In: Enkin MW, Keirse MJNC, Renfrew MJ, et al, eds. *Pregnancy and childbirth module. Cochrane database of systematic reviews.* Cochrane updates on disk, Issue 2, 1994. Oxford: Update Software. Search date and primary sources not stated.
24. De Jong PR, Johanson RB, Baxen P, et al. Randomised trial comparing the upright and supine positions for the second stage of labour. *Br J Obstet Gynaecol* 1997;104:567–571.
25. Eason E, de Jong P. Randomised trial comparing the upright and supine positions for the second stage of labour. *Br J Obstet Gynaecol* 1999;106:291–292.
26. Gupta JK, Nikodem VC. Woman's position during the second stage of labour. In: The Cochrane Library, Issue 4, 2000. Oxford: Update Software. Search date March 1999; primary sources Cochrane Pregnancy and Childbirth Group Trials Register; Cochrane Controlled Trials Register.
27. Nikodem VC. Sustained (Valsalva) vs exhalatory bearing down in 2nd stage of labour. In: Enkin MW, Keirse MJNC, Renfrew MJ, et al, eds. *Pregnancy and childbirth module.* In: The Cochrane Library, Issue 2, 1994. Oxford: Update Software. Search date October 1993; primary sources Cochrane Pregnancy and Childbirth Database, Medline, plus handsearch of specialist journals, conference proceedings.
28. Kettle C, Johanson RB. Absorbable synthetic vs catgut suture material for perineal repair. In: The Cochrane Library, Issue 4, 2000. Oxford: Update Software. Search date 1999; primary source Cochrane Pregnancy and Childbirth Group Trials Register.
29. Kettle C, Johanson RB. Continuous versus interrupted sutures for perineal repair. In: Cochrane Library, Issue 4, 2000. Oxford: Update Software. Search date 1999; primary source Cochrane Pregnancy and Childbirth Group Specialised Register of Controlled Trials.
30. Gordon B, Mackrodt C, Fern E, et al. The Ipswich Childbirth Study: 1. A randomised evaluation of two stage postpartum perineal repair leaving the skin unsutured. *Br J Obstet Gynaecol* 1998;105:435–440.
31. Lundquist M, Olsson A, Nissen E, Norman M. Is it necessary to suture all lacerations after a vaginal delivery? *Birth* 2000;27:79–85.

Chris Kettle
Midwifery Research Fellow, North Staffordshire Hospital (NHS Trust) and Keele University, Stoke-on-Trent, UK

Competing interests: The author has received a grant from the Iolanthe Midwifery Research Trust and support from Ethicon Ltd, which enabled her to carry out a randomised controlled trial of perineal management — The Methods or Materials Study (MOMS).

Search date November 2000: expanded this issue

Lelia Duley

INTERVENTIONS

PREVENTION

Beneficial

Unknown effectiveness

TREATMENT

Beneficial

Likely to be beneficial

Unknown effectiveness

**To be covered in future issues of
*Clinical Evidence***

Interventions in women with
pre-existing hypertension

Treatment for postpartum
hypertension

See glossary, p 993

Key Messages

- One systematic review of many RCTs has found that antiplatelet drugs (mainly aspirin) reduce the risk of pre-eclampsia by 15%. One systematic review of RCTs has found that calcium supplementation reduces the relative risk of pre-eclampsia by about a third.

- We found insufficient evidence on the effects of fish oil, or of evening primrose oil plus fish oil or calcium, or of other dietary interventions, on the risk of pre-eclampsia and preterm birth.

- It is unclear whether women with mild to moderate hypertension during pregnancy benefit from antihypertensive drugs.

- For women with severe hypertension during pregnancy, antihypertensive drugs will lower blood pressure, but we found no reliable evidence that any one agent is substantially better than another.

- We found insufficient evidence to assess the effects of hospital admission, bed rest, or day care compared with outpatient care.

- We found evidence that magnesium sulphate may reduce the risk of developing eclampsia, but other possible benefits and harms are unclear. These are being addressed by an ongoing trial.

- One large systematic review has found that magnesium sulphate is the best choice of anticonvulsant for treatment of eclampsia.

- More efficient systems need to be developed to assess severe adverse events (likely to be rare), particularly for drugs widely used during pregnancy. They should include monitoring of events for both the woman and child.

DEFINITION   Hypertension during pregnancy may be associated with one of several conditions. **Pregnancy induced hypertension** is a rise in blood pressure, without proteinuria, during the second half of pregnancy. **Pre-eclampsia** is a multisystem disorder, unique to pregnancy, which is usually associated with raised blood pressure and proteinuria. It rarely presents before 20 weeks' gestation. **Eclampsia** is one or more convulsions in association with the syndrome of pre-eclampsia. **Pre-existing hypertension** is known hypertension before pregnancy, or raised blood pressure before 20 weeks' gestation. It may be essential hypertension or, less commonly, secondary to underlying disease.[1]

INCIDENCE/   Pregnancy induced hypertension affects 10% of pregnancies, and
PREVALENCE pre-eclampsia complicates 2–8%.[2] Eclampsia occurs in about one in 2000 deliveries in developed countries.[3] In developing countries, estimates of the incidence of eclampsia vary from one in 100 to one in 1700.[4,5]

AETIOLOGY/   The cause of pre-eclampsia is unknown. It is likely to be multifac-
RISK FACTORS torial and may result from deficient placental implantation during the first half of pregnancy.[6] Pre-eclampsia is more common among women likely to have a large placenta, such as those with multiple pregnancy, and among women with medical conditions associated with microvascular disease, such as diabetes, hypertension, and collagen vascular disease.[7,8] Other risk factors include genetic susceptibility, increased parity, and older maternal age.[9] Cigarette smoking seems to be associated with a lower risk of pre-eclampsia, but this potential benefit is outweighed by an increase in adverse outcomes such as low birth weight, placental abruption, and perinatal death.[10]

PROGNOSIS The outcome of pregnancy in women with pregnancy induced hypertension alone is at least as good as that for normotensive pregnancies.[7,11] However, once pre-eclampsia develops, morbidity and mortality rise for both mother and child. For example, perinatal mortality for women with severe pre-eclampsia is double that for normotensive women.[7] Perinatal outcome is worse with early gestational hypertension.[7,9,11] Perinatal mortality also increases in women with severe essential hypertension.[12]

AIMS To delay or prevent the development of pre-eclampsia and eclampsia, and to improve outcomes for women and their children. Once pre-eclampsia has occurred, to minimise morbidity and mortality for the woman and her child, and to ensure that health service resources are used appropriately.

OUTCOMES **For the woman:** Rates of pre-eclampsia (proteinuria and hypertension), eclampsia, death, severe morbidity (such as renal failure, coagulopathy, cardiac failure, liver failure, and stroke), placental abruption, and caesarean section; use of resources (such as dialysis, ventilation, admission to intensive care, or length of stay); adverse effects of treatment. **For the child:** Rates of death, intrauterine growth restriction, prematurity, and severe morbidity (such as intraventricular haemorrhage, respiratory distress syndrome, or asphyxia); measures of infant and child development (such as cerebral palsy or significant learning disability); use of resources (such as admission to special care nursery, ventilation, length of stay in hospital, and special needs in the community); adverse effects of treatment.

METHODS *Clinical Evidence* update search and appraisal November 2000. The methods are described in greater detail in the relevant Cochrane reviews. The author also searched the register of trials held by the Cochrane Pregnancy and Childbirth Group.

QUESTION **What are the effects of preventive interventions in women at high risk of pre-eclampsia?**

OPTION **ANTIPLATELET DRUGS**

One systematic review of many large RCTs has found that antiplatelet drugs (mainly aspirin) are associated with reduced relative risk of pre-eclampsia (15%), death of the baby (14%), and prematurity (8%), with no significant difference in other important outcomes. Two large aspirin trials that followed children to age 12–18 months have found that aspirin is safe in the short to medium term.

Benefits: We found one systematic review of antiplatelet agents (search date 1999, 41 RCTs, over 32 000 women) and one subsequent RCT.[13,14] **Versus placebo/no antiplatelet drug:** The systematic review found that antiplatelet agents reduced pre-eclampsia (RR 0.85, 95% CI 0.78 to 0.92), premature delivery (before 37 completed weeks; RR 0.92, 95% CI 0.88 to 0.97), and baby deaths (RR 0.86, 95% CI 0.77 to 0.98). There were no clear effects on other important outcomes. There was no effect of starting treatment before 20 weeks, and no differences between women at high and low risk. The benefit was greatest for women given more than

75 mg aspirin daily. The subsequent small RCT compared ozagrel hydrochloride with placebo, but was too small for any reliable conclusions.[14] **Versus each other:** Trials comparing one antiplatelet agent with another were too small for reliable conclusions.[13]

Harms:
The systematic review found no evidence that aspirin increased the risk of bleeding for mother or baby.[13] Two large RCTs that followed up children to age 12–18 months found no differences between the children of mothers given aspirin or placebo.[15,16]

Comment:
Almost all studies used low dose aspirin (50–75 mg), and most were placebo controlled. The trials included women with a variety of risk factors, including a history of previous early onset disease, diabetes, or chronic hypertension, and were conducted in different countries in the developed and developing world.

OPTION	MATERNAL CALCIUM SUPPLEMENTATION

One systematic review of 10 RCTs found that calcium supplementation (≥ 1 g/day) versus placebo reduces the risk of pre-eclampsia and hypertension by 30% and the risk of having a baby with birthweight under 2500 g by 17%. There was no significant effect on the risk of caesarean delivery, preterm delivery, or death of the baby.

Benefits:
We found one systematic review of calcium supplementation (search date 2000, 10 RCTs, 7173 women).[17] **Versus placebo:** In the 10 RCTs, calcium (mainly 2 g daily) significantly reduced the risk of pre-eclampsia (196/3412 [6%] with calcium supplementation v 287/3452 [8%] with placebo; RR 0.70, 95% CI 0.58 to 0.83; NNT 40, 95% CI 28 to 77). Subgroup analysis found the strongest effect was for high risk women (8/266 [3%] with calcium supplementation v 47/291 [16%] with placebo for high risk women, compared with 188/3146 [6%] with calcium supplementation v 240/3161 [8%] with placebo for low risk women); and for women with low dietary calcium (27/907 [3%] with calcium supplementation v 90/935 [10%] with placebo for low dietary calcium compared with 169/2505 [7%] with calcium supplementation v 197/2517 [8%] with placebo for normal dietary calcium). Calcium supplementation significantly reduced the risk of having a baby with birthweight under 2500 g (RR 0.83, 95% CI 0.71 to 0.98; NNT 67, 95% CI 36 to 1000). There was little evidence of effect on the risk of caesarean delivery, preterm delivery, or death of the baby. **Calcium and evening primrose oil versus placebo:** One small trial (48 women) did not provide sufficient evidence for reliable conclusions.[18]

Harms:
No adverse events were reported in these trials.[17] One large study followed a subgroup of 518 children for 7 years and found no harms associated with long term use of calcium supplementation by their mothers.

Comment:
Most trials in the systematic review were of good quality and included a wide range of women. They were conducted largely in the USA and South America. They included mainly women at low risk with adequate dietary calcium, so the number of women in the category who would benefit most from calcium supplementation was small. Several studies reported that adherence to treatment was between

60–90%. The proportion of women taking 90–100% of all allocated treatment was low (20% in one study).

| OPTION | OTHER DIETARY INTERVENTIONS |

We found insufficient evidence on the effects of fish oil, or of evening primrose oil plus fish oil or calcium, on the risk of pre-eclampsia and preterm birth. One RCT found that fish oil was associated with increased risk of post-term delivery and postpartum haemorrhage. One systematic review of two RCTs has found that reduced salt intake (to 20–50 mmol/day) or supplementation with magnesium does not reduce the risk of pre-eclampsia or its complications. One RCT has found that supplementation with vitamins C and E reduces the risk of pre-eclampsia. One small RCT has found that supplementation with protein, fish oil and calcium, plus rest in the left lateral position, reduces the risk of pre-eclampsia compared with iron supplementation alone.

Benefits:
Fish and evening primrose oil: We found no systematic review. We found six RCTs of fish and evening primrose oil that were too small to draw reliable conclusions.[19–24] **Protein, fish oil and calcium, plus rest in left lateral position:** We found one RCT (74 women with a positive roll over test [see glossary, p 993] at 28–29 weeks).[25] It compared protein (25 mg), fish oil (300 mg), and calcium (300 mg) three times a week plus 15 minutes rest in the left lateral position twice daily versus ferrous sulphate (105 mg) three times a week. It found a reduced risk of pre-eclampsia in the multiple supplements group (2/37 [5%] with multiple supplements v 16/37 [46%] with iron alone; RR 0.12, 95% CI 0.03 to 0.51; NNT 3, 95% CI 2 to 6). It was too small for reliable conclusions on other outcomes. **Reduced salt versus normal or high salt:** We found one systematic review (2 RCTs, 600 women) comparing reduced salt with normal dietary salt.[26] Although these trials were too small for reliable conclusions, together they did not provide any substantive evidence that reducing salt intake during pregnancy affected pre-eclampsia (RR 1.11, 95% CI 0.46 to 2.66). **Magnesium:** We found one systematic review (2 RCTs, 474 women) reporting pre-eclampsia. The RCTs were too small for reliable conclusions.[27] **Vitamins C and E:** We found one RCT (283 high risk women) that found a reduced risk of pre-eclampsia with vitamin C (1000 mg/day) and vitamin E (400 IU/day) compared with placebo (11/141 [8%] with vitamins v 24/142 [17%] with placebo; RR 0.46, 95% CI 0.24 to 0.91; NNT 11, 95% CI 8 to 61).[28] The study was too small to provide reliable evidence about effects on other important outcomes.

Harms:
Fish oil: One RCT (533 women) found that fish oil compared with either olive oil or no supplement produced an insignificant increase in post-term delivery (RR 1.19, 95% CI 0.73 to 1.93) and postpartum haemorrhage (RR 1.21, 95% CI 0.76 to 1.92).[29] These outcomes were not reported in the other smaller studies. **Fish oil and evening primrose oil:** Vomiting was more commonly reported in the oil treated group, but numbers were not given.[23] No other adverse events were reported. **Evening primrose oil:** These studies were too small for reliable conclusions. **Reduced salt:** We found no evidence of harmful effects in the trials.[26] **Magnesium:** There was no significant difference between the groups in the number of reported adverse effects (RR 0.84, 95% CI 0.65 to 1.08).[27]

Pre-eclampsia and hypertension

Vitamins C and E: We found little evidence about the safety of these vitamins at the high doses used in the RCT.[28]

Comment: The fish oil trials may have been difficult to blind, because of the distinctive taste of fish oil. One study found that olive oil provided better masking than a no oil placebo.[29] The trials of salt restriction were conducted in the Netherlands, where advice to restrict salt intake during pregnancy has been routine for many years. Such advice is no longer widespread elsewhere. An updated systematic review of fish oil for prevention of pre-eclampsia will be available soon.

| OPTION | OTHER PHARMACOLOGICAL INTERVENTIONS | New |

We found two small RCTs. One compared atenolol versus placebo, the other compared glyceryl trinitrate patches versus placebo. Both were too small for any reliable conclusions.

Benefits: **Atenolol versus placebo:** We found one small RCT (68 women), which found no significant reduction in the risk of pre-eclampsia with atenolol (100 mg daily) (1/28 [4%] with atenolol v 5/28 [18%] with placebo; RR 0.20, 95% CI 0.02 to 1.60).[30] **Glyceryl trinitrate versus placebo:** One small RCT (40 women) found no significant difference between glyceryl trinitrate patches versus placebo (RR 1.13, 95% CI 0.35 to 3.60), but the confidence interval was wide.[31]

Harms: The RCT (68 women) of atenolol versus placebo found that mean birthweight was significantly lower with atenolol for a subgroup of primiparous women (mean difference 440 g, $P = 0.02$).[30]

Comment: Although the possible benefits of atenolol for prevention of pre-eclampsia remain unclear, the reduction in birthweight may be real. Concerns about the possible harmful effects of atenolol on fetal growth and development have been discussed for some time (see harms of antihypertensive agents, p 990).[32,33]

| QUESTION | What are the effects of interventions in women who develop hypertension during pregnancy? |

| OPTION | BED REST/HOSPITAL ADMISSION VERSUS DAY CARE |

We found inadequate evidence about hospital admission, bed rest, or day care versus outpatient care or normal activities in hospital.

Benefits: **Bed rest/hospital admission:** We found two systematic reviews of hospital admission.[34,35] The first compared hospital admission with outpatient clinic assessment for non-proteinuric hypertension (search date 1993, 3 trials, 408 women), and found no significant difference for any major outcome.[34] The second review (search date 1993, 2 RCTs, 145 women with proteinuric hypertension) compared bed rest in hospital versus normal ambulation in hospital, but the trials were too small for any reliable conclusions.[35] **Day care versus outpatient clinic assessment:** We found one RCT (54 women), but it was too small for reliable conclusions.[36]

Harms: It has been suggested that hospital admission increases the risk of venous stasis, thromboembolic disease, or infection, but we found no evidence in this context. In the trial of day care units, women preferred not to be admitted to hospital. We found no evidence from the other trials about the views of women and their families.

Comment: Trials of hospital admission and bed rest in hospital were conducted before widespread introduction of day care assessment units. Women with hypertension during pregnancy are now often seen in day care units, but only one small trial has compared day care assessment with assessment in an outpatient clinic.

OPTION ANTIHYPERTENSIVE AGENTS

Two systematic reviews have found evidence from many small RCTs that antihypertensive agents may reduce the chance of developing severe hypertension by more than half. The effects of antihypertensive agents on pre-eclampsia and on perinatal death are unclear. We found insufficient evidence for reliable conclusions about any other important outcomes, and few trials reported on hospital admission and use of health service resources.

Benefits: We found two systematic reviews and one subsequent RCT. The first systematic review (search date 1994, 23 small RCTs, > 2600 women).[37] The second systematic review (search date 1997, 8 RCTs, 991 women) included only studies that compared β blockers with no antihypertensive drug.[38] The small subsequent RCT (33 women) comparing alternative antihypertensive drugs found no significant differences in the risk of pre-eclampsia.[39] **Versus placebo or no antihypertensive:** The only effect was a reduced risk of developing severe hypertension (RR 0.40, 95% CI 0.27 to 0.58), which was not reflected in other, more substantive outcomes (pre-eclampsia: RR 0.81, 95% CI 0.58 to 1.14; perinatal death: RR 0.59, 95% CI 0.31 to 1.10).[37] **Versus other antihypertensive agents:** The trials comparing one drug with another were too small for reliable conclusions.

Harms: Antihypertensive drugs seem to be well tolerated during pregnancy, but adverse effects have not been reported in many RCTs. All antihypertensive drugs cross the placenta, but few trials reported possible adverse effects for the baby. The baby's risk of being small for its gestational age was increased if a β blocker was used to control the mother's hypertension (RR 1.34, 95% CI 1.01 to 1.79, 13 RCTs, 1382 women).[40] Meta regression within a systematic review suggested that lowering blood pressure for women with mild or moderate hypertension may increase the risk of having a baby that is small for its gestational age.[41]

Comment: The RCTs were too small to exclude beneficial effects of antihypertensive agents. The trials had problems with their methods. Many were not placebo controlled, and few attempted to blind blood pressure measurement. Many important outcomes were reported by only a few studies. We found little evidence about adherence to treatment. One systematic review (6 RCTs in women with pre-existing chronic hypertension) found that the effects of antihypertensive agents were similar to those for women with pregnancy induced hypertension.[37] An updated systematic review of antihypertensive drugs for mild to moderate hypertension will be available soon.[42]

Pre-eclampsia and hypertension

QUESTION	What are the effects of interventions in women who develop severe pre-eclampsia or very high blood pressure during pregnancy?

OPTION	ANTIHYPERTENSIVE DRUGS FOR VERY HIGH BLOOD PRESSURE

One systematic review found no evidence of a difference in the control of blood pressure by various antihypertensive drugs, with the possible exceptions of diazoxide and ketanserin, which seem less effective. Studies were too small for any further conclusions about relative effects of different agents.

Benefits: We found one systematic review (search date 1998, 14 trials, 1200 women), which compared many agents (including hydralazine, labetalol, nifedipine, diazoxide, and ketanserin) mainly with hydralazine.[43] All reduced blood pressure, but there was no significant evidence that any one was better than another.

Harms: The use of ketanserin is associated with more persistent high blood pressure than hydralazine (RR 8.44, 95% CI 2.05 to 34.7), and labetalol is associated with less hypotension requiring treatment than diazoxide (RR 0.06, 95% CI 0.00 to 0.99).[43] Hypotension may compromise fetoplacental blood flow. Only four RCTs reported adverse effects, and frequency varied from 5–50%. Antihypertensives cross the placenta, but we found little evidence about effects on the baby.

Comment: Women in these studies had blood pressures high enough to merit immediate treatment, and many also had proteinuria or "severe pre-eclampsia". The trials were small and reported few outcomes other than control of blood pressure. In most trials there was no blinding after trial entry.

OPTION	PLASMA VOLUME EXPANSION

One systematic review of three small RCTs of plasma volume expansion versus no expansion found insufficient evidence for reliable conclusions, although the results suggest that benefit is unlikely.

Benefits: We found one systematic review (search date 1999, 3 RCTs, 61 women) evaluating colloid solutions compared with placebo or no infusion. The RCTs were too small for reliable conclusions but suggest that plasma volume expansion is not beneficial.[44]

Harms: RCTs found a non-significant increase in the risk of caesarean section (RR 1.46, 95% CI 0.75 to 2.85), and a non-significant increase in the need for additional treatment (RR 1.51, 95% CI 0.73 to 3.11) with the use of plasma volume expansion compared with placebo or no infusion.

Comment: These three RCTs all used a colloid rather than crystalloid solution. Systematic reviews of plasma volume expansion in critically ill men and non-pregnant women have found an increased mortality with albumin (a colloid) when compared with either no expansion or crystalloid.[45,46]

OPTION	ANTIOXIDANTS

We found insufficient evidence on the effects of antioxidants.

Benefits: We found no systematic review but one RCT (56 women) evaluating combined vitamin E, vitamin C, and allopurinol versus placebo.[47] It was too small for reliable conclusions to be drawn.

Harms: We found insufficient evidence for reliable conclusions.

Comment: Women in this study had severe pre-eclampsia at 24–32 weeks' gestation.

OPTION	PROPHYLACTIC ANTICONVULSANTS FOR WOMEN WITH SEVERE PRE-ECLAMPSIA

One systematic review of 10 RCTs has found that prophylactic anticonvulsants may reduce the risk of eclampsia, but it provides little evidence about effects on other important outcomes. Limited evidence from case control studies suggests that *in utero* exposure to magnesium sulphate may reduce the risk of cerebral palsy, but it is possible that such exposure may increase infant mortality.

Benefits: We found one systematic review (search date 2000, 10 RCTs, 3747 women).[48] **Magnesium sulphate versus placebo or no anticonvulsant:** Four RCTs (1249 women) found reduction in the risk of eclampsia that did not quite reach significance (RR 0.33, 95% CI 0.11 to 1.02). There were no clear effects on other reported outcomes. Limited evidence from case control studies suggests that magnesium sulphate may reduce the risk of cerebral palsy for babies weighing less than 1500 g by as much as 80%.[49,50] One small RCT (59 women) compared diazepam with no anticonvulsant; it was too small for any reliable conclusions. **Magnesium sulphate versus phenytoin or diazepam:** Five RCTs (2439 women) found that magnesium sulphate was better than phenytoin for preventing eclampsia (RR 0.05, 95% CI 0.00 to 0.84), but there was insufficient evidence for reliable conclusions about the differential effect compared with diazepam.[48]

Harms: We found only one RCT (135 women), which reported maternal adverse effects of anticonvulsants. It found a significant increase in flushing (RR 3.81, 95% CI 2.22 to 6.53), and a non-significant increase in slurred speech (RR 3.04, 95% CI 0.13 to 73).[48] Compared with phenytoin, magnesium sulphate was associated with an increased risk of caesarean section (RR 1.21, 95% CI 1.05 to 1.41; NNH 29, 95% CI 12 to 84). One small trial evaluated magnesium sulphate for preventing and treating preterm labour in women who did not have pre-eclampsia. It found an increase in infant mortality for babies born to these women, many of whom had very low birthweight.[51]

Comment: The quality of these RCTs was average to poor. Most trials included women with severe pre-eclampsia. One small study recruited women with mild pre-eclampsia. A large international trial (the Magpie trial) comparing magnesium sulphate with placebo for women with pre-eclampsia is under way (L Duley, personal communication, 2000).

| OPTION | AGGRESSIVE MANAGEMENT FOR SEVERE EARLY ONSET PRE-ECLAMPSIA |

Two RCTs found that a policy of expectant, or conservative, management for severe early onset pre-eclampsia may have substantive benefits for the baby. There was insufficient evidence for reliable conclusions about possible effects for the woman.

Benefits: We found no systematic review but two small RCTs (133 women) that, taken together, found expectant management to be associated with reduced risk of respiratory distress syndrome in the baby (RR 2.30, 95% CI 1.39 to 3.81).[52,53] The trials were too small for any reliable conclusions on the effect on perinatal mortality or on maternal morbidity.

Harms: Expectant care aims to gain additional time *in utero* for the baby, but could increase morbidity for the women. We found insufficient evidence for reliable conclusions about possible effects of expectant management on maternal morbidity.

Comment: The women in these trials were at 28–34 weeks' gestation. A systematic review is in preparation (D Churchill, personal communication, 2000).

| OPTION | CHOICE OF ANALGESIA DURING LABOUR   New |

We found one RCT comparing intravenous patient controlled analgesia during labour with epidural analgesia.

Benefits: We found one RCT (105 women) comparing intravenous patient controlled analgesia versus epidural analgesia.[54] Mean pain scores were significantly lower with an epidural but the clinical importance of the difference is unclear. The trial was too small for a reliable conclusion about other outcomes. We found no RCTs of other forms of intrapartum analgesia for this group of women.

Harms: Neonatal naloxone was more likely to be given following intravenous patient controlled analgesia (28/52 [54%] with intravenous patient controlled analgesia v 5/53 [9%] with epidural analgesia; RR 5.71, 95% CI 2.39 to 13.64; NNH 3, 95% CI 2 to 4). No other neonatal outcomes were reported.

Comment: The drug used for patient controlled analgesia was not stated.

| QUESTION | What is the best choice of anticonvulsant for women with eclampsia? |

Systematic reviews have found that magnesium sulphate is better than phenytoin, diazepam, or lytic cocktail for the prevention of further fits in women with eclampsia. Although the effects on maternal mortality are not statistically significant, all three reviews found trends towards a reduced risk associated with magnesium sulphate.

Benefits: **Versus diazepam:** We found one systematic review (search date 1999, 5 RCTs, 1236 women).[55] Magnesium sulphate reduced both maternal mortality (RR 0.59, 95% CI 0.36 to 1.00) and further fits (RR 0.45, 95% CI 0.35 to 0.58) more than diazepam. There was no evidence of any differential effects on any other reported outcome. **Versus phenytoin:** We found one systematic review (search date 1999, 4 RCTs, 845 women).[56] Magnesium sulphate versus phenytoin reduced the risks of further fits (RR 0.32, 95% CI 0.20 to 0.49), pneumonia (RR 0.44, 95% CI 0.24 to 0.79), requirement for ventilation (RR 0.66, 95% CI 0.49 to 0.90), and admission to intensive care (RR 0.67, 95% CI 0.50 to 0.89).[56] Fewer babies died or stayed in a special baby care unit for more than 7 days (RR 0.77, 95% CI 0.63 to 0.95). The lower maternal death rate with magnesium sulphate compared with phenytoin was not significant, but the confidence interval was wide and a clinically important effect could not be excluded (RR 0.50, 95% CI 0.24 to 1.05). **Versus lytic cocktail:** We found two RCTs (198 women) comparing magnesium sulphate with lytic cocktail (see glossary, p 993).[57,58] Magnesium sulphate was better than lytic cocktail for preventing further fits (RR 0.09, 95% CI 0.03 to 0.24). It was also associated with a lower risk of pneumonia (RR 0.08, 95% CI 0.02 to 0.42), and of respiratory depression (RR 0.12, 95% CI 0.02 to 0.91).

Harms: **Versus diazepam:** We found no good evidence from RCTs about harms. **Versus phenytoin:** Clinical experience suggests that magnesium sulphate is safer than phenytoin. **Versus lytic cocktail:** Magnesium sulphate seems to be considerably safer than lytic cocktail.

Comment: Most information about the comparisons with diazepam and phenytoin comes from one large multicentre trial, in which adherence to treatment was 99%. The lytic cocktail trials were conducted in India. Women with both antepartum and postpartum eclampsia were included.

GLOSSARY

Lytic cocktail A mixture of pethidine, chlorpromazine, and promethazine.
Roll over test A test in which a woman lies on her left side for 15 minutes after which blood pressure is recorded. She then rolls into the supine position and, after 5 minutes, blood pressure is measured again. A rise in diastolic blood pressure in the supine position of more than 20 mmHg is defined as abnormal. The value of this test has been questioned.

Substantive changes since last issue

Other dietary interventions One new RCT[25] found that supplementation with protein, fish oil and calcium, plus rest in the left lateral position, reduced the risk of pre-eclampsia compared with iron supplementation alone.
Antihypertensive treatment One new RCT;[40] this was too small for reliable conclusions.

REFERENCES

1. Gifford RW, August P, Chesley LC, et al. National high blood pressure education program working group report on high blood pressure in pregnancy. *Am J Obstet Gynecol* 1990;163(5 Pt 1):1691–1712.

2. WHO international collaborative study of hypertensive disorders of pregnancy. Geographic variation in the incidence of hypertension in pregnancy. *Am J Obstet Gynecol* 1988;158:80–83.

3. Douglas K, Redman C. Eclampsia in the United Kingdom. *BMJ* 1994;309:1395–1400.

4. Crowther CA. Eclampsia at Harare maternity hospital. An epidemiological study. *S Afr Med J* 1985;68:927–929.

5. Bergström S, Povey G, Songane F, et al. Seasonal incidence of eclampsia and its relationship to meteorological data in Mozambique. *J Perinat Med* 1992;20:153–158.

6. Roberts JM, Redman CWG. Pre-eclampsia: more than pregnancy-induced hypertension. *Lancet* 1993;341:1447–1451.

7. Taylor DJ. The epidemiology of hypertension during pregnancy. In: Rubin PC, ed. *Hypertension in Pregnancy*. Amsterdam: Elsevier Science, 1988: 223–240.

8. Sibai BM, Caritis S, Hauth J. Risks of preeclampsia and adverse neonatal outcomes among women with pregestational diabetes mellitus. National Institute of Child Health and Human Development Network of Maternal-Fetal Medicine Units. *Am J Obstet Gynecol* 2000;182: 364–369.

9. MacGillivray I. *Pre-eclampsia. The hypertensive disease of pregnancy*. London: WB Saunders, 1983.

10. Conde-Agudelo A, Althabe F, Belizan JM, Kafury-Goeta AC. Cigarette smoking during pregnancy and risk of preeclampsia: a systematic review. *Am J Obstet Gynecol* 1999;181:1026–1035. Search date 1998; primary sources Medline, Embase, Popline, Cinahl, Lilacs, and hand searches of proceedings of international meetings on pre-eclampsia and reference lists of retrieved articles.

11. Chamberlain GVP, Philip E, Howlett B, Masters K. *British births*. London: Heinemann, 1970.

12. Sibai B, Lindheimer M, Hauth J, et al. Risk factors for preeclampsia, abruptio placentae, and adverse neonatal outcomes among women with chronic hypertension. *N Engl J Med* 1998;339: 667–671.

13. Knight M, Duley L, Henderson-Smart D, et al. The effectiveness and safety of antiplatelet agents for the prevention and treatment of pre-eclampsia. In: The Cochrane Library, Issue 4, 2000. Oxford: Update Software. Search date 1999; primary sources Cochrane Pregnancy and Childbirth Group Trials Register; conference proceedings.

14. Seki H, Kuromaki K, Takeda S, Kinoshita K, Satoh K. Trial of prophylactic administration of TXA2 synthetase inhibitor, ozagrel hydrochloride, for pre-eclampsia. *Hypertens Pregnancy* 1999;18:157–164.

15. Grant A, Farrell B, Heineman J, et al. Low dose aspirin in pregnancy and early childhood development: follow up of the collaborative low dose aspirin study in pregnancy. *Br J Obstet Gynaecol* 1995;102:861–868.

16. Parazzini F, Bortolus R, Chatenoud L, Restelli S, Benedetto C. Follow-up of children in the Italian study of aspirin in pregnancy. *Lancet* 1994;343: 1235.

17. Atallah AN, Hofmeyr GJ, Duley L. Calcium supplementation during pregnancy to prevent hypertensive disorders and related adverse outcomes. In: The Cochrane Library, Issue 4, 2000. Oxford: Update Software. Search date 2000; primary sources Cochrane Pregnancy and Childbirth Group Trials Register.

18. Herrera JA, Arevalo-Herrera M, Herrera S. Prevention of pre-eclampsia by linoleic acid and calcium supplementation: a randomized controlled trial. *Obstet Gynecol* 1998;91:585–590.

19. Salvig JD, Olsen SF, Secher NJ. Effects of fish oil supplementation in late pregnancy on blood pressure: a randomised controlled trial. *Br J Obstet Gynaecol* 1996;103:529–533.

20. Onwude JL, Lilford RJ, Hjartardottir H, et al. A randomised double blind placebo controlled trial of fish oil in high risk pregnancy. *Br J Obstet Gynaecol* 1995;102:95–100.

21. Bulstra-Ramakers MTE, Huisjes HJ, Visser GHA. The effects of 3 g eicosapentaenoic acid daily on recurrence of intrauterine growth retardation and pregnancy induced hypertension. *Br J Obstet Gynaecol* 1994;102:123–126.

22. Laivuori H, Hovatta O, Viinikka L, et al. Dietary supplementation with primrose oil or fish oil dose not change urinary excretion of prostacyclin and thromboxane metabolites in pre-eclamptic women. *Prostaglandins Leukot Essent Fatty Acids* 1993;49:691–694.

23. D'Almeida A, Carter JP, Anatol A, Prost C. Effects of a combination of evening primrose oil (gamma linolenic acid) and fish oil (eicosapentaenoic + docahexaenoic acid) versus magnesium, and versus placebo in preventing pre-eclampsia. *Women Health* 1992;19:117–131.

24. Moodley J, Norman RJ. Attempts at dietary alteration of prostaglandin pathways in the management of pre-eclampsia. *Prostaglandins Leukot Essent Fatty Acids* 1989;37:145–147.

25. Herrera JA. Nutritional factors and rest reduce pregnancy-induced hypertension and pre-eclampsia in positive roll-over test primigravidas. *Int J Gynaecol Obstet* 1993;41:31–35.

26. Duley L, Henderson-Smart D. Reduced salt intake compared to normal dietary salt, or high intake, during pregnancy. In: The Cochrane Library, Issue 4, 2000. Oxford: Update Software. Search date 1999; primary sources Cochrane Pregnancy and Childbirth Group Trials Register.

27. Makrides M, Crowther C. Magnesium supplementation during pregnancy. In: The Cochrane Library, Issue 4, 2000. Oxford: Update Software. Search date 1998; primary sources Cochrane Pregnancy and Childbirth Group Trials Register.

28. Chappell LC, Seed PT, Briley AL, et al. Effect of antioxidants on the occurrence of pre-eclampsia in women at increased risk: a randomised trial. *Lancet* 1999;354:810–816.

29. Olsen SF, Sorensen JD, Secher NJ, et al. Randomised controlled trial of effect of fish oil supplementation on pregnancy duration. *Lancet* 1992;339:1003–1007.

30. Easterling TR, Brateng D, Schucker B, Brown Z, Millard SP. Prevention of preeclampsia: a randomized trial of atenolol in hyperdynamic patients before onset of hypertension. *Obstet Gynecol* 1999; 93:725–733.

31. Lees C, Valensise H, Black R, et al. The efficacy and fetal-maternal cardiovascular effects of transdermal glyceryl trinitrate in the prophylaxis of pre-eclampsia and its complications: a randomized double blind placebo controlled trial. *Ultrasound Obstet Gynaecol* 1998;12:334–338.

32. Butters L, Kennedy S, Rubin PC. Atenolol in essential hypertension during pregnancy. *BMJ* 1990;301:587–589.

33. Churchill D, Bayliss H, Beevers G. Fetal growth restriction. *Lancet* 1999;355:1366–1363.

34. Duley L. Hospitalisation for non-proteinuric pregnancy hypertension. In: Keirse MJNC, Renfrew MJ, Neilson JP, et al, eds. *Pregnancy and childbirth module*. In: The Cochrane Library, Issue 2, 1995. Oxford: Update Software. Search date 1993; primary sources Cochrane Pregnancy and Childbirth Group Trials Register.

35. Duley L. Strict bed rest for proteinuric hypertension in pregnancy. In: Keirse MJNC, Renfrew MJ, Neilson JP, et al, eds. *Pregnancy and childbirth module*. In: The Cochrane Library, Issue 4, 1995. Oxford: Update Software. Search date

1993; primary sources Cochrane Pregnancy and Childbirth Group Trials Register.

36. Tuffnell DJ, Lilford RJ, Buchan PC, et al. Randomised controlled trial of day care for hypertension in pregnancy. *Lancet* 1992;339: 224–227.

37. Duley L. Any antihypertensive therapy for pregnancy hypertension. In: Keirse MJNC, Renfrew MJ, Neilson JP, et al, eds. *Pregnancy and childbirth module*. In: The Cochrane Library, Issue 2, 1995. Oxford: Update Software. Search date 1994; primary sources Cochrane Pregnancy and Childbirth Group Trials Register.

38. Magee LA, Elran E, Bull SB, Logan A, Koren G. Risks and benefits of beta-receptor blockers for pregnancy hypertension: overview of the randomized trials. *Eur J Obstet Gynecol Reprod Biol* 2000; 88:15–26. Search date 1997; primary sources Medline, Embase, hand searches of reference lists, *Hypertension and Pregnancy* journal 1992–1997, and a standard toxicology text.

39. Rudnicki M, Frolich A, Pilsgaard K, et al. Comparison of magnesium and methyldopa for the control of blood pressure in pregnancies complicated with hypertension. *Gynecol Obstet Invest* 2000;49:231–235.

40. Magee L, Duley L. Oral beta-blockers for mild to moderate hypertension during pregnancy. In: The Cochrane Library, Issue 4, 2000. Oxford: Update Software. Search date 2000; primary data source Cochrane Pregnancy and Childbirth Group Trials Register.

41. Von Dadelszen P, Ornstein MP, Bull SB, Logan AG, Koren G, Magee LA. Fall in mean arterial pressure and fetal growth restriction in pregnancy hypertension: a meta-analysis. *Lancet* 2000;355: 87–92. Search date 1997; primary sources Medline, Embase, hand searches of reference lists, *Hypertension and Pregnancy* 1992–1997, and a standard toxicology text.

42. Abalos E, Duley L, Henderson-Smart D, Steyn W. Antihypertensive drug therapy for mild to moderate hypertension during pregnancy [protocol]. In: The Cochrane Library, Issue 4, 2000. Oxford: Update Software.

43. Duley L, Henderson-Smart D. Drugs for rapid treatment of very high blood pressure during pregnancy. In: The Cochrane Library, Issue 4, 2000. Oxford: Update Software. Search date 1998; primary sources Cochrane Pregnancy and Childbirth Group Trials Register.

44. Duley L, Williams J, Henderson-Smart D. Plasma volume expansion for severe pre-eclampsia. In: The Cochrane Library, Issue 4, 2000. Oxford: Update Software. Search date 1999; primary sources Cochrane Pregnancy and Childbirth Group Trials Register.

45. The Albumin Reviewers (Alderson P, Bunn F, Li Wan Po L, Roberts I, Schierhout I). Human albumin solution for resuscitation and volume expansion in critically ill patients. In: The Cochrane Library, Issue 4, 2000. Oxford: Update Software. Search date 1999; primary sources Cochrane Injuries Group Trials Register, Cochrane Controlled Trials Register, Medline, Embase, Bids Scientific and Technical Proceedings, hand searches of reference lists of trials and review articles, and personal contacts with authors of identified trials.

46. Alderson P, Schierhout G, Roberts I, Bunn F. Colloids versus crystalloids for fluid resuscitation in critically ill patients. In: The Cochrane Library, Issue 4, 2000. Oxford: Update Software. Search date 1999; primary sources Cochrane Clinical Trials Register, Medline, Bids Index to Scientific and Technical Proceedings, and reference lists of trials and review articles.

47. Gülmezoglu AM, Hofmeyr GJ, Oosthuizen MMJ. Antioxidants in the treatment of severe preeclampsia: a randomized explanatory study. *Br J Obstet Gynecol* 1997;104:689–696.

48. Duley L, Gülmezoglu AM, Henderson-Smart D. Anticonvulsants for women with pre-eclampsia. In: The Cochrane Library, Issue 4, 2000. Oxford: Update Software. Search date 2000; primary sources Cochrane Pregnancy and Childbirth Group Trials Register.

49. Nelson K, Grether JK. Can magnesium sulfate reduce the risk of cerebral palsy in very low birthweight infants? *Pediatrics* 1995;95:263–269.

50. Schendel DE, Berg CJ, Yeargin-Allsopp M, et al. Prenatal magnesium sulfate exposure and the risk of cerebral palsy or mental retardation among very low-birth-weight children aged 3 to 5 years. *JAMA* 1996;276:1805–1810.

51. Mittendorf R, Covert R, Boman J, et al. Is tocolytic magnesium sulphate associated with increased total paediatric mortality? *Lancet* 1997;350: 1517–1518.

52. Odendaal HJ, Pattinson RC, Bam R, et al. Aggressive or expectant management for patients with severe preeclampsia between 28–34 weeks gestation: a randomized controlled trial. *Obstet Gynecol* 1990;76:1070–1075.

53. Sibai BM, Mercer BM, Schiff E, et al. Aggressive versus expectant management of severe preeclampsia at 28–32 weeks' gestation: a randomized controlled trial. *Am J Obstet Gynecol* 1994;171:818–822.

54. Hogg B, Owen J, Shih G, Vincent R, Chestnut D, Hauth JC. A randomised trial of intrapartum analgesia in women with severe pre-eclampsia. *Am J Obstet Gynecol* 2000;182:148.

55. Duley L, Henderson-Smart D. Magnesium sulphate versus diazepam for eclampsia. In: The Cochrane Library, Issue 4, 2000. Oxford: Update Software. Search date 1999; primary sources Cochrane Pregnancy and Childbirth Group Trials Register.

56. Duley L, Henderson-Smart D. Magnesium sulphate versus phenytoin for eclampsia. In: The Cochrane Library, Issue 4, 2000. Oxford: Update Software. Search date 1999; primary sources Cochrane Pregnancy and Childbirth Group Trials Register.

57. Bhalla AK, Dhall GI, Dhall K. A safer and more effective treatment regimen for eclampsia. *Aust NZ J Obstet Gynaecol* 1994;34:144–148.

58. Jacob S, Gopalakrishnan K, Lalitha K. Standardised clinical trial of magnesium sulphate regime in comparison with M K K. Menon's lytic cocktail regime in the management of eclampsia. The 27th British Congress of Obstetrics and Gynaecology [abstract 303], London, 1995.

Lelia Duley
Obstetric Epidemiologist
Institute of Health Sciences
Oxford UK

Competing interests: None declared.

Preterm birth

Search date January 2001

Bridgette Byrne and John Morrison

INTERVENTIONS

Key Messages

In women at high risk of preterm delivery

- A subgroup analysis in one systematic review of placebo controlled RCTs has found that antibiotic treatment of bacterial vaginosis during pregnancy decreases the incidence of preterm delivery in women who have had a previous preterm delivery.

- RCTs, carried out in a range of countries, found no evidence that enhanced antenatal care reduces the risk of preterm delivery.

- One large RCT has found that, in women presumed to have cervical incompetence, prophylactic cervical cerclage significantly reduces preterm birth (less than 33 weeks' gestation). It found that 25 women would need to undergo cerclage to prevent one additional preterm delivery.

In women with preterm premature rupture of membranes

- One systematic review of RCTs has found that, in women with preterm premature rupture of membranes, antibiotics prolong pregnancy and reduce the risk of neonatal infection. The review found no significant reduction in perinatal mortality, but this may have been because most trials did not include administration of antenatal corticosteroids.

- One systematic review found limited evidence from one small RCT that amnioinfusion was associated with improved neonatal outcomes.

In threatened preterm labour

- One systematic review of RCTs has found that tocolytics significantly prolong pregnancy but do not improve perinatal mortality or neonatal morbidity. Tocolytics were associated with a significant increase in adverse maternal events. Two subsequent RCTs have found that the oxytocin receptor antagonist atosiban is an effective tocolytic with minimal maternal side effects.

In preterm delivery

- Systematic reviews of RCTs have found:
  - Antenatal treatment with glucocorticoids reduces the risk of respiratory distress syndrome, neonatal mortality, infant mortality, and intraventricular haemorrhage in preterm infants.
  - Treatment with thyrotropin releasing hormone (TRH) plus corticosteroids before preterm delivery is not associated with better neonatal outcomes than corticosteroids alone. There were significantly more maternal and fetal adverse events with TRH.
  - Evidence of a benefit from antibiotics in women in preterm labour with intact membranes. The benefit was prolongation of pregnancy, reduced incidence of maternal infection, and necrotising enterocolitis. However, antibiotics were associated with an increase in perinatal mortality.

DEFINITION Preterm or premature birth is defined by the World Health Organization as delivery of an infant before 37 completed weeks of gestation.[1] There is no set lower limit to this definition, but 23–24 weeks' gestation is widely accepted,[1] which approximates to an average fetal weight of 500 g.

INCIDENCE/ PREVALENCE Preterm birth occurs in about 5–10% of all births in developed countries,[2–4] but in recent years the incidence seems to have increased in some countries, particularly the USA.[5] We found little reliable evidence for less developed countries that used the exact definition of premature birth. The rate in northwestern Ethiopia has been reported to vary between 11.3–21.8% depending on the age group studied, being highest in teenagers.[6]

AETIOLOGY/ RISK FACTORS About 30% of preterm births are unexplained and spontaneous.[4,7,8] The two strongest risk factors for idiopathic preterm labour are low socioeconomic status and previous preterm delivery. Multiple pregnancy accounts for about another 30% of cases.[4,7] Other known risk factors include genital tract infection, preterm premature rupture of the membranes, antepartum haemorrhage, cervical incompetence, and congenital uterine abnormalities, which collectively account for about 20–25% of cases. The remaining cases (15–20%) are attributed to elective preterm delivery secondary to hypertensive disorders of pregnancy, intrauterine fetal growth restriction, congenital abnormalities, and medical disorders of pregnancy.[4,5,7,8]

PROGNOSIS Preterm labour usually results in preterm birth. One systematic review (search date not stated) of tocolysis versus placebo found that about 27% of preterm labours spontaneously resolved, and about 70% progressed to preterm delivery.[9] Observational studies have found that one preterm birth significantly raises the risk of another in a subsequent pregnancy.[10]

AIMS To prevent preterm birth; to prolong the interval between threatened preterm labour and delivery; and to optimise the condition of the fetus in preparation for delivery in order to improve neonatal outcome.

OUTCOMES The main clinical outcome is improved neonatal outcome, as indicated by perinatal mortality, neonatal mortality and morbidity (incidence of respiratory distress syndrome, intraventricular haemorrhage, necrotising enterocolitis, neonatal sepsis, and neonatal convulsions). Proxy outcomes include duration of pregnancy, number of hours or days between onset of labour and delivery, and number of deliveries before 37 completed weeks of gestation. An additional clinical outcome is incidence of maternal adverse effects.

METHODS *Clinical Evidence* update search and appraisal January 2001. In addition, the author performed a detailed search of the Cochrane Library and Medline from 1966 using the following terms: preterm delivery, preterm labour, perinatal mortality, respiratory distress syndrome, TRH, corticosteroids, tocolysis, and cervical cerclage.

QUESTION What are the effects of preventive interventions in women at high risk of preterm delivery?

OPTION ANTIBIOTIC TREATMENT OF BACTERIAL VAGINOSIS IN PREGNANCY

One systematic review of placebo controlled RCTs and a subsequent large placebo controlled RCT found that antibiotic treatment of bacterial vaginosis during pregnancy did not significantly alter the rate of preterm delivery. However, limited evidence from a subgroup analysis in the systematic review of women who had a previous preterm delivery, found that treatment for bacterial vaginosis versus placebo significantly reduced the risk of preterm delivery.

Benefits: We found one systematic review (search date 1998, 5 RCTs, 1508 women) comparing one or more antibiotic regimens versus placebo.[11] It found fewer cases of preterm delivery after treatment for bacterial vaginosis than after placebo, but the difference was not significant (OR 0.78, 95% CI 0.60 to 1.02). In the subgroup of women who had a previous preterm birth (3 RCTs, 303 women), the reduced risk of preterm birth was significant (OR 0.37, 95% CI 0.23 to 0.60). A subsequent RCT (1953 women with bacterial vaginosis in a general obstetric population) found no significant difference in preterm delivery in women receiving treatment with metronidazole versus placebo (OR 1.0, 95% CI 0.8 to 1.2).[12]

Harms: Adverse effects were addressed in 1757 of the 1953 (90%) participating women. Adverse effects were more common in women taking antibiotics for bacterial vaginosis (side effects 21.6% with metronidazole v 9.1% with placebo; gastrointestinal adverse effects 19.7% with metronidazole v 7.5% with placebo; vomiting 9.7% with metronidazole v 2.8% with placebo; requirement of treatment for vaginal yeast 12.0% with metronidazole v 4.9% with placebo).[12] Withdrawals varied between 1–17% for the various treatment and placebo groups in the six trials.

Comment: The quality of the RCTs was generally good; all RCTs provided data on withdrawals.[11,12]

OPTION ENHANCED ANTENATAL CARE FOR SOCIALLY DEPRIVED WOMEN AND OTHER HIGH RISK GROUPS

RCTs, carried out in a range of countries, found no evidence that enhanced antenatal care (see glossary, p 1007) reduces the risk of preterm delivery.

Benefits: We found no systematic review. We found nine RCTs. All RCTs (carried out in Europe, USA, and Latin America; number of high risk women ranging from 150–2200) found no significant difference between enhanced and normal antenatal care.[13–21]

Harms: No adverse effects were reported.

Comment: The definition of enhanced prenatal care varied.[13–19] Examples of enhanced prenatal care include increased number of antenatal visits, a bed rest programme including rest periods three times daily, home visits by midwives, fortnightly social worker counselling sessions, nutritional education, and counselling by a psychologist. We found no evidence of superiority of one particular intervention.

OPTION PROPHYLACTIC CERVICAL CERCLAGE IN WOMEN AT RISK OF CERVICAL INCOMPETENCE

One large RCT has found that, in women presumed to have cervical incompetence, prophylactic cervical cerclage (see glossary, p 1007) significantly reduces preterm birth (less than 33 weeks' gestation). Twenty five women would need to undergo cerclage to prevent one additional preterm delivery.

Benefits: We found no systematic review. We found one multicentre RCT (1292 women) comparing the effect of cerclage versus no cerclage

Pregnancy and childbirth

on the incidence of delivery before 33 weeks' gestation and before 37 weeks' gestation, and the vital status of the baby after delivery.[22] All women had a history of early delivery or cervical surgery, and their obstetrician was uncertain whether to advise cerclage or not. Cerclage significantly reduced the rate of delivery before 33 weeks' gestation (83/647 [13%] with cerclage v 110/645 [17%] with no cerclage; RR 0.75, 95% CI 0.57 to 0.98; NNT 24, 95% CI 14 to 275). There was no significant difference in the rate of deliveries occurring between weeks 33 and 36.

Harms: Insertion of cervical sutures doubled the risk of puerperal pyrexia (24/415 [6%] with cerclage v 11/405 [3%] with no cerclage; RR 2.13, 95% CI 1.06 to 4.15; NNT 33, 95% CI 12 to 607).[22] Information about puerperal pyrexia was collected only after 360 women had been recruited to the trial.

Comment: The commonest indication for entry to the trial was a history of preterm delivery or second trimester miscarriage (74% of the cerclage group, 70% of the controls).[20]

| QUESTION | What are the effects of interventions to improve outcome after preterm premature rupture of the membranes? |

| OPTION | ANTIBIOTICS |

One systematic review has found that, in women with preterm premature rupture of membranes (see glossary, p 1007), antibiotics prolong pregnancy and reduce the risk of neonatal infection. The review found no significant reduction in perinatal mortality (see glossary, p 1007), but this may have been because of the fact that most trials did not include administration of antenatal corticosteroids.

Benefits: We found one systematic review (search date 1999, 12 RCTs, 1599 women with preterm premature rupture of membranes) comparing antibiotics versus placebo (see table 1, p 1009).[23] Antibiotics reduced the number of babies born within 48 hours of randomisation (5 RCTs, 140/513 [27%] with antibiotics v 207/545 [38%] with placebo; OR 0.6, 95% CI 0.46 to 0.77), the number of babies born within 7 days (4 RCTs, 287/483 [59%] with antibiotics v 393/508 [77%] with placebo; OR 0.43, 95% CI 0.33 to 0.57), the risk of chorioamnionitis (11 RCTs, 125/795 [16%] with antibiotics v 209/814 [26%] with placebo; OR 0.54, 95% CI 0.42 to 0.69), and the risk of neonatal infection (11 RCTs, 86/775 [11%] with antibiotics v 127/ 799 [16%] with placebo; OR 0.62, 95% CI 0.45 to 0.86). However, there was no significant reduction in risk of perinatal death or necrotising enterocolitis (see comment below). Pooled data from the trials found lower risk of abnormal brain scan and respiratory distress syndrome among babies exposed to antibiotics, but these also did not reach significance.

Harms: Adverse effects were looked for in the trials, and none were reported.[23]

Comment: Most of the trials did not include antenatal administration of corticosteroids, which may explain the lack of beneficial effect on neonatal mortality. All but one of the trials gave data on withdrawals, which was always less than 20%. Various different antibiotic regimens were used in the studies, including use of one of the following: erythromycin, benzylpenicillin, ampicillin, piperacillin, and clindamycin.[23]

| OPTION | AMNIOINFUSION |

One systematic review found limited evidence from one small RCT that amnioinfusion (see glossary, p 1007) improves neonatal outcomes after preterm premature rupture of the membranes.

Benefits: We found one systematic review (search date 1998, 1 RCT, 66 women) comparing amnioinfusion versus no amnioinfusion (see table 2, p 1010).[24] No significant difference in rates of caesarean section, low Apgar scores, neonatal death, or endometritis were detected. Amnioinfusion was associated with fewer severe fetal heart rate decelerations per hour during the first stage of labour (mean difference −1.20, 95% CI −1.83 to −0.57) and higher mean umbilical artery pH values (umbilical artery pH difference 0.11, 95% CI 0.08 to 0.14).

Harms: Adverse effects were looked for in the trials, and none were reported.

Comment: The trial was too small to detect clinically important changes of some of the outcomes (rates of caesarean section, neonatal death, and infectious morbidity), and had shortcomings in methods used (unspecified method of random assignment of women; blinding of treatment not possible).

| QUESTION | What are the effects of treatments in threatened preterm labour? |

| OPTION | TOCOLYTICS |

One systematic review of RCTs has found that β mimetics, indomethacin, atosiban, and ethanol are associated with a significant prolongation of pregnancy for women in threatened preterm labour (see glossary, p 1007) but with no evidence of improved perinatal mortality or neonatal morbidity. A subsequent RCT found that the oxytocin receptor antagonist atosiban appears to be as effective as other tocolytics, but is associated with less maternal side effects. Its safety and efficacy before 28 weeks' gestation merits further investigation.

Benefits: **Tocolytics:** We found one systematic review (search date 1998)[25] and two subsequent RCTs.[26,27] The systematic review (18 RCTs, 2785 women in preterm labour) comparing different tocolytic drugs (β mimetics, magnesium sulphate, indomethacin, atosiban, and ethanol) versus placebo or no tocolytic.[25] Three trials included women with ruptured membranes. The most frequently evaluated specific tocolytic agent was ritodrine (5 RCTs). There was heterogeneity in the effects between different types of tocolytics, and therefore its effects should not be considered as a group. Tocolytics that significantly delay delivery following the onset of preterm labour for greater than 24 hours, 48 hours, and 7 days when compared with placebo (or to no treatment) include β mimetics, indometha-cin, atosiban, and ethanol. **β Mimetics:** The review found non-significant differences with placebo or no treatment for perinatal death (8 trials, 62/682 [9%] with β mimetics v 48/604 [8%] with placebo or no treatment; OR 1.08, 95% CI 0.72 to 1.62), respiratory distress syndrome (6 trials, 117/639 [18%] with β mimetics v 140/565 [25%] with placebo or no treatment; OR 0.76, 95% CI 0.57 to 1.01), birth weight < 2500 g (5 trials, 332/601 [50%] with β mimetics v 332/525 [63%] with placebo or no treatment; OR 0.79, 95% CI 0.61 to 1.01), patent ductus arteriosus, necrotizing enterocolitis, intraventricular haemorrhage, seizures, hypoglyce-mia, or neonatal sepsis. **Magnesium sulphate:** The review found non-significant differences with placebo or no treatment for perina-tal death (4 trials, 11/169 [7%] with magnesium sulphate v 7/182 [4%] with placebo or no treatment; OR 1.83, 95% CI 0.70 to 4.77), respiratory distress syndrome (3 trials, 22/139 [16%] with magne-sium sulphate v 22/153 [14%] with placebo or no treatment; OR 1.83, 95% CI 0.70 to 4.77). No differences were found for birth weight less than 2500 g, patent ductus arteriosus, necrotizing enterocolitis, intraventricular haemorrhage, seizures, hypoglyce-mia, or neonatal sepsis. However, the number of newborns assessed for the later outcomes was small. **Indomethacin:** The review found no significant differences with placebo or no treatment for perinatal death, respiratory distress syndrome, bronchopulmo-nary dysplasia, necrotizing enterocolitis, neonatal sepsis, or low birth weight. These outcomes have to be approached with care as the number of assessed newborns was small. **Atosiban:** One trial (114 newborns) included in the systematic review assessed the effect of atosiban. It found no significant differences in the inci-dence of respiratory distress syndrome, patent ductus arteriosus, and hypoglycemia. The results should be interpreted with caution as the trial was too small to rule out a significant difference. One subsequent RCT (247 women) compared the oxytocin antagonist atosiban versus ritodine.[26] It found that atosiban was as effective as ritodrine in delaying delivery for 48 hours (107/126 [85%] with atosiban v 105/121 [87%] with ritodrine; OR 1.01, 95% CI 0.48 to 1.10) and 7 days (92/126 [73%] with atosiban v 92/ 121 [76%] with ritodrine; OR 0.94, 95% CI 0.49 to 1.79) following the onset of preterm labour. However, women taking ritodine had significantly more adverse effects (see harms below).[26] The second subsequent RCT compared atosiban with placebo. It found that for pregnancies at 28 weeks or over, atosiban prolonged pregnancy for up to 24 hours (150/203 [74%] with atosiban v 128/221 [58%] with pla-cebo; RR 1.28, 95% CI 1.11 to 1.47; NNT 7, 95% CI 4 to 15), 48 hours (140/203 [69%] with atosiban v 122/221 [55%] with pla-cebo; RR 1.25, 95% CI 1.08 to 1.45; NNT 8, 95% CI 5 to 23), and 7 days (131/203 [65%] with atosiban v 105/220 [48%] with placebo; RR 1.35, 95% CI 1.14 to 1.60; NNT 6, 95% CI 4 to 14) with minimal maternal side effects.[27]

Harms:　In the systematic review,[25] **β mimetics** were associated with sig-nificant adverse maternal side effects namely chest pain (2 RCTs, 39/406 [10%] with β mimetics v 3/408 [1%] with placebo or no treatment; OR 6.2, 95% CI 3.3 to 11.5), palpitations (3 RCTs, 200/420 [18%] with β mimetics v 19/423 [4%] with placebo or no treatment; OR 10.2, 95% CI 7.4 to 13.9), dyspnoea (2 RCTs, 55/406 [14%] with β mimetics v 4/408 [1%] with placebo or no treatment; OR 6.6, 95% CI 3.9 to 11.2), tremor (1 RCT, 138/352 [39%] with β mimetics v 13/356 [4%] with placebo or no treatment; OR 8.3, 95% CI 5.8 to 11.9), nausea (1 RCT, 72/352 [20%] with β mimetics v 42/356 [12%] with placebo or no treatment; OR 1.9, 95% CI 1.3 to 2.8), vomiting (2 RCTs, 48/366 [13%] with β mimetics v 29/371 [8%] with placebo or no treatment; OR 1.79, 95% CI 1.1 to 2.9), headache (2 RCTs, 84/366 [24%] with β mimetics v 22/371 [6%] with placebo or no treatment; OR 4.0, 95% CI 2.6 to 6.0), hyperglycaemia (1 RCT, 106/352 [30%] with β mimetics v 37/356 [10%] with placebo or no treatment; OR 3.4, 95% CI 2.4 to 4.9), hypokalemia (1 RCT, 138/352 [39%] with β mimetics v 23/356 [6%] with placebo or no treatment; OR 6.4, 95% CI 4.5 to 9.1), and frequently these side effects necessitated discontinuation of treatment (3 RCTs, 25/88 [32%] with β mimetics v 0/86 with placebo or no treatment; OR 11.5, 95% CI 4.8 to 27.5). **Magnesium sulphate** was associated with a significant increase in the need to discontinue treatment (3 RCTs, 10/137 [7%] with magnesium sulphate v 0/144 with placebo or no treatment; OR 8.36, 95% CI 2.36 to 29.61). **Indomethacin** was associated with an increased incidence of postpartum haemorrhage (1 RCT, 7/16 [44%] with indomethacin v 2/18 [11%] with placebo or no treatment; OR 5.1, 95% CI 1.1 to 22.9), and a non-significant increase in nausea (1 RCT, 2/18 [11%] with indomethacin v 0/18 with placebo or no treatment; OR 7.8, 95% CI 0.5 to 130.5) and chorioamnionitis (1 RCT, 2/15 [13%] with indomethacin v 0/15 with placebo or no treatment; OR 7.9, 95% CI 0.5 to 133.3). **Atosiban** was associated with an increased incidence of nausea in women (2 RCTs, 33/306 [11%] with atosiban v 15/307 [5%] with placebo or no treatment; OR 2.3, 95% CI 1.3 to 4.1), but there was no increased vomiting (2 RCTs, 10/306 [3%] with atosiban v 13/307 [4%] with placebo or no treatment; OR 0.8, 95% CI 0.3 to 1.8). Chest pain (2 RCTs, 3/306 [1%] with atosiban v 13/307 [4%] with placebo or no treatment; OR 0.3, 95% CI 0.1 to 0.8) and dyspnoea (1 RCT, 1/250 [0.4%] with atosiban v 7/251 [3%] with placebo or no treatment; OR 0.8, 95% CI 0.3 to 1.8) were significantly less likely to occur in patients receiving atosiban compared with controls. The RCT comparing atosiban with ritodrine[26] found increased neonatal morbidity in women with multiple births who received atosiban. There was an increased incidence of respiratory distress syndrome (17/39 [44%] with atosiban v 5/28 [18%] with ritodrine; RR 2.44, 95% CI 1.02 to 5.83; NNH 3, 95% CI 2 to 33), apnoea (11/39 [28%] with atosiban v 4/28 [14%] with ritodrine; RR 1.97, 95% CI 0.70 to 5.57), patent ductus arteriosus (5/39 [13%] with atosiban v 0/28 with ritodrine; ARR +0.13, 95% CI −0.01 to +0.27), and bradycardia (4/39 [10%] with atosiban v 1/28 [4%] with ritodrine; RR 2.87, 95% CI 0.34 to 24.33). The numbers of multiple births included in the study were small. Multiple pregnancies less than 28 weeks gestation were more common in the atosiban group (4/126 [3.2%] in women randomised to receive atosiban v 1/121 [0.8%] women randomised to receive ritodrine). Logistic regression of multiple pregnancies population showed that neither atosiban nor ritodrine correlated with length of stay at the intensive care unit (P = 0.88), but an inverse correlation with gestational age and time at enrolment was found. Injection site reactions were a problem with prolonged use of atosiban (110/250 [44%] with atosiban v 58/251 [23%] with placebo; RR 1.90, 95% CI 1.46 to 2.48; NNH 4, 95% CI 3 to 7) necessitating significantly higher discontinuation of treatment in the women receiving atosiban (16%) than in women receiving placebo (4%).[27]

Comment: False preterm labour presents a problem in analysis of effects of tocolytic agents. However, in 15 of the 17 trials included in the systematic review, the definition of preterm labour used for entry into the study included cervical dilatation, effacement, or change in the cervical condition in addition to uterine contractions. This would minimise the potential confounding effect of spurious preterm labour. Combining results for all tocolytics was reasonable, based on the lack of evidence of the merits of one tocolytic over another.[28] The confidence intervals for delivery before 37 weeks' gestation were wide and included the possibility of a large positive effect.[25] Tocolytic rescue with ritodrine was used in the RCT comparing atosiban with placebo.[27] In the second RCT,[27] 24 of 246 (10%) women randomised to receive atosiban and 13 of 255 (5%) women randomised to receive placebo were recruited at less than 26 weeks' gestation. This may have contributed to a higher incidence of fetal–infant death at less than 26 weeks' gestation in the atosiban group (10/27 [37%] v 0/16 [0%]).

QUESTION What are the effects of interventions to improve outcome in preterm delivery?

OPTION CORTICOSTEROIDS BEFORE PRETERM DELIVERY

One systematic review has found that antenatal treatment with glucocorticoids significantly reduces the risk of respiratory distress syndrome, neonatal mortality, infant mortality, and intraventricular haemorrhage in preterm infants.

Benefits: We found one systematic review (search date 1996, 18 RCTs, > 3700 babies).[29] The RCTs compared corticosteroids (betamethasone, dexamethasone, or hydrocortisone) versus placebo or no treatment in women before anticipated preterm delivery (elective or after spontaneous onset of preterm labour). The review found that treatment with antenatal corticosteroids significantly reduced rates of respiratory distress syndrome (18 trials, 292/1885 women with corticosteroids v 439/1850 women with placebo or no treatment; OR 0.53, 95% CI 0.44 to 0.63). In the subgroup of neonates delivered before 28 weeks' gestation, there was no significant difference (3 trials, 7/17 [41%] with corticosteroids v 18/31 [58%] with placebo or no treatment; OR 0.64, 95% CI 0.16 to 2.50). Differences for respiratory distress syndrome in babies delivered within less than 24 hours (45/176 [26%] with corticosteroids v 57/173 [40%] with placebo or no treatment; OR 0.70, 95% CI 0.43 to 1.16) or less than 48 hours (3/23 [13%] v 6/19 [32%] on control; OR 0.34, 95% CI 0.08 to 1.47) were non-significant. A significant reduction in respiratory distress syndrome was seen only 48 hours after receiving corticosteroids. For babies born between

24 hours and 7 days after treatment, there was a significant reduction in respiratory distress syndrome (44/382 [12%] v 87/346 [25%] on control; OR 0.38, 95% CI 0.25 to 0.57). There was no significant effect in neonates delivered more than 7 days after treatment. Significant reductions in respiratory distress were seen with both betamethasone and dexamethasone but not with hydrocortisone. The sex of the neonate had no effect on treatment response. The small numbers of evaluable neonates from twin pregnancies did not allow a confident statement about the effects in multiple pregnancy. Antenatal corticosteroids were significantly associated with reduced neonatal mortality (14 trials, 129/1770 with corticosteroids v 204/1747 with placebo or no treatment; OR 0.6, 95% CI 0.48 to 0.75), and risk of intraventricular haemorrhage (diagnosed at autopsy: 7/446 with corticosteroids v 23/417 with placebo or no treatment, OR 0.29, 95% CI 0.14 to 0.61; diagnosed by ultrasound: 47/300 with corticosteroids v 77/296 with placebo or no intervention, OR 0.48, 95% CI 0.32 to 0.72). Antenatal corticoids did not significantly reduce the rates of necrotising enterocolitis (17/587 [3%] with corticosteroids v 27/567 [5%] with placebo or no treatment; OR 0.59, 95% CI 0.32 to 1.09) or chronic lung disease (38/204 [19%] with corticosteroids v 25/207 [12%] with placebo or no treatment; OR 1.57, 95% CI 0.87 to 2.84).

Harms: There was no strong evidence of any adverse effects of corticosteroids in these trials. Subgroup analysis in one trial suggested that corticosteroids might predispose to fetal death in hypertensive women. No deaths were observed in this subgroup in the other three trials for which data were available.[29]

Comment: The fact that the beneficial effect of corticosteroids on respiratory distress syndrome was not significant at less than 28 weeks' gestation may be because of the small numbers available for analysis at this gestation. No trials addressed the potentially harmful effects of repeated doses of antenatal corticosteroids, or whether one form of corticosteroid was more harmful than another, as a recent retrospective cohort study involving 883 babies delivered between 24 and 31 weeks' gestation suggests.[30]

OPTION	THYROTROPIN RELEASING HORMONE BEFORE PRETERM DELIVERY

One systematic review of RCTs found that treatment with TRH and corticosteroids before preterm delivery was not associated with better neonatal outcomes than corticosteroids alone. There were significantly more maternal and fetal adverse events with TRH.

Benefits: We found one systematic review (search date 1999, 11 RCTs in > 4500 women).[31] Seven trials compared TRH plus steroids versus steroids alone and analysed by intention to treat. TRH plus steroids versus steroids alone had no significant effect on gestational age at delivery, admission to the neonatal intensive care unit, respiratory distress syndrome, need for oxygen supplementation at 28 days, intraventricular haemorrhage, necrotising enterocolitis, and perinatal mortality.

Harms: In babies who received TRH plus steroids versus steroids alone, there was an increased risk of low Apgar score at 5 minutes (OR

1.8, 95% CI 1.03 to 1.29) and an increased requirement for assisted ventilation (OR 1.16, CI 1.03 to 1.29). One study included in the review[31] reported at 12 month follow up, an increase in motor delay (RR 1.31, 95% CI 1.09 to 1.56), motor impairment (RR 1.51, 95% CI 1.01 to 2.24), sensory impairment (RR 1.97, 95% CI 1.10 to 3.53), and social delay (RR 1.25, 95% CI 1.03 to 1.51). Antenatal TRH was associated with a significant rise in maternal blood pressure (risk of an increase of 25 mmHg in systolic blood pressure; 1 RCT, 36/506 [7%] with TRH plus steroids v 20/505 [4%] with steroids alone, RR 1.8, 95% CI 1.05 to 3.06), and a 15 mmHg increase in diastolic blood pressure (1 RCT, 115/506 [23%] with TRH plus steroids v 71/505 [14%] with steroids alone, RR 1.62, 95% CI 1.24 to 2.12). Other maternal adverse effects included nausea (3 RCTs, 303/1175 [26%] with TRH plus steroids v 77/1195 [6%] with steroids alone, RR 3.92, 95% CI 3.13 to 4.92), vomiting (1 RCT, 40/506 [8%] with TRH plus steroids v 17/505 [3%] with steroids alone, RR 2.35, 95% CI 1.35 to 4.09), lightheadedness (1 RCT, 139/506 [27%] with TRH plus steroids v 80/505 [16%] with steroids alone, RR 1.73, 95% CI 1.36 to 2.22), urgency of micturition (1 RCT, 115/506 [23%] with TRH plus steroids v 48/505 [10%] with steroids alone, RR 2.39, 95% CI 1.75 to 3.27), and facial flushing (3 RCTs, 397/1252 [32%] with TRH plus steroids v 149/1271 [12%] with steroids alone, RR 2.67, 95% CI 2.26 to 3.16).[31]

Comment: Corticosteroids were administered in all trials but the TRH regimens varied between studies.

OPTION	ANTIBIOTICS IN PRETERM LABOUR WITH INTACT MEMBRANES

One systematic review has found that antibiotics versus placebo or no antibiotics significantly prolongs pregnancy, with a reduction in maternal infectious morbidity and necrotising enterocolitis when antibiotics were used to treat women in preterm labour with intact membranes. However, antibiotics significantly increased perinatal mortality (see glossary, p 1007).

Benefits: We found one systematic review (search date 1997, 10 RCTs) comparing single antibiotics in two trials, combinations in eight trials, versus placebo or no antibiotics in preterm labour with intact membranes.[32] All trials used similar definitions of preterm labour, including uterine contractions and cervical dilatation. The antibiotics were ampicillin, erythromycin, metronidazole, sulbactam, mezlocillin, clavulonic acid, clindamycin, and ceftizoxime. Antibiotics were associated with prolongation of pregnancy of 5.4 days, 95% CI 0.9 to 9.8 days. Antibiotics significantly reduced the incidence of maternal infection (OR 0.59, 95% CI 0.36 to 0.97) and necrotising enterocolitis (OR 0.33, 95% CI 0.13 to 0.88) in the group that received antibiotics. Differences for neonatal sepsis (OR 0.67, 95% CI 0.42 to 1.07), mean birth weight, respiratory distress syndrome, or intraventricular haemorrhage were not statistically significant.

Harms: Antibiotics were associated with increased perinatal mortality (8 trials, 12/481 [2.5%] with antibiotics v 3/486 [0.6%] with no antibiotics; OR 3.36, 95% CI 1.21 to 9.32), a finding that persisted when only deaths related to prematurity were included (OR 2.74, 95% CI 1.02 to 7.35).[32]

Comment: The trials were of good quality (9 out of 10 were double blind and placebo controlled). Data for the impact of antibiotics on prolongation of pregnancy could only be analysed in four of the 10 studies. The definition of neonatal sepsis was not consistent and, therefore, the rate of neonatal sepsis varied significantly between each trial. Tocolytics and corticosteroids were administered in all but one trial.[32] Multiple pregnancies were excluded in seven of 10 trials.

GLOSSARY

Amnioinfusion Infusion of physiological saline or Ringers lactate through a catheter transabdominally or transcervically into the amniotic cavity.

Cervical cerclage Insertion of a cervical suture, using non-absorbable suture material, circumferentially around the cervix. May be done transvaginally or transabdominally.

Enhanced antenatal care Includes various programmes of increased medical, midwifery, psychological, social, and nutritional support during pregnancy.

Perinatal Refers to the period after 24 weeks' gestation and includes the first 7 days of postnatal life for the neonate.

Preterm labour Onset of labour (regular uterine contractions with cervical effacement and dilatation) in the preterm period.

Preterm premature rupture of membranes Leakage of amniotic fluid from the amniotic cavity during the preterm period owing to rupture of the fetal membranes.

Substantive changes since last issue

Antibiotic treatment of bacterial vaginosis in pregnancy New RCT;[12] conclusion unchanged.

Thyrotropin releasing hormone before preterm delivery Systematic review updated;[31] harms section includes some additional clinical outcomes.

Antibiotics in preterm labour with intact membranes Systematic review updated;[32] conclusions unchanged.

REFERENCES

1. Morrison JJ, Rennie JM. Clinical, scientific and ethical aspects of fetal and neonatal care at extremely preterm periods of gestation. Br J Obstet Gynaecol 1997;104:1341–1350.
2. Rush RW, Keirse MJNC, Howat P, et al. Contribution of preterm delivery to perinatal mortality. BMJ 1976;2:965–968.
3. Creasy RK. Preterm birth prevention: Where are we? Am J Obstet Gynecol 1993;168:1223–1230.
4. Burke C, Morrison JJ. Perinatal factors and preterm delivery in an Irish obstetric population. J Perinat Med 2000;28:49–53.
5. Goldenberg RL, Rouse DJ. Prevention of premature birth. N Engl J Med 1998;339:313–320.
6. Kumbi S, Isehak A. Obstetric outcome of teenage pregnancy in northwestern Ethiopia. East Afr Med J 1999;76:138–140.
7. Iannucci TA, Tomich PG, Gianopoulos JG. Etiology and outcome of extremely low-birth-weight infants. Am J Obstet Gynecol 1996;174:1896–1902.
8. Main DM, Gabbe SG, Richardson D, et al. Can preterm deliveries be prevented? Am J Obstet Gynecol 1985;151:892–898.
9. King JF, Grant A, Keirse MJNC, et al. β-mimetics in preterm labour: an overview of the randomised controlled trials. Br J Obstet Gynaecol 1988;95:

211–222. Search date not stated; primary sources Oxford Database of Perinatal Trials, hand searches of reference lists, and personal contacts.
10. Keirse MJNC, Rush RW, Anderson AB, et al. Risk of preterm delivery and/or abortion. Br J Obstet Gynaecol 1978;85:81–85.
11. Brocklehurst P, Hannah M, McDonald H. Interventions for treating bacterial vaginosis in pregnancy. In: The Cochrane Library, Issue 4, 2000. Oxford: Update Software. Search date July 1998; primary sources Cochrane Pregnancy and Childbirth Group Trials Register, Cochrane Controlled Trial Registers.
12. Carey JC, Klebanoff MA, Hauth JC, et al. Metranidazole to prevent preterm delivery in pregnant women with asymptomatic bacterial vaginosis. N Engl J Med 2000;342:534–540.
13. Spencer B, Thomas H, Morris J. A randomized controlled trial of the provision of a social support service during pregnancy; the South Manchester Family Worker project. Br J Obstet Gynaecol 1989; 96:281–288.
14. Mueller-Heubach E, Reddick D, Barrett B, et al. Preterm birth prevention: evaluation of a prospective controlled randomized trial. Am J Obstet Gynecol 1989;160:1172–1178.

15. Goldenberg R, Davis R, Copper R, et al. The Alabama birth prevention project. *Obstet Gynecol* 1990;75:933–939.

16. Blondel B, Breart G, Glado J, et al. Evaluation of the home-visiting system for women with threatened preterm labour. Results of a randomized controlled trial. *Eur J Obstet Gynaecol Reprod Biol* 1990;34:47–58.

17. Villar J, Farnot U, Barros F, et al. A randomized trial of psychosocial support during high-risk pregnancies. *N Engl J Med* 1992;327:1266–1271.

18. Collaborative Group on Preterm Birth Prevention. Multicenter randomized controlled trial of a preterm birth prevention program. *Am J Obstet Gynecol* 1993;169:352–366.

19. Moore ML, Meis PJ, Ernest JM, et al. A randomized trial of nurse intervention to reduce preterm and low birth weight births. *Obstet Gynecol* 1998;91:656–661.

20. Olds DL, Henderson CR Jr, Tatelbaum R, et al. Improving the delivery of prenatal care and outcomes of pregnancy: a randomized trial of nurse home visitation. *Pediatrics* 1986;77:16–28.

21. Koniak-Griffin D, Anderson NL, Verzemnieks I, et al. A public health nursing early intervention program for adolescent mothers: outcomes from pregnancy through 6 weeks postpartum. *Nursing Res* 2000;49:130–138.

22. MRC/RCOG Working Party on Cervical Cerclage. Final report of the Medical Research Council/Royal College of Obstetricians and Gynaecologists Multicentre Randomised Trial of Cervical Cerclage. *Br J Obstet Gynaecol* 1993;100:516–523.

23. Kenyon S, Boulvain M. Antibiotics for preterm premature rupture of membranes. In: The Cochrane Library, Issue 4, 2000 Oxford: Update Software. Search date 1999; primary source Cochrane Pregnancy Childbirth Group Trials Register.

24. Hofmeyr GJ. Amnioinfusion for preterm rupture of membranes. In: The Cochrane Library, Issue 4, 2000 Oxford: Update Software. Search date 1998; primary sources Cochrane Pregnancy and Childbirth Group Trials Register and Cochrane Register of Controlled Trials.

25. Gyetvai K, Hannah ME, Hodnett ED, et al. Tocolytics for preterm labor: A systematic review. *Obstet Gynecol* 1999;94:869–877. Search date 1998; primary sources Medline and Cochrane Register of Controlled Trials.

26. Moutquin J-M, Sherman D, Cohen H, et al. Double-blind, randomized, controlled trial of atosiban and ritodrine in the treatment of preterm labour: A multicenter effectiveness and safety study. *Am J Obstet Gynecol* 2000;182:1191–1199.

27. Romero R, Sibai BM, Sanchez-Ramos L, et al. An oxytocin receptor antagonist (atosiban) in the treatment of preterm labor: a randomized, double-blind, placebo-controlled trial with tocolytic rescue. *Am J Obstet Gynecol* 2000;182;1173–1183.

28. Hannah M, Amankwah K, Barret J, et al. The Canadian consensus on the use of tocolytics for preterm labour. *J SOGC* 1995;17:1089–1115.

29. Crowley P. Prophylactic corticosteroids for preterm birth. In: The Cochrane Library, Issue 4, 2000. Oxford: Update Software. Search date 1996; primary sources Cochrane Pregnancy and Childbirth Group Trials Register.

30. Baud O, Foix-L'Helias L, Kaminski M, et al. Antenatal glucocorticoid treatment and cyctic periventricular leokomalacia in very premature infants. *N Engl J Med* 1999;341:1190–1196.

31. Crowther CA, Alfirevic Z, Haslam RR. Prenatal thyrotropin-releasing hormone (TRH) for preterm birth. In: The Cochrane Library, Issue 4, 2000 Oxford: Update Software. Search date 1999; primary source Cochrane Pregnancy and Childbirth Group Trials Register.

32. King J, Flenady V. Antibiotics for preterm labour with intact membranes. In: The Cochrane Library, Issue 4, 2000 Oxford: Update Software. Search date 1997; primary sources Cochrane Pregnancy and Childbirth Group Trials Register, personal contacts, and hand searches of reference lists.

Bridgette Byrne

Lecturer in Obstetrics and Gynaecology
University College Dublin
Coombe Womens Hospital
Dublin
Ireland

John Morrison

Professor of Obstetrics and Gynaecology
Clinical Science Institute
University College Hospital
Galway
Ireland

Competing interests: None declared.

TABLE 1 The effects of antibiotics after premature preterm rupture of membranes: results of placebo controlled RCTs (see text, p 1000).[23]

Outcome	Absolute risks		ARR (95% CI)	OR (95% CI)	NNT (95% CI)
	Antibiotic	Control			
Born within 48 hours of rupture	140/513 (27%)	207/545 (38%)	11% (6% to 16%)	0.6 (0.46 to 0.77)	9 (6 to 17)
Born within 7 days of rupture	283/483 (59%)	364/508 (72%)	14% (8% to 21%)	0.54 (0.41 to 0.70)	7 (5 to 13)
Chorioamnionitis	122/736 (17%)	188/763 (25%)	8% (4% to 11%)	0.61 (0.47 to 0.79)	12 (9 to 24)
Neonatal infection	86/775 (11%)	127/799 (16%)	5% (2% to 8%)	0.62 (0.45 to 0.86)	18 (12 to 52)
Perinatal death	50/700 (7%)	53/732 (7%)	0.1% (−3% to +2%)	0.98 (0.66 to 1.47)	–
Necrotising enterocolitis	43/611 (7%)	48/644 (7.5%)	0.4% (−2.9% to +2.7%)	0.93 (0.61 to 1.44)	–

| TABLE 2 | Effects of amnioinfusion after premature preterm rupture of membranes: results of RCT (see text, p 1001).[24] |

| Outcome | Absolute risks | | OR (95% CI) |
	Antibiotic	Control	
Caesarean section	2/29	7/32	0.31 (0.08 to 1.26)
Low Apgar scores	1/29	4/32	0.31 (0.05 to 1.88)
Neonatal death	1/29	2/32	0.55 (0.06 to 5.56)
Endometritis	2/29	3/32	0.03 (0.05 to 2.89)

Search date September 2000: expanded this issue

Christopher Cates and Mark FitzGerald

INTERVENTIONS

*No direct randomised evidence available, but highly likely to be effective. Trials unlikely to be conducted.

See glossary, p 1024

Respiratory disorders

In people with chronic asthma

- RCTs have found that regular use of short acting inhaled agonists provides no additional clinical benefits and may worsen asthma control in people with mild intermittent asthma.

- RCTs have found that, in people with mild persistent asthma, low doses of inhaled corticosteroids improve asthma more than placebo or regular β_2 agonists.

- One systematic review and one additional RCT have found that, in people with asthma that is poorly controlled on inhaled corticosteroids, adding long acting, inhaled β_2 agonists improves symptoms and lung function. We found no evidence that regular use of long acting β_2 agonists causes deterioration in asthma control.

- RCTs have found that leukotriene antagonists added to short acting β_2 agonists alone significantly reduce asthma symptoms and β_2 agonist use more than placebo. One systematic review found no significant difference in the rate of exacerbations between leukotriene antagonists versus inhaled corticosteroids, but inhaled corticosteroids significantly increased quality of life, lung function, and symptom control.

In people with acute exacerbations of asthma

- One systematic review found no difference in efficacy between β_2 agonists delivered by spacer device/holding chamber versus nebulisers.

- Two systematic reviews have found that systemic corticosteroids taken at the start of an acute exacerbation reduce rates of admission and relapse, although one recent systematic review found no significant difference in the rates of admission. There was no significant difference between oral corticosteroids versus inhaled or intramuscular corticosteroids. We found no evidence on the optimal dose or duration of treatment.

- One large RCT has found that continuous treatment with short acting β_2 agonists improves FEV_1 more than as needed treatment. Other smaller RCTs found no significant difference.

- We found conflicting evidence from RCTs of intravenous short acting β_2 agonists versus nebulised short acting β_2 agonists in acute exacerbations. Intravenous administration was associated with more adverse effects.

- One systematic review and one subsequent RCT have found that combining short acting β_2 agonists with ipratropium bromide significantly reduces hospital admissions, and improves lung function in people with more severe acute asthma.

- There is a strong consensus that oxygen should be a key component of acute treatment. We found no RCTs of oxygen therapy. Clinical monitoring and case control studies have found that people with near fatal asthma suffer from significant hypoxaemia.

- Subgroup analysis from one systematic review suggests that intravenous magnesium sulphate may reduce rates of hospital admission in people with severe acute asthma. One small subsequent RCT found that nebulised magnesium sulphate improved peak expiratory flow rate (PEFR) significantly more than saline.

- We found no RCT of mechanical ventilation, but clinical experience, historical cohort studies, and case-series suggest that it is likely to reduce death rates in near fatal asthma.

- One non-systematic review has found that specialist care is more effective than generalist care for people with acute exacerbations of asthma.

- One systematic review has found that asthma self management involving asthma education reduces hospital admission, unscheduled visits to physicians, and days off work.

DEFINITION	Asthma is characterised by dyspnoea, cough, chest tightness, wheezing, variable airflow obstruction, and airway hyperresponsiveness. The diurnal variation of PEFR is increased in people with asthma. **Chronic asthma** is defined here as asthma requiring maintenance treatment. Asthma is classified differently in the USA and UK (see table 1, p 1027): where necessary, the text specifies the system of classification used.[1,2] **Acute asthma** is defined here as an exacerbation of underlying asthma requiring urgent or emergency treatment.
INCIDENCE/ PREVALENCE	Reported prevalence of asthma is increasing worldwide. About 10% of people have suffered an attack of asthma.[3,4]
AETIOLOGY/ RISK FACTORS	Most people with asthma are atopic; exposure to certain stimuli initiates inflammation and structural changes in airways, causing airway hyperresponsiveness and variable airflow obstruction, which in turn cause most asthma symptoms. Stimuli include environmental allergens, occupational sensitising agents, and respiratory viral infections.[5,6]
PROGNOSIS	**Chronic asthma:** In people with mild asthma, prognosis is good and progression to severe disease is rare. However, as a group, people with asthma lose lung function faster than those without asthma, although less quickly than people without asthma who smoke.[7] People with persistent asthma can improve with treatment. However, for reasons not clearly understood, some people (possibly up to 5%) have severe disease that responds poorly to treatment. These people are most at risk of morbidity and death from asthma. **Acute asthma:** About 10–20% of people presenting to the emergency department with asthma are admitted to hospital. Of these, fewer than 10% receive mechanical ventilation,[8,9] although previous ventilation is associated with a 19-fold increased risk of ventilation for a subsequent episode.[10] It is unusual for people to die unless they have suffered respiratory arrest before reaching hospital.[11] One prospective study of 939 people discharged from emergency care found that 17% (95% CI 14% to 20%) relapsed by 2 weeks.[12]
AIMS	To minimise or eliminate symptoms; to maximise lung function; to prevent exacerbations; to minimise the need for medication; to minimise adverse effects of treatment; and to provide enough information and support to facilitate self management of asthma.
OUTCOMES	Symptoms (daytime and nocturnal); lung function (PEFR and FEV_1 — see glossary, p 1024); need for rescue medication such as inhaled β_2 agonists; variability of flow rates; activities of daily living; adverse effects of treatment.
METHODS	*Clinical Evidence* update search and appraisal September 2000, using the following key words for the acute sections: acute asthma, therapy, β agonists, oxygen, corticosteroids, anticholinergics, mechanical ventilation, magnesium sulphate, and asthma education. Additional sources identified by experts.

Respiratory disorders

Christopher Cates

OPTION REGULAR VERSUS AS NEEDED USE OF SHORT ACTING, INHALED β_2 AGONISTS IN ADULTS WITH MILD, INTERMITTENT ASTHMA

RCTs have found that regular use of short acting inhaled β_2 agonists in people with mild, intermittent asthma provides no additional clinical benefits, compared with as needed use, and may worsen asthma control.

Benefits: We found no systematic review. We found several RCTs comparing regular versus as needed inhaled salbutamol (see glossary, p 1024). The most recent RCT (983 people with asthma in a general practice setting, 90% using regular inhaled corticosteroids) compared as needed versus regular salbutamol (400 µg four times daily).[13] At 1 year, it found no significant difference between regular versus as needed salbutamol in the rate of exacerbations (RR 0.96, 95% CI 0.8 to 1.15) or in morning PEFR. Evening PEFR was significantly higher with regular salbutamol (difference 10.3 l/ minute, 95% CI 6.7 to 14.0), and as a consequence diurnal variation (see glossary, p 1024) was also higher (difference 3.3%, 95% CI 2.5% to 4.1%).[13] Another RCT (255 people with mild, intermittent asthma taking inhaled β agonists only) compared regular versus as needed salbutamol.[14] At 16 weeks, there was no significant difference between the groups in symptoms, quality of life, airflow obstruction, or frequency of exacerbations. People taking regular salbutamol used more medication than those taking it as needed (total salbutamol 9.3 v 1.6 puffs/day), and experienced significantly greater variability in PEFR (see glossary, p 1024) and methacholine responsiveness. earlier placebo controlled, double blind crossover trial (64 people taking inhaled or oral corticosteroids and/or inhaled cromoglycate if usually required) found that of the 57 people who had better control during active treatment periods, most did better with as needed versus regular treatment (40 v 17). In addition, five of the six severe exacerbations occurred in people taking regular versus as needed fenoterol.[15] Exacerbations were not prevented by inhaled corticosteroids.

Harms: Two case control studies found an association between increased asthma mortality, and overuse of inhaled short acting β_2 agonists.[16,17] The evidence does not establish causality, as overusing β_2 agonists to treat frequent symptoms may simply indicate severe, uncontrolled asthma in high risk individuals. Other RCTs found that regular use of inhaled β_2 agonists was associated with transient rebound deterioration in airway hyperresponsiveness after stopping the medication,[18] and increased allergen induced bronchoconstriction.[19] Tremor was commonly reported, but tolerance developed with more frequent use.[20]

Comment: In the most recent RCT, 33% of people randomised did not complete the trial, reducing the power of the RCT to detect a significant difference between regular versus as needed salbutamol.[13]

| OPTION | LOW DOSES OF INHALED CORTICOSTEROIDS IN PEOPLE WITH MILD, PERSISTENT ASTHMA |

RCTs have found that, in people with mild, persistent asthma, low doses of inhaled corticosteroids (250–500 µg of beclomethasone dipropionate or equivalent) significantly improve symptoms and lung function more than placebo or regular β_2 agonists. We found no evidence of clinically important adverse effects in adults.

Benefits:
Versus placebo: We found no systematic review. We found seven placebo controlled RCTs (1000 adults and adolescents with mild, persistent asthma, using US classification; see table 1, p 1027) evaluating low doses of inhaled budesonide,[21–24] beclomethasone,[25,26] and triamcinolone.[26–28] They all found significant improvement in lung function, symptoms, and short acting bronchodilator use compared with placebo. **Versus β_2 agonists:** We found one systematic review (search date not stated, 5 small RCTs, 141 adults with mild persistent asthma using regular inhaled corticosteroids, ≤ 2 drugs to control asthma).[29] It found that inhaled corticosteroids significantly improved lung function (overall weighted effect size for PEFR 0.59, 95% CI 0.32 to 0.84). One RCT not included in the review (103 adults with mild asthma, diagnosed within 12 months, not using oral corticosteroids) found that inhaled budesonide 1200 µg/day versus inhaled β_2 agonists persistently and significantly improved all outcomes over 2 years (no CI available).[30]

Harms:
We found no published evidence that low doses of inhaled corticosteroids (< 1000 µg/day of beclomethasone dipropionate or equivalent) cause important systemic effects in adults.[31] Although posterior subcapsular cataracts occur more frequently in people taking oral corticosteroids,[32] most studies in adults provide no evidence that inhaled corticosteroids increase the risk once the confounding effect of oral corticosteroids is removed.[33] However, one recent population based, case control study suggested that, in older people, inhaled high dose beclomethasone dipropionate was associated with a slightly greater risk of nuclear cataracts (RR 1.5, 95% CI 1.2 to 1.9) and posterior subcapsular cataracts (RR 1.9, 95% CI 1.3 to 2.8).[34] We found no published reports of an increased risk of osteoporosis or fractures. Inhaled corticosteroids can cause oral candidiasis, dysphonia, and bruising, but these are troublesome in fewer than 5% of people.[35,36]

Comment:
The results of the systematic review should be interpreted with caution as the few small RCTs included neither consistently measured PEFR at the same time of the day nor reported morning and evening PEFRs.[29] The case control study on cataract formation did not allow for the confounding effect of allergy,[34] which is also a risk factor for cataract development.[37]

| OPTION | ADDITION OF LONG ACTING INHALED β_2 AGONISTS IN PEOPLE WHOSE ASTHMA IS POORLY CONTROLLED BY INHALED CORTICOSTEROIDS |

One systematic review and one additional RCT have found that, in people with poorly controlled asthma, adding regular doses of long acting, inhaled β_2 agonists to inhaled corticosteroids improves symptoms and lung function. Unlike regular use of short acting β_2 agonists, regular use of long acting β_2 agonists has not been linked to deterioration in asthma control. We found no good evidence relating to their effect on mortality.

Benefits: **Versus placebo:** We found no systematic review. We found two RCTs (506 and 217 people with moderate, persistent asthma, which was not controlled on inhaled corticosteroids 250–2000 µg/day beclomethasone or equivalent)[38,39] comparing regular, long acting inhaled β_2 agonists versus placebo. These trials found that twice daily salmeterol or formoterol improved quality of life scores, PEFR, and FEV_1 more than placebo. Exacerbation rates were not significantly different between the two groups in either trial. **Versus increased use of inhaled corticosteroids:** We found one systematic review[40] and one additional RCT.[41] The review (search date 1999, 9 double blind RCTs, 3685 people with symptomatic asthma on their current dose of inhaled steroids, duration 3–6 months) compared adding salmeterol versus increased use of inhaled corticosteroids (at least double the usual dose). It found that morning PEFR was significantly higher with salmeterol (3 months: WMD in PEFR 22 l/minute, 95% CI 15 to 30, P < 0.001; 6 months: WMD 28 l/minute, 95% CI 19 to 36). Salmeterol versus higher dose corticosteroids significantly increased days without symptoms (WMD at 6 months: 15, 95% CI 12 to 18) and nights without symptoms (WMD at 6 months: 5, 95% CI 3 to 7). Salmeterol versus higher dose corticosteroids also significantly reduced the need for rescue medication. No increase in asthma exacerbations of any severity was found in the salmeterol group.[40] The additional RCT (852 people taking low to moderate dose inhaled corticosteroids) found that additional twice daily formoterol plus as needed terbutaline versus no additional treatment significantly improved symptoms and lung function, and reduced exacerbations.[41] Exacerbations were reduced further by a fourfold increase in daily dosage of inhaled corticosteroid, and further still by combined, higher dose of budesonide plus formoterol.

Harms: Several studies have found that people taking regular doses of long acting, inhaled β_2 agonists develop tolerance to protection against bronchoconstriction,[42–44] and may develop a tremor. Short acting inhaled β_2 agonists are associated with deterioration in asthma control and increased risk of death.[15–17] Regular use of long acting inhaled β_2 agonists has not been linked to deterioration in asthma control.

Comment: We found no RCTs or other studies with sufficient power to assess the effect of regular use of long acting inhaled β_2 agonists on death rates.[45]

LEUKOTRIENE ANTAGONISTS IN ADULTS WITH MILD TO MODERATE, PERSISTENT ASTHMA New

RCTs have found that leukotriene antagonists versus placebo added to β_2 agonists significantly reduce asthma symptoms and β_2 agonist use. One systematic review found no significant difference in the rate of exacerbations between leukotriene antagonists versus inhaled corticosteroids, but inhaled corticosteroids significantly increased quality of life, lung function, and symptom control.

Benefits: **Versus placebo:** We found no systematic review. We found three RCTs (1300 adults with asthma taking β_2 agonists alone), which compared the addition of leukotriene antagonists versus placebo for 13 weeks.[46–48] The RCTs found consistently that zafirlukast (20 mg twice daily) versus placebo significantly reduced daytime and night time asthma symptoms, and β_2 agonist use. The largest RCT (762 people)[46] found that zafirlukast versus placebo significantly reduced daytime symptoms, night time awakenings, and β_2 agonist use (zafirlukast v placebo: 3.9 v 3.1 puffs per day; $P < 0.01$). Morning FEV_1 was significantly increased in people taking zafirlukast (morning FEV_1 improved by 7% v 3%, $P < 0.01$).[46]

Versus inhaled corticosteroids: We found one systematic review (search date 1999, 8 RCTs, > 2000 adults with asthma),[49] and one subsequent RCT.[50] The review compared various leukotriene antagonists with inhaled corticosteroids for 6–12 weeks. Doses of corticosteroids were equivalent to beclomethasone 250 µg to 400 µg daily. The review found no significant difference between leukotriene antagonists versus corticosteroids in the number of people with exacerbations who required systemic steroids (4 RCTs, RR 1.3, 95% CI 0.9 to 1.9). However, corticosteroids versus leukotriene antagonists significantly improved lung function (FEV_1: 3 RCTs, SMD 0.3, 95% CI 0.2 to 0.4), morning PEFR (3 RCTs, SMD 0.4, 95% CI 0.2 to 0.5), quality of life (3 RCTs, WMD 0.3, 95% CI 0.1 to 0.4), symptoms (3 RCTs, SMD 0.3, 95% CI 0.2 to 0.4), night awakenings (2 RCTs, WMD 0.6, 95% CI 0.3 to 0.9), and reduced the need for rescue β_2 agonists (3 RCTs, SMD 0.3, 95% CI 0.2 to 0.4).[49] The subsequent RCT (451 adults with asthma, previously treated with β_2 agonists alone) compared fluticasone 88 mg with zafirlukast 20 mg, both twice daily for 12 weeks.[50] The RCT found results consistent with the systematic review for exacerbations, lung function, day and night symptoms, and use of rescue β_2 agonists.

Harms: In the RCT comparing zafirlukast versus placebo, the incidence of adverse effects (predominantly pharyngitis and headache) was similar in both groups (350/514 [68%] v 160/248 [65%]).[46] The systematic review found that adverse effects were not significantly different with leukotriene antagonist versus corticosteroids, but leukotriene antagonists significantly increased the risk of "withdrawals for any cause" (RR 1.4, 95% CI 1.1 to 1.9), and "withdrawals due to adverse effects" (RR 1.9, 95% CI 1.1 to 3.3).[49]

Comment: The systematic review found that few RCTs providing results about specific outcomes and included few unpublished trials. The results should therefore be interpreted cautiously.

| QUESTION | What are the effects of treatments for acute asthma? |

Mark FitzGerald

| OPTION | SPACER DEVICES/HOLDING CHAMBERS VERSUS NEBULISERS FOR DELIVERING β_2 AGONISTS |

One systematic review of RCTs found no difference in efficacy between nebulisers and holding chambers with metered dose inhalers for delivering β_2 agonists in people with acute but not life threatening asthma.

Benefits:
We found one systematic review (search date 1999, 13 RCTs, non-hospitalised adults and children with acute asthma) comparing holding chambers plus metered dose inhalers versus nebulisation for delivering β_2 agonists.[51] Results in adults and children were analysed separately (see asthma in children, p 189). In adults, there was no significant difference in rates of hospital admission (OR 1.12, 95% CI 0.45 to 2.76), length of time spent in the emergency department (WMD +0.02 hours, 95% CI –0.40 to +0.44 hours), or in PEFR or FEV_1. There was still no significant difference when the three studies involving the most severely affected people (FEV_1 < 30% predicted) were included (WMD for FEV_1 holding chamber v nebuliser –1.5% predicted, 95% CI –8.3% to +5.3%). Symptoms were measured on different scales and findings could not be combined.

Harms:
The review found no significant difference in heart rates between the two methods (WMD with holding chamber v nebuliser +1.6% of baseline, 95% CI –2.4% to +5.5% of baseline).

Comment:
The review found no evidence of publication bias. To overcome possible dose confounding, the review was confined to studies that used multiple treatment doses titrated against the individuals' responses. As studies excluded people with life threatening asthma, results may not generalise to such people.

| OPTION | ORAL CORTICOSTEROIDS IN ACUTE ASTHMA |

Two systematic reviews have found that systemic corticosteroids taken at the start of an acute exacerbation reduce rates of admission and relapse, and the need for additional β_2 agonists, without increasing adverse effects. One systematic review found no significant difference in rates of hospital admission. There was no significant difference between oral corticosteroids versus inhaled or intramuscular corticosteroids. We found no evidence on the optimal dose or duration of treatment.

Benefits:
Rates of admission: We found three systematic reviews.[52-54] The most recent systematic review (search date 2000, 7 RCTs, 1204 people)[52] compared oral versus inhaled corticosteroids and found no significant difference in the admission rate (2 RCTs, OR 1.0, 95% CI 0.4 to 2.5). The second systematic review (search date 1997, 7 RCTs in about 320 people) compared oral corticosteroids versus placebo (4 RCTs), oral versus intramuscular corticosteroids (2 RCTs), and intramuscular corticosteroids versus placebo (1 RCT).[53]

It found that systemic corticosteroids given during an acute asthma exacerbation reduced the number of relapses requiring additional care (first week: RR v placebo 0.39, 95% CI 0.21 to 0.74; NNT 10. First 21 days: RR 0.47, 95% CI 0.25 to 0.89) and reduced hospital admissions (RR 0.35, 95% CI 0.13 to 0.95). Corticosteroids reduced the use of β_2 agonists (WMD −3.3 activations/day, 95% CI −5.5 to −1.0). The review found no clear difference between intramuscular and oral corticosteroids. The third, earlier systematic review (search date 1991, 5 RCTs, 422 people) compared systemic corticosteroids versus placebo.[54] It also found that early use of systemic corticosteroids reduced hospital admissions and relapses in both adults and children (OR of hospital admission in adults for corticosteroids v placebo: 0.47, 95% CI 0.27 to 0.79). **Stopping treatment:** We found no systematic review. One RCT (35 people admitted to hospital with acute asthma) compared tapering of prednisolone over a week versus abrupt cessation. It found that 0.5–1 mg/kg a day for 10 days was effective and, once asthma control was re-established, could be stopped without tapering.[55] **Optimal dose and duration of treatment:** We found no systematic review or RCTs. The optimal duration of treatment is likely to depend on the individual, the severity of the exacerbation, and use of concomitant medications.

Harms: Systemic corticosteroids can cause the same adverse effects in asthma as in other diseases, even when administered for a short time (see asthma in children, p 189).

Comment: We found no reliable evidence about the role of oral corticosteroids in acute asthma after admission to hospital, nor is it likely that a placebo controlled RCT would be conducted in acute severe asthma. One RCT (413 adults presenting to general practitioners with acute asthma) found no difference in rates of treatment failure between a short course of oral steroids and a high dose of inhaled fluticasone.[56]

OPTION	CONTINUOUS VERSUS AS NEEDED SHORT ACTING β_2 AGONISTS FOR ACUTE ASTHMA

One RCT has found that continuous versus as needed β_2 agonists in acute asthma is associated with greater improvement in FEV_1. Other smaller RCTs found no significant difference. In adults with more severe airflow obstruction, RCTs consistently found that continuous nebulised treatment improved outcome more than intermittent treatment.

Benefits: We found no systematic review. We found seven RCTs.[9,57–62] The first, larger RCT (99 people) found that, in a subgroup of 69 people with more severe asthma, continuous aerosol delivery versus as needed delivery increased PEFR at 120 minutes (296 l/minute, 95% CI 266 to 329 with continuous v 244 l/minute, 95% CI 216 to 272 with as needed delivery).[57] Hospital admissions were also significantly lower with continuous delivery (11/35 [28%] v 19/34 [57%], P = 0.03). The *post hoc* nature of the analysis weakens these results. One RCT (38 people) found no significant difference in FEV_1 improvement between continuous and as needed salbutamol. Subgroup analysis found a greater improvement in FEV_1 with continuous treatment in people with lower initial FEV_1.[59] Another

RCT (165 people) compared four regimens of salbutamol in a factorial design: high (1.5 mg) versus standard (0.5 mg) doses, and continuous versus as needed delivery. It found greater improvement in FEV_1 at 2 hours with continuous versus as needed delivery at both high and standard doses.[61]

Harms: Commonly reported, mild adverse effects associated with frequent dosing include tachycardia, tremor, and headache. Metabolic upsets are less common, and include hypokalemia. One RCT found the highest rate of adverse effects with high dose as needed treatment. The most common adverse effect was tremor (24% as needed high dose, 20% continuous high dose, 9.3% hourly standard dose, and 2.5% continuous standard dose).[61]

Comment: We also found one RCT (46 adults in hospital), which addressed the slightly different, but related question of regular nebulised salbutamol (5 mg every 4 hours) versus on demand salbutamol (2.5–5 mg).[63] It found that on demand dosage was significantly associated with shorter hospital stay (3.7 days v 4.7 days), reduced number of nebulisations (geometric mean 7.0 v 14, P = 0.003), and fewer palpitations (P = 0.049).

OPTION   INTRAVENOUS VERSUS NEBULISED DELIVERY OF SHORT ACTING β_2 AGONISTS FOR ACUTE ASTHMA

RCTs found conflicting evidence on the effect of intravenous versus nebulised salbutamol. Intravenous salbutamol was associated with more adverse effects.

Benefits: We found no systematic review, and conflicting results from three RCTs comparing intravenous versus nebulised salbutamol.[64–66] The largest trial (76 people who had not responded to nebulised salbutamol after 30 minutes) compared nebulised treatment at 30 minutes and 2 hours versus intravenous salbutamol. It found greater bronchodilation in the intravenous group (FEV_1 improved by 25% with intravenous v 14% with nebulised salbutamol; difference 11%, 95% CI 2.4% to 19%).[66] The second, multicentre RCT (47 people) found that nebulised salbutamol (total 10 mg) was more effective than intravenous salbutamol (0.5 mg) over 1 hour (19/22 responded with nebulised v 12/25 with intravenous salbutamol, P = 0.006).[64] The third RCT (16 people) found no significant difference in FEV_1, but greater self reported improvement in symptoms among those treated with inhaled salbutamol.[65]

Harms: All trials found more adverse effects with intravenous delivery.[64–66] In the largest RCT, two of 39 people in the intravenous group withdrew because of tachyardia.[66] In the nebulised salbutamol group none withdrew because of adverse effects, but three people withdrew because of lack of effect.

Comment: None.

OPTION   ADDITION OF IPRATROPIUM BROMIDE TO β_2 AGONISTS IN ACUTE ASTHMA

One systematic review and one subsequent RCT have found that combining short acting β_2 agonists with ipratropium bromide significantly reduces hospital admissions, and improves lung function in people with more severe acute asthma.

Benefits: We found one systematic review (search date 1999, 5 RCTs evaluating hospital admissions)[67] and one subsequent RCT.[68] The review compared salbutamol plus inhaled ipratropium bromide versus salbutamol alone, and found that the addition of ipratropium significantly reduced hospital admissions (OR 0.62, 95% CI 0.44 to 0.88; NNT 18, 95% CI 11 to 77). Meta-analysis of the four trials that evaluated people with severe airflow obstruction ($FEV_1 < 35\%$) found that additional treatment with ipratropium bromide improved FEV_1 over 90 minutes (effect size 0.38, 95% CI 0.05 to 0.67). The subsequent RCT (180 people with acute asthma, mean $FEV_1 < 50\%$) compared salbutamol plus placebo versus salbutamol plus ipratroprium.[68] It found that the addition of ipratropium significantly improved PEFR (difference in improvement with ipratroprium v placebo: 21%, 95% CI 2.6% to 38%), and FEV_1 (difference in improvement with ipratroprium v placebo: 48%, 95% CI 20% to 76%). People taking ipratropium were significantly less likely to require hospital admission at the end of the 3 hour trial period (20% v 39%, P = 0.01).

Harms: Addition of ipratropium bromide had no significant effect on adverse effects.[68]

Comment: None.

<hr>

OPTION	OXYGEN

We found no systematic review or RCTs of oxygen in acute asthma. However, experience and pathophysiology suggest that its role is vital in acute asthma. Small RCTs found mixed evidence that combining oxygen with helium may improve PEFR.

Benefits: **Oxygen alone:** We found no systematic review and no RCTs. **Oxygen with helium:** We found three RCTs of combined helium (70% or 80%) and oxygen (30% or 20%) in adults with acute asthma.[69–71] One RCT included 27 people; PEFR < 250 l/minute despite treatment, pulsus paradoxus (see glossary, p 1024) > 15 mmHg. Breathing a helium–oxygen mixture (80 : 20) compared with breathing room air alone reduced pulsus paradoxus and improved peak flow (results presented only as a graph).[69] The second RCT (23 people) found the helium–oxygen combination versus 30% oxygen increased PEFR (58% with helium–oxygen v 10% with oxygen).[70] The third RCT (205 people) found no evidence of benefit from helium plus oxygen, but it was limited by a brief intervention (15 minutes), single blinding, and inclusion of people with mild to moderate acute asthma.[71]

Harms: We found no evidence of adverse effects associated with oxygen alone or with helium–oxygen in acute asthma.

Comment: The most severe stages of acute asthma are respiratory failure, cardiopulmonary arrest, and death.[10,11] Studies of near fatal asthma suggest that hypoxia rather than arrhythmias account for asthma deaths. It seems reasonable that supplemental oxygen should continue to form a critical part of management even though we found no RCTs providing direct evidence for this. Peak flow readings vary depending on the viscosity of the gas being delivered (helium is less dense than oxygen, so non-standardised measures of peak flow will increase relative to air, even if the mixture has no effect on airway narrowing). It was not clear in all studies whether peak flow readings were standardised for air and for helium–oxygen mixtures.

| OPTION | INTRAVENOUS MAGNESIUM SULPHATE |

Valid subgroup analysis from one systematic review suggests that, in people with more severe acute asthma, adding intravenous magnesium sulphate to usual treatment may reduce rates of hospital admission. One small subsequent RCT found that nebulised magnesium sulphate improved PEFR significantly more than saline.

Benefits: We found one systematic review (search date 1999, 5 RCTs in adults, 3 RCTs in children, 665 people),[72] and one subsequent RCT.[73] The review compared the addition of intravenous magnesium sulphate versus placebo with usual treatment, and found no significant difference in hospital admissions (OR 0.31, 95% CI 0.09 to 1.02). Prespecified subgroup analysis of adults with more severe airflow obstruction (sample size not given; $FEV_1 < 30\%$ at presentation, failure to respond to initial treatment, or failure to improve beyond 60% in FEV_1 after 1 hour) found that those receiving magnesium sulphate had better PEFR and reduced rates of hospital admission. The subsequent RCT (35 people) compared salbutamol plus saline versus salbutamol plus magnesium sulphate through a nebuliser. It found that magnesium sulphate versus saline significantly increased PEFR (increase in PEFR after 10 minutes: 61% v 31%; difference 30%, 95% CI 3 to 56%; P = 0.03).[73]

Harms: We found no significant adverse effects associated with treatment.

Comment: Further studies are needed to clarify the role of intravenous magnesium sulphate in acute asthma. Two of the studies involved treatment with aminophylline and one with ipratropium, both of which have been found to affect hospital admission rates without affecting the degree of airflow obstruction.[74] The subgroup analysis involved intergroup and intragroup analyses specified before the trial was conducted, and so provides reasonably strong evidence of an effect.

| OPTION | MECHANICAL VENTILATION |

We found no RCTs comparing mechanical ventilation versus no ventilation for severe acute asthma. Evidence from cohort studies and case series support its use, despite a high level of morbidity related to the intervention.

Benefits: We found no systematic reviews or RCTs.

Harms: Mechanical ventilation is associated with hypotension, barotrauma, infection, and myopathy, especially when prolonged paralysis is required with muscle relaxants and systemic corticosteroids.[75] Adverse effects reported in one retrospective study of 88 episodes of mechanical ventilation were hypotension (20%), pulmonary barotrauma (14%), and arrhythmias (10%).[76]

Comment: Experience suggests that mechanical ventilation is a life saving intervention needed by a small minority of people with severe acute asthma. Cohort studies[77,78] and one case series[79] found fewer deaths with controlled hypoventilation compared with ventilation in which carbon dioxide levels were normalised (for which historical cohorts and case series have reported mortality rates of 7.5–23%).[76,80–82] Non-invasive ventilation has been used in people with acute exacerbations of chronic obstructive lung disease,[83] but requires prospective validation in people with acute asthma. Future research should focus on delivery of bronchodilators, optimal use of muscle relaxants, and dose of corticosteroids.

OPTION   SPECIALIST VERSUS GENERALIST CARE

Non-randomised trials suggest that specialist care is more effective than generalist care.

Benefits: We found no systematic review and no RCTs. One non-systematic review of controlled trials (search date 1999) found that "expert based" care was associated with improved outcomes.[84] One trial quasi-randomised people (based on day of attendance) referred from the emergency department to specialist care versus routine general medical follow up.[85] It found that people receiving specialist care were significantly less likely to wake at night (OR 0.24, 95% CI 0.11 to 0.52), suffer relapse requiring emergency admission by 6 months (for one admission RR 0.56, 95% CI 0.34 to 0.95; for two admissions RR 0.3, 95% CI 0.16 to 0.6), or suffer multiple relapses. They were more likely to use inhaled corticosteroids (OR 3.6, 95% CI 1.9 to 6.6) and cromolyn (RR 2.2, 95% CI 1.9 to 2.5).

Harms: We found no harms associated with specialist versus generalist care.

Comment: None.

OPTION   ASTHMA EDUCATION FOR PEOPLE WITH ACUTE ASTHMA

One systematic review of RCTs has found that education to facilitate self management of asthma in adults reduces hospital admission, unscheduled visits to the doctor, and days off work.

Benefits: We found one systematic review (search date 1999, 22 RCTs) of adult self management of asthma.[86] The review found that education about asthma to facilitate self management, whether initiated from a specialist or generalist setting, significantly reduced the risk of hospital admission (RR 0.62, 95% CI 0.41 to 0.96; NNT 38, 95% CI 20 to 382), unscheduled visits to the doctor (RR 0.74, 95% CI 0.63 to 0.90; NNT 12, 95% CI 8 to 36), and days off work (RR 0.75, 95% CI 0.63 to 0.90; NNT 7, 95% CI 5 to 13). Best results were achieved in people who had written care plans.

Harms: None reported.

Comment: None.

GLOSSARY

Diurnal variation A characteristic of people with asthma is increased variation in peak flow rates and FEV_1 during the day. The diurnal variation is sometimes expressed as the difference between maximum and minimum values expressed as a fraction of the maximum value.

Forced expiratory volume in 1 second (FEV_1) The volume breathed out in the first second of forceful blowing into a spirometer, measured in litres.

Peak expiratory flow rate (PEFR) The maximum rate that gas is expired from the lungs when blowing into a peak flow meter or a spirometer. It is measured at an instant, but the units are expressed as litres per minute.

Pulsus paradoxus A measure of the severity of asthma based on the difference in systolic pressure during inspiration and expiration. The blood pressure normally falls a little during inspiration ($< 10\,mmHg$), but in acute severe asthma (and in some other conditions) the fall of systolic pressure in inspiration is greater.

Salbutamol A short acting β_2 agonist known as albuterol in the USA.

Substantive changes since last issue

Regular versus as needed short acting β_2 agonists New RCT;[13] conclusions unchanged.

Addition of long acting β_2 agonists New systematic review;[40] conclusions unchanged.

Oral corticosteroids New systematic review;[52] conclusions unchanged.

Continuous versus as needed β_2 agonists Two new RCTs;[9,62] conclusions unchanged.

Addition of ipratropium to β_2 agonists New RCT;[67] conclusions unchanged.

Intravenous magnesium sulphate New RCT;[73] conclusions unchanged.

REFERENCES

1. National Heart, Blood and Lung Institute. National Asthma Education and Prevention Program. Expert Panel Report 2. Guidelines for the Diagnosis and Management of Asthma. NIH Publication No. 97–4051;July 1997:20.
2. British Thoracic Society Guidelines. *Thorax* 1997; 52:S1–S2.
3. Kaur B, Anderson HR, Austin J, et al. Prevalence of asthma symptoms, diagnosis, and treatment in 12–14 year old children across Great Britain (international study of asthma and allergies in childhood, ISAAC UK). *BMJ* 1998;316:118–124.
4. Woolcock AJ, Peat JK. Evidence for an increase in asthma world-wide. *Ciba Found Symp* 1997;206: 122–134.
5. Duff AL, Platts-Mills TA. Allergens and asthma. *Pediatr Clin North Am* 1992;39:1277–1291.
6. Chan-Yeung M, Malo JL. Occupational asthma. *N Engl J Med* 1995;333:107–112.
7. Lange P, Parner J, Vestbo J, Schnohr P, Jensen G. A 15-year follow-up study of ventilatory function in adults with asthma. *N Engl J Med* 1998;339: 1194–1200.
8. FitzGerald JM, Grunfeld A. Acute life-threatening asthma. In: FitzGerald JM, Ernst PP, Boulet LP, O'Byrne PM, eds. *Evidence based asthma management.* Decker, 2000:233–244.
9. Nahum A, Tuxen DT. Management of asthma in the intensive care unit. In: FitzGerald JM, Ernst PP, Boulet LP, O'Byrne PM, eds. *Evidence based asthma management.* Decker, 2000:245–261.
10. Turner MT, Noertjojo K, Vedal S, Bai T, Crump S, FitzGerald JM. Risk factors for near-fatal asthma: a case control study in patients hospitalised with acute asthma. *Am J Respir Crit Care Med* 1998; 157:1804–1809.
11. Molfino NA, Nannini A, Martelli AN, Slutsky AS. Respiratory arrest in near fatal asthma. *N Engl J Med* 1991;324:285–288.
12. Emmerman CL, Woodruff PG, Cydulka RK, Gibbs MA, Pollack CV, Camargo CA Jr. Prospective multi-center study of relapse following treatment for acute asthma among adults presenting to the emergency department. *Chest* 1999;115:919–927.
13. Dennis SM, Sharp SJ, Vickers MR, et al. Regular inhaled salbutamol and asthma control: the TRUST randomised trial. *Lancet* 2000;355:1675–1679.
14. Drazen JM, Israel E, Boushey HA, et al. Comparison of regularly scheduled with as-needed use of albuterol in mild asthma. Asthma clinical research network. *N Engl J Med* 1996;335:841–847.
15. Sears MR, Taylor DR, Print CG, et al. Regular inhaled β-agonist treatment in bronchial asthma. *Lancet* 1990;336:1391–1396.
16. Spitzer WO, Suissa S, Ernst P, et al. The use of β-agonists and the risk of death and near death from asthma. *N Engl J Med* 1992;326:501–506.
17. Crane J, Pearce N, Flatt A, et al. Prescribed fenoterol and death from asthma in New Zealand, 1981–1983: case-control study. *Lancet* 1989;1: 917–922.
18. Kerrebijn KF, van Essen-Zandvliet EE, Neijens HJ. Effect of long-term treatment with inhaled corticosteroids and β-agonists on the bronchial responsiveness in children with asthma. *J Allergy Clin Immunol* 1987;79:653–659.
19. Cockcroft DW, McParland CP, Britto SA, Swystun VA, Rutherford BC. Regular inhaled salbutamol and airway responsiveness to allergen. *Lancet* 1993;342:833–837.

20. Ahrens RC. Skeletal muscle tremor and the influence of adrenergic drugs. *J Asthma* 1990;27: 11–20.

21. O'Byrne PM, Cuddy L, Taylor DW, Birch S, Morris J, Syrotiuk J. The clinical efficacy and cost benefit of inhaled corticosteroids as therapy in patients with mild asthma in primary care practice. *Can Respir J* 1996;3:169–175.

22. Kemp J, Wanderer AA, Ramsdell J, Southern DL, et al. Rapid onset of control with budesonide turbuhaler in patients with mild-to-moderate asthma. *Ann Allergy Asthma Immunol* 1999;82: 463–471.

23. Busse WW, Chervinsky P, Condemi J, et al. Budesonide delivered by Turbuhaler is effective in a dose-dependent fashion when used in the treatment of adult patients with chronic asthma. *J Allergy Clin Immunol* 1998;101:457–463.

24. McFadden ER, Casale TB, Edwards TB, et al. Administration of budesonide once daily by means of turbuhaler to subjects with stable asthma. *J Allergy Clin Immunol* 1999;104:46–52.

25. Nathan RA, Pinnas JL, Schwartz HJ, Grossman J, et al. A six-month, placebo-controlled comparison of the safety and efficacy of salmeterol or beclomethasone for persistent asthma. *Ann Allergy Asthma Immunol* 1999;82:521–529.

26. Bronsky E, Korenblat P, Harris AG, Chen R. Comparative clinical study of inhaled beclomethasone dipropionate and triamcinolone acetonide in persistent asthma. *Ann Allergy* 1998; 80:295–302.

27. Bernstein DI, Cohen E, Ginchansky E, Pedinoff AJ, Tinkelman DG. A multicenter, placebo-controlled study of twice daily triamcinolone acetonide (800 μg per day) for the treatment of patients with mild-to-moderate asthma. *J Allergy Clin Immunol* 1998;101:433–438.

28. Ramsdell JW, Fish L, Graft D, et al. A controlled trial of twice daily triamcinolone oral inhaler in patients with mild-to-moderate asthma. *Ann Allergy* 1998;80:385–390.

29. Hatoum HT, Schumock GT, Kendzierski DL. Meta-analysis of controlled trials of drug therapy in mild chronic asthma: the role of inhaled corticosteroids. *Ann Pharmacother* 1994;28: 1285–1289. Search date not given; primary source Medline.

30. Haahtela T, Jarvinen M, Tuomo K, et al. Comparison of a β₂ antagonist, terbutaline, with an inhaled corticosteroid, budesonide, in newly detected asthma. *N Engl J Med* 1991;325:388–392.

31. Barnes PJ, Pedersen S, Busse WW. Efficacy and safety of inhaled corticosteroids: new developments. *Am J Respir Crit Care Med* 1998; 157:1–53.

32. Weusten BL, Jacobs JW, Bijlsma JW. Corticosteroid pulse therapy in active rheumatoid arthritis. *Semin Arthritis Rheum* 1993;23:183–192.

33. Toogood JH, Markov AE, Baskerville JC, Dyson C. Association of ocular cataracts with inhaled and oral steroid therapy during long-term treatment of asthma. *J Allergy Clin Immunol* 1993;91:571–579.

34. Cumming RG, Mitchell P, Leeder SR. Use of inhaled corticosteroids and the risk of cataracts. *N Engl J Med* 1997;337:8–14.

35. Toogood JH, Jennings B, Greenway RW, Chuang L. Candidiasis and dysphonia complicating beclomethasone treatment of asthma. *J Allergy Clin Immunol* 1980;65:145–153.

36. Roy A, Levlanc C, Paquette L, Ghezzo H, Cote J, Malo JL. Skin bruising in asthmatic subjects treated with high doses of inhaled steroids: frequency and association with adrenal function. *Eur Respir J* 1996;9:226–231.

37. Eckerskorn U, Hockwin O, Müller-Breitenkamp R, Chen TT, Knowles W, Dobbs RE. Evaluation of cataract-related risk factors using detailed classification systems and multivariate statistical methods. *Dev Ophthalmol* 1987;15:82–91.

38. Kemp JP, Cook DA, Incaudo GA, et al. Salmeterol improves quality of life in patients with asthma requiring inhaled corticosteroids. *J Allergy Clin Immunol* 1998;101:188–195.

39. FitzGerald JM, Chapman KR, Della Cioppa G, et al. Sustained bronchoprotection, bronchodilatation, and symptom control during regular formoterol use in asthma of moderate or greater severity. *J Allergy Clin Immunol* 1999;103:427–435.

40. Shrewsbury S, Pyke S, Britton M. Meta-analysis of increased dose of inhaled steroid or addition of salmeterol in symptomatic asthma (MIASMA). *BMJ* 2000;320:1368–1373. Search date September 1999; primary sources Medline; Embase; and GlaxoWellcome databases.

41. Pauwels RA, Lofdahl C-G, Postma DS, O'Byrne PM, Barnes PJ, Ullman A. Effect of inhaled formoterol and budesonide on exacerbations of asthma. *N Engl J Med* 1997;337:1405–1411.

42. Cheung D, Timmers MC, Zwinderman AH, Bel EH, Dijkman JH, Sterk PJ. Long-term effects of a long-acting β₂-adrenoceptor agonist, salmeterol, on airway hyperresponsiveness in patients with mild asthma. *N Engl J Med* 1992;327:1198–1203.

43. O'Connor BJ, Aikman SL, Barnes PJ. Tolerance to the nonbronchodilating effects of inhaled β₂-agonists in asthma. *N Engl J Med* 1992;327: 1204–1208.

44. Nelson JA, Strauss L, Skowronski M, Ciufo R, Novak R, McFadden ER Jr. Effect of long-term salmeterol treatment on exercise-induced asthma. *N Engl J Med* 1998;339:141–146.

45. Castle W, Fuller R, Hall J, Palmer J. Serevent nationwide surveillance study: comparison of salmeterol with salbutamol in asthmatic patients who require regular bronchodilator treatment. *BMJ* 1993;306:1034–1037.

46. Fish JE, Kemp JP, Lockey RF, et al. Zafirlukast for symptomatic mild-to-moderate asthma: A 13-week multicenter study. *Clin Ther* 1997;19: 675–690.

47. Suissa S, Dennis R, Ernst P, Sheehy O, Wood-Dauphinee S. Effectiveness of the leukotriene receptor antagonist zafirlukast for mild-to-moderate asthma. A randomized, double-blind, placebo-controlled trial. *Ann Intern Med* 1997; 126:177–183.

48. Nathan RA, Bernstein JA, Bielory L, Bonuccelli CM, Calhoun WJ. Zafirlukast improves asthma symptoms and quality of life in patients with moderate reversible airflow obstruction. *Allergy Clin Immunol* 1998;102:935–942.

49. Ducharme FM, Hicks GC. Anti-leukotriene agents compared to inhaled corticosteroids in the management of recurrent and/or chronic asthma. In: The Cochrane Library, Issue 3, 2000. Oxford: Update Software. Search date 1999; primary sources Medline, Embase, Cinahl.

50. Bleecker ER, Welch MJ, Weinstein SE, et al. Low-dose inhaled fluticasone propionate versus oral zafirlukast in the treatment of persistent asthma. *J Allergy Clin Immunol* 2000;105:1123–1229.

51. Cates C. Holding chambers versus nebulisers for β agonist treatment of acute asthma. In: The Cochrane Library, Issue 3, 2000. Search date February 1999; primary sources Cochrane Airways Review Group Register of Trials, Cochrane Controlled Trials Register, bibliographies of all included papers, and authors of included studies.

52. Edmonds ML, Camargo CA Jr, Saunders LD, Brenner BE, Rowe, BH. Inhaled steroids in acute asthma following emergency department

discharge. In: The Cochrane Library, Issue 3, 2000. Oxford: Update Software. Search date April 1999; primary sources Cochrane Airways Review Group Trials Register, and handsearching of 20 respiratory journals.

53. Rowe BH, Spooner CH, Duchrame FM, Bratzlaff JA, Bota GW. Corticosteroids for preventing relapse following acute exacerbations of asthma. In: The Cochrane Library, Issue 3, 2000. Oxford: Update Software. Search date 1997; primary sources Cochrane Airways Review Group, Asthma and Wheeze RCT Register.

54. Rowe BH, Keller JL, Oxman AD. Effectiveness of steroid therapy in acute exacerbations of asthma: a meta-analysis. Am J Emerg Med 1992;10:301–310. Search date 1991; primary sources Medline 1966 to 1991; Science Citation Index 1980 to 1990; review articles; textbooks; experts and primary authors.

55. O'Driscoll BR, Kalra S, Wilson M, Pickering CA, Carroll KB, Woodcock AA. Double-blind trial of steroid tapering in acute asthma. Lancet 1993; 341:324–327.

56. Levy ML, Stevenson C, Maslen T. Comparison of a short course of oral prednisone and fluticasone propionate in the treatment of adults with acute exacerbations of asthma in primary care. Thorax 1996;51:1087–1092.

57. Rudnitsky GS, Eberlein RS, Schoffstall JM, Mazur JE, Spivey WH. Comparison of intermittent and continuously nebulized albuterol for treatment of asthma in an urban emergency department. Ann Emerg Med 1993;22:1842–1846.

58. Resiner C, Kotch A, Dworkin G. Continuous versus frequent intermittent nebulisations of albuterol in acute asthma: a randomized, prospective study. Ann Allergy Asthma Immunol 1995;75:41–47.

59. Lin RY, Sauter D, Newman T, Sirleaf J, Walters J, Tavakol M. Continuous versus intermittent nebulization in the treatment of acute asthma. Ann Emerg Med 1993;22:1847–1853.

60. Khine H, Fuchs SM, Saville AL. Continuous vs intermittent nebulized albuterol for emergency management of asthma. Acad Emerg Med 1969; 3:1019–1024.

61. Shrestha M, Bidadi K, Gourlay S, Hayes J. Continuous vs intermittent albuterol, at high and low doses, in the treatment of severe acute asthma in adults. Chest 1996;110:42–47.

62. Nouira S, Marghili S, Elatrous S, et al. Nebulized salbutamol in acute severe asthma: a comparison of two initial doses. Clin Intensive Care 1999;10: 227–232.

63. Bradding P, Rushby I, Scullion J, Morgan MDL. As required versus regular nebulized salbutamol for the treatment of acute severe asthma. Eur Respir J 1997;13:290–294.

64. Salmeron S, Brochard L, Mal H, et al. Nebulized versus intravenous albuterol in hypercapnoeic acute asthma. A multi-center, double blind, randomized study. Am J Respir Crit Care Med 1994;149:1466–1470.

65. Lawford P, Jones BJM, Milledge JS. Comparison of intravenous and nebulized salbutamol in the initial treatment of severe asthma. BMJ 1978;1:84.

66. Cheong B, Reynolds SR, Rajan G, Ward MJ. Intravenous β-agonist in acute severe asthma. BMJ 1988;297:448–450.

67. Rodrigo G, Rodrigo C, Burschtin O. Ipratropium bromide in acute adult severe asthma: a meta-analysis of randomized controlled trials. Am J Med 1999;107:363–370. Search date April 1999; primary sources Medline 1978 to 1999; Current Contents; Science Citation Index; review articles; experts; pharmaceutical manufacturer; Medical Editor's Trial Amnesty Register; and hand searched references.

68. Rodrigo GJ, Rodrigo C. First-line therapy for adult patients with acute asthma receiving multiple dose protocol of ipratropium bromide plus albuterol in the emergency department. Am J Respir Crit Care Med 2000;161:1862–1868.

69. Manthous CA, Hall JB, Caputo MA, et al. Heliox improves pulsus paradoxus and peak expiratory flow in non-intubated patients with severe asthma. Am J Respir Care Crit Care Med 1995;151:310–314.

70. Kass JE, Terregino CA. The effect of heliox in acute severe asthma: a randomized controlled trial. Chest 1999;116:296–300.

71. Henderson SO, Acharay P, Kilaghbian T, Perez J, Korn CS, Chan LS. Use of heliox-driven nebulized therapy in the treatment of acute asthma. Ann Emerg Med 1999;33:141–146.

72. Rowe BH, Bretzlaff JA, Bourdon C, Bota GW, Camargo CA Jr. Magnesium sulfate for treating acute asthmatic exacerbations of acute asthma in the emergency department. In: The Cochrane Library, Issue 3, 2000. Oxford: Update Software. Search date 1999; primary sources Cochrane Airways Review Group Trials Register; review articles; textbooks; experts; primary authors of included studies and hand searched references.

73. Nannini LJ, Pendino JC, Corna RA, Mannarino S, Quispe R. Magnesium sulfate as a vehicle for nebulized salbutamol in acute asthma. Am J Med 2000;108:193–197.

74. FitzGerald JM. Commentary: intravenous magnesium in acute asthma. Evid Based Med Sep/Oct 1999;4:138.

75. Behbehani NA, Al-Mane FD, Yachkova Y, Pare PD, FitzGerald JM. Myopathy following mechanical ventilation for acute severe asthma: the role of muscle relaxants and corticosteroids. Chest 1999; 115:1627–1631.

76. Williams TJ, Tuxen DV, Sceinkestel CD, Czarny D, Bowes G. Risk factors for morbidity in mechanically ventilated patients with acute severe asthma. Am Rev Respir Dis 1992;146:607–615.

77. Darioli R, Perret C. Mechanical controlled hypoventilation in status asthmaticus. Am Rev Respir Dis 1984;129:385–387.

78. Menitove SM, Godring RM. Combined ventilator and bicarbonate strategy in the management of status asthmaticus. Am J Med 1983;74:898–901.

79. Higgins B, Greening AP, Crompton GK. Assisted ventilation in severe acute asthma. Thorax 1986; 41:464–467.

80. Lam KN, Mow BM, Chew LS. The profile of ICU admissions for acute severe asthma in a general hospital. Singapore Med J 1992;33:460–462.

81. Mansel JK, Stogner SW, Petrini MF, Norman JR. Mechanical ventilation in patients with acute severe asthma. Am J Med 1990;89:42–48.

82. Lim TK. Status asthmaticus in a medical intensive care unit. Singapore Med J 1989;30:334–338.

83. Keenan SP, Brake D. An evidence based approach to non invasive ventilation in acute respiratory failure. Crit Care Clin 1998;14:359–372.

84. Bartter T, Pratter MR. Asthma: better outcome at a lower cost? The role of the expert in the care system. Chest 1996;110:1589–1596.

85. Zeiger RS, Heller S, Mellon MH, Wald J, Falkoff R, Schatz M. Facilitated referral to asthma specialist reduces relapses in asthma emergency room visits. J Allergy Clin Immunol 1991;87:1160–1168.

86. Gibson PG, Coughlan J, Wilson AJ, et al. Self-management education and regular practitioner review for adults with asthma. The Cochrane Library Issue 3, 2000. Search date 1999; primary sources Cochrane Airways Group Trials Register, and hand searched references.

Christopher Cates
General Practitioner
Manor View Practice
Bushey
UK

Mark FitzGerald
Respiratory Physician
Vancouver General Hospital
Vancouver
Canada

Competing interests: CC, none declared. MF has received honoraria for lectures and research funds from GlaxoSmithKline, Merck, AstraZeneca, Novartis, Boehringer Ingelheim, Byk Canada, Schering Canada, and 3M.

TABLE 1	Classification of severity for chronic asthma (see text, p 1013).

In the USA[1]

Asthma is classified by symptoms of severity. Using this system, even people with mild, intermittent asthma can develop severe exacerbations if exposed to appropriate stimuli.

Mild intermittent asthma	Symptoms less than weekly with normal or near normal lung function.
Mild persistent asthma	Symptoms more than weekly but less than daily with normal or near normal lung function.
Moderate persistent asthma	Daily symptoms with mild to moderate variable airflow obstruction.
Severe asthma	Daily symptoms and frequent night symptoms, and moderate to severe variable airflow obstruction.

In the UK[2]

Chronic asthma in ambulatory settings is graded according to the amount of medication required to keep symptoms controlled. People are classified according to whether, for symptom control, they need:

Step 1	Occasional β agonists for symptomatic relief.
Step 2	In addition, regular, inhaled anti-inflammatory agents (such as inhaled corticosteroids, cromoglycate, or nedocromil).
Step 3	In addition, high-dose inhaled corticosteroids or low dose inahled steroids plus long-acting inhaled β_2 bronchodilator.
Step 4	In addition, high-dose inhaled corticosteroids plus regular bronchodilators.
Step 5	In addition, regular oral corticosteroids.

Chronic obstructive pulmonary disease

Search date October 2000

Huib Kerstjens and Dirkje Postma

QUESTIONS

INTERVENTIONS

Key Messages

Short term effects of treatment

- RCTs have found evidence of short term benefit from oral steroids, inhaled anticholinergic drugs, and inhaled β_2 agonists. The short term benefits of anticholinergic drugs and β_2 agonists are not seen in all people with chronic obstructive pulmonary disease (COPD). RCTs found that the two agents combined are slightly more effective than either alone.

- RCTs found no evidence of short term benefit from inhaled corticosteroids.

- Small, short term RCTs of theophyllines found some evidence of benefit, but the usefulness of these drugs is limited by adverse effects and the need for frequent monitoring of blood concentrations.

Long term effects of treatment

- One systematic review found some evidence of reduction in mortality in people with hypoxaemia from long term treatment with oxygen.

- We found insufficient evidence on the long term effects of maintenance treatment with antibiotics, oral steroids, inhaled β_2 agonists, or theophyllines.

- RCTs of inhaled anticholinergic drugs or inhaled steroids provide no clear evidence of an effect on disease course.
- Two systematic reviews of RCTs have found that mucolytics significantly reduce the frequency of exacerbations.

DEFINITION COPD is characterised by airflow obstruction caused by chronic bronchitis or emphysema. Emphysema is abnormal permanent enlargement of the air spaces distal to the terminal bronchioles, accompanied by destruction of their walls and without obvious fibrosis. Chronic bronchitis is chronic cough or mucus production for at least 3 months in at least 2 successive years when other causes of chronic cough have been excluded.[1]

INCIDENCE/ PREVALENCE COPD mainly affects middle aged and elderly people. It is one of the leading causes of morbidity and mortality worldwide. In the USA, it affects about 14 million people and is the fourth leading cause of death. Both morbidity and mortality are rising. Estimated prevalence in the USA has risen by 41% since 1982, and age adjusted death rates rose by 71% between 1966 and 1985. All cause age adjusted mortality declined over the same period by 22% and mortality from cardiovascular diseases by 45%.[1]

AETIOLOGY/ RISK FACTORS COPD is largely preventable. The main cause is exposure to cigarette smoke. COPD is rare in lifetime non-smokers (estimated incidence 5% in three large representative US surveys from 1971 to 1984), in whom exposure to environmental tobacco smoke will explain at least some disease.[2,3] Other proposed causes include airway hyperresponsiveness, air pollution, and allergy.[4-6]

PROGNOSIS The airway obstruction is usually progressive in those who continue to smoke. Progression results in early disability and shortened survival. Smoking cessation reverts decline in lung function to values of non-smokers.[7] Many people will use medication chronically for the rest of their lives, with the need for increased doses and additional drugs during exacerbations.

AIMS To alleviate symptoms; to prevent exacerbations; to preserve optimal lung function; and to improve activities of daily living, quality of life, and survival.[8]

OUTCOMES Short and long term changes in lung function, including changes in forced expiratory volume in one second (FEV_1); exercise tolerance; peak expiratory flow rate (PEF); frequency, severity, and duration of exacerbations; symptom scores for dyspnoea; quality of life; and survival.

METHODS This review deals only with treatment of stable COPD and not with treatment of acute exacerbations. *Clinical Evidence* update search and appraisal October 2000. Because we were interested in the maintenance treatment of stable COPD, we did not include single dose or single day cumulative dose response trials.

Chronic obstructive pulmonary disease

QUESTION	What are the short term and long term effects of maintenance treatment in stable COPD?

OPTION	INHALED ANTICHOLINERGIC DRUGS

RCTs using a range of methods found that anticholinergic drugs achieved short term bronchodilation and symptomatic relief in people with COPD. One large RCT found no evidence that long term treatment with inhaled anticholinergic drugs improved long term prognosis in COPD.

Benefits:
We found no systematic review comparing anticholinergic drugs with placebo. **Short term treatment:** We found many small placebo controlled RCTs using different methods and end points. Most included at least some measure of airways obstruction and found a significant effect of ipratropium.[9–12] We found one large RCT (276 people) comparing ipratropium 36 µg four times daily versus placebo or versus salmeterol for 12 weeks.[13] The FEV_1 for people using ipratropium improved significantly from baseline but results against placebo were only presented graphically. We found two subsequent RCTs comparing a long acting (up to 24 hours) anticholinergic drug, tiotropium 18 µg once daily versus placebo or versus ipratropium.[14,15] The first RCT (169 people) compared tiotropium versus placebo for 4 weeks. It found that tiotropium versus placebo significantly improved FEV_1 in the first 6 hours after treatment (mean improvement in FEV_1: 0.13 litres v –0.02 litres with placebo, $P < 0.05$), and significantly increased trough FEV_1 24 hours after the last dose (mean FEV_1: +0.07 litres v –0.03 litres with placebo, $P < 0.05$).[14] The second RCT (288 people, average age 65 years) compared tiotropium 18 µg once daily versus ipratropium 40 µg four times daily for 13 weeks.[15] It found that tiotropium versus ipratropium significantly increased FEV_1 (mean FEV_1 6 hours after treatment on first day: 0.24 litres v 0.18 litres with ipratropium; difference 0.06 litres, 95% CI 0.02 to 0.09 litres), and significantly increased mean trough FEV_1 (0.15 litres v 0.01 litres with ipratropium; difference 0.13 litres, 95% CI 0.09 to 0.18). **Long term treatment:** We found one RCT in 5887 men and women smokers aged 35–60 with spirometric signs of early COPD (FEV_1 75% predicted).[7] Three interventions were compared over a 5 year period: usual care; an intensive 12 session smoking cessation programme combining behaviour modification and use of nicotine gum; and the same smoking intervention programme plus ipratropium three times daily. The addition of ipratropium had no significant effect on decline in FEV_1. Decline in FEV_1 was significantly slower in people in the smoking cessation group (5 year mean cumulative decline in prebronchodilator FEV_1: usual care 249 ml, 95% CI 236 to 262 ml; smoking programme plus ipratropium 188 ml, 95% CI 175 to 200 ml; smoking programme plus placebo 172 ml, 95% CI 159 to 185 ml).

Harms:
One RCT (233 people with asthma or COPD) found that continuous (as opposed to as needed) treatment with bronchodilators (both ipratropium and fenoterol) resulted in faster decline in lung function.[16] This result has not been found in other trials. In the RCT of long term treatment, serious adverse events (cardiac symptoms,

hypertension, skin rashes, and urinary retention) occurred in 1.2% of people taking ipratropium versus 0.8% taking placebo.[7] Dry mouth was the most common mild adverse event. The RCT comparing tiotropium versus ipratroprium found no significant difference in the occurrence of a dry mouth (14.7% with tiotropium v 10.3% with ipratropium).[15]

Comment: Over a 5 year period, there was no evidence that people developed tachyphylaxis to the bronchodilating effect of ipratropium.[7]

OPTION	INHALED β_2 AGONISTS

Short term RCTs found that short and long acting inhaled β_2 agonists achieved bronchodilation and symptomatic relief in many people. The effects of long term treatment with β_2 agonists on disease progression have not yet been adequately evaluated.

Benefits: **Short term treatment with short acting β_2 agonists:** We found no systematic review. We found over 100 placebo controlled RCTs. Most of these found improved symptoms and some bronchodilatory effect, the magnitude of which depended partly on whether participants were selected on the basis of having irreversible airways obstruction. One RCT (985 people with severe COPD) found a significant increase in lung function in up to half of participants.[17] Ten out of 17 trials assessing walking distance as a measure of exercise capacity found a significant improvement with short acting β_2 agonists. **Short term treatment with long acting β_2 agonists:** We found one systematic review (search date 1998, 3 RCTs of salmeterol)[18] and two subsequent RCTs.[13,19] All found significant improvements in either symptoms, lung function, or quality of life. The first RCT in the review (674 people) compared salmeterol 50 µg versus 100 µg doses twice daily for 16 weeks and found a significant increase in FEV_1 in both treatment groups (50 µg: WMD 0.10 litres, 95% CI 0.05 to 0.15 litres; 100 µg: WMD 0.12 litres, 95% CI 0.06 to 0.17 litres).[20] Quality of life improved significantly in the group taking the lower but not the higher dose compared with placebo.[21] The second RCT, a crossover trial in 63 smokers, found significant increases in morning FEV_1 after 4 weeks of treatment with salmeterol 50 µg twice daily compared with placebo (mean treatment difference 12 ml, 95% CI 6 ml to 17 ml). Evening values were not significantly different from placebo.[22] The third RCT (29 people) found that significantly fewer people taking salmeterol 50 µg daily were scored as moderately dyspnoeic or worse (OR 0.60, 95% CI 0.40 to 0.88). There was no significant difference in the mean change from baseline in the 6 minute walking distance (WMD +1.9 m, 95% CI −15.4 m to +19.3 m).[23] The systematic review found no trials of formoterol.[18] The first subsequent RCT (278 people), which compared salmeterol 42 µg twice daily versus placebo for 12 weeks, found that salmeterol significantly improved the average FEV_1.[13] The second subsequent RCT (97 people) compared salmeterol 50 µg twice daily versus placebo over 12 weeks.[19] There was a significant improvement with salmeterol in morning and evening peak flow rates, and in FEV_1 (mean improvement as a percentage of the predicted FEV_1: 5% v 1%, P < 0.01), and day time but not night time symptoms. In the same study, no improvement in quality of life was found with salmeterol compared with placebo.[24] **Long term treatment:** We found no systematic review or RCTs looking at reduction of decline in lung function with inhaled β_2 agonists compared with placebo.

Harms:

In people with asthma, β_2 agonists have been linked to increased risk of death, worsened asthma control, and deterioration in lung function.[25] We found no evidence for people with COPD. One RCT (223 people with asthma or COPD) found that continuous (as opposed to as needed) treatment with bronchodilators (ipratropium bromide as well as fenoterol) resulted in faster decline in lung function.[16] We found no other studies of β_2 agonists in COPD addressing this possibility. We found no systematic review on frequency of adverse effects of β_2 agonists in COPD. The most common immediate adverse effect is tremor, which is usually worse in the first few days of treatment. High doses of β_2 agonists can cause a fall in plasma potassium, dysrhythmias, and reduced arterial oxygen tension.[26] Extra caution is warranted for use in people with pre-existing cardiac arrhythmias and hypoxaemia.[27] One trial comparing salmeterol versus placebo over 12 weeks found no increase in any adverse events, but allowed rescue salbutamol.[13]

Comment:

The measured improvement in lung function does not seem to reflect the symptomatic improvement that can occur in some people when taking β_2 agonists. Long term placebo controlled RCTs of β_2 agonists, looking at adverse effects such as decline in lung function or worsened COPD control, are ethically difficult because of their beneficial effects in the short term.

OPTION   **ANTICHOLINERGICS PLUS INHALED β_2 AGONISTS**

RCTs found that combining a β_2 agonist with an anticholinergic drug provided small additional bronchodilation compared with either drug alone.

Benefits:

We found no systematic review. **With short acting inhaled β_2 agonists:** We found six RCTs (705, 195, 652, 863, and 357 people, one article combined the results from two RCTs) comparing the addition of ipratropium versus standard dose short acting inhaled β_2 agonists for 2 weeks to 3 months in people with stable COPD.[28-32] All found significant improvements in FEV_1 of about 25% with the combination compared with either drug alone. **With long acting inhaled β_2 agonists:** One RCT (94 people) evaluated a long acting β_2 agonist, salmeterol 50 µg twice daily versus salmeterol 50 µg twice daily plus ipratropium 40 µg four times daily for 12 weeks.[19] It found the combination versus the β_2 agonist alone significantly improved FEV_1 (mean improvement as a percentage of predicted FEV_1: 8% v 5%, P < 0.01), and evening but not morning peak flow rates. It found no significant difference in day time or night time symptoms. Quality of life was found to improve more with the combination than with salmeterol alone.[24]

Harms:

The trials found no significant differences in adverse effects between the groups.

Comment: None.

We found conflicting evidence from RCTs on the effects of inhaled β_2 agonists versus anticholinergics.

Benefits: We found no systematic review. **Short term treatment:** Several RCTs with different methods and outcomes have compared ipratropium bromide versus a β_2 agonist. They used different methods and found conflicting results. **Long term treatment:** One non-systematic review pooled data from seven RCTs (1445 people) of ipratropium bromide versus various short acting β_2 agonists for 90 days.[33] Lung function measurements were performed after withholding bronchodilators for at least 12 hours. There was a significantly greater mean improvement in FEV_1 with ipratropium bromide than with the β_2 agonists (28 ml increase v 1 ml decrease, $P < 0.05$). We found one additional trial (411 people) comparing the long acting β_2 agonist salmeterol (42 µg) twice daily versus ipratropium (36 µg) four times daily during 12 weeks' treatment.[13] It found a significant improvement in average FEV_1 with salmeterol treatment compared with ipratropium at weeks 4 and 8 ($P < 0.005$), but not at weeks 0 and 12.

Harms: Although adverse effects associated with β_2 agonists such as tremor and dysrhythmias seem to be more frequent than the adverse clinical events associated with anticholinergics, the review provided no evidence.[33] The RCT comparing salmeterol versus ipratropium versus placebo found no significant difference in adverse events.[13]

Comment: A residual effect of the anticholinergic drugs cannot be ruled out, limiting the interpretation of a favourable effect of anticholinergic drugs compared with β_2 agonists. It has been suggested that older people experience greater bronchodilator response with anticholinergic drugs than with β_2 agonists, but we found no evidence for this.

We found limited evidence from small RCTs of a small bronchodilatory effect of theophyllines in people with COPD. Adverse effects are frequent.

Benefits: We found no systematic review. **Short term treatment:** We found one non-systematic review (published in 1995, 11 small RCTs) of theophyllines in people with COPD.[34] These evaluated treatment periods ranging from 1 week to 2 months and found changes in FEV_1 ranging from 0–20%, with equally varied effects on exercise capacity and symptoms. **Long term treatment:** We found no RCTs.

Harms: The RCTs did not report adverse effects. The therapeutic range for theophyllines is small with blood concentrations of 10–15 mg/litre required for optimal effects. Well documented adverse effects include nausea, diarrhoea, headache, irritability, seizures, and cardiac arrhythmias. These may occur within the therapeutic range.[35]

Comment: Non-bronchodilator effects of theophylline have been found in laboratory settings, including effects on respiratory muscles and improved right ventricular function. Clinical significance has not been established. Anti-inflammatory effects have been claimed in asthma, especially at lower dosages, but have not been measured in COPD. One RCT found little value from the use of "n of 1" trials to determine objective individualised treatment effects.[36]

OPTION ORAL CORTICOSTEROIDS

One systematic review of short term RCTs has found that steroids versus placebo significantly improves lung function. We found no RCT of the effects of long term treatment on lung function. We found evidence of potentially serious adverse effects.

Benefits: **Short term treatment:** We found one systematic review (search date 1989, 15 RCTs), which compared oral steroids with placebo in stable COPD.[37] Treatment usually lasted 2–4 weeks. Data pooling from the 10 RCTs that met all inclusion criteria found that a 20% or greater improvement in baseline FEV_1 occurred significantly more often in people taking oral corticosteroids than those on placebo (WMD 10%, 95% CI 2% to 18%). When the other five RCTs were included, the difference in effect size was 11% (95% CI 4% to 18%). **Long term treatment:** We found no long term RCTs examining the effects of oral steroids on decline in lung function.

Harms: Many reviews have described the considerable harms of systemic corticosteroids, including osteoporosis and induction of diabetes.[38]

Comment: None.

OPTION INHALED CORTICOSTEROIDS

Short term RCTs found no evidence of benefit of inhaled corticosteroids. Large RCTs of at least 6 months have found that inhaled steroids increase FEV_1 during the first 3–6 months of use, but found no subsequent effect on decline of lung function. Two studies also found a reduction in exacerbation frequency and an improvement in health status.

Benefits: **Short term treatment:** We found no systematic review. We found 10 placebo controlled RCTs shorter than 6 months summarised in one non-systematic review.[39] Nine short term trials (10 days to 10 weeks, 10–127 people) found no significant benefit in lung function (FEV_1) with inhaled steroids. None of the trials measuring airway hyperresponsiveness to histamine found a change. **Long term treatment:** We found one systematic review (search date 1996, 3 long term placebo controlled RCTs of inhaled steroids, 197 people treated for 2–2.5 years)[40] and four large subsequent RCTs.[41–44] The systematic review found that, at 2 years, people on inhaled steroids had significantly greater rate of improvement in prebronchodilator FEV_1 compared with placebo (WMD 34 ml/year, 95% CI 5 to 63 ml/year). There was no significant difference in rate of improvement of postbronchodilator FEV_1 (WMD +39 ml/year, 95% CI –6 to +84 ml/year) or in the frequency of exacerbations. The first subsequent RCT (281 people), comparing 6 months' treatment with fluticasone versus placebo found a significant reduction in moderate and severe exacerbations (86% v 60%, P < 0.001) but not mild exacerbations. Fluticasone versus placebo also significantly improved lung function (adjusted baseline daily peak expiratory flow 15 litres/minute v 2 litres/minute on placebo, P < 0.001) and 6 minute walking distance (adjusted mean change in distance walked 27 m v 8 m, P = 0.03).[41] The second RCT (290 people with mild airways obstruction, FEV_1 86% of predicted) found that budesonide (800 µg plus 400 µg daily for 6 months followed by 400 µg twice daily for 30 months) versus placebo had no significant effect on decline in lung function or exacerbation frequency.[42] The third RCT (1277 people, mean FEV_1 77% of predicted; 912 completed the trial) compared 800 µg budesonide daily versus placebo for 3 years.[43] In the first 6 months of the study, FEV_1 improved at the rate of 17 ml a year in the budesonide group compared with a decline of 81 ml a year in the placebo group (P < 0.001). However, there was no effect on subsequent decline. The fourth RCT (751 people with more severe COPD, FEV_1 50% of predicted) compared fluticasone 500 µg twice daily for 3 years versus placebo.[44] It found no effect on decline in lung function but there was a 25% reduction in exacerbation rate (from 1.32 per year on placebo to 0.99 on fluticasone). It also found a significant reduction in the deterioration of quality of life with fluticasone compared with placebo.[44]

Harms: Extrapolation from studies in people with asthma is of limited value, as people with COPD are generally at higher risk for osteoporosis because of age, menopausal status, inactivity, and cigarette smoking.[38] One RCT (1277 people) reported skin bruising in 10% of people taking budesonide versus 4% taking placebo.[43] Newly diagnosed hypertension, bone fractures, postcapsular cataracts, myopathy, and diabetes occurred in less than 5% of people, with no significant difference between the groups.[43]

Comment: The finding of improved quality of life in one trial is preliminary.[44] A large North American RCT is underway (AS Buist, personal communication, 1999).

OPTION   ORAL VERSUS INHALED STEROIDS

We found limited evidence from RCTs suggesting that oral prednisolone is more effective than inhaled beclomethasone in people with mild to moderate COPD.

Benefits: We found no systematic review. **Short term treatment:** We found three RCTs comparing oral prednisolone versus inhaled beclomethasone (12, 83, 107 people).[45–47] All were double blind placebo controlled crossover trials, with treatment periods of 2 weeks. One small RCT found no significant difference between the number of people responding to either or both treatments.[45] The other two trials found greater benefit with oral versus inhaled steroids. One found that FEV_1 rose from 0.65 to 1 litres on prednisolone versus 0.63 to 0.81 litres on beclomethasone (P < 0.01). The other found that the proportion of participants responding to oral treatment was significantly higher (39/107 [36%] v 26/107 [24%], P < 0.05).[46,47] **Long term treatment:** We found no RCTs.

Harms: None of the RCTs reported adverse effects.

Comment: The smallest RCT recruited only people known to be responsive to oral steroids, and did not report severity of COPD.[46] The other two

RCTs included people with COPD of more than 5 years' duration and FEV_1 less than 70% predicted.[45,47] All trials excluded people with evidence of reversible airflow obstruction.

OPTION	MUCOLYTIC DRUGS

Two systematic reviews of RCTs have found that long term treatment with mucolytics versus placebo significantly reduces the frequency and duration of exacerbations.

Benefits: **Long term treatment:** We found two systematic reviews.[48,49] The first systematic review (search date 1999) identified 15 double blind placebo controlled RCTs.[48] Mucolytics were associated with a significant reduction in the average number of exacerbations (WMD 0.105 exacerbations per month, 95% CI 0.10 to 0.11), days of disability (WMD 0.65 days per month, 95% CI 0.61 to 0.69), and days on antibiotics (WMD 0.68 days per month, 95% CI 0.64 to 0.71). Most of the trials were in people with mild COPD. Two trials in people with severe COPD ($FEV_1 < 50\%$) found greater reductions in exacerbation frequency (WMD compared with placebo 0.14 per month, CI not given). The review found a small but significant improvement in lung function compared with placebo (WMD in FEV_1 compared with mucolytics 0.06 litres, 95% CI 0.08 litres to 0.04 litres; WMD in forced vital capacity 0.04 litres, 95% CI 0.06 litres to 0.02 litres). However, this finding should be interpreted with caution because it was based on only three trials that reported FEV_1 and four trials that reported vital capacity, and there was considerable heterogeneity in the studies. There was no significant difference between N-acetylcysteine and other mucolytics as a group. The second systematic review (search date 1995, 9 RCTs) compared N-acetylcysteine with placebo.[49] Seven of the RCTs were included in the first review.[48] It found an overall weighted effect size of 1.37 (95% CI 1.25 to 1.5), corresponding to a 23% reduction in exacerbations compared with placebo.

Harms: The first systematic review found no differences between mucolytics and placebo in the total number of adverse events.[46] Adverse effects of N-acetylcysteine were mainly mild gastrointestinal complaints.

Comment: In both reviews there was significant heterogeneity between the RCTs, and symptom scores could not be pooled.[48,49] The effect of N-acetylcysteine in slowing the decline in lung function is being examined in a large European multicentre study (PNR Dekhuijzen, personal communication, 1999).

OPTION	ANTIBIOTICS

We found no RCTs of antibiotics in long term treatment of stable COPD.

Benefits: **Long term treatment:** We found one systematic review (search date 1994), which identified no RCTs of antibiotics as long term treatment in stable COPD.[50]

Harms: The adverse effects of antibiotics vary between agents and individuals.

Comment: None.

| OPTION | DOMICILIARY OXYGEN TREATMENT |

We found limited evidence that domiciliary oxygen treatment improves survival in people with COPD and hypoxaemia. One RCT found that continuous treatment was more effective than nocturnal treatment.

Benefits: **Long term treatment:** We found one systematic review (search date 1999, 4 RCTs) and one additional RCT comparing domiciliary oxygen treatment versus control treatment.[51] Results could not be aggregated because of differences in trial design and participant selection. One 5 year RCT (87 people), which compared oxygen for at least 15 hours versus no oxygen, found that domiciliary oxygen significantly reduced mortality (OR 0.42, 95% CI 0.18 to 0.98).[52] The second RCT (38 people) compared nocturnal domiciliary oxygen versus room air in people with arterial desaturation at night. It found no difference in mortality at 3 years (figures not given).[53] The third trial (135 people) compared oxygen versus no oxygen in people with moderate hypoxaemia and found no significant difference in survival at 3 years (HR 0.92, 95% CI 0.57 to 1.47).[54] The fourth RCT (203 people) compared continuous versus nocturnal domiciliary oxygen treatment. Continuous oxygen was associated with significant reduction in mortality over 24 months (OR 0.45, 95% CI 0.25 to 0.81).[55] The additional RCT (76 people with moderate day time hypoxaemia [7.4–9.2 kPa] and significant nocturnal desaturation) compared 2 years of nocturnal oxygen therapy with placebo.[56] It found no significant difference in survival.

Harms: No adverse effects of domiciliary oxygen have been reported. Administration is cumbersome.

Comment: Only one of the studies was double blinded. Domiciliary oxygen treatment seems to be more effective in people with severe hypoxaemia (arterial $Po_2 < 8.0$ kPa) than in people with moderate hypoxaemia or those who have arterial desaturation only at night.

Substantive changes since last issue

Inhaled anticholinergic drugs Two new RCTs;[14,15] conclusion unchanged.

REFERENCES

1. American Thoracic Society. Standards for the diagnosis and care of patients with chronic obstructive pulmonary disease: ATS statement. *Am J Respir Crit Care Med* 1995;152 (5 pt 2) (suppl): 77–120.

2. Whittemore AS, Perlin SA, DiCiccio Y. Chronic obstructive pulmonary disease in lifelong nonsmokers: results from NHANES. *Am J Public Health* 1995;85:702–706.

3. Brunekreef B, Fischer P, Remijn B, van der Lende R, Schouten JP, Quanjer PH. Indoor air pollution and its effects on pulmonary function of adult non-smoking women: III passive smoking and pulmonary function. *Int J Epidemiol* 1985;14: 227–230.

4. Rijcken B, Weiss ST. Longitudinal analyses of airway responsiveness and pulmonary function decline. *Am J Respir Crit Care Med* 1996;154 (6 pt 2) (suppl):246–249.

5. Dockery DW, Brunekreef B. Longitudinal studies of air pollution effects on lung function. *Am J Respir Crit Care Med* 1996;154 (6 pt 2) (suppl):250–256.

6. O'Connor GT, Sparrow D, Weiss ST. The role of allergy and non-specific airway hyperresponsiveness in the pathogenesis of chronic obstructive pulmonary disease: state of the art. *Am Rev Respir Dis* 1989;140:225–252.

7. Anthonisen NR, Connett JE, Kiley JP, et al. Effects of smoking intervention and the use of an inhaled anticholinergic bronchodilator on the rate of decline of FEV_1: the lung health study. *JAMA* 1994;272:1497–1505.

8. Siafakas NM, Vermeire P, Pride NB, et al. Optimal assessment and management of chronic obstructive pulmonary disease (COPD): a consensus statement of the European Respiratory Society. *Eur Respir J* 1995;8:1398–1420.

9. Braun SR, McKenzie WN, Copeland W, Kingman L, Ellersieck M, Knight GJ. A comparison of the effect of ipratropium bromide and albuterol in the treatment of chronic obstructive airway disease. *Arch Intern Med* 1989;149:544–547.

10. Higgins BG, Powell RM, Cooper S, Tattersfield AE. Effect of salbutamol and ipratropium bromide on airway calibre and bronchial reactivity in asthma

Chronic obstructive pulmonary disease

and chronic bronchitis. *Eur Respir J* 1991;4:415–420.

11. Ikeda A, Nishimura K, Koyama H, Izumi T. Bronchodilating effects of combined therapy with clinical dosages of ipratropium bromide and salbutamol for stable COPD: comparison with ipratropium bromide alone. *Chest* 1995;107:401–405.

12. Ikeda A, Nishimura K, Koyama H, Izumi T. Comparative dose-response study of three anticholinergic agents and fenoterol using a metered dose inhaler in patients with chronic obstructive pulmonary disease. *Thorax* 1995;50:62–66.

13. Mahler DA, Donohue JF, Barbee RA, et al. Efficacy of salmeterol xinafoate in the treatment of COPD. *Chest* 1999;115:957–965.

14. Littner MR, Ilowite JS, Tashkin DP, et al. Long-acting bronchodilation with once-daily dosing of tiotropium (Spiriva) in stable chronic obstructive pulmonary disease. *Am J Respir Crit Care Med* 2000;161:1136–1142.

15. Van Noord JA, Bantje TA, Eland ME, Korducki L, Cornelissen PJ. A randomised controlled comparison of tiotropium and ipratropium in the treatment of chronic obstructive pulmonary disease. The Dutch Tiotropium Study Group. *Thorax* 2000;55:289–294.

16. Van Schayck CP, Dompeling E, van Herwaarden CLA, et al. Bronchodilator treatment in moderate asthma or chronic bronchitis: continuous or on demand? A randomised controlled study. *BMJ* 1991;303:1426–1431.

17. Anthonisen NR, Wright EC, IPPB Trial Group. Bronchodilator response in chronic obstructive pulmonary disease. *Am Rev Respir Dis* 1986;133:814–819.

18. Appleton S, Smith B, Veale A, Bara A. Regular long-acting beta-2 adrenoceptor agonists in stable chronic obstructive airways disease. In: The Cochrane Library, Issue 1, 2000. Oxford: Update Software. Search date October 1998; primary sources Cochrane Airways Group Register to October 1998; hand searched references; and pharmaceutical companies contacted for unpublished studies.

19. Van Noord JM, de Munck DR, Bantje TA, Hop WC, Akveld ML, Bommer, AM. Long-term treatment of chronic obstructive pulmonary disease with salmeterol and the additive effect of ipratropium. *Eur Respir J* 2000;15:878–885.

20. Boyd G, Morice AH, Pounsford JC, Siebert M, Peslis N, Crawford C. An evaluation of salmeterol in the treatment of chronic obstructive pulmonary disease (COPD). *Eur Respir J* 1997;10:815–821.

21. Jones PW, Bosh TK. Quality of life changes in COPD patients treated with salmeterol. *Am J Respir Crit Care Med* 1997;155:1283–1289.

22. Ulrik CS. Efficacy of inhaled salmeterol in the management of smokers with chronic obstructive pulmonary disease: a single centre randomised, double blind, placebo controlled, crossover study. *Thorax* 1995;50:750–754.

23. Grove A, Lipworth BJ, Reid P, et al. Effects of regular salmeterol on lung function and exercise capacity in patients with chronic obstructive airways disease. *Thorax* 1996;51:689–693.

24. Rutten van Molken M, Roos B, van Noord JA. An empirical comparison of the St George's Respiratory Questionnaire (SGRQ) and the Chronic Respiratory Disease Questionnaire (CRQ) in a clinical trial setting. *Thorax* 1999;54:995–1003.

25. O'Byrne PM, Kerstjens HAM. Inhaled β_2-agonists in the treatment of asthma. *N Engl J Med* 1996;335:886–888.

26. Hall IP, Tattersfield AE. Beta-agonists. In: Clark TJH, Godfrey S, Lee TH, eds. *Asthma*. 3rd ed.

London: Chapman and Hall Medical, 1992:341–365.

27. Cazzola M, Imperatore F, Salzillo A, et al. Cardiac effects of formoterol and salmeterol in patients suffering from COPD with preexisting cardiac arrhythmias and hypoxemia. *Chest* 1998;114:411–415.

28. Friedman M, Serby C, Menjoge S, Wilson JD, Hilleman DE, Witek TJ Jr. Pharmoeconomic evaluation of a combination of ipratropium plus albuterol compared with ipratropium alone and albuterol alone in COPD. *Chest* 1999:115:635–641.

29. Levin DC, Little KS, Laughlin KR, et al. Addition of anticholinergic solution prolongs bronchodilator effect of beta 2 agonists in patients with chronic obstructive pulmonary disease. *Am J Med* 1996;100(1A;suppl):40–48.

30. Combivent Inhalation Solution Study Group. Routine nebulized ipratropium and albuterol together are better than either alone in COPD. *Chest* 1997;112:1514–1521.

31. Gross N, Tashkin D, Miller R, Oren J, Coleman W, Linberg S. Inhalation by nebulization of albuterol-ipratropium combination (Dey combination) is superior to either agent alone in the treatment of chronic obstructive pulmonary disease. Dey combination solution study group. *Respiration* 1998;65:354–362.

32. Campbell S. For COPD a combination of ipratropium bromide and albuterol sulfate is more effective than albuterol base. *Arch Intern Med* 1999;159:156–160.

33. Rennard SI, Serby CW, Ghafouri M, Johnson PA, Friedman M. Extended therapy with ipratropium is associated with improved lung function in patients with COPD: a retrospective analysis of data from seven clinical trials. *Chest* 1996;110:62–70.

34. Calverley PMA. Symptomatic bronchodilator treatment. In: Calverley PMA, Pride N, eds. *Chronic obstructive pulmonary disease*. London: Chapman and Hall, 1995:419–446.

35. Ramsdell J. Use of theophylline in the treatment of COPD. *Chest* 1995;107(suppl):206–209.

36. Mahon JL, Laupacis A, Hodder RV, et al. Theophylline for irreversible chronic airflow limitation: a randomized study comparing n of 1 trials to standard practice. *Chest* 1999;115:38–48.

37. Callahan CM, Dittus RS, Katz BP. Oral corticosteroid therapy for patients with stable chronic obstructive pulmonary disease: a meta-analysis. *Ann Intern Med* 1991;114:216–223. Search date 1989; primary sources Medline 1966 to 1989.

38. McEvoy CE, Niewoehner DE. Adverse effects of corticosteroid therapy for COPD: a critical review. *Chest* 1997;111:732–743.

39. Postma DS, Kerstjens HAM. Are inhaled glucocorticosteroids effective in chronic obstructive pulmonary disease? *Am J Respir Crit Care Med* 1999;160 (5 pt 2):66–71.

40. Van Grunsven PM, van Schayck CP, Derenne JP, et al. Long term effects of inhaled corticosteroids in chronic obstructive pulmonary disease: a meta-analysis. *Thorax* 1999;54:714–729. Search date 1996; primary sources Medline 1983 to 1996; Biosis 1991 to 1996; Online Contents 1993 to 1996; GLin 1982 to 1996; Cochrane Library; Embase 1993 to 1996.

41. Paggiaro PL, Dahle R, Bakran I, Frith L, Hollingworth K, Efthimou J. Multicentre randomised placebo-controlled trial of inhaled fluticasone propionate in patients with chronic obstructive pulmonary disease. *Lancet* 1998;351:773–780.

42. Vestbo J, Sorensen T, Lange P, Brix A, Torre P, Viskum K. Long-term effect of inhaled budesonide in mild and moderate chronic obstructive pulmonary disease: a randomised controlled trial. *Lancet* 1999;353:1819–1823.

43. Pauwels RA, Lofdahl CG, Laitinen LA, et al. Long-term treatment with inhaled budesonide in persons with mild chronic obstructive pulmonary disease who continue smoking. European Respiratory Society study on chronic obstructive pulmonary disease. *N Engl J Med* 1999;340: 1948–1953.

44. Burge PS, Calverley PM, Jones PW, Spencer S, Anderson JA, Maslen TK. Randomised, double blind, placebo controlled study of fluticasone propionate in patients with moderate to severe chronic obstructive pulmonary disease: the ISOLDE trial. *BMJ* 2000;320:1297–1303.

45. Robertson AS, Gove RI, Wieland GA, Burge PS. A double-blind comparison of oral prednisolone 40 mg/day with inhaled beclomethasone dipropionate 1500 g/day in patients with adult onset chronic obstructive pulmonary disease. *Eur J Respir Dis* 1986;69(suppl 146):565–569.

46. Shim CS, Williams MH. Aerosol beclomethasone in patients with steroid-responsive chronic obstructive pulmonary disease. *Am J Med* 1985; 78:655–658.

47. Weir DC, Gove RI, Robertson AS, Burge PS. Corticosteroid trials in non-asthmatic chronic airflow obstruction: a comparison of oral prednisolone and inhaled beclomethasone dipropionate. *Thorax* 1990;45:112–117.

48. Poole PJ, Black PN. Mucolytic agents for chronic bronchitis or chronic obstructive pulmonary disease. In: The Cochrane Library, Issue 1, 2000. Oxford: Update Software. Search date May 1999; primary sources Cochrane Airways Group Register to May 1999; and hand searched references.

49. Grandjean EM, Berthet P, Ruffmann R, Leuenberger P. Efficacy of oral long-term N-acetylcysteine in chronic bronchopulmonary disease: a meta-analysis of published double-blind, placebo-controlled clinical trials. *Clin Ther* 2000;22:209–221. Search date 1995; primary sources Medline; hand searches of reference list; and personal contact with two experts.

50. Saint S, Bent S, Vittinghoff E, Grady D. Antibiotics in chronic obstructive pulmonary disease exacerbations: a meta-analysis. *JAMA* 1995;273: 957–960. Search date 1994; primary sources Medline 1966 to May 1994; hand searched Index Medicus up to 1966.

51. Crockett AJ, Moss JR, Cranston JM, Alpers JH. Domiciliary oxygen in chronic obstructive pulmonary disease. In: The Cochrane Library, Issue 1, 2000. Oxford: Update Software. Search date April 1999; primary sources Cochrane Airways Group Register.

52. Medical Research Council Working Party. Long term domiciliary oxygen therapy in chronic hypoxic cor pulmonale complicating chronic bronchitis and emphysema. *Lancet* 1981;1:681–686.

53. Fletcher EC, Luckett RA, Goodnight-White S, Miller CC, Qian W, Costarangos-Galarza C. A double-blind trial of nocturnal supplemental oxygen for sleep desaturation in patients with chronic obstructive pulmonary disease and a daytime PaO_2 above 60 mm Hg. *Am Rev Respir Dis* 1992; 145:1070–1076.

54. Gorecka D, Gorzelak K, Sliwinski P, Tobiasz M, Zielinski J. Effect of long-term oxygen therapy on survival in patients with chronic obstructive pulmonary disease with moderate hypoxaemia. *Thorax* 1997;52:674–679.

55. Nocturnal Oxygen Therapy Trial Group. Continuous or nocturnal oxygen therapy in hypoxemic chronic obstructive lung disease: a clinical trial. *Ann Intern Med* 1980;93:391–398.

56. Chaouat A, Weitzenblum E, Kessler R, Charpentier C, Enrhart M, Schott R, et al. A randomized trial of nocturnal oxygen therapy in chronic obstructive pulmonary disease patients. *Eur Respir J* 1999; 14:1002–1008.

Huib Kerstjens
Pulmonary Physician

Dirkje Postma
Professor of Pulmonary Medicine

University Hospital Groningen
Groningen
The Netherlands

Competing interests: Both authors have received funding from the following manufacturers: AstraZeneca, the manufacturer of budesonide, terbutaline, formoterol; Glaxo Wellcome, the manufacturer of beclomethasone, salbutamol, salmeterol, and fluticasone; Boehringer Ingelheim, the manufacturer of fenoterol, ipratropium bromide, and tiotropium bromide; and Novartis, the manufacturer of formoterol. DP has also received funding from Zambon, the manufacturer of N-acetylcysteine.

Community acquired pneumonia

Search date October 2000

Thomas Marrie

QUESTIONS

INTERVENTIONS

TREATMENT

Likely to be beneficial

Unknown effectiveness

Unlikely to be beneficial

PREVENTION

Beneficial

Likely to be beneficial

Unknown effectiveness

To be covered in future issues of *Clinical Evidence*

Other antiviral treatments

Covered elsewhere in this issue

Antivirals for influenza, p 490

Key Messages

Treatment

- One systematic review found no evidence of a difference between most oral antibiotics in people in outpatient settings with community acquired pneumonia, when local microbial sensitivities are taken into account.

- We found no strong evidence supporting new over older antibiotics for people admitted to hospital, nor of any particular combination of antibiotics for use in intensive care.

- RCTs in immunocompetent people in hospital found no evidence of a difference in effectiveness between intravenous antibiotics and oral antibiotics. Intravenous antibiotics were associated with longer hospital stays.

- One RCT has found that bottle blowing physiotherapy significantly reduces hospital stay.

- One multicentre retrospective review has found that prompt administration of antibiotics improves survival.

- We found no evidence that critical pathway guidelines improve clinical outcomes in community acquired pneumonia. One multicentre RCT has found that a critical pathway guideline improves process outcomes: more people treated at home, fewer hospital bed days for people managed, fewer days on intravenous antibiotics, and more frequent use of one class of antibiotics.

Prevention

- One systematic review of cohort studies, and three subsequent RCTs, have found evidence that influenza vaccine reduces risk of influenza and death in elderly people.

- RCTs of pneumococcal vaccine have found mixed results. One systematic review found that vaccination with currently available pneumococcal vaccines did not protect against death. It also found that pneumococcal vaccine was associated with increased protection in young, fit adults (but not older adults at high risk) against pneumococcal pneumonia. Subsequent RCTs found no evidence of benefit in older adults. Subgroup analysis suggested a benefit in older adults at high risk of pneumonia.

DEFINITION	Community acquired pneumonia is pneumonia contracted in the community rather than in hospital.
INCIDENCE/ PREVALENCE	In the northern hemisphere, community acquired pneumonia affects about 12 of 1000 people a year, particularly during winter and at the extremes of age (incidence: < 1 year old 30–50/1000 per year; 15–45 years 1–5/1000 a year; 60–70 years 10–20/1000 a year; 71–85 years 50/1000 a year).[1–6]
AETIOLOGY/ RISK FACTORS	Over 100 microorganisms have been implicated, but most cases are caused by *Streptococcus pneumoniae* (see table 1, p 1049).[4–7] Smoking is probably an important risk factor.[8]
PROGNOSIS	Severity varies from mild to life threatening illness within days of the onset of symptoms. One systematic review (search date 1995) of prognosis studies for community acquired pneumonia found overall mortality to be 13.7%, ranging from 5.1% for ambulant people to 36.5% for people requiring intensive care.[9] The following prognostic factors were significantly associated with mortality: male sex (OR 1.3, 95% CI 1.2 to 1.4); pleuritic chest pain (OR 0.5, 95% CI 0.3 to 0.8, i.e. lower mortality); hypothermia (OR 5, 95% CI 2.4 to 10.4); systolic hypotension (OR 4.8, 95% CI 2.8 to 8.3); tachypnoea (OR 2.9, 95% CI 1.7 to 4.9); diabetes mellitus (OR 1.3, 95% CI 1.1 to 1.5); neoplastic disease (OR 2.8, 95% CI 2.4 to 3.1); neurologic disease (OR 4.6, 95% CI 2.3 to 8.9); bacteraemia (OR 2.8, 95% CI 2.3 to 3.6); leukopenia (OR 2.5, 95% CI 1.6 to 3.7); and multilobar radiographic pulmonary infiltrates (OR 3.1, 95% CI 1.9 to 5.1).
AIMS	**Treatment:** To cure infection; to prevent death in seriously ill people; to alleviate symptoms; to enable a return to normal activities; and to prevent recurrence. **Prevention:** To prevent pneumonia and death.

Community acquired pneumonia

OUTCOMES	Clinical cure (defined as return to premorbid health status); relief of symptoms; admission to hospital; complications (empyema, endocarditis, lung abscess); death; adverse effects of antibiotics (allergy, diarrhoea, colitis); adverse effects of procedures (endotracheal intubation, central vascular lines).
METHODS	*Clinical Evidence* update search and appraisal October 2000.

QUESTION Which antibiotics should be used in outpatient settings?

OPTION NEW VERSUS OLD ANTIBIOTICS

One systematic review found no evidence that newer antibiotics have an advantage over older antibiotics, such as broad spectrum penicillins, in outpatient settings.

Benefits:	We found one systematic review (search date not stated, 9 RCTs comparing different oral antibiotics in outpatient settings).[10] Five trials had fewer than 100 participants, the other trials included between 118 and 267 people (total 1164 people). Antibiotics tested were amoxicillin with and without clavulanate; macrolides; first, second, and third generation cephalosporins; and quinolones. Cure or improvement was reported in over 90% of trial participants.
Harms:	Antibiotics can cause allergic reactions (including anaphylaxis), rash, gastrointestinal intolerance (nausea, vomiting, diarrhoea), vaginal or oral candidiasis, and *Clostridium difficile* diarrhoea (including pseudomembranous colitis). Frequency of adverse effects varies with the antibiotic used.
Comment:	None.

QUESTION Which treatments should be used in people admitted to hospital?

OPTION NEW VERSUS OLD ANTIBIOTICS

RCTs found no evidence of a significant difference in effectiveness between new and older antibiotics in people with community acquired pneumonia admitted to hospital. However, most trials were small and were designed to show equivalence between treatments rather than superiority of one over another.

Benefits:	We found no systematic review. **Second generation cephalosporin versus broad spectrum penicillin:** We found several RCTs, all too small, too old, or both, to be reliable given the changing sensitivity of organisms to antibiotics. **Quinolones versus high dose amoxycillin:** We found one multicentre double blind RCT (329 people in hospital in France, South Africa, and Switzerland) comparing sparfloxacin versus amoxycillin.[11] Early discontinuation of the drug (days 3, 4, or 5) occurred in fewer people treated with sparfloxacin versus amoxycillin (2.4% v 7.9%; no CIs given). It found no significant difference in clinical cure rates (AR 84% with sparfloxacin v AR 85% with amoxycillin). **Quinolones versus second and third generation cephalosporins:** We found one double blind

RCT (226 people, half of whom had been admitted to hospital) comparing oral levofloxacin versus intravenous ceftriaxone followed by oral cefuroxime.[12] Clinical cure was greater with levofloxacin compared with cephalosporins (AR 96.5% v AR 90.4%; ARR 6.1%, 95% CI 1.3% to 10.7%).

Harms: See harms of new versus old antibiotics in outpatient settings, p 1042.

Comment: Although detection of penicillin resistant and multidrug resistant S pneumoniae is commonly reported, it is hard to enrol people with this infection in randomised studies. One study was carried out in areas with high prevalence of penicillin resistant S pneumoniae.[11] However, only eight of 135 isolates tested were resistant to penicillin and none showed high level resistance. The trials in uncomplicated pneumonia may not apply to people with comorbidities such as meningitis.[13] There are also concerns about macrolide-resistant S pneumoniae but, so far, treatment failure in ambulatory people with community acquired pneumonia is uncommon.[14] We found one retrospective review of 12 945 people in hospital (≥65 years old) with community acquired pneumonia. It found that initial treatment with a second generation cephalosporin plus a macrolide, a non-pseudomonal third generation cephalosporin plus a macrolide, or a fluoroquinolone alone, was associated with lower mortality at 30 days than treatment with β-lactam/β-lactamase inhibitor plus a macrolide, and an aminoglycoside plus another agent.[15] However, the results should be interpreted with caution as they may not account for confounding factors. There have been case reports of failure of azithromycin to cure multidrug resistant bacteraemic pneumococcal pneumonia.[16] One retrospective cohort study found that people infected with penicillin resistant S pneumoniae were at greater risk of death in hospital (RR 2.1, 95% CI 1 to 4.3) and suppurative complications (RR 4.5, 95% CI 1 to 19.3). From national surveillance data, mortality after the first 4 days in hospital was significantly associated with resistant pneumonia.[17] However, these results should be interpreted with caution as they may not account for confounding factors.

| OPTION | INTRAVENOUS VERSUS ORAL ANTIBIOTICS |

RCTs have found that, in immunocompetent people admitted to hospital who are not suffering life threatening illness, intravenous antibiotics are no more effective than oral antibiotics, and are associated with increased length of hospital stay.

Benefits: We found no systematic review. We found two RCTs comparing oral with intravenous antibiotics in people admitted to hospital with community acquired pneumonia. The first included 541 people with lower respiratory tract infections, two fifths of whom had chest radiographs that were compatible with pneumonia.[18] People were excluded if they had life threatening infection or were immunocompromised. Participants were randomised to 7 days of treatment with oral co-amoxiclav versus intravenous co-amoxiclav for 3 days followed by oral co-amoxiclav versus intravenous cefotaxime for 3 days followed by oral cefuroxime. At discharge there was no significant difference in cure rates or mortality among the three groups, but hospital stay was significantly shorter in those on oral treatment than in those on intravenous treatment (P < 0.001). The second RCT (73 people, no intention to treat analysis) compared intravenous versus oral cefuroxime.[19] Participants were randomised to 2 days of intravenous followed by 8 days of oral treatment (group 1) versus 5 days of each treatment (group 2) versus 10 days of intravenous treatment (group 3). The only significant difference was in the length of hospital stay (6 days with group 1 v 8 days with group 2 v 11 days with group 3, no CI or P values given).

Harms: None reported.

Comment: Intravenous antibiotics are needed in people who cannot take oral medication because of severe nausea or vomiting, or who are bacteraemic or in septicaemic shock. A follow up study (96 people admitted to hospital with community acquired pneumonia) found that people could be switched from intravenous to oral antibiotics when they had been afebrile for 8 hours, symptoms of cough and shortness of breath were improving, white blood counts were returning to normal, and they could tolerate oral medication.[20]

OPTION   BOTTLE BLOWING

One RCT has found that bottle blowing physiotherapy plus early mobilisation versus early mobilisation alone significantly reduces hospital stay.

Benefits: We found no systematic review. We found one RCT (145 people in hospital with community acquired pneumonia).[21] People were randomised to three groups: early mobilisation; early mobilisation and encouragement to sit up 10 times a day and take 20 deep breaths; and early mobilisation and encouragement to sit up 10 times a day and blow bubbles through a plastic tube for 20 breaths into a bottle containing 10 cm of water. Mean hospital stay in the three groups was 5.3, 4.6, and 3.9 days (P = 0.01 for early mobilisation compared with bottle blowing).

Harms: None reported.

Comment: Neither study participants nor clinicians could be blinded to the intervention.

QUESTION   Which treatments should be used in people with community acquired pneumonia receiving intensive care?

OPTION   DIFFERENT COMBINATIONS OF ANTIBIOTICS

We found no good evidence supporting any particular antibiotic combination in this setting.

Benefits: We found no systematic review and no RCTs comparing one combination of antibiotics with another in intensive care units.

Harms: We found no good evidence.

Comment: Using a combination of antibiotics is regarded as current best practice.

| OPTION | PROMPT VERSUS DELAYED ANTIBIOTIC TREATMENT |

Retrospective studies have found that prompt administration of antibiotics improve survival.

Benefits: We found no systematic review and no prospective studies. One multicentre retrospective review (medical records of ≥ 14 000 people aged 65 years or older who were severely ill with community acquired pneumonia) found that administering antibiotics within 8 hours of admission to hospital was associated with lower 30 day mortality (OR 0.90, 95% CI 0.75 to 0.96).[22] Another retrospective study (39 people with serologically confirmed Legionnaires' Disease) examined outcome and time to start of treatment.[23] For the 10 people who died, the median delay between diagnosis of pneumonia and start of erythromycin was 5 days (range 1–10 days), and for those who survived it was 1 day (range 1–5 days, P < 0.001).

Harms: None reported.

Comment: It would probably be regarded as unethical to perform an RCT of delayed antibiotic treatment.

| QUESTION | What are the effects of guidelines on the treatment of community acquired pneumonia? |

We found no evidence that guidelines improve clinical outcomes in community acquired pneumonia. One multicentre RCT has found that a critical pathway guideline improves process outcomes: more people treated at home; fewer hospital bed days for people managed; fewer days on intravenous antibiotics; and more frequent use of one class of antibiotics.

Benefits: We found one multicentre trial with cluster randomisation (9 teaching and 10 community hospitals, 1743 people presenting to emergency rooms) in Canada.[24] People who were immunosuppressed, people with active tuberculosis, people with cystic fibrosis, pregnant or lactating women, people with alcohol addiction, and people with chronic renal failure were excluded. Intervention hospitals (9 hospitals) used a critical pathway guideline for treating pneumonia (consisting of an admission guideline based on a severity of illness scoring system, a guideline for switching from intravenous to oral antibiotic therapy, a discharge guideline, and treatment with the antibiotic levofloxacin). Treatment at control hospitals (10 hospitals) consisted of usual care. The two groups did not significantly differ in quality of life (short form 36 physical component score), occurrence of complications, re-admission, or mortality. Intervention hospitals admitted fewer people at low risk (31% v 49%, P = 0.01), used fewer bed days per person managed (4.4 v 6.1, P = 0.04), administered 1.7 fewer days of intravenous antibiotic therapy (4.6 v 6.3 days, P = 0.01), and were more likely to use only one class of antibiotic (64% v 27%, P < 0.001).

Harms: None identified.

Comment: The effects might be larger than observed because people admitted to hospitals using the critical pathway guideline were at higher risk, so might have been expected to spend longer in hospital. The trial did not identify which components of the critical pathway guideline were beneficial.

Community acquired pneumonia

QUESTION What are the effects of preventive interventions?

OPTION INFLUENZA VACCINE

One systematic review of cohort studies, and three RCTs, have found that influenza vaccination reduces the risk of influenza and death in elderly people.

Benefits:
We found one systematic review (published in 1995, 20 cohort studies),[25] and three additional RCTs.[27–29] The pooled estimate for prevention of pneumonia was an absolute risk reduction of 53% (95% CI 35% to 66%) and for prevention of death 68% (95% CI 56% to 76%). Analysis of an administrative database ($\geq 25\,000$ people aged ≥ 64) suggested that influenza vaccination reduced the rate of admission to hospital for pneumonia and influenza by 48–57% (P < 0.01).[26] We found one double blind RCT (over 1800 people aged 60 years or over) comparing split viron vaccine versus saline solution.[27] At 5 months' follow up, the incidence of clinical influenza was significantly lower with vaccine than placebo (AR 17/927 [2%] v AR 31/911 [3%]; RR 0.53, 95% CI 0.39 to 0.73). One double blind RCT (324 elderly residents of nursing homes) compared trivalent inactivated parenteral vaccine with or without intranasal live attenuated cold adapted vaccine. It found that live vaccine provided additional protection against influenza A (rates of documented influenza were 9/162 [AR 5.5%] v 24/169 [AR 14.2%]; RRR 61%, 95% CI 18% to 82%).[28] One RCT (12 geriatric care hospitals) found that vaccination of healthcare workers in geriatric long term care facilities reduced total mortality of elderly residents from 17% to 10% during one winter.[29]

Harms:
Local adverse effects included pain and tenderness at the site of injection. Guillain-Barré syndrome was rare. It complicated one in 100 000 vaccinations during the national immunisation programme against swine influenza in the USA in 1976, during which 45 million people were vaccinated.[30]

Comment:
Reduction of rates of influenza does not necessarily imply reduction in rates of pneumonia.

OPTION PNEUMOCOCCAL VACCINE

RCTs of pneumococcal vaccine have found mixed results. One systematic review found evidence that available pneumococcal vaccines do not protect against death. It also found that pneumococcal vaccine protected young fit adults (but not older adults at high risk) against pneumococcal pneumonia. Subsequent RCTs found no evidence of benefit in older adults. Subgroup analysis suggests benefit in older adults at high risk of pneumonia.

Benefits:
We found one systematic review (search date 1991, 9 RCTs with 12 direct comparisons of vaccines v control, 40 431 people)[31] and two subsequent RCTs.[29,32] The review found that in adults at low risk (immunocompetent, aged < 55 years, no other chronic medical conditions), vaccination offered significant protection against confirmed pneumococcal pneumonia (positive S pneumoniae cultures) (OR v no vaccine 0.32, 95% CI 0.22 to 0.46). Meta-analysis found no evidence

of benefit in adults at high risk (people aged > 55 years, with one or more chronic medical conditions or immunosuppresssed: OR 1.23, 95% CI 0.28 to 5.43). It found no significant protection against other outcomes (all cause pneumonia, bronchitis, or death). The first subsequent double blind RCT (691 middle aged and elderly people admitted to hospital with community acquired pneumonia) compared a 23-valent pneumococcal capsular polysaccharide vaccine versus placebo.[32] It found no significant protective effect against subsequent pneumococcal pneumonia (RR 0.78, 95% CI 0.40 to 1.51) or all cause pneumonia (RR 0.83, 95% CI 0.58 to 1.12). The second RCT (2837 nursing home residents) compared pneumococcal and influenza vaccines versus influenza vaccine only.[29] All participants were followed for 3 years for development of radiologically confirmed pneumonia. Pneumococcal cause was defined serologically. No significant protection from pneumococcal pneumonia was found in the study group as a whole (RR v influenza vaccine alone 0.85, 95% CI 0.50 to 1.43).[33] However, there was significant protection in the subgroup with risk factors for contracting pneumonia: those who were immunocompromised; had received immunosuppressive treatment within 1 year before vaccination; had cancer, systemic connective tissue diseases, alcohol dependence, heart or lung disease; or were institutionalised or permanently bedridden (RR 0.41, 95% CI 0.18 to 0.94).

Harms: Injections often caused discomfort at the injection site. No other harms reported.

Comment: A fifth of healthy elderly adults (mean age 71 years) do not have an antibody response to vaccination.[34] New conjugate pneumococcal vaccines are being evaluated. These have been shown to be immunogenic in infants and have decreased the rate of carriage of resistant strains of S pneumoniae.[35,36] One recent retrospective cohort study (1898 elderly members of a staff healthcare organisation) found that pneumococcal vaccination was associated with lower risks of admission to hospital for pneumonia (adjusted RR 0.57, 95% CI 0.38 to 0.84) and for death (adjusted RR 0.71, 95% CI 0.56 to 0.91).[37] The study found evidence of an additive effect for people who received both pneumococcal and influenza vaccinations during the influenza season (RR 0.28, 95% CI 0.14 to 0.58 for admission to hospital for pneumonia and influenza; RR 0.18, 95% CI 0.11 to 0.31 for death).

REFERENCES

1. Foy HM, Cooney MK, Allan I, Kenny GE. Rates of pneumonia during influenza epidemics in Seattle, 1964–1975. JAMA 1979;241:253–258.

2. Murphy TF, Henderson FW, Clyde WA, Collier AM, Denny FW. Pneumonia: an 11 year study in a pediatric practice. Am J Epidemiol 1981;113:12–21.

3. McConnochie KM, Hall CB, Barker WH. Lower respiratory tract illness in the first two years of life: epidemiologic patterns and costs in a suburban pediatric practice. Am J Public Health 1988;78:34–39.

4. Porath A, Schlaeffer F, Lieberman D. The epidemiology of community-acquired pneumonia among hospitalized adults. J Infect 1997;34:41–48.

5. Jokinen C, Heiskanen L, Juvonen H, et al. Incidence of community-acquired pneumonia in the population of four municipalities in eastern Finland. Am J Epidemiol 1993;137:977–988.

6. Houston MS, Silverstein MD, Suman VJ. Risk factors for 30-day mortality in elderly patients with lower respiratory tract infection. Arch Intern Med 1997;157:2190–2195.

7. Bartlett JG, Mundy LM. Community-acquired pneumonia. N Engl J Med 1995;333:1618–1624.

8. Almirall J, Gonzalez CA, Balanco X, Bolibar I. Proportion of community-acquired pneumonia attributable to tobacco smoking. Chest 1999;116:375–379.

9. Fine MJ, Smith MA, Carson CA, et al. Prognosis and outcomes of patients with community-acquired pneumonia: a meta-analysis. JAMA 1995;274:134–141. Search date June 1995; primary sources Medline, and handsearching of reference lists.

10. Pomilla PV, Brown RB. Outpatient treatment of community-acquired pneumonia in adults. Arch

Intern Med 1994;154:1793–1802. Search date not given; primary sources Medline.

11. Aubier M, Verster R, Regamey C, Geslin, Vercken J-B, and the Sparfloxacin European Study Group. Once-daily sparfloxacin versus high-dosage amoxicillin in the treatment of community-acquired, suspected pneumococcal pneumonia in adults. Clin Infect Dis 1998;26:1312–1320.

12. File TM Jr, Segreti J, Dunbar L, et al. A multicenter, randomized study comparing the efficacy and safety of intravenous and/or oral levofloxacin versus ceftriaxone and/or cefuroxime axetil in treatment of adults with community-acquired pneumonia. Antimicrob Agents Chemother 1997; 41:1965–1972.

13. Friedland IR, McCracken GH Jr. Management of infections caused by antibiotic-resistant Streptococcus pneumoniae. N Engl J Med 1994; 331:377–382.

14. Siegel RE. The significance of serum vs. tissue levels of antibiotics in the treatment of penicillin-resistant Streptococcus pneumoniae and community-acquired pneumonia. Are we looking in the wrong place? Chest 1999;116:535–538.

15. Gleason PP, Meehan TP, Fine JM, et al. Associations between initial antimicrobial therapy and medical outcomes for hospitalized elderly patients with pneumonia. Arch Intern Med 1999; 159:2562–2572.

16. Siegel RE. The significance of serum vs. tissue levels of antibiotics in the treatment of penicillin-resistant Streptococcus pneumoniae and community-acquired pneumonia. Are we looking in the wrong place? Chest 1999;116:535–538.

17. Leikin DR, Schuchat A, Kolczak M, et al. Mortality from invasive pneumococcal pneumonia in the era of antibiotic resistance, 1995–1997. Am J Public Health 2000;90:223–229.

18. Chan R, Hemeryck L, O'Regan M, Clancy C, Feely J. Oral versus intravenous antibiotics for community-acquired lower respiratory tract infection in a general hospital: open randomised controlled trial. BMJ 1995;310:1360–1362.

19. Siegel RE, Halperin NA, Almenoff PL, Lee A, Greene JG. A prospective randomized study of inpatient IV antibiotics for community-acquired pneumonia: the optimal duration of therapy. Chest 1996;110:965–971.

20. Ramirez JA, Ahkee S. Early switch from intravenous antimicrobials to oral clarithromycin in patients with community acquired pneumonia. Infect Med 1997;14:319–323.

21. Bjorkqvist M, Wiberg B, Bodin L, Barany M, Holmberg H. Bottle-blowing in hospital-treated patients with community-acquired pneumonia. Scand J Infect Dis 1997;29:77–82.

22. Meehan TP, Fine MJ, Krumholz HM, et al. Quality of care, process, and outcomes in elderly patients with pneumonia. JAMA 1997;278:2080–2084.

23. Heath CH, Grove DI, Looke DFM. Delay in appropriate therapy of Legionella pneumonia associated with increased mortality. Eur J Clin Microbiol Infect Dis 1966;15:286–290.

24. Marrie TJ, Lau CY, Wheeler SL, et al. A controlled trial of a critical pathway for treatment of community-acquired pneumonia. JAMA 2000; 283:749–755.

25. Gross PA, Hermogenes AW, Sacks HS, Lau J, Levandowski RA. The efficacy of influenza vaccine in elderly persons: a meta-analysis and review of the literature. Ann Intern Med 1995;123:518–527. Search date not stated; primary source Medline.

26. Nichol KL, Margolis KL, Wuorenma J, Von Sternberg T. The efficacy and cost effectiveness of vaccination against influenza among elderly persons living in the community. N Engl J Med 1994;331:778–784.

27. Govaert TM, Thijs CT, Masurel N, Sprenger MJW, Dinant GJ, Knottnerus JA. The efficacy of influenza vaccination in elderly individuals: a randomized double-blind placebo-controlled trial. JAMA 1994; 272:1661–1665.

28. Treanor JJ, Mattison HR, Dumyati G, et al. Protective efficacy of combined live intranasal and inactivated influenza A virus vaccines in the elderly. Ann Intern Med 1992;117:625–633.

29. Potter J, Stott DJ, Roberts MA, et al. Influenza vaccination of health care workers in long-term-care hospitals reduces the mortality of elderly patients. J Infect Dis 1997;175:1–6.

30. Betts RF. Influenza virus. In: Mandell GL, Bennett JE, Dolin R, eds. Principles and practice of infectious diseases. 4th edn. New York: Churchill Livingstone, 1995.

31. Fine MJ, Smith MA, Carson CA, et al. Efficacy of pneumococcal vaccination in adults: a meta-analysis of randomized controlled clinical trials. Arch Intern Med 1994;154:2666–2677. Search date 1991; primary source Medline; hand searching of bibliographies of retrieved articles; and contact with key researchers and manufacturers.

32. Ortqvist A, Hedlund J, Burman L-A, et al, and Swedish Pneumococcal Vaccination Study Group. Randomised trial of 23-valent penumococcal capsular polysaccharide vaccine in prevention of pneumonia in middle-aged and elderly people. Lancet 1998;351:399–403.

33. Koivula I, Sten M, Leinonen M, Makela PH. Clinical efficacy of par pneumococcal vaccine in the elderly: a randomized, single-blind population-based trial. Am J Med 1997;103:281–290.

34. Rubins JB, Puri AKG, Loch J, et al. Magnitude, duration, quality and function of pneumococcal vaccine responses in elderly adults. J Infect Dis 1998;178:431–440.

35. Mbelle N, Wasas A, Huebner R, Kimura A, Chang I, Klugman K. Immunogenicity and impact on carriage of 9-valent pneumococcal conjugate vaccine given to infants in Soweto, South Africa. Proceedings of the 37th Interscience Conference on Antimicrobial Agents and Chemotherapy; 1997 September. Toronto, Herndon VA: ASM Press, 1997.

36. Gesner M, Desidero D, Kim M, et al. Streptococcus pneumoniae in human immunodeficiency virus type 1 infected children. Pediatr Infect Dis J 1994;13:697–703.

37. Nichol KL, Baken L, Wuorenma J, Nelson A. The health and economic benefits associated with pneumococcal vaccination in elderly people with chronic lung disease. Arch Intern Med 1999;159: 2437–2442.

Thomas Marrie

Professor and Chair, Department of Medicine, University of Alberta, Edmonton, Canada

Competing interests: The author has received a research grant from Bayer, and has spoken at events sponsored by Bayer, Janssen Ortho, Pfizer, and Abbott.

TABLE 1 Causes of community acquired pneumonia (see text, p 1041).

	USA (% of participants)*	UK (% of participants)†	Susceptibility (laboratory results)‡
Streptococcus pneumoniae	20–60	60–75	25% penicillin resistant, sensitive to quinolones
Haemophilus influenzae	3–10	4–5	30% ampicillin resistant, sensitive to cephalosporins or amoxicillin/clavulanic acid
Staphylococcus aureus	3–5	1–5	Methicillin resistant S aureus rare as cause of community acquired pneumonia
Chlamydia pneumoniae	4–6	–	Sensitive to macrolides, tetracyclines, quinolones
Mycoplasma pneumoniae	1–6	5–18	Sensitive to macrolides, tetracyclines, quinolones
Legionella pneumophila	2–8	2–5	Sensitive to macrolides, tetracyclines, quinolones
Gram-negative bacilli	3–10	Rare	
Aspiration	6–10	–	
Viruses	2–15	8–16	

*Pooled data from 15 published reports from North America;[7] †Data from British Thoracic Society;[7] ‡Susceptibility data from recent studies.

Lung cancer

Search date January 2001: expanded this issue

Alan Neville

QUESTIONS

INTERVENTIONS

NON-SMALL CELL LUNG CANCER
Beneficial

Likely to be beneficial

Unknown effectiveness

Unlikely to be beneficial

SMALL CELL LUNG CANCER
Beneficial

Trade off between benefits and harms

Unknown effectiveness

See glossary, p 1058

Key Messages

Non-small cell lung cancer

- One systematic review has found that, in people with completely resected stage 2 and 3 disease, postoperative cisplatinum based chemotherapy does not improve survival compared with surgery alone. We found limited evidence from two small RCTs that preoperative chemotherapy improved survival in people with technically resectable stage 3A disease.

- Systematic reviews and additional RCTs have found that, in people with unresectable stage 3 non-small cell lung cancer, combining thoracic irradiation with chemotherapy improves survival compared with radiotherapy alone. We found insufficient evidence about effects on quality of life.

- We found insufficient evidence from RCTs on the effects of hyperfractionation (including CHART — see glossary, p 1058) versus conventional fractionation in people with stage 3 non-small cell lung cancer.

- Systematic reviews have found a survival benefit with chemotherapy regimens containing cisplatin compared with best supportive care in people with stage 4 non-small cell lung cancer. Limited evidence from RCTs suggests that chemotherapy may improve quality of life compared with best supportive care. One systematic review and subsequent RCTs found conflicting evidence on the effects of single versus combined chemotherapy. We found insufficient evidence to assess the effects of second line chemotherapy.

Small cell lung cancer

- We found no good evidence on standard cisplatin or doxorubicin based chemotherapy versus other chemotherapy regimens.

- Two systematic reviews have found that adding thoracic irradiation to chemotherapy improves survival in people with limited stage small cell lung cancer. The best timing, dose, and fractionation of radiation remain uncertain.

- One systematic review of irradiation in people in complete remission found that prophylactic cranial irradiation improves survival and reduces the risk of developing brain metastases. Long term cognitive dysfunction following cranial irradiation has been described, but longer follow up studies are needed to assess its significance and importance.

- RCTs have found that oral etoposide improves survival significantly less than combination chemotherapy, but is less toxic in the short term. We found no evidence that it offers significantly better quality of life.

DEFINITION	Lung cancer or bronchogenic carcinoma is an epithelial cancer arising from the bronchial surface epithelium or bronchial mucous glands (see table 1, p 1061).
INCIDENCE/ PREVALENCE	Lung cancer is the leading cause of cancer death in both men and women, affecting about 100 000 men and 80 000 women annually in the USA, and about 40 000 men and women in the UK. Small cell lung cancer constitutes about 20–25% of all lung cancers, the remainder being non-small cell lung cancers, of which adenocarcinoma is now the most prevalent form.[1]
AETIOLOGY/ RISK FACTORS	Smoking remains the major preventable risk factor, accounting for about 80–90% of all cases.
PROGNOSIS	Lung cancer has an overall 5 year survival rate of 10–12%.[2] At the time of diagnosis, 10–15% of people with lung cancer have localised disease. Of these, half will have died at 5 years despite potentially curative surgery. Over half of people have metastatic disease at the time of diagnosis. For those with initially unresectable non-small cell lung cancer, combined treatment with radiotherapy and chemotherapy followed by surgery has achieved modest improvements in 5 year survival.[2] Prognosis depends on the stage of disease. In people with small cell cancer, those with limited stage disease who undergo combined chemotherapy and mediastinal irradiation have a median survival of 18–24 months, whereas those with extensive stage disease who are given palliative chemotherapy have a median survival of 10–12 months. About 5–10% of people with small cell lung cancer present with central nervous system involvement, and half develop symptomatic brain metastases by 2 years. Of these, only half respond to palliative radiation, and their

median survival is less than 3 months. People with non-small cell cancer who undergo surgery have a 5 year survival of 60–80% for stage 1 disease and 25–50% for stage 2 disease.[2]

AIMS   To cure disease; to prolong life; to improve quality of life; and to provide palliation, with minimum adverse effects of treatment.

OUTCOMES   Survival; clinical response rates; disease related symptoms; adverse effects of treatment; quality of life. Despite recent progress in the development of valid instruments, measuring quality of life in people with lung cancer remains a serious challenge.[3,4]

METHODS   *Clinical Evidence* update search and appraisal January 2001.

QUESTION   **What are the effects of treatments for non-small cell lung cancer?**

OPTION   PRE AND POSTOPERATIVE CHEMOTHERAPY IN NON-SMALL CELL LUNG CANCER   New

One systematic review has found that, in people with completely resected stage 2 and 3 disease, postoperative cisplatinum based chemotherapy does not improve survival compared with surgery alone. We found limited evidence from two small RCTs that preoperative chemotherapy improved survival in people with technically resectable stage 3A disease.

Benefits: **Postoperative chemotherapy:** We found one systematic review (search date 1995, 8 RCTs, 1394 people with resected stages 1–3 non-small cell lung cancer)[5] and one subsequent RCT.[6] The review compared postoperative cisplatin based chemotherapy versus surgery alone, and found that adjuvant chemotherapy did not significantly increase survival at 5 years (HR for death with chemotherapy v no chemotherapy: 0.87, 95% CI 0.74 to 1.02, P = 0.08; ARR for death at 5 years +5%, 95% CI −1% to +10%).[6] The subsequent RCT (488 people with completely resected stage 2 or 3A non-small cell lung cancer) compared postoperative radiotherapy with or without cisplatin plus etoposide.[6] It found no significant difference in survival between groups (median survival 38.8 months for radiotherapy alone v 37.9 months for radiotherapy plus chemotherapy, P = 0.56). **Preoperative chemotherapy:** We found two small RCTs (60 people each, with technically resectable stage 3A disease) of preoperative chemotherapy versus no chemotherapy.[7,8] A pooled analysis of these trials found that preoperative chemotherapy versus no chemotherapy significantly improved 2 year survival (OR 0.18, 95% CI 0.06 to 0.51, P = 0.001).[9]

Harms: Many adjuvant chemotherapy studies were published before serotonin receptor antagonist antiemetics were available. One trial (269 people) found that only 53% of people completed all four courses of cyclophosphamide, adriamycin, and cisplatin. Mild to severe gastrointestinal toxicity was reported in 88% of people.[10] A second RCT reported similar toxicity.[11]

Comment: Most of the chemotherapy regimens in the postoperative studies are no longer used, and trials examining newer agents are needed. Larger trials of preoperative chemotherapy in people with stage 3A non-small cell lung cancer are also needed.

THORACIC RADIATION ADDED TO CHEMOTHERAPY FOR UNRESECTABLE STAGE 3 NON-SMALL CELL LUNG CANCER

Systematic reviews and additional RCTs have found that, in people with unresectable stage 3 non-small cell lung cancer, combining thoracic irradiation with chemotherapy improves survival compared with radiotherapy alone. We found insufficient evidence about effects on quality of life.

Benefits: We found three systematic reviews[5,12,13] and two additional RCTs[14,15] comparing thoracic irradiation plus chemotherapy versus radiotherapy alone in people with unresected stage 3 non-small cell lung cancer. The first review (search date 1995, 22 RCTs, 3033 people, range 48–353) found a pooled hazard ratio for mortality of 0.90 (95% CI 0.83 to 0.97), with an absolute survival benefit associated with combined treatment of 3% at 2 years.[5] The second review (search date 1995, 14 RCTs, 1887 people) found that adding a cisplatin based regimen to radiotherapy was associated with a significant reduction in mortality at 1 and 2 years (pooled OR at 1 year 0.76, 95% CI 0.6 to 0.9; at 2 years 0.7, 95% CI 0.5 to 0.9).[12] The third review (search date 1995, 14 RCTs, 2589 people) found similar results.[13] We found two additional RCTs. The first (458 people) compared 2 months of cisplatin and vinblastine followed by standard radiotherapy versus either standard or hyperfractionated radiotherapy alone. It found that combined therapy significantly improved 5 year survival compared with hyperfractionated therapy (8% v 6%, P = 0.04), and compared with standard therapy (8% v 5%, P = 0.04).[14] The second RCT (446 people) compared radical radiotherapy with versus without of up to four cycles of mitomycin, ifosfamide, and cisplatin. It found no significant difference in survival (median survival 11.7 months with combined treatment v 9.7 months with radiotherapy alone).[15]

Harms: The reviews gave no information on long term adverse effects of treatment.

Comment: We found insufficient evidence about effects on quality of life.

HYPERFRACTIONATED RADIATION THERAPY FOR UNRESECTABLE STAGE 3 NON-SMALL CELL LUNG CANCER New

We found insufficient evidence from RCTs on the effects of CHART (see glossary, p 1058) or hyperfractionation versus conventional fractionation in people with stage 3 non-small cell lung cancer.

Benefits: **Hyperfractionation:** We found one systematic review (search date 1999, 3 RCTs, 442 people) comparing standard hyperfractionation (not CHART) versus conventional radiotherapy. It found no significant difference in 2 year survival (OR 0.67, 95% CI 0.42 to 1.07, P = 0.09).[16] **CHART:** We found no systematic review or RCTs exclusively in people with stage 3 non-small cell lung cancer. One RCT (563 people with non-small cell lung cancer; 61% with stage 3A or 3B; 39% with stage 1 or stage 2) compared CHART versus conventional radiotherapy.[17] It found that CHART significantly improved 2 year survival compared with conventional radiotherapy (AR 29% v 20% with conventional radiotherapy, HR 0.78, 95% CI 0.65 to 0.94, P = 0.008), and improved local tumour control (HR for local control 0.79, 95% CI 0.63 to 0.98, P = 0.03).

Harms: Additional evidence on adverse effects were published subsequent to the RCT on CHART.[18] Significantly more people receiving CHART versus conventional radiotherapy had cough (P = 0.01), shortness of breath (P = 0.03), and dizziness (P = 0.03). There was no significant difference in long term morbidity.[17,18]

Comment: RCTs comparing CHART versus conventional radiotherapy versus chemotherapy plus radiotherapy in people with stage 3 non-small cell lung cancer are in progress.[16]

OPTION	CHEMOTHERAPY IN STAGE 4 NON-SMALL CELL LUNG CANCER

Systematic reviews have found a survival benefit with chemotherapy regimens containing cisplatin compared with best supportive care in people with stage 4 non-small cell lung cancer. Limited evidence from RCTs suggests that chemotherapy may improve quality of life compared with best supportive care. One systematic review and subsequent RCTs found conflicting evidence on the effects of single versus combined chemotherapy. We found insufficient evidence to assess the effects of second line chemotherapy.

Benefits: **First line chemotherapy:** We found five systematic reviews,[4,5,19–21] which addressed survival in people with stage 4 non-small cell lung cancer. The most recent review (search date 2000, 11 RCTs, 1190 people with advanced disease) compared supportive care versus supportive care plus chemotherapy.[21] It found that, in older trials (from the 1970s), long term alkylating agents did not significantly improve survival (death with supportive care plus chemotherapy v supportive alone; HR 1.26, 95% CI 0.96 to 1.66, P = 0.095). However, cisplatin containing regimens significantly reduced the risk of death at 1 year (HR 0.73 for death with combined treatment v supportive care alone, P < 0.0001), and increased median survival (5.5 v 4 months). It is not possible to deduce from these studies to what extent the observed effects are due to the cisplatin or to all the other drugs in the combinations studied. We found four RCTs, which compared single agent chemotherapy versus best supportive care, and assessed effects on quality of life.[22–25] Chemotherapeutic agents used were vinorelbine (191 people aged over 70),[22] gemcitabine (300 people),[23] docetaxel (207 people),[24] and paclitaxel (157 people).[25] Overall, the trials consistently found that chemotherapy improved quality of life compared with best supportive care. **Single agent versus combined chemotherapy:** We found one systematic review (search date 1996, 25 RCTs, 5156 people)[26] and four subsequent RCTs.[27–30] The review found that overall, platinum analogue or vinorelbine-containing combination chemotherapy did not significantly improve 1 year survival compared with platinum analogue or vinorelbine alone (RR 1.10, 95% CI 0.94 to 1.43).[26] The first subsequent RCT (120 people with advanced disease aged > 70 years) found that gemcitabine plus vinorelbine improved survival compared with vinorelbine alone (at 14 months median follow up, median survival 29 weeks with combined treatment v 18 weeks, P < 0.01).[27] The second RCT (522 chemotherapy-naive people) found that gemcitabine plus cisplatin versus cisplatin alone significantly improved survival (median survival 9.1 months with combination treatment v 7.6 months, P = 0.004).[28] The third RCT (415 people) found a similar result for cisplatin plus vinorelbine versus cisplatin alone (median survival 8 months with combination v 6 months, P = 0.002).[29] The fourth RCT found no significant difference for median survival between cisplatin plus etoposide versus gemcitabine (median survival 6.6 months with gemcitabine v 7.6 months with cisplatin plus etoposide).[30] **Second line chemotherapy:** We found one systematic review (search date not stated, 34 single agent studies and 24 combination regimen studies),[31] and two subsequent RCTs.[32,33] The review found that results from RCTs were conflicting, and that studies differed in their definition of people considered sensitive or refractory to treatment. The first subsequent RCT (104 people) found that docetaxel versus supportive care significantly improved 1 year survival (37% with docetaxel v 11% with supportive care, P = 0.003).[32] The second RCT (373 people who had previously received cisplatin based chemotherapy) comparing docetaxel versus vinorelbine or isofosfamide found no significant difference in median survival.[33]

Harms: Some studies have reported improvement in lung cancer symptoms with chemotherapy, but over 50% of advanced lung cancer patients treated with chemotherapy reported alopecia, and gastrointestinal and haematological toxicity.[34] One non-systematic review found greater toxicity in patients with Eastern Cooperative Oncology Group performance status 3 or 4 (see glossary, p 1058).[35]

Comment: People with Eastern Cooperative Oncology Group performance status 3 or 4 have usually been excluded from RCTs of lung cancer chemotherapy. Carboplatin has comparable activity to, but a better toxicity profile than, cisplatin in patients with stage 4 non-small cell lung cancer.[36] Newer agents such as vinorelbine, gemcitabine, irinotecan, paclitaxel, and docetaxel produce objective responses in more than 20% of people with advanced lung cancer, and are being studied prospectively alone or in combination with cisplatin or carboplatin in RCTs.[36] For people with stage 4 non-small cell lung cancer, treatment options consist of either chemotherapy or symptomatic care, including palliative radiation. Measuring quality of life in people with lung cancer remains a serious challenge.

QUESTION   **What are the effects of treatments for small cell lung cancer?**

OPTION   STANDARD CHEMOTHERAPY VERSUS OTHER REGIMENS

We found no good evidence comparing standard cisplatin or doxorubicin based chemotherapy with other drug regimens.

Benefits: We found no systematic review and no large scale RCT. One RCT (229 people) comparing dose intense treatment versus standard chemotherapy found no significant difference in progression free survival (median 0.66 years in each group), or overall survival (0.98 v 0.91 years).[37]

Harms: Except in people with widespread extensive stage disease, adverse effects of chemotherapy were of short duration. One RCT found that dose intense treatment increased toxic deaths (deaths related to toxicity 9/110 [8%] with dose intense treatment v 1/109 [1%] with standard chemotherapy; ARI 7%, 95% CI 2% to 14%; RR 8.9, 95% CI 1.1 to 69; NNH 14; 95% CI 7 to 60).[37]

Comment: Standard chemotherapy for both limited and extensive stage disease comprised 4–6 cycles of etoposide plus cisplatin, or a regimen that alternates three cycles of etoposide plus cisplatin with three cycles of cyclophosphamide, doxorubicin, and vincristine.[38] Thoracic irradiation was given to people responding to high dose treatment and by discretion to people on standard dose treatment.

OPTION   **ADDING THORACIC IRRADIATION TO CHEMOTHERAPY IN LIMITED STAGE SMALL CELL LUNG CANCER**

Two systematic reviews of RCTs have found that adding thoracic irradiation to chemotherapy improves survival in people with limited stage small cell lung cancer. The best timing, dose, and fractionation of radiation remains uncertain.

Benefits: We found two systematic reviews of adding thoracic irradiation to chemotherapy in people with limited stage small cell lung cancer. The first review (search date 1992, 13 RCTs, 2573 people, range 52–426 people) found 3 year survival was significantly higher with radiation plus chemotherapy versus chemotherapy alone (15% v 10%, P = 0.001).[39] The second review (search date not stated, 11 RCTs, 10 of which were common to the first review, 1911 people) pooled data from nine of the RCTs (1521 people) and found that local control was achieved in 50% with radiation versus 25% with chemotherapy alone (ARR 25%, 95% CI 17% to 34%).[40] **Timing of radiation:** We found one systematic review (search date 1999, 4 RCTs, 927 people), which added early versus late thoracic radiotherapy to chemotherapy,[41] and one additional RCT.[42] The review found no significant difference in 5 year survival (30% v 15%, P = 0.03).[42] **Dose:** We found one RCT (333 people) comparing standard dose radiotherapy (25 Gy over 2 weeks) versus high dose radiotherapy (37.5 Gy over 3 weeks).[43] It found no significant difference in overall survival between the groups. **Fractionation:** We found two RCTs.[44,45] One RCT found that hyperfractionation (twice daily treatment) versus conventional fractionation significantly improved 5 year survival (26% with hyperfractionation v 16% with conventional fractionation, P = 0.04).[44] The second RCT found no significant difference in 3 year survival (34% with 50.4 Gy in 28 fractions daily v 29% with 48 Gy in 32 fractions twice daily, P = 0.46).[45]

Harms: The risk of treatment related death was more than twice as high in people given thoracic irradiation compared with those receiving chemotherapy alone (29/884 [3.3%] v 12/841 [1.4%]; OR 2.54,

95% CI 1.90 to 3.18).[40] The incidence of oesophagitis was also higher in those treated with twice daily irradiation.[44]

Comment: Interest in adding thoracic irradiation derives from the observation that local recurrence in the chest is a major cause of first treatment failure and carries an extremely poor prognosis. A non-systematic review found that median survival in limited stage disease has improved over the past 10 years from 14–16 months to 20–24 months.[46] The causes of this improvement have not been established but may include the early use of radiation plus chemotherapy rather than improvements in either modality alone.[47] The RCTs of timing used different methods and do not provide strong evidence. The different results from the three RCTs on early versus late concurrent radiotherapy may be explained by different rates of early toxicity from treatment and different rates of relapse in the central nervous system.

OPTION	PROPHYLACTIC CRANIAL IRRADIATION IN LIMITED STAGE SMALL CELL LUNG CANCER

One systematic review of RCTs of irradiation in people in complete remission found that prophylactic cranial irradiation improves survival and reduces the risk of developing brain metastases. Long term cognitive dysfunction following cranial irradiation has been described, but longer follow up studies are needed to assess its significance and importance.

Benefits: We found one systematic review (search date not stated, 7 RCTs, 987 people) of cranial irradiation for people with small cell lung cancer in complete remission.[48] The review identified RCTs that used individual participant data. Of the people studied, 12% in the irradiation group and 17% in the control group had extensive stage disease at presentation. Meta-analysis found that cranial irradiation significantly improved survival (RR of death at 3 years 0.84, 95% CI 0.73 to 0.97, corresponding to a 5.4% increase in survival) and increased disease-free survival (RR of recurrence or death at 3 years 0.75, 95% CI 0.65 to 0.86). Subgroup analysis identified survival benefit only for men and not for women, but the difference in survival was not significant ($P = 0.07$). The cumulative incidence of brain metastases was decreased (RR 0.46, 95% CI 0.38 to 0.57). Larger doses of radiation led to a greater decrease in brain metastases ($P = 0.02$), but did not influence survival significantly ($P = 0.89$).

Harms: Whether prophylactic cranial irradiation leads to neuropsychological sequelae could not be addressed in the meta-analysis because adequate assessments were carried out in only two of the seven trials. These and other studies found that 24–60% of participants may have neuropsychological problems before treatment,[48] and other studies have not accounted for potential confounding factors such as age, tobacco use, paraneoplastic syndromes, and neurotoxic chemotherapy effects.[48]

Comment: The clinical significance of cognitive impairment after prophylactic cranial irradiation remains unclear.

| OPTION | ORAL ETOPOSIDE IN EXTENSIVE STAGE SMALL CELL LUNG CANCER |

RCTs have found that oral etoposide improves survival signicantly less than combination chemotherapy. Etoposide is less toxic in the short term, but we found no evidence that it offers significantly better quality of life.

Benefits: We found no systematic review. Several RCTs have compared oral etoposide versus chemotherapy. One RCT (155 people with extensive stage disease) compared oral etoposide 100 mg daily for 5 days versus combination chemotherapy. Survival was significantly higher with combination chemotherapy than with etoposide at 1 year (19.3% v 9.8%, P < 0.05). There was no significant difference in median survival (5.9 v 4.8 months) and there were conflicting results on quality of life. Nausea was worse with combination chemotherapy (P < 0.01), but pain, appetite, general wellbeing, and mood were worse with oral etoposide (P < 0.001). Palliation of lung cancer symptoms was of shorter duration with etoposide (P < 0.01).[49]

Harms: Acute nausea and vomiting were worse with combined intravenous chemotherapy, but there was no significant difference in overall quality of life.[49] Treatment related symptoms were worse with combination chemotherapy (P < 0.01).

Comment: Because treatment of extensive stage disease is palliative, and because age has been identified as a prognostic factor in small cell lung cancer, studies have looked at outcomes in elderly people with limited and extensive stage disease, and in people of all ages with a poor prognosis. Although small cell lung cancer is relatively sensitive to chemotherapy, extensive stage disease remains incurable. Median survival with treatment is 10–12 months, and as yet has been unaffected by high dose combination chemotherapy. Because of its lower toxicity, etoposide may be considered for elderly people with extensive stage disease or people with a poor prognosis.

GLOSSARY

Continuous, hyperfractionated, accelerated radiotherapy (CHART) Radiotherapy given at a rate of two or more radiation fractions a day (each of smaller dose than conventionally fractionated doses). The number of fractions a week is gradually increased to shorten overall duration of therapy.

Performance status Expression used to describe functional status or wellness of participants in studies of cancer. There are two widely accepted scales: the Eastern Cooperative Oncology Group scale (0 = no symptoms; 1 = symptomatic but no extra time in bed; 2 = in bed less than 50% of the day, no work, can care for self; 3 = in bed more than 50% of day, not bedridden, minimal self care; 4 = completely bedridden), and the Karnofsky Scale of symptoms and disability (from 100% = no symptoms to 0% = dead).

Substantive changes since last issue

Thoracic radiation added to chemotherapy for unresectable stage 3 nonsmall cell lung cancer Two additional RCTs;[14,15] conclusions unchanged.

First line chemotherapy for stage 4 non-small cell lung cancer Updated systematic review;[21] conclusions unchanged.

First line chemotherapy for stage 4 non-small cell lung cancer Four RCTs;[22–25] conclusions updated.

Single agent versus combined chemotherapy for stage 4 non-small cell lung cancer One new systematic review and subsequent RCTs;[26–30] conclusions updated.

Second line chemotherapy for stage 4 non-small cell lung cancer New systematic review[31] and one subsequent RCT;[33] conclusions updated.

Timing and sequencing of radiation in limited stage small cell lung cancer New systematic review replaces previous RCTs;[41] conclusions unchanged.

Dose and fractionation of radiation in limited stage small cell lung cancer Additional RCTs;[43,45] conclusions unchanged.

REFERENCES

1. Travis WD, Travis LB, Devesa SS. Lung cancer. *Cancer* 1995;75(suppl 1):191–202.
2. Ihde DC, Pass HI, Glatstein E. Lung cancer. In: DeVita VT Jr, Hellman S, Rosenberg SA, eds. *Cancer, principles and practice of oncology*, 5th ed. Philadelphia: Lippincott-Raven, 1997;849–959.
3. Montazeri A, Gillis CR, McEwen J. Quality of life in people with lung cancer: a review of literature from 1970 to 1995. *Chest* 1998;113:467–481.
4. Grilli R, Oxman AD, Julian JA. Chemotherapy for advanced non-small cell lung cancer: how much benefit is enough? *J Clin Oncol* 1993;11:1866–1872. Search date 1991; primary source Medline 1970 to 1991.
5. Non-Small Cell Lung Cancer Collaborative Group. Chemotherapy in non-small cell lung cancer: a meta-analysis using update individual patient data from 52 randomized clinical trials. *BMJ* 1995; 311:899–909. Search date 1995; primary sources Medline; Cancer CD; hand search of meetings abstracts, bibliographies of books and specialist journals; consultation of trials registers of National Cancer Institute, UK Coordinating Committee for Cancer Research, and the Union Internationale Contre le Cancer.
6. Keller SM, Adak S, Wagner H, et al. A randomized trial of postoperative adjuvant therapy in patients with completely resected stage II or IIIA non-small-cell lung cancer. *N Engl J Med* 2000;343:1217–1222.
7. Rosell R, Gomez-Codina J, Camps C, et al. A randomized trial comparing preoperative chemotherapy plus surgery alone in patients with non-small-cell lung cancer. *N Engl J Med* 1994; 330:153–158.
8. Roth JA, Atkinson EN, Fossella F, et al. Long-term follow-up of patients enrolled in a randomized trial comparing perioperative chemotherapy and surgery with surgery alone in resectable stage IIIA non-small-cell lung cancer. *Lung Cancer* 1998;21:1–6.
9. Goss G, Paszat L, Newman T, et al. Use of preoperative chemotherapy with or without postoperative radiotherapy in technically resectable stage IIIA non-small cell lung cancer. *Cancer Prev Control* 1998;2:32–39.
10. Feld R, Rubinstein L, Thomas PA, Lung Cancer Study Group. Adjuvant chemotherapy with cyclophosphamide, doxorubicin, and cisplatin in patients with completely resected stage I non-small-cell lung cancer. *J Natl Canc Inst* 1993;85:299–306.
11. Niiranen A, Niitamo-Korhonen S, Kouri M, et al. Adjuvant chemotherapy after radical surgery for non-small cell lung cancer: A randomized study. *J Clin Oncol* 1992;10:1927–1932.
12. Marino P, Preatoni A. Randomized trials of radiotherapy alone versus combined chemotherapy and radiotherapy in stages IIIa and IIIb non small cell lung cancer. *Cancer* 1995;76: 593–601. Search date 1995; primary sources Medline and manual search of references of review articles and abstracts.
13. Pritchard RS, Anthony SP. Chemotherapy plus radiotherapy compared with radiotherapy alone in the treatment of locally advance, unresectable, non-small-cell lung cancer. *Ann Intern Med* 1996; 125:723–729. Search date 1995; primary sources Medline, plus manual search of references of review articles and abstracts.
14. Sause W, Kolesar P, Taylor S, et al. Final results of phase III trial in regionally advanced unresectable non-small cell lung cancer: Radiation Therapy Oncology Group, Eastern Cooperative Oncology Group, and Southwest Oncology Group. *Chest* 2000;117:358–364.
15. Cullen MH, Billingham CM, Woodroffe AD, et al. Mitomycin, ifosfamide, and cisplatin in unresectable non-small cell lung cancer: effects on survival and quality of life. *J Clin Oncol* 1999; 17:3188–3194.
16. Yu E, Lochrin C, Dixon P, et al. Altered fractionation of radical radiation therapy in the management of unresectable non-small-cell lung cancer. *Curr Oncol* 2000;7:98–109.
17. Saunders M, Dische S, Barrett A, et al. Continuous, hyperfractionated, accelerated radiotherapy (CHART) versus conventional radiotherapy in non-small cell lung cancer: mature data from the randomised multicentre trial. *Radiother Oncol* 1999;52:137–148.
18. Bailey AJ, Parmar MKB, Stephens RJ. Patient-reported short-term and long-term physical and psychological symptoms: results of the continuous hyperfractionated accelerated radiotherapy (CHART) randomized trial in non-small cell lung cancer. *J Clin Oncol* 1998;16:3082–3093.
19. Souquet PJ, Chauvin F, Boissel JP, et al. Polychemotherapy in advanced non small cell lung cancer: a meta-analysis. *Lancet* 1993;342:19–21. Search date not given; manual and computerised search of medical journals.
20. Marino P, Pampallona S, Preatoni A, et al. Chemotherapy versus supportive care in advanced non-small cell lung cancer: results of a meta-analysis of the literature. *Chest* 1994;106:861–865. Search date not given; primary sources Medline and manual search of references from review articles and abstracts.
21. Non-Small Cell Lung Cancer Collaborative Group. Chemotherapy for non-small cell lung cancer. In: The Cochrane Library, Issue 4, 2000. Search date February 2000; primary sources Medline, Cancerlit, handsearching, and discussion with trialists..
22. Elderly Lung Cancer Vinorelbine Study Group. Effects of vinorelbine on quality of life and survival

of elderly patients with non-small cell lung cancer. *J Natl Cancer Inst* 1999;91:66–72.

23. Anderson H, Hopwood P, Stephens RJ, et al. Gemcitabine plus best supportive care (BSC) versus BSC in inoperable non-small cell lung cancer in a randomised trail with quality of life as the primary outcome. *Br J Cancer* 2000;83:447–453.

24. Roszkowski K, Pluzanska A, Krzakowski M, et al. A Multicenter, randomised phase III study of docetaxel plus best supportive care versus best supportive care in chemo-naive patients with metastatic or non-resectable localised non-small cell lung cancer (NSCLC). *Lung Cancer* 2000;27: 145–157.

25. Ranson M, Davidson N, Nicolson M, et al. Randomised trial of paclitaxel plus supportive care versus supportive care for patients with advanced non-small cell lung cancer. *J Natl Cancer Inst* 2000;92:1074–1080.

26. Lilenbaum RC, Langenberg P, Dickersin K. Single agent versus combination chemotherapy in patients with advanced non-small cell lung cancer: a meta-analysis of response, toxicity and survival. *Cancer* 1998;82:116–126. Search dates and primary sources Medline 1976 to 1995; Embase 1974 to 1996; handsearching of references; physician data query from the National Cancer Institute; and expert consultation.

27. Frasci G, Lorusso V, Panza N, et al. Gemcitabine plus vinorelbine versus vinorelbine alone in elderly patients with advanced non-small cell lung cancer. *J Clin Oncol* 2000;18:2529–2536.

28. Sandler AB, Nemunaitis J, Denham C, et al. Phase III trial of gemcitabine plus cisplatin versus cisplatin alone in patients with locally advanced or metastatic non-small cell lung cancer. *J Clin Oncol* 2000;18:122–130.

29. Wozniak AG, Crowley JJ, Balcerzak SP, et al. Randomised trial comparing cisplatin with cisplatin plus vinorelbine in the treatment of advanced non-small cell lung cancer: a Southwest Oncology Group study. *J Clin Oncol* 1998;16:2459–2465.

30. Bokkel-Huinink WW, Bergman B, Chemaissani A, et al. Single-agent gemcitabine: an active and better tolerated alternative to standard cisplatin-based chemotherapy in locally advanced or metastatic non-small cell lung cancer. *Lung Cancer* 1999;26:85–94.

31. Huisman C, Smit EF, Postmus PE. Second-line chemotherapy in relapsing or refractory non-small cell lung cancer: a review. *J Clin Oncol* 2000;18: 3722–3730. Search date not stated; primary sources Medline and hand searches of the past five conference abstracts of the American Society of Clinical Oncology, European Cancer Conference, and the European Society of Medical Oncology.

32. Shepherd FA, Dancey J, Ramlau, et al. Prospective randomized trial of docetaxel versus best supportive care in patients with non-small-cell lung cancer previously treated with platinum-based chemotherapy. *J Clin Oncol* 2000;18: 2095–2103.

33. Fossella FV, DeVore R, Kerr RN. Randomized phase III trial of docetaxel versus vinorelbine or ifosfamide in patients with advanced non-small cell lung cancer previously treated with platinum-containing regimens. *J Clin Oncol* 2000;18:2354–2362.

34. Le Chevalier T, Brisgand D, Douillard J-Y, et al. Randomised study of vinorelbine and cisplatin versus vindesine and cisplatin versus vinorelbine alone in advanced non-small cell lung cancer:

results of a European multicenter trial including 612 people. *J Clin Oncol* 1994;12:360–367.

35. Bunn PA Jr, Kelly K. New chemotherapeutic agents prolong survival and improve quality of life in non-small cell lung cancer: a review of literature and future directions. *Clin Cancer Res* 1998;16:27–33.

36. Bunn PA Jr. Review of therapeutic trials of carboplatin in lung cancer. *Semin Oncol* 1989;16: 27–33.

37. Murray N, Livingston RB, Shepherd FA, et al. Randomised study of CODE versus alternating CAV/EP for extensive-stage small-cell lung cancer: an intergroup study of the National Cancer Institute of Canada clinical trials group and the Southwest oncology group. *J Clin Oncol* 1999;17: 2300–2308.

38. Murray N. New drugs for small cell lung cancer. *Oncology* 1997;11:38–42.

39. Pignon JP, Arriagada R, Ihde DC, et al. A meta-analysis of thoracic radiotherapy for small-cell lung cancer. *N Engl J Med* 1992;327:1618–1624. Search date 1992; primary sources Medline and hand search of proceedings of key oncology meetings.

40. Warde P, Payne D. Does thoracic irradiation improve survival and local control in limited-stage small cell carcinoma of the lung? A meta-analysis. *J Clin Oncol* 1992;10:890–895. Search date not given; primary sources Medline and Cancerline.

41. Okawara G, Gagliardi A, Evans WK, et al. The role of thoracic radiotherapy as an adjunct to standard chemotherapy in limited-stage small-cell lung cancer. *Curr Oncol* 2000;7:162–172.

42. Jeremic B, Shibamoto Y, Acimovic L, et al. Initial versus delayed accelerated hyperfractionated radiation therapy and concurrent chemotherapy in limited small-cell lung cancer. A randomised study. *J Clin Oncol* 1997;15:893–900.

43. Coy P, Hodson I, Payne DG, et al. The effect of dose of thoracic irradiation on recurrence in patients with limited stage small cell lung cancer. Initial results of a Canadian Multicentre Randomized Trial. *Int J Radiat Oncol Biol Phys* 1988;14:219–226.

44. Turrisi AT, Kim K, Blum R, et al. Twice-daily compared with once-daily thoracic radiotherapy in limited small-cell lung cancer treated concurrently with cisplatin and etoposide. *N Engl J Med* 1999; 340:265–271.

45. Bonner JA, Sloan JA, Shanahan TG, et al. Phase III comparison of twice-daily split-course irradiation versus once-daily irradiation for patients with limited stage small-cell lung carcinoma. *J Clin Oncol* 1999;17:2681–2691.

46. Kumar P. The role of radiotherapy in the management of limited-stage small cell lung cancer: past, present, and future. *Chest* 1997; 112(suppl):259–265.

47. Murray N, Coy P, Pater JL, et al. Importance of timing for thoracic irradiation in the combined modality treatment of limited-stage small cell lung cancer. *J Clin Oncol* 1993;11:336–344.

48. Auperin A, Arriagada R, Pignon J-P, et al. Prophylactic cranial irradiation for people with small-cell lung cancer in complete remission. *N Engl J Med* 1999;341:476–484. Search date not given; primary sources Medline, CancerLit, Excerpta Medica, and Biosis.

49. Souhami RL, Spiro SG, Rudd RM, et al. Five day oral etoposide treatment for advanced small cell lung cancer: randomized comparison with intravenous chemotherapy. *J Natl Cancer Inst* 1997;89:577–580.

Alan Neville

Professor, McMaster University, Hamilton, Canada

Competing interests: None declared.

TABLE 1 Staging lung cancer (see text, p 1051).

Non-small cell lung cancer

Stage	Definition*	5 year survival (%)
1	T1–T2, N0, M0	55–75
2	T1–T2, N1, M0	25–50
3A	T3, N0–N1, M0 or T1–T3, N2, M0	20–40
3B	T4, any N, M0 or any T, N3, M0	≤5
4	Any M1	≤5

Small cell lung cancer

Stage	Definition	Median survival
Limited stage disease	Tumour confined to the same side of the chest, supraclavicular lymph nodes, or both	18–24 months†
Extensive stage disease	Defined as anything beyond limited stage	10–12 months‡

*M, metastases; N, nodes; T, tumour; †with combined chemotherapy and mediastinal irradiation; ‡with palliative chemotherapy.

Spontaneous pneumothorax

Search date December 2000

John Cunnington

INTERVENTIONS

Key Messages

Treatment

- We found insufficient evidence to determine whether any intervention is more effective than none for spontaneous pneumothorax.

- Two small RCTs have found that resolution is more rapid with chest tube drainage than needle aspiration, but people treated with needle aspiration required less analgesia and spent less time in hospital.

- One small RCT found no difference in duration of tube drainage between small and standard sized chest tubes, but for people with larger pneumothoraces successful resolution was more likely with larger tubes.

- One small RCT found no difference in rate of resolution when one way valves were compared with drainage bottles with an underwater seal, but people treated with one way valves required less analgesia and spent less time in hospital.

- One small RCT found no difference in rate of resolution whether chest tube drainage bottles were connected to suction or not.

Preventing recurrence

- Two RCTs and one non-randomised trial have found that chemical pleurodesis reduces the rate of recurrence of spontaneous pneumothorax. The studies found that pleurodesis can be painful and may increase time spent in hospital.

- We found insufficient evidence to inform decisions on whether pleurodesis should take place after the first, second, or subsequent episodes of spontaneous pneumothorax.

- We found insufficient evidence on the effects of surgical versus chemical pleurodesis. One small RCT has found that video-assisted thorascopic surgery versus thoracotomy significantly reduces hospital stay. The rate of recurrence was not significantly different, but limited evidence does not exclude a clinically significant difference.

DEFINITION	A pneumothorax is air in the pleural space. A spontaneous pneumothorax occurs when there is no provoking factor, such as trauma, surgery, or diagnostic intervention. It implies a leak of air from the lung parenchyma through the visceral pleura into the pleural space.
INCIDENCE/ PREVALENCE	Incidence is about seven in 100 000 for men and one in 100 000 for women.[1] Smoking increases the likelihood of spontaneous pneumothorax by 22 times for men and 8 times for women. A dose response relationship has been observed.[2]
AETIOLOGY/ RISK FACTORS	Spontaneous pneumothorax can be primary (generally occurring in young fit people and thought to be due to a congenital abnormality of the pleura, a subpleural apical bleb) or secondary (owing to underlying lung disease, typically occurring in older people with emphysema or pulmonary fibrosis).
PROGNOSIS	Death from spontaneous pneumothorax is rare and in some cases a consequence of tension pneumothorax. Morbidity with pain and dyspnoea is common. Published recurrence rates vary, but one cohort study found that, after a first episode of primary spontaneous pneumothorax, 23% of people suffered a recurrence within 5 years, most within a year.[3] Recurrence rates had been thought to increase substantially after the first recurrence, but one case control study of military personnel found that 28% of men with a first spontaneous pneumothorax had a recurrence; 23% of the 28% had a second recurrence; and only 14% of that 23% had a third recurrence, giving a total recurrence rate of 35%.[4]
AIMS	To reduce morbidity; to restore normal function as quickly as possible; to prevent recurrence and mortality, with minimum adverse effects.
OUTCOMES	Rate of successful resolution of spontaneous pneumothorax; time to full expansion; duration of hospital stay; time off work; harmful effects of treatments (pain, surgical emphysema, wound and pleural space infection); and rate of recurrence.
METHODS	*Clinical Evidence* update search and appraisal December 2000. Most of the literature comprised uncontrolled case series. We found no systematic reviews.

QUESTION   What are the effects of treatments?

OPTION   NEEDLE ASPIRATION

Limited data from one small RCT provided no good evidence of a difference between needle aspiration and observation. Two small RCTs found faster resolution with chest tube drainage than with needle

aspiration, but no evidence of a difference in recurrence rate, mortality, or rate of return to normal function. One of the trials found that people treated with needle aspiration experienced less pain and spent less time in hospital than those treated with chest tube drainage.

Benefits: We found no systematic review. **Versus observation:** We found one small RCT (21 people) comparing needle aspiration versus no treatment.[5] It found that there may have been more rapid re-expansion in the treatment group (3.2 weeks v 1.6 weeks; insufficient information for reliable statistical analysis). **Versus chest tube drainage:** We found two small RCTs, both reporting higher success rates with chest tube drainage. The first RCT found that more people treated with chest tube drainage versus needle aspiration had resolution of the pneumothorax (0/38 v 28/35 people, time frame not given). The other seven people required subsequent chest tube drainage.[6] There was no significant difference in recurrence rate at 1 year. The second RCT reported success (resolution of the pneumothorax within 24 hours) in significantly more people treated with chest tube drainage versus needle aspiration (26/28 [93%] v 22/33 [67%], P = 0.01).[7] There was no significant difference in recurrence rate. The study was not designed to show a difference in duration of hospital stay because chest tube drainage was done on admission whereas in most cases needle aspiration was performed after 3 days of observation in hospital.

Harms: We found no reports of harmful effects of needle aspiration. **Versus chest tube drainage:** In one RCT, people treated with needle aspiration versus chest tube drainage experienced significantly less pain on daily total pain scores during their hospital stay (total pain with needle aspiration 2.7, 95% CI 1.6 to 3.8 v 6.7, 95% CI 5.5 to 7.9) and spent an average of 2 days less in hospital (3.2 days v 5.3 days, P = 0.005).[6]

Comment: The RCT of needle aspiration versus simple observation[5] is consistent with a large case series in which 74% (88/119) of spontaneous pneumothoraces presenting to an outpatient chest clinic were managed successfully without intervention or hospital admission.[8]

OPTION   CHEST TUBE DRAINAGE

We found insufficient evidence on the effects of chest tube drainage compared with observation. Two small RCTs found faster resolution with chest tube drainage than needle aspiration but no evidence of a difference in recurrence rate, mortality, or rate of return to normal function. Chest tube drainage caused more pain and longer hospital stay. Limited data provided no evidence that larger tubes reduce duration of drainage, but suggested that they increase success rates in people with large pneumothoraces.

Benefits: We found no systematic review. **Versus observation:** We found no sufficiently large RCTs. **Versus needle aspiration:** See option, p 1063. **Different sized tubes:** We found no RCTs. One non-randomised trial in 44 people compared small gauge (8 French) catheters versus standard chest tubes.[9] There was no significant difference in duration of drainage between groups. In people with large pneumothoraces (> 50% lung volume), successful resolution was more likely with standard chest tubes than catheters (100% v 57%, P < 0.05). No such difference was reported in people with small (< 50%) pneumothoraces.

Harms: **Versus needle aspiration:** In one RCT, people treated with chest tube drainage versus needle aspiration experienced significantly more pain on daily and total pain scores during their hospital stay (total pain with chest tube drainage 6.7, 95% CI 5.5 to 7.9 v 2.7, 95% CI 1.6 to 3.8) and spent an average of 2 days less in hospital (3.2 days v 5.3 days, P = 0.005).[6] Small gauge chest tubes are easier to insert and may cause less pain and morbidity. Conventional chest tubes versus catheters significantly increased the risk of subcutaneous emphysema (9/23 v 0/21, P < 0.05).[9]

Comment: None.

OPTION ONE WAY VALVES ON CHEST TUBES

One small RCT found no significant difference in rates of resolution between one way valves and drainage bottles with underwater seals, but the trial was too small to rule out a clinically important difference. People treated with one way valves required less analgesia and spent less time in hospital.

Benefits: We found no systematic review. We found one RCT in 30 people with spontaneous pneumothorax and respiratory distress, comparing a 13 French chest tube connected to a one way valve versus a 14 French chest tube connected to a drainage bottle with an underwater seal.[10] It found no significant difference in rates of resolution between the groups, but people treated with a one way valve required significantly less analgesia (29% v 77%, P = 0.027).

Harms: The RCT found that, compared with drainage using an under water seal, there was no significant difference in the rate of complications.[10]

Comment: One way valves often allow people to be treated at home. All people treated with drainage bottles were treated in hospital compared with only 30% of those treated with one way valves (P < 0.01).[10]

OPTION CHEST TUBE DRAINAGE PLUS SUCTION

One RCT found no significant difference in rate of resolution regardless of whether chest tube drainage bottles were connected to suction or not. However, the trial was too small to rule out a clinically important difference.

Benefits: We found no systematic review. We found one RCT (53 people) comparing chest tube drainage using an underwater seal only versus drainage with suction. Suction pressures ranged from 8–20 cm H_2O.[11] There was no significant difference in rate of success, defined as full lung expansion within 10 days (57% with suction v 50% without).

Harms: We found no reports of adverse effects due to suction.

Comment: We found one RCT comparing suction versus no suction in 80 people with traumatic pneumothorax, but because the mechanism of injury is different the results should not be extrapolated to spontaneous pneumothorax.[12]

Spontaneous pneumothorax

QUESTION **What are the effects of interventions to prevent recurrence?**

OPTION **CHEMICAL PLEURODESIS**

Two RCTs have found that chemical pleurodesis reduces the rate of recurrence of spontaneous pneumothorax. RCTs found that treatment can be painful. We found conflicting evidence about the effect of pleurodesis on the duration of hospital stay compared with chest tube drainage alone. We found no reliable evidence about the optimal timing of pleurodesis.

Benefits: We found no systematic review. We found two RCTs. One unblinded RCT (229 men) compared chest tube insertion plus intrapleural instillation of tetracycline (113 people, mean follow up 34 months) versus chest tube insertion alone (116 people, mean follow up 29 months).[13] The recurrence rate was 25% in the tetracycline group and 41% in the control group (P = 0.02). There was no significant difference in length of hospital stay or 5 year survival (40 deaths in the tetracycline group v 42 in controls). The other RCT (96 people treated with a chest tube) compared three groups: no further treatment; tetracycline pleurodesis; and talc pleurodesis.[14] Mean follow up was 4.6 years. The recurrence rate was significantly higher in people receiving no treatment versus talc pleurodesis (36% v 8%, P < 0.05), and was 13% in the tetracycline group. **Versus surgical pleurodesis:** See option below. **Optimal timing of pleurodesis:** We found no systematic reviews, RCTs, or high quality cohort studies comparing pleurodesis undertaken at different times (after the first, second, or subsequent episodes of spontaneous pneumothorax).

Harms: In the first unblinded RCT, 58% of people reported intense chest pain on injection of tetracycline.[13] The trial found no effect on pulmonary function at 2 years' follow up.[13] In a similar prospective, controlled, but not randomised, study, the duration of hospital stay was significantly longer for the tetracycline group than for the other two groups (mean 10 days v 4 days, P < 0.01).[15]

Comment: If the 5 year recurrence rate after a first pneumothorax is about 28%, there may be little reason to undertake pleurodesis with the first episode.[4] Although it has generally been thought that pleurodesis is warranted after the second or third episode, this convention may be questionable if only 23% of this 28% will have a second recurrence and only 14% of that 23% will have a third recurrence.[4] Even though the probability of success with pleurodesis is high, clinicians will have to weigh the likelihood of recurrence against the morbidity associated with the procedure.

OPTION **SURGICAL PLEURODESIS**

We found insufficient evidence on the effects of surgical versus chemical pleurodesis. One small RCT has found that video-assisted thorascopic surgery versus thoracotomy significantly reduces hospital stay. The rate of recurrence was not significantly different, but limited data do not exclude a clinically significant difference.

Benefits: We found no systematic review. **Versus chemical pleurodesis:** We found no RCTs. We found one non-randomised prospective study (see comment). **Video-assisted thorascopic surgery:** We found one RCT (60 people with primary spontaneous pneumothorax, either first recurrence or non-resolving first episode) that compared video-assisted thorascopic surgery versus thoracotomy.[16] Video-assisted surgery versus thoracotomy significantly reduced the need for analgesia and hospital stay (hospital stay 6.5 v 10.7 days, P < 0.0001). There was no significant difference in the rate of recurrence after 3 years (3/30 [10%] people after thorascopic surgery v 0/30 [0%] after thoracotomy; ARR 10%, 95% CI 7% to 20%).

Harms: We found no good information on harms.

Comment: The RCT was too small to exclude a clinically significant difference in recurrence rate between thorascopic surgery and thoracotomy. One non-randomised prospective study compared tetracycline pleurodesis (78 people) versus thoracotomy (28 people).[15] The mean follow up was 45 months. It found no significant difference in recurrence rate (chemical pleurodesis 9%, 8 treatment failures, 4 lost to follow up; thoracotomy 0%, P = 0.13). Compared with chemical pleurodesis, morbidity and time lost from work is likely to increase with thoracotomy, and decrease with video-assisted thorascopic surgery. However, we found no good studies comparing chemical pleurodesis with either technique.

Substantive changes since last issue

Surgical pleurodesis New RCT;[16] conclusion unchanged.

REFERENCES

1. Melton LJ, Hepper NG, Offord KP. Incidence of spontaneous pneumothorax in Olmsted County, Minnesota: 1950–1974. Am Rev Respir Dis 1979;120:1379–1382.
2. Bense L, Eklung G, Wiman LG. Smoking and the increased risk of contracting spontaneous pneumothorax. Chest 1987;92:1009–1012.
3. Lippert HL, Lund O, Blegvad S, et al. Independent risk factors for cumulative recurrence rate after first spontaneous pneumothorax. Eur Respir J 1991;4:324–331.
4. Voge VM, Anthracite R. Spontaneous pneumothorax in the USAF aircrew population: a retrospective study. Aviat Space Environ Med 1986;57:939–949.
5. Flint K, Al-Hillawi AH, Johnson NM. Conservative management of spontaneous pneumothorax. Lancet 1984;1:687–688.
6. Harvey J, Prescott RJ. Simple aspiration versus intercostal tube drainage for spontaneous pneumothorax in patients with normal lungs. British Thoracic Society Research Committee. BMJ 1994;309:1338–1339.
7. Andrivet P, Djedaini K, Teboul JL, et al. Spontaneous pneumothorax. Comparison of thoracic drainage vs immediate or delayed needle aspiration. Chest 1995;108:335–339.
8. Stradling P, Poole G. Conservative management of spontaneous pneumothorax. Thorax 1966;21:145–149.
9. Kang YJ, Koh HG, Shin JW, et al. The effect of 8 French catheter and chest tube on the treatment of spontaneous pneumothorax. Tuber Respir Dis 1996;43:410–419.
10. Roggla M, Wagner A, Brunner C, et al. The management of pneumothorax with the thoracic vent versus conventional intercostal tube drainage. Wien Klin Wochenschr 1996;108:330–333.
11. So SY, Yu DYC. Catheter drainage of spontaneous pneumothorax: suction or no suction, early or late removal? Thorax 1982;37:46–48.
12. Davis JW, Mackersie RC, Hoyt DB, et al. Randomized study of algorithms for discontinuing tube thoracostomy drainage. J Am Coll Surg 1994;179:553–557.
13. Light RW, O'Hara VS, Moritz TE, et al. Intrapleural tetracycline for the prevention of recurrent spontaneous pneumothorax. Results of a Department of Veterans Affairs cooperative study. JAMA 1990;264:2224–2230.
14. Almind M, Lange P, Viskum K. Spontaneous pneumothorax: comparison of simple drainage, talc pleurodesis, and tetracycline pleurodesis. Thorax 1989;44:627–630.
15. Alfageme I, Moreno L, Huertas C, Vargas A, Hernandez J, Beiztegui A. Spontaneous pneumothorax. Long-term results with tetracycline pleurodesis. Chest 1994;106:347–350.
16. Ayed AK, Al-Din HJ. Video-assisted thoracoscopy versus thoracotomy for primary spontaneous pneumothorax: A randomized controlled trial. Med Principles Pract 2000;9:113–118.

John Cunnington

Associate Professor, Medicine McMaster University, Hamilton, Ontario, Canada

Competing interests: None declared.

Upper respiratory tract infection

Search date May 2000

Paul Glasziou and Chris Del Mar

INTERVENTIONS

Key Messages

- We found no evidence that antibiotics have a clinically important effect on colds uncomplicated by secondary infection. Systematic reviews have found a minimal to modest effect of antibiotics in acute bronchitis, pharyngitis, and sinusitis. Antibiotics can prevent non-suppurative complications of β haemolytic streptococcal pharyngitis, but in developed societies such complications are rare.

- RCTs have found that β agonists reduce the duration of cough in acute bronchitis.

- One systematic review of RCTs has found that vitamin C reduces duration of symptoms in undifferentiated colds. However, the beneficial effect is small and may be explained by publication bias.

- One systematic review found inconsistent evidence on the effects of zinc gluconate.

- We found limited evidence from one systematic review of RCTs that some preparations of echinacea may be superior to placebo for treatment and prevention of cold, but we found insufficient evidence to recommend a specific product.

- One systematic review of RCTs found conflicting evidence for the efficacy of steam inhalation.
- One systematic review of RCTs found evidence for limited short term benefit of decongestants but no evidence of benefit with longer term use.
- One systematic review of RCTs found evidence that antihistamines reduce runny nose and sneezing.

DEFINITION	Upper respiratory tract infection involves inflammation of the respiratory mucosa from the nose to the lower respiratory tree, not including the alveoli. In addition to malaise, it causes localised symptoms that constitute several overlapping syndromes: sore throat (pharyngitis); rhinorrhoea (common cold); facial fullness and pain (sinusitis); and cough (bronchitis).
INCIDENCE/ PREVALENCE	Upper respiratory tract infections, nasal congestion, throat complaints, and cough are responsible for 11% of general practice consultations in Australia.[1] Each year, children suffer about five such infections, and adults two to three.[1]
AETIOLOGY/ RISK FACTORS	Infective agents include over 200 viruses (with 100 rhinoviruses) and several bacteria. Transmission is mostly through hand to hand contact with subsequent passage to the nares or eyes, rather than, as commonly perceived, through droplets in the air.[2]
PROGNOSIS	Upper respiratory tract infections are usually self limiting. Although they cause little mortality or serious morbidity, upper respiratory tract infections are responsible for considerable discomfort, lost work, and medical costs. Clinical patterns vary and overlap between infective agents. In addition to nasal symptoms, half of sufferers experience sore throat and 40% experience cough. Symptoms peak within 1–3 days and generally clear by 1 week, although cough often persists.[2]
AIMS	To relieve symptoms and to prevent suppurative and non-suppurative complications of bacterial infection, with minimal adverse effects from treatments.
OUTCOMES	Cure rate, duration of symptoms, incidence of complications, incidence of adverse effects of treatment.
METHODS	*Clinical Evidence* search and appraisal May 2000.

QUESTION What are the effects of treatments?

OPTION ANTIBIOTICS

We found no evidence that antibiotics have a clinically important effect on undifferentiated colds. Systematic reviews have found a minimal to modest effect of antibiotics in acute bronchitis, pharyngitis, and sinusitis. Antibiotics can prevent non-suppurative complications of β haemolytic streptococcal pharyngitis, but in industrialised countries, such complications are rare.

Benefits: **Colds:** We found two systematic reviews. The first, identifying seven RCTs in acute upper respiratory infections without complications, found no effect of antibiotics on general improvement or cure (RR 0.95; 95% CI 0.70 to 1.25).[3] The second (identifying 12 RCTs of antibiotics in children) found no change in clinical outcomes in the six trials with adequate data (RR 1.01; 95% CI 0.90 to 1.13) or in complications or progression (RR 0.71; 95% CI 0.45 to 1.12).[4] Similarly, one recent RCT in 314 adults comparing co-amoxiclav (375 mg three times daily) versus placebo found no overall difference in "cure" rates.[5] However, in the 61 people (20%) who were found to have positive sputum cultures for *Haemophilus influenzae, Moraxella catarrhalis,* or *Streptococcus pneumoniae,* there was a significant difference in recovery of 27% with co-amoxiclav versus 4% with placebo at 5 days. If such people could be identified at first consultation, then treating four of these people with antibiotic rather than placebo would result in one more recovery at 5 days (NNT 4, no CI given). **Cough:** We found one systematic review (updated in 1997), which identified eight RCTs comparing doxycycline (4 RCTs), erythromycin (3 RCTs), and trimethoprim/sulfamethoxazole (1 RCT) versus placebo in 750 people (aged 8 to > 65 years).[6] People receiving antibiotics were less likely to report feeling unwell at a follow up visit (OR for reporting feeling unwell at follow up antibiotics *v* placebo 0.42, 95% CI 0.22 to 0.82), although the review reported only significant results, which may have led to optimistic bias. There was a small but significant difference in time to return to work or usual activities (WMD 0.74 days earlier with antibiotics *v* placebo; 95% CI 0.16 to 1.32). **Sore throat:** We found one systematic review (updated in 1998), which identified 18 controlled trials in 9189 people with sore throat.[7] The combined effects from six trials found that antibiotics reduced the risk of rheumatic fever compared with no antibiotic (RR 0.28, 95% CI 0.19 to 0.40). There were too few events to detect any possible protective effect of antibiotics against acute glomerulonephritis (2/1459 cases among controls *v* 0/1625 treated with antibiotics). Suppurative complications were also significantly reduced (otitis media RR 0.23, 95% CI 0.12 to 0.45; quinsy RR 0.19, 95% CI 0.08 to 0.47). Acute sinusitis was not significantly reduced (RR 0.33, 95% CI 0.07 to 1.65). To prevent one case of otitis media, 30 children or 145 adults suffering from sore throat would need to be treated. Antibiotics shortened symptom duration but by a mean of only about 8 hours overall. **Sinusitis:** We found one systematic review, published in 1998, which identified six RCTs comparing antibiotics versus placebo in 761 people with sinusitis.[8] It found that antimicrobial agents (amoxicillin in 3 trials, other agents in 3 trials) were effective in treating uncomplicated acute sinusitis. Symptoms improved or disappeared in 69% of people on placebo, compared with nearly 84% with antibiotics (RRR for symptoms not improving or disappearing compared with placebo 46%, 95% CI 21% to 63%). The same review analysed head to head trials of different antibiotics and found no advantage for other antibiotics over amoxicillin.

Harms: Adverse effects such as nausea, vomiting, headache, skin rash, or vaginitis were more common on antibiotics than placebo. For example, in the bronchitis review the absolute risk increase for adverse effects was 6% (95% CI 0.1% to 12%), or a rate of one extra adverse effect per 16 people treated. We found no evidence of the size of the risk of antibiotic resistance or pseudomembranous colitis.

Comment: Because most upper respiratory tract infections are viral, the potential benefit from antibiotics is limited. Until rapid identification of those likely to benefit is possible, the modest effects seen in trials must be weighed against the adverse effects of antibiotics, costs, and potential for inducing antibiotic resistance.

OPTION β AGONISTS

We found that β agonists reduce the duration of cough in acute bronchitis compared with placebo or erythromycin, although we found limited evidence that this beneficial effect may only be in people with bronchial hyperresponsiveness, wheeze, or airflow limitation.

Benefits: We found no systematic review. Two RCTs in people with acute bronchitis have compared erythromycin versus the β agonist, salbutamol, and one RCT compared fenoterol versus placebo.[9-11] In the first study, 59% on liquid salbutamol compared with 12% on erythromycin were not coughing at 7 days.[9] In the second study, 39% on inhaled salbutamol compared with 9% on erythromycin were not coughing.[10] These absolute risk reductions of 47% and 30% mean two to three people need to be treated for one less person to be coughing at the end of 1 week. A subgroup analysis of the fenoterol trial found that benefits may be confined to people with bronchial hyperresponsiveness, wheezes, or baseline $FEV_1 < 80\%$ of predicted.[11]

Harms: Short term use of a β agonist may cause tachycardia and anxiety.

Comment: The cough associated with acute bronchitis is self limiting, so treatment is for symptomatic relief. Hence it is important to consider the degree of disturbance caused and people's preferences and interpretation of cough.

OPTION VITAMIN C

One systematic review of RCTs found evidence that vitamin C reduces the duration of symptoms in people with upper respiratory tract infections. However, the beneficial effect is small and may be explained by publication bias.

Benefits: We found one systematic review, updated in 1998.[12-14] This identified 30 RCTs comparing vitamin C with placebo for prophylaxis and treatment of colds. Three RCTs used 1 g or more daily of vitamin C taken at symptom onset. Duration of symptoms was half a day less (WMD 0.55 days per cold episode, 95% CI 0.17 to 0.92), representing about 15% fewer symptomatic days per episode.

Harms: The studies of treatment found no difference in adverse effects potentially caused by vitamin C.

Comment: The beneficial effect reported in the review was small and might be explained by publication bias.

OPTION ZINC

One systematic review of RCTs found no clear evidence that zinc gluconate or acetate is beneficial in people with upper respiratory tract infections.

Upper respiratory tract infection

Benefits: We found one systematic review, which identified seven RCTs comparing zinc (gluconate or acetate) versus placebo for the treatment of colds.[15] Symptoms were unchanged at 3 and 5 days, but there was a relative reduction of 31% at 7 days (NNT 7, 95% CI 5 to 15). However the 7-day results showed statistically significant heterogeneity, which may be due to the zinc formulation, the type of virus, or to other, unknown factors.

Harms: Adverse outcomes were not systematically reviewed, but individual trials found that nausea, altered taste, dry mouth, abdominal pain, and headache were increased in the zinc group.

Comment: None.

OPTION   ECHINACEA

One recent systematic review of RCTs suggests that some preparations of echinacea may be better than placebo for cold treatment and prevention, but we found insufficient evidence to recommend a specific echinacea product for treating or preventing common colds.

Benefits: **Treatment:** We found one systematic review (search date 1998, 8 RCTs).[16] All trials were double blind except one, which was single blind. The review found most trials to be of poor quality. Quantitative data could only be extracted for two trials on duration of illness, for three trials for runny nose, and for five trials for a summary symptom score. Data pooling was not possible because of trial heterogeneity. There were nine comparisons (8 versus placebo and, in 1 trial, an additional comparison of high versus low dose treatment) from the eight trials. Six comparisons found significantly better results associated with echinacea. One trial found significant results for a subgroup only and two trials found no difference after treatment.[16]
Prevention: The systematic review identified eight trials, with a total of almost 4000 participants.[16] The trials varied considerably in quality of methods and preparation used and so results were not combined. Of the five placebo controlled treatment trials, two found a significantly lower incidence of infection in the treatment group. One of these had large loss to follow up. The other trials found a non-significant reduction in the rate of infection. Data pooling found that significantly fewer people had one infection episode after taking echinacea (167/571 v 292/566; OR 0.36, 95% CI 0.28 to 0.46). The three uncontrolled trials all found a significant benefit, but were not randomised or blinded.

Harms: Three of the eight treatment trials and four of the eight prevention trials reported adverse events. These were generally infrequent and not significantly different between echinacea and placebo. However, outside the trials, anaphylaxis has been reported with echinacea.[17]

Comment: Echinacea is not a single product. There are more than 200 different preparations based upon different plants, different parts of the plant (roots, herbs, whole plant), and different methods of extraction. None of the trials were published in a Medline listed journal. The weakness of trial methods and differences in interventions make drawing conclusive evidence of effectiveness impossible. Large studies may not be done because echinacea is not patentable and each producer controls a small share of the market. The authors of the systematic review received personal information about several unpublished studies that they were not able to include.

OPTION   STEAM INHALATION

One systematic review of six RCTs found conflicting evidence for the efficacy of steam inhalation.

Benefits: Steam inhalation at 40–47° has been evaluated in several trials, with conflicting results. Six RCTs (319 people) were included in a systematic review, search dates 1966–1998.[18] Some suggest benefit, and none found any harm. Benefits included increased patency of the nose following exposure to hot, humid steam.

Harms: The trials found no evidence of harms. There may be a danger from spilling very hot water and from nosocomial infections related to humidifier units.

Comment: None.

OPTION   DECONGESTANTS

One systematic review of four RCTs found evidence for limited short term benefit following a single dose but no evidence of benefit with longer use of decongestants for symptomatic relief.

Benefits: We found one systematic review (search dates 1966 to 1999, 4 RCTs, 246 adults).[19] It found that in the common cold a single dose of nasal decongestant was only moderately effective (reducing subjective symptom scores by 13%) for the short term relief of congestion in adults. We found no evidence of benefit after repeated use over several days.

Harms: Information about harms was not sought actively or reported in RCTs.

Comment: There were no trials undertaken in children.

OPTION   ANTIHISTAMINES

One systematic review of nine RCTs in adults found evidence that antihistamines produce small clinical benefits for the symptoms of runny nose and sneezing.

Benefits: One well conducted systematic review of previously unpublished individual patient data from nine RCTs (1757 people) of antihistamines against placebo found antihistamines reduced the symptoms of runny nose and sneezing for the first 2 days of both natural and experimentally induced colds.[20] The effects were small. On a severity scale ranging from 0 (no symptoms) to 3.0 or 4.0 (severe symptoms), antihistamines reduced the score by 0.25 (95% CI 0.12 to 0.73) for runny nose on days 1 and 2, and 0.14 (95% CI 0.0 to 0.3) for sneezing on day 1 and 0.3 (95% CI 1.5 to 4.5) on day 2.

Upper respiratory tract infection

Harms: Harms were not actively sought in RCTs, but are known to include drowsiness and dry mouth.

Comment: None.

REFERENCES

1. Fry J, Sandler G. *Common diseases. Their nature, prevalence and care*. Dordrecht, The Netherlands: Kluwer Academic, 1993.

2. Lauber B. The common cold. *J Gen Intern Med* 1996;11:229–236.

3. Arroll B, Kenealy T. The use of antibiotics versus placebo in the common cold. In: The Cochrane Library, Issue 1, 2000. Oxford: Update software. Search date 1998; primary sources Cochrane Controlled Trials Register; Medline; Embase; Family Medicine Database; reference lists in articles; principal investigators.

4. Fahey T, Stocks N, Thomas T. Systematic review of the treatment of upper respiratory tract infection. *Arch Dis Child* 1998;79:225–230. Search date not given; primary sources Medline; Embase; Science Citation Index; Cochrane Controlled Trials Register; authors of published RCTs; drug manufacturers; and hand search references.

5. Kaiser L, Lew D, Hirschel B, et al. Effects of antibiotic treatment in the subset of common-cold patients who have bacteria in nasopharyngeal secretions. *Lancet* 1996;347:1507–1510.

6. Becker L, Glazier R, McIsaac W, Smucny J. Antibiotics for acute bronchitis. In: The Cochrane Library, Issue 1, 2000. Oxford: Update software. Search date 1997; primary sources Medline 1966 to 1996; Embase 1974 to 1996; Science Citation Index 1989 to 1996; hand search of reference lists of relevant trials, textbooks, and review articles.

7. Del Mar CB, Glasziou PP. Antibiotics for the symptoms and complications of sore throat. In: The Cochrane Library, Issue 1, 2000. Oxford: Update software. Search date 1998; primary sources Index Medicus 1945 to 1965; Medline 1966 to 1997; Cochrane Library 1997 issue 4; hand search of reference lists of relevant articles.

8. De Ferranti SD, Ionnidis JPA, Lau J, et al. Are amoxycillin and folate inhibitors as effective as other antibiotics for acute sinusitis? A meta-analysis. *BMJ* 1998;317:632–637. Search date May 1998; primary sources Medline 1966 to May 1998; manual search of Excerpta Medica; recent abstracts for Interscience Conference on Antimicrobial Agents and Chemotherapy 1993 to 1997; and references of all trials, review articles, and special issues for additional studies.

9. Hueston WJ. A comparison of albuterol and erythromycin for the treatment of acute bronchitis. *J Fam Pract* 1991;33:476–480.

10. Hueston WJ. Albuterol delivered by metered-dose inhaler to treat acute bronchitis. *J Fam Pract* 1994;39:437–440.

11. Melbye H, Aasebo U, Straume B. Symptomatic effect of inhaled fenoterol in acute bronchitis: a placebo-controlled double-blind study. *Fam Pract* 1991;8:216–222.

12. Douglas RM, Chalker EB, Treacy B. Vitamin C for preventing and treating the ommon cold. In: The Cochrane Library, Issue 2, 1998. Oxford: Update Software. Search date not given; primary sources reviews by Kleinjen and Hemila.[13,14]

13. Kleijnen J, ter Riet G, Knipschild PG. Vitamin C and the common cold; review of a megadoses literature (in Dutch). *Ned Tijdschr Geneeskd* 1989;133:1532–1535. Search date 1998; primary sources Medline 1963 to 1988, and hand searched references.

14. Hemila H. Vitamin C and the common cold. *Br J Nutr* 1992;67:3–16. Search date not given; primary sources not given.

15. Marshall I. Zinc in the treatment of the common cold. In: The Cochrane Library, Issue 1, 2000. Oxford: Update software. Search date December 1997; primary sources Medline, Embase, The Cochrane Library, hand searched journals.

16. Melchart D, Linde K, Fischer P, Kaesmayr J. Echinacea for the prevention and treatment of the common cold. In: The Cochrane Library, Issue 1, 2000. Oxford: Update software. Search date 1998; primary sources Medline 1966 to 1998; Embase 1991 to 1998; database of the Cochrane Acute Respiratory Infections Group; database of the Cochrane Field Complementary Medicine; database Phytodok; bibliographies of existing reviews, personal communications.

17. Mullins RJ. Echinacea associated anaphylaxis. *Med J Aust* 1998;168:170–171.

18. Singh M. Heated, humidified air for the common cold. In: The Cochrane Library, Issue 2, 2000. Oxford: Update Software. Search date 1999; primary sources Medline; Embase; Current Contents and hand search of review articles and reference lists and contact with manufacturers.

19. Taverner D, Bickford L, Draper M. Nasal decongestants for the common cold. In: The Cochrane Library, Issue 2, 2000. Oxford: Update Software. Search date 1999; primary sources Medline; Embase; Current Contents; Cochrane Acute Respiratory Infectious Group's trials register, and hand search of reference lists and personal contacts with known investigators and pharmaceutical companies.

20. D'Agostino RB Sr, Weintraub M, Russell HK, et al. The effectiveness of antihistamines in reducing the severity of runny nose and sneezing: a meta-analysis. *Clin Pharmacol Ther* 1998;64:579–96. Search date not given; primary sources Medline, FDA unpublished clinical trials.

Paul Glasziou
Professor of Evidence-Based Medicine

Chris Del Mar
Professor of General Practice
University of Queensland
Brisbane, Australia

Competing interests: None declared.

Search date November 2000

M Joesoef and George Schmid

INTERVENTIONS

TREATMENT
Beneficial
Antianaerobic treatment in
symptomatic non-pregnant
women 1077

Likely to be beneficial
Antianaerobic treatment in
pregnant women who have had
a previous preterm birth . . .1078
Oral antianaerobic treatment
before surgical abortion . . .1080

Unknown effectiveness
Antianaerobic treatment in low-risk
pregnancy 1078

Antianaerobic treatment before
gynaecological procedures .1080

PREVENTING RECURRENCE
Likely to be ineffective or harmful
Treating pregnant women with
intravaginal clindamycin
cream 1079
Treating pregnant women without
bacterial vaginosis 1079
Treating a woman's one steady
male sexual partner 1080

To be covered in future issues of
Clinical Evidence
Screening in pregnancy

Key Messages

- Bacterial vaginosis may resolve spontaneously.

In non-pregnant women

- One systematic review found no significant difference in cure rates between oral and intravaginal antianaerobic drugs. Another systematic review has found that a 7 day course of twice daily oral metronidazole is more effective than a single 2 g dose. Limited evidence from RCTs found no significant difference in cure rates between oral clindamycin and oral metronidazole, and no difference between once and twice daily dosing with intravaginal metronidazole gel.

In pregnant women

- Limited evidence from a subgroup analysis in a systematic review has found that in pregnant women who have had a previous preterm birth, oral anti-anaerobic treatment for bacterial vaginosis reduces the risk of premature delivery. The systematic review and subsequent RCTs found no benefit from antianaerobic treatment for bacterial vaginosis in pregnant women without previous preterm delivery.

- Two RCTs found a higher risk of preterm delivery before 34 weeks in women without bacterial vaginosis who received intravaginal clindamycin cream or oral metronidazole and erythromycin.

- Two RCTs found a higher risk of preterm delivery and low birth weight in women with bacterial vaginosis who received intravaginal clindamycin cream.

Preventing recurrence

- One systematic review has found that, in women with one steady male sexual partner, treating the partner with an oral antianaerobic agent does not reduce the woman's risk of recurrence.

Before procedures

- Two RCTs found that antianaerobic treatment for bacterial vaginosis in women about to undergo surgical abortion reduces the risk of pelvic inflammatory disease.
- We found no evidence on the effects of treatment of women with bacterial vaginosis about to undergo other gynaecological procedures, including abdominal hysterectomy, caesarean section, or insertion of an intrauterine contraceptive device.

DEFINITION	Bacterial vaginosis is a microbial disease characterised by an alteration in the bacterial flora of the vagina from a predominance of *Lactobacillus* species to high concentrations of anaerobic bacteria. Diagnosis requires three out of four features: the presence of clue cells; a homogenous discharge adherent to the vaginal walls; pH of vaginal fluid greater than 4.5; and a "fishy" amine odour of the vaginal discharge before or after addition of 10% potassium hydroxide. The condition is asymptomatic in 50% of infected women. Women with symptoms have an excessive white to grey, or malodorous vaginal discharge, or both; the odour may be particularly noticeable during sexual intercourse.
INCIDENCE/ PREVALENCE	Bacterial vaginosis is the most common infectious cause of vaginitis, being about twice as common as candidiasis.[1] Prevalences of 10–61% have been reported among unselected women from a range of settings.[2] Data on incidence are limited but one study found that, over a 2 year period, 50% of women using an intrauterine contraceptive device had at least one episode, as did 20% of women using oral contraceptives.[3] Bacterial vaginosis is particularly prevalent in lesbians.[4]
AETIOLOGY/ RISK FACTORS	The cause is not understood fully. Risk factors include new or multiple sexual partners[1,3,5] and early age of sexual debut,[6] but no causative microorganism has been shown to be transmitted between partners. Use of an intrauterine contraceptive device[3] and douching[5] have also been reported as risk factors. Infection seems to be most common around the time of menstruation.[7]
PROGNOSIS	The course of bacterial vaginosis varies and is poorly understood. Without treatment, symptoms may persist or resolve in both pregnant and non-pregnant women. Recurrence after treatment occurs in about a third of women. The condition is associated with complications of pregnancy: low birth weight; preterm birth (pooled OR from 10 cohort studies: 1.8, 95% CI 1.5 to 2.6);[8] preterm labour; premature rupture of membranes; late miscarriage; chorioamnionitis (48% v 22%, OR 2.6, 95% CI 1.0 to 6.6);[9] endometritis after normal delivery (8.2% v 1.5%, OR 5.6, 95% CI 1.8 to 17.2);[10] endometritis after caesarean section (55% v 17%, OR 5.8, 95% CI 3.0 to 10.9);[11] and surgery to the genital tract. Women who have had a previous premature delivery are especially at risk of complications in pregnancy, with a sevenfold increased risk of preterm birth (AR 24/428 [5.6%] in all women v 10/24 [41.7%] in women with a previous preterm birth).[12] Bacterial vaginosis may also enhance HIV acquisition and transmission.[13]

AIMS   To alleviate symptoms and to prevent complications relating to childbirth, termination of pregnancy, and gynaecological surgery, with minimal adverse effects; and to reduce adverse neonatal outcomes.

OUTCOMES   Preterm delivery; puerperal and neonatal morbidity and mortality; clinical or microbiological cure rates, usually at 1–2 weeks or 4 weeks after completing treatment.

METHODS   *Clinical Evidence* update search and appraisal November 2000. In addition the authors searched Medline (keywords: bacterial vaginosis, non-specific vaginosis, clindamycin, metronidazole) from 1988 to September 1998, and also used information from drug manufacturers.

QUESTION	What are the effects of different antianaerobic regimens in non-pregnant women with symptomatic bacterial vaginosis?

One systematic review found no significant difference in cure rates between oral and intravaginal antianaerobic drugs. Another systematic review has found that a 7 day course of twice daily oral metronidazole is more effective than a single 2 g dose. Limited evidence from RCTs found no significant difference in cure rates between oral clindamycin and oral metronidazole, and no difference between once and twice daily dosing with intravaginal metronidazole gel.

Benefits: **Oral versus intravaginal antianaerobic treatment:** We found one systematic review (search date 1996, 5 RCTs) comparing oral and intravaginal formulations of metronidazole and clindamycin,[14] and one subsequent RCT.[15] Three RCTs were in symptomatic non-pregnant women and two were in symptomatic and asymptomatic non-pregnant women. There was no significant difference in cumulative cure rates 5–10 days after completing treatment (86% for oral metronidazole 500 mg twice daily for 7 days v 85% for clindamycin vaginal cream 5 g at bedtime for 7 days v 81% for metronidazole vaginal gel 5 g twice daily for 5 days). Four weeks after completing treatment, the cumulative cure rates were 78% for oral metronidazole versus 82% for clindamycin vaginal cream versus 71% for metronidazole vaginal gel. The subsequent RCT (233 women) of clindamycin vaginal cream versus oral metronidazole supports the conclusion of the systemic review of no significant difference in cure rates between clindamycin cream and oral metronidazole (68.1% v 66.7%).[15] **Different oral antianaerobic regimens:** We found one systematic review (search date 1996, 4 RCTs) comparing metronidazole 500 mg twice daily for 7 days versus a single 2 g dose of metronidazole.[14] Cumulative cure rates 3–4 weeks after completing treatment were 82% and 62% ($P < 0.05$). We found one additional RCT (143 symptomatic non-pregnant women) comparing oral metronidazole 500 mg twice daily for 7 days versus oral clindamycin 300 mg twice daily for 7 days.[16] It found no significant difference in cure rates within 7–10 days of starting treatment (women cured: AR 46/49 [94%] with clindamycin v 48/50 [96%] with metronidazole; RR 0.98, 95% CI 0.89 to

1.07). A quarter of women were lost to follow up. **Different intravaginal antianaerobic regimens:** One RCT (514 women) found no significant difference in effectiveness between once daily versus twice daily dosing of intravaginal metronidazole gel (AR 118/207 [57%] with once daily gel v 129/209 [62%] with twice daily gel; RR 0.92, 95% CI 0.79 to 1.08).[17] **Recurrence:** One RCT (139 women) found that recurrence occurred in 30% of women after 12 weeks' treatment with clindamycin vaginal cream whose partner received placebo versus 32% of women whose partner received clindamycin capsules.[18] In another RCT (61 people, 19 withdrew), more than 50% of women taking clindamycin vaginal cream versus oral metronidazole had recurrent bacterial vaginosis 2 months after treatment.[19] We found no good studies of maintenance regimens for recurrent bacterial vaginosis.

Harms: The review of different oral antianaerobic regimens found that adverse effects occurred in a quarter to two thirds of women taking oral metronidazole, including mild to moderate nausea/dyspepsia, unpleasant metallic taste, headache, and dizziness.[14] Infrequent adverse effects from oral clindamycin included heartburn, nausea, vomiting, diarrhoea, constipation, headache, dizziness, and vertigo; the trials gave no data on frequency. Intravaginal clindamycin has been associated, rarely, with mild to severe colitis[20] and vaginal candidiasis. The RCT of once versus twice daily intravaginal metronidazole gel found no significant difference in frequency of adverse effects.[17] Yeast vulvovaginitis may be less common with intravaginal than with oral metronidazole (4% for intravaginal[21] v 8–22% for oral[22]).

Comment: Intravaginal administration reduces systemic absorption and systemic adverse effects. Some women may prefer oral medication because it is more convenient. Generic oral metronidazole is the most cost effective treatment for bacterial vaginosis.[23]

QUESTION   **What are the effects of treatments in pregnant women with bacterial vaginosis?**

One systematic review of antianaerobic treatment of bacterial vaginosis during pregnancy found that antibiotics versus placebo reduced the incidence of preterm delivery, but the difference was not significant. Subgroup analysis in women with bacterial vaginosis who had a previous preterm delivery found that oral antianaerobic treatment significantly reduced the risk of preterm delivery. Subsequent RCTs found no significant difference between antianaerobic treatment versus placebo in the rate of preterm birth in women with bacterial vaginosis.

Benefits: We found one systematic review (updated 1998, 5 RCTs, 1508 women)[24] and three subsequent RCTs comparing one or more antibiotic regimens versus placebo.[25–27] The review found that women taking antibiotics versus placebo had reduced risk of preterm delivery, but the result did not quite reach significance (144/985 [14.6%] with antibiotics v 136/891 [15.3%] with placebo; OR 0.78, 95% CI 0.6 to 1.02). However, in the subgroup of women who had a previous preterm birth, the risk of preterm delivery was significantly less (57/187 [30%] with antibiotics v 58/116 [50%] with placebo; OR 0.37, 95% CI 0.23 to 0.60; NNT 4, 95% CI 3 to

8).[24] The first subsequent large RCT (1953 pregnant women) with asymptomatic bacterial vaginosis) compared oral metronidazole versus placebo and found no significant difference in the risk of preterm birth (116/953 [12.2%] with metronidazole v 121/966 [12.5%] with placebo; RR 0.97, 95% CI 0.76 to 1.23).[25] In the subgroup of women who had a previous preterm birth, there was no significant difference in preterm birth (30/101 [30%] with metronidazole v 26/109 [24%] with placebo; RR 1.24, 95% CI 0.78 to 1.84).[25] The second RCT (129 evaluable pregnant women with bacterial vaginosis) comparing intravaginal clindamycin cream (5 g at bedtime for 7 days) versus placebo found no significant difference in preterm birth (9/60 [15%] with clindamycin v 5/69 [7%] with placebo; RR 2.1, 95% CI 0.7 to 5.0), or in low birth weight babies (8/59 [14%] with clindamycin v 3/69 [4%] with placebo; RR 3.1, 95% CI 0.9 to 11.2).[26] A small subgroup analysis of a third RCT (168 women) comparing clindamycin cream versus placebo found no significant difference in rates of preterm birth (before 34 weeks' gestation) between groups (1/11 [9.1%] with clindamycin cream v 1/11 [9.1%] with placebo) and in women without bacterial vaginosis (9/72 [13%] with clindamycin cream v 3/74 [4%] with placebo; RR 3.1, 95% CI 0.9 to 10.9).[27]

Harms: Adverse effects occurred in 4% of women receiving antibiotics for bacterial vaginosis. **In women without bacterial vaginosis:** Two RCTs[27,28] found an increase in preterm birth (before 34 weeks' gestation) in a subgroup of women without bacterial vaginosis who received intravaginal clindamycin cream[27] or oral metronidazole and erythromycin.[28] For the first RCT, differences between groups did not reach statistical significance (AR 6/62 [9.7%] with clindamycin v 1/64 [1.6%] with placebo; recalculation by *Clinical Evidence*: ARI 8.1%, 95% CI −0.3% to +46%; RR 6.2, 95% CI 0.79 to 31).[27] A subgroup analysis of the second RCT found no significant difference for preterm birth before 37 weeks' gestation (AR 56/254 [22%] with metronidazole and erythromycin v 26/104 [25%] with placebo; RR 0.88, 95% CI 0.57 to 1.3), but found a significant difference for preterm birth before 34 weeks' gestation (AR 34/254 [13%] with metronidazole and erythromycin v 5/104 [5%] with placebo; RR 2.8, 95% CI 1.2 to 6.0; NNH 12, 95% CI 4 to 136).[28] Two trials[26,29] found an increase in preterm birth and low birth weight of women with bacterial vaginosis who received intravaginal clindamycin cream. In both trials, the increase was not statistically significant. In the second trial, the rate of preterm birth (< 32 weeks' gestation) was higher with clindamycin cream than with placebo (AR 16/340 [4.7%] with clindamycin v 9/341 [2.6%] with placebo; OR 1.8, 95% CI 0.8 to 4.2). The rate of low birth weight was higher with clindamycin (AR 30/334 [9%] for clindamycin cream v 23/338 [6.8%] for placebo; OR 1.3, 95% CI 0.8 to 2.4).[29]

Comment: The average quality of the trials in the systematic review was good. All trials reported loss to follow up between 1% and 17% for the various treatment groups.[24] Results from the two subsequent RCTs conflict with those of the systematic review. The subgroup analysis for the third trial had a small sample size.

Does treating male partners prevent recurrence?

One systematic review found that, in women with one steady male sexual partner, treating the partner with an oral antianaerobic agent does not reduce the woman's risk of recurrence.

Benefits: We found one systematic review (search date not stated, 5 RCTs) with a variety of treatment regimens and populations.[30] It found that treatment of a sexual partner with metronidazole or clindamycin had no significant effect on recurrence rates.

Harms: No harmful effects were reported.

Comment: The lack of evidence of effectiveness of both metronidazole and clindamycin suggests that anaerobes are unlikely to be the sole pathogenic agents linking bacterial vaginosis with sexual intercourse.

QUESTION   What are the effects of treatment before gynaecological procedures?

In women with bacterial vaginosis who are about to undergo surgical abortion, two RCTs found that oral or intravaginal antianaerobic treatment reduced the risk of pelvic inflammatory disease. We found no RCTs on the effects of treatment before other gynaecological procedures, including insertion of intrauterine contraceptive devices.

Benefits: We found no systematic review. **Before surgical abortion:** We found two RCTs. The first RCT (174 women with bacterial vaginosis) compared oral metronidazole 500 mg three times daily for 10 days versus placebo in women about to undergo surgical abortion.[31] Fewer women taking metronidazole developed pelvic inflammatory disease than those taking placebo, although the result did not quite reach significance (AR 3/84 [3.6%] with metronidazole v 11/90 [12.2%] with placebo; RR 0.29, 95% CI 0.08 to 1.01; NNT 12, 95% CI 6 to 279). The second RCT (1655 women) compared intravaginal clindamycin cream versus placebo in women about to undergo surgical abortion. It found that clindamycin significantly reduced the risk of post abortion infection (recalculation by *Clinical Evidence*: post abortion infection AR 3/181 [1.7%] with clindamycin cream v 12/181 [6.6] with placebo; RR 0.25, 95% CI 0.07 to 0.87; NNT 20, 95% CI 10 to 125).[32] **Before gynaecological surgery:** Bacterial vaginosis is associated with an increased risk of endometritis after caesarean section and vaginal cuff cellulitis after abdominal hysterectomy,[11,33] but we found no RCTs of antianaerobic treatment in women before such surgery. **Before insertion of an intrauterine contraceptive device:** Bacterial vaginosis has been associated with pelvic inflammatory disease (see pelvic inflammatory disease, p 1123) in women using intrauterine contraceptive devices,[3] but we found no RCTs of antianaerobic treatment in women with bacterial vaginosis before insertion of these devices.

Harms: The RCTs provided no information on adverse effects.[31]

Comment: None.

Substantive changes since last issue

Antianaerobic treatments in non-pregnant women New RCT;[15] conclusions unchanged.

Treating male partners New systematic review;[30] conclusions unchanged.

Treatment before surgery New RCT;[31] conclusions unchanged.

REFERENCES

1. Barbone F, Austin H, Louv WC, Alexander WJ. A follow-up study of methods of contraception, sexual activity, and rates of trichomoniasis, candidiasis, and bacterial vaginosis. *Am J Obstet Gynecol* 1990;163:510–514.
2. Mead PB. Epidemiology of bacterial vaginosis. *Am J Obstet Gynecol* 1993;169:446–449.
3. Avonts D, Sercu M, Heyerick P, et al. Incidence of uncomplicated genital infections in women using oral contraception or an intrauterine device: a prospective study. *Sex Transm Dis* 1990;17:23–29.
4. Berger BJ, Kolton S, Zenilman JM, et al. Bacterial vaginosis in lesbians: a sexually transmitted disease. *Clin Infect Dis* 1995;21:1402–1405.
5. Hawes SE, Hillier SL, Benedetti J, et al. Hydrogen peroxide-producing lactobacilli and acquisition of vaginal infections. *J Infect Dis* 1996;174:1058–1063.
6. Hillier SL, Nugent RP, Eschenbach DA, et al. Association between bacterial vaginosis and preterm delivery of a low-birth-weight infant. *N Engl J Med* 1995;333:1737–1742.
7. Schwebke JR, Morgan SC, Weiss HL. The use of sequential self-obtained vaginal smears for detecting changes in the vaginal flora. *Sex Transm Dis* 1997;24:236–239.
8. Flynn CA, Helwig AL, Meurer LN. Bacterial vaginosis in pregnancy and the risk of prematurity: a meta-analysis. *J Fam Pract* 1999;48:885–892.
9. Hillier SL, Martius J, Krohn MA, et al. Case-control study of chorioamnionic infection and chorioamnionitis in prematurity. *N Engl J Med* 1988;319:972–975.
10. Newton ER, Prihoda TJ, Gibbs RS. A clinical and microbiologic analysis of risk factors for puerperal endometritis. *Obstet Gynecol* 1990;75:403–406.
11. Watts D, Krohn M, Hillier S, Eschenbach DA. Bacterial vaginosis as a risk factor for postcesarean endometritis. *Obstet Gynecol* 1990; 75:52–58.
12. McDonald HM, O'Loughlin JA, Vigneswaran R, et al. Impact of metronidazole therapy on preterm birth in women with bacterial vaginosis flora (*Gardnerella vaginalis*): a randomised, placebo controlled trial. *Br J Obstet Gynaecol* 1997;104:1391–1397.
13. Schmid G, Markowitz L, Joesoef R, Koumans E. Bacterial vaginosis and HIV infection [editorial]. *Sex Transm Infect* 2000;76:3–4.
14. Joesoef MR, Schmid GP. Bacterial vaginosis: review of treatment options and potential clinical indications for therapy. *Clin Infect Dis* 1999; 28(suppl 1):72–79. Search date 1996; primary sources Medline, hand searches of text books about sexually transmitted diseases, meeting abstracts, and contact with drug manufacturers.
15. Paavonen J, Mangioni C, Martin MA, Wajszczuk CP. Vaginal clindamycin and oral metronidazole for bacterial vaginosis: a randomized trial. *Obstet Gynecol* 2000;96:256–260.
16. Greaves WL, Chungafung J, Morris B, Haile A, Townsend JL. Clindamycin versus metronidazole in the treatment of bacterial vaginosis. *Obstet Gynecol* 1988;72:799–802.
17. Livengood CH, Soper DE, Sheehan KL, et al. Comparison of once daily and twice daily dosing of 0.75% metronidazole gel in the treatment of bacterial vaginosis. *Sex Transm Dis* 1999;26:137–142.
18. Colli E, Landoni M, Parazzini F. Treatment of male partners and recurrence of bacterial vaginosis: a randomised trial. *Genitourin Med* 1997;73:267–270.
19. Sobel JD, Schmitt C, Meriwether C. Long-term follow-up of patients with bacterial vaginosis treated with oral metronidazole and topical clindamycin. *J Infect Dis* 1993;167:783–784.
20. Trexler MF, Fraser TG, Jones MP. Fulminant pseudomembranous colitis caused by clindamycin phosphate vaginal cream. *Am J Gastroenterol* 1997;92:2112–2113.
21. Hillier SL, Lipinski C, Briselden AM, Eschenbach DA. Efficacy of intravaginal 0.75% metronidazole gel for the treatment of bacterial vaginosis. *Obstet Gynecol* 1993;81:963–967.
22. Schmitt C, Sobel JD, Meriwether C. Bacterial vaginosis: treatment with clindamycin cream versus oral metronidazole. *Obstet Gynecol* 1992; 79:1020–1023.
23. Ransom SB, McComish JF, Greenberg R, Tolford DA. Oral metronidazole vs. metrogel vaginal for treating bacterial vaginosis. Cost-effectiveness evaluation. *J Reprod Med* 1999;44:359–362.
24. Brocklehurst P, Hannah M, McDonald H. The management of bacterial vaginosis in pregnancy. In: The Cochrane Library, Issue 1, 2000. Oxford: Update Software. Most recent substantive amendment/search date July 1998; primary sources Cochrane Pregnancy and Childbirth Group Trials Register.
25. Carey JC, Klebanoff MA, Hauth JC, et al. Metronidazole to prevent preterm delivery in pregnant women with asymptomatic bacterial vaginosis. *N Engl J Med* 2000;342:534–540.
26. McGregor JA, French JI, Jones W, et al. Bacterial vaginosis is associated with prematurity and vaginal fluid mucinase and sialidase: results of a controlled trial of topical clindamycin cream. *Am J Obstet Gynecol* 1994;170:1048–1059.
27. Vermeulen GM, Bruinse HW. Prophylactic administration of clindamycin 2% vaginal cream to reduce the incidence of spontaneous preterm birth in women with an increased recurrence risk: a randomized placebo-controlled double-blind trial. *Br J Obstet Gynaecol* 1999;106:652–657.
28. Hauth JC, Goldenberg RL, Andrews WW, DuBard MB, Copper RL. Reduced incidence of preterm delivery with metronidazole and erythromycin in women with bacterial vaginosis. *N Engl J Med* 1995;333:1732–1736.
29. Joesoef MR, Hillier SL, Wiknjosastro G, et al. Intravaginal clindamycin treatment for bacterial vaginosis: effect on preterm delivery and low birth weight. *Am J Obstet Gynecol* 1995;173:1527–1531.
30. Hamrick M, Chambliss ML. Bacterial vaginosis and treatment of sexual partners. *Arch Fam Med* 2000;9:647–648. Search date not stated; primary sources Medline, and The Cochrane Library.
31. Larsson PG, Platz-Christensen JJ, Thejls H, Forsum U, Pahlson C. Incidence of pelvic inflammatory disease after first-trimester legal abortion in

women with bacterial vaginosis after treatment with metronidazole: a double-blind, randomized study. *Am J Obstet Gynecol* 1992;166:100–103.

32. Larsson PG, Platz-Christensen JJ, Dalaker K, et al. Treatment with 2% clindamycin vaginal cream prior to first trimester surgical abortion to reduce signs of postoperative infection: a prospective, double-blinded, placebo-controlled, multicenter study. *Acta Obstet Gynecol Scand* 2000;79:390–396.

33. Soper DE, Bump RC, Hurt WG. Bacterial vaginosis and trichomoniasis vaginitis are risk factors for cuff cellulitis after abdominal hysterectomy. *Am J Obstet Gynecol* 1990;163:1016–1021.

M Joesoef
Medical Epidemiologist

George Schmid
Medical Epidemiologist

National Center for HIV, STD and TB
Prevention
Atlanta
USA

Competing interests: None declared.

Search date September 2000

Nicola Low and Frances Cowan

INTERVENTIONS

IN MEN AND NON-PREGNANT WOMEN

Beneficial

Likely to be beneficial

Unknown effectiveness

Unlikely to be beneficial

IN PREGNANT WOMEN

Likely to be beneficial

Unknown effectiveness

To be covered in future issues of *Clinical Evidence*

Non-gonococcal urethritis and
mucopurulent cervicitis
Screening for genital chlamydial
infection

Covered elsewhere in this issue

Pelvic inflammatory disease,
p 1123
Partner notification, p 1117

Key Messages

- Short term microbiological cure is the outcome used in most trials, but this may not mean eradication of *Chlamydia trachomatis*. Long term cure rates have not been studied extensively because of high default rates and difficulty in distinguishing persistent infection from reinfection due to re-exposure.

In men and non-pregnant women

- Small RCTs with short term follow up and high withdrawal rates have found that multiple dose regimens of tetracyclines (doxycycline, tetracycline) and macrolides (rosaramicin) achieve microbiological cure in at least 95% of people with genital chlamydia. Erythromycin (daily dose 2 g) is likely to be beneficial. Ciprofloxacin is unlikely to be beneficial. We found limited evidence on the effectiveness of other antibiotics. We found no differences in microbiological cure rates between men and women or between those with proven or presumed infection.

- A meta-analysis of short term RCTs has found that a single dose of azithromycin may be as effective in achieving microbiological cure of *C trachomatis* as a 7 day course of doxycycline. Rates of adverse effects were similar.

Genital chlamydial infection

In pregnant women

- Two systematic reviews have found that both amoxicillin and erythromycin are likely to be effective in achieving microbiological cure.

- One small RCT found that clindamycin and erythromycin had a similar effect on cure rates.

- One systematic review has found that a single dose of azithromycin is more effective in achieving microbiological cure of C trachomatis than a 7 day course of erythromycin.

DEFINITION	Uncomplicated genital chlamydia is a sexually transmitted infection of the urethra in men and of the endocervix, urethra, or both, in women that has not ascended to the upper genital tract. Infection is asymptomatic in up to 80% of women, but may cause non-specific symptoms, including vaginal discharge and intermenstrual bleeding. Infection in men causes urethral discharge and urethral irritation or dysuria, but may also be asymptomatic in up to half of cases.[1]
INCIDENCE/ PREVALENCE	Genital chlamydia is the commonest bacterial sexually transmitted infection in developed countries. In the USA, over 642 000 cases of chlamydia were reported in 2000.[2] The prevalence of uncomplicated genital chlamydia in women attending general practice surgeries in the UK is reported to be 3–5%.[3] Prevalence is highest in young adults. Reported rates in 15–19 year old women are about 800 per 100 000 in the UK,[4] 1000 per 100 000 in Sweden,[1] and 2500 per 100 000 in the USA.[5]
AETIOLOGY/ RISK FACTORS	Infection is caused by the bacterium C trachomatis serotypes D–K. It is transmitted primarily through sexual intercourse.
PROGNOSIS	Untreated chlamydial infection may persist asymptomatically in women for at least 15 months[6] and for an unknown period in men. In women, untreated chlamydial infection that ascends to the upper genital tract causes pelvic inflammatory disease in an estimated 30–40% of women[7] (see pelvic inflammatory disease, p 1123). Tubal infertility has been found to occur in about 11% of women after a single episode of pelvic inflammatory disease, and the risk of ectopic pregnancy is increased six to sevenfold.[8] Ascending infection in men causes epididymitis, but evidence that this causes male infertility is limited.[9] Maternal to infant transmission can lead to neonatal conjunctivitis and pneumonitis in 30–40% of cases.[1] Chlamydia may coexist with other genital infections and may facilitate transmission and acquisition of HIV infection.[1]
AIMS	To eradicate C trachomatis; to prevent the development of upper genital tract infection; and to prevent further sexual transmission, with minimal adverse effects of treatment.
OUTCOMES	Microbiological cure rate (calculated as the percentage of people attending a follow up visit at least 1 week after the end of antibiotic treatment who had a negative test for C trachomatis); adverse effects of treatment, including effects on the fetus; short term microbiological cure may not mean eradication of C trachomatis but long term cure rates have not been studied extensively because of high default rates and difficulty in distinguishing persistent infection from reinfection due to re-exposure; pelvic inflammatory disease; infertility.

METHODS *Clinical Evidence* update search and appraisal September 2000. All relevant systematic reviews and masked clinical trials were included. We present the range of cure rates (with exact binomial confidence intervals) or, if there was no evidence of statistical heterogeneity between trials, the summary cure rate (95% confidence intervals) weighted by the standard error. Summary rates do not include cure rates of 100% because the standard error cannot be computed if there are no treatment failures. Where two or more trials compared the same regimens with no evidence of statistical heterogeneity, we used a fixed effects meta-analysis to calculate the summary odds ratio with 95% confidence intervals. Trial quality was assessed in terms of randomisation, blinding, and numbers of withdrawals from analysis.[10] Trials with methodological limitations have been included but relevant problems are mentioned in the text. **Categorising interventions:** We considered a regimen beneficial if the summary cure rate from two or more RCTs was 95% or greater, as previously suggested,[11] and if the lower confidence limit was also above 90%. There were insufficient data to differentiate reinfections from persistent infections. We considered regimens to be likely (or unlikely) to be beneficial on the basis of positive (or negative) results from two or more RCTs, of unknown effectiveness if there was only one RCT, or if results were conflicting.

QUESTION	What are the effects of antibiotic treatment for men and non-pregnant women with uncomplicated genital chlamydial infection?

OPTION	MULTIPLE DOSE REGIMENS

Small RCTs, with short term follow up and high withdrawal rates, have found that tetracyclines (doxycycline, tetracycline) and macrolides (rosaramicin) achieve microbiological cure in 95% or more cases of genital chlamydia. We found no differences in microbiological cure rates between men and women or between those with proven or presumed infection. We found limited evidence on the effectiveness of other macrolides, quinolones, and penicillins.

Benefits: We found no systematic review. We found 22 RCTs reported to be double blind or with blinded outcome assessment comparing 19 different antibiotic regimens (see table on website www.clinicalevidence.org).[12–33] Results were similar in men and women and in populations with proven and presumed infection, so data were combined. **Doxycycline:** We found 11 RCTs (1434 men and women) comparing doxycycline with another antibiotic.[12–14,16–23] The cure rate was 100% in six trials and the weighted average 98% (95% CI 96% to 99%) in the other five. We found no trials comparing different regimens for doxycycline, but the most frequent schedule (in 6 trials) was 100 mg twice daily for 7 days. **Tetracycline:** The summary cure rate in four trials (201 men and women) comparing tetracycline hydrochloride 500 mg four times daily for 7 days versus another antibiotic was 97% (95% CI 94% to 99%).[24–27] Our meta-analysis of three trials[25–27] found that rates of treatment failure with rosaramicin compared with tetracycline were similar (OR 1.5, 95% CI 0.5 to 4.4). **Erythromycin:** Cure rates with erythromycin stearate 1 g daily for 7 days (3 trials, 191 participants) ranged from 77–95%,[30–32] and with erythromycin 2 g daily for 7 days (2 trials, 40 participants) from 94–100%.[29,32] **Ciprofloxacin:** In two trials (190 men and women), the cure rate for ciprofloxacin ranged from 63–92%.[20,21] Our meta-analysis found that failure of microbiological cure was more frequent with ciprofloxacin than doxycycline (OR 5.0, 95% CI 1.2 to 10.0). A variety of other antibiotics were studied in single trials (see table on website www.clinicalevidence.org). No trial measured the effect of antibiotics on pelvic inflammatory disease or infertility.

Harms: Reported adverse effects varied widely between trials but were mostly gastrointestinal (see table on website www.clinicalevidence.org).

Comment: Most trials were conducted in sexually transmitted diseases clinics where follow up is difficult; in seven of 14 trials with available data, more than 15% of randomised participants were not included in the analysis.[15,22,29–33] Most trials were small (three had fewer than 40 participants with chlamydia)[16,24,29] and many antibiotic regimens were compared so it is difficult to draw conclusions about relative efficacy. Only five trials reported that sexual partners of participants were offered treatment. Amoxicillin and ampicillin have not been adequately assessed in the treatment of genital chlamydia infection (see table on website www.clinicalevidence.org) because *in vitro* studies suggest that amoxicillin does not eradicate *C trachomatis*,[34] raising the concern that infection may persist and recrudesce *in vivo*.

| OPTION | SINGLE DOSE VERSUS MULTIPLE DOSE REGIMENS |

A meta-analysis of short term RCTs has found that a single dose of azithromycin may be as effective in achieving microbiological cure of *C trachomatis* as a 7 day course of doxycycline. Rates of adverse effects were similar.

Benefits: We found one systematic review (search date 1996, 9 blinded and unblinded RCTs, 1800 people) comparing azithromycin 1 g as a single dose versus doxycycline 100 mg twice daily for 7 days in participants with proven or presumed genital chlamydia.[35] Data about laboratory diagnosed infection were available for five trials (554 men and women). Cure rates for azithromycin ranged from 90–100% and for doxycycline from 93–100%. Microbiological failure tended to be more frequent with azithromycin than with doxycycline, but this did not reach statistical significance (AR 22/301 v 10/253; OR recalculated from data in the paper 1.8, 95% CI 0.9 to 3.9; P = 0.11).

Harms: Short term adverse effects of both azithromycin and doxycycline were reported to be mild.

Comment: Azithromycin can be given in a single dose as directly observed therapy. More comparisons of azithromycin and doxycycline are needed to rule out a clinically important difference between them.

QUESTION	What are the effects of treatment for pregnant women with uncomplicated genital chlamydial infection?

OPTION	MULTIPLE DOSE REGIMENS

Two systematic reviews of RCTs have found that both amoxicillin and erythromycin are likely to be effective in achieving microbiological cure of genital chlamydia in pregnant women. One small RCT found that clindamycin and erythromycin had a similar effect on cure rates.

Benefits: We found two systematic reviews, (search date 1998[36] and search date not stated[37]), the most recent of which (11 blinded and unblinded trials, 1449 people)[36] included all studies in the earlier review. **Erythromycin and amoxicillin:** Both achieved high rates of microbiological cure (cure rates 182/199 [91%] with amoxicillin 500 mg three times daily for 7 days v 163/191 [85%] with erythromycin 500 mg four times daily for 7 days; OR for failure of cure with amoxicillin compared with erythromycin 0.54, 95% CI 0.28 to 1.02, P = 0.059); and treatment with any antibiotic was better than placebo (OR for failure of cure 0.06, 95% CI 0.03 to 0.12). **Clindamycin:** One small RCT found no significant difference in cure rates between clindamycin and erythromycin (38/41 [93%] v 31/37 [84%]).

Harms: Rates of adverse effects were similar for clindamycin and erythromycin, but adverse effects sufficient to stop treatment were less frequent with amoxicillin than erythromycin (OR 0.16, 95% CI 0.09 to 0.30). None of the trials gave information on adverse clinical outcomes in the offspring.

Comment: We found no long term follow up data.

OPTION	SINGLE VERSUS MULTIPLE DOSE REGIMENS

One systematic review of RCTs has found that, in pregnant women, a single dose of azithromycin is as effective in achieving microbiological cure of *C trachomatis* as a 7 day course of erythromycin.

Benefits: We found one systematic review (search date 1998, 4 non-blinded RCTs, 290 pregnant women) comparing a single dose of azithro-mycin 1 g versus erythromycin 500 mg four times daily for 7 days. Failure of microbiological cure was less frequent with azithro-mycin than erythromycin (11/145 [8%] v 27/145 [19%], OR 0.38, 95% CI 0.19 to 0.74).[36] There was no significant difference in the rate of premature delivery (OR 0.73, 95% CI 0.24 to 2.20).

Harms: The RCTs found that azithromycin was associated with fewer adverse effects. Fetal anomaly was reported in one infant in each group.[36] Effects of azithromycin in pregnancy have not been extensively studied.

Comment: None.

REFERENCES

1. Holmes KK, Sparling PF, Mårdh PA, et al, eds. *Sexually transmitted diseases*. 3rd edition. New York: McGraw Hill Inc, 1999.
2. Anonymous. Notifiable diseases/deaths in selected cities weekly information. *MMR Morb Mortal Wkly Rep* 2001;49:1168.
3. Stokes T. Screening for chlamydia in general practice: a literature review and summary of the evidence (review). *J Public Health Med* 1997;19: 222–232.
4. http://www.phls.co.uk/facts/STI/EpidOfSTIsInE&W-chlamydia.htm Last accessed 13 March 2001.
5. *Sexually Transmitted Disease Surveillance, 1999.* US Department of Health and Human Services, Public Health Service. Atlanta. Centers for Disease Control and Prevention (CDC), September 2000.
6. McCormack WM, Alpert S, McComb DE, Nichols RL, Semine DZ, Zinner SH. Fifteen-month follow-up study of women infected with *Chlamydia trachomatis*. *N Engl J Med* 1979;300:123–125.
7. Cates W Jr, Rolfs RT Jr, Aral SO. Sexually transmitted diseases, pelvic inflammatory disease, and infertility: an epidemiologic update. *Epidemiol Rev* 1990;12:199–220.
8. Weström L, Bengtsson LP, Mårdh PA. Incidence, trends, and risks of ectopic pregnancy in a population of women. *BMJ* 1981;282:15–18.
9. Ness RB, Markovic N, Carlson CL, Coughlin MT. Do men become infertile after having sexually transmitted urethritis? An epidemiologic examination [review]. *Fertil Steril* 1997;68:205–213.
10. Chalmers I, Adams M, Dickersin K, et al. A cohort study of summary reports of controlled trials. *JAMA* 1990;263:1401–1405.
11. Clinical Effectiveness Group. National guideline for the management of *Chlamydia trachomatis* genital tract infection. *Sex Transm Infect* 1999;75(suppl 1):4–8.
12. Nilsen A, Halsos A, Johansen A, et al. A double blind study of single dose azithromycin and doxycycline in the treatment of chlamydial urethritis in males. *Genitourin Med* 1992;68:325–327.
13. Steingrímsson Ó, Ólafsson JH, Thórarinsson H, Ryan RW, Johnson RB, Tilton RC. Single dose azithromycin treatment of gonorrhea and infections caused by *C trachomatis* and *U urealyticum* in men. *Sex Transm Dis* 1994;21:43–46.
14. Stamm WE, Hicks CB, Martin DH, et al. Azithromycin for empirical treatment of the nongonococcal urethritis syndrome in men. A randomized double-blind study. *JAMA* 1995;274: 545–549.
15. Brihmer C, Mårdh PA, Kallings I, et al. Efficacy and safety of azithromycin versus lymecycline in the treatment of genital chlamydial infections in women. *Scand J Infect Dis* 1996;28:451–454.
16. Stein GE, Mummaw NL, Havlichek DH. A preliminary study of clarithromycin versus doxycycline in the treatment of nongonococcal urethritis and mucopurulent cervicitis. *Pharmacotherapy* 1995;15:727–731.
17. Romanowski B, Talbot H, Stadnyk M, Kowalchuk P, Bowie WR. Minocycline compared with doxycycline in the treatment of nongonococcal urethritis and mucopurulent cervicitis. *Ann Intern Med* 1993; 119:16–22.
18. Boslego JW, Hicks CB, Greenup R, et al. A prospective randomized trial of ofloxacin vs. doxycycline in the treatment of uncomplicated male urethritis. *Sex Transm Dis* 1988;15:186–191.
19. Phillips I, Dimian C, Barlow D, et al. A comparative study of two different regimens of sparfloxacin versus doxycycline in the treatment of non-gonococcal urethritis in men. *J Antimicrob Chemother* 1996;37(suppl A):123–134.
20. Hooton TM, Rogers ME, Medina TG, et al. Ciprofloxacin compared with doxycycline for nongonococcal urethritis. Ineffectiveness against *Chlamydia trachomatis* due to relapsing infection. *JAMA* 1990;264:1418–1421.
21. Jeskanen L, Karppinen L, Ingervo L, Reitamo S, Happonen HP, Lassus A. Ciprofloxacin versus doxycycline in the treatment of uncomplicated urogenital *Chlamydia trachomatis* infections. A double-blind comparative study. *Scand J Infect Dis Suppl* 1989;60:62–65.
22. McCormack WM, Dalu ZA, Martin DH, et al. Double-blind comparison of trovafloxacin and doxycycline in the treatment of uncomplicated Chlamydial urethritis and cervicitis. Trovafloxacin Chlamydial Urethritis/Cervicitis Study Group. *Sex Transm Dis* 1999;26:531–536.
23. Lassus AB, Virrankoski T, Reitamo SJ, et al. Pivampicillin versus doxycycline in the treatment of chlamydial urethritis in men. *Sex Transm Dis* 1990;17:20–22.
24. Lassus A, Juvakoski T, Kanerva L. Comparison between rifampicin and tetracycline in the treatment of nongonococcal urethritis in males with special reference to *Chlamydia trachomatis*. *Eur J Sex Transm Dis* 1984;2:15–7.
25. Lassus A, Allgulander C, Juvakoski T. Efficacy of rosaramicin and tetracycline in chlamydia-positive and -negative nongonococcal urethritis. *Eur J Sex Transm Dis* 1982;1:29–31.
26. Juvakoski T, Allgulander C, Lassus A. Rosaramicin and tetracycline treatment in *Chlamydia trachomatis*-positive and -negative nongonococcal urethritis. *Sex Transm Dis* 1981;8:12–15.
27. Brunham RC, Kuo CC, Stevens CE, Holmes KK. Therapy of cervical chlamydial infection. *Ann Intern Med* 1982;97:216–219.
28. Batteiger BE, Zwickl BE, French ML, Jones RB. Women at risk for gonorrhea: comparison of rosaramicin and ampicillin plus probenecid in the eradication of *Neisseria gonorrhoeae*, *Chlamydia trachomatis* and genital mycoplasmas. *Sex Transm Dis* 1985;12:1–4.
29. Robson HG, Shah PP, Lalonde RG, Hayes L, Senikas VM. Comparison of rosaramicin and erythromycin stearate for treatment of cervical infection with *Chlamydia trachomatis*. *Sex Transm Dis* 1983;10:130–134.
30. Worm AM, Hoff G, Kroon S, Petersen CS, Christensen JJ. Roxithromycin compared with erythromycin against genitourinary chlamydial infections. *Genitourin Med* 1989;65:35–38.
31. Worm AM, Avnstorp C, Petersen CS. Erythromycin against Chlamydia trachomatis infections. A double blind study comparing 4- and 7-day treatment in men and women. *Dan Med Bull* 1985;32:269–271.
32. Linnemann CCJ, Heaton CL, Ritchey M. Treatment of *Chlamydia trachomatis* infections: comparison of 1- and 2-g doses of erythromycin daily for seven days. *Sex Transm Dis* 1987;14:102–106.
33. Paavonen J, Kousa M, Saikku P, Vartiainen E, Kanerva L, Lassus A. Treatment of nongonococcal urethritis with trimethoprim-sulphadiazine and with placebo. A double-blind partner-controlled study. *Br J Venereal Dis* 1980;56:101–104.
34. Kuo CC, Wang SP, Grayston JT. Antimicrobial activity of several antibiotics and a sulfonamide against *Chlamydia trachomatis* organisms in cell culture. *Antimicrob Agents Chemother* 1977;12:80–83.

35. Chlamydial STD treatment. *Bandolier* 1996;28: 4–6. Search date 1996; primary source Medline 1990 to 1996. http://www.jr2.ox.ac.uk/bandolier/band28/b28–4.html Last accessed 13 March 2001.

36. Brocklehurst P, Rooney G. Interventions for treating genital *Chlamydia trachomatis* infection in pregnancy. In: The Cochrane Library, Issue 4, 1999. Oxford: Update Software. Search date 1998; primary sources Cochrane Pregnancy and

Childbirth Review Group Specialised Register of Controlled Trials, and Cochrane Controlled Trials Register.

37. Turrentine MA, Newton ER. Amoxicillin or erythromycin for the treatment of antenatal chlamydial infection: a meta-analysis. *Obstet Gynecol* 1995;86:1021–1025. Search date not stated; primary sources Medline and Cochrane Pregnancy and Childbirth Database.

Nicola Low
Department of Social Medicine
University of Bristol
Bristol
UK

Frances Cowan
Department of Sexually Transmitted
Diseases
Royal Free and University College
Medical School
London
UK

Competing interests: FC has received research and symposium funding from Glaxo Wellcome in relation to HSV research. NL, none declared.

Genital herpes

Search date October 2000

Anna Wald

INTERVENTIONS

Beneficial

Oral antiviral treatment in first episodes 1092

Oral antiviral treatment taken at the start of a recurrence. . .1093

Daily oral antiviral treatment in people with high rates of recurrence. 1093

Likely to be beneficial

Daily oral antiviral treatment in late pregnancy (36 or more weeks of gestation) in women with a history of genital herpes . . .1096

Unknown effectiveness

Psychotherapy to reduce recurrence. 1094

Condoms and other interventions to prevent sexual transmission 1095

Serological screening and counselling in late pregnancy 1096

Oral antiviral treatment in people with HIV infection. 1096

Likely to be ineffective or harmful

Abdominal delivery in women with genital lesions at term 1095

To be covered in future issues of *Clinical Evidence*

Type-specific herpes simplex virus (HSV) serological assays for diagnosis of HSV-2 infection

Key Messages

Treating first and recurrent episodes of genital herpes

- RCTs have found that oral antiviral treatment reduces the duration of symptoms, lesions, and viral shedding in first and recurrent episodes of genital herpes, and that daily treatment reduces rates of recurrence and may improve quality of life.

- RCTs found no evidence of significant differences in effectiveness or adverse events between aciclovir, valaciclovir, and famciclovir.

- We found only limited evidence of an effect of antiviral treatment versus placebo for genital herpes in people with HIV infection.

Preventing transmission of herpes simplex virus

- Limited evidence from a prospective cohort study suggests that condom use may decrease the risk of sexual transmission of herpes simplex virus (HSV) type 2. Other interventions aimed at preventing transmission (antiviral treatment and immunisation) have not been adequately studied.

- The highest risk of mother to baby transmission is in women newly infected with genital herpes in late pregnancy. We found inadequate evaluation of interventions to prevent infection in late pregnancy (such as serological screening and counselling).

- We found that the effect of abdominal delivery on mother to baby transmission has not been adequately evaluated. The procedure carries the risk of increased maternal morbidity and mortality.

- Limited evidence from RCTs suggests that antiviral treatment may reduce the number of pregnant women with genital lesions at term. Because women with genital lesions at term are usually offered abdominal deliveries, antiviral treatment may reduce the rate of abdominal delivery.

DEFINITION	Genital herpes is an infection with HSV-1 or HSV-2, causing ulceration in the genital area. HSV infections can be defined on the basis of virological and serological findings. Types of infection include: **first episode primary infection**, which is HSV in a person without prior HSV-1 or HSV-2 antibodies; **first episode non-primary infection**, which is HSV-2 in a person with prior HSV-1 antibodies or vice-versa; **first recognised recurrence**, which is HSV-2 (or HSV-1) in a person with prior HSV-2 (or HSV-1) antibodies; and **recurrent genital herpes**, which is caused by reactivation of latent HSV.
INCIDENCE/ PREVALENCE	Genital herpes infections are among the most common sexually transmitted diseases. Seroprevalence studies show that 22% of adults in the USA have HSV-2 antibodies.[1] A UK study found that 23% of adults attending sexual medicine clinics and 7.6% of blood donors in London had antibodies to HSV-2.[2]
AETIOLOGY/ RISK FACTORS	Both HSV-1 and HSV-2 can cause a first episode of genital infection, but HSV-2 is more likely to cause recurrent disease.[3] Most people with HSV-2 infection are not aware that they have genital herpes, as their symptoms are mild. However, these people can pass on the infection to sexual partners and newborns.[4,5]
PROGNOSIS	Sequelae of HSV infection include neonatal HSV, opportunistic infections in immunocompromised people, recurrent genital ulceration, and psychosocial morbidity. HSV-2 infection is associated with an increased risk of HIV transmission and acquisition. The most common neurological complications are aseptic meningitis (reported in about a quarter of women during primary infection) and urinary retention. The absolute risk of neonatal infection is high (41%, 95% CI 26% to 56%) in babies born to women who acquire infection near the time of labour[6,7] and low (< 3%) in women with established infection, even in those who have a recurrence at term. About 15% of neonatal infections result from postnatal transmission from oral lesions.
AIMS	To reduce the morbidity of the first episode; to reduce the risk of recurrent disease after a first episode; and to prevent further transmission, with minimal adverse effects of treatment.
OUTCOMES	Severity and duration of symptoms; healing time; duration of viral shedding; recurrence rates; psychosocial morbidity; rates of transmission; and adverse effects of treatment.

METHODS *Clinical Evidence* update search and appraisal October 2000, using the terms herpes simplex virus, aciclovir, valaciclovir, famciclovir, cidofovir, trifluridine, and neonatal herpes. We also included preliminary results of clinical trials published in the abstracts of the Interscience Conference on Antimicrobial Agents and Chemotherapy and International Society for STD Research. We also contacted experts in the field and makers of antiviral drugs to identify completed studies that were undergoing peer review, but which had not yet been published.

| QUESTION | What are the effects of antiviral treatment in people with a first episode of genital herpes? |

RCTs have found that oral antiviral treatment decreases the duration of lesions, symptoms, and viral shedding, and prevents neurological complications in people with first episode genital herpes. Oral treatment is more convenient than intravenous and more effective than topical treatment. Limited data provide no evidence that oral antiviral treatment reduces the rate of recurrence compared with placebo. RCTs found no evidence of a significant difference in clinical or biological variables of a first episode of genital herpes between aciclovir, valaciclovir, and famciclovir.

Benefits: We found no systematic review. **Immediate effects:** We found several RCTs (350 men and women) of oral aciclovir for the treatment of first episode genital herpes. Compared with placebo, aciclovir (200 mg 5 times daily) decreased the duration of viral shedding (2 v 10 days), pain (5 v 7 days), time to healing of lesions (8 v 14 days), and prevented formation of new lesions. Neurological complications (aseptic meningitis and urinary retention) were also reduced. Numbers were small so no firm estimates of effectiveness were available.[8–12] **Different regimens:** In one international trial of 643 healthy adults with first episode genital herpes, oral valaciclovir (1000 mg twice daily) was compared with oral aciclovir (200 mg 5 times daily) for 10 days.[13] No significant differences were noted between the two medications in terms of any clinical or virological variables. Another RCT (951 adults with first episode genital herpes) compared three different doses of oral famciclovir (125, 250, or 500 mg three times daily) versus oral aciclovir (200 mg 5 times daily).[14] No significant differences were found. **Recurrence rates:** A meta-analysis of two small placebo controlled RCTs (61 people) found no significant difference in time to recurrence or frequency of recurrence between people given oral aciclovir and those given placebo.[15] **Systemic versus topical treatment:** We found no direct randomised comparisons of oral, intravenous, or topical antiviral treatment. Comparison of results from different trials performed at one institution suggests that systemic treatment is more effective than topical.[16]

Harms: Adverse effects (mostly headache and nausea) were rare and frequency was similar for aciclovir, valaciclovir, famciclovir, and placebo.

Comment: Oral aciclovir has the advantage of convenience over intravenous aciclovir.[16]

QUESTION What interventions reduce the impact of recurrence?

OPTION ANTIVIRAL TREATMENT AT THE START OF RECURRENCE

RCTs have found that oral antiviral treatment taken at the start of a recurrence reduces the duration of lesions, symptoms, and viral shedding in people with recurrent genital herpes.

Benefits:
We found one systematic review (search date 1997, 4 RCTs, 3393 people).[17] **Famciclovir versus placebo:** One RCT (467 people with recurrent genital herpes) found that oral famciclovir versus placebo (125–500 mg twice daily) significantly reduced the duration of lesions (5 v 4 days) and viral shedding (3 v 2 days). **Valaciclovir versus placebo:** Another RCT (987 people with recurrent genital herpes) found that self initiated oral valaciclovir (500 or 1000 mg twice daily) for 5 days versus placebo decreased the episode duration (4 v 6 days) and viral shedding (2 v 4 days), and increased the rate of aborted recurrences (31% v 21%). **Valaciclovir versus aciclovir:** The other two RCTs (1939 people) found no significant difference between oral valaciclovir and aciclovir. **Aciclovir versus placebo:** Several RCTs in more than 650 healthy adults with recurrent genital herpes were identified in a non-systematic review published in 1990.[18] These evaluated 5 days of oral aciclovir (200 mg 5 times daily or 800 mg twice daily), started at the first sign of recurrence. Compared with placebo, treatment decreased the period of viral shedding (1 v 2 days) and duration of lesions (5 v 6 days).

Harms:
Adverse effects (mostly headache and nausea) were rare, and frequency was similar for aciclovir, valaciclovir, famciclovir, and placebo.

Comment:
The benefit was found to be greater if the person with recurrent herpes initiated treatment at the first symptom or sign of a recurrence.[19] People can learn to recognise recurrences early on and should have an adequate supply of medication at home.

OPTION DAILY MAINTENANCE ANTIVIRAL TREATMENT

RCTs have found that daily maintenance treatment with oral antiviral agents reduces the frequency of recurrences and viral shedding in people with genital herpes. Daily treatment may also improve psychosocial function.

Benefits:
Recurrence rates: We found one systematic review (search date 1997, 4 RCTs).[17] Two RCTs evaluated treatment for 1 year. In one RCT (1479 people), freedom from recurrence was reported in 40–50% of people who received valaciclovir (500 or 1000 mg once daily), valaciclovir (250 mg twice daily), or aciclovir (400 mg twice daily) compared with 5% who received placebo.[20] In the other RCT (455 people), the median time to first recurrence was 11 months with famciclovir (250 mg twice daily) and 1.5 months with placebo.[21] One non-systematic review (published in 1990) identified several placebo controlled RCTs of aciclovir.[18] Most participants had a history of frequent recurrence (≥ 6 per year). Daily aciclovir was

associated with reduced recurrence rate (74–93%) and duration of recurrences (3.5 v 5 days).[18] Of 210 adults in one trial who completed 5 years of continuous treatment with aciclovir (400 mg twice daily), 53–70% were free of recurrence each year.[22] The first year of this trial was a double blind placebo controlled RCT in 1146 adults. Those on aciclovir had significantly fewer recurrences during the first year (1.7 v 12.5, P < 0.0001). **Viral shedding:** We found one RCT that evaluated the effect of daily maintenance treatment versus placebo on viral shedding in women with recently acquired genital HSV-2 infection. Women obtained swabs for viral cultures daily for 70 days while receiving aciclovir (400 mg twice daily) or placebo.[23] Viral shedding was reduced by 95% with aciclovir on days with reported lesions and by 94% on days without lesions. **Psychosocial morbidity:** We found one RCT (1479 people) that evaluated the effect of daily oral antiviral treatment on a genital herpes quality of life scale.[24] Participants receiving daily aciclovir or valaciclovir had significantly greater mean improvements from baseline than those receiving placebo.[25]

Harms: Daily treatment with aciclovir, famciclovir, and valaciclovir was well tolerated. People taking aciclovir have been followed for up to 7 years, and those taking famciclovir and valaciclovir for up to 1 year. Nausea and headache were infrequent, and participants rarely discontinued treatment because of adverse effects. We found no studies evaluating whether daily maintenance treatment increases high risk sexual behaviour. We found no evidence that daily treatment with aciclovir results in emergence of aciclovir resistant HSV during or after stopping treatment in healthy adults.[26]

Comment: Viral shedding is an intermediate outcome, but may be important to people with herpes as it reflects the risk of transmitting infection.

OPTION   PSYCHOTHERAPY

We found that the effects of psychotherapy on the rate of genital herpes recurrence have not yet been adequately studied.

Benefits: We found one systematic review (search date 1991), which identified six poor quality studies of psychotherapeutic interventions in 69 participants (4 studies had < 10 participants).[27] Interventions varied from hypnotherapy and progressive muscle relaxation to cognitive therapy and multifaceted intervention. In the largest study, 31 people with four or more recurrences a year were randomly assigned to psychosocial intervention, social support, or waiting list. Participants receiving psychosocial intervention had significantly lower recurrence rates (6 recurrences a year) compared with the pretreatment frequency (11 a year), and with the other groups (11 a year).

Harms: No adverse effects were noted.

Comment: Small numbers of people, inadequate controls, and subjective and retrospective assessment of recurrence frequency at baseline, limit the usefulness of these studies. Controlled studies that include prospective clinical evaluation of disease activity are needed.

QUESTION   What interventions prevent transmission of HSV?

OPTION   CONDOMS, ANTIVIRAL TREATMENT, IMMUNISATION

Limited evidence from one non-randomised study suggests that condom use may decrease the risk of sexual transmission of HSV-2. Other interventions have not been adequately studied.

Benefits: **Condoms:** We found no RCTs. In a prospective study of 528 couples discordant for HSV-2 infection and followed for 18 months, the use of condoms was associated with lower risk of HSV-2 acquisition (adjusted RR of acquiring HSV infection when using condoms in less than 25% of sexual acts versus more than 25% was 3.9, 95% CI 1.1 to 13.6). Only 61% of couples ever used condoms during the study and only 7.6% used them consistently. One person acquired HSV-2 despite consistent condom use (A Wald, et al, personal communication, 1999).[28]
Antiviral treatment: We found no direct evidence that treatment reduces HSV transmission in serologically discordant couples. However, RCTs have shown that daily antiviral treatment decreases the frequency of clinical and subclinical viral shedding (see text, p 1093).
Immunisation: No effective vaccines are currently available.

Harms: As for individual interventions.

Comment: Controlled trials of condoms for prevention of HSV-2 transmission are unlikely to be done. Even with routine counselling, many couples do not regularly use condoms.

OPTION   ABDOMINAL DELIVERY TO PREVENT NEONATAL HERPES

We found insufficient evidence for the effect of abdominal delivery on the risk of neonatal herpes. The procedure carries the risk of increased maternal morbidity and mortality.

Benefits: We found no systematic review and no RCTs that assessed the effects of abdominal delivery on the risk of mother to child transmission of HSV. In the Netherlands, women with recurrent genital herpes at delivery have been allowed vaginal birth since 1987. This policy has not resulted in an increase of neonatal herpes: 26 cases from 1981–1986, and 19 cases from 1987–1991.[7]

Harms: Abdominal delivery is associated with significant maternal morbidity and mortality. It has been estimated that, for every two neonatal deaths from HSV infection prevented by abdominal delivery, one maternal death may be caused.[29]

Comment: Countries vary in their approach to obstetric management of women with recurrent genital herpes at term. In the USA and the UK, these women are advised to undergo abdominal delivery, with its attendant risks to the mother. The absolute risk of neonatal infection is high (AR 41%, 95% CI 26% to 56%) in babies born to women who acquired infection near the time of labour[6,7] and low (AR < 3%) in women with established infection, even in those who have recurrence at term. Most women who acquired infection towards the end of pregnancy are undiagnosed, and most cases of neonatal HSV infection are acquired from women without a history of genital herpes. The available evidence suggests that efforts to prevent neonatal HSV infection should focus on preventing the acquisition of infection in late pregnancy.

OPTION　**ANTIVIRAL TREATMENT DURING PREGNANCY**

We found limited evidence from one systematic review of RCTs suggesting that aciclovir reduces the rate of genital lesions at term in women with first or recurrent episodes of genital HSV during pregnancy. We found that adverse effects have not been adequately studied.

Benefits:　We found one systematic review (search date 1996). This identified three studies, including two RCTs, of daily aciclovir versus placebo in 210 pregnant women near term with genital herpes.[7] The studies differed in terms of the dose and duration of aciclovir and the populations enrolled. Abdominal delivery was performed in women with genital lesions at term. All three studies found lower rates of abdominal delivery in women treated with aciclovir, although in two studies the effect was not significant (AR of abdominal delivery 4/21 [19%] in women receiving aciclovir v 10/15 [40%] in women receiving placebo, RR 0.48, 95% CI 0.17 to 1.30;[30] AR of abdominal delivery 6/46 [13%] in women receiving aciclovir v 15/46 [33%] in women receiving no treatment, RR 0.4, 95% CI 0.17 to 0.94, NTT 6, 95% CI 3 to 43,[31] and AR of abdominal delivery 7/31 [23%] in women receiving aciclovir v 10/32 [31%] in women receiving placebo, RR 0.72, 95% CI 0.32 to 1.66).[32]

Harms:　No adverse effects for women or newborns were reported, but the number of women was small. Rare adverse events, such as an increase in asymptomatic viral shedding or aciclovir related obstructive uropathy in the newborns, would be difficult to detect.

Comment:　None.

OPTION　**SEROLOGICAL SCREENING AND COUNSELLING TO PREVENT ACQUISITION OF HSV DURING PREGNANCY**

We found insufficient evidence about the effects of serological screening and counselling during pregnancy on infection rates.

Benefits:　We found no systematic review or RCTs that assessed either serological screening with type specific assays to identify women at risk for HSV acquisition in late pregnancy, or counselling to avoid genital–genital and oral–genital contact in late pregnancy.

Harms:　We found insufficient evidence.

Comment:　None.

QUESTION　**What are the effects of treatments in people with genital herpes and HIV infection?**

OPTION　**ANTIVIRAL TREATMENTS**

We found only limited evidence of the effect of antiviral treatment for genital herpes in people with HIV infection. However, evidence from other settings suggests that antivirals may be effective treatment of genital herpes in immunocompromised people.

Benefits: We found no systematic review and no RCTs on the treatment of the first episode of genital herpes in people with HIV infection. **Treatment of recurrence:** We found two RCTs. One RCT (193 people on stable anti-retroviral therapy) compared famciclovir (500 mg twice daily) with aciclovir (400 mg 5 times daily) for 1 week.[33] No difference was found between the two drugs in mucocutaneous recurrence of HSV. The other (467 people) compared valaciclovir (1 g twice daily) to aciclovir (200 mg 5 times daily) for 5 days.[34] No significant differences between the two drugs were found. **Prevention of recurrence:** We found two RCTs. One crossover RCT (48 people with antibodies to HIV and HSV; 38 with a history of genital herpes) compared famciclovir with placebo over 8 weeks.[35] The conclusions of this study are difficult to interpret (see comment below). The other RCT (1062 people with a median CD4 count of 320/mm^3) compared valaciclovir (500 mg twice daily) versus valaciclovir (1000 mg once daily) versus aciclovir (400 mg twice daily) over 1 year.[36] It found no significant difference between either dose of valaciclovir versus aciclovir, although recurrence was less likely with valaciclovir (500 mg twice daily) than with the valaciclovir (1000 mg once daily) (82% v 71% recurrence free at 48 weeks, $P < 0.05$).

Harms: Adverse effects (mostly headache and nausea) occurred with similar frequency with aciclovir, valaciclovir, and famciclovir. Thrombotic microangiopathy, which has been reported in people receiving valaciclovir (8 g daily), has not been reported among 713 HIV infected persons who received oral valaciclovir in daily doses ranging from 250–1000 mg for up to 1 year (A Wald, personal communication, 2000).

Comment: Three of the four RCTs did not have a placebo control. Most studies to date have compared new treatments with aciclovir, rather than placebo. The crossover trial of famciclovir versus placebo was difficult to interpret because the dropout rate was high. Although we found only limited evidence of an effect of antivirals for treatment of genital herpes in people with HIV infection, there was a consensus that antiviral treatment may be helpful, based on evidence from immunocompromised people who do not have HIV. Aciclovir has been found effective in immunocompromised populations. With the availability of effective treatments for HIV, trials of antiviral (anti-HSV) versus placebo may now be conducted. A trial of valaciclovir versus placebo is now in progress (A Wald, 2000, personal communication). In HIV infected people, there is a markedly increased rate of HSV viral shedding.[37] HIV has been recovered from genital herpes lesions.[38] We found no evidence about the effect of daily antiviral therapy on transmission of HIV to sexual partners.

REFERENCES

1. Fleming DT, McQuillan GM, Johnson RE, et al. Herpes simplex virus type 2 in the United States, 1976 to 1994. N Engl J Med 1997;337:1105–1111.

2. Cowan FM, Johnson AM, Ashley R, et al. Antibody to herpes simplex virus type 2 as serological marker of sexual lifestyle in populations. BMJ 1994;309:1325–1329.

3. Benedetti J, Corey L, Ashley R. Recurrence rates in genital herpes after symptomatic first-episode infection. Ann Intern Med 1994;121:847–854.

4. Mertz GJ, Schmidt O, Jourden JL, et al. Frequency of acquisition of first-episode genital infection with herpes simplex virus from symptomatic and asymptomatic source contacts. Sex Transm Dis 1985;12:33–39.

5. Whitley RJ, Kimberlin DW, Roizman B. Herpes simplex viruses. Clin Infect Dis 1998;26:541–553.

6. Brown ZA, Selke SA, Zeh J, et al. Acquisition of herpes simplex virus during pregnancy. N Engl J Med 1997;337:509–515.

Genital herpes

7. Smith J, Cowan FM, Munday P. The management of herpes simplex virus infection in pregnancy. Br J Obstet Gynaecol 1998;105:255–268. Search date 1996; primary source Medline.

8. Nilsen AE, Aasen T, Halsos AM, et al. Efficacy of oral acyclovir in treatment of initial and recurrent genital herpes. Lancet 1982;2:571–573.

9. Corey L, Fife K, Benedetti JK, et al. Intravenous acyclovir for the treatment of primary genital herpes. Ann Intern Med 1983;98:914–921.

10. Mertz G, Critchlow C, Benedetti J, et al. Double-blind placebo-controlled trial of oral acyclovir in the first episode genital herpes simplex virus infection. JAMA 1984;252:1147–1151.

11. Mindel A, Adler MW, Sutherland S, et al. Intravenous acyclovir treatment for primary genital herpes. Lancet 1982;2:697–700.

12. Bryson YJ, Dillon M, Lovett M, et al. Treatment of first episodes of genital herpes simplex virus infections with oral acyclovir: a randomized double-blind controlled trial in normal subjects. N Engl J Med 1983;308:916–1920.

13. Fife KH, Barbarash RA, Rudolph T, et al. Valaciclovir versus acyclovir in the treatment of first-episode genital herpes infection: results of an international, multicenter, double-blind randomized clinical trial. Sex Transm Dis 1997;24: 481–486.

14. Loveless M, Harris W, Sacks S. Treatment of first episode genital herpes with famciclovir. Programs and abstracts of the 35th Interscience Conference on Antimicrobial Agents and Chemotherapy. San Francisco, California, 1995.

15. Corey L, Mindel A, Fife KH, et al. Risk of recurrence after treatment of first episode genital herpes with intravenous acyclovir. Sex Transm Dis 1985;12:215–218.

16. Corey L, Benedetti J, Critchlow C, et al. Treatment of primary first-episode genital herpes simplex virus infections with acyclovir: results of topical, intravenous and oral therapy. J Antimicrob Chemother 1983;12(suppl B):79–88.

17. Wald A. New therapies and prevention strategies for genital herpes. Clin Infect Dis 1999;28:S4–13. Search date not stated; primary source Medline.

18. Stone K, Whittington W. Treatment of genital herpes. Rev Infect Dis 1990;12(suppl 6):610–619.

19. Reichman RC, Badger GJ, Mertz GJ, et al. Treatment of recurrent genital herpes simplex infections with oral acyclovir: a controlled trial. JAMA 1984;251:2103–2107.

20. Reitano M, Tyring S, Lang W, et al. Valaciclovir for the suppression of recurrent genital herpes simplex virus infection: a large-scale dose range finding study. J Infect Dis 1998;178:603–610.

21. Diaz-Mitoma F, Sibbald RG, Shafran SD. Oral famciclovir for the suppression of recurrent genital herpes: a randomized controlled trial. JAMA 1998; 280:887–892.

22. Goldberg L, Kaufman R, Kurtz T, et al. Continuous five-year treatment of patients with frequently recurring genital herpes simplex virus infection with acyclovir. J Med Virol 1993(suppl 1);45–50.

23. Wald A, Zeh J, Barnum G, et al. Suppression of subclinical shedding of herpes simplex virus type 2 with acyclovir. Ann Intern Med 1996;124:8–15.

24. Doward LC, McKenna SP, Kohlmann T, et al. The international development of the RGHQoL: a quality of life measure for recurrent genital herpes. Qual Life Res 1998;7:143–153.

25. Patel R, Tyring S, Strand A, et al. Impact of suppressive antiviral therapy on the health related quality of life of patients with recurrent genital herpes infection. Sex Transm Infect 1999;75: 398–402.

26. Fife KH, Crumpacker CS, Mertz GJ. Recurrence and resistance patterns of herpes simplex virus following stop of ≥ 6 years of chronic suppression with acyclovir. J Infect Dis 1994;169:1338–1341.

27. Longo D, Koehn K. Psychosocial factors and recurrent genital herpes: a review of prediction and psychiatric treatment studies. Int J Psychiatry Med 1993;23:99–117. Search date 1991; primary sources Psychological Abstracts, Medline, and hand searches of referee lists.

28. Corey L, Langenberg AG, Ashley R, et al. Recombinant glycoprotein vaccine for the prevention of genital HSV-2 infection: two randomized controlled trials. Chiron HSV Vaccine Study Group. JAMA 1999;282:331–340.

29. Randolph A, Washington A, Prober C. Cesarean delivery for women presenting with genital herpes lesions. JAMA 1993;270:77–82.

30. Scott LL, Sanchez PJ, Jackson GL, Zeray F, Wendel Jr GD. Acyclovir suppression to prevent cesarean delivery after first-episode genital herpes. Obstet Gynecol 1996;87:69–73.

31. Stray-Pedersen B. Acyclovir in late pregnancy to prevent neonatal herpes simplex [Letter] [see comments]. Lancet 1990;336:756.

32. Brocklehurst P, Kinghorn G, Carney O, et al. A randomised placebo controlled trial of suppressive acyclovir in late pregnancy in women with recurrent genital herpes infection. Br J Obstet Gynaecol 1998;105:275–280.

33. Romanowski B, Aoki FY, Martel AY, Lavender EA, Parsons JE, Saltzman RL. Efficacy and safety of famciclovir for treating mucocutaneous herpes simplex infection in HIV-infected individuals. Collaborative Famciclovir HIV Study Group. AIDS 2000;14:1211–1217.

34. Schacker T, International Valaciclovir Study Group. Valaciclovir as acute treatment for recurrent ano-genital herpes in immunocompromised (HIV positive) individuals. 13th International Society for STD Research. Denver, Colorado, 1999.

35. Schacker T, Hu HL, Koelle DM, et al. Famciclovir for the suppression of symptomatic and asymptomatic herpes simplex virus reactivation in HIV-infected persons. A double-blind, placebo-controlled trial. Ann Intern Med 1998;128:21–28.

36. Gold J, Bell A, Valaciclovir International HSV Study Group. Valaciclovir prevents herpes simplex virus recurrences in HIV-infected individuals – a double-blind controlled trial. Programs and abstracts of the 20th International Congress of Chemotherapy. Sydney, Australia, 1997.

37. Schacker T, Zeh J, Hu HL, et al. Frequency of symptomatic and asymptomatic HSV-2 reactivations among HIV-infected men. J Infect Dis 1998;178:1616–1622.

38. Schacker T, Ryncarz A, Goddard J, et al. Frequent recovery of HIV from genital herpes simplex virus lesions in HIV infected persons. JAMA 1998;280: 61–66.

Anna Wald

Assistant Professor of Medicine and Epidemiology, University of Washington
Seattle, USA

Competing interests: The author has received a fee from Glaxo Wellcome, SmithKline Beecham, Wyeth Lederle Vaccines and Paediatrics, Merck Sharpe & Dohme, and from Glaxo Wellcome for consultancy.

INTERVENTIONS

Key Messages

- We found five treatments that were compared with placebo. Podophyllotoxin, imiquimod, and intralesional interferon have been found to be significantly more effective in the clearance of warts compared with placebo, but data on recurrence are lacking. Placebo controlled RCTs of topical interferon give conflicting results, and those of systemic interferon show no evidence of benefits.

- We found no RCTs comparing placebo with cryotherapy, electrosurgery, surgical excision, or laser surgery.

- We found no clear evidence that one treatment is superior to another.

- Topical 5-fluorouracil, and bi- and trichloroacetic acid have not been adequately evaluated.

- We found no evidence that treatment of external genital warts decreases infectivity, and the preventive effects of condoms have not been adequately evaluated.

DEFINITION	External genital warts are benign epidermal growths on the external perianal and perigenital region. There are four morphological types: condylomatous, keratotic, papular, and flat warts.
INCIDENCE/ PREVALENCE	In 1996, external and internal genital warts accounted for over 180 000 initial visits to private physicians' offices in the USA, about 60 000 fewer than were reported for 1995.[1] In the USA, 1% of sexually active men and women aged 18–49 years are estimated to have external genital warts.[2]
AETIOLOGY/ RISK FACTORS	External genital warts are caused by the human papillomavirus (HPV). Although more than 70 types of HPV have been identified, most external genital warts in immunocompetent people are caused by HPV types 6 and 11.[3,4] HPV infections and, more specifically, external genital warts are sexually transmissible.
PROGNOSIS	Clinical trials found that recurrences are frequent and may necessitate repeated treatment. Without treatment, external genital warts may remain unchanged, may increase in size or number, or may completely resolve. They rarely, if ever, progress to cancer.[5] Juvenile laryngeal papillomatosis, a rare and sometimes life threatening condition, occurs in children of women with a history of genital warts. Its rarity makes it hard to design studies that can evaluate whether treatment in pregnant women alters the risk.[6,7]
AIMS	To eliminate symptomatic warts from the external genitalia, to prevent recurrence, and to avoid sequelae, with minimal adverse effects.
OUTCOMES	Wart clearance (generally accepted as complete eradication of warts from the treated area); recurrence; sequelae; adverse effects of treatment; quality of life; transmission.
METHODS	*Clinical Evidence* search and appraisal from 1985 to May 2000. We also performed selected Medline searches for papers published before 1985. Other data came from abstract booklets, conference proceedings, references identified from bibliographies of pertinent articles and books, and manufacturers of therapeutic agents. This review is limited to systematic reviews of RCTs and subsequent RCTs, unless no RCTs were found for a particular treatment. This limitation may have biased the review in favour of newer and heavily marketed treatments.

QUESTION   What are the effects of non-surgical treatments?

OPTION   PODOPHYLLOTOXIN

RCTs have found that podophyllotoxin is more effective than placebo.

Benefits:
We found no systematic review. **Versus placebo:** Data from eight placebo controlled RCTs in a total of 1035 people found that, within 16 weeks of treatment, podophyllotoxin was more effective than placebo (wart clearance occurred in 45–77% of people on treatment; RR of clearance v placebo between 2.0, 95% CI 0.9 to 4.3,[8] and 48, 95% CI 3.0 to 773).[9–15] **Recurrence rates:** RCTs of 0.5% cream or solution found recurrence rates ranging from 4%[15] to 33%.[9] One RCT in 57 people of 0.5% podophyllotoxin solution as

prophylaxis against recurrence of external genital warts (initially treated in an open label study) found fewer recurrences among people taking placebo.[16] **Versus podophyllin:** Five RCTs compared podophyllotoxin versus podophyllin.[17–21] They found no significant difference in wart clearance (RRs for podophyllin v podophyllotoxin between 0.7, 95% CI 0.4 to 1.12 and 1.7, 95% CI 0.9 to 3.2).[20] One RCT used a 2% solution in a limited study of self treatment for penile warts and found no significant difference with podophyllotoxin versus podophyllin (RR for podophyllin v podophyllotoxin 0.6, 95% CI 0.3 to 1.3).[21]

Harms: Safety during pregnancy is unknown. Podophyllotoxin does not contain the mutagenic flavonoid compounds, quercetin and kaempherol, that are contained in podophyllin resin preparations.[22] Local inflammation or irritation, erosion, burning, pain, and itching are reported in most trials. Balanoposthitis,[23,24] dyspareunia, bleeding, scarring, and insomnia are reported rarely.[8] One large RCT reported burning and inflammation in 75% and bleeding in 25% of treated people.[12] Although rare, preputial tightening has been reported.[17]

Comment: RCTs examined the efficacy of podophyllotoxin solutions more often than cream preparations, but cream or gel preparations may be easier to apply than solutions. This and other differences may cause variable efficacy.

OPTION   IMIQUIMOD

RCTs have found that imiquimod is more effective at clearing warts than placebo.

Benefits: We found no systematic review. **Versus placebo:** We found two RCTs in a total of 968 people. Wart clearance within 3 months occurred twice as often with 1% cream as placebo (clearance rate 37–56% with imiquimod v 0–56% with placebo; RR 1.9, 95% CI 1.1 to 3).[25,26] For 5% cream, clearance was 13 times greater than with placebo (RR 13, 95% CI 4.2 to 40.2.[26] **Recurrence:** No recurrences were reported in people using 1% cream, but recurrences were reported in 13–19% of participants treated with 5% cream.[25,26] This compared to 10% among placebo treated participants in one study.[25]

Harms: One RCT reported local itching, erythema, and burning in more than 15% of people, and irritation, tenderness, ulceration, and pain in less than 10%.[26]

Comment: None.

OPTION   CRYOTHERAPY

RCTs have found that cryotherapy is as effective as podophyllin at clearing warts, trichloroacetic acid, and electrosurgery. We found no trials comparing cryotherapy with placebo. One RCT found that recurrence rates were similar after cryotherapy and electrosurgery. Cryotherapy has been used successfully in pregnancy.

Benefits: We found no systematic review. **Versus placebo:** We found no RCTs. **Versus other treatments:** We found six comparative RCTs:

two compared cryotherapy plus interferon versus cryotherapy alone;[27,28] the other four compared cryotherapy versus podophyllin,[29] trichloroacetic acid,[30,31] or electrosurgery.[29,32] **Clearance:** Four RCTs reported 63–88% clearance 3 months or more after cryotherapy.[29–32] Although one trial found cryotherapy was more effective than podophyllin after six treatments (RR of wart clearance compared with podophyllin 1.9, 95% CI 1.4 to 2.6), there was no significant difference in wart clearance 3 months after treatment (RR 1.4, 95% CI 0.9 to 2.2), suggesting merely a difference in speed of effect.[29] Two of the trials found no significant difference between cryotherapy and trichloroacetic acid at the end of treatment or 3 months later (RRs 1.1, 95% CI 0.8 to 1.5,[30] and 0.9, 95% CI 0.8 to 1.1).[31] Two trials found that electrosurgery was slightly more effective than cryotherapy (RRs of wart clearance with electrosurgery v cryotherapy at the end of treatment: 1.2, 95% CI 1.1 to 1.3, and after 3 months 1.4, 95% CI 1.0 to 2.0).[29,32] **Recurrence:** One trial found no significant difference in recurrence rates between cryotherapy and electrosurgery (21% v 22%).[29]

Harms: Discomfort, ulceration, and scabbing were reported in nearly a fifth of people after cryotherapy.[29,32] One RCT reported local infection in one of 86 people taking cryotherapy versus none of 149 people taking podophyllin resin or electrosurgery.[29]

Comment: One case series of 34 pregnant women who received three or fewer treatments of cryotherapy found no subsequent infection or premature rupture of membranes.[33]

OPTION   PODOPHYLLIN

RCTs have found that podophyllin resin is as effective as most other treatments, but is less effective than surgical excision. We found no trials comparing podophyllin with placebo.

Benefits: We found no systematic review. **Versus placebo:** We found no RCTs. **Versus other treatments:** We found 13 RCTs: four compared podophyllin versus podophyllotoxin,[17–20] one versus cryotherapy,[28] one versus electrosurgery,[29] three with and without interferon,[34–36] one with and without trichloroacetic acid,[37] two versus surgical excision,[37,38] and one compared alternative doses of podophyllin.[39] **Clearance:** None of the four trials comparing podophyllin with podophyllotoxin found a significant difference in wart clearance (RRs ranging between 0.7, 95% CI 0.4 to 1.1[18] and 1.7, 95% CI 0.9 to 3.2[20]). The trials comparing cryotherapy or electrosurgery versus podophyllin found no significant difference 3 months after treatment (RR for both comparison treatments 1.4, 95% CI 0.9 to 2.1).[29] One RCT found that podophyllin and intralesional interferon together were more effective than podophyllin alone for clearance 3 weeks after treatment (RR 2.0, 95% CI 1.1 to 3.6), however, it found no significant difference at 11 weeks (RR 2.3 95% CI 0.9 to 5.8).[35] Two RCTs found that podophyllin was less effective than surgical excision (RRs 0.3, 95% CI 0.2 to 0.7; and 0.5, 95% CI 0.2 to 0.9).[37,38] **Recurrence:** Two RCTs found that recurrence was more frequent with podophyllin versus surgical excision (60–65% v 19–29% after surgery).[37,38]

Harms: Eight RCTs reported pain, erythema, irritation, and tenderness in 3–17% of participants treated with podophyllin.[17,18,20,29,34,35,37,38] Skin burns (1–3%[37,38]), bleeding (4%[38]), and erosion or ulcerations (1%[18]–11%[34]) were also reported. Faecal incontinence (4%[38]) and preputial tightening (1%[17]) were reported rarely.

Comment: Safety during pregnancy is unknown. Podophyllin may contain the mutagenic flavonoid compounds, quercetin and kaempherol.[22]

OPTION   BI- AND TRICHLOROACETIC ACID

We found inadequate evidence to evaluate the efficacy of bi- and trichloroacetic acid.

Benefits: We found no systematic review. **Versus placebo:** We found no RCTs. **Versus other treatments:** We found two RCTs comparing trichloroacetic acid versus cryotherapy in 192 participants. These found no significant difference in wart clearance (RRs of trichloro-acetic acid v cryotherapy 1.1, 95% CI 0.8 to 1.5 and 0.9, 95% CI 0.8 to 1.1).[30,31] We also reviewed one RCT in 73 people comparing trichloroacetic acid plus podophyllin versus podophyllin alone.[40] Participants were followed for 3 months. The trial found no significant difference in wart clearance between the two groups.

Harms: Insufficient data are available to comment on possible harms.

Comment: Small numbers of participants and inadequate study designs make it difficult to evaluate effectiveness. In pregnant women, only case series are available: 31 of 32 pregnant women treated with trichloroacetic acid showed wart clearance, and 2 of 31 showed recurrence.[41] The evidence is inadequate to evaluate adverse effects of trichloroacetic acid in pregnancy.

OPTION   TOPICAL INTERFERON

Three RCTs found increased wart clearance with topical interferon versus placebo.

Benefits: We found no systematic review. **Versus placebo:** We found three RCTs in 223 men and women. Complete wart clearance 4 weeks after treatment occurred in more people using interferon versus placebo (6% v 3%, no P value given;[42] 73% v 10%, P < 0.0001;[43] 90% v 20%, no P value given[11]). About a third of each group in the first study had cleared their warts by 16 weeks.[42] Recurrence rates were not evaluated. **Versus podophyllotoxin:** One of the trials also compared topical interferon versus podophyllotoxin, and found that interferon was significantly more effective than podophyllotoxin about 4 weeks after treatment (RR compared with podophyllotoxin 1.5, 95% CI 1.03 to 1.63).[11] **As adjuvant to other treatment:** One RCT compared recombinant β interferon at two doses plus CO_2 laser versus CO_2 laser alone, electrotherapy, and liquid nitrogen. Recurrences occurred in 62% of participants (21/36) treated with 1 million IU interferon, in 54% (19/35) treated with 150 000 IU interferon, and 75% (27/36) treated with placebo.[44]

Harms: One placebo controlled study reported local burning and itching in 39% of treated people.[42] Another RCT reported fever, headache, and itching in 18% of people treated with interferon.[11]

Comment: Differences in the RCTs' findings may be attributable to the preparations used; one preparation was incorporated into a methyl cellulose aqueous base[42] and the other was instilled into a cream base.[11]

RCTs have found that intralesional injection of interferon is more effective than placebo.

Benefits: We found no systematic review. We found eight placebo controlled trials,[45–53] and one RCT comparing interferon plus podophyllin versus podophyllin alone (1000 people).[35] Doses and follow up intervals varied. Two of the placebo controlled RCTs randomised treatment to lesions rather than to people.[48,50] Complete wart clearance was reported in 17–63% of participants on intralesional interferon within 8–20 weeks of treatment. **Versus placebo:** In studies using 1 MU/ml, intralesional interferon was between twofold (95% CI 0.8 to 4.6)[49] and 3.5 fold (95% CI 1.4 to 8.8)[46] more likely to achieve complete wart clearance than placebo. One RCT found no significant difference for complete wart clearance between 1 MU/ml intralesional interferon and placebo. However, it found a twofold improvement if complete and partial responders were grouped together for analysis (RR of clearance 2.3, 95% CI 1.2 to 4.3).[53] **Added to podophyllin:** One RCT found that podophyllin and intralesional interferon together were more effective than podophyllin alone 3 weeks after treatment (RR 2.0, 95% CI 1.1 to 3.6), however, no significant difference was observed at 11 weeks (RR 2.3, 95% CI 0.9 to 5.8).[35]

Harms: Flu like symptoms (dizziness, fever, malaise, myalgia, nausea and vomiting, headache, and pain) were reported in 0–100% of participants. Eight of nine studies reported local irritation and one reported hypopigmentation among treated individuals.[53] Several studies reported a fall in white cell counts,[35,45–47,49–52] thrombocytopenia (1%),[45] and raised serum aspartate transaminase concentrations (6%)[35] in people on interferon.

Comment: None.

RCTs have found no evidence that systemic interferon is more effective than placebo, and it is associated with a range of adverse effects.

Benefits: We found no systematic review. We found 16 RCTs in 1992 men and women: six placebo controlled trials, two trials that compared systemic interferon versus podophyllin or diathermocoagulation, and eight trials that evaluated its use with one or more adjunct therapies.[27,28,54–67] **Clearance:** Fourteen of the trials reported wart clearance within 3 months of treatment in 17–67% of participants. However, four trials comparing systemic interferon with placebo found no significant difference in rates of wart clearance.[55–60] One study found that people taking systemic interferon showed greater wart clearance than placebo treated people, which was significant at 8 weeks of follow up (51% v 29%, P < 0.05), but no difference was detected 12 months after treatment.[59] **Recurrence:** Recurrence rates varied from 9–69%.[27,55,57,67]

Harms: Flu like symptoms were reported at variable frequencies; headache, fatigue and malaise, myalgia, nausea and vomiting, fever, chills, and dizziness were reported in 0.5–100% of participants on interferon.[27,28,54–62,64,65,67–69] Anaphylactic reaction occurred in 2% of participants in one RCT,[62] leukopenia in 6–28%,[57,64,65] thrombocytopenia in 3–4%,[57,65] and raised liver enzymes in 3%.[57,68] Bronchospasm and depression were rarely reported (in 1 of 97 participants for each symptom in one trial).[27]

Comment: None.

OPTION   TOPICAL 5-FLUOROURACIL

Topical 5-fluorouracil has not yet been adequately evaluated in the treatment of external genital warts.

Benefits: We found no systematic review or RCTs.

Harms: One case series of 1% solution reported minor local erosions (48%), urinary meatus erosions (5%), vulvar irritation (10%), burning (10%), and dysuria (4%).[70]

Comment: We found three case series in 224 men and women treated with 1% and 5% cream and solution preparations in various doses.[70–72] Wart clearance was reported in 10–50% of participants within 3 months of treatment. Only one study reported recurrence rates based on data from only 20 of its 49 participants; recurrences were noted in 10.[71] 5-fluorouracil has teratogenic and mutagenic properties. Safety in pregnancy is not known. Exposure to 5-fluorouracil during pregnancy has been reported rarely, with no untoward outcomes.[73,74]

QUESTION   What are the effects of surgical treatments?

OPTION   ELECTROSURGERY

Limited evidence from RCTs suggests that electrosurgery is more effective than intramuscular and subcutaneous interferon. We found no trials comparing electrosurgery with no treatment.

Benefits: We found no systematic review. **Clearance:** We found no RCTs versus no or sham treatment and found three RCTs comparing electrosurgery versus interferon, cryotherapy, or podophyllin resin in 482 men and women.[29,32,62] Complete wart clearance was reported in 61–94% of participants 3–6 weeks after treatment. Electrosurgery was more effective than intramuscular interferon (RR v intramuscular 3.3, 95% CI 1.8 to 5.9), or subcutaneous interferon (RR v subcutaneous 6.9, 95% CI 2.8 to 17.1).[62] One RCT found that electrosurgery was more effective than podophyllin resin 4 weeks after treatment (RR 2.3, 95% CI 1.7 to 3.0), but this difference ceased to be significant after 3 months (RR 1.4, 95% CI 0.9 to 2.1).[29] Two studies found that electrosurgery was slightly more effective than cryotherapy within 3–4 weeks of treatment (RRs

1.2, 95% CI 1.1 to 1.3[29]; and 1.4, 95% CI 1.0 to 2.0[32]). One of these trials followed people for 3 months, after which time this difference ceased to be significant (RR 1.0, 95% CI 0.8 to 1.2).[29]
Recurrence: One trial found recurrence in 22% of participants after electrosurgery versus 21% after cryotherapy and 44% using podophyllin resin.[29]

Harms: Pain and local irritation were reported in 17% of treated participants.[29]

Comment: None.

OPTION   SURGICAL EXCISION

RCTs have found that surgical (scissor) excision is as effective as laser surgery and more effective than podophyllin. We found no trials comparing surgical excision with no treatment.

Benefits: We found no systematic review. **Clearance:** We found no RCTs versus no treatment or sham treatment, but found three RCTs comparing surgical excision versus CO_2 laser[75] or podophyllin.[38,37] Within 1 year of treatment, complete wart clearance occurred in 35–72% of people treated with surgical excision. Two studies found that podophyllin was less effective than surgery for clearance (RRs of clearance 0.3, 95% CI 0.2 to 0.7[38]; and 0.5, 95% CI 0.2 to 0.9[37]). One trial found no significant difference in clearance between laser and conventional surgery (RR 1.2, 95% CI 0.6 to 2.4).[75] **Recurrence:** Recurrence occurred in 19–29% of excision treated participants versus 60–65% of those treated with podophyllin.[38,37] The trial comparing conventional and laser surgery found no significant difference in recurrence rates between the two treatments.[75]

Harms: All surgically treated participants experienced pain. Scar formation (9%)[75] and bleeding (37%)[38] were less frequent.

Comment: None.

OPTION   LASER SURGERY

One RCT found limited evidence of a difference in wart clearance or recurrence rates between laser and conventional surgery. We found no trials comparing laser surgery with no treatment.

Benefits: We found no systematic review. We found no RCT versus no or sham treatment, three RCTs in 285 people evaluating laser surgery plus interferon versus laser alone,[64–66] and one RCT in 50 people comparing laser surgery versus conventional surgical excision.[75] **Clearance:** Complete wart clearance was reported in 23–52% of participants within 36 months of laser surgery. This was not significantly different from clearance after conventional surgery (RR for laser v conventional surgery 1.2, 95% CI 0.6 to 2.4).[75] **Recurrence:** Recurrence was reported in 60–77% of participants after laser surgery.[64,66,75] This did not differ significantly from recurrence rates with conventional surgery.[75]

Harms: The RCT comparing laser with conventional surgery found no significant difference in the rate of local scar formation (28% after laser surgery v 9% after conventional surgery, $P > 0.2$).[75] Post-operative pain was reported equally in both groups.

Comment: We found two case series of laser surgery, which included 47 pregnant women.[41,76] These reported premature rupture of membranes in 2 of 32 women, prolonged rupture of membranes in 1 of 32, the need for postoperative suprapubic catheterisation in 7 of 32, pyelonephritis in 1 of 32, prolonged healing time in 1 of 52, and rectal perforation with secondary abscess in 1 of 52.

QUESTION	Does treatment of external genital warts or the use of barrier contraceptives prevent transmission of HPV?

We found insufficient evidence about barrier contraceptives or treatment of external genital warts to prevent transmission of human papillomavirus (HPV).

Benefits: We found no controlled studies about the effects of barrier contraceptives or treatment of external genital warts on the rate of transmitting HIV.

Harms: None reported.

Comment: Penetrative intercourse may not be required for transmission of HPV infection, and it is unclear whether sexual contact with any infected and uninfected perigenital tissues is sufficient to cause external genital warts.

REFERENCES

1. US Department of Health and Human Services, Public Health Service. Division of STD Prevention. *Sexually transmitted disease surveillance*. Atlanta: Centers for Disease Control and Prevention, 1996.
2. Koutsky LA, Galloway DA, Holmes KK. Epidemiology of genital human papillomavirus infection. *Epidemiol Rev* 1988;10:122–163.
3. Gissmann L, zur Hausen H. Partial characterization of viral DNA from human genital warts (condylomata acuminata). *Int J Cancer* 1980;25:605–609.
4. Gissmann L, Boshart M, Durst M, Ikenberg H, Wagner D, zur Hausen H. Presence of human papillomavirus in genital tumors. *J Invest Dermatol* 1984;83(suppl 1):26–28.
5. IARC Working Group on Evaluation of Carcinogenic Risks to Humans. *IARC monographs on the evaluation of carcinogenic risks to humans: human papillomaviruses*. Lyon, France: World Health Organization, International Agency for Research on Cancer, 1995.
6. Bonnez W, Kashima HK, Leventhal B, et al. Antibody response to human papillomavirus (HPV) type 11 in children with juvenile-onset recurrent respiratory papillomatosis (RRP). *Virology* 1992; 188:384–387.
7. Hallden C, Majmudar B. The relationship between juvenile laryngeal papillomatosis and maternal condylomata acuminata. *J Reprod Med* 1986;31:804–807.
8. Greenberg MD, Rutledge LH, Reid R, Berman NR, Precop SL, Elswick RK, Jr. A double-blind, randomized trial of 0.5% podofilox and placebo for the treatment of genital warts in women. *Obstet Gynecol* 1991;77:735–739.
9. Beutner KR, Conant MA, Friedman-Kien AE, et al. Patient-applied podofilox for treatment of genital warts. *Lancet* 1989;i:831–834.
10. Kirby P, Dunne King D, Corey L. Double-blind randomized clinical trial of self-administered podofilox solution versus vehicle in the treatment of genital warts. *Am J Med* 1990;88:465–469.
11. Syed TA, Khayyami M, Kriz D, et al. Management of genital warts in women with human leukocyte interferon-α vs podophyllotoxin in cream: a placebo-controlled, double-blind, comparative study. *J Mol Med* 1995;73:255–258.
12. Tyring S, Edwards L, Cherry LK, et al. Safety and efficacy of 0.5% podofilox gel in the treatment of anogenital warts. *Arch Dermatol* 1998;134:33–38.
13. Von Krogh G, Hellberg D. Self-treatment using a 0.5% podophyllotoxin cream of external genital condylomata acuminata in women. A placebo-controlled, double-blind study. *Sex Transm Dis* 1992;19:170–174.
14. Von Krogh G, Szpak E, Andersson M, Bergelin I. Self-treatment using 0.25%–0.50% podophyllotoxin-ethanol solutions against penile condylomata acuminata: a placebo-controlled comparative study. *Genitourin Med* 1994;70:105–109.
15. Syed TA, Lundin S, Ahmad SA. Topical 0.3% and 0.5% podophyllotoxin cream for self-treatment of condyloma acuminata in women: a placebo-controlled, double-blind study. *Dermatology* 1994; 189:142–145.
16. Bonnez W, Elswick RK, Jr, Bailey-Farchione A, et al. Efficacy and safety of 0.5% podofilox solution in the treatment and suppression of anogenital warts. *Am J Med* 1994;96:420–425.
17. Edwards A, Atma-Ram A, Thin RN. Podophyllotoxin 0.5% v podophyllin 20% to treat penile warts. *Genitourin Med* 1988;64:263–265.
18. Hellberg D, Svarrer T, Nilsson S, Valentin J. Self-treatment of female external genital warts with

0.5% podophyllotoxin cream (Condyline) vs weekly applications of 20% podophyllin solution. *Int J STD AIDS* 1995;6:257–261.

19. Kinghorn GR, McMillan A, Mulcahy F, Drake S, Lacey C, Bingham JS. An open, comparative, study of the efficacy of 0.5% podophyllotoxin lotion and 25% podophyllotoxin solution in the treatment of condylomata acuminata in males and females. *Int J STD AIDS* 1993;4:194–199.

20. Lassus A, Haukka K, Forsstrom S. Podophyllotoxin for treatment of genital warts in males: a comparison with conventional podophyllin therapy. *Eur J Sex Transm Dis* 1984;2:31–33.

21. White, DJ, Billingham C, Chapman S, et al. Podophyllin 0.5% or 2.0% v podophyllotoxin 0.5% for self treatment of penile warts: a double blind randomised study. *Genitourin Med* 1997;73:184–187.

22. Petersen CS, Weismann K. Quercetin and kaempferol: an argument against the use of podophyllin? *Genitourin Med* 1995;71:92–93.

23. Von Krogh G. Topical self-treatment of penile warts with 0.5% podophyllotoxin in ethanol for four or five days. *Sex Transm Dis* 1987;14:135–140.

24. Von Krogh G. Penile condylomata acuminata: an experimental model for evaluation of topical self-treatment with 0.5–1.0% ethanolic preparations of podophyllotoxin for three days. *Sex Transm Dis* 1981;8:179–186.

25. Edwards L, Ferenczy A, Eron L, et al. Self-administered topical 5% imiquimod cream for external anogenital warts. *Arch Dermatol* 1998;134:25–30.

26. Beutner KR, Spruance SL, Hougham AJ, Fox TL, Owens ML, Douglas JM, Jr. Treatment of genital warts with an immune-response modifier (imiquimod). *J Am Acad Dermatol* 1998;38(2 pt 1):230–239.

27. Eron LJ, Alder MB, O'Rourke JM, Rittweger K, DePamphilis J, Pizzuti DJ. Recurrence of condylomata acuminata following cryotherapy is not prevented by systemically administered interferon. *Genitourin Med* 1993;69:91–93.

28. Handley JM, Horner T, Maw RD, Lawther H, Dinsmore WW. Subcutaneous interferon α 2a combined with cryotherapy vs cryotherapy alone in the treatment of primary anogenital warts: a randomised observer blind placebo controlled study. *Genitourin Med* 1991;67:297–302.

29. Stone KM, Becker TM, Hadgu A, Kraus SJ. Treatment of external genital warts: a randomised clinical trial comparing podophyllin, cryotherapy, and electrodesiccation. *Genitourin Med* 1990;66:16–19.

30. Abdullah AN, Walzman M, Wade A. Treatment of external genital warts comparing cryotherapy (liquid nitrogen) and trichloroacetic acid. *Sex Transm Dis* 1993;20:344–345.

31. Godley MJ, Bradbeer CS, Gellan M, Thin RN. Cryotherapy compared with trichloroacetic acid in treating genital warts. *Genitourin Med* 1987;63:390–392.

32. Simmons PD, Langlet F, Thin RN. Cryotherapy versus electrocautery in the treatment of genital warts. *Br J Venereal Dis* 1981;57:273–274.

33. Bergman A, Bhatia NN, Broen EM. Cryotherapy for treatment of genital condylomata during pregnancy. *J Reprod Med* 1984;29:432–435.

34. Condylomata International Collaborative Study Group. A comparison of interferon alfa-2a and podophyllin in the treatment of primary condylomata acuminata. *Genitourin Med* 1991;67:394–399.

35. Douglas JM Jr, Eron LJ, Judson FN, et al. A randomized trial of combination therapy with intralesional interferon α 2b and podophyllin versus podophyllin alone for the therapy of anogenital warts. *J Infect Dis* 1990;162:52–59.

36. Potkul RK, Lancaster WD, Kurman RJ, Lewandowski G, Weck PK, Delgado G. Vulvar condylomas and squamous vestibular micropapilloma. Differences in appearance and response to treatment. *J Reprod Med* 1990;35:1019–1022.

37. Khawaja HT. Podophyllin versus scissor excision in the treatment of perianal condylomata acuminata: a prospective study. *Br J Surg* 1989;76:1067–1068.

38. Jensen SL. Comparison of podophyllin application with simple surgical excision in clearance and recurrence of perianal condylomata acuminata. *Lancet* 1985;2:1146–1148.

39. Simmons PD. Podophyllin 10% and 25% in the treatment of ano-genital warts: a comparative double-blind study. *Br J Venereal Dis* 1981;57:208–209.

40. Gabriel G, Thin RN. Treatment of anogenital warts. Comparison of trichloroacetic acid and podophyllin versus podophyllin alone. *Br J Venereal Dis* 1983;59:124–126.

41. Schwartz DB, Greenberg MD, Daoud Y, Reid R. Genital condylomas in pregnancy: use of trichloroacetic acid and laser therapy. *Am J Obstet Gynecol* 1988;158(6 pt 1):1407–1416.

42. Keay S, Teng N, Eisenberg M, Story B, Sellers PW, Merigan TC. Topical interferon for treating condyloma acuminata in women. *J Infect Dis* 1988;158:934–939.

43. Syed TA, Ahmadpour OA: Human leukocyte derived interferon-α in a hydrophilic gel for the treatment of intravaginal warts in women: a placebo-controlled, double-blind study. *Int J STD AIDS* 1998;9:769–772.

44. Gross G, Rogozinski T, Schofer H, et al. Recombinant interferon β gel as an adjuvant in the treatment of recurrent genital warts: results of a placebo-controlled double blind study of 120 patients. *Dermatology* 1998;196:330–334.

45. Eron LJ, Judson F, Tucker S, et al. Interferon therapy for condyloma acuminata. *N Engl J Med* 1986;315:1059–1064.

46. Friedman-Kien AE, Eron LJ, Conant M, et al. Natural interferon alfa for treatment of condylomata acuminata. *JAMA* 1988;259:533–538.

47. Friedman-Kien A. Management of condyloma acuminata with Alferon N injection, interferon alfa-n3 (human leukocyte derived). *Am J Obstet Gynecol* 1995;172(4 pt 2):1359–1368.

48. Monsonego J, Cessot G, Ince SE, Galazka AR, Abdul-Ahad AK. Randomised double-blind trial of recombinant interferon-β for condyloma acuminatum. *Genitourin Med* 1996;72:111–114.

49. Reichman RC, Oakes D, Bonnez W, et al. Treatment of condyloma acuminatum with three different interferons administered intralesionally: a double-blind, placebo-controlled trial. *Ann Intern Med* 1988;108:675–679.

50. Scott GM, Csonka GW. Effect of injections of small doses of human fibroblast interferon into genital warts: a pilot study. *Br J Venereal Dis* 1979;55:442–445.

51. Vance JC, Bart BJ, Hansen RC, et al. Intralesional recombinant α-2 interferon for the treatment of patients with condyloma acuminatum or verruca plantaris. *Arch Dermatol* 1986;122:272–277.

52. Welander CE, Homesley HD, Smiles KA, Peets EA. Intralesional interferon alfa-2b for the treatment of genital warts. *Am J Obstet Gynecol* 1990;162:348–354.

53. Bornstein J, Pascal B, Zarfati D, et al. Recombinant human interferon-β for condyloma acuminata: a randomized, double-blind, placebo

controlled study of intralesional therapy. *Int J STD AIDS* 1997;8:614–621.

54. Armstrong DK, Maw RD, Dinsmore WW, et al. A randomised, double-blind, parallel group study to compare subcutaneous interferon α-2a plus podophyllin with placebo plus podophyllin in the treatment of primary condylomata acuminata. *Genitourin Med* 1994;70:389–393.

55. Armstrong DK, Maw RD, Dinsmore WW, et al. Combined therapy trial with interferon α-2a and ablative therapy in the treatment of anogenital warts. *Genitourin Med* 1996;72:103–107.

56. Condylomata International Collaborative Study Group. Recurrent condylomata acuminata treated with recombinant interferon alfa-2a: a multicenter double-blind placebo-controlled clinical trial. *JAMA* 1991;265:2684–2687.

57. Condylomata International Collaborative Study Group. Recurrent condylomata acuminata treated with recombinant interferon α-2a: a multicenter double-blind placebo-controlled clinical trial. *Acta Derm Venereol* 1993;73:223–226.

58. Gall SA, Constantine L, Koukol D. Therapy of persistent human papillomavirus disease with two different interferon species. *Am J Obstet Gynecol* 1991;164(1 pt 1):130–134.

59. Olmos L, Vilata J, Rodriguez Pichardo A, Lloret A, Ojeda A, Calderon MD. Double-blind, randomized clinical trial on the effect of interferon-β in the treatment of condylomata acuminata. *Int J STD AIDS* 1994;5:182–185.

60. Reichman RC, Oakes D, Bonnez W, et al. Treatment of condyloma acuminatum with three different interferon-α preparations administered parenterally: a double-blind, placebo-controlled trial. *J Infect Dis* 1990;162:1270–1276.

61. Condylomata International Collaborative Study Group. A comparison of interferon alfa-2a and podophyllin in the treatment of primary condylomata acuminata. *Genitourin Med* 1991;67:394–399.

62. Benedetti Panici P, Scambia G, Baiocchi G, Perrone L, Pintus C, Mancuso S. Randomized clinical trial comparing systemic interferon with diathermocoagulation in primary multiple and widespread anogenital condyloma. *Obstet Gynecol* 1989;74(3 pt 1):393–397.

63. Bonnez W, Oakes D, Bailey-Farchione A, et al. A randomized, double-blind, placebo-controlled trial of systemically administered interferon-α, -β, or -γ in combination with cryotherapy for the treatment of condyloma acuminatum. *J Infect Dis* 1995; 171:1081–1089.

64. Condylomata International Collaborative Study Group. Randomized placebo-controlled double-blind combined therapy with laser surgery and systemic interferon-α 2a in the treatment of anogenital condylomata acuminatum. *J Infect Dis* 1993;167:824–829.

65. Petersen C, Bjerring P, Larson J, et al. Systemic interferon α-2b increases the cure rate in laser treated patients with multiple persistent genital warts: a placebo-controlled study. *Genitourin Med* 1991;67:99–102.

66. Reid R, Greenberg MD, Pizzuti DJ, Omoto KH, Rutledge LH, Soo W. Superficial laser vulvectomy. V. Surgical debulking is enhanced by adjuvant systemic interferon. *Am J Obstet Gynecol* 1992; 166:815–820.

67. Bonnez W, Oakes D, Bailey-Farchione A, et al. A randomized, double blind trial of parenteral low dose versus high dose interferon β in combination with cryotherapy for treatment of condyulomata acuminatum. *Antiviral Res* 1997;35:41–52.

68. Kirby PK, Kiviat N, Beckman A, Wells D, Sherwin S, Corey L. Tolerance and efficacy of recombinant human interferon γ in the treatment of refractory genital warts. *Am J Med* 1988;85:183–188.

69. Reichman RC, Micha JP, Weck PK, et al. Interferon α-n1 (Wellferon) for refractory genital warts: efficacy and tolerance of low dose systemic therapy. *Antiviral Res* 1988;10(1–3):41–57.

70. Von Krogh G. The beneficial effect of 1% 5-fluorouracil in 70% ethanol on therapeutically refractory condylomas in the preputial cavity. *Sex Transm Dis* 1978;5:137–140.

71. Krebs H. Treatment of extensive vulvar condylomata acuminata with topical 5-fluorouracil. *South Med J* 1990;83:761–764.

72. Haye KR. Treatment of condyloma acuminata with 5 per cent 5-fluorouracil (5-FU) cream [letter]. *Br J Vener Dis* 1974;50:466.

73. Dreicer R, Love RR. High total dose 5-fluorouracil treatment during pregnancy. *Wis Med J* 1991;90: 582–583.

74. Van Le L, Pizzuti DJ, Greenberg M, Reid R. Accidental use of low-dose 5-fluorouracil in pregnancy. *J Reprod Med* 1991;36:872–874.

75. Duus BR, Philipsen T, Christensen JD, Lundvall F, Sondergaard J. Refractory condylomata acuminata: a controlled clinical trial of carbon dioxide laser versus conventional surgical treatment. *Genitourin Med* 1985;61:59–61.

76. Kryger-Baggesen N, Falck Larsen J, Hjortkjaer Pedersen P. CO_2 laser treatment of condylomata acuminata. *Acta Obstet Gynecol Scand* 1984;63: 341–343.

DJ Wiley
Assistant Professor in Residence
School of Nursing, Primary Care
University of California
Los Angeles, California
USA

Karl Beutner
Associate Clinical Professor
Department of Dermatology University
of California
San Francisco, California
USA

Competing interests: KB has been reimbursed for speaking at symposia, paid a fee for speaking and organising education, performing clinical trials, and consulting by Oclassem Dermatologics, a division of Watson Pharmaceuticals, 3M Pharmaceuticals, Epitome Pharmaceuticals, Matrix Pharmaceuticals, Puntose Pharmaceuticals, and ISIS Pharmaceuticals. DJW has been a consultant to 3M Pharmaceuticals and has received research funding from Merck and Co.

Gonorrhoea

Search date January 2001

John Moran

INTERVENTIONS

Beneficial
Single dose regimens using selected fluoroquinolones, selected cephalosporins, or spectinomycin in uncomplicated infection 1112
Single dose regimens using selected cephalosporins or spectinomycin in uncomplicated infection in pregnant women 1113

Likely to be beneficial
Selected injectable fluoroquinolones or selected injectable cephalosporins in disseminated infection* . . .1113

Unknown effectiveness
Dual treatment for gonorrhoea and chlamydia infections in all people diagnosed with gonorrhoea 1114

*Based only on non-RCT evidence and consensus.

Key Messages

- One systematic review of RCTs in people with uncomplicated gonococcal infection has found that single drug regimens using selected fluoroquinolones, selected cephalosporins, or spectinomycin are highly effective and safe. Resistance to penicillins, sulphonamides, and tetracyclines is now widespread.
- We found little evidence on treatment in pregnant women. Two RCTs found that antibiotics were effective in pregnant women. We found no reports of serious adverse effects.
- We found no recent trials evaluating treatments for disseminated gonococcal infection, but found no reports of treatment failures.
- Dual treatment for gonorrhoea and chlamydia infections is based on theory and expert opinion rather than on evidence from clinical trials. The balance between benefits and harms varies with the prevalence of co-infection in each population.

DEFINITION

Gonorrhoea is caused by infection with *Neisseria gonorrhoeae*. In men, uncomplicated urethritis is the most common manifestation, with dysuria and urethral discharge. Less typically, signs and symptoms are mild and indistinguishable from chlamydial urethritis. In women, the most common manifestation is cervicitis, which produces symptoms (e.g. vaginal discharge, lower abdominal discomfort, and dyspareunia) in only half of cases. Co-infection with chlamydia is reported in 20–40% of people.[1]

INCIDENCE/ PREVALENCE

Between 1975 and 1997, the incidence of reported gonorrhoea in the USA fell by 74%, reaching a level in 1997 of 122 of 100 000 people; since then it has increased by 9% to 133 of 100 000 people.[2] In the UK, diagnoses of gonorrhoea have increased since 1994, reaching 39 of 100 000 males and 17 of 100 000 females in 1999.[3] In poor communities, rates may be higher: the estimated incidence in people aged 15–59 years living in three inner London boroughs in 1994–1995 was 138 of 100 000 women and 292 of 100 000 men.[4] Rates are highest in younger people. In the USA in 1999, incidence was highest in women aged 15–19 years (738/ 100 000) and men aged 20–24 years (585/100 000).[2]

AETIOLOGY/ RISK FACTORS

Most infections result from penile-vaginal, penile-rectal, or penile-pharyngeal contact. An important minority of infections are transmitted from mother to child during birth, which can cause ophthalmia neonatorum. Less common are ocular infections in older children and adults as a result of sexual exposure, poor hygiene, or the medicinal use of urine.

PROGNOSIS

The natural history of untreated gonococcal infection is spontaneous resolution after weeks or months of unpleasant symptoms. During this time, there is a substantial likelihood of transmission to others and of complications developing in the infected individual.[5] Symptoms in most men are severe enough to cause them to seek treatment, but an estimated 1–3% of infected men remain asymptomatic. These men, and men who are infectious but not yet symptomatic, are largely responsible for spread of the disease. In many women, the lack of readily discernible signs or symptoms of cervicitis means that infections go unrecognised and untreated. An unknown proportion of untreated infections causes local complications, including lymphangitis, periurethral abscess, bartholinitis, and urethral stricture; epididymitis in men; and in women involvement of the uterus, fallopian tubes, or ovaries causing pelvic inflammatory disease (see pelvic inflammatory disease, p 1123). It is the association of gonorrhoea with pelvic inflammatory disease — a major cause of secondary infertility, ectopic pregnancy, and chronic pelvic pain — that makes gonorrhoea an important public health issue. Manifestations of disseminated infection are petechial or pustular skin lesions; asymmetrical arthropathies, tenosynovitis or septic arthritis; and, rarely, meningitis or endocarditis.

AIMS

To relieve symptoms; avoid complications; and prevent further transmission, with minimal adverse effects of treatment.

OUTCOMES

Microbiological cure rates (number of infected people or infected sites culture negative 1–14 days after treatment, divided by number of infected people or infected sites cultured 1–14 days after treatment).

METHODS *Clinical Evidence* update search and appraisal January 2001. Key words: gonorrhoea and *N gonorrhoeae* infections, plus search of references of key articles and books. Studies were excluded if they defined possible treatment failures as "reinfections", if they did not use end points based on microbiological cure, or if they were based on drug regimens unlikely to be of general use (e.g. those using antibiotic regimens that are toxic, or to which resistance is now widespread).[6]

> **QUESTION** What are the effects of treatments for uncomplicated infections in men and non-pregnant women?

One systematic review has found that modern antimicrobial agents other than penicillin and tetracycline achieve cure rates of 97% or higher. Cure rates are lower (≤ 80%) for pharyngeal infection. Most regimens cause few adverse effects. Resistance is now widespread to penicillins, tetracyclines, and sulphonamides.

Benefits: **Uncomplicated urogenital, rectal, and pharyngeal infections:** We found one systematic review (search date 1993). It identified studies published from 1981 to 1993 that used a single dose regimen based on an antimicrobial other than a β lactamase sensitive penicillin or a tetracycline.[6] The data comprised 24 383 evaluable people or infections, of which 96.7% were cured on the basis of culture results. Sites of infection, when specified, included the cervix, urethra, rectum, and pharynx. Comparison of cure rates by site of infection found that cure rates were over 95% for all sites except the pharynx, for which they were about 80% (see table 1, p 1116).[7] **Eye infections:** We found no systematic review or RCTs. the only recent published study of the treatment of gonococcal conjunctivitis, all 12 participants responded well to a single 1 g dose of ceftriaxone.[8]

Harms: Single dose regimens using fluoroquinolones, third generation and extended spectrum cephalosporins, or spectinomycin are generally safe and well tolerated. The most important adverse effects are rare hypersensitivity reactions. Minor adverse effects are most troublesome for the 800 mg cefixime regimen,[9,10] and the 2 g azithromycin regimen;[11] both cause frequent gastrointestinal upset. All the other doses found effective are associated with a low incidence of adverse outcomes. The ceftriaxone and spectinomycin regimens require intramuscular injection. One large observational cohort study of azithromycin, cefixime, ciprofloxacin, and ofloxacin "in everyday use" found few serious adverse effects.[12] Quinolones may cause arthropathy in animals. No evidence of joint toxicity has been observed in clinical use, even with prolonged, multiple dose regimens used for the management of children with cystic fibrosis.[13–17] Resistance is now widespread for all penicillins, sulphonamides, and tetracyclines, but has not been reported widely for fluoroquinolones, third generation and extended spectrum cephalosporins, or spectinomycin (see table 2, p 1116).

Comment: There is good agreement between antigonococcal activity of antimicrobials *in vitro* and their efficacy in clinical trials. The large number of people evaluated in a range of settings means the results can be generalised. Single dose regimens may make adherence more likely.

What are the effects of treatments for uncomplicated infections in pregnant women?

Two RCTs found that antibiotic treatment in pregnancy was effective. We found no reports of serious adverse effects.

Benefits: We found one systematic review (2 RCTs, 1 fully published, 329 women)[18] addressing treatments of gonococcal infection during pregnancy. One of the RCTs (267 pregnant women with positive cultures for gonorrhoea) compared amoxicillin with probenecid, spectinomycin, and ceftriaxone regimens. Eradication rates ranged from 89% to 97%. Single dose ceftriaxone 250 mg cured 95.2% (95% CI 89.2% to 98.5%) of rectal and cervical infections and 100% (95% CI 54.1% to 100%) of pharyngeal infections; spectinomycin 2 g cured 97.0% (95% CI 91.5% to 99.4%) of rectal and cervical infections and 83.3% (95% CI 35.9% to 99.6%) of pharyngeal infections. The second RCT (62 women with endocervical gonorrhoea) compared ceftriaxone intramuscularly versus cefixime orally. It found that eradication rates were similar in the two groups (AR 28/30 [93%] with ceftriaxone 125 mg v 31/32 [97%] with cefixime 400 mg; RR 2.1, 95% CI 0.2 to 14).[18]

Harms: The systematic review reported vomiting after treatment in only one of the 267 women included in one trial.[18] Little information on other adverse effects was available. Because quinolones cause arthropathy in animals, their use is not recommended in pregnancy, although we found no reports of adverse effects of quinolones on pregnancy outcome in humans. A single, multicentre, prospective, controlled study of 200 exposed women found no evidence of adverse effects.[19] We found no evidence that the non-quinolone regimens listed above are less safe or less well tolerated by pregnant women than by men or non-pregnant women.

Comment: None.

What are the effects of treatments for disseminated gonococcal infection?

We found no recent trials evaluating treatment for disseminated gonococcal infection. However, we found no reports of treatment failure.

Benefits: We found no systematic review and no studies of the treatment of disseminated gonococcal infection published in the last 10 years.

Harms: We found no reports of adverse effects of these drugs in this context.

Comment: More than a hundred clinical trials involving over 20 000 people have found that many single dose antimicrobial regimens cure uncomplicated infections more than 90% of the time.[6] Given the protracted natural history without treatment, this evidence suggests that treatment with these antimicrobial regimens is beneficial. Which regimens are most beneficial cannot be determined precisely because placebo controlled RCTs have not been performed. However, analysis of available trials supports the consensus that the most effective regimens are those using selected third generation or expanded spectrum cephalosporins and, except where resistance is common, those using selected fluoroquinolones or spectinomycin. We found no RCTs of antibiotic treatment in complicated gonorrhoea, but there is a strong consensus supporting the view that the most effective treatments for these conditions are multidose regimens using injectable cephalosporins or quinolones. Although we found no published data establishing the efficacy of this treatment, we found no reports of treatment failures.

QUESTION **What are the effects of dual treatment for gonorrhoea and chlamydia infection?**

Dual treatment with an antimicrobial effective against *Chlamydia trachomatis* is based on theory and expert opinion rather than evidence. The balance between benefits and harms from controlled trials will vary with the prevalence of co-infection in each population.

Benefits: We found no systematic review or RCTs.

Harms: We found no good evidence on the harms of dual treatment. Treatment for chlamydia can cause mild gastrointestinal distress, and there is the possibility that using a second drug could stimulate the emergence or spread of resistance in *Neisseria* or other bacteria.

Comment: Routine dual treatment has been advocated and implemented for the last 10 years, and is believed to have two potential benefits. First, it is believed by some to have contributed to the decline in the prevalence of chlamydia infection observed in some populations. We found no evidence for any direct effect of dual treatment on chlamydia prevalence. Other factors may have contributed to reduced chlamydia prevalence (including widespread screening for asymptomatic chlamydia infection and changes in sexual behaviour), making it difficult to attribute decreases in the prevalence of chlamydia infection to any specific cause. Secondly, routine dual treatment may retard the spread of resistant gonococcal strains. Limited data from case reports support this belief. In the past, chlamydia testing was often unavailable, expensive, time consuming, and not highly sensitive, whereas dual treatment with a tetracycline, such as doxycycline, was safe and inexpensive. Chlamydia testing has now become more widely available, more affordable, quicker, and more sensitive, and the prevalence of chlamydia has fallen in some populations. Nevertheless, chlamydia is still found in 20–40% of people with gonorrhoea in many clinics.[1]

REFERENCES

1. Centers for Disease Control and Prevention. 1998 Guidelines for the treatment of sexually transmitted diseases. *Morb Mortal Wkly Rep* 1998;47(RR-1):60.

2. Division of STD Prevention, Centers for Disease Control and Prevention, Sexually transmitted diseases surveillance, 1999. Atlanta: US Department of Health and Human Services. 2000. http://www.cdc.gov/nchstp/dstd/Stats_trends/1999SurvRpt.htm

3. PHLS, DHSS and PS, Scottish ISD(D)5 Collaborative Group. Trends in sexually transmitted infections in the United Kingdom, 1990 to 1999. London: Public Health Laboratory Service, 2000. http://www.phls.co.uk/facts/STI/sti.htm

4. Low N, Daker-White G, Barlow D, Pozniak AI. Gonorrhoea in inner London: results of a cross-sectional study. *BMJ* 1997;314:1719–1723.

5. Hook EW, Handsfield HH. Gonococcal infections in the adult. In: Holmes KK, Mardh P-A, Sparling PF, et al, eds. *Sexually Transmitted Diseases* 3rd ed. New York: McGraw-Hill, 1999.

6. Moran JS, Levine WC. Drugs of choice for the treatment of uncomplicated gonococcal infections. *Clin Infect Dis* 1995;20(suppl 1):47–65. Search date 1993; primary sources Medline 1981–1993; reference lists from retrieved articles; abstracts from the annual Interscience Conference on Antimicrobial Agents and Chemotherapy and the meeting of the International Society for Sexually

Transmitted Disease Research 1990–1993.

7. Moran JS. Treating uncomplicated *Neisseria gonorrhoeae* infections: is the anatomic site of infection important? *Sex Transm Dis* 1995;22:39–47.

8. Haimovici R, Roussel TJ. Treatment of gonococcal conjunctivitis with single-dose intramuscular ceftriaxone. *Am J Ophthalmol* 1989;107:511–514.

9. Handsfield HH, McCormack WM, Hook EW III, et al. The Gonorrhea Treatment Study Group. A comparison of single-dose cefixime with ceftriaxone as treatment for uncomplicated gonorrhea. *N Engl J Med* 1991;325:1337–1341.

10. Megran DW, LeFebvre K, Willets V, Bowie WR. Single-dose oral cefixime versus amoxicillin plus probenecid for the treatment of uncomplicated gonorrhea in men. *Antimicrob Agents Chemother* 1990;34:355–357.

11. Handsfield HH, Dalu ZA, Martin DH, et al. Azithromycin Gonorrhea Study Group. Multicenter trial of single-dose azithromycin vs. ceftriaxone in the treatment of uncomplicated gonorrhea. *Sex Transm Dis* 1994;21:107–111.

12. Wilton LV, Pearce GL, Mann RD. A comparison of ciprofloxacin, norfloxacin, ofloxacin, azithromycin and cefixime examined by observational cohort studies. *Br J Clin Pharmacol* 1996;41:277–284.

13. Green SD. Indications and restrictions of fluoroquinolone use in children. *Br J Hosp Med* 1996;56:420–423.

14. Grenier B. Use of fluoroquinolones in children. An overview. *Adv Antimicr Antineopl Chemother* 1992;11–2:135–140.

15. Schaad UB. Use of quinolones in children and articular risk. *Arch Pediatr* 1996;3:183–184.

16. Hampel B, Hullmann R, Schmidt H. Ciprofloxacin in pediatrics: worldwide clinical experience based on compassionate use. Safety report. *Pediatr Infect Dis J* 1997;16:127–129.

17. Warren RW. Rheumatologic aspects of pediatric cystic fibrosis patients treated with fluoroquinolones. *Pediatr Infect Dis J* 1997;16:118–122.

18. Brocklehurst P. Interventions for treating gonorrhoea in pregnancy (Cochrane Review). In: The Cochrane Library, Issue 1, 2001. Oxford: Update Software. Search date 1998; primary sources Cochrane Pregnancy and Childbirth Group Register, Cochrane Controlled Trials register.

19. Loebstein R, Addis A, Ho E, et al. Pregnancy outcome following gestational exposure to fluoroquinolones: a multicenter prospective controlled study. *Antimicrob Agents Chemother* 1998;42:1336–1339.

20. Ye SZ. Survey on antibiotic sensitivity of Neisseria gonorrhoeae strains isolated in China, 1987–1992. *Sex Transm Dis* 1994;21:237–240.

21. Guoming L, Qun C, Shengchun W. Resistance of Neisseria gonorrhoeae epidemic strains to antibiotics: report of resistant isolates and surveillance in Zhanjiang, China: 1998–1999. *Sex Transm Dis* 2000;27:115–118.

22. The WHO Western Pacific Region Gonococcal Antimicrobial Surveillance Programme. Surveillance of antibiotic resistance in Neisseria gonorrhoeae in the WHO Western Pacific Region, 1999. *Commun Dis Intell* 2000;24:269–271.

23. Forsyth A, Moyes A, Young H. Increased ciprofloxacin resistance in gonococci isolated in Scotland. *Lancet* 2000;356:1984–1985.

John Moran
Medical Epidemiologist
Centers for Disease
Control and Prevention
Atlanta
USA

Competing interests: None declared.

TABLE 1 Effectiveness of selected single-dose regimens in published clinical trials[6] and updated to 2000 (see text, p 1112).

Drug and dose	Pharyngeal infections		Urogenital and rectal infections	
	% cured	95% CI	% cured	95% CI
Ceftriaxone 250 mg	98.8	94.2 to 100	99.2	98.8 to 99.5
Ciprofloxacin 500 mg	97.2	85.5 to 100	99.8	98.7 to 100
Ceftriaxone 125 mg	93.7	84.5 to 98.2	99.1	98.7 to 99.8
Ciprofloxacin 250 mg	89.0	82.3 to 95.8	99.2	98.6 to 99.8
Spectinomycin 2 g	51.8	38.7 to 64.9	98.2	97.6 to 99.0
Azithromycin 2 g	100	82.3 to 100	99.2	97.3 to 99.9
Ofloxacin 400 mg	88.0	68.8 to 97.5	98.4	97.2 to 99.8
Cefixime 800 mg	80.0	51.9 to 95.7	98.4	95.9 to 99.6
Cefixime 400 mg	100	63.1 to 100	97.4	96.0 to 98.8

Data have been updated to include those from eligible studies published between 1993 and 2000. Only those regimens that are available in the USA and have been shown in published studies to cure more than 95% of uncomplicated urogenital and rectal infections (with a lower 95% confidence limit > 95%) have been selected.

TABLE 2 Reported resistance of N gonorrhoeae to antimicrobials (see text, p 1112).

Drug	Resistance
Sulphonamides	Widespread
Penicillins	Widespread
Tetracyclines	Widespread
Third generation cephalosporins (e.g. ceftriaxone, cefixime)	Two reports from China[20,21]
Spectinomycin	Rare
Quinolones	Parts of Asia: common[22] USA: in 1999, resistance to ciprofloxacin was reported in 0.2% of isolates from the mainland and in 14% of isolates from Hawaii[2] UK: rare reports of imported fluoroquinolone resistant N gonorrhoeae[23] Australia, New Zealand, and Pacific Islands: 0–14%[22]

Search date November 2000

Catherine Mathews, Nicol Coetzee, Merrick Zwarenstein and Sally Guttmacher

QUESTIONS

Effects of different partner notification strategies in different groups of people.....................................1118

How to improve the effectiveness of patient referral...........1121

Effects of allowing people to choose type of partner notification . . .1122

INTERVENTIONS

Likely to be beneficial

Provider referral (versus patient referral in some sexually transmitted diseases).....1118

Contract referral (as effective as provider referral in people with syphilis) 1120

Adding telephone reminders and contact cards to patient referral 1121

Unknown effectiveness

Patient referral 1118

Contract referral (in sexually transmitted diseases other than syphilis) 1119,1120

Outreach assistance 1121

Educational videos 1121

Different types of healthcare professionals...........1121

Allowing patient choice 1122

See glossary, p 1122

Key Messages

- We found limited evidence on acceptability of different strategies of partner notification.

- We found no good evidence on the effects of partner notification on relationships between patients and partners and, in particular, on the rate of violence, abuse, and abandonment of patient or partner.

- We found no studies comparing the effects of an intervention across different groups, such as people with different diseases or combinations of diseases, or people from different settings.

- RCTs comparing different partner notification strategies have found that provider referral is more effective than patient referral in HIV and chlamydia infections, and that in people with syphilis there is no significant difference between provider and contract referral.

- One RCT has found that adding telephone reminders and contact cards improves patient referral compared with counselling alone. We found insufficient evidence about other methods, such as educational videos.

- We found insufficient evidence on the effects of giving people choice about which type of partner notification should be used.

Partner notification

DEFINITION Partner notification is a process whereby the sexual partners of people with a diagnosis of sexually transmitted infection are informed of their exposure to infection. The main methods are patient referral, provider referral, contract referral, and outreach assistance.

INCIDENCE/ PREVALENCE A large proportion of people with sexually transmitted infections will have neither symptoms nor signs of infection. For example, 22–68% of men with gonorrhoea who were identified through partner notification were asymptomatic.[1] Partner notification is one of the two strategies to reach such individuals, the other strategy being screening. Managing infection in people with more than one current sexual partner is likely to have the greatest impact on the spread of sexually transmitted infections.[2]

AIMS To prevent complications of infection in the partner; to prevent transmission to others; to prevent reinfection; and to identify social networks of people practising risky sexual behaviours.

OUTCOMES Partners identified; partners notified; partners presenting for care; partners testing positive; partners treated; rates of reinfection in the patient; incidence of sexually transmitted diseases in the population; harms to patient or partner, such as domestic violence and abuse; ethical outcomes (patient autonomy versus beneficence).

METHODS *Clinical Evidence* update search and appraisal November 2000. We included RCTs comparing at least two alternative partner notification strategies and in which randomisation was appropriate, patient follow up was greater than 80%, participants were analysed in the groups to which they were assigned, and the groups were similar at the start of the trial. The outcome used in this summary was the absolute difference between the ratio of partners identified, notified, presenting for care, testing positive, or treated per index case.

QUESTION **What are the effects of different partner notification strategies in different groups of people?**

OPTION IN PEOPLE WITH HIV INFECTION

One RCT found that, for people with HIV infection, provider referral results in more partners being notified than patient referral.

Benefits: We found one systematic review (search date not stated),[3] which identified only one RCT; we found no subsequent RCTs. **Provider versus patient referral:** The RCT (162 people who tested positive for HIV) compared provider referral (see glossary, p 1122) with patient referral (see glossary, p 1122). It was conducted at three public health departments in North Carolina, USA. Of those approached, the 46% who agreed to participate in the study were mostly men (69%), of whom most were homosexual or bisexual (76%). Provider referral significantly increased the likelihood that partners would be notified (AR 78/157 [50%] for the provider referral group v 10/153 [7%] for the patient referral group; RR 7.6, 95% CI 6.3 to 8.9; NNT 3, 95% CI 2 to 3). Thus, three patients would have to be offered provider referral, compared with using patient referral, for one additional partner to be notified. One group in the USA tried to compare contract referral (see glossary, p 1122) with provider referral, but contamination between comparison groups made this impossible.[4] The results were therefore analysed as a cohort study without comparison groups, where all patients were assigned to provider referral. The study included 1070 people, who reported having had 8633 partners in the past year. Of these partners, 1035 were successfully located, of whom 248 had previously tested positive for HIV, 560 were tested by the disease intervention specialist, 69 refused testing, and 158 were located by record search only. Of the 560 partners tested, 122 tested positive. **Contract referral:** We found no RCTs evaluating contract referral in people with HIV infection. **Outreach assistance:** See glossary, p 1122. We found one RCT (63 people with HIV who were injecting drug users) comparing patient referral with outreach assistance.[5]

Harms: People's reluctance to disclose their HIV status to partners (see comment below) suggests expectation of harms from doing so. These and other potential harms are poorly understood.

Comment: The number of partners notified is an intermediate outcome. The number of infections in partners that are prevented or treated has not been evaluated. Thus, the true benefits and harms of HIV partner notification are unknown. **Rates of disclosure:** A descriptive study of 276 people attending for initial primary care for HIV infection in the USA found that 40% of the respondents had not disclosed their HIV status to all partners over the preceding 6 months.[6] Individuals with more than one partner were significantly less likely to disclose to all partners. Only 42% of the non-disclosers reported that they used condoms all the time, which indicates that many partners were at risk of HIV infection. Another descriptive study conducted in the USA found that, even after repeated individual counselling of people with HIV infection and a 6 month opportunity to disclose HIV status, 30% had not informed any of their past partners, and 29% had not informed any of their present partners.[7] Additional results to the paper by Levy and Fox[5] are expected to be published soon (C Mathews, personal communication, 2001).

OPTION	IN PEOPLE WITH GONORRHOEA AND CHLAMYDIA

Two RCTs have found that, for people with gonorrhoea, contract referral is no better at identifying partners with positive culture than patient referral. For people with chlamydia, one RCT found that provider referral increases the proportion of partners notified and of positive partners detected per patient compared with patient referral.

Benefits: We found one systematic review (search date not stated), which identified two RCTs of partner notification in people with gonorrhoea and one in people with non-gonococcal urethritis.[3] We found no subsequent studies that met our inclusion criteria. **Gonorrhoea:** The two RCTs (2085 people with gonorrhoea) compared patient referral with contract referral. A meta-analysis found no significant difference in the proportion of partners with positive gonorrhoea culture per patient (ARR 5%, 95% CI −10% to

+21%).[3] **Chlamydia:** The RCT in people with non-gonococcal urethritis compared patient referral with provider referral in 678 people. It found that provider referral significantly increased the proportion of partners assessed per patient (ARR for non-assessment 52%, 95% CI 44% to 59%). In this study, provider referral also significantly increased the proportion of partners with positive culture per index patient (ARR 6%, 95% CI 2% to 10%). Provider referral was six times as costly per partner with positive culture. Provider referral would have to be offered to two index patients with non-gonococcal urethritis for one additional partner to be assessed (NNT 2, 95% CI 1 to 2) and to 17 index patients to identify one additional partner with a positive culture (NNT 17, 95% CI 10 to 50). These findings are likely to underestimate the effectiveness of patient referral, as partners referred by index patients may have been assessed elsewhere.[3]

Harms: These are poorly understood.

Comment: A cohort study (265 urban, adolescent girls attending a clinic in Alabama, USA) found that, given the choice, people with gonorrhoea or chlamydia are about as likely to choose provider referral as patient referral.[8]

| OPTION | IN PEOPLE WITH SYPHILIS |

One large RCT found that provider referral was no more effective than contract referral, when people receiving the contract referral option were given only 2 days in which to notify their partners. We found no RCTs evaluating patient referral.

Benefits: We found no systematic review. We found one RCT (1966 people diagnosed with syphilis) in three US states.[9] It compared the proportion of partners per patient who were located, tested, tested positive, and treated, using three types of referral process: contract referral (patients were given 2 days to notify partners themselves, before disease intervention specialists would notify them); provider referral (immediate notification by an intervention specialist); and provider referral with the option of a blood test (immediate notification by an intervention specialist who had the option of performing a blood test if he or she thought that the partner would not seek medical attention despite being notified of exposure). In the three groups: 1.2, 1.1, and 1.1 partners per patient were located; 0.92, 0.87, and 0.86 were tested; and 0.67, 0.61, and 0.62 were treated (confidence intervals not reported).

Harms: These are poorly understood.

Comment: In this trial, the investigators had no way of determining whether disease intervention specialists began actively seeking partners in the contract referral group before waiting 2 days.[9] The use of disease intervention specialists is an approach that may not be generalisable outside the USA.

| QUESTION | What can be done to improve the effectiveness of patient referral? |

One RCT has found that adding telephone reminders and contact cards improves patient referral compared with counselling alone. One RCT found no difference between different kinds of healthcare professional. We found insufficient evidence about other methods, such as educational videos.

Benefits: We found one systematic review (search date not stated), which identified two published RCTs and one unpublished RCT. All were in people with gonococcal or chlamydial infections.[3] We found no subsequent studies that met our inclusion criteria. **Counselling plus referral cards and telephone follow up:** One RCT (65 people from a university clinic in the USA) compared the use of counselling plus referral cards and telephone follow up of the index case with counselling alone. The referral card was to be given to the partner or to be used in preparing to speak to the partner. It contained the patient's diagnosis to facilitate treatment of the partner and a message exhorting the partner to seek treatment. The addition of referral cards and telephone follow up significantly increased the number of partners presenting for care per patient identified (ARR for failure to present 34%, 95% CI 13% to 56%). A referral card and telephone follow up would have to be offered to only three patients for one additional partner to present for care (NNT 3, 95% CI 2 to 8). The trial also evaluated adding a $3 incentive to the referral card. Charges for clinic visits for patients and partners would be waived following successful recruitment of partners for treatment. This had no effect on the number of partners presenting for care.[3] **Different health professionals:** One RCT found that there was no difference between patient referral using nurses who did not ask for partners' names and gave referral letters, and disease intervention specialists who took partners' names but no contact details, in terms of the number of partners with positive cultures who were identified (ARR 0.1%, 95% CI –3% to +3%).[3] **Information pamphlets:** One unpublished RCT, conducted in the USA, investigated the use of information pamphlets compared with a routine counselling interview. Providing patients with information pamphlets was slightly less effective than the interview and significantly reduced the number of partners presenting for care per index patient (ARR for failing to present –5%, 95% CI –7% to –3%). The two strategies were equally effective in terms of the number of partners identified with a positive culture per patient. However, the RCT combined two interventions: different health professionals and asking for partners' names, either of which may have affected the results.[3] **Optional outreach assistance:** We found one RCT comparing patient referral with a choice between patient referral and outreach assistance.[5] The 60 patients who returned for their test results named an average of 2.4 partners each, and no differences were found in the ratio of partners named per patient by treatment group. Of those in the outreach assisted group, 82% chose to have the outreach team notify at least one partner, and the team was asked to notify 71% of all partners named by this group. **Educational videos:** We found no RCTs.

Harms: None reported.

Partner notification

Comment: Contact cards seem to be easily generalised to other settings. Telephone reminders may not be possible in countries with poorly developed telecommunication systems.

QUESTION **What are the effects of allowing people to choose the type of partner notification?**

We found insufficient evidence on the effects of giving people choice about which type of partner notification should be used compared with assigning them to one or other type.

Benefits: We found no systematic review. We found one RCT comparing patient referral with a choice between patient referral and outreach assistance.[5]

Harms: These are poorly understood.

Comment: None.

GLOSSARY

Contract referral (also referred to as conditional referral) Index patients are encouraged to inform their partners, with the understanding that health service personnel will notify those partners who do not visit the health service within a contracted time period.

Outreach assistance At the request of patients, partners are notified by members of an outreach team indigenous to the community, who do not disclose the name of the patient to the partners.

Patient referral Health service personnel encourage index patients to inform partners directly of their possible exposure to sexually transmitted infections.

Provider referral Third parties (usually health service personnel) notify partners identified by index patients.

REFERENCES

1. Holmes KK, Mardh PA, Sparling PF, Weisner PJ, eds. *Sexually Transmitted Diseases*, 2nd edn. New York: McGraw-Hill, 1990:1083.
2. Fenton KA, Peterman TA. HIV partner notification: taking a new look. *AIDS* 1997;11:1535–1546.
3. Oxman AD, Scott EAF, Sellors JW, et al. Partner notification for sexually transmitted diseases: an overview of the evidence. *Can J Public Health* 1994;85:127–132. Search date not stated; primary sources Medline, Embase, SciSearch, hand searching of five key journals, personal contact with 80 key experts.
4. Toomey KE, Peterman TA, Dicker LW, Zaidi AA, Wroten JE, Carolina J. Human immunodeficiency virus partner notification. *Sex Transm Dis* 1998; 25:310–316.
5. Levy JA, Fox SE. The outreach-assisted model of partner notification with IDUs. *Public Health Rep* 1998;113(suppl 1):160–169.
6. Stein MD, Freedberg KA, Sullivan LM, et al. Sexual ethics: disclosure of HIV-positive status to partners. *Arch Intern Med* 1998;158:253–257.
7. Perry SW, Card CAL, Moffatt M, Ashman T, Fishman B, Jacobsberg LB. Self-disclosure of HIV infection to sexual partners after repeated counseling. *AIDS Educ Prev* 1994;6:403–411.
8. Oh MK, Boker JR, Genuardi FJ, Cloud GA, Reynolds J, Hodgens JB. Sexual contact tracing in adolescent chlamydial and gonococcal cervicitis cases. *J Adolesc Health* 1996;18:4–9.
9. Peterman TA, Toomey KE, Dicker LW, Zaidi AA, Wroten JE, Carolina J. Partner notification for syphilis: a randomized, controlled trial of three approaches. *Sex Transm Dis* 1997;24:511–518.

Catherine Mathews
Senior Scientist, Health Systems Unit
South African Medical Research
Council, University of Cape Town
Cape Town, South Africa

Merrick Zwarenstein
Director, Health Systems
Research Unit
Medical Research Council
Tygerberg, South Africa

Nicol Coetzee
Senior Lecturer and Consultant
Department of Public Health
University of Cape Town
Cape Town, South Africa

Sally Guttmacher
Department of Health Studies
New York University
New York, USA
Competing interests: None declared.

Search date December 2000

Jonathan Ross

QUESTIONS

INTERVENTIONS

Key Messages

- We found no good evidence comparing empirical treatment with antibiotics (before receiving results of microbiological tests) versus delaying treatment until test results are available.

- One systematic review has found that several regimens of parenteral followed by oral antibiotic treatment are effective in relieving the short term symptoms and signs of pelvic inflammatory disease (PID).

- We found no good evidence on the optimal duration of treatment, or on oral versus parenteral treatment.

Pelvic inflammatory disease

DEFINITION   Pelvic inflammatory disease (PID) is inflammation and infection of the upper genital tract in women, typically involving the fallopian tubes, ovaries, and surrounding structures.

INCIDENCE/   The exact incidence of PID is unknown because the disease cannot
PREVALENCE be diagnosed reliably from clinical symptoms and signs.[1–3] Direct visualisation of the fallopian tubes by laparoscopy is the best single diagnostic test, but it is invasive and not used routinely in clinical practice. PID is the most common gynaecological reason for admission to hospital in the USA, accounting for 49 of 10 000 recorded hospital discharges. However, since most PID is asymptomatic, this figure almost certainly underestimates true prevalence.[1,4]

AETIOLOGY/   Factors associated with PID mirror those for sexually transmitted
RISK FACTORS infections: young age, reduced socioeconomic circumstances, African/Afro-Caribbean ethnicity, lower educational attainment, and recent new sexual partner.[2,5,6] Most cases seem to result from ascending infection from the cervix. Initial epithelial damage caused by bacteria (especially *Chlamydia trachomatis* and *Neisseria gonorrhoeae*) allows the opportunistic entry of other organisms. Isolates from the upper genital tract are polymicrobial, including *Mycoplasma hominis* and anaerobes.[7] The spread of infection to the upper genital tract may be influenced by vaginal douching, instrumentation of the cervix, and using contraceptives.[8–11]

PROGNOSIS   PID has high morbidity; about 20% of affected women become infertile, 20% develop chronic pelvic pain, and 10% of those who conceive have an ectopic pregnancy.[2] We found no placebo controlled trials of antibiotic treatment. Uncontrolled observations suggest that clinical symptoms and signs resolve in a significant number of untreated women.[12] Repeated episodes of PID are associated with a four to sixfold increase in the risk of permanent tubal damage.[13]

AIMS   To alleviate the pain and systemic malaise associated with infection; to achieve microbiological cure; to prevent development of permanent tubal damage with associated sequelae, such as chronic pelvic pain, ectopic pregnancy, and infertility; and to prevent the spread of infection to others.

OUTCOMES   Incidence and severity of acute symptoms and signs; microbiological cure of the upper genital tract; incidence of chronic pelvic pain, ectopic pregnancy, and infertility; rate of transmission to others.

METHODS   *Clinical Evidence* update search and appraisal December 2000.

QUESTION Should suspected PID be treated empirically or should treatment be delayed until the results of microbiological investigations are known?

OPTION EMPIRICAL ANTIBIOTIC TREATMENT

We found no evidence to support or refute empirical treatment for suspected PID.

Benefits: We found no systematic review or RCTs comparing empirical versus delayed treatment.

Harms: We found no reliable evidence on harms.

Comment: Because there are no reliable clinical diagnostic criteria for PID, early empirical treatment is common.[3] The positive predictive value of a clinical diagnosis is 65–90% compared with laparoscopy.[1-3] The absence of infection from the lower genital tract, where samples are usually taken, does not exclude PID,[2] and so may not influence the decision to treat.

QUESTION   How do different antimicrobial regimens compare?

One systematic review has found that several regimens of parenteral followed by oral antibiotic treatment are effective in resolving the acute symptoms and signs associated with PID (see table 1, p 1127). We found no good evidence on the optimal duration of treatment, or comparing oral versus parenteral treatment.

Benefits: We found one systematic review (search date 1992),[14] which was subsequently updated (search date 1997).[15] These reviews answer different questions and cover different aspects. They both identified 26 studies of 16 antimicrobial regimens in 1925 women with PID. The identified studies included case series, and it is not possible from the aggregated data published in the reviews to ascertain how many studies were RCTs. Inclusion criteria were a diagnosis of PID (clinical, microbiological, laparoscopic, or by endometrial biopsy) and microbiological testing for *C trachomatis* and *N gonorrhoeae*. The reviews found antibiotics were effective in relieving the symptoms associated with PID, with clinical and microbiological cure rates of 90–100% (see table 1, p 1127). **Duration of treatment:** The duration of treatment was not addressed, although the most common treatment period was 14 days. **Oral versus parenteral treatment:** The reviews did not analyse outcomes by oral or parenteral route of administration. Most regimens started with parenteral treatment and continued with oral treatment at different points. Two RCTs (249 and 72 women) compared oral ofloxacin versus parenteral cefoxitin and doxycycline. The trials found no significant difference in cure rates among groups (clinical cure rates about 95% for all treatments).[16,17]

Harms: The harms associated with treatment were not specifically addressed by the systematic reviews.[14,15] In two RCTs reporting adverse effects, withdrawal from treatment was uncommon (2/20 for doxycycline/metronidazole; 0/20 for perfloxacin/metronidazole; 0/16 for ciprofloxacin).[18,19]

Comment: We found little evidence about long term sequelae of PID, adverse effects of treatment, treatment of PID of differing severity, the effect of ethnicity, or the relevance of tracing sexual contacts. See partner notification, p 1117. The risks of tubal occlusion and subsequent infertility relate to the severity of PID prior to starting therapy,[20] and clinical improvement may not translate into preserved fertility.[21,22] Two papers are awaiting translation and will be considered in a future issue of *Clinical Evidence*.

REFERENCES

1. Morcos R, Frost N, Hnat M, Petrunak A, Caldito G. Laparoscopic versus clinical diagnosis of acute pelvic inflammatory disease. *J Reprod Med* 1993; 38:53–56.

2. Metters JS, Catchpole M, Smith C, et al. *Chlamydia trachomatis: summary and conclusions of CMO's expert advisory group.* London: Department of Health, 1998.

3. Centers for Disease Control. *1998 guidelines for treatment of sexually transmitted diseases.* Bethesda, Maryland: CDC, 1998. http://www.cdc.gov/epo/mmwr/preview/mmwrhtml/00050909.htm.

4. Velebil P, Wingo PA, Xia Z, Wilcox LS, Peterson HB. Rate of hospitalization for gynecologic disorders among reproductive-age women in the United States. *Obstet Gynecol* 1995;86:764–769.

5. Simms I, Catchpole M, Brugha R, Rogers P, Mallinson H, Nicoll A. Epidemiology of genital Chlamydia trachomatis in England and Wales. *Genitourin Med* 1997;73:122–126.

6. Grodstein F, Rothman KJ. Epidemiology of pelvic inflammatory disease. *Epidemiology* 1994;5:234–242.

7. Bevan CD, Johal BJ, Mumtaz G, Ridgway GL, Siddle NC. Clinical, laparoscopic and microbiological findings in acute salpingitis: report on a United Kingdom cohort. *Br J Obstet Gynaecol* 1995;102:407–414.

8. Wolner-Hanssen P, Eschenbach DA, Paavonen J, et al. Association between vaginal douching and acute pelvic inflammatory disease. *JAMA* 1990; 263:1936–1941.

9. Jacobson L, Westrom L. Objectivized diagnosis of acute pelvic inflammatory disease. Diagnostic and prognostic value of routine laparoscopy. *Am J Obstet Gynecol* 1969;105:1088–1098.

10. Kelaghan J, Rubin GL, Ory HW, Layde PM. Barrier-method contraceptives and pelvic inflammatory disease. *JAMA* 1982;248:184–187.

11. Wolner-Hanssen P, Eschenbach DA, Paavonen J, et al. Decreased risk of symptomatic chlamydial pelvic inflammatory disease associated with oral contraceptive use. *JAMA* 1990;263:54–59.

12. Curtis AH. Bacteriology and pathology of fallopian tubes removed at operation. *Surg Gynecol Obstet* 1921;33:621.

13. Hillis SD, Owens LM, Marchbanks PA, Amsterdam LF, MacKenzie WR. Recurrent chlamydial infections increase the risks of hospitalization for ectopic pregnancy and pelvic inflammatory disease. *Am J Obstet Gynecol* 1997;176:103–107.

14. Walker CK, Kahn JG, Washington AE, Peterson HB, Sweet RL. Pelvic inflammatory disease: metaanalysis of antimicrobial regimen efficacy. *J Infect Dis* 1993;168:969–978. Search date 1992; primary sources Medline 1966–1992, and bibliographies from reviews, textbooks, and references.

15. Walker CK, Workowski KA, Washington AE, Soper DE, Sweet RL. Anaerobes in pelvic inflammatory disease: implications for the Centers for Disease Control and Prevention's guidelines for treatment of sexually transmitted diseases. *Clin Infect Dis* 1999;28(suppl):29–36. Search date 1997; primary sources Medline 1966–1997, and bibliographies from reviews, textbooks, and references.

16. Martens MG, Gordon S, Yarborough DR, Faro S, Binder D, Berkeley A. Multicenter randomized trial of ofloxacin versus cefoxitin and doxycycline in outpatient treatment of pelvic inflammatory disease. Ambulatory PID Research Group. *South Med J* 1993;86:604–610.

17. Wendel GD, Cox SM, Bawdon RE, Theriot SK, Heard MC, Nobles BJ. A randomized trial of ofloxacin versus cefoxitin and doxycycline in the outpatient treatment of acute salpingitis. *Am J Obstet Gynecol* 1991;164:1390–1396.

18. Witte EH, Peters AA, Smit IB, et al. A comparison of pefloxacin/metronidazole and doxycycline/metronidazole in the treatment of laparoscopically confirmed acute pelvic inflammatory disease. *Eur J Obstet Gynecol Reprod Biol* 1993;50:153–158.

19. Heinonen PK, Teisala K, Miettinen A, Aine R, Punnonen R, Gronroos P. A comparison of ciprofloxacin with doxycycline plus metronidazole in the treatment of acute pelvic inflammatory disease. *Scand J Infect Dis Suppl* 1989;60:66–73.

20. Soper DE, Brockwell NJ, Dalton HP. Microbial etiology of urban emergency department acute salpingitis: treatment with ofloxacin. *Am J Obstet Gynecol* 1992;167:653–660.

21. Buchan H, Vessey M, Goldacre M, Fairweather J. Morbidity following pelvic inflammatory disease. *Br J Obstet Gynaecol* 1993;100:558–562.

22. Brunham RC, Binns B, Guijon F, et al. Etiology and outcome of acute pelvic inflammatory disease. *J Infect Dis* 1988;158:510–517.

Jonathan Ross
Honorary Senior Lecturer
University of Birmingham
Birmingham
UK

Competing interests: None declared.

TABLE 1	Cure rates for the antibiotic treatment of acute PID: aggregated data from systematic reviews of RCTs and case series (see text, p 1125).[14,15]

Drug regimen	Number of studies	Number of women	Cure rate (%) clinical/ microbiological*
Inpatient treatment (initially parenteral switching to oral)			
Clindamycin + aminoglycoside	11	470	91/97
Cefoxitin + doxycycline	8	427	91/98
Cefotetan + doxycycline	3	174	95/100
Ceftizoxime + tetracycline	1	18	88/100
Cefotaxime + tetracycline	1	19	94/100
Ciprofloxacin	4	90	94/96
Ofloxacin	1	36	100/97
Sulbactam/ampicillin + doxycycline	1	37	95/100
Co-amoxiclav	1	32	93/-
Metronidazole + doxycycline	2	36	75/71
Outpatient treatment (oral unless indicated otherwise)			
Cefoxitin (im) + probenecid + doxycycline	3	219	89/93
Ofloxacin	2	165	95/100
Co-amoxiclav	1	35	100/100
Sulbactam/ampicillin	1	36	70/70
Ceftriaxone (im) + doxycycline	1	64	95/100
Ciprofloxacin + clindamycin	1	67	97/94

im, intramuscular; *N gonorrhoeae, C trachomatis*, or both, when detected in lower genital tract.

Search date May 2000

Fay Crawford, Rachel Hart, Sally EM Bell-Syer, David J Togerson
Philip Young and Ian Russell

QUESTIONS

INTERVENTIONS

Beneficial

Likely to be beneficial

Unknown effectiveness

To be covered in future issues of
    Clinical Evidence
Oral antifungal treatments

Key Messages

- Systematic reviews of RCTs have found strong evidence that topical treatments, including allylamines, azoles, undecenoic acid, and tolnaftate, increase cure rates in fungal skin infections of the foot compared with placebo (NNT 2).
- We found no evidence of significant differences in efficacy between individual allylamines or individual azoles.
- One systematic review of RCTs has found that topical allylamines produce a faster response than azoles but the cure rates are similar.
- Single RCTs found that topical ciclopiroxolamine and griseofulvin were more effective than placebo.
- We found no evidence about the effectiveness of topical treatments for fungal nail infections.

DEFINITION   Athlete's foot is a cutaneous fungal infection that causes the skin to itch, flake, and fissure. Nail involvement is characterised by ungual thickening and discolouration.

INCIDENCE/   In the UK, athlete's foot is present in about 15% of the general
PREVALENCE   population,[1] and 1.2 million people have fungally infected toe nails.[2]

AETIOLOGY/   Swimming pool users and industrial workers may have increased
RISK FACTORS   risk of fungal foot infection. However, one survey found fungal foot infection in only 8.5% of swimmers, with the highest incidence (20%) in men aged 16 years and over.[1]

PROGNOSIS   Fungal infections of the foot are not life threatening in people with normal immunity, but in some people they cause persistent symptoms. Others are apparently oblivious of persistent infection. The infection can spread to other parts of the body and to other individuals.

AIMS   To control symptoms and prevent recurrence, with minimal adverse effects.

OUTCOMES   Rates of fungal eradication, shown by negative microscopy and culture, and resolution of clinical signs and symptoms at follow up.

METHODS   We searched Medline, Embase, and the Cochrane Controlled Trials Register to May 2000 for systematic reviews and subsequent RCTs (all languages). Studies were excluded if foot specific data could not be extracted. We excluded studies that did not use microscopy and culture (skin infections) or culture (nail infections) for diagnosis and as an outcome measure.

QUESTION   What are the effects of topical antifungals for athlete's foot?

OPTION   TOPICAL ALLYLAMINES

A systematic review of RCTs has found that allylamines are more effective than placebo in curing fungal skin infections. It found insufficient evidence comparing different allylamines with one another. Allylamines produce a faster response than azoles but the cure rates are similar.

Benefits: We found one systematic review (search date May 1999).[3,4]
                Versus placebo: The review identified 12 RCTs comparing topical allylamines versus placebo for 1–4 weeks in 1433 people with fungal infections of the foot.[3,4] Follow up was 6–8 weeks. Topical allylamines reduced the risk of treatment failure assessed by culture or microscopy (AR 27% v 80% for placebo; ARR 54%, 95% CI 48% to 58%; RRR 67%, 95% CI 61% to 73%; NNT 2 at 6 weeks). **Different allylamines:** The systematic review identified one small RCT that compared different allylamines (n = 60).[3] It found no significant difference between naftifine versus terbinafine (AR of treatment failure 75% v 81% for terbinafine; ARR 5%, 95% CI –17% to +21%). **Versus topical azoles:** See topical azoles, p 1130.

Harms: The systematic review did not report frequency of adverse effects.[3] We found few reports of local irritation in any of the trials.

Comment: The systematic review assessed the quality of reporting in the trials. Out of a possible 12 points, the mean quality score for all 72 included studies was 6.3. Few demographic details of participants were reported.[3]

OPTION	TOPICAL AZOLES

A systematic review of RCTs has found that azole creams administered for 4–6 weeks increase cure rate compared with placebo. We found no evidence of differences in efficacy between individual azoles. Allylamines produce a faster response than azoles but the cure rates are similar.

Benefits: We found one systematic review (search date 1999).[3,4] **Versus placebo:** The review identified 17 placebo controlled RCTs in 1259 people with fungal skin infections of the foot. Intervention lasted for 4–6 weeks and follow up ranged from 6–10 weeks. Azoles reduced the risk of failure to cure, determined by culture or microscopy (AR 126/664 [19%] with azoles, 362/595 [61%] with placebo; ARR 42%, 95% CI 38% to 48%; RRR 69%, 95% CI 62% to 75%; NNT 2 to achieve one extra cure, 95% CI 2 to 3). **Different azoles:** The systematic review identified 12 RCTs in 584 people with fungal infection of the foot comparing one azole against another over 3–4 weeks and with follow up over 3–10 weeks. No consistent difference was found. **Versus topical allylamines:** The systematic review identified 12 RCTs (n = 1487) that compared at least 4 weeks of azole treatment with 1–6 weeks of topical allylamine treatment in people with fungal infections of the foot. It found that after 3–12 weeks of follow up, allylamines reduced the risk of treatment failure compared with azoles (AR of treatment failure with allylamines 146/773 [19%] v 224/714 [31%] for azoles; ARR 13%, 95% CI 9% to 16%; RRR 40%, 95% CI 27% to 51%; NNT 8, 95% CI 6 to 12). Four included RCTs found that a 1 week course of allylamines produced similar cure rates as a 4 week course of azoles (AR of treatment failure 53/464 [11%] for 1 week allylamine, 71/448 [16%] for 4 weeks azole; ARR 4.4%, 95% CI 0% to 8%).[3,4]

Harms: The systematic review did not report frequency of adverse effects with topical azoles. We found few reports of local irritation of the feet.

Comment: The trials comparing allylamines and azoles were not consistent in their results; four non-English language RCTs found no evidence of a difference between allylamines and azoles.

OPTION	OTHER TOPICAL AGENTS

A systematic review of RCTs has found that topical undecenoic acid and tolnaftate are more effective than placebo (NNT 2). Single RCTs found that topical ciclopiroxolamine and griseofulvin cured more than placebo.

Benefits: We found one systematic review (search date May 1999).[3,4] **Topical ciclopiroxolamine versus placebo:** The review identified one RCT comparing ciclopiroxolamine with placebo in 144 people with fungal skin infection of the foot for 4 weeks, with 6 weeks' follow up. Ciclopiroxolamine reduced the risk of treatment failure (AR 31/71 [44%] for ciclopiroxolamine, 67/73 [92%] for placebo; ARR 48%, 95% CI 25% to 69%; RRR 52%, 95% CI 27% to 75%; NNT 2, 95% CI 1 to 4). **Topical griseofulvin versus placebo:** The review identified one RCT in 94 people, which found that griseofulvin reduced the risk of treatment failure compared with placebo (AR 9/47 [19%] for griseofulvin, 31/47 [66%] for placebo; ARR 47%, 95% CI 28% to 58%; RRR 71%, 95% CI 43% to 87%; NNT 2, 95% CI 2 to 4). **Topical undecenoic acid versus placebo:** The review identified four RCTs in 223 people, which found that undecenoic acid reduced the risk of treatment failure compared with placebo (AR 40/123 [33%] with undecenoic acid, 81/103 [79%] with placebo; ARR 46%, 95% CI 32% to 58%; RRR 59%, 95% CI 40% to 73%; NNT 2, 95% CI 2 to 3). **Topical tolnaftate versus placebo:** The review identified three RCTs in 148 people, which found that tolnaftate for 4 weeks was more effective than placebo at 5–8 weeks' follow up (AR 20/78 [26%] for tolnaftate v 49/70 [70%] for placebo; ARR 44%, 95% CI 29% to 56%; RRR 63%, 95% CI 41% to 79%; NNT 2, 95% CI 2 to 4).

Harms: The systematic review did not report frequency of adverse effects.

Comment: None.

QUESTION   What are the effects of topical antifungals for nail infections?

We found insufficient evidence on the effects of topical antifungal agents in people with frequently infected toenails.

Benefits: We found one systematic review (search date May 1999, 2 RCTs, n = 36 and n = 117) comparing topical treatments for toenail infections. The review found insufficient evidence to draw conclusions.[3,4]

Harms: We found no evidence.

Comment: Neither trial included in the systematic review reported blinding of outcome assessment. The smaller trial did not report the method of randomisation.[3,4]

REFERENCES

1. Gentles JC, Evans EGV. Foot infections in swimming baths. *BMJ* 1973;3:260–262.

2. Roberts DT. Prevalence of dermatophyte onychomycosis in the UK: results of an omnibus survey. *Br J Dermatol* 1992;126(suppl 39):23–27.

3. Crawford F, Hart R, Bell-Syer S, Torgerson D, Young P, Russell I. Topical treatments for fungal infections of the skin and nails of the foot. In: The Cochrane Library, Issue 1, 2000. Oxford: Update Software. Search date May 1999; primary sources Medline 1966 to May 1999; Embase 1980 to May 1999; Cinahl to May 1999; Cochrane Controlled Trials Register 1966 to May 1999; Science Citation Index (no search dates given); Biosis (no search dates given); CAB-Health to 1997; Healthstar to 1997; DARE to 1997; the

NHS Economic Evaluation Database to 1997; Econlit to 1997; hand searched references and key journals, and pharmaceutical companies contacted.

4. Hart R, Bell-Syer EM, Crawford F, Torgerson DJ, Young P, Russell I. Systematic review of topical treatments for fungal infections of the skin and nails of the feet. *BMJ* 1999;319:79–82. Search date 1997; primary sources Medline to 1997; Embase to 1997; Cinahl to 1997; Cochrane Controlled Trials Register to 1997; CAB—Health to 1997; Healthstar to 1997; BIDS to 1997; DARE to 1997; the NHS Economic Evaluation Database to 1997; Econlit to 1997; hand searched references and key journals, and pharmaceutical companies contacted.

Fay Crawford
MRC Fellow

University of York
York
UK

Rachel Hart
Research Podiatrist

University of Wales Institute
Cardiff
UK

Sally EM Bell-Syer
Research Fellow

David J Torgerson
Senior Research Fellow

Philip Young
Lecturer

Ian Russell
Professor of Health Sciences

University of York
York
UK

Competing interests: None declared.

Search date January 2001

Carolyn Charman

QUESTIONS

INTERVENTIONS

Key Messages

Treatments

- Small RCTs have found that topical corticosteroids provide symptomatic relief and are safe in the short term. We found little good information on their long term adverse effects or on effects (if any) on the natural history of atopic eczema.

- Three RCTs provide no evidence that routinely adding antimicrobial agents to topical steroid preparations provides additional benefit. However, only two of the trials studied people with clinically infected eczema.

- Limited evidence from two RCTs suggests that adding emollients to topical steroid treatment improves symptoms and signs more than topical steroids alone.

- We found insufficient evidence on the effects of wet wrap or other forms of bandaging.

- We found limited evidence suggesting that controlling house dust mite reduces severity of symptoms, especially in people with positive mite radioallergosorbent test (RAST) scores and in children, but only if very low levels are achieved. One RCT found that bedding covers were the most effective method of control.

■ We found insufficient evidence that dietary manipulation in adults or children reduces symptom severity.

Prevention in predisposed infants

■ We found insufficient evidence that either prolonged breast feeding or maternal dietary manipulation during lactation protects against eczema in infants with a family history of atopy.

Avoidance of provoking factors

■ We found no evidence that avoidance of animals, detergents containing enzymes, all washing detergents, or vaccinations is beneficial in atopic eczema.

■ We found limited evidence suggesting that the roughness of clothing textiles is a more important factor for skin irritation than the type of fabric (cotton or polyester).

DEFINITION	Atopic eczema (atopic dermatitis) is an inflammatory skin disease characterised by an itchy erythematous poorly demarcated skin eruption with a predilection for skin creases.[1]
INCIDENCE/ PREVALENCE	Atopic eczema affects 15–20% of school children in the UK and 2–3% of adults.[2] Prevalence has increased substantially over the past 30 years,[3] possibly because of environmental and lifestyle changes.
AETIOLOGY/ RISK FACTORS	Aetiology is believed to be multifactorial. Recent interest has focused on airborne allergens (house dust mites, pollen, animal dander), outdoor pollution, climate, diet, and prenatal/early life factors such as infections.
PROGNOSIS	Although there is currently no cure, several interventions can help to control symptoms. Atopic eczema clears in 60–70% of children by their early teens, although relapses may occur.
AIMS	To reduce the risk of atopic eczema in predisposed infants and children; to minimise the impact of the disease on quality of life.
OUTCOMES	Severity of symptoms (pruritus, sleep disturbance) and signs (erythema, oozing/crusting, lichenification, cracking, oedema/ papulation, excoriation, and dryness); quality of life; area of skin involvement. Trials used a range of atopic eczema scoring systems, including SCORAD (scoring of atopic dermatitis), SASSAD (six area six sign atopic dermatitis severity score), Rajka and Langeland scoring system, and the dermatology life quality index.
METHODS	*Clinical Evidence* update search and appraisal January 2001. Because of the limited studies available for many questions, we included some with shortcomings in methods, which we mention in the text.

QUESTION What are the effects of treatments in adults and children?

OPTION TOPICAL STEROIDS

Small, short term, placebo controlled RCTs have found that topical corticosteroids applied for 1–4 weeks improve atopic eczema. We found little good information on their long term effects. No systemic effects have been reported in short term RCTs or in one longer term cohort study. Volunteer studies have found that potent topical steroid preparations cause skin thinning after twice daily application for up to 6 weeks, although skin thickness returns to normal within 4 weeks of stopping treatment. Topical steroids provide symptomatic relief while used, but their effect on the natural history of atopic eczema is unknown.

Benefits: We found no systematic review. **Versus placebo:** We found 10 double blind RCTs comparing topical steroids versus placebo cream (vehicle) in children and adults with atopic eczema.[4–13] All the studies found significant improvement with steroid compared with placebo (see table 2, p 1145). **Versus each other:** We found 35 additional double blind RCTs in children and adults with atopic eczema, which compared a variety of topical steroids with each other. These found significant improvements in 22–100% of people after 1–6 weeks of treatment. **Prevention of relapse:** One RCT (54 adults with atopic eczema that had "completely healed" with a 4 week course of a potent topical steroid) compared fluticasone propionate versus placebo. It found that application of fluticasone propionate on 2 consecutive days a week for 16 weeks significantly maintained improvement compared with clinical deterioration in people receiving placebo.[14]

Harms: No serious systemic effects or cases of skin atrophy were reported in these short term RCTs, nor in a longer cohort study in 14 pre-pubertal children (median treatment 6.5 years with mild to moderate potency topical steroids). Minor adverse effects such as burning, stinging, irritation, folliculitis, hypertrichosis, contact dermatitis, and pigmentary disturbances occurred in less than 10% of patients. **Skin thinning:** In the RCT examining prevention of relapse in people with atopic eczema, no histological evidence of skin atrophy was noted after 16 weeks of applying a potent steroid compared with placebo twice weekly to healed lesions.[14] We found no further RCTs looking at skin thinning in people with atopic eczema. Four small RCTs in healthy volunteers (12 people) used ultrasound to evaluate skin thickness.[15–18] Significant skin thinning occurred after 1 week with clobetasol 17-propionate 0.05% twice daily, and after 3 weeks with twice daily triamcinolone acetate 0.1%, and betamethasone 17-valerate 0.1%. All preparations were used for up to 6 weeks, and skin thinning reversed within 4 weeks of stopping treatment. No significant thinning was reported with hydrocortisone prednicarbate twice daily, or mometasone furoate once daily after 6 weeks.

Comment: Studies that did not specify the type of eczema, or those that included other dermatoses in the overall analysis, were excluded. The RCTs used different clinical scoring systems, making it difficult to compare results.

Three RCTs found no evidence that combinations of topical antimicrobial agents and steroids are better than topical steroids alone in improving the clinical signs and symptoms of atopic eczema. Only two of the trials studied people with clinically infected eczema.

Benefits: We found no systematic review. **Versus topical steroid alone:** We found three RCTs comparing topical antimicrobial/steroid combinations versus topical steroid alone in people with atopic dermatitis.[19–21] The RCTs found no significant improvement in clinical signs and symptoms after betamethasone valerate/fusidic acid,[20] hydrocortisone acetate/fusidic acid,[19] or betamethasone valerate/gentamicin[21] compared with topical steroid alone. **Versus each other:** We found five further RCTs (34–207 people) comparing different topical steroid/antimicrobial preparations with each other in people with clinically infected eczema (atopic eczema not specified).[22–26] These found clinical improvement in 54–95% of participants, with no significant difference between the various preparations with respect to improvement in clinical signs and symptoms. People treated with fusidic acid/hydrocortisone showed a more rapid clinical response than those treated with miconazole/ hydrocortisone, and bacteriological responses to betamethasone/ fusidic acid and fucidic acid/hydrocortisone were superior to those with betamethasone/clioquinol and miconazole/hydrocortisone, respectively.

Harms: Overall, the RCTs reported minor adverse effects comprising itching, stinging, burning, and irritation in fewer than 2% of people.

Comment: Only two of the studies specified a degree of infection in most participants at recruitment.[20,21] One of these also included people with contact dermatitis in the overall analysis, and the use of left/right comparisons within individual participants may have reduced the difference between groups because of systemic absorption of the antimicrobial agent.[20]

Two RCTs found that adding an emollient to a topical corticosteroid regimen further improved clinical signs and symptoms of atopic eczema. One comparative study also found improvements in atopic eczema when emollients were used in combination with topical steroids.

Benefits: We found no systematic review. **As adjunct to topical steroids:** One RCT (80 children and adults with mild to moderate atopic eczema) assessed adding moisturising cream three times daily to a topical corticosteroid regimen (desonide 0.05%) applied twice daily.[27] It found additional significant improvement in people receiving the emollient after 3 weeks (70% v 55%), with 96% of people preferring treatment with the emollient and topical steroid than with topical steroid alone. Another RCT (50 people with atopic eczema) compared two different emollients (cream and lotion) applied once daily as an adjunct to once daily hydrocortisone 2.5% cream. After 3 weeks, a significant improvement in signs and symptoms was noted with both treatment regimens.[28] One further controlled clinical trial (25 children, randomisation not mentioned) found no significant difference between once daily emollient cream plus once daily hydrocortisone 2.5% cream, and twice daily hydrocortisone 2.5% cream; both treatment regimens produced no significant difference in signs and symptoms after 3 weeks.[29]

Harms: Minor adverse effects, such as a burning sensation, were reported in fewer than 2% of people.

Comment: Many of the studies located in our search did not specify the type of eczema, or included people with other forms of eczema, so were excluded from this review. We have not included studies looking at bath additives.

| OPTION | WET WRAP DRESSINGS AND BANDAGING |

We found insufficient evidence on the effects of wet wrap or other forms of bandaging in people with atopic eczema.

Benefits: We found no systematic review or RCTs.

Harms: Enhanced topical steroid absorption and adverse effects have been found with earlier forms of wet wrap dressings (see glossary, p 1142). Mean serum cortisol concentrations were depressed significantly after treatment in the 30 erythrodermic children described (see comment below) returning to normal after 2 weeks.[30]

Comment: One uncontrolled study used wet wrap dressings in 30 children with acute erythrodermic eczema.[30] All children responded well to treatment after 2–5 days, with no relapses 2 weeks later (no quantitative results given). Another uncontrolled study in 21 children with chronic severe atopic eczema treated with wet wrap dressings twice per week or less for 3 months found that in all children the eczema improved after starting treatment and sleep disturbance was reduced. Most parents reported a reduction in topical steroid requirements (no quantitative results given).[31] As both studies were uncontrolled, the improvement may have been attributable to the additional medical or nursing input during the study rather than to an effect of the wet wraps.

| OPTION | CONTROL OF HOUSE DUST MITE |

One small RCT found that extreme reduction in dust levels (achieved by synthetic mattress covers, acaricidal spraying, and high filtration vacuuming) reduced eczema severity score. It is impossible to tell from this evidence how many people might benefit and for how long. The clinical relevance of the reduced severity score is uncertain. Bedding covers seem to be the most effective intervention for reducing levels in the home (see table 1, p 1144).

Benefits: We found no systematic review. We found two RCTs, and one controlled clinical trial that did not mention randomisation. One double blind RCT (24 atopic adults and 24 atopic children > 7 years old, skin prick and RAST status not specified) compared bed covers made of a breathable synthetic material plus benzyltannate spray and high filtration vacuuming, versus cotton bedcovers plus placebo spray and standard vacuum cleaners. After 6 months there was a significantly greater reduction in eczema severity scores on active treatment compared with placebo (mean difference in severity score [maximum 108 units] 4.3 units, 95% CI 1.3 to 7.3). This was associated with a 98% reduction in mean mattress dust load compared with 16% in the placebo group (P = 0.002) and a 91% and 76% reduction in the concentration of mite allergen Der p1 on bedroom and living room carpet, compared with 89% (P = 0.94) and 38% (P = 0.27) in the placebo group.[32] The second RCT (20 atopic dermatitis patients, aged 12–47 years with positive skin prick and RAST tests to house dust mite), comparing natamycin or placebo spray with or without vacuuming, found no correlation between improvement in clinical score and lowered mite numbers. The study was small and the maximum reduction in mite numbers in mattresses was only 68%.[33] One controlled trial (51 people with atopic eczema, randomisation not mentioned) found, in 30 people with positive mite RAST scores, induction of an itch free period and prolonged remission after 3 weeks in a "clean room" with reduced dust levels. (Der p1 levels were not measured). Neither an itch free period nor prolonged remission were seen in the 11 people with negative RAST scores treated in a similar environment, or in the 10 controls with positive mite RAST scores treated in an ordinary hospital room.[34]

Harms: No harmful effects were reported in the trials.

Comment: Additional, small, uncontrolled studies have suggested a beneficial effect of mite reduction measures on symptoms, although mite or allergen levels were not quantified. The use of bedding covers seems to be the simplest and most effective measure to reduce house dust mite levels in the home (see table 1, p 1145).

| OPTION | DIETARY MANIPULATION |

We found insufficient evidence about dietary manipulation, such as exclusion of egg and cow's milk in children with atopic eczema. We found no good evidence that dietary manipulation alters the severity of eczema in adults.

Benefits: **In infants:** We found one systematic review (search date 1995, 1 RCT, 17 breast fed infants with atopic eczema). It assessed the effect of excluding allergenic foods, such as cow's milk and eggs, from the mother's diet. It found no effect on eczema severity.[35] However, soya milk, which is potentially allergenic itself, was used as a cow's milk substitute in this trial. **In children:** We found no systematic review. We found two double blind crossover RCTs evaluating the effects of an egg and milk exclusion diet in unselected children with eczema. Both used potentially allergenic soya based milk substitute during the trial period.[36,37] One RCT (20 children aged 2–8 years) found a significant improvement in eczema severity (14/20 treated children improved v 1/20 controls).[36] The other trial (40 children and young adults) found no significant effect.[38] One further RCT evaluated the effect of an egg exclusion diet in 55 children with proven sensitivity to eggs (positive RAST). The mean reduction in surface area affected by eczema was significantly greater in the group receiving dietary advice (from 19.6% to 10.9%) versus controls (from 21.9% to 18.9%). The mean improvement in severity score in the diet group (from 33.9 to 24) was also significantly greater than in controls (from 36.7 to 33.5).[38] Double blind placebo controlled food challenges have been used to identify people with food allergy, but the clinical relevance of positive reactions (which may include gastrointestinal, respiratory, or cutaneous symptoms) to subsequent eczema control is unclear. One retrospective diagnostic study examined hypersensitivity reactions up to 48 hours after double blind, placebo controlled food challenges in 107 children aged 5 months to 12 years with moderate to severe atopic dermatitis and a history suggestive of food allergy. This study found positive reactions in 81% of children, with 70% of reactions occurring within 2 hours. Egg and cow's milk accounted for 83% of the positive reactions.[39] In three further studies, double blind, placebo controlled food challenges caused hypersensitivity reactions (all within 2 hours of the challenge) in 63% of children with moderate to severe atopic eczema (320 children), and in 33–39% of children with mild to severe atopic eczema (211 children). Egg, milk, and peanut accounted for 67–78% of the reactions. The effect of subsequent dietary elimination was studied in only 27 of these children. This showed a greater improvement in children on exclusion diets than in non-randomly selected controls, using a crude scoring system.[40] We found one RCT (85 children, 46 evaluable) that looked at a "few foods diet", in which all but a handful of foods were excluded. It found no significant benefit on eczema severity.[41] **In adults:** We found no systematic review but found two RCTs.[37,42] The first crossover RCT studied adults and children separately. It found no significant improvement in eczema severity with an egg and cow's milk exclusion diet in 18 adults, although potentially allergenic soya milk was used as a cow's milk substitute.[37] The second RCT (33 adults, 25 evaluable) found no significant benefit of an elemental diet (containing amino acids, essential fatty acids, glucose, trace elements, sorbic acid, and vitamins) on eczema severity.[42]

Harms: Calcium, protein, and calorie deficiency are risks of dairy free diets in children.

Comment: The clinical relevance of changes in severity scores obtained in many studies is unknown. We have not included studies looking at the role of food additives, fatty acid supplementation, or trace elements in eczema.

QUESTION	What are the effects of preventive interventions in predisposed infants?

OPTION	PROLONGED BREAST FEEDING IN PREDISPOSED INFANTS

We found limited observational evidence suggesting that exclusive breast feeding for at least 5 months reduces the risk of eczema in infants with a family history of atopy.

Benefits: We found no systematic review or RCTs. One 17 year prospective cohort study (236 healthy infants) found that those who were breast fed exclusively for more than 6 months had a significantly lower prevalence of eczema at 1 year (all infants) and 3 years (infants with a family history of atopy) than those breast fed for less than 1 month and weaned onto cow's milk formula.[43] It found no reduction in the prevalence of eczema in infants who were intermittently breast fed for 2–6 months. Two prospective studies compared prevalence of eczema in exclusively breast fed infants and in non-breast fed infants (non-breast fed infants were randomised to different formulae).[44,45] In infants with a family history of atopy, those who were exclusively breast fed for an average of 5 months had a significantly lower prevalence of eczema at 18 months compared with non-breast fed infants randomised to soya or cow's milk, but not compared with those randomised to whey hydrolysate or casein hydrolysate. One further prospective study that randomised non-breast fed infants to different formulae found a significantly lower incidence of eczema at 3 years in infants breast fed for 6–13 months (8.1%) compared with those fed conventional adapted formula (23.7%) but a comparable incidence to those fed hydrolysed milk formula (10%). All infants were given hypoantigenic weaning diet.[46]

Harms: We found no evidence of harms associated with prolonged breast feeding.

Comment: Much of the available evidence was limited by poor methodology, for example selection and information bias, short duration of breast feeding, and inadequate control for confounding factors such as introducing supplemental milk or solid foods. Prolonged self selected breast feeding may be associated with unknown protective factors, leading to bias.

OPTION   **MATERNAL DIETARY RESTRICTION DURING LACTATION**

We found limited evidence from one systematic review of poor quality trials that maternal dietary restriction during lactation may protect against the development of eczema in infants with a family history of atopy.

Benefits: We found one systematic review (search date 1995, 3 poor quality RCTs).[47] It found a lower prevalence of eczema in breast fed infants whose mothers took antigen avoidance diets compared with those on normal diets during lactation.

Harms: None reported.

Comment: All three trials were limited by poor methods, therefore the results should be interpreted with caution.[47]

What are the effects of avoidance of provoking factors in adults and children?

OPTION CLOTHING TEXTILES

Two small RCTs found that, in people with atopic eczema, the roughness of clothing textiles is a more important factor for skin irritation than the type of textile fibre (synthetic or natural). Polyester and cotton of similar textile fineness seem to be equally well tolerated. We found no evidence on the long term effect of different textiles on the severity of atopic eczema.

Benefits: We found no systematic review but found two small RCTs. The first double blind RCT (20 people with atopic eczema and 20 healthy controls; mean age 25 years) compared cotton and polyester shirts of different fabric structure and coarseness at rest and after exercise to induce sweating.[48] All fabrics were tolerated less well when sweating, in people with eczema and in healthy controls. Comfort ratings for the fabrics did not differ significantly between the two groups. Knitted fabrics (polyester or cotton) were better tolerated than woven fabrics (all polyester). Of the knitted fabrics, polyester was as well tolerated by people with eczema as the comparable cotton shirt of similar textile fineness. At rest, people with eczema tolerated the less coarse knitted polyester better than the other polyester knitted fabrics, although there was no significant difference during exercise. Of the woven fabrics, the finer polyester was better tolerated by people with eczema than the coarser fabrics, both at rest and during exercise, although controls showed no significant difference. The second crossover RCT (24 women with atopic eczema, aged 15–20 years, with a history of wool irritation) compared the effects of two different wool fibres on itching.[49] Wool induced itching was more frequent after 12 hours with the coarser 36 μm wool fibre (16 women) than with the 20 μm wool fibre (9 women). Visible skin changes were seen in six women as a result of the thin fibre wool and 11 women with the thick fibre wool, disappearing within 24 hours in all cases.

Harms: With the exception of short term skin irritation, no harmful effects were reported in these trials.

Comment: None.

OPTION WASHING DETERGENTS

One RCT found no evidence that washing detergents that contain enzymes had a significant provoking effect on eczema severity compared with washing detergents without enzymes. We found no studies looking at the effect of avoidance of all contact with washing detergents.

Benefits: We found no systematic review. **Biological versus non-biological detergents:** We found one double blind crossover RCT (25 people with atopic eczema, aged 17–59 years), which compared washing detergents with or without enzymes.[50] It found no significant differ-ence in clinical disease severity (using SCORAD scale), subjective symptoms, or corticosteroid use between the two groups after using each detergent for 1 month. **Avoidance of all washing detergents:** We found no RCTs.

Harms: No harmful effects were reported in this trial.

Comment: None.

OPTION VACCINATION/IMMUNISATION

We found no evidence about the effects of vaccination on atopic eczema severity.

Benefits: We found no systematic reviews or RCTs.

Harms: One observational study in 134 allergic children (with atopic eczema, asthma, or cows milk allergy) reported transient mild generalised urticaria and fever in two children with atopic eczema within 24 hours of vaccination.[51]

Comment: The study found that the lowest rate of positive skin prick tests to measles, mumps, and rubella vaccine was in the 68 children with atopic eczema (4% positive), compared with the 47 children with asthma (9% positive), and the 11 children with cow's milk allergy (18% positive).[51] The 64 children with atopic eczema who were subsequently vaccinated had no serious reactions, although the long term effect on eczema severity was not studied.

OPTION ANIMAL CONTACT

We found no good evidence on the effects of avoiding animal contact on the severity of atopic eczema.

Benefits: We found no systematic review, RCTs, or cohort studies of the effects of avoiding animals or removing the family pet on the severity of atopic eczema.

Harms: We found no evidence.

Comment: Observational studies have suggested that keeping pets is associated with an increased prevalence of atopic eczema. Following removal of animals from the home it may take many months for the allergen load to decrease because of widespread distribution in carpets and soft furnishings.

GLOSSARY

Wet wrap dressings Wet occlusive tubifast dressings that are applied over topical steroid or emollient.

REFERENCES

1. Williams HC, Burney PGJ, Pembroke AC, Hay RH. The UK working party's diagnostic criteria for atopic dermatitis. III. Independent hospital validation. *Br J Dermatol* 1994;131:406–417.
2. Kay J, Gawkrodger DJ, Mortimer MJ, Jaron AG. The prevalence of childhood atopic eczema in a general population. *J Am Acad Dermatol* 1994;30:35–39.
3. Williams HC. Is the prevalence of atopic dermatitis increasing? *Clin Exp Dermatol* 1992;17:385–391.
4. Lawlor F, Black AK, Greaves M. Prednicarbate 0.25% ointment in the treatment of atopic dermatitis: A vehicle-controlled double-blind study. *J Dermatol Treat* 1995;6:233–235.
5. Roth HL, Brown EP. Hydrocortisone valerate. Double-blind comparison with two other topical steroids. *Cutis* 1978;21:695–698.
6. Maloney JM, Morman MR, Stewart DM, et al. Clobetasol propionate emollient 0.05% in the

treatment of atopic dermatitis. *Int J Dermatol* 1998;37:128–144.

7. Sears HW, Bailer JW, Yeadon A. Efficacy and safety of hydrocortisone buteprate 0.1% cream in patients with atopic dermatitis. *Clin Ther* 1997; 19:710–719.

8. Vanderploeg DE. Betamethasone dipropionate ointment in the treatment of psoriasis and atopic dermatitis: a double-blind study. *South Med J* 1976;69:862–863.

9. Lupton ES, Abbrecht MM, Brandon ML. Short-term topical corticosteroid therapy (halcinonide ointment) in the management of atopic dermatitis. *Cutis* 1982;30:671–675.

10. Stalder JF, Fleury M, Sourisse M, et al. Local steroid therapy and bacterial skin flora in atopic dermatitis. *Br J Dermatol* 1994;131:536–540.

11. Sefton J, Loder JS, Kyriakopoulos AA. Clinical evaluation of hydrocortisone valerate 0.2% ointment. *Clin Ther* 1984;6:282–293.

12. Wahlgren CF, Hägermark O, Bergström R, Hedin B. Evaluation of a new method of assessing pruritus and antipruritic drugs. *Skin Pharmacol* 1988;1:3–13.

13. Sudilovsky A, Muir JG, Bocobo FC. A comparison of single and multiple applications of Halcinonide cream. *Int J Dermatol* 1981;20:609–613.

14. Van der Meer JB, Glazenburg EJ, Mulder PGH, et al. The management of moderate to severe atopic dermatitis in adults with topical fluticasone propionate. *Br J Dermatol* 1999;140:1114–1121.

15. Kerscher MJ, Hart H, Korting HC, Stalleicken D. In vivo assessment of the atrophogenic potency of mometasone furoate, a newly developed chlorinated potent topical glucocorticoid as compared to other topical glucocorticoids old and new. *Int J Clin Pharmacol Ther* 1995;33:187–189.

16. Kerscher MJ, Korting HC. Comparative atrophogenicity potential of medium and highly potent topical glucocorticoids in cream and ointment according to ultrasound analysis. *Skin Pharmacol* 1992;5:77–80.

17. Kerscher MJ, Korting HC. Topical glucocorticoids of the non-fluorinated double-ester type. *Acta Derm Venereol* 1992;72:214–216.

18. Korting HC, Vieluf D, Kerscher M. 0.25% prednicarbate cream and the corresponding vehicle induce less skin atrophy than 0.1% betamethasone-17-valerate cream and 0.05% clobetasol-17-propionate cream. *Eur J Clin Pharmacol* 1992;42:159–161.

19. Ramsay CA, Savoie JM, Gilbert M, et al. The treatment of atopic dermatitis with topical fusidic acid and hydrocortisone acetate. *J Eur Acad Dermatol Venereol* 1996;7(suppl 1):15–22.

20. Hjorth N, Schmidt H, Thomsen K. Fusidic acid plus betamethasone in infected or potentially infected eczema. *Pharmatherapeutica* 1985;4:126–131.

21. Wachs GN, Maibach HI. Co-operative double-blind trial of an antibiotic/corticoid combination in impetiginized atopic dermatitis. *Br J Dermatol* 1976;95:323–328.

22. Hill VA, Wong E, Corbett MF, Menday AP. Comparative efficacy of betamethasone/clioquinol (Betnovate-C) cream and betamethasone/fusidic acid (Fucibet) cream in the treatment of infected hand eczema. *J Dermatol Treat* 1998;9:15–19.

23. Poyner TF, Dass BK. Comparative efficacy and tolerability of fusidic acid/hydrocortisone cream (Fucidin H cream) and miconazole/hydrocortisone cream (Daktacort cream) in infected eczema. *J Eur Acad Dermatol Venereol* 1996;7(suppl 1):23–30.

24. Meenan FOC. A double-blind comparative study to compare the efficacy of Locoid C with Tri-Adcortyl in children with infected eczema. *Br J Clin Pract* 1988;42:200–202.

25. Jaffe GV, Grimshaw JJ. A clinical trial of hydrocortisone/potassium hydroxyquinolone sulphate (Quinocort) in the treatment of infected eczema and impetigo in general practice. *Pharmatherapeutica* 1986;4:628–636.

26. Wilkinson JD, Leigh DA. Comparative efficacy of betamethasone and either fusidic acid or neomycin in infected or potentially infected eczema. *Curr Ther Res* 1985;38:177–182.

27. Hanifin JM, Hebert AA, Mays SR, et al. Effects of a low-potency corticosteroid lotion plus a moisturizing regimen in the treatment of atopic dermatitis. *Curr Ther Res* 1998;59:227–233.

28. Kantor I, Milbauer J, Posner M, et al. Efficacy and safety of emollients as adjunctive agents in topical corticosteroid therapy for atopic dermatitis. *Today Ther Trend* 1993;11:157–166.

29. Lucky AW, Leach AD, Laskarzewski P, Wenck H. Use of an emollient as a steroid-sparing agent in the treatment of mild to moderate atopic dermatitis in children. *Pediatr Dermatol* 1997;14:321–324.

30. Goodyear HM, Spowart K, Harper JI. 'Wet wrap' dressings for the treatment of atopic eczema in children. *Br J Dermatol* 1991;125:604.

31. Mallon E, Powell S, Bridgman A. 'Wet-wrap' dressings for the treatment of atopic eczema in the community. *J Dermatol Treat* 1994;5:97–98.

32. Tan B, Weald D, Strickland I, Frieman PS. Double-blind controlled trial of effect of house dust-mite allergen avoidance on atopic dermatitis. *Lancet* 1996;347:15–18.

33. Colloff MJ, Lever RS, McSharry C. A controlled trial of house dust mite eradication using natamycin in homes of patients with atopic dermatitis: effect on clinical status and mite populations. *Br J Dermatol* 1989;121:199–208.

34. Sanda T, Yasue T, Oohashi M, Yasue A. Effectiveness of house dust-mite allergen avoidance through clean room therapy in patients with atopic dermatitis. *J Allergy Clin Immunol* 1992;89:653–657.

35. Kramer MS. Maternal antigen avoidance during lactation for infants with atopic eczema. In: The Cochrane Library, Issue 4, 2000. Oxford: Update Software. Search date 1995; primary sources The Cochrane Pregnancy and Childbirth Group Trials Register, and contact with authors of studies.

36. Atherton DJ, Sewell M, Soothill JF, Wells RS, Chilvers CE. A double-blind controlled crossover trial of an antigen avoidance diet in atopic eczema. *Lancet* 1978;1:401–403.

37. Neild VS, Marsden RA, Bailes JA, Bland JM. Egg and milk exclusion diets in atopic eczema. *Br J Dermatol* 1986;114:117–123.

38. Lever R, MacDonald C, Waugh P, Aitchison T. Randomised controlled trial of advice on an egg exclusion diet in young children with atopic eczema and sensitivity to eggs. *Pediatr Allergy* 1998;9:13–19.

39. Niggemann B, Sielaff B, Beyer K, Binder C, Wahn U. Outcome of double-blind, placebo-controlled food challenge tests in 107 children with atopic dermatitis. *Clin Exp Allergy* 1999;29:91–96.

40. Sampson HA, McCaskill CM. Food hypersensitivity and atopic dermatitis: evaluation of 113 patients. *J Pediatr* 1985;107:669–675.

41. Mabin DC, Sykes AE, David TJ. Controlled trial of a few foods diet in severe atopic eczema. *Arch Dis Child* 1995;73:202–207.

42. Munkvad M, Danielsen L, Høj L, et al. Antigen-free diet in adult patients with atopic dermatitis. *Acta Derm Venereol* 1984;64:524–528.

43. Saarinen UM, Kajosaari M. Breast-feeding as prophylaxis against atopic disease: prospective

follow-up study until 17 years old. *Lancet* 1995; 346:1065–1069.

44. Chandra RK. Five year follow up of high risk infants with a family history of allergy. *J Pediatr Gastroenterol Nutr* 1997;24:380–388.

45. Chandra RK, Shakuntla P, Hamed A. Influence of maternal diet during lactation and use of formula feeds on development of atopic eczema in high risk infants. *BMJ* 1989;299:228–230.

46. Marini A, Agostoi M, Motta G, Mosca F. Effects of a dietary and environmental prevention programme on the incidence of allergic symptoms in high atopic risk infants: three years follow-up. *Acta Paediatr* 1996;414(suppl):1–22.

47. Kramer MS. Maternal antigen avoidance during lactation in women at high risk for atopic offspring. In: The Cochrane Library, Issue 4, 2000. Oxford: Update Software. Search date 1995; primary sources The Cochrane Pregnancy and Childbirth Group Trials Register and contact with authors of studies.

48. Diepgen TL, Salzer B, Tepe A, Hornstein OP. A study of skin irritations caused by textiles under standardized sweating conditions in patients with atopic eczema [in German]. *Melliand Deutsch/English* 1995;12:E268–E269.

49. Bendsöe N, Björnberg A, Åsnes H. Itching from wool fibres in atopic dermatitis. *Contact Dermatitis* 1987;17:21–22.

50. Andersen PH, Bindslev-Jensen C, Mosbech H, et al. Skin symptoms in patients with atopic dermatitis using enzyme-containing detergents. *Acta Derm Venereol* 1998;78:60–62.

51. Juntunen-Backman K, Peltola H, Backman A, Salo OP. Safe immunisation of allergic children against measles, mumps and rubella. *Am J Dis Child* 1987;141:1103–1105.

Carolyn Charman
Research Fellow in Dermatology
Queen's Medical Centre
Nottingham
UK

Competing interests: None declared.

TABLE 1	**Methods for reducing house dust mite levels: results of controlled trials (see text, p 1137).**

Methods	Results*
Mattress, pillow and duvet covers (micro-porous or polyurethane coated)	Very effective (3 RCTs). Dust mite allergen levels 1–25% of control levels after 3–12 months; 44–98% reduction in dust load after 3 months.
Washing bedding at 55°C	Effective (2 RCTs). Reduces levels of dust mite allergen by > 95% and kills 100% of mites.
Removal of carpets and curtains	Unknown.
Acaricides (e.g. benzyl benzoate)	Conflicting results from RCTs — better when used on carpets than on mattresses. Effect may be short lived.
Intensive vacuuming	Small effect on mite levels in mattresses (1 RCT, 1 crossover trial) but not correlated with improvement in symptoms, possibly because conventional rather than high filtration cleaners may increase levels of airborne mite allergens, which may aggravate atopic disease (1 RCT in 16 rooms).
Air filters and dehumidifiers	Conflicting results from RCTs.

*Trials have tended to use a combination of control measures, making it difficult to see which measures were responsible for beneficial effects.

TABLE 2 Topical steroids versus placebo in atopic eczema: results of RCTs* (see text, p 1135).[4-13]

	Number of participants (age in years)	Outcome
Prednicarbate ointment, 0.25% twice daily for 4 weeks.[4]	51 (18–60)	Reduced dermatitis: 87% active treatment, 8% controls. Significantly reduced patient-assessed pruritis on active treatment.
Hydrocortisone valerate cream, 0.2% three times daily for 2 weeks.[5]	20 (2–75)	Excellent or better: 75% active treatment, 20% controls.
Clobetasol propionate cream, 0.05% twice daily for 4 weeks.[6]	81 (≥12)	Good, excellent, or clear: 82% active treatment, 29% controls.
Hydrocortisone buteprate cream, 0.1% once daily for 2 weeks.[9]	194 (17–76)	Excellent or good: 69% active treatment, 26% controls.
Betamethasone dipropionate ointment, 0.05% twice daily for 3 weeks.[8]	36 (2–63)	Good or excellent: 94% active treatment, 13% controls.
Halcinonide ointment, 0.1% three times daily for 2 weeks.[7]	233 (2–67)	Good or excellent: 85% active treatment, 44% controls.
Desonide cream, once daily for 1 week.[10]	40 (0.4–15)	Improvement or resolution: 67% active treatment, 16% controls.
Hydrocortisone valerate, 0.2% ointment twice daily for 2 weeks.[11]	64 (>12)	Disease severity score: 70% reduction with active treatment, 15% controls.
Betamethasone dipropionate, twice daily for 4 days.[12]	30 (19–57)	Itch free on days 3–4: 36% active treatment, 22% controls.
Halcinonide cream, 0.1% twice daily for 3 weeks.[13]	58 (0.8–86)	57% of people achieved a better response with active treatment than control treatment ("better response" was not defined).

*Confidence intervals not reported.

Cellulitis and erysipelas

Search date February 2001

Andrew Morris

QUESTIONS

INTERVENTIONS

Likely to be beneficial

Unknown effectiveness

To be covered in future issues of *Clinical Evidence*
Role of prophylactic antibiotics in reducing risk of recurrent disease

Key Messages

- We found little RCT evidence on the treatment of cellulitis and erysipelas.
- We found no evidence on the effect of routine microbiological investigations on clinical outcomes.
- We found no placebo controlled trials of antibiotics.
- We found no good evidence on the effects of oral versus intravenous antibiotics, on combinations of antibiotics, on optimal duration of treatment, or on the effects of treating predisposing factors on recurrence.

DEFINITION Cellulitis is a spreading bacterial infection of the dermis and subcutaneous tissues. It manifests as local signs of inflammation such as warmth, erythema, pain, and lymphangitis, and, frequently, systemic upset with fever and leucocytosis. Erysipelas differs from cellulitis in that it tends to be more superficial, with a clearly demarcated edge. The lower limb is by far the commonest site, but any area can be affected.

INCIDENCE/ PREVALENCE We found no specific data on the incidence of cellulitis. However, in the UK in 1991, cellulitis and abscess infections were responsible for 158 consultations per 10 000 person years at risk. In 1985, skin and subcutaneous tissue infections resulted in 29 820 hospital admissions and a mean occupancy of 664 hospital beds each day.[1,2]

AETIOLOGY/ RISK FACTORS The commonest infective organisms in adults are *Streptococci* (particularly *S pyogenes*) and *Staphylococcus aureus*.[3] In children, *Haemophilus influenzae* is a frequent cause. Several risk factors for erysipelas/cellulitis have been identified in a case control study (167 cases and 294 controls): lymphoedema (OR 71.2, 95% CI 5.6 to 908), leg ulcer (OR 62.5, 95% CI 7.0 to 556), toe web intertrigo (OR 13.9, 95% CI 7.2 to 27.0), and traumatic wounds (OR 10.7, 95% CI 4.8 to 23.8).[4]

PROGNOSIS Cellulitis can spread through the blood stream and lymphatics. A retrospective case note study of people admitted to hospital with cellulitis found that systemic symptoms such as fever and leucocytosis were present in up to 42% of cases at presentation.[5] Lymphatic involvement can lead to obstruction and damage that predisposes to recurrent cellulitis. Recurrence can occur rapidly or after months or years. One study found that 29% of people with erysipelas had a recurrent episode within 3 years.[6] Local necrosis and abscess formation can also occur. It is not known whether the prognosis of erysipelas differs from that of cellulitis. We found no evidence about factors that predict recurrence, or a better or worse outcome. We found no good evidence on the prognosis of untreated cellulitis.

AIMS To reduce the severity and duration of infection; to relieve pain and systemic symptoms; to restore the skin to its premorbid state; to prevent recurrence; and to minimise adverse effects of treatment.

OUTCOMES Duration and severity of symptoms (pain, swelling, erythema, fever); clinical cure (defined as the absence of pain, swelling, and erythema); recurrence rate; adverse effects of treatment. We found no standard scales of severity in cellulitis or erysipelas.

METHODS *Clinical Evidence* update search and appraisal February 2001. Where we found no RCTs we included observational studies.

Cellulitis and erysipelas

| QUESTION | What are the effects of routine microbiological investigations? |

We found no good evidence.

Benefits: We found no systematic reviews, RCTs, or observational studies that addressed the impact of routine microbiological investigations on clinical outcomes.

Harms: Two small prospective studies reported no adverse effects.[7,8]

Comment: Two small prospective studies found that routine microbiological investigations had low diagnostic yields except where a primary lesion (e.g. leg ulcer) was present.[7,8]

| QUESTION | What are the effects of antibiotics? |

We found no good evidence evaluating antibiotics versus placebo, oral versus intravenous antibiotics, different combinations of antibiotics, or different durations of treatment. Small RCTs found cure rates of about 70% for all antibiotics evaluated (penicillin, flucloxacillin, ceftriaxone, and roxithromycin).

Benefits: We found no systematic review. **Antibiotics versus placebo:** We found no placebo controlled RCTs. **Oral versus intravenous antibiotics:** We found one small quasi randomised trial (73 people with erysipelas in hospital, assigned alternately to each group) of oral versus intravenous penicillin.[9] Inclusion criteria were no suspected septicemia and a temperature greater than 38.5 °C on admission. It found no significant difference in clinical efficacy. However, clinical efficacy was assessed by indirect measures (temperature fall, length of hospital stay, and absence from work), and no results were provided on relapse rates. **Combinations of antibiotics:** We found no RCTs of combinations of antibiotics. **Different antibiotic regimens:** We found two RCTs comparing different antibiotic regimens.[10,11] One small unblinded RCT (58 people with moderate to severe cellulitis — defined as cellulitis requiring parenteral antibiotics) compared intravenous flucloxacillin (1 g every 6 hours for a mean of 9 days) versus ceftriaxone (1 g daily for 7 days).[10] Only 45 people (78%) completed the study. It found no significant difference in the rate of clinical cure (complete resolution of all signs and symptoms). More people achieved clinical success (cure or improvement) with ceftriaxone, but the difference did not quite reach significance (16/22 [72%] with flucloxacillin v 22/23 [96%] with ceftriaxone; ARR +23%, 95% CI −0.4% to +73%). The trial provided no data on relapse rates. The second RCT (69 people with erysipelas) compared oral roxithromycin versus intravenous followed by oral penicillin.[11] Inclusion criteria were a white blood cell count greater than 10×10^9/litre and a body temperature greater than 38 °C. Mean treatment duration in both groups was 13 days (range 2–29). It found no significant difference in cure rates between treatments (29/38 [76%] with penicillin v 26/31 [84%] with roxithromycin; ARR +7.6%, 95% CI −7.7% to +35%). **Short versus long courses of antibiotics:** We found no RCTs comparing different durations of treatment.

Harms: Out of 22 people treated with flucloxacillin, three had nausea and vomiting, two had diarrhoea, and one had abdominal pain.[10] Out of

23 people treated with ceftriaxone, two had diarrhoea and vomiting and one had vaginal candidiasis.[10] Drug related rashes occurred in two out of 38 people receiving penicillin, although no adverse effects were reported in 31 people receiving roxithromycin.[11] Adverse events occurred in 15 people taking oral penicillin (exanthem 4, diarrhoea 7, abscess 4) and in 10 people taking intravenous penicillin (exanthem 2, diarrhoea 4, cannula phlebitis 4).[9]

Comment: We found several RCTs of antibiotics in people with a range of skin infections, including cellulitis, but none analysed the subgroup with cellulitis separately.[12-16] The trials of different antibiotics were too small to detect clinically important differences.[10,11] The first trial defined moderate to severe cellulitis as cellulitis requiring parenteral antibiotics.[10] It gave no information on what factors were used to assess the need for parenteral antibiotics.

QUESTION Does the treatment of predisposing factors reduce disease recurrence?

We found no evidence on the effects of treatment of predisposing factors on disease recurrence.

Benefits: We found no systematic reviews, RCTs, or observational studies answering this question.

Harms: We found no good evidence.

Comment: Although there is a consensus that successful treatment of the predisposing factors reduces the risk of developing erysipelas/cellulitis (see aetiology, p 1147), we found no evidence to support this.

REFERENCES

1. Office of Population Censuses and Surveys. *Morbidity statistics from general practice. Fourth National Study.* HMSO 1992 (series MB5):272.
2. Hospital in-patient inquiry. HMSO 1985 (series MB4):16,28.
3. Bernard P, Bedane C, Mounier M, et al. Streptococcal cause of erysipelas and cellulitis in adults. *Arch Dermatol* 1989;125:779–782.
4. Dupuy A, Benchikhi H, Roujeau J-C, et al. Risk factors for erysipelas of the leg (cellulitis): case-control study. *BMJ* 1999;318:1591–1594.
5. Aly AA, Roberts NM, Seipol K, MacLellan DG. Case survey of management of cellulitis in a tertiary teaching hospital. *Med J Aust* 1996;165:553–556.
6. Jorup-Ronstrom C, Britton S. Recurrent erysipelas: predisposing factors and costs of prophylaxis. *Infection* 1987;15:105–106.
7. Hook EW, Hooton TM, Horton CA, et al. Microbiologic evaluation of cutaneous cellulitis in adults. *Arch Intern Med* 1986;146:295–297.
8. Leppard BJ, Seal DV, Colman G, Hallas G. The value of bacteriology and serology in the diagnosis of cellulitis and erysipelas. *Br J Dermatol* 1985; 112:559–567.
9. Jorup-Ronstrom C, Britton A, Gavlevik K, et al. The course, costs and complications of oral versus intravenous penicillin therapy of erysipelas. *Infection* 1984;12:390–394.

10. Vinen J, Hudson B, Chan B, Fernandes C. A randomized comparative study of once-daily ceftriaxone and 6-hourly flucloxacillin in the treatment of moderate to severe cellulitis. Clinical efficacy, safety and pharmacoeconomic implications. *Clin Drug Invest* 1996;12:221–225.
11. Bernard P, Plantin P, Roger H, et al. Roxithromycin versus penicillin in the treatment of erysipelas in adults: a comparative study. *Br J Dermatol* 1992; 127:155–159.
12. Neldner KH. Double-blind randomized study of oral temafloxacin and cefadroxil in patients with mild to moderately severe bacterial skin infections. *Am J Med* 1991;91(suppl 6A):111–114.
13. Nolen TM, Conetta BJ, Durham SJ, Wilber RB. Treatment of mild to moderate skin and skin-structure infections. *Infect Med* 1992;9(suppl C):56–67.
14. Wachs G, Rogan MP, Cefprozil Multicentre Study Group. Cefprozil vs. Erythromycin for mild to moderate skin and skin-structure infections. *Infect Med* 1992;9(suppl E):57–65.
15. Nolen TM. Clinical trials of cefprozil for treatment of skin and skin structure infections: review. *Clin Infect Dis* 1992;14(suppl 2):255–263.
16. Perez-Ruvalcaba JA, Quintero-Perez NP, Morales-Reyes JJ, et al. Double-blind comparison of Ciprofloxacin with Cefotaxime in the treatment of skin and skin structure infections. *Am J Med* 1987;82(suppl 4A):242–246.

Andrew Morris
Specialist Registrar in Dermatology, University Hospital, Nottingham, UK
Competing interests: None declared.

Skin disorders

Chronic plaque psoriasis

Search date January 2001: expanded this issue

Luigi Naldi and Berthold Rzany

QUESTIONS

INTERVENTIONS

To be covered in future issues of *Clinical Evidence*

Tacrolimus, anti CD4 monoclonal antibody, cytokine blocking agents

See glossary, p 1162

Key Messages

- We found no good evidence on the effects of non-drug treatments.
- We found that topical treatments have been evaluated only in the short term, with few comparative RCTs. We found no good evidence on the value of maintenance treatment with topical treatments or on methods for assessing individuals' preferences and satisfaction.
- RCTs have found that ultraviolet B (UVB) phototherapy and psoralen plus ultraviolet A (PUVA) are effective in clearing psoriasis and in its long term maintenance. Long term treatment with PUVA carries a risk of squamous cell carcinoma.
- RCTs have found that cyclosporin clears psoriasis, but we found little evidence of its value as maintenance treatment. Toxicity makes treatment unacceptable to many people.

© Clinical Evidence 2001;5:1150–1164.

- We found limited evidence on the long term effects of other systemic treatments (etretinate, acitretin, methotrexate, and fumaric acid derivatives) and no comparative RCTs.

DEFINITION	Chronic plaque psoriasis is a chronic inflammatory skin disease characterised by well demarcated erythematous scaly patches on the extensor surfaces of the body and scalp. The lesions may itch, sting, and occasionally bleed. Dystrophic nail changes are found in more than a third of people with chronic plaque psoriasis, and psoriatic arthropathy occurs in 1–3%. The condition waxes and wanes with wide variations between and within individuals. Other varieties of psoriasis include guttate, inverse, pustular, and erythrodermic psoriasis. This review deals only with treatments for chronic plaque psoriasis.
INCIDENCE/ PREVALENCE	Psoriasis affects 1–2% of the general population. It is believed to be less frequent in people from Africa and Asia, but we found no convincing epidemiological data.[1]
AETIOLOGY/ RISK FACTORS	Genetic and environmental factors are both important. About a third of people with psoriasis have a family history of psoriasis, but physical trauma, acute infection, and selected medications (e.g. lithium salts and β blockers) are commonly viewed as triggers. A few observational studies have linked the onset or relapse of psoriasis with stressful life events and personal habits, including cigarette smoking and, less consistently, alcohol consumption. Others have found an association of psoriasis with body mass index and an inverse association with the intake of fruit and vegetables.
PROGNOSIS	We found no long term prognostic studies. With the exception of erythrodermic and acute generalised pustular psoriasis (severe conditions affecting less than 1% of people with psoriasis and requiring intensive hospital care), psoriasis is not known to affect mortality. Psoriasis may substantially affect quality of life.[2] At present there is no cure for psoriasis.
AIMS	To achieve short term suppression of symptoms and long term modulation of disease severity; to improve quality of life, with minimal adverse effects of treatment.
OUTCOMES	State of lesions over time; use of routine treatments; duration of remission; patient satisfaction and autonomy; disease related quality of life; adverse effects of treatment. We found no documented evidence that clinical activity scores, such as the Psoriasis Area Severity Index (PASI) (see glossary, p 1162), are reliable proxies for these outcomes. Many clinical studies provide no explicit criteria for severity.[3]
METHODS	*Clinical Evidence* update search and appraisal January 2001. In addition, we hand searched a number of dermatological and medical journals for the years 1976–1996 as a project of the European Dermatoepidemiology Network. These were the *Journal of Investigative Dermatology, British Journal of Dermatology, Dermatology, Acta Dermo-Venereologica, Archives of Dermatology, Journal of the American Academy of Dermatology, Annales de Dermatologie et de Vénéréologie, Giornale Italiano di Dermatologia e Venereologia, Hautarzt, British Medical Journal, Lancet, Journal of the American Medical Association,* and *New England Journal of Medicine.*

We found no good evidence on the effects of non-drug treatments. A few interventions have been tested in small RCTs.

Benefits: We found no systematic review. **Heliotherapy:** We found one RCT (2 year crossover design, 95 people), which compared 4 weeks of supervised heliotherapy versus no intervention.[4] Heliotherapy significantly improved psoriasis and reduced use of routine treatment in the year after heliotherapy by 30%. **Sunbeds:** We found one small RCT (38 people with chronic stable plaque psoriasis) comparing UVA light versus placebo (visible light).[5] In each person, one side of the body was exposed to UVA light and the other to placebo. The trial found a small improvement in the modified Psoriasis Area and Severity Score (mean PASI score 3.9 UVA treated side v 4.2 placebo treated side, $P = 0.04$). **Fish oil supplementation:** We found six RCTs, which reported conflicting results. The largest RCT (145 people) found no significant benefit from fish oil versus corn oil.[6] **Oral vitamin D:** One RCT (50 people) found no significant difference in effectiveness between oral cholecalciferol and placebo.[7] **Stress reduction:** We found two small RCTs, which found that psychological interventions to reduce stress improved psoriasis. The largest RCT (51 people) found slight but significant improvement in psoriasis activity scores.[8] **Lifestyle change:** We found no RCTs of smoking cessation or dietary change in people with psoriasis. **Antistreptococcal treatments:** We found one systematic review of antistreptococcal interventions for guttate and chronic plaque psoriasis (search date 1999, 1 RCT, 20 people).[9] The review found no evidence that tonsillectomy (or antibiotics) versus placebo is beneficial. **Thermal baths:** We found no good quality RCTs. We found one poor quality RCT (50 people), which compared thermal bath (oligometallic, bicarbonate, calcium, and magnesium rich water) versus tap water bath.[10] Clinical improvement occurred in more people having a thermal bath versus a tap water bath (64% v 11%). **Acupuncture:** We found one RCT (56 people), which found no significant difference between classic acupuncture and sham (placebo) acupuncture.[11]

Harms: We found no good evidence on harms.

Comment: As several trigger and perpetuating factors for psoriasis have been recognised, including physical trauma, acute infections, smoking, diet, and stress, there is good reason to believe that disease severity could be modulated by non-drug treatments. However, we found no good evidence on the effects of non-drug treatments.

OPTION   **EMOLLIENTS AND KERATOLYTICS**

We found no clear evidence on the effects of emollients and keratolytics.

Benefits: We found two systematic reviews of emollients and keratolytics[12,13] and five additional RCTs. One systematic review (search date 1994, 4 RCTs, 245 people) found that capsaicin versus other treatments had a beneficial effect on itching, scaling, and erythema.[13] However, there was significant unexplained heterogeneity in the results from individual trials. The other systematic review (search date 1999, 10 RCTs) evaluated *aloe vera* for a large variety of conditions, including psoriasis. The review found no clear evidence of effectiveness, but did not exclude the possibility of a clinically important effect.[12] The largest of the additional RCTs (43 people) found that emollients temporarily improved psoriasis when they were combined with UVB radiation.[14]

Harms: Local irritation and contact dermatitis have been reported with emollients and keratolytics.

Comment: Emollients and keratolytics are usually used as adjuncts to other treatments.

OPTION	TARS

Small RCTs found conflicting results on the effects of tars.

Benefits: We found no systematic review. We found one small RCT (18 people), which found that coal tar was more effective than the emollient base in improving disease activity scores.[15] Four small RCTs found conflicting results on the added efficacy of coal tar when combined with UVB exposure and dithranol (see Ingram regimen, p 1157).

Harms: Smell, staining, and burning are the main adverse effects of coal tar.

Comment: None.

OPTION	DITHRANOL

Small RCTs have found that dithranol improves chronic plaque psoriasis more than placebo. The best evidence on its effects relates to its use in the Ingram regimen (see Ingram regimen, p 1157).

Benefits: **Versus placebo:** We found no systematic review. We found two small RCTs, which found that dithranol was more effective than placebo in improving psoriasis. **Conventional versus short contact treatment:** One survey of published studies (search date 1989, 22 small RCTs) compared conventional dithranol treatment versus dithranol short contact treatment (shorter contact time at higher concentrations).[16] It found no significant differences, but the trials were too small to rule out clinically important differences.

Harms: Smell, staining, and burning are the main adverse effects of dithranol.

Comment: Few trials examined patient satisfaction, so it remains unclear whether short contact treatment is easier and more convenient for people at home compared with conventional dithranol treatment.

Chronic plaque psoriasis

OPTION **TOPICAL STEROIDS**

RCTs have found that topical steroids improve psoriasis in the short term.

Benefits: We found no systematic review. **Clearance:** More than 30 short term, mainly small, vehicle controlled RCTs, often involving within-person comparisons, found that topical mid to high potency steroids temporarily improved psoriatic lesions. The study duration was usually no longer than 8 weeks and improvement was judged mainly in terms of reduced erythema and scaling. The largest parallel group RCTs have evaluated the more recently developed molecules (such as mometasone). **Maintenance:** One RCT (90 people with one target area cleared or nearly cleared of psoriasis by betamethasone dipropionate) found better control at 6 months by topical steroids applied once a week than by placebo (AR for maintenance of clearance in the target area 60% v 20%).[17] **Occlusive dressings:** Twelve small RCTs, mostly using people as their own controls, found that occlusive polyethylene or hydrocolloid dressings enhanced clinical activity.

Harms: Topical steroids may cause striae and atrophy, which increase with clinical potency and use of occlusive dressings. Continuous use may lead to adrenocortical suppression,[18] and case reports suggest that severe flares of the disease may occur on withdrawal. Diminishing clinical response with repeated use (tachyphylaxis) has been described, but we found no estimates of its frequency.

Comment: As the RCT assessed only maintenance value within the target area, the results may not generalise to clinical practice.[17]

OPTION **VITAMIN D DERIVATIVES**

One systematic review of RCTs and long term uncontrolled studies have found that calcipotriol improves plaque psoriasis compared with placebo and is at least as effective as topical steroids, coal tars, and dithranol. The review found that calcipotriol monotherapy causes more irritation than potent topical steroids. Only limited evidence is available for other vitamin D derivatives, including tacalcitol, maxacalcitol, and calcitriol.

Benefits: We found one systematic review (search date 1999, 37 RCTs, 6038 people)[19] and an additional seven RCTs of calcipotriol. **Versus placebo:** The review identified eight RCTs, which found benefit in people with mild to moderately severe plaque psoriasis (mean difference in the percentage change in severity index was 44%, 95% CI 28% to 60%). Long term uncontrolled studies found that treatment gains were maintained in about 70% of people for as long as the treatment was continued.[20] **Versus each other:** We found six RCTs comparing calcipotriol versus another vitamin D derivative. Five were of tacalcitol, the largest of which (287 people) found that tacalcitol once daily was slightly less effective than calcipotriol twice daily in clearing psoriasis.[21] Another RCT (144 people) found that maxacalcitol once daily compared favourably with calcipotriol once daily (55% v 46% of patients reporting large improvement or clearance). However, the established dosage of calcipotriol is twice daily.[22] **Versus topical steroids:** In four short term comparative RCTs, the largest one involving 345 people, calcipotriol was either as effective or slightly more effective than topical steroids.[23] **Versus dithranol short contact treatment:** Four RCTs, the largest one involving 478 people,[24] found that calcipotriol was either as effective or slightly more effective than dithranol short contact treatment. However, one recent RCT (171 people) found that, of people who initially improved on treatment, more stayed in remission with dithranol than with calcipotriol.[25] One RCT (114 people) found no significant difference between twice daily calcitriol ointment and short contact therapy.[26] The treatment acceptability was rated as good by 47% with calcitriol and only 22% with dithranol. Twenty eight people (24%) terminated the study prematurely. **Versus coal tar:** Two RCTs, the largest one involving 122 people,[27] found that calcipotriol was more effective than coal tar. **With other treatments:** Five RCTs, the largest one involving 169 people, found that a combination of calcipotriol with topical steroids provided better clearance and maintenance.[28]

Harms: The review found that calcipotriol monotherapy caused more irritation than potent topical steroids (NNH 10, 95% CI 6 to 34).[19] Perilesional irritation from calcipotriol has been reported in as many as 25% of people, the face and skin folds being more susceptible. In the short term, the combination of a topical steroid may reduce the incidence of skin irritation.[29] Hypercalcaemia and hypercalciuria are dose related adverse effects.

Comment: There is a consensus that the dosage of calcipotriol should be limited to 100 g a week.

OPTION   TOPICAL RETINOIDS (TAZAROTENE)

RCTs have found that tazarotene improves chronic plaque psoriasis in the short term compared with placebo. One RCT has found that tazarotene plus topical steriods versus calcipotriol improves short term outcomes.

Benefits: We found no systematic review. **Versus placebo:** Three vehicle controlled RCTs found that tazarotene was effective in chronic plaque psoriasis. In the largest RCT (318 evaluable people), clinical response was judged after 12 weeks of treatment to be good, excellent, or completely cleared in 60% on tazarotene 0.1%, 50% on tazarotene 0.05%, and 30% on vehicle control (RRR for tazarotene 0.1% compared with placebo 43%, 95% CI 30% to 60%).[30] **Versus steroids:** One RCT (275 evaluable people) found that tazarotene was nearly as effective in clearing psoriasis as the high potency topical steroid flucinonide.[31] **Plus steroids:** Three RCTs, the largest one involving 398 people, found that topical mid or high potency steroids added to tazarotene, or alternated on a daily basis with tazarotene, increased the response rate compared with tazarotene alone.[32,33] **Versus calcipotriol:** One RCT (120 people) compared tazarotene 0.1% in conjunction with topical mometasone furoate 0.1% once daily, versus calcipotriol 0.005% twice daily for 8 weeks.[34] The trial found significant improvements with the tazarotene and mometasone combination versus calcipotriol for the number of people showing marked improvement (≥ 75% global improvement) after 2 weeks, and for scaling, erythema and percentage of body surface coverage after 4 weeks. It found no significant difference in the number of people attaining complete or almost complete clearance (≥90% clearance) at any time during follow up.

Harms: The RCTs found that some perilesional irritation was reported in most people. Addition of steroids reduced the incidence of patient withdrawals and treatment related adverse effects.[32,33]

Comment: Tazarotene is contraindicated in women who are, or intend to become, pregnant as it is potentially teratogenic.

QUESTION What are the effects of treatments with ultraviolet light?

OPTION PHOTOTHERAPY

RCTs have found that phototherapy improves psoriasis in the short term and when used as maintenance treatment. We found no good evidence that narrow band phototherapy is better than broad band.

Benefits: We found no systematic review. **Clearance:** We found two RCTs comparing UVB with PUVA.[35,36] The first RCT (183 people with moderate to severe psoriasis) found no significant difference in clearance rates between PUVA and UVB radiation (88% for PUVA v 80% for UVB; RRR for non-clearance with PUVA compared with broad band UVB radiation +38%, 95% CI −22% to +71%).[35] Subgroup analysis found that UVB radiation was significantly less effective in people with more than 50% body involvement. The second RCT (100 people) found that clearance was achieved in more people treated with PUVA compared with narrow band UVB (84% v 63%).[36] **Maintenance:** One RCT examined the maintenance value of weekly treatment with UVB phototherapy after initial clearance. Of the 165 people enrolled, 104 (63%) were cleared of their symptoms. More than 50% of people in the maintenance group were still clear 181 days after initial clearance compared with 28% in the control group (RRR for relapsing at 181 days 33%, 95% CI 8% to 59%).[37] **Narrow versus broad band phototherapy:** We found only three small, short term, self controlled RCTs, the largest one involving 23 people.[38]

Harms: UVB radiation may increase photoageing and the risk of skin cancer. A recent systematic review (search date 1996) concluded that it was unlikely that the excess risk of non-melanoma skin cancer associated with UVB radiation exceeded 2% a year.[39]

Comment: None.

OPTION PUVA

RCTs have found effective clearance and long term maintenance with conventional PUVA treatment (i.e. oral 8-methoxypsoralen plus UVA radiation). Long term treatment carries the risk of squamous cell carcinoma, reported in a quarter of people.

Benefits: We found no systematic review. We found 17 RCTs. **Clearance:** One RCT (224 people) compared PUVA treatment versus an inpatient Ingram regimen (see glossary, p 1162) in people with at least 10% of body surface area involved.[40] The trial found clearance rates of 91% with PUVA versus 82% with the Ingram regimen. Another RCT (85 people with skin types I and II — see glossary, p 1162) found that the clearance rate was lower with the minimal phototoxic dose regimen compared with the skin type regimen (see glossary, p 1162) (67.5% v 95%).[41] **Maintenance:** The largest RCT (1005 people whose psoriasis had been cleared by PUVA) found that maintenance treatment reduced relapse at 18 months (AR of flares 27% with treatment once a week, 34% with treatment once every 3 weeks, and 62% with no treatment; RRR for relapse with once weekly treatment v no treatment 56%, 95% CI 44% to 68%).[42] **Different regimens:** At least eight small RCTs have looked at different combinations of ultraviolet radiation and systemic or topical treatments, including UVA plus 5-methoxypsoralen, UVA plus bath water delivered psoralen (bath PUVA), and psoralen plus UVB. The trials found no significant difference from conventional PUVA treatment, but they were probably too small to exclude a clinically important difference.

Harms: The best evidence on chronic toxicity comes from an ongoing study of more than 1300 people who first received PUVA treatment in 1975.[43,44] The study found a dose dependent increased risk of squamous cell carcinoma, basal cell carcinoma, and possibly malignant melanoma compared with the risk in the general population. A recent systematic review of eight additional studies (search date 1998) has confirmed the findings concerning non-melanoma skin cancer.[45] Premature photoageing is another expected adverse effect. After less than 15 years, about a quarter of people exposed to 300 or more treatments of PUVA had at least one squamous cell carcinoma of the skin, with particularly high risk for people with skin types I and II. In people who wear UVA opaque glasses for 24 hours after psoralen ingestion, the risk of cataract development seems negligible. A combined analysis of two cohort studies (944 people treated with bath PUVA) excluded a threefold excess risk of squamous cell carcinoma after a mean follow up of 14.7 years, suggesting that bath PUVA is possibly safer than conventional PUVA.[46]

Comment: People receiving PUVA need close monitoring for acute toxicity and cutaneous carcinogenic effects.

OPTION   COMBINATION REGIMENS

One RCT has found that the Ingram regimen was of similar effectiveness to PUVA in clearing moderate to severe psoriasis. We found no good evidence on effectiveness of the Goeckerman treatment.

Benefits: We found no systematic review. **Ingram regimen:** One RCT (224 people) compared an inpatient Ingram regimen (dithranol concentration 0.01–1.0%) versus PUVA in people with at least 10% of body surface involvement. It found that clearance rates were 82% (95% CI 77% to 89%) with the Ingram regimen compared with 91% (95% CI 86% to 96%) with PUVA.[40] Five small RCTs, the largest one involving 53 people,[47] found conflicting results on the added efficacy of dithranol when combined with UVB exposure. However, the trials were too small to rule out a clinically important difference. **Goeckerman treatment:** We found no good evidence on the effects of combining coal tar and UVB radiation. **Other combinations:** We found five RCTs, which assessed the combination of calcipotriol with UVB radiation or PUVA, but the results were conflicting.[48–51] The largest RCT (164 people) found that fewer UVB treatments were required to achieve clearance in people receiving calcipotriol plus UVB compared with UVB alone (median number of UVB treatments required with calcipotriol plus UVB was 22 v 25 with UVB alone; no statistical analysis for a continuous variable was reported).[48]

Harms: Adverse effects vary with the treatments being combined. Local irritation often occurs.

Comment: None.

QUESTION What are the effects of systemic drug treatments?

OPTION ORAL RETINOIDS (ETRETINATE AND ACITRETIN)

We found limited evidence that oral retinoids may achieve complete clearance in a small proportion of people with plaque psoriasis. We found no good evidence about the effects of oral retinoids as maintenance treatment. Adverse effects lead to discontinuation of treatment in 10–20% of patients. Teratogenicity in females make oral retinoids less acceptable.

Benefits: We found no systematic review (although there has been one of oral retinoids in psoriatic arthropathy).[52] **Versus placebo:** We found seven RCTs comparing etretinate (0.2–1.2 mg/kg per day) versus placebo or conventional therapy. The trials reported wide differences in effects, with clearance found in 15–90% of participants. Differences may be explained by different entry criteria, outcome measures, or treatment schedules. Intention to treat analysis was not performed, and the withdrawal rates were high (10–30%). The largest RCT (97 people) was a crossover placebo controlled study with four phases, each lasting 3 months.[53] A total of 74 people (76%) completed all the study phases. Analysis of the first phase (completed by 95 people) found that etretinate improved clinical outcomes versus placebo (AR of clinically significant improvement 16% with etretinate v 6% with placebo, RRR 16%, 95% CI 10% to 22%). **Versus each other:** Four RCTs compared etretinate and acitretin (0.5–1.0 mg/kg per day). The largest (168 people) found similar benefits but a higher rate of mucocutaneous adverse effects with acitretin, especially hair loss and scaling of palms and soles. There was a higher withdrawal rate with acitretin (acitretrin 12% v etretinate 5%).[54] **In combination with other treatments:** Nine RCTs found that the combination of PUVA or UVB and retinoids accelerated response and therefore reduced the cumulative ultraviolet exposure and retinoid dosage. The largest RCT (82 people) compared UVB plus acitretin (35 mg reducing to 25 mg after the first 4 weeks) versus UVB plus placebo in severe psoriasis.[55] After 8 weeks, combination treatment improved response rate compared with control (AR for 75% or more reduction in psoriasis severity index 60% with combination v 24% with control group; RRR 47%, 95% CI 34% to 60%). One RCT (135 people) compared the combination of calcipotriol and acitretin versus acitretin alone.[56] It found a higher clearance rate with the combination therapy (clearance with combination 67% v 41% with acitretin alone; RRR 44%, 95% CI 38% to 50%). The withdrawal rates were 21% with combination and 35% with control. **Different types of psoriasis:** In subgroup analyses of the above mentioned RCTs and two further small RCTs,[57,58] pustular and erythrodermic psoriasis seemed to be more responsive to etretinate and acitretin than plaque psoriasis. **Maintenance:** We found one small RCT (36 people) of 1 year duration comparing low dose etretinate (half of the maximum dose tolerated) versus placebo, after clearance with combined PUVA and etretinate.[59] Etretinate reduced relapse rate compared with placebo (relapse rate was 6/16 [37%] with etretinate v 15/20 [75%] with placebo; RRR 50%, 95% CI 22% to 78%).

Harms: Most people experience mucocutaneous adverse effects, such as dry skin, cheilitis, and conjunctivitis. Increased serum cholesterol and triglyceride concentrations occurred in about half of the people. Low grade hepatotoxicity was observed in about 1% of people treated with etretinate.[60] Occasionally, acute hepatitis occurred as a purported idiosyncratic hypersensitivity reaction. Radiographic evidence of extraspinal tendon and ligament calcifications has been documented. In one cohort study, a quarter of 956 people treated with etretinate attributed a joint problem or its worsening to the drug.[60] Etretinate is a known teratogen and may be detected in the plasma for 2–3 years after treatment stops. Acitretin can undergo esterification to etretinate.

Comment: Women of childbearing age are given effective contraception for 1 month before starting etretinate and acitretin, throughout treatment, and after stopping treatment for at least 3 years because it is potentially teratogenic. Etretinate is no longer available in many countries.

OPTION	METHOTREXATE

Limited evidence from one small RCT suggests that methotrexate improves skin lesions in psoriasis. Non-randomised data suggest that clearance can be maintained as long as treatment is continued. About half of people relapse within 6 months of stopping treatment. Long term treatment carries the risk of serious adverse effects, especially liver fibrosis, reported in about a third of people.

Benefits: We found no systematic review (although there has been one in psoriatic arthropathy).[52] **Clearance:** We found one small RCT (37 people). It found that methotrexate reduced psoriatic surface area involvement compared with placebo after 12 weeks (P = 0.04).[61] **Maintenance:** We found no RCTs. In one uncontrolled series (113 people with severe psoriasis), maintenance treatment with low dose methotrexate (weekly dose not exceeding 15 mg) provided satisfactory control of skin lesions in 81% of people (mean treat-

duration 8 years). When treatment was stopped, 45% of people experienced a full relapse within 6 months.[62]

Harms: In the uncontrolled case series mentioned above, treatment was stopped in 33 of 113 people (29%) because of adverse effects.[62] The most serious acute reaction, particularly in elderly people, is dose related myelosuppression. In the long term, major adverse events included liver fibrosis and pulmonary toxicity. One systematic review found that about 28% (95% CI 24% to 32%) of people taking long term methotrexate for psoriasis and rheumatoid arthritis developed liver fibrosis of histological grade 1 or higher on liver biopsy, whereas 5% developed advanced liver disease (histological grade IIIB or IV).[63] The risk was dose related and increased with increased alcohol consumption. A limitation of the systematic review was the lack of untreated control groups. Pulmonary disease associated with methotrexate has been described as an acute or chronic interstitial pneumonitis.[64] Adverse pulmonary effects of treatment are considered much rarer in psoriasis than in rheumatoid arthritis, but we found no published evidence to support this claim. Several drug interactions that increase methotrexate toxicity have been described (e.g. with sulphonamides). Methotrexate seems to double the risk of developing squamous cell carcinoma in people exposed to PUVA and may be an independent in people with psoriatic arthritis risk factor for this cancer.[43] A higher risk of lymphoproliferative diseases in long term users has been suggested by a few case reports. On the basis of data from a large case series (248 people), the cumulative incidence of lymphoma is not expected to be much higher than 1%.[65]

Comment: People using methotrexate are closely monitored for liver toxicity,[66] and advised to limit their consumption of alcohol. The most reliable test of liver damage remains needle biopsy of the liver. It is rare for life threatening liver disease to develop with the first 1.0–1.5 g of methotrexate.

| OPTION | CYCLOSPORIN AND OTHER IMMUNOSUPPRESSIVE DRUGS |

RCTs have found that cyclosporin clears psoriasis, especially at higher doses, although toxicity is high and causes many people to withdraw from continuous long term treatment. We found little evidence about the effects of other immunosuppressive drugs, such as tacrolimus.

Benefits: We found no systematic review. **Clearance:** Six dose-finding, placebo controlled RCTs found that cyclosporin temporarily controlled psoriasis. A pooled analysis based on five European dose-finding studies used individual data from 457 people. Success (defined as activity score reduction ≥ 75%) was more likely with higher initial daily doses of cyclosporin (24% achieved success with 1.25 mg/kg per day; 52% with 2.5–3 mg/kg per day; 88% with 5 mg/kg per day).[67] Most people relapsed within weeks after stopping treatment. One RCT (309 people) found a more rapid response with a microemulsion formulation than with the usual oil-in-water emulsion.[68] **Maintenance:** Three RCTs have assessed different maintenance schedules.[69–71] In one study, 61 people who had achieved clearance during an induction phase were randomised to 1.5 or

3.0 mg/kg a day cyclosporin or placebo.[69] At 4 months' follow up, there had been no relapse in 57% of the 3 mg/kg group compared with 21% of the 1.5 mg/kg group and 5% of the placebo group (RRR for relapse in the 3 mg/kg group compared with placebo 55%, 95% CI 30% to 80%). **Speed of discontinuation:** Another RCT (400 people) compared abrupt versus tapered discontinuation of a microemulsion formulation of cyclosporin (starting dose 2.5 mg/kg per day) after clearance was achieved or after a maximum of 12 weeks' treatment (short course treatment). The median time to relapse was significantly less in people stopping abruptly (109 days v 113 days, P = 0.04). Participants were followed up for at least 1 year during which time they were allowed to use as many treatment courses as necessary (intermittent short course treatment). A total of 259 people (65%) received two treatment courses and 117 (29%) three treatment courses.[71] **Versus other treatments:** One RCT (210 people) compared cyclosporin 2.5 mg/kg a day versus etretinate 0.5 mg/kg a day. After 10 weeks, 47% of the people taking cyclosporin and 10% taking etretinate showed a reduction of more than 80% in skin involvement.[72] **Different types of psoriasis:** One small RCT (58 people) found that low dose (1–2 mg/kg per day) cyclosporin was effective maintenance treatment in palmoplantar pustulosis.[73]

Harms: In a follow up study of 122 consecutive people treated for 3–76 months at a dose not exceeding 5 mg/kg a day, 104 people discontinued treatment.[74] Of these, 55 stopped treatment because of adverse effects, which included renal dysfunction in 34 people (28%) and hypertension in 23 people (19%). One RCT (400 people) found that intermittent treatment with a microemulsion formulation for 1 year was well tolerated and produced no clinically significant change of blood pressure or creatinine concentration.[71] Long term follow up studies are needed to confirm this finding.

Comment: Renal function should be monitored. The long term safety profile has yet to be defined. Evidence about the effects of other immunosuppressive drugs remains inconclusive.

| OPTION | FUMARIC ACID DERIVATIVES |

We found limited evidence of short term effectiveness but high rates of acute adverse effects. We found no evidence on the value of fumaric acid derivatives as maintenance treatment.

Benefits: We found no systematic review. We found five RCTs. The largest RCT (100 people) found a response, ranging from slight improvement to complete clearance, in 71% of those treated with esters of fumaric acid (maximum dose 1290 mg ester mixture per day) compared with 18% in the placebo group.[75]

Harms: The safety profile is poorly defined. Acute adverse effects, including flushing and gastrointestinal symptoms, have been reported in as many as 75% of people.[75] Eosinophilia is often observed, and we found a few case reports of drug induced tubular nephropathy.[76]

Comment: The largest RCT had a high withdrawal rate (48%).[75]

Chronic plaque psoriasis

GLOSSARY

Goeckerman treatment A daily application of coal tar followed by UVB irradiation.

Ingram regimen A daily coal tar bath, UVB irradiation, and dithranol.

Psoriasis Area and Severity Index (PASI score) Composite score grading severity of psoriasis in six body regions according to erythema, scaling, thickness, and the total area of skin affected.

Skin types A clinical classification of an individual's burning and tanning tendencies. Usually ranges from skin phototype I (which always burns and never tans) to skin phototype VI (marked constitutive pigmentation).

Skin type regimen and minimal phototoxic dose regimen The four parameters of PUVA are the dose of psoralen, the frequency of treatment, the initial dose of UVA, and the incremental UVA dose. The initial and incremental UVA doses are described by at least two regimens. In the minimal phototoxic dose regimen, the initial UVA dose is a fraction of the minimal phototoxic dose. Weekly increments in dose occur until a maximum dose is reached. In the skin type regimen, the initial dose is based on skin phototype. Weekly dose increments are decreased if erythema develops.

Substantive changes since last issue

Sunbeds New RCT;[5] conclusion unchanged.

Thermal baths New poor quality RCT;[10] conclusion unchanged.

Vitamin D derivatives New RCT;[26] conclusion unchanged.

Topical retinoids New RCT;[34] conclusion unchanged.

Oral retinoids Study with weak methods removed; conclusion unchanged.

REFERENCES

1. Naldi L. Psoriasis. In: Williams HC, Strachan DP, eds. *The challenge of dermato-epidemiology.* Boca Raton: CRC Press, 1997;175–190.

2. O'Neill P, Kelly P. Postal questionnaire of disability in the community associated with psoriasis. *BMJ* 1996;313:919–921.

3. Petersen LJ, Kristensen JK. Selection of patients for psoriasis clinical trials: a survey of the recent dermatological literature. *J Dermatol Treat* 1992; 3:171–176.

4. Snellman E, Aromaa A, Jansen CT, et al. Supervised four-week heliotherapy alleviates the long-term course of psoriasis. *Acta Derm Venereol* 1993;73:388–392.

5. Turner RJ, Walshaw D, Diffey BL, Farr PM. A controlled study of ultraviolet A sunbed treatment of psoriasis. *Br J Dermatol* 2000;143:957–963.

6. Soyland E, Funk J, Rajka G, et al. Effect of dietary supplementation with very-long-chain n-3 fatty acids in patients with psoriasis. *N Engl J Med* 1993;328:1812–1816.

7. Siddiqui MA, Al Khawajah MM. Vitamin D and psoriasis: a randomised double-blind placebo-controlled study. *J Dermatol Treat* 1990;1:243–245.

8. Zachariae R, Oster H, Bjerring P, Kragballe K. Effects of psychologic intervention on psoriasis: a preliminary report. *J Am Acad Dermatol* 1996;34:1008–1015.

9. Owen CM, Chalmers RJG, O'Sullivan T, Griffiths CEM. Antistreptococcal interventions for guttate and chronic plaque psoriasis. In: The Cochrane Library, Issue 2, 2000. Oxford: Update Software. Search date November 1999; primary sources Cochrane Clinical Trials Register, Medline, Embase, Salford Database of Psoriasis Trials, European Dermato-Epidemiology Network Psoriasis Trials Database.

10. Zumiani G, Zanoni M, Agostini G. Evaluation of the efficacy of Comano thermal baths water versus tap water in the treatment of psoriasis. *G Ital Dermatol Venereol* 2000;135:259–263.

11. Jerner B, Skogh M, Vahlquist A. A controlled trial of acupuncture in psoriasis: no convincing effect. *Acta Derm Venereol* 1997;77:154–156.

12. Zhang WY, Li Wan Po A. The effectiveness of topically applied capsaicin: a meta-analysis. *Eur J Clin Pharmacol* 1994;46:517–522. Search date 1994; primary sources BIDS, Medline.

13. Vogler BK, Ernst E. Aloe vera: a systematic review of its clinical effectiveness. *Br J Gen Pract* 1999; 49:823–828. Search date May 1998; primary sources Medline 1966 to May 1998; Embase 1980 to May 1998; Biosis 1985 to May 1998; and Cochrane Library, Issue 2, 1998.

14. Berne B, Blom I, Spangberg S. Enhanced response of psoriasis to UVB therapy after pretreatment with a lubrificating base. *Acta Derm Venereol* 1990;70:474–477.

15. Kanzler MH, Gorsulowsky DC. Efficacy of topical 5% liquor carbonis detergens vs. its emollient base in the treatment of psoriasis. *Br J Dermatol* 1993;129:310–314.

16. Naldi L, Carrel CF, Parazzini F, et al. Development of anthralin short-contact therapy in psoriasis: survey of published clinical trials. *Int J Dermatol* 1992;31:126–130. Search date 1989; primary sources Medline, Index Medicus, Excerpta Medica.

17. Katz HI, Prawer SE, Medansky RS, et al. Intermittent corticosteroid treatment of psoriasis: a double-blind multicenter trial of augmented betamethasone dipropionate ointment in a pulse dose treatment regimen. *Dermatologica* 1991; 183:269–274.

18. Wilson L, Williams DI, Marsh SD. Plasma corticosteroid levels in outpatients treated with topical steroids. *Br J Dermatol* 1973;88:373–380.

19. Ashcroft DM, Li Wan Po A, Williams HC, Griffiths CEM. Systematic review of comparative efficacy

and tolerability of calcipotriol in treating chronic plaque psoriasis. *BMJ* 2000;320:963–967. Search date January 1999; primary sources Medline, Embase, Cochrane Controlled Trials Register, BIDs, hand searches of reference lists, and manufacturer of calcipotriol contacted.

20. Ramsay CA, Berth-Johnes J, Brundin J, et al. Long-term use of topical calcipotriol in chronic plaque psoriasis. *Dermatology* 1994;189:260–264.

21. Veien NK, Bjerke JR, Rossmann-Ringdahl I, Jakobsen HB. Once daily treatment of psoriasis with tacalcitol compared with twice daily treatment with calcipotriol: a double-blind trial. *Br J Dermatol* 1997;137:581–586.

22. Barker JN, Ashton RE, Marks R, et al. Topical maxacalcitol for the treatment of psoriasis vulgaris: a placebo controlled, double-blind, dose-finding study with active comparator. *Br J Dermatol* 1999;141:274–278.

23. Kragballe K, Gjertsen BT, De Hoop D, et al. Double-blind, right/left comparison of calcipotriol and betamethasone valerate in treatment of psoriasis vulgaris. *Lancet* 1991;337:193–196.

24. Berth-Jones J, Chu AC, Dodd WAH, et al. A multicentre, parallel-group comparison of calcipotriol ointment and short-contact therapy in chronic plaque psoriasis. *Br J Dermatol* 1992; 127:266–271.

25. Christensen OB, Mork NJ, Ashton R, Daniel F, Anehus S. Comparison of a treatment phase and a follow-up phase of short contact dithranol and calcipotriol in outpatients with chronic plaque psoriasis. *J Dermatol Treat* 1999;10:261–265.

26. Hutchinson PE, Marks R, White J. The efficacy, safety, and tolerance of calcitriol 3 mcgr/g ointment in the treatment of plaque psoriasis. A comparison with short-contact therapy. *Dermatology* 2000;201:139–245.

27. Pinheiro N. Comparative effects of calcipotriol ointment (50 micrograms/g) and 5% coal tar/2% allantoin/0.5% hydrocortisone cream in treating plaque psoriasis. *Br J Clin Pract* 1997;51:16–19.

28. Ruzicka T, Lorenz B. Comparison of calcipotriol monotherapy and a combination of calcipotriol and betamethasone valerate after 2 weeks' treatment with calcipotriol in the topical therapy of psoriasis vulgaris: a multicentre, double-blind, randomized study. *Br J Dermatol* 1998;138:254–258.

29. Kragballe K, Barnes L, Hamberg K, et al. Calcipotriol cream with or without concurrent topical corticosteroid in psoriasis. Tolerability and efficacy. *Br J Dermatol* 1998;139:649–654.

30. Weinstein GD, Krueger GG, Lowe NJ, et al. Tazarotene gel, a new retinoid, for topical therapy of psoriasis: vehicle-controlled study of safety, efficacy, and duration of therapeutic effect. *J Am Acad Dermatol* 1997;37:85–92.

31. Lebwohl M, Ast E, Callen JP, et al. Once-daily tazarotene gel versus twice-daily fluocinonide cream in the treatment of plaque psoriasis. *J Am Acad Dermatol* 1998;38:705–711.

32. Lebwohl MG, Breneman DL, Goffe BS, et al. Tazarotene 0.1% gel plus corticosteroid cream in the treatment of plaque psoriasis. *J Am Acad Dermatol* 1998;39:590–596.

33. Gollnick H, Menter A. Combination therapy with tazarotene plus a topical corticosteroid for the treatment of plaque psoriasis. *Br J Dermatol* 1999;140(suppl):18–23.

34. Guenther LC, Poulin YP, Pariser DM. A comparison of tazarotene 0.1% gel once daily plus mometasone furoate 0.1% cream once daily versus calcipotriene 0.005% ointment twice daily in the treatment of plaque psoriasis. *Clin Ther* 2000;22:1225–1238.

35. Boer J, Hermans J, Schothorst AA, Suurmond D. Comparison of phototherapy (UVB) and photochemotherapy (PUVA) for clearing and maintenance therapy of psoriasis. *Arch Dermatol* 1984;120:52–57.

36. Gorden PM, Diffey BL, Mathews JN, Farr PM. A randomised comparison of narrow-band TL-01 phototherapy for psoriasis. *J Am Acad Dermatol* 1999;41:728–732.

37. Stern RS, Armstrong RB, Anderson TF, et al. Effect of continued ultraviolet B phototherapy on the duration of remission of psoriasis. A randomized study. *J Am Acad Dermatol* 1986;15:546–552.

38. Storbeck K, Holzle E, Schurer N, et al. Narrow-band UVB (311 nm) versus conventional broad-band UVB with and without dithranol in phototherapy for psoriasis. *J Am Acad Dermatol* 1993;28:227–231.

39. Pieternel CM, Pasker-de-Jong M, Wielink G, et al. Treatment with UV-B for psoriasis and nonmelanoma skin cancer. A systematic review of the literature. *Arch Dermatol* 1999;135:834–840. Search date 1996; primary sources Medline, Biosis, Online Contents.

40. Rogers S, Marks J, Shuster S, et al. Comparison of photochemotherapy and dithranol in the treatment of chronic plaque psoriasis. *Lancet* 1979;i:455–458.

41. Kirby B, Buckley DA, Rogers S. Large increments in psoralen-ultraviolet A (PUVA) therapy are unsuitable for fair skinned individuals with psoriasis. *Br J Dermatol* 1999;140:661–666.

42. Melski JW, Tanenbaum L, Parrish JA, et al. Oral methoxsalen photochemotherapy for the treatment of psoriasis. A cooperative clinical trial. *J Invest Dermatol* 1977;68:328–324.

43. Stern RS, Laird N. The carcinogenic risk of treatments for severe psoriasis. Photochemotherapy follow-up study. *Cancer* 1994;73:2759–2764.

44. Stern RS, Nichols KT, Vakeva LH. Malignant melanoma in patients treated for psoriasis with methoxsalen (psoralen) and ultraviolet A radiation. *N Engl J Med* 1997;336:1041–1045.

45. Stern RS, Lunder EJ. Risk of squamous cell carcinoma and methoxsalen (psoralen) and UV-A radiation (PUVA). A meta-analysis. *Arch Dermatol* 1998;134:1582–1585. Search date 1998; primary sources Medline, Healthstar, Aidsline, Cancerlit.

46. Hannuksela-Svahn A, Sigurgeirsson B, Pukkala E, et al. Trioxsalen bath PUVA did not increase the risk of squamous cell skin carcinoma and cutaneous malignant melanoma in a joint analysis of 944 Swedish and Finnish patients with psoriasis. *Br J Dermatol* 1999;141:497–501.

47. Paramsothy Y. Effect of UVB therapy and a coal tar bath on short contact dithranol treatment for psoriasis. *Br J Dermatol* 1988;118:783–789.

48. Ramsay CA, Schwartz BE, Lowson D, et al. Calcipotriol cream combined with twice weekly broad-band UVB phototherapy: a safe, effective and UVB-sparing antipsoriatic combination treatment. The Canadian Calcipotriol and UVB Study Group. *Dermatology* 2000;200:17–24.

49. Kragballe K. Combination of topical calcipotriol (MC 903) and UVB radiation for psoriasis vulgaris. *Dermatologica* 1990;181:211–214.

50. Frappaz A, Thivolet J. Calcipotriol in combination with PUVA: a randomized double-blind placebo study in severe psoriasis. *Eur J Dermatol* 1993;3:351–354.

51. Molin L. Topical calcipotriol with phototherapy for psoriasis. The results of two randomized trials and a review of the literature. Calcipotriol-UVB Study Group. *Dermatology* 1999;198:375–381.

52. Jones G, Crotty M, Brooks P. Psoriatic arthritis. An overview of therapy and toxicity. In: The Cochrane Library, Issue 3, 2000. Oxford: Update Software. Search date February 2000; primary sources Medline, Excerpta Medica, Cochrane Clinical Trials Register.

53. Lassus A. Systemic treatment of psoriasis with an oral retinoic acid derivative (Ro 10–9359). Br J Dermatol 1980;102:195–202.

54. Kragballe K, Jansen CT, Bjerke JR, et al. A double-blind comparison of acitretin and etretinate in the treatment of severe psoriasis. Results of a Nordic multicentre study. Acta Derm Venereol 1989;69: 35–40.

55. Ruzicka T, Sommerburg C, Braun-Falco O, et al. Efficiency of acitretin in combination with UV-B in the treatment of severe psoriasis. Arch Dermatol 1990;126:482–486.

56. Van de Kerkhof PC, Cambazard F, Hutchinson PE, et al. The effect of addition of calcipotriol ointment (50 micrograms/g) to acitretin therapy in psoriasis. Br J Dermatol 1998;138:84–89.

57. Lassus A, Lauharanta J, Juvakoski T, Kanerva L. Efficacy of etretinate (Tigason) in clearing and prevention of relapse of palmoplantar pustulosis. Dermatologica 1983;166:215–219.

58. White SI, Puttick L, Marks JM. Low-dose etretinate in the maintenance of remission of palmoplantar pustular psoriasis. Br J Dermatol 1986;115:577–582.

59. Dubertret L, Chastang C, Beylot C, et al. Maintenance treatment of psoriasis by Tigason: a double-blind randomized clinical trial. Br J Dermatol 1985;113:323–330.

60. Stern RS, Fitzgerald E, Ellis CN, et al. The safety of etretinate as long-term therapy for psoriasis. Results of the etretinate follow-up study. J Am Acad Dermatol 1995;33:44–52.

61. Wilkens RF, Williams HJ, Ward JR, et al. Randomized, double-blind, placebo controlled trial of low-dose pulse methotrexate in psoriatic arthritis. Arthritis Rheum 1984;27:376–381.

62. Van Dooren-Greebe RJ, Kuijpers AL, Mulder J, et al. Methotrexate revisited: effects of long-term treatment of psoriasis. Br J Dermatol 1994;130: 204–210.

63. Whiting-O'Keefe QE, Fye KH, Sack KD. Methotrexate and histologic hepatic abnormalities. Am J Med 1991;90:711–716. Search date and primary sources not stated.

64. Cottin V, Tebib J, Souquet PJ, Bernard JP. Pulmonary function in patients receiving long-term low-dose methotrexate. Chest 1996;109:933–938.

65. Nyfors A, Jensen H. Frequency of malignant neoplasms in 248 long-term methotrexate-treated psoriatics. A preliminary study. Dermatologica 1983;167:260–261.

66. Roenigk HH, Auerbach R, Maibach H, Weinstein G, Lebwohl M. Methotrexate in psoriasis: consensus conference. J Am Acad Dermatol 1998;38:478–485.

67. Timonen P, Friend D, Abeywickrama K, et al. Efficacy of low-dose cyclosporin A in psoriasis: results of dose finding studies. Br J Dermatol 1990;122(suppl 36):33–39.

68. Koo J. A randomized double-blind study comparing the efficacy, safety and optimal dose of two formulations of cyclosporin, Neoral and Sandimmun in patients with severe psoriasis. OLP302 Study Group. Br J Dermatol 1998;139: 88–95.

69. Shupack J, Abel E, Bauer E, et al. Cyclosporin as maintenance therapy in patients with severe psoriasis. J Am Acad Dermatol 1997;36:423–432.

70. Ellis CN, Fradin MS, Hamilton TA, Voorhees JJ. Duration of remission during maintenance cyclosporin therapy for psoriasis. Arch Dermatol 1995;131:791–795.

71. Ho V, Griffiths CEM, Albrecht G, et al. Intermittent short courses of cyclosporin (Neoral) for psoriasis unresponsive to topical therapy: a 1-year multicentre, randomized study. Br J Dermatol 1999;141:283–291.

72. Mahrle G, Schulze HJ, Fraber L, et al. Low-dose short-term cyclosporin versus etretinate: improvement of skin, nail, and joint involvement. J Am Acad Dermatol 1995;32:78–88.

73. Erkko P, Granlund H, Remitz A, et al. Double-blind placebo-controlled study of long-term low-dose cyclosporin in the treatment of palmoplantar pustulosis. Br J Dermatol 1998;139:997–1004.

74. Grossman RM, Chevret S, Abi-Rached J, Blanchet F, Dubertret L. Long-term safety of cyclosporin in the treatment of psoriasis. Arch Dermatol 1996; 132:623–629.

75. Altmeyer PJ, Matthes U, Pawlak F, et al. Antipsoriatic effect of fumaric acid derivatives. Results of a multicenter double-blind study in 100 patients. J Am Acad Dermatol 1994;30:977–981.

76. Mrowietz U, Christophers E, Altmeyer P. Treatment of psoriasis with fumaric acid esters: results of a prospective multicentre study. Br J Dermatol 1998;138:456–460.

Luigi Naldi
Dermatologist
Ospedali Riuniti Bergamo
Bergamo
Italy

Berthold Rzany
Dermatologist
Klinik für Dermatologie
Universitätsklinikum Mannheim
Mannheim
Germany

Competing interests: The research activities of the Italian Group for Epidemiologic Research in Dermatology, which is coordinated by one of the authors (LN), have been supported by grants from Glaxo Wellcome, Roche, Novartis, Schering and Schering-Plough. BR, none declared.

Search date January 2001

Ian Burgess

QUESTIONS

INTERVENTIONS

Key Messages

- We found limited evidence from two systematic reviews of RCTs that chemical insecticides are effective.
- We found no good evidence on combing or alternative treatments.

DEFINITION	Head lice are obligate ectoparasites of socially active humans. They infest the scalp, causing itching, and attach their eggs to the hair shafts. Infestation can be diagnosed only by finding living lice. Eggs glued to hairs, whether hatched (nits) or unhatched, are not proof of active infection, because eggs may retain a viable appearance for weeks after death.
INCIDENCE/ PREVALENCE	We found no data on incidence and no recent published prevalence data from any developed country. Anecdotal reports suggest that prevalence has increased in the last 4–5 years in most communities in the UK and USA.
AETIOLOGY/ RISK FACTORS	Observational studies indicate that infections occur most frequently in school children, although there is no proof of a link with school attendance. We found no evidence that lice prefer clean hair to dirty hair.
PROGNOSIS	The infection is essentially harmless. Sensitisation reactions to louse saliva and faeces may result in localised irritation and erythema. Secondary infection of scratches may occur. Lice have been identified as primary mechanical vectors of scalp pyoderma caused by streptococci and staphylococci usually found on the skin.[1]
AIMS	To eliminate infestation by killing or removing all head lice and their eggs.
OUTCOMES	Treatment success is given as the percentage of people completely cleared of head lice. A clinically important difference between treatments might be a more than 20% difference in the numbers of people successfully treated. There are no standard criteria for judging treatment success. Trials used different methods, and in many cases the method was not stated.
METHODS	The initial search was performed by the Cochrane Infectious Diseases Group at the Liverpool School of Tropical Medicine for a systematic review compiled in July 1998.[2] *Clinical Evidence* update search and appraisal January 2001.

QUESTION What are the effects of treatment for head lice?

OPTION INSECTICIDE BASED PHARMACEUTICAL PRODUCTS

We found two systematic reviews of small, poor quality RCTs of insecticide based pharmaceutical products. One review of three RCTs found that permethrin and malathion were more effective than placebo, and synergised pyrethrins and permethrin were of similar effectiveness. An earlier systematic review found permethrin more effective than lindane. All RCTs had flaws in methodology.

Benefits: We found two systematic reviews.[2,3] The first (search date 1995, 7 RCTs, 1808 people) of 11 insecticide products, including lindane, carbaryl, malathion, permethrin, and other pyrethroids in various vehicles.[3] Two RCTs found that only permethrin produced clinically significant differences in the rate of treatment success; both compared lindane (1% shampoo) versus permethrin (1% cream rinse). Permethrin was found to be more effective (lindane *v* permethrin;

OR for not clearing head lice 15.2, 95% CI 8.0 to 28.8). The subsequent systematic review (search date 1998) set stricter criteria for RCTs and rejected all but three trials.[2] It excluded both studies on which the earlier review was based. One RCT (63 people) found that, after 7 days, permethrin (1% cream rinse) versus placebo was more effective against headlice (29/29 people had no headlice with permethrin v 3/34 with placebo; RR 11.3, 95% CI 3.9 to 33.4). Two weeks after permethrin treatment, more people had no headlice compared with placebo (28/29 v 2/24; RR 16.4, 95% CI 4.3 to 63.1). One RCT (115 people) compared malathion (0.5% alcoholic lotion) with the vehicle base as placebo. At 1 week, more people treated with malathion versus placebo had no headlice (62/65 v 21/47; RR 2.1, 95% CI 1.6 to 3.0). One RCT (22 people) of synergised pyrethrin (0.16% mousse) versus permethrin (1% cream rinse) found that at 6 days, more people treated with pyrethrin had no lice compared with permethrin (17/19 v 3/3; RR 0.89, 95% CI 0.8 to 1.0).

Harms: Only minor adverse effects have been reported for most insecticides. The exception is lindane, where there are extensive reports of effects related to overdosing (treatment of scabies), and absorption (treatment of head lice). Transdermal passage of lindane occurs during treatment of headlice,[4] but we found no reports of adverse effects in this setting. We found no confirmed reports of adverse effects from the organophosphate, malathion, when used therapeutically.

Comment: Follow up for 6 days is inadequate, as the eggs take at least 7 days to hatch. The three trials included in the most recent systematic review were conducted in developing countries, where insecticide treatments were not regularly available.[2] This may have resulted in greater efficacy, because the insects have not been subjected to any kind of selection pressure. No RCT has yet considered that a pediculicide's formulation might affect its activity. Studies in vitro suggest that other components of products (e.g. terpenoids and solvents) may be more effective pediculicides than the insecticide itself.[5] Resistance to one or more insecticides is now common.[6-8]

OPTION	MECHANICAL REMOVAL OF LICE OR VIABLE EGGS BY COMBING

We found insufficient evidence on the effects of combing.

Benefits: We found no systematic reviews that evaluated lice removal by combing, or nit combing to remove eggs. We found one new community based RCT (72 people), comparing "Bug-busting" (wet combing with conditioner) with two applications of 0.5% malathion, 7 days apart. Seven days after treatment, more people taking malathion had no lice compared with "Bug-busting" (31/40 v 12/32; RR 2.8, 95% CI 1.5 to 5.2).[9] We found two RCTs comparing different pediculicides in combination with nit combing, but neither included a non-combing control group.[10,11]

Harms: We found no evidence of harms apart from discomfort.

Comment: The RCT[9] was designed to be a pragmatic RCT (see glossary, p 1168) with results that are applicable to normal practice.

| OPTION | HERBAL TREATMENTS AND AROMATHERAPY |

We found no good evidence on the effects of these alternative treatments.

Benefits: We found no systematic reviews, RCTs, or cohort studies evaluating herbal treatments or aromatherapy.

Harms: We found no evidence of harms.

Comment: None.

GLOSSARY

Pragmatic RCT An RCT designed to provide results that are directly applicable to normal practice (compared to explanatory trials that are intended to clarify efficacy under ideal conditions). Pragmatic RCTs recruit a population that is representative of those who are normally treated, allow normal compliance with instructions (by avoiding incentives and by using oral instructions with advice to follow manufacturers instructions), and analyse results by "intention to treat" rather than by "on treatment" methods.[9]

REFERENCES

1. Taplin D, Meinking TL. Infestations. In: Schachner LA, Hansen RC, eds. *Pediatric dermatology*, vol 2. New York: Churchill Livingstone, 1988:1465–1493.
2. Dodd C. Head lice treatment. In: The Cochrane Library, Issue 4, 2000. Oxford: Update Software. Search date May 1998; primary sources CCTR, Medline, Embase, BIDS SC, BIOSIS, Toxline.
3. Vander Stichele RH, Dezeure EM, Bogaert MG. Systematic review of clinical efficacy of topical treatments for head lice. *BMJ* 1995;311:604–608. Search date March 1995; primary sources Medline, International Pharmaceutical Abstracts, Science Citation Index.
4. Ginsburg CM, Lowry W. Absorption of gamma benzene hexachloride following application of Kwell shampoo. *Pediatr Dermatol* 1983;1:74–76.
5. Burgess I. Malathion lotions for head lice: a less reliable treatment than commonly believed. *Pharm J* 1991;247:630–632.
6. Burgess IF, Brown CM, Peock S, et al. Head lice resistant to pyrethroid insecticides in Britain [letter]. *BMJ* 1995;311:752.
7. Pollack RJ, Kiszewski A, Armstrong P, et al. Differential permethrin susceptibility of head lice sampled in the United States and Borneo. *Arch Pediatr Adolesc Med* 1999;153:969–973.
8. Lee SH, Yoon KS, Williamson M, et al. Molecular analyses of *kdr*-like resistance in permethrin-resistant strains of head lice, *Pediculus capitis*. *Pestic Biochem Physiol* 2000;66:130–143.
9. Roberts RJ, Casey D, Morgan DA, et al. Comparison of wet combing with malathion for treatment of head lice in the UK: a pragmatic randomised controlled trial. *Lancet* 2000;356:540–544.
10. Bainbridge CV, Klein GI, Neibart SI, et al. Comparative study of the clinical effectiveness of a pyrethrin-based pediculicide with combing versus a permethrin-based pediculicide with combing. *Clin Pediatr (Phila)* 1998;37:17–22.
11. Clore ER, Longyear LA. A comparative study of seven pediculicides and their packaged nit combs. *J Pediatr Health Care* 1993;7:55–60.

Ian Burgess
Director
Medical Entomology Centre
Cambridge
UK

Competing interests: The author has been a consultant to several companies involved in development and marketing of pediculicides and has received payment for professional services, including development of educational materials.

Search date December 2000

Graham Worrall

INTERVENTIONS

Key Messages

Prevention

- Limited evidence from RCTs suggests that prophylactic oral aciclovir may reduce the frequency and severity of attacks, but the optimal timing and duration of treatment is uncertain.

- We found no good evidence on the effects of topical antiviral agents used as prophylaxis.

- One small RCT has found that ultraviolet sunscreen reduces the rate of herpes recurrence.

Treatment

- RCTs have found that oral aciclovir marginally reduces the duration of symptoms and pain of first time and recurrent herpes labialis.

- We found limited evidence of benefit from RCTs for the use of topical antiviral agents early in an attack.

- One RCT has found that topical tetracaine used early in an attack reduces time to scab loss.

DEFINITION	Herpes labialis is a mild self limiting infection with herpes simplex virus type 1 (HSV-1). It causes pain and blistering on the lips and perioral area (cold sores); fever and constitutional symptoms are rare. Most people have no warning of an attack, but some experience a recognisable prodrome.
INCIDENCE/ PREVALENCE	Herpes labialis accounts for about 1% of primary care consultations in the UK each year; 20–40% of people have experienced cold sores at some time.[1]
AETIOLOGY/ RISK FACTORS	Herpes labialis is caused by HSV-1. After the primary infection, which usually occurs in childhood, the virus is thought to remain latent in the trigeminal ganglion.[2] A variety of factors, including exposure to bright sunlight, fatigue, or psychological stress, can precipitate a recurrence.
PROGNOSIS	In most people, herpes labialis is a mild, self limiting illness. Recurrences are usually shorter and less severe than the initial attack. Healing is usually complete in 7–10 days without scarring.[3] Rates of reactivation are unknown. Herpes labialis can cause serious illness in immunocompromised patients.
AIMS	To reduce the frequency and severity of recurrent attacks; to speed healing of lesions; and to reduce pain, with minimal adverse effects.
OUTCOMES	Severity of symptoms, time to healing, rate of recurrence, adverse effects of treatment.
METHODS	*Clinical Evidence* update search and appraisal December 2000 using keywords herpes labialis, treatment, prevention, prophylaxis, controlled trial, and effectiveness.

QUESTION   What are the effects of interventions aimed at preventing attacks?

OPTION   ORAL/TOPICAL ANTIVIRAL AGENTS

We found limited evidence from RCTs that prophylactic oral aciclovir reduced the frequency and severity of attacks. It is not clear whether prophylaxis should be continuous or restricted to high risk periods. We found no good evidence on the effects of topical antiviral agents.

Benefits: We found no systematic review. **Topical antiviral agents:** We found no good quality RCTs. **Oral antiviral agents:** We found four double blind placebo controlled RCTs. The first (147 American skiers with a history of herpes labialis precipitated by ultraviolet [UV] light) found that people given prophylactic oral aciclovir (200 mg five times daily for 5 days beginning 7 days before UV exposure) suffered significantly fewer attacks and shorter duration of symptoms (P < 0.05).[4] The second (239 Canadian skiers) found no significant difference between aciclovir 800 mg twice daily, starting on the day before exposure to ultraviolet light for 37 days, versus placebo.[5] The third (20 people with recurrent herpes labialis) found that aciclovir 400 mg twice daily for 4 months led to 53% fewer clinical recurrences and 71% fewer virus culture positive recurrences (P = 0.05).[6] The fourth RCT (248 adults with a history of sun induced recurrent herpes labialis) compared three different dosages of famciclovir (125 mg, 250 mg, and 500 mg) versus placebo.[7] Treatment was given three times a day for 5 days beginning 48 hours after exposure to artificial UV light. There was no significant difference in the number of lesions in the four groups, but increasing the dose of famciclovir significantly reduced the mean size (P = 0.04) and duration of lesions, in a dose response relation. Compared with placebo, the 500 mg dose reduced the mean time to healing by 2 days (P < 0.01).

Harms: See harms under the effects of antiviral treatment for the first attack, below.

Comment: None.

OPTION   SUNSCREEN

Two small RCTs have found that sunscreen reduces the rate of herpes recurrence.

Benefits: We found no systematic review. We found two small randomised double blind crossover trials,[8,9] both of which found that sunscreen significantly reduced the rate of recurrence. The first (38 people with a history of recurrent herpes) found that 71% suffered recurrence with placebo versus 0% with sunscreen (P < 0.001; NNT 1.4, 95% CI 1.2 to 2).[8] The second trial (19 people) comparing sunscreen versus placebo found that significantly more people taking placebo suffered recurrence (11/19 [58%] with placebo v 1/19 [5.2%] with sunscreen, P < 0.01; NNT 2, 95% CI 1.2 to 6).[9]

Harms: None reported.

Comment: None.

QUESTION   What are the effects of antiviral treatment for the first attack of herpes labialis?

We found no good evidence on the effects of topical agents on the duration or severity of symptoms of the first attack of herpes labialis. Limited evidence from small RCTs in children suggests that oral aciclovir may marginally reduce duration of pain and time to healing.

Benefits: We found no systematic review. **Topical antiviral agents:** We found no RCTs. **Oral antiviral agents:** We found two small RCTs, both of which found a beneficial effect.[10,11] One double blind RCT (20 children having their first attack) compared oral aciclovir 200 mg five times daily versus placebo.[10] Mean duration of pain was reduced from 5.0 to 4.3 days, and mean duration of excess salivation was reduced from 5.0 to 3.3 days (P < 0.05). The second RCT (72 children aged 1–6 years with gingivostomatitis of less than 3 days duration) compared oral aciclovir 15 mg/kg five times daily for 7 days versus placebo. Time to healing was reduced from 10 to 4 days, a mean reduction of 6 days (95% CI 4 to 8 days).[11] We found no RCTs in adults.

Harms: Topical aciclovir causes rash, pruritus, and irritation in some people, but no more frequently in trials than placebo.[12–14] It has also caused head and tail abnormalities in fetal rats, but we found no recorded cases of teratogenicity in humans. Oral aciclovir is excreted in breast milk. Aciclovir has been used to treat pregnant women with genital herpes, and one systematic review of three studies found no evidence of adverse effects in women or newborn children[14] (see antiviral treatment during pregnancy under genital herpes, p 1096). However, the evidence is limited, and clinically significant adverse effects cannot be ruled out.

Comment: Research in this area is difficult because people do not usually consult clinicians until after they have had several attacks of herpes labialis.

QUESTION Do treatments taken at the beginning or during a recurrent attack reduce the duration or severity of symptoms?

OPTION ORAL/TOPICAL ANTIVIRAL AGENTS

We found limited evidence of benefit from RCTs for the use of topical antiviral agents early in an attack.

Benefits: We found no systematic review. **Topical antiviral agents:** We found several trials of antiviral cream, which reported mixed results.[12,13,15–20] The largest RCT (double blind, 2209 people) compared penciclovir cream 2 hourly for 4 days versus placebo.[18] Penciclovir cream reduced healing times by 0.7 days and duration of pain by 0.6 days (CIs could not be calculated from the published report). One small RCT (31 people aged over 17 years with recurrent herpes labialis) with three parallel arms compared 5% aciclovir cream (10 people) versus 5% aciclovir in a liposomal carrier (12 people) versus the drug free vehicle (9 people). The mean time to crusting of the lesions was significantly reduced for aciclovir in liposomal carrier versus drug free carrier (1.6 days for aciclovir in liposomes v 4.8 days for control, P < 0.05) but not for aciclovir cream versus the drug free carrier (4.3 days for aciclovir cream v 4.8 days for control).[20] Fifteen of the participants then took part in a crossover study in which they received the two forms of aciclovir (in random order) separated by a washout period of at least 1 month. Again, the time to crusting of lesions was shorter with aciclovir in liposomes than for aciclovir cream (1.8 v 3.5 days, P < 0.05). Too few people experienced pain to analyse the impact of the preparations on discomfort. A further double blind RCT (534 people) compared 1% penciclovir cream versus placebo.[21] It found that penciclovir reduced the mean healing time of lesions from 8.8 to 7.6 days (P < 0.01). **Oral antiviral agents:** We found two RCTs. One double blind RCT (174 adults with recurrent herpes labialis) compared oral aciclovir 400 mg five times daily for 5 days versus placebo.[22] Oral aciclovir taken early in the attack (when the person first experienced tingling), reduced the duration of symptoms from 12.5 to 8.1 days (CIs could not be calculated from the published report). If treatment was initiated later (when the vesicular rash appeared), there was no benefit compared with placebo. A second double blind RCT (149 people) compared oral aciclovir within 12 hours of onset of symptoms versus placebo.[23] It found a significant but clinically small effect; oral aciclovir reduced healing time by 0.98 days and duration of pain by 0.04 days (P < 0.05).

Harms: See harms under the effects of antiviral treatment for the first attack, p 1171.

Comment: We found no RCTs comparing early versus delayed intervention, so no firm conclusions regarding timing of treatment can be drawn.

OPTION   **TOPICAL ANAESTHETIC AGENTS**

One RCT of topical tetracaine has found that use early in an attack reduces time to scab loss. We found insufficient evidence on the effects of other agents.

Benefits: We found no systematic review. One double blind RCT (72 people) found that 1.8% tetracaine cream versus placebo, applied six times daily until scab loss occurred, significantly reduced mean time to scab loss from 7.2 to 5.1 days (P = 0.002), and increased a composite symptom benefit index from 5.9 to 7.3 (P = 0.036).[24]

Harms: None reported.

Comment: See comment under antiviral agents for recurrent attacks above.

REFERENCES

1. Hodgkin K. *Towards earlier diagnosis: a guide to general practice*. London: Churchill Livingstone 1973:129.
2. Baringer SR, Swoveland P. Recovery of herpes simplex virus from human trigeminal ganglions. *N Engl J Med* 1973;288:648–650.
3. Baker C, Crumpacker CS, Schnipner LE. The natural history of recurrent facial-oral infections with the herpes simplex virus. *J Infect Dis* 1978;138:897–905.
4. Raborn GW, Martel AY, Grace MG, McGaw WT. Oral acyclovir in prevention of herpes labialis: a randomized, double-blind, placebo controlled trial. *Oral Surg Oral Med Oral Pathol Oral Radiol Endod* 1998;85:55–59.
5. Spruance SL, Stewart JC, Rowe NH, et al. Treatment of recurrent herpes simplex labialis with oral acyclovir. *J Infect Dis* 1990;161:185–190.
6. Raborn WG, McGraw WT, Grace M, Tyrell LD, Samuels SM. Oral acyclovir and herpes labialis: a randomized, double-blind, placebo-controlled study. *J Am Dental Assoc* 1987;115:38–42.
7. Spruance SL, Rowe NH, Raborn GW, et al. Peroral famciclovir in the treatment of experimental ultraviolet radiation-induced herpes simplex labialis: a double-blind, dose-ranging, placebo-controlled, multicenter trial. *J Infect Dis* 1999;179:303–310.
8. Rooney JF, Bryson Y, Mannix ML, Dillon M, et al. Prevention of ultraviolet-light-induced herpes labialis by sunscreen. *Lancet* 1991;338:1419–1421.
9. Duteil L, Queille-Roussel C, Loesche C, Verschoore M. Assessment of the effect of a sunblock stick in the prevention of solar-simulating ultraviolet light-induced herpes labialis. *J Dermatol Treat* 1998;9:11–14.
10. Ducoulombier H, Cousin J, DeWilde A. La stomato-gingivite herpetique de l'enfant: essai a contolle aciclovir versus placebo (in French). *Ann Pediatr* 1988;35:212–216.
11. Amir J, Harel L, Smetana Z, Varsano I. Treatment of herpes simplex gingivostomatitis with aciclovir in children: a randomised double blind placebo controlled trial. *BMJ* 1997;314:1800–1803.
12. Raborn GW, Martel WT, Grace M, Percy UJ, Samuels S. Herpes labialis treatment with acyclovir modified aqueous cream: a double-blind randomized trial. *Oral Surg Oral Med Oral Pathol* 1989;67:676–679.
13. Fiddian AP, Ivanyi L. Topical acyclovir in the management of recurrent herpes labialis. *Br J Dermatol* 1983;109:321–326.
14. Smith J, Cowan FM, Munday P. The management of herpes simplex virus infection in pregnancy. *Br J Obstet Gynaecol* 1998;105:255–268. Search date 1996; primary sources Medline 1983 to 1996, and hand searched references.
15. Van Vloten WA, Swart RNJ, Pot F. Topical acyclovir therapy in patients with recurrent orofacial herpes simplex infections. *J Antimicrob Chemother* 1993;12(suppl B):89–93.
16. Shaw M, King M, Best JM. Failure of acyclovir ointment in treatment of recurrent herpes labialis. *BMJ* 1985;291:79.
17. Spruance SL, Schnipper LE, Overcall JC. Treatment of herpes simplex labialis with topical acyclovir in polyethylene glycol. *J Infect Dis* 1982;146:85–90.
18. Spruance SL, Rea TL, Thoming C, Tucker R, Saltzman R, Boon R. Penciclovir cream for the treatment of herpes simplex labialis. *JAMA* 1997;277:1374–1379.
19. Raborn GW, McGraw WT, Grace MG, Houle L. Herpes labialis treatment with acyclovir 5 per cent

ointment. *Sci J* 1989;55:135–137.

20. Horwitz E, Pisanty S, Czerninski R, Helser M, Eliav E, Touitou E. A clinical evaluation of a novel liposomal carrier for acyclovir in the topical treatment of recurrent herpes labialis. *Oral Surg Oral Med Oral Pathol* 1999;87:700–705.
21. Boon R, Goodman JJ, Martinez J, Marks GL, Gamble M, Welch C. Penciclovir cream for the treatment of sunlight-induced herpes simplex labialis: a randomized, double-blind, placebo-controlled trial. Penciclovir Cream Herpes Labialis Study Group. *Clin Ther* 2000;22:76–90.
22. Spruance SL, Hammil ML, Hoge WS, Davis G, Mills J. ACV prevents reactivation of herpes labialis in skiers. *JAMA* 1988;260:1597–1599.
23. Rooney JF, Strauss SE, Mannix ML, et al. Oral acyclovir to suppress frequently recurrent herpes labialis: a double-blind, placebo controlled trial. *Ann Intern Med* 1993;118:268–272.
24. Kaminester LH, Pariser RJ, Pariser, et al. A double-blind, placebo-controlled study of topical tetracaine in the treatment of herpes labialis. *J Am Acad Dermatol* 1999;41:996–1001.

Graham Worrall
Associate Professor of Family Medicine
Memorial University of Newfoundland
Whitbourne
Canada

Competing interests: None declared.

Search date May 2000

Thomas Crosby, Malcolm Mason and David Crosby

QUESTIONS

INTERVENTIONS

Likely to be beneficial
Primary excision 1177

Trade off between benefits and harms
Adjuvant alfa-2_b interferon. . .1178

Unknown effectiveness
Sunscreens in prevention. . . .1177
Other adjuvant treatments . . .1179

Unlikely to be beneficial
Radical primary excision (no better than less radical surgery) . .1177
Elective lymph node dissection 1178

To be covered in future issues of Clinical Evidence
Screening people at high risk
Treatment of metastatic malignant melanoma

Key Messages

- We found insufficient evidence on the preventive effect of sunscreens.
- RCTs have found narrow primary excision to be as effective as wide excision in terms of overall survival and probably local recurrence. Narrow excision reduces the need for skin grafting.
- RCTs have found that elective lymph node dissection offers no advantage in overall survival compared with surgery deferred until clinical recurrence.
- We found insufficient evidence on the effects of adjuvant treatments, although limited evidence from one RCT suggests that alfa-2_b interferon may improve survival in high risk people.

Malignant melanoma: non-metastatic

DEFINITION
Cutaneous malignant melanoma is a tumour derived from melanocytes in the basal layer of the epidermis. After undergoing malignant transformation, it becomes invasive by penetrating into and beyond the dermis.

INCIDENCE/ PREVALENCE
Incidence in developed countries has increased by 50% in the past 20 years. Incidence varies in different populations (see table 1, p 1181), and is about 10-fold higher in white than in non-white populations. Despite the rise in incidence, mortality has plateaued and even fallen in some populations (e.g. in women and young men in Australia).[1,2] During the same period there has been a sixfold increase in the incidence of melanoma *in situ,* suggesting earlier detection.

AETIOLOGY/ RISK FACTORS
The number of common, atypical, and dysplastic naevi on a person's body correlates closely with the risk of developing malignant melanoma. A genetic predisposition probably accounts for 5–10% of all cases. Although the risk of developing malignant melanoma is higher in fair skinned white populations living close to the equator, the relation between sun exposure, sunscreen use, and skin type is not clear cut. Exposure to excessive sunlight and severe sunburn in childhood are associated with an increased risk of developing malignant melanoma in adult life. However, people do not necessarily develop tumours at sites of maximum exposure to the sun.

PROGNOSIS
The prognosis of early malignant melanoma (stages I–III) (see table 2, p 1182) relates to the depth of invasion of the primary lesion, the presence of ulceration, and involvement of the regional lymph nodes, the prognosis worsening with the number of nodes involved.[3] A person with a thin lesion (Breslow depth < 0.75 mm) and without lymph node involvement has a 3% risk of developing metastases and a 95% chance of surviving 5 years.[4] If regional lymph nodes are macroscopically involved there is a 20–50% chance of surviving 5 years. Most studies have shown a better prognosis in women and in people with lesions on the extremities compared with those with lesions on the trunk.

AIMS
To prevent melanoma; to detect melanoma earlier; to minimise mutilating surgical treatment while still achieving cure of local disease; to optimise quality of life; and to eradicate occult micrometastatic disease, with minimum adverse effects.

OUTCOMES
Prevention: Rates and severity of sunburn (proxy measure); incidence of malignant melanoma; mortality from malignant melanoma. **Primary excision:** Local recurrence; overall survival; requirement for skin grafting. **Lymph node dissection and adjuvant treatment:** Overall survival; disease free survival; quality of life; morbidity of disease treatment, or both.

METHODS
Clinical Evidence search and appraisal May 2000, plus search of reference lists of all review articles found, and the main oncological and dermatological textbooks.

QUESTION   Does the use of sunscreens help to prevent malignant melanoma?

OPTION   SUNSCREENS

We found no RCTs assessing the effect of sunscreens on the incidence of, or mortality from, malignant melanoma. The correct use of sunscreen, however, seems a sensible measure to avoid excessive exposure to sunlight.

Benefits: We found no systematic review. Although one RCT found that sunscreens reduced the incidence or progression of solar keratosis,[5] we found no similar evidence for malignant melanoma. Retrospective case control studies and questionnaire based surveys, all of which have potential biases and confounding factors, have found conflicting results.[6–8] One case control study found that adults with melanoma were less likely to have been protected from sunlight as children,[7] whereas some questionnaire based surveys found no such effect.[6,8]

Harms: Sunscreens can irritate the skin and cause allergic contact dermatitis. Some questionnaire based surveys have suggested that sunscreen may have contributed to the development of malignant melanoma.[6,8] A possible mechanism for this suggestion may be that since some sunscreens protect predominantly against ultraviolet B (UVB, which induces sunburn), people may spend more time exposed to higher doses of ultraviolet A (UVA). One placebo controlled RCT found that a sunscreen with a high sun protection factor (SPF 30) was associated with significantly longer recreational sun exposure.[9]

Comment: Although we found no prospective evidence, it would seem reasonable to take sensible precautions to avoid excessive exposure to sunlight, particularly in children and fair skinned individuals. Sunscreens may have a role if used appropriately (sun protection factor of at least 15 and a star rating for UVA protection of 3–4), rather than being used to prolong the time spent in direct sunlight.

QUESTION   Is there an optimal margin for primary excision of melanoma of different Breslow thicknesses?

RCTs have found that more radical local surgery (4–5 cm excision margins) provides no greater benefit than less radical surgery (1–2 cm excision margins).

Benefits: **Radical local surgery versus less radical surgery:** We found no systematic review. We found three RCTs in people with thin (< 1 mm) and intermediate thickness (1–4 mm) malignant melanoma.[10–12] The first trial randomised 612 people with lesions < 2 mm thick to surgical excision with either 1 or 3 cm margins.[10] The second trial randomised 486 people with intermediate thickness lesions (1–4 mm) to either 2 or 4 cm margins. The remaining trial randomised 769 people with lesions 0.8–2.0 mm to either 2 or 5 cm margins.[12] None of the trials found that wide margins reduced local recurrence rates or increased overall survival compared with narrow excision margins.

Malignant melanoma: non-metastatic

Harms: Narrower excision margins reduced skin grafting (in one RCT by 75%), anaesthetic requirements, and inpatient stay.[10] Narrow margin surgery can usually be performed on outpatient day surgery lists. Of concern is the possibility of higher local recurrence rates using 1 cm margins for tumours 1–2 mm. One RCT in 612 people comparing narrow margin with wide margin surgery reported three local recurrences, all in people with tumours 1–2 mm treated with narrow (1 cm) margin excision; local cure was achieved in two people with further surgery.[10] Although not measured, there is potential for psychological and physical morbidity associated with further surgery after local recurrence.

Comment: The evidence relating to survival is good but we found no good evidence relating to quality of life or physical and psychological morbidity caused by extent of surgery or local recurrence.

QUESTION Does elective lymph node dissection improve outcomes in people with clinically uninvolved lymph nodes?

RCTs found no benefit from elective lymph node dissection in people with clinically uninvolved lymph nodes, although an effect within particular subgroups cannot be ruled out.

Benefits: We found no systematic review. We found four RCTs comparing elective lymph node dissection with surgery deferred until the time of clinical recurrence in a total of 1718 people with no clinical evidence of lymph node metastases.[13–16] None of the studies showed a significant overall survival benefit for people receiving elective lymph node dissection. Retrospective subgroup analyses found non-significant trends in favour of elective lymph node dissection in certain groups of people (those with intermediate thickness tumours, especially those under 60 years of age), but such analyses are subject to bias.

Harms: Lymph node dissection has several complications. In one retrospective case series, these included temporary seroma (17%), wound infection (9%), wound necrosis (3%), and lymphoedema (20%).[17]

Comment: In about 20% of people who do not have clinically apparent lymph node involvement, the lymph nodes will contain occult micrometastases. None of the RCTs gave data on morbidity and quality of life in people undergoing lymph node dissection. An alternative to elective lymph node dissection, sentinel lymph node excision, which can accurately determine the specific nodes draining the primary lesion and their involvement with metastatic disease,[18] is currently being evaluated in clinical trials.

QUESTION Does adjuvant treatment improve prognosis after curative surgery of cutaneous malignant melanoma and at what stage?

OPTION ALFA-2$_B$ INTERFERON

RCTs have found that alfa-2$_b$ interferon extends the time to relapse and, in high doses, may improve survival in high risk people. However, toxicity and withdrawal rates are high. Less toxic regimens for interferon treatment are being evaluated.

Benefits: We found no systematic review. **High dose:** We found one RCT comparing high dose alfa-2$_b$ interferon (20 MIU/m^2 per day intravenously for 1 month, followed by 10 MIU/m^2 three times a week subcutaneously for 11 months) versus observation in 287 people with primary lesions greater than 4 mm or resectable stage III disease.[19] At a median of 6.9 years of follow up, an intention to treat analysis found a significant improvement in disease free survival (median 1.7 v 1.0 years) and overall survival (median 3.8 v 2.8 years, CIs not given in the report). A retrospective analysis of this study by the authors showed prolonged quality of life-adjusted survival in people receiving interferon alfa. The significance of this gain varied with the values assigned by people for the impact of treatment toxicity and time with relapsed disease.[20] Preliminary results at a median of 4.3 years of follow up of a larger study of 642 people failed to confirm a survival benefit for high or low dose adjuvant alfa interferon.[21] **Low dose:** We found two RCTs. Both of these studies were performed in people with stage II melanoma (primary tumours > 1.5 mm and lymph node negative). One RCT compared low dose interferon (3 MIU three times a week for 18 months) versus surgery alone in 499 people. It showed a significant extension of the relapse free interval and a trend towards extension of overall survival (HR for relapse free survival 0.75, 95% CI 0.57 to 0.98, P = 0.038; HR for overall survival 0.72, 95% CI 0.51 to 1.0, P = 0.059).[22] The second trial randomised 311 people to receive interferon alfa-2$_b$ (3 MIU given daily for 3 weeks and three times per week for 12 months) or observation after excision of their primary tumour. At 41 months follow up there was a prolonged relapse free survival (P = 0.02, CIs not reported) but no effect on overall survival.[23]

Harms: Interferons commonly cause malaise, fevers, and flu-like symptoms. In the RCT described above, high dose alfa interferon also caused significant (> grade 3) myelosuppression in 24% of people, hepatotoxicity in 15% (including 2 deaths), and neurotoxicity in 28%. At 11 months, only 25% of participants were receiving more than 80% of the planned dose.[19] In the trial of low dose interferon, 10% of people suffered significant toxicity.[22]

Comment: RCTs investigating the effects of more tolerable alfa interferon regimens are underway.

OPTION   OTHER ADJUVANT TREATMENTS

We found no evidence of benefit in terms of survival with other adjuvant treatments (non-specific immunotherapy and chemotherapy); surveillance, specific immunotherapy, hormones, coumarin, retinoids have not been evaluated adequately.

Benefits: We found no systematic review. We found 60 RCTs of adjuvant systemic treatment. Most were too small or too short term to detect a clinically significant benefit, and involved heterogeneous groups of participants (see table 3, p 1182). **Non-specific immunostimulation:** A total of 24 RCTs (mainly small, ranging from 26 to 400 people) evaluated non-specific immunostimulation with agents such as bacille Calmette-Guérin and *Corynebacterium parvum*.

These found no beneficial effect on survival, although most trials were too small to exclude a beneficial effect. **Active specific immunostimulation:** Results from RCTs are awaited, but small pilot studies in single institutions found encouraging results compared with historical controls, especially from allogeneic tumour cell vaccines, viral oncolysates, gangliosides, or melanoma associated peptide vaccines. **Chemotherapy:** About 15 RCTs (mostly small, ranging from 15 to 258 people) compared single agent cytotoxic agents, especially dacarbazine, chemo-immunotherapy, and multi-agent cytotoxic treatments versus placebo. No beneficial effect on survival was found. The regimen believed to be most powerful in advanced disease—cisplatin, bischloroethylnitrosourea, dacarbazine, and tamoxifen (the Dartmouth regimen)—has not yet been tested in RCTs. **Hormones, coumarins, retinoids:** Several small RCTs of hormones (megesterol acetate) and coumarins found mixed results. Several small RCTs all found no benefit from retinoids. **Surveillance:** We found no RCTs. Retrospective studies found that people presented with symptomatic recurrent disease regardless of whether they were taking part in an intensive follow up programme.[24] Thinner lesions (< 0.76 mm) may require longer surveillance as recurrences peak between 5 and 10 years.[25]

Harms: Certain types of immunostimulation may be associated with flu-like symptoms such as fevers, arthralgias, and rigors. Chemotherapy toxicities are well known and include nausea and vomiting, myelosuppression, and alopecia, depending on the cytotoxic agents used. Hormonal therapy can cause weight gain and lead to an increased risk of thromboembolism. Long term adverse effects of retinoids are less well known, but they may possibly be carcinogenic in certain circumstances. Although surveillance can do little physical harm, the possibility of inducing anxiety has not been excluded.

Comment: None.

REFERENCES

1. Giles GG, Armstrong BK, Burton RC, et al. Has mortality from melanoma stopped rising in Australia? Analysis of trends between 1931 and 1994. *BMJ* 1996;312:1121–1125.

2. Armstrong BK, Kricker A. Cutaneous melanoma. *Cancer Surv* 1994;19–20:219–240.

3. Balch CM, Soong SJ, Shaw HM, et al. An analysis of prognostic factors in 8500 patients with cutaneous melanoma. In: Balch CM, Houghton Anilton GW, Sober AJ, Soong SJ, eds. *Cutaneous melanoma*, 2nd ed. New York: Ellis Horwood, 1992.

4. Balch CM, Smalley RV, Bartolucci AA, et al. A randomised prospective clinical trial of adjuvant *C. parvum* immunotherapy in 260 patients with clinically localized melanoma (stage I): prognostic factor analysis and preliminary results of immunotherapy. *Cancer* 1982;49:1079–1084.

5. Thompson SC, Jolley D, Marks R. Reduction of solar keratoses by regular sunscreen use. *N Engl J Med* 1993;329:1147–1151.

6. Autier P, Dore J-F, Lejeune FJ, et al. Sun protection in childhood or early adolescence and reduction of melanoma risk in adults: an EORTC case-control study in Germany, Belgium and France. *J Epidemiol Biostat* 1998;1:51–57.

7. Holly EA, Aston DA, Cress RD, et al. Cutaneous melanoma in women. *Am J Epidemiol* 1995;141:923–933.

8. Wolf P, Quehenberger F, Mullegger R, et al. Phenotypic markers, sunlight-related factors and sunscreen use in patients with cutaneous melanoma: an Austrian case-control study. *Melanoma Res* 1998;8:370–378.

9. Autier P, Dore JF, Negrier S, et al. Sunscreen use and duration of sun exposure: a double-blind, randomized trial. *J Natl Cancer Inst* 1999;91:1304–1309.

10. Veronesi U, Cascinelli N, Adamus J, et al. Thin stage I primary cutaneous malignant melanoma: comparison of excision with margins of 1 or 3 cm. *N Engl J Med* 1988;318:1159–1162.

11. Balch CM, Urist MM, Karakousis CP, et al. Efficacy of 2 cm surgical margins for intermediate-thickness melanomas (1 to 4 mm): results of a multi-institutional randomized surgical trial. *Ann Surg* 1993;218:262–267.

12. Ringborg U, Anderron R, Eldh J, et al. Resection margins of 2 versus 5 cm for cutaneous malignant melanoma with a tumour thickness of 0.8 to 2.0 mm: randomized study by the Swedish melanoma study group. *Cancer* 1996;77:1809–1814.

13. Balch CM, Soong SJ, Bartolucci AA, et al. Efficacy of an elective regional lymph node dissection of 1–4 mm thick melanomas for patients 60 years of age and younger. *Ann Surg* 1996;224:255–263.

14. Cascinelli N, Morabito A, Santinami M, et al. Immediate or delayed dissection of regional nodes in patients with melanoma of the trunk: a randomised trial. WHO Melanoma Programme. *Lancet* 1998;351:793–796.

15. Sim FH, Taylor WF, Ivins JC, et al. A prospective randomized study of the efficacy of routine elective lymphadenectomy in management of malignant melanoma: preliminary results. *Cancer* 1978;41:948–956.

16. Veronesi U, Adamus J, Bandiera DC, et al. Inefficacy of immediate node dissection in stage I melanoma of the limbs. *N Engl J Med* 1977;297: 627–630.

17. Baas PC, Schraffordt KH, Koops H, et al. Groin dissection in the treatment of lower-extremity melanoma: short-term and long-term morbidity. *Arch Surg* 1992;127:281–286.

18. Ross MI. Surgical management of stage I and II melanoma patients: approach to the regional lymph node basin. *Semin Surg Oncol* 1996;12: 394–401.

19. Kirkwood JM, Strawderman MH, Erstoff MS, et al. Interferon alfa-2_b adjuvant therapy of high-risk resected cutaneous melanoma: The eastern cooperative oncology group trial EST 1684. *J Clin Oncol* 1996;14:7–17.

20. Cole BF, Gelber RD, Kirkwood JM, et al. Quality-of-life-adjusted survival analysis of high-risk resected cutaneous melanoma: the eastern cooperative oncology group study. *J Clin Oncol* 1996;14: 2666–2673.

21. Kirkwood JM, Ibrahim J, Sondak V, et al. Preliminary analysis of the E1690/S9111/C9190 intergroup postoperative adjuvant trial of high- and low-dose IFN-2_b (HDI and LDI) in high risk primary or lymph node metastatic melanoma. *Proc ASCO* 1999;18 (abstract 2072)

22. Grob JJ, Dreno B, de la Salmoniere P, et al. Randomised trial of interferon alpha-2_a as adjuvant therapy in resected primary melanoma thicker than 1.5 mm without clinically detectable node metastases. French cooperative group on melanoma. *Lancet* 1998;351:1905–1910.

23. Pehamberger H, Peter Soyer H, Steiner A, et al. Adjuvant interferon alfa-2_a treatment in resected primary stage II cutaneous melanoma. *J Clin Oncol* 1998;16:1425–1429.

24. Shumate CR, Urist MM, Maddox WA. Melanoma recurrence surveillance: patient or physician based? *Ann Surg* 1995;221:566–559.

25. Rogers GS, Kopf AW, Rigel DS, et al. Hazard-rate analysis in stage I malignant melanoma. *Arch Dermatol* 1986;122:999–1002.

Thomas Crosby
Consultant Clinical Oncologist

Malcolm Mason
Professor of Clinical Oncology

Velindre Hospital
Cardiff
UK

David Crosby
Consultant Surgeon
Cardiff Community Healthcare Trust
Cardiff
UK
Competing interests: None declared.

TABLE 1	Melanoma incidence and mortality in different populations (see text, p 1176).[2]

Population	Incidence (per 100 000 people)	New cases per year	Deaths per year
Asian/Oriental	0.2	NA	NA
United Kingdom	8	4000	1500
United States	12	32 000	6700
Caucasians in Queensland, Australia	40	NA	NA

NA, not available.

TABLE 2 Stage of malignant melanoma and 5 year survival (see text, p 1176).[3]

Stage	Description	Approx 5 year survival (%)
I	Primary tumour < 0.75 mm (T1) or > 0.75–1.5 mm (T2). No lymphadenopathy (N0).	95
II	Primary tumour > 1.5–4 mm (T3). No lymphadenopathy (N0).	50–70
III	Primary tumour > 4 mm or satellite(s) within 2 cm, lymphadenopathy < 3 cm (N1) or > 3 cm/in transit metastasis (N2). No metastases (M0).	20–50
IV	Presence of metastases (M1).	0–5

TABLE 3 Effects of non-cytokine adjuvant treatment (see text, p 1179).

Intervention	Example	Evidence
Non-specific immunotherapy	BCG Corynebacterium parvum	Many RCTs have found no evidence of improved overall or disease free survival
Active specific immunotherapy	Melanoma cell vaccines Viral oncolysates Defined antigen vaccines Dendritic cells	No evidence from RCTs (although some are under way)
Chemotherapy	Single agents Combination treatments	RCTs reported no evidence of benefit. The most powerful regimen (DTIC, cisplatin, BCNU, and tamoxifen) has not been evaluated in RCTs
Others	Hormones (megesterol acetate) Coumarin Retinoids	Small RCTs reported survival benefit from hormones and coumarin, but not from retinoids. Findings have not yet been replicated in larger studies
Surveillance	Follow up programme (e.g. every 3 months for first 2 years)	Standard management for stage I (thin lesions < 0.76 mm). Thinner lesions may require longer follow up to detect later relapses. Has not been evaluated in RCTs

BCG, Bacille Calmette-Guérin; BCNU, bischloroethylnitrosourea; DTIC, dimethyltriazeno-imidazole carboxamide (dacarbazine).

Search date May 2000

Godfrey Walker and Paul Johnstone

INTERVENTIONS

Key Messages

- One systematic review of mainly small RCTs has found that topical permethrin and gamma benzene hexachloride are effective in the treatment of scabies. However, gamma benzene hexachloride has been linked to rare reports of serious adverse effects.

- We found limited evidence from two RCTs suggesting that crotamiton is safe but less effective than permethrin.

- We found insufficient evidence on the effects of other topical agents (malathion, benzyl benzoate, and sulphur compounds). Case series have found that malathion achieves cure rates of over 80%, but its safety has not been assessed adequately.

- We found insufficient evidence on the effects of oral ivermectin. It is known to be safe in young adults from its use in onchocerciasis, but its safety in children and elderly people is uncertain.

DEFINITION	Scabies is an infestation of the skin by the mite *Sarcoptes scabiei*.[1] Typical sites of infestation are skin folds and flexor surfaces. In adults, the most common sites are between the fingers and on the wrists, although infection may manifest in elderly people as a diffuse truncal eruption. In infants and children, the face, scalp, palms, and soles are also often affected.
INCIDENCE/ PREVALENCE	Scabies is a common public health problem with an estimated prevalence of 300 million cases worldwide, mostly affecting people in developing countries where prevalence can exceed 50%.[2] In industrialised countries, it is most common in institutionalised communities. Case studies suggest that epidemic cycles occur every 7–15 years and that these partly reflect the population's immune status.
AETIOLOGY/ RISK FACTORS	Scabies is particularly common where there is social disruption, overcrowding with close body contact, and limited access to water.[3] Young children, immobilised elderly people, people with HIV/AIDS, and other medically and immunologically compromised people are predisposed to infestation and have particularly high mite counts.[4]
PROGNOSIS	Scabies is not life threatening, but the severe, persistent itch and secondary infections may be debilitating. Occasionally, crusted scabies develops. This form of the disease is resistant to routine treatment and can be a source of continued reinfestation and spread to others.
AIMS	To eliminate the scabies mites and ova from the skin; to cure pruritus (itching); to prevent reinfestation; to prevent spread to other people.
OUTCOMES	Number of visible burrows and papular and vesicular eruptions; presence of mites, ova, or faecal pellets in skin scrapings under a magnifying lens or microscope; pruritus. Outcomes should be assessed 28–30 days after start of treatment, which is the time it takes for lesions to heal and for any eggs and mites to reach maturity if treatment fails.
METHODS	In preparing a systematic review,[5] we searched for all RCTs of pharmaceutical preparations, both topical and oral, using the Cochrane Controlled Trials Register, Medline and Embase, using standardised search strategies, and by direct approaches to pharmaceutical companies and experts in the field. A *Clinical Evidence* search and appraisal was performed in May 2000. Of the five trials of different topical treatments that we identified, four used gamma benzene hexachloride (lindane) as one of the comparators. Gamma benzene hexachloride has been off the market in the UK since 1995 because of concern about possible adverse effects.

QUESTION   What are the effects of topical treatments?

OPTION   PERMETHRIN

One systematic review of RCTs has found that permethrin is effective in the treatment of scabies, with a parasitic cure rate of about 90%. Two small trials found that it was more effective than crotamiton. A larger trial found no difference compared with gamma benzene hexachloride, although non-trial data suggest that permethrin is less toxic.

Benefits: We found one systematic review (search date 1997),[5] which identified four RCTs.[6–9] **Permethrin versus crotamiton:** Two RCTs in a total of 194 adults and children compared topical permethrin versus crotamiton.[6,7] Permethrin was associated with significantly higher clinical cure rates in both trials (OR for failed clinical cure with permethrin v crotamiton 0.21, 95% CI 0.10 to 0.47).[5] Only one of the RCTs evaluated parasitic cure rates.[7] It also found permethrin to be significantly more effective (OR for failed parasitic cure with permethrin v crotamiton 0.21, 95% CI 0.08 to 0.53). The same RCT found no significant difference in patients' reports of pruritus (OR for itch persistence with permethrin v with crotamiton 0.38, 95% CI 0.12 to 1.19).[7] **Permethrin versus gamma benzene hexachloride:** The systematic review[5] found three RCTs comparing permethrin versus gamma benzene hexachloride, all using the same drug concentrations.[6,8,9] Two trials in a total of 152 adults and children found permethrin to be more effective than gamma benzene hexachloride.[6,9] The largest trial, with 467 participants,[8] found no significant difference between the two treatments (OR for failed parasitic cure with permethrin v gamma benzene hexachloride 0.68, 95% CI 0.34 to 1.36). This trial also reported patient assessed outcome, with a result in favour of permethrin (OR for itch persistence with permethrin v gamma benzene hexachloride 0.65, 95% CI 0.44 to 0.96). **Permethrin versus ivermectin:** We found one additional RCT that compared topical permethrin with ivermectin, but details were insufficient to report results in this issue. The RCT will be reported fully in a subsequent issue.[10]

Harms: One RCT reported five serious adverse effects, two in the permethrin group (rash and possible diarrhoea) and three in the gamma benzene hexachloride group (pruritic rash, papules, and diarrhoea).[8] During 1990–1995, six adverse events were reported per 100 000 units distributed in the USA (one central nervous system adverse effect reported per 500 000 units of permethrin distributed).[11] Resistance to permethrin seems to be rare.[11]

Comment: None.

OPTION **GAMMA BENZENE HEXACHLORIDE**

One systematic review of RCTs has found that gamma benzene hexachloride is effective in the treatment of scabies, but we found rare reports of convulsions and other adverse effects.

Benefits: We found one systematic review,[5] which identified three RCTs comparing gamma benzene hexachloride versus other topical agents.[6,8,9] We also found one subsequent RCT comparing gamma benzene hexachloride versus ivermectin.[12] **Gamma benzene hexachloride versus crotamiton:** One RCT in 100 adults and children found no significant difference in clinical cure rates (OR for failed clinical cure with crotamiton v gamma benzene hexachloride 0.41, 95% CI 0.15 to 1.10).[6] **Gamma benzene hexachloride versus permethrin:** See permethrin above. **Gamma benzene hexachloride versus ivermectin:** One RCT in 53 adults referred to hospital with scabies found no significant difference in clinical cure rates at 15 days (risk of being cured AR 14/26 [54%] with ivermectin v 13/27 [48%] with gamma benzene hydrochloride; ARI 6%, 95% CI −20% to +31%; RR 1.1, 95% CI 0.7 to 1.9) or at 29 days (risk of being cured AR 18/26 [69%] with ivermectin v 23/27 [85%] with gamma benzene hexachloride; ARI 16%, 95% CI −7% to +37%; RR 0.8, 95% CI 0.6 to 1.1).[12]

Harms: The RCTs reported no severe adverse effects. Case reports and data from the WHO collaborating Centre for International Drug Monitoring included reports of rare severe adverse effects (e.g. convulsions and aplastic anaemia), particularly when gamma benzene hexachloride was applied to people with extensive skin disease and to children.[13,14] Summary reports from 47 countries suggest that gamma benzene hexachloride is more toxic than other preparations. Four convulsions were reported in people on benzyl benzoate, one on crotamiton, 38 on gamma benzene hexachloride, two on malathion, and six on permethrin. Deaths reported on benzyl benzoate were nil, crotamiton one, gamma benzene hexachloride one, malathion nil, and permethrin five.[15] Resistance has been reported in many countries.[16]

Comment: Gamma benzene hexachloride has been off the market in the UK since 1995 because of concern about possible adverse effects. The evidence linking gamma benzene hexachloride with convulsions is suggestive but not conclusive. Summary reports are influenced by how much the products are used for the treatment of scabies and other infestations, and the quality of reporting. Safety data from trials and observational studies need to be summarised, particularly regarding additional risks in infants and pregnant women.

OPTION   CROTAMITON

One systematic review of RCTs found no evidence of a difference between crotamiton and gamma benzene hexachloride, but found crotamiton to be less effective than permethrin.

Benefits: We found one systematic review,[5] which identified two RCTs comparing crotamiton versus other topical agents.[6,7] **Crotamiton versus permethrin:** See benefits of permethrin, p 1185. **Crotamiton versus gamma benzene hexachloride:** See benefits of gamma benzene hexachloride, p 1185.

Harms: We found limited data on the toxicity of crotamiton, but reports of serious adverse effects are rare.[13] There have been a few reports of resistance (see above).[13]

Comment: None.

OPTION   MALATHION

We found insufficient evidence. Cure rates of over 80% have been reported in case series.

Benefits: We found one systematic review, which identified no RCTs comparing malathion with any other drug treatments.[5] Case series suggest that malathion is effective in curing infestation with scabies, with a cure rate at 4 weeks of over 80%.[17,18]

Harms: No important adverse events have been reported.

Comment: The safety data from trials and observational studies need to be summarised, particularly with regard to additional risks in infants and pregnant women.

OPTION BENZYL BENZOATE

We found insufficient evidence from RCTs. Cure rates of about 50% have been reported in non-randomised trials.

Benefits: We found one systematic review and one additional RCT. **Benzyl benzoate versus ivermectin:** The review (search date 1997)[5] identified one small RCT in 44 adults and children that compared benzyl benzoate versus oral ivermectin.[19] This found no significant difference between the two treatments (see text, p 1188). **Benzyl benzoate versus sulphur ointment:** One RCT compared benzyl benzoate and sulphur ointment in 158 adults and children identified in a house to house survey of a semi-urban area of India.[20] There was no significant difference between the number with apparently cured lesions by 8 days (AR 68/89 [76%] with benzyl benzoate v 45/69 [65%] with sulphur ointment; RR cure 1.17, 95% CI 0.95 to 1.33) or by 14 days (AR 81/89 [91%] v 67/69 [97%]; RR 0.94, 95% CI 0.86 to 1.01).

Harms: About a quarter of people treated with benzyl benzoate reported a transient increase in pruritus and dermatitis.[19]

Comment: Non-randomised trials suggest benzyl benzoate has variable effectiveness (as low as 50%).[21–23] The low cure rate may be related to concentration of the preparation and resistance of the mite to benzyl benzoate.

OPTION SULPHUR COMPOUNDS

We found insufficient evidence.

Benefits: We found one RCT comparing sulphur ointment with benzyl benzoate (see benzyl benzoate above).[20]

Harms: Use of sulphur was associated with increased local irritation in about a quarter of cases.[13]

Comment: None.

QUESTION What are the effects of systemic treatments?

OPTION IVERMECTIN

We found inadequate evaluation of ivermectin in RCTs. Experience of its use in onchocerciasis suggests that it is safe in younger adults, but no such experience exists for children, and there have been reports of increased risk of death in elderly people.

Benefits: We found one systematic review,[5] which identified two RCTs comparing ivermectin with other topical agents.[19,24] We also found one subsequent RCT comparing ivermectin with gamma benzene hexachloride.[12] **Ivermectin versus placebo:** One RCT in 55 young adults and children aged over 5 years found oral ivermectin significantly more effective than placebo (clinical cure after 7 days AR 23/29 [79%] with ivermectin v 4/26 [15%] with placebo; ARI 64%, 95% CI 39% to 78%; RR 5.2, 95% CI 2.1 to 12.9; NNT 2, 95% CI 1 to 3).[24] **Ivermectin versus benzyl benzoate:** One RCT in 44 adults and children found no significant difference in clinical cure rates at 30 days (clinical cure AR 16/23 [70%] with ivermectin v 10/21 [48%] with benzyl benzoate; ARI 22%, 95% CI −7% to +46%; RR 1.5, 95% CI 0.9 to 2.5).[19] **Ivermectin versus gamma benzene hexachloride:** See benefits of gamma benzene hexachloride, p 1185. **Ivermectin versus permethrin:** See benefits of permethrin, p 1185.

Harms: The three RCTs were too small to give adequate data on harms.[12,19,24] Ivermectin has been used widely in adults with onchocerciasis; even with repeated doses, serious adverse effects have been rare.[25,26] There are no good data on its safety in children. An increased risk of death has been reported among elderly people taking ivermectin for scabies in a long term care facility.[27] It is not clear whether this was caused by ivermectin, or interactions with other scabicides (including gamma benzene hexachloride and permethrin) or other treatments such as psychoactive drugs. Other studies reported no such complications from its use in elderly people.[28]

Comment: Case series suggest that ivermectin may be effective when included in the treatment of hyperkeratotic crusted scabies (also known as Norwegian scabies),[29,30] and in people with concomitant HIV disease.[4]

REFERENCES

1. Meinking TL, Taplin D. Infestations. In: Schachner LA, Hansen RC, eds. *Pediatric dermatology*. New York: Churchill Livingston, 1995.

2. Stein DH. Scabies and pediculosis. *Curr Opin Pediatr* 1991;3:660–666.

3. Green M. Epidemiology of scabies. *Epidemiol Rev* 1989;11:126–150.

4. Meinking TL, Taplin D, Hermida JL, Pardo R, Kerddel FA. The treatment of scabies with ivermectin. *N Engl J Med* 1995;333:26–30.

5. Walker GJA, Johnstone PW. Treating scabies. In: The Cochrane Library, Issue 4, 1999. Oxford: Update Software. Search date 1997; primary sources Medline 1966 to 1997; Embase 1974 to 1997; records of military trials from UK, USA, Russia; and specialist register of the Cochrane Diseases Group.

6. Amer M, El-Gharib I. Permethrin versus crotamiton and lindane in the treatment of scabies. *Int J Dermatol* 1992;31:357–358.

7. Taplin D, Meinking TL, Chen JA, Sanchez R. Comparison of crotamiton 10% cream (Eurax) and permethrin 5% cream (Elimite) for the treatment of scabies in children. *Pediatr Dermatol* 1990;7:67–73.

8. Schultz MW, Gomez M, Hansen RC, et al. Comparative study of 5% permethrin cream and 1% lindane lotion for the treatment of scabies. *Arch Dermatol* 1990;126:167–170.

9. Taplin D, Meinking TL, Porcelain SL, Castilero PM, Chen JA. Permethrin 5% dermal cream: a new treatment for scabies. *J Am Acad Dermatol* 1986;15:995–1001.

10. Usha, V. and Gopalakrishnan Nair, TV. A comparative study of oral ivermectin and topical permethrin cream in the treatment of scabies. *J Am Acad Dermatol* 2000;42:236–240.

11. Meinking TL, Taplin D. Safety of permethrin vs lindane for the treatment of scabies. *Arch Dermatol* 1996;132:959–962.

12. Chouela EN, Abeldano AM, Pellerano G, et al. Equivalent therapeutic efficacy and safety of ivermectin and lindane in the treatment of human scabies. *Arch Dermatol* 1999;135:651–655.

13. Elgart ML. A risk-benefit assessment of agents used in the treatment of scabies. *Drug Saf* 1996;14:386–393.

14. McLeod WA. Acute lindane poisoning [letter]. *Can Med Assoc J* 1978;118:123–125.

15. WHO Collaborating Centre for International Drug Monitoring. Reported adverse reactions to ectoparasiticodes, including scabicides, insecticides and repellents. Uppsala, Sweden. January 1998.

16. Brown S, Belcher J, Brady W. Treatment of ectoparasitic infections: review of the English-language literature. *Clin Infect Dis* 1995;20(suppl 1):104–109.

17. Hanna NF, Clay JC, Harris JRW. Sarcoptes scabiei infestation treated with malathion liquid. *Br J Vener Dis* 1978;54:354.

18. Thianprasit M, Schuetzenberger R. Prioderm lotion in the treatment of scabies. *Southeast Asian J Trop Med Public Health* 1984;15:119–120.

19. Glaziou P, Cartel JL, Alzieu P, Moulia-Pelat JP, Martin PMV. Comparison of ivermectin and benzyl

benzoate for treatment of scabies. *Trop Med Parasitol* 1993;44:331–332.

20. Gulati PV, Singh KP. A family based study on the treatment of scabies with benzyl benzoate and sulphur ointment. *Indian J Dermatol Venereol Lepr* 1978;44:269–273.

21. Burgess I, Robinson RJF, Robinson J, Maunder JW, Hassan Z. Aqueous malathion 0.5% as a scabicide: clinical trial. *BMJ* 1986;292:1172.

22. Kaur GA, Nadeswary K. Field trials on the management of scabies in Jengka Triangle, Pahang. *Med J Malaysia* 1980;35:14–21.

23. Haustein UF, Hlawa B. Treatment of scabies with permethrin versus lindane and benzyl benzoate. *Acta Derm Venereol* 1989;69:348–351.

24. Macotela-Ruiz E, Pena-Gonzalez G. Tratamiento de la escabiasis con ivermectina por via oral. *Gac Med Mex* 1993;129:201–205.

25. Pacque M, Munoz B, Greene BM, et al. Safety of and compliance with community-based ivermectin therapy. *Lancet* 1990;335:1377–1380.

26. De Sole G, Remme J, Awadzi K, et al. Adverse reactions after large-scale treatment of onchocerciasis with ivermectin: combined results from eight community trials. *Bull World Health Organ* 1989;67:707–719.

27. Barkwell R, Shields S. Deaths associated with ivermectin treatment of scabies. *Lancet* 1997; 349:1144–1145.

28. Diazgranados JA, Costa JL. Deaths after ivermectin treatment. *Lancet* 1997;349:1698.

29. Sullivan JR, Watt G, Barker B. Successful use of ivermectin in the treatment of endemic scabies in a nursing home. *Australas J Dermatol* 1997;38: 137–140.

30. Aubin F, Humbert P. Ivermectin for crusted (Norwegian) scabies. *N Engl J Med* 1995;332:612.

Godfrey Walker
WHO Adviser in Reproductive Health
UNFPA Country Support Team for
Central and South Asia
Kathmandu
Nepal

Paul Johnstone
Director of Public Health,
Visiting Professor in Public Health
University of Teeside
Middlesborough
UK
Competing interests: None declared.

Squamous cell carcinoma of the skin: non-metastatic

Search date October 2000: new for this issue

Adèle Green and Robin Marks

INTERVENTIONS

Likely to be beneficial
Sunscreen in prevention (regular versus discretionary use) . .1192

Unknown effectiveness
Primary excision (unknown optimal margin of excision) 1193
Micrographically controlled (Mohs') surgery (unknown benefit compared with standard surgical excision) 1193
Radiotherapy after surgery (unknown benefit compared with surgery alone) 1194

See glossary, p 1194

Key Messages

- One RCT found limited evidence that daily sunscreen compared with placebo sunscreen reduces the incidence of new solar keratoses.
- One RCT found limited evidence that daily compared with discretionary use of sunscreen in adults prevents squamous cell carcinoma.
- We found no good evidence of an optimal margin for primary excision of squamous cell carcinoma.
- We found no good evidence comparing micrographically controlled (Mohs') surgery versus standard surgery as primary treatment.
- We found no good evidence comparing radiotherapy after surgery versus surgery alone in preventing local recurrence.

DEFINITION Cutaneous squamous cell carcinoma is a malignant tumour of committed keratinocytes arising in the epidermis, showing histological evidence of dermal invasion.

INCIDENCE/ PREVALENCE Incidence rates are often derived from special surveys because few cancer registries routinely collect notifications of squamous cell carcinoma of the skin. Incidence rates on exposed skin vary markedly round the world according to skin colour and latitude, and range from negligible rates in black populations and white populations living at very high latitudes, to rates of about 1000 per 100 000 in white residents of tropical Australia.[1]

AETIOLOGY/ RISK FACTORS People with fair skin colour who sunburn easily without tanning, people with xeroderma pigmentosum (see glossary, p 1194),[2–4] and those who are immunosuppressed[5] are susceptible to squamous cell carcinoma. The strongest environmental risk factor for squamous cell carcinoma is chronic sun exposure. Cohort and case control studies have found that clinical signs of chronic skin damage, especially solar keratoses, are also determinants of cutaneous squamous cell carcinoma.[3,4] For example, the risk of squamous cell carcinoma in people with the propensity to severe sunburn or with a history of multiple sunburns is three times greater than in people with no such propensity. In people with multiple solar keratoses (> 15), the risk of squamous cell carcinoma is 10–15 times greater than in people with no solar keratoses.[3,4]

PROGNOSIS Relates to location and size of tumour, histological pattern, depth of invasion, perineural involvement, and whether the person is immunosuppressed.[6,7] A worldwide review of 95 case series, each comprising at least 20 people, found the overall metastasis rate for squamous cell carcinoma on the ear is 11% and on the lip 14%, compared with an average over all sites of 5%.[7] A review of 71 case series found that lesions less than 2 cm in diameter compared with lesions greater than 2 cm have more than twice the local recurrence rate (6% v 16%), and three times the rate of metastasis (8% v 23%).[7]

AIMS To prevent the occurrence of squamous cell carcinoma; to achieve cure by eradicating local disease including microinvasive disease; and to reduce mortality.

OUTCOMES **Prevention:** Incidence of cutaneous squamous cell carcinoma; mortality from squamous cell carcinoma. **Primary excision:** Local recurrence; survival; cosmetic outcome. **Radiotherapy after surgery:** Local recurrence; regional recurrence; survival.

METHODS *Clinical Evidence* search and appraisal October 2000, and supplementary search of reference lists of all identified review articles and relevant sections of dermatology textbooks.

Squamous cell carcinoma of the skin: non-metastatic

Skin disorders

QUESTION Does the use of sunscreen help to prevent cutaneous squamous cell carcinoma?

Adèle Green

One RCT found significantly fewer new solar keratoses with daily sunscreen versus placebo sunscreen. One RCT found a 40% reduction in the incidence of squamous cell carcinoma with daily application of sunscreen to the head and neck, arms, and hands compared with discretionary application.

Benefits: We found no systematic review. **Versus placebo:** One RCT (588 people with previous solar keratoses) found a significant decrease in new solar keratoses after 7 months use of daily sunscreen versus placebo (mean 1.6 v 2.3 new lesions per person; RR 0.62, 95% CI 0.54 to 0.71), and a significantly greater chance of lesion remission (OR 1.5, 95% CI 1.3 to 1.8).[8] **Daily versus discretionary use:** One community based RCT (1621 adults in a subtropical Australian community) compared daily use of a sunscreen (sun protection factor 15+) versus sunscreen use at their usual discretionary rate.[9] People allocated to daily use of sunscreen were told to apply it to the head, neck, arms, and hands every morning and reapplication was advised after heavy sweating, bathing, or long sun exposure. They were reminded every 3 months by research staff when sunscreen supplies were replenished. There was a significantly lower incidence of squamous cell carcinoma tumours after 4.5 years (22 people with 28 new squamous cell carcinomas with daily sunscreen use v 25 people with 46 new squamous cell carcinomas with discretionary sunscreen use; RR 0.61, 95% CI 0.46 to 0.81). Subgroup analysis found no significant difference between those with a history of skin cancer and those without.[9]

Harms: Daily sunscreen use in two RCTs caused contact allergy in a small proportion of users (< 10%)[10] and skin irritation in a variable proportion of users (2–15%).[9,10] No people tested were allergic to the active ingredients of sunscreen, whereas irritant reactions both to active sunscreen and the control base cream were observed in the placebo controlled RCT.[8] The RCT of regular versus discretionary use found that daily sunscreen use was not associated with greater sun exposure, including recreational exposure.[9] However, another RCT among young adults who used sunscreen while intentionally exposing themselves to the sun ("sunbathing") found that use of a sun protection factor 30 sunscreen compared with a sun protection factor 10 sunscreen was associated with significantly longer exposure times.[11]

Comment: In a long term prevention trial using skin cancer as the outcome, placebo sunscreen may be regarded as unethical. It would also be difficult to mask treatment allocation.

QUESTION What is the optimal margin for primary excision of cutaneous squamous cell carcinoma?

Robin Marks

We found insufficient evidence relating size of primary excision margin to local recurrence rate.

Benefits: We found no systematic reviews or RCTs assessing different excision margins at any sites measuring local recurrence.

Harms: Although we found no quantified evidence, it is thought that with all kinds of surgery there is potential for tissue destruction and scarring, particularly of vital structures such as eyelids, lip margins, and, motor and sensory nerves.

Comment: One prospective case series using Mohs' surgery (see glossary, p 1194) related excision margins to histological extension of the tumour and found a 95% clearance rate of squamous cell carcinomas less than 2 cm in diameter with a margin of 4 mm of normal skin, and a 96% clearance rate of tumours greater than 2 cm with a margin of 6 mm.[12] The sites of scalp, ears, eyelid, nose, and lip were found to have more deeply invasive tumours. Numerous case series suggest that primary excision of cutaneous squamous cell carcinoma has a likelihood of local recurrence varying from 5–20% depending on tumour size, site, histopathological differentiation, perineural involvement, and depth of invasion.[7,13–18]

QUESTION Does micrographically controlled (Mohs') surgery result in lower rates of local recurrence than standard primary excision?

We found insufficient evidence.

Benefits: We found no RCTs comparing Mohs' surgery with standard surgical excision.

Harms: Although we found no quantified evidence, it is thought that with all kinds of surgery there is potential for tissue destruction and scarring particularly of vital structures such as eyelids, lip margins, and motor and sensory nerves.

Comment: A review of case series since 1940 suggested a local recurrence rate of 3% for Mohs' surgery compared with 8% for primary excision of cutaneous squamous cell carcinoma. However, the evidence must be treated with caution because of differing study quality, the long time period covered, and potential differences between cases referred to Mohs' surgery and those treated with non-Mohs' surgery.[7] A site specific comparison found lower 5 year local recurrence rates after Mohs' surgery for primary squamous cell carcinoma of the lip (2% v 16%) and of the ear (5% v 19%).[7]

QUESTION Does radiotherapy after surgery effect local recurrence of cutaneous squamous cell carcinoma?

Adèle Green

We found insufficient evidence.

Benefits: We found no systematic reviews and no RCTs.

Harms: Although not measured, there is the potential for long term scar deterioration with post-radiation depigmentation, and gradual development of chronic radio-dermatitis, including telangiectasiae, thinning of the skin, and hyperkeratosis (see glossary, p 1194).

Comment: In rare instances squamous cell carcinomas cannot be excised completely and these have recurrence rates of over 50%.[19,20] Case series of inadequately excised squamous cell carcinomas, especially those with microscopic perineural invasion (see glossary, p 1194) found at time of curative surgery, have reported recurrence rates of 20–25% after 5 years when surgery was followed by radiotherapy.[21,22]

GLOSSARY

Hyperkeratosis Increased scaling on the surface of the skin.

Micrographically controlled (Mohs') surgery Does not use standard excision margins as the basis for achieving tumour clearance. The visible tumour and a thin margin of apparently normal skin are removed, mapped, and examined microscopically using a specialised sectioning technique at the time of surgery, and the surgery continues until there is microscopic confirmation of complete tumour clearance, at which stage the wound is closed.[23]

Perineural invasion Tumour IK nerve.

Radio-dermatitis Chronic non-malignant changes in the skin due to excessive radiation.

Telangiectasiae Dilated small blood vessels that form a small focal red lesion in the skin.

Xeroderma pigmentosum An inherited disorder with defective repair of DNA damage caused by ultraviolet radiation, resulting in sun related skin cancers of all types at a very early age.

REFERENCES

1. Buettner PG, Raasch BA. Incidence rates of skin cancer in Townsville, Australia. *Int J Cancer* 1998; 78:587–593.

2. Bouwes Bavinck JN, Claas FH, Hardie DR, Green A, Vermeer BJ, Hardie IR. The risk of skin cancer in renal transplant recipients in Queensland, Australia: a follow-up study. *Transplantation* 1996; 15:715–711.

3. English DR, Armstrong BK, Kricker A, Winter MG, Heenan PJ, Randell PL. Demographic characteristics, pigmentary and cutaneous risk factors for squamous cell carcinoma: a case-control study. *Int J Cancer* 1998;76:628–634.

4. Green A, Battistutta D, Hart V, Leslie D, Weedon D, the Nambour Study Group. Skin cancer in a subtropical Australian population: incidence and lack of association with occupation. *Am J Epidemiol* 1996;144:1034–1040.

5. Kraemer KH, Lee MM, Andrews AD, Lambert WC. The role of sunlight and DNA repair in melanoma and nonmelanoma skin cancer. The xeroderma

pigmentosum paradigm. *Arch Dermatol* 1994; 130:1018–1021.

6. Johnson TM, Rowe DE, Nelson BR, Swanson NA. Squamous cell carcinoma of the skin (excluding lip and oral mucosa). *J Am Acad Dermatol* 1992;26: 467–484.

7. Rowe DE, Carroll RJ, Day CL. Prognostic factors for local recurrence, metastasis, and survival rates in squamous cell carcinoma of the skin, ear, and lip. *J Am Acad Dermatol* 1992;26:976–990.

8. Thompson SC, Jolley D, Marks R. Reduction of solar keratoses by regular sunscreen use. *N Engl J Med* 1993;329:1147–1151.

9. Green A, Williams G, Neale R, et al. Daily sunscreen application and betacarotene supplementation in prevention of basal cell and squamous-cell carcinomas of the skin: a randomised controlled trial. *Lancet* 1999;354: 723–729.

10. Foley P, Nixon R, Marks R, Frowen K, Thompson S. The frequency of reactions to sunscreens: results of a longitudinal population-based study on the

regular use of sunscreens in Australia. *Br J Dermatol* 1993;128:512–518.

11. Autier P, Dore JF, Negrier S, et al. Sunscreen use and duration of sun exposure: a double blind randomised trial. *J Natl Cancer Inst* 1999;15: 1304–1309.

12. Brodland DG, Zitelli JA. Surgical margins for excision of primary cutaneous squamous cell carcinoma. *J Am Acad Dermatol* 1992;27:241–248.

13. de Visscher JGAM, Botke G, Schakenradd JACM, van der Waal I. A comparison of results after radiotherapy and surgery for stage 1 squamous cell carcinoma of the lower lip. *Head Neck* 1999: 526–530.

14. Ashby MA, Smith J, Ainslie J, McEwan L. Treatment of nonmelanoma skin cancer at a large Australian Center. *Cancer* 1989;6:1863–1871.

15. Eroglu A, Berberoglu U, Berreroglu S. Risk factors related to locoregional recurrence in squamous cell carcinoma of the skin. *J Surg Oncol* 1996;61: 124–130.

16. McCombe D, MacGill, Ainslie J, Beresford J, Matthews J. Squamous cell carcinoma of the lip: A retrospective review of the Peter MacCallum Cancer Institute experience 1979–88. *Aust NZ J Surg* 2000;70:358–361.

17. Yoon M, Chougule P, Dufresne R, Wanebo HJ. Localised carcinoma of the external ear is an unrecognised aggressive disease with a high propensity for local regional recurrence. *Am J Surg* 1992;164:574–577.

18. Zitsch RP, Park CW, Renner GJ, Rea JL. Outcome analysis for lip carcinoma. *Otolaryngol Head Neck Surg* 1995;113:589–596.

19. Glass RL, Perez-Mesa C. Management of inadequately excised epidermoid carcinoma. *Arch Surg* 1974;108:50–51.

20. Glass RL, Spratt JS, Perez-Mesa C. The fate of inadequately excised epidermoid carcinoma of the skin. *Surg Gynaecol Obstet* 1966;122:245–248.

21. Shimm DS, Wilder RB. Radiation therapy for squamous cell carcinoma of the skin. *Am J Clin Oncol* 1991;14:381–386.

22. McCord MW, Mendenhall WM, Parsons JT, et al. Skin cancer of the head and neck with clinical perineural invasion. *Int J Radiat Oncol Biol Phys* 2000;47:89–93.

23. Holmkvist KA, Roenigk RK. Squamous cell carcinoma of the lip treated with Mohs' micrographic surgery: outcome at 5 years. *J Am Acad Dermatol* 1998;38:960–966.

Adèle Green
Professor
Queensland Institute
of Medical Research
Brisbane
Australia

Robin Marks
Professor
University of Melbourne
Melbourne
Australia

Competing interests: AG, none declared. RM has undertaken studies in association with 3M Pharmaceuticals on the value of topically applied Imiquimod in the management of actinic (solar) keratoses and basal cell carcinoma.

Breast cancer: metastatic

Search date January 2001: expanded this issue

Stephen Johnston and Justin Stebbing

QUESTIONS

INTERVENTIONS

Beneficial

Hormone Therapy

Tamoxifen in oestrogen receptor
positive disease 1198

Combined gonadorelin analogues
and tamoxifen in premenopausal
women New 1200

Selective aromatase inhibitors as
second line therapy in
postmenopausal women. . .1202

Chemotherapy

Anthracycline based regimens
(CAF) containing
doxorubicin 1204

Classical combination
chemotherapy (CMF) 1204

For bone metastasis

Radiotherapy plus appropriate
analgesia* 1209

*For central nervous system
metastases*

Radiotherapy for spinal cord
compression* 1210

Adding high dose steroids to
radiotherapy in spinal cord
compression* 1211

Likely to be beneficial

Selective aromatase inhibitors as
first line hormonal therapy in
postmenopausal
women New 1201

New cytotoxic drugs in
anthracycline resistant disease
(such as taxanes and
semisynthetic vinca
alkaloids) 1207

Bisphosphonates 1208

Radiotherapy to control cerebral
and choroidal
metastases* 1211

**Trade off between benefits and
harms**

Progestins (beneficial in women with
bone pain or anorexia) 1199

Ovarian ablation in premenopausal
women (versus tamoxifen) . .1200

Likely to be ineffective or harmful

Progestins (versus tamoxifen). .1199

High dose chemotherapy
(versus conventional
chemotherapy) 1206

**To be covered in future issues of
*Clinical Evidence***

Combined anthracyclines and
taxanes for first line
chemotherapy

Biological therapy for HER-2
positive tumours with
trastuzumab

Supportive care (analgesics,
antiemetics, steroids)

* Not based on RCT evidence
See glossary, p 1212

Key Messages

RCTs have found:

- Benefit from tamoxifen in the first line treatment of women with oestrogen receptor positive metastatic breast cancer.
- Survival benefit from combined ovarian ablation with gonadorelin analogue with tamoxifen compared with gonadorelin analogue alone in premenopausal oestrogen receptor positive metastatic breast cancer.
- Survival benefit (and acceptable toxicity profile) from selective aromatase inhibitors in postmenopausal women who have relapsed during or after treatment with tamoxifen.
- Overall survival benefit with combination chemotherapy regimens (particularly those containing an anthracycline, such as doxorubicin) compared with single drug regimens.
- No evidence that high dose chemotherapy confers additional survival benefit compared with standard dose chemotherapy.
- Limited survival benefit from second line chemotherapy, but no good evidence on its impact on quality of life compared with best supportive care.
- Benefit from bisphosphonates in terms of reduced skeletal complications with minimal toxicity in women with bone metastases secondary to metastatic breast cancer.
- Benefit from radiotherapy in women with symptoms from bone or spinal metastases, and probable benefit in those with cerebral or choroidal metastases.

DEFINITION Metastatic or advanced breast cancer is the presence of disease at distant sites such as the bone, liver, or lung. It is not treatable by primary surgery and is currently considered incurable. Symptoms may include pain from bone metastases, breathlessness from spread to the lung, and nausea or abdominal discomfort from liver involvement.

INCIDENCE/ PREVALENCE Metastatic breast cancer causes up to 500 000 deaths worldwide per year (46 000 in the USA and 15 000 in the UK).[1] The true prevalence of metastatic disease is much higher because some women live with the disease for many years.

AETIOLOGY/ RISK FACTORS The risk of metastatic disease relates to known prognostic factors in the original primary tumour. These factors include oestrogen receptor negative disease, primary tumours 3 cm or more in diameter, and axillary node involvement—recurrence occurred within 10 years of adjuvant chemotherapy (see glossary, p 1212) for early breast cancer in 60–70% of node positive women and 25–30% of node negative women in one large systematic review.[2]

PROGNOSIS Most women who develop metastatic breast cancer will ultimately die of their disease. Prognosis depends on age, extent of disease, and oestrogen receptor status. There is also evidence that overexpression of the product of the HER2/neu oncogene, which occurs in about a third of women with metastatic breast cancer, is associated with a worse prognosis.[3] A short disease free interval (see glossary, p 1212) (e.g. less than 1 year) between surgery for early breast cancer and developing metastases suggests that the recurrent disease is likely to be resistant to the drug used for adjuvant treatment (see glossary, p 1212).[4] In women who receive no treatment for metastatic disease, the median survival from diagnosis of metastases is 12 months.[5] The choice of first line treatment (see glossary, p 1213) (hormonal or chemotherapy) is based on a variety of clinical factors (see glossary, p 1212 and table 1, p 1217).[6-9]

AIMS To relieve symptoms, prolong life, and improve quality of life, with minimal adverse effects.

OUTCOMES Symptoms; progression free survival; overall objective response rate; complete response; partial response (see glossary, p 1213); duration of response; disease stabilisation; time to progression of disease (progression defined as more than a 25% increase in lesion size or the appearance of new lesions); quality of life;[10] improvement in performance status (according to validated scales of daily functioning/activity[11]); adverse effects and toxicity of treatment;[12] and overall survival. Response to treatment is a surrogate outcome measure for assessing the effects of treatment on survival or quality of life. The link between clinical and proxy outcomes has not been clearly validated. Women who respond to treatment are more likely to experience improved symptomatic relief, performance status, and survival.[13-15] One recent prospective study of 300 women with metastatic breast cancer showed that there was a significant relationship between improvement and objective response for three symptoms in particular: cancer pain, shortness of breath, and abnormal mood. Symptom improvement was greatest in those people who had a complete or partial response.[16]

METHODS *Clinical Evidence* update search and appraisal January 2001. We looked for good systematic reviews of RCTs that used the outcome measures listed above. Where we found no good systematic reviews, we selected relevant randomised phase III trials using these outcomes. Data presented only in abstract form were discarded. Response to treatment is often assessed in an unblinded fashion, introducing the possibility of bias. Few trials of acceptable quality reported data on symptoms or quality of life.

| QUESTION | What are the effects of first line treatments? |

| OPTION | ANTIOESTROGENS (TAMOXIFEN) |

RCTs have found that antioestrogens such as tamoxifen (see glossary, p 1213) are effective in prolonging remission in women with oestrogen receptor positive metastatic breast cancer.

Benefits: We found no systematic review. Non-systematic reviews published in 1987 and 1991 identified 86 RCTs in 5353 women with metastatic breast cancer unselected for oestrogen receptor status. The overall objective response rate to tamoxifen was 34%. Disease stabilisation was achieved in a further 20%, and overall the median duration of response was 12–18 months.[6,7] The likelihood of responding to tamoxifen was highest (60–70%) in postmenopausal women with oestrogen receptor positive disease(see comment below).[8,9] **Versus ovarian ablation in premenopausal women:** See ovarian ablation in premenopausal women, p 1200.

Harms: **Minor adverse effects:** Tamoxifen is well tolerated in women with metastatic breast cancer; fewer than 3% of women discontinued tamoxifen as a result of toxicity.[17] Reported adverse effects included minor gastrointestinal upset (8%), hot flushes (27%), and menstrual disturbance in premenopausal women (13%).[18] **Tumour flare:** During the first few weeks of treatment, tumour flare occurred in fewer than 5% of women. For those with bone metastases, this may result in increased pain or symptomatic hypercalcaemia. **Relapse:** Most women who initially respond to tamoxifen eventually progress and develop acquired resistance to tamoxifen, although they may still respond to further hormonal interventions.[19]

Comment: The choice of first line treatment (hormonal or chemotherapy) is based on a variety of clinical factors (see table 1, p 1217).[6–9] **Anti-oestrogens:** An emerging problem is that many women have already received adjuvant tamoxifen for early breast cancer, or have developed metastatic disease while still on tamoxifen, and are thus considered resistant to it. Effective second line (see glossary, p 1213) hormonal drugs such as selective aromatase inhibitors (see glossary, p 1212) are now used after tamoxifen failure (see selective aromatase inhibitors in postmenopausal women, p 1202), and RCTs have compared these drugs with tamoxifen as first line treatment (see selective aromatase inhibitors first line therapy, p 1201). New non-steroidal antioestrogens (toremifene, idoxifene, raloxifene) and steroidal antioestrogens (fulvestrant) are more selective than tamoxifen and may have fewer long term adverse effects. RCTs comparing some of these drugs with tamoxifen as first line hormonal treatment in metastatic breast cancer are in progress. So far, one RCT in 658 women has found no evidence of clear clinical superiority of toremifene over tamoxifen.[20] **Oestrogen receptor status:** Tamoxifen is a competitive oestrogen receptor antagonist, and adjuvant tamoxifen has been found to have no effect in women with early breast cancer that is oestrogen receptor negative (systematic review of 55 RCTs in 37 000 women).[21] We found no RCTs comparing outcomes in women with oestrogen receptor positive disease versus those whose oestrogen receptor status was unknown (oestrogen receptor negative women were excluded from most trials).

OPTION   **PROGESTINS (MEDROXYPROGESTERONE; MEGESTROL)**

RCTs have found that progestins (see glossary, p 1213) are as effective as tamoxifen in first line treatment of metastatic breast cancer, but they are not as well tolerated. Specific beneficial effects can make progestins useful in women with bone pain or anorexia.

Benefits: We found one systematic review (search date 1991, 7 RCTs, 801 women with metastatic breast cancer) comparing medroxyprogesterone acetate versus tamoxifen. This found no significant difference in response rates (35–54%), remission rates, or survival between the two groups.[22] Benefits of progestins included an analgesic effect (assessed using questionnaires), especially on painful bone metastases,[23] increased appetite, weight gain, and a feeling of wellbeing. A more recent RCT (166 women) found that the rate of response of bone metastases was significantly higher with medroxyprogesterone than with tamoxifen (33% v 13%, P = 0.01), although there was no significant difference in survival.[24]

Harms: Women taking medroxyprogesterone experienced more adverse effects than women taking tamoxifen.[25] These were common at higher doses and included nausea (14%), weight gain (56%), vaginal bleeding (10%), and exacerbation of hypertension. In women with lymphangitis carcinomatosis, progestins may exacerbate symptoms of breathlessness.[26]

Comment: In view of the lack of evidence of greater benefit, and the evidence of greater harm, progestins are reserved for second or third line hormonal treatment in women with advanced breast cancer who have not responded to tamoxifen. Specific groups of women may benefit from earlier use, such as those with painful bone metastases and anorexia.

OPTION   OVARIAN ABLATION IN PREMENOPAUSAL WOMEN

RCTs found no evidence in premenopausal women that ovarian ablation is more effective than tamoxifen in response to treatment or survival. It is associated with substantial adverse effects.

Benefits: **Versus tamoxifen:** We found one systematic review (seach date not stated, 4 RCTs, 220 premenopausal women) comparing tamoxifen versus ovarian ablation (carried out by either surgery or irradiation).[27] There was no significant difference between treatments in terms of response rate, response duration, or survival. A subsequent RCT (39 premenopausal women) comparing initial treatment with tamoxifen or ovarian ablation confirmed these findings (OR for progressive disease (see glossary, p 1213) 0.71, 95% CI 0.37 to 1.38; median survival 2.35 years with tamoxifen, 2.46 years with ovarian ablation, P = 0.98; OR for death 1.07, 95% CI 0.55 to 2.06).[28] **Different methods of ovarian ablation:** We found no good systematic review. We found two RCTs comparing gonadorelin analogues (see glossary, p 1213) versus surgical ovariectomy or irradiation. They found no significant difference in survival between treatments.[29,30]

Harms: Adverse effects include hot flushes (75% with gonadorelin analogues, 46% with surgical ovariectomy) and "tumour flare" (16% with gonadorelin analogues).[29] In addition, surgical ovariectomy requires an operation and anaesthetic in someone with an incurable disease.

Comment: None.

OPTION   COMBINED GONADORELIN ANALOGUES PLUS TAMOXIFEN AS FIRST LINE HORMONAL THERAPY IN PREMENOPAUSAL WOMEN   New

Stephen Johnston

One meta-analysis has found that, in pre-menopausal women, combined therapy with a gonadorelin analogue and tamoxifen is more effective than gonadorelin analogue alone.

Benefits: We found one meta-analysis (4 RCTs, 506 women), which found a significant improvement in both progression free survival (HR 0.70, 95% CI 0.58 to 0.85, P = 0.0003) and overall survival (HR 0.78, 95% CI 0.63 to 0.96, P = 0.02) for combined endocrine therapy with gonadorelin analogues plus tamoxifen compared with a gonadorelin analogue alone.[31] The overall response rate was also significantly higher for combined therapy (OR 0.67, P = 0.03).

Harms: Although the meta-analysis did not analyse differences in tolerability, in the largest of the individual trials there was no difference in the incidence of expected hormonal effects (hot flushes, vaginal discharge) for the combined therapy versus gonadorelin analogues alone.

Comment: This is the first time that combined endocrine therapy in metastatic breast cancer has been shown to be beneficial over single agent therapy. Attention is now turning to see if there is any additional benefit for complete oestrogen deprivation in premenopausal women using ovarian ablation with gonadorelin analogues combined with aromatase inhibitors.

OPTION	SELECTIVE AROMATASE INHIBITORS AS FIRST LINE HORMONAL THERAPY IN POSTMENOPAUSAL WOMEN New

Stephen Johnston and Justin Stebbing

Two RCTs have found that the aromatase inhibitor anastrozole is at least as effective as tamoxifen as first line therapy in metastatic postmenopausal breast cancer.

Benefits: We found no systematic review. We found two RCTs comparing anastrozole versus tamoxifen.[32,33] The larger RCT (668 women) showed no difference in time to disease progression (HR 0.99, 95% CI 0.86 to 1.12) or response rate (32.9% anastrozole v 32.6% tamoxifen).[32] The smaller RCT (353 women) showed a significant benefit for anastrozole in prolonging time to progression (HR 1.44, 95% CI 1.16 to 1.82).[33] There are no data from either trial on the effect on survival.

Harms: In both trials, the incidence of thromboembolic events was less in women receiving anastrozole than in those receiving tamoxifen (4.8 v 7.3% and 4.1% v 8.2%, respectively).[32,33] In addition, there were fewer reported events of vaginal bleeding (1.2 % with anastrazole v 3.8% with tamoxifen,[32] and 1.2% with anastrazole v 2.4% with tamoxifen.[33])

Comment: The final published results of two large RCTs with the aromatase inhibitors letrozole or exemestane versus tamoxifen are awaited, although preliminary published data in abstract form from both trials have suggested that response rates and time to disease progression were superior compared with tamoxifen for both letrozole (H Mouridsen, personal communication, 2001) and exemestane (R Paridaeens, personal communication, 2001).

| QUESTION | What are the effects of second line hormonal treatments in women who have not responded to tamoxifen? |

| OPTION | PROGESTINS |

RCTs have found that progestins are less effective in second line treatment than selective aromatase inhibitors (see glossary, p 1212) and have more adverse effects.

Benefits: **Versus selective aromatase inhibitors:** See selective aromatase inhibitors in postmenopausal women below.

Harms: **Versus selective aromatase inhibitors:** See selective aromatase inhibitors in postmenopausal women below.

Comment: In women who are not responding to tamoxifen, progestins may have a role in increasing feelings of wellbeing and relieving anorexia.

| OPTION | SELECTIVE AROMATASE INHIBITORS IN POSTMENOPAUSAL WOMEN |

RCTs have found that, in postmenopausal women with metastatic breast cancer who have relapsed on adjuvant tamoxifen or progressed during first line treatment with tamoxifen, the selective aromatase inhibitors anastrozole, letrozole, and exemestane prolong survival with minimal adverse effects. The evidence suggests that selective aromatase inhibitors are significantly more effective and better tolerated than previous standard second line treatment with a progestin or the non-selective aromatase inhibitor aminoglutethimide, and are most effective in oestrogen receptor positive women.

Benefits: We found no systematic review. **Anastrozole versus progestins:** A meta-analysis of the only two randomised phase III trials comparing anastrozole versus megestrol (764 postmenopausal women with metastatic breast cancer unresponsive to tamoxifen, median age 65 years, 70% oestrogen receptor positive, 30% oestrogen receptor status unknown) found no significant difference in objective response rates (10.3% v 7.9%) or in the proportion of women whose disease was stabilised for 6 months (25.1% v 26.1%).[34] A subsequent analysis after a median of 31 months' follow up found a significant improvement in overall survival with anastrozole (HR 0.78, P = 0.02), with an absolute improvement in 2 year survival from 46.3% to 56.1% (P = 0.02) and an improvement in median survival of 4 months (from 22.5 to 26.7 months).[35] **Exemestane versus progestins:** Exemestane is currently being evaluated in phase III trials.[36] One RCT (769 women) found that median survival time was significantly longer with exemestane (median not reached) than with megestrol (123 weeks; P = 0.039), as were the median duration of overall success (complete response/partial response or stable disease ≥24 weeks; 60.1 v 49.1 weeks; P = 0.025), and time to tumour progression (20.3 v 16.6 weeks; P = 0.037).[37] Compared with megestrol, there were similar or greater improvements in pain control, tumour related signs and symptoms, and quality of life with exemestane.[37] **Letrozole versus progestins or aminoglutethimide:** Two large RCTs compared letrozole 0.5 mg or

2.5 mg versus megestrol (551 women[38]) and aminoglutethimide (555 women[39]). Both trials were in postmenopausal women with metastatic breast cancer unresponsive to tamoxifen (median age 64–65 years, 55% oestrogen receptor positive, 45% oestrogen receptor status unknown). Letrozole was significantly more effective; compared with megestrol, letrozole 2.5 mg was associated with a significantly higher response rate (HR 1.82, 95% CI 1.02 to 3.25, P = 0.04), longer duration of response (HR 0.42, 95% CI 0.2 to 0.86, P = 0.02), and longer time to treatment failure (HR 0.77, 95% CI 0.61 to 0.99, P = 0.04).[38] Compared with aminoglutethimide, letrozole achieved better overall survival (HR 0.64, 95% CI 0.49 to 0.85, P = 0.002) and time to progression (HR 0.72, 95% CI 0.57 to 0.92, P = 0.008).[39]

Harms: The selective aromatase inhibitors were generally well tolerated and associated with fewer adverse events than with aminoglutethimide or progestins. **Anastrozole:** In the RCTs, anastrozole 1 mg was associated with a higher incidence of minor gastrointestinal disturbance (nausea or change in bowel habit) than megestrol (29% v 21%, P = 0.005) but a significantly lower incidence of greater than 5% gain in weight (13% v 34%, P < 0.0001).[34] **Exemestane:** In the RCTs, more women treated with progestin had adverse events (45.8% v 39.1%). The most frequently reported adverse events in the women treated with exemestane were low grade hot flushes (12.6%), nausea (9.2%), and fatigue (7.5%). In the RCT against megestrol, both drugs were well tolerated, although grade 3 or 4 weight changes (> 10% weight gain) were more common with megestrol (17.1% v 7.6%; P = 0.001).[37] **Letrozole:** Compared with megestrol, letrozole 2.5 mg was associated with a significantly lower incidence of serious cardiovascular adverse events (2% v 11%) and greater than 5% weight gain (19% v 30%).[38] Compared with aminoglutethimide, letrozole 2.5 mg had a significantly lower incidence of skin rash (3% v 11%) and serious drug related adverse events (0% v 3%).[39]

Comment: The greater efficacy and tolerability of anastrozole, and letrozole over megestrol acetate or aminoglutethimide means that they are now considered the agents of choice as second line hormonal treatment in postmenopausal women no longer responding to tamoxifen. An ongoing RCT is comparing anastrozole versus letrozole in this context (C Rose et al, personal communication, 1999). A trial conducted in 2000 has evaluated the activity of exemestane in metastatic breast cancer after failure of non-steroidal aromatase inhibitors.[40] A total of 241 people were enrolled; 56% had received aminoglutethimide, 19% anastrozole, and 17% letrozole. Exemestane produced objective responses in 6.6% of treated women, including 8.1% and 4.8% of women after failure of treatment with aminoglutethimide and other non-steroidal aromatase inhibitors (anastrozole, letrozole, vorozole), respectively, and an overall success rate (complete response plus partial response plus no change for 24 weeks or longer) of 24.3%. People who do not respond to anastrozole or letrozole may respond to exemestane.

Women's health

OPTION | COMBINATION CHEMOTHERAPY

We found no RCTs comparing combination chemotherapy (see glossary, p 1212) versus no chemotherapy in women with metastatic breast cancer (see comment, p 1205). Trials comparing one type of chemotherapy versus another found that first line chemotherapy was associated with an objective tumour response in 40–60% of women, with a median response duration of 6–12 months irrespective of menopausal or oestrogen receptor status. A small proportion of women achieve complete remission, which may persist for an extended length of time (see high dose chemotherapy, p 1206).

Benefits: **Versus best supportive care:** We found no systematic review and no RCTs comparing first line chemotherapy versus palliative (best supportive) care in women with metastatic breast cancer. **Different chemotherapy regimens:** We found one systematic review (189 RCTs, 31 510 women) evaluating different chemotherapy and endocrine regimens.[17] **"Classical" versus modified CMF:** In the largest RCT (254 postmenopausal women with metastatic breast cancer who had received no prior chemotherapy), the classical CMF (see glossary, p 1212) regimen was more effective than a modified version in which all three drugs were given intravenously every 3 weeks (response rate 48% v 29%, P = 0.03; median survival 17 v 12 months, P = 0.016).[41] One RCT (133 women who had received no prior chemotherapy) found that standard dose CMF was also significantly more effective than low dose CMF, both in response rate (30% v 11%, P = 0.03) and symptom control.[42] **CAF versus CMF:** One systematic review (search date not stated), found that regimens containing doxorubicin versus other regimens had better response rate, time to progression, and survival.[43] However, two RCTs comparing CAF (see glossary, p 1212) versus non-anthracycline based regimens (CMF) found no evidence of improved survival.[44,45] **Standard versus modified CAF regimens:** Two large multicentre trials of CAF (containing doxorubicin) versus FEC (see glossary, p 1212), a modified anthracycline based regimen containing epirubicin, found no significant difference in response rates (263 women, response rate 52% v 50%;[46] 497 women, response rate 56% v 54%[47]). An RCT in 249 women comparing standard CAF (containing doxorubicin) versus a modified better tolerated anthracycline based regimen containing mitoxantrone found that the regimen containing doxorubicin was associated with significantly longer time to progression (3.2 v 5.3 months, P = 0.03) and longer median survival (10.9 v 15.2 months, P = 0.003).[48]

Harms: The toxicity profiles of different combination chemotherapy regimens vary. In RCTs, anthracycline based regimens (CAF) and non-anthracycline based regimens (CMF) are equally associated with haematological toxicity,[45] but CAF is more likely to be associated with alopecia (34% v 22%) and severe nausea and vomiting (17% v 7%, P = 0.05). Other studies reported the incidence of greater than grade 3 alopecia (complete hair loss) to be 55–61%

with CAF, which is significantly higher than with either mitoxantrone or epirubicin (FEC).[47,48] In one of the trials comparing CAF versus FEC, FEC was associated with fewer episodes of ≥ grade 2 neutropenia (10% v 13.1%), and significantly lower rates of nausea and vomiting (7.8% v 13.3%, P < 0.01), and no cardiotoxicity (8 women taking CAF discontinued treatment because of cardiac dysfunction compared with none taking FEC).[46]

Comment: The optimal duration of chemotherapy for metastatic breast cancer is unknown, although a more recent systematic review (65 publications reporting 97 treatment comparisons) has found that more rather than fewer cycles of chemotherapy given at appropriate doses improved survival (ratio of median survivals 1.23, 95% CI 1.01 to 1.49, P = 0.01).[49] The choice of first line treatment (hormonal or chemotherapy) is based on a variety of clinical factors (see table 1, p 1217).[6-9] In one RCT, 231 women undergoing first line treatment (60% oestrogen receptor positive, remainder unknown) were randomised to receive either chemotherapy (CAF) or chemotherapy plus hormonal therapy (see glossary, p 1213) (CAF plus tamoxifen and fluoxymesterone). The response rates were similar, although time to treatment failure was slightly longer for women who received chemohormonal therapy compared with chemotherapy alone (13.4 months v 10.3 months, P = 0.087). The effect on time to treatment failure was just significant for women who were oestrogen receptor positive compared with those who were negative (17.4 v 10.3 months, P = 0.048). The oestrogen receptor status had no effect on overall survival.[50] The choice of a specific drug or regimen is based on what drugs have already been given as adjuvant treatment, together with the likelihood of benefit balanced against a given drug's adverse effects and tolerability profile. Retrospective series in sequential decades (from 1950 to 1980) have compared the survival of women from the time of diagnosis with metastatic breast cancer. They suggest that the introduction of chemotherapy has improved median survival by about 9 months (from 12 months without treatment to 21 months with treatment).[5,51] This median survival conceals a bimodal distribution of benefit, with the 40–60% of women who respond to treatment achieving survival of 1 year or greater, and the non-responders experiencing little or no survival benefit. Fifteen year follow up of women with metastatic breast cancer treated with standard dose FAC (see glossary, p 1212) chemotherapy found that 263/1581 achieved complete remission and had a median time to progression of 2 years, and that 19% of these women remained free of disease at 5 years.[15] With the increasing use of adjuvant chemotherapy,[52] more women who develop metastatic disease will have received combination chemotherapy. In the treatment of metastatic breast cancer, better quality of life scores predict better outcome (this is not the case in adjuvant treatment).[53] In one RCT (283 women with metastatic breast cancer) evaluating quality of life as a primary end point no significant differences were found between women randomised to receive either docetaxel or sequential methotrexate and 5-fluorouracil. This suggests that choice of treatment should be based on expected clinical effect.[54] This may influence the likelihood of response to further treatment.[4,55] An emerging problem is a subgroup of women with good performance status who have not responded to anthracycline based combination chemotherapy (anthracycline resistance — see glossary, p 1212) as first line treatment for metastatic disease, or who have relapsed within a few months of adjuvant chemotherapy. For these women relapsing after adjuvant anthracyclines, emerging evidence suggests that single agent taxanes (see glossary, p 1213) are the treatment of choice as first line therapy. Equally, for women who have not received anthracyclines, current RCTs are evaluating the benefit of adding taxanes to anthracyclines as first line chemotherapy (see benefits of second line chemotherapy, p 1207).

OPTION	HIGH DOSE VERSUS STANDARD DOSE CHEMOTHERAPY

One RCT found no evidence that high dose chemotherapy improves time to progression or overall survival.

Benefits: We found no systematic review. We found one RCT (533 women aged 18–60 who had complete or partial response to induction chemotherapy). It compared high dose chemotherapy (single course of high doses of carboplatin, thiotepa, and cyclophosphamide) plus hematopoietic stem cell rescue versus prolonged course of monthly conventional dose chemotherapy (cyclophosphamide, methotrexate, and fluorouracil). It found no significant difference in overall survival at 3 years (32%, 95% CI 21% to 42% v 38%, 95% CI 26% to 50%) or in median progression free survival (9.6 months v 9.0 months, CI not given).[56]

Harms: Although haematological support with colony stimulating growth factors (see glossary, p 1212) has lessened complications from high dose chemotherapy, non-haematological toxicity to the gastrointestinal tract and nervous system remain dose limiting. There is a recognised mortality with high dose chemotherapy (3%), although this is lower than in the early days of this approach.

Comment: Fifteen year follow up of women with metastatic breast cancer treated with standard dose FAC chemotherapy found that 263 of 1581 women achieved a complete response and had a median time to progression of 2 years, and that 19% of these women remained free of disease at 5 years.[15] Any long term remissions associated with high dose chemotherapy in metastatic disease must be interpreted in the context of these figures. Five RCTs are in progress and full results from RCTs published as abstracts are awaited. It remains to be seen if certain women, for example those with a complete response after standard dose chemotherapy, may benefit from high dose treatment as a "coup de grace" for any remaining cancer cells. Several RCTs have found that inadequate doses of chemotherapy produce an inadequate response, and that once adequate doses are achieved, further dose escalation within the limits of haematological toxicity produces no further benefit.[57,58]

The response rates to further chemotherapy when women relapse after standard dose chemotherapy are generally poor, with objective response rates of only 20–30%, and median durations of response ranging from 3–6 months. New cytotoxic drugs, in particular the taxanes and semi-synthetic vinca alkaloids, are associated with higher response rates, especially in anthracycline resistant disease.

Benefits: We found no systematic review and no RCTs comparing treatment with no treatment. **Taxanes:** One non-systematic review of RCTs and other studies concluded that, in women with anthracycline resistant disease, second line treatment with paclitaxel was associated with response rates ranging from 6–48%.[59] The taxane paclitaxel has been compared in two RCTs with both doxorubicin (331 women)[60] and CMF based chemotherapy (209 women).[61] The response rates were higher with doxorubicin than paclitaxel (41% v 25%, P = 0.003), yet compared with CMF based chemotherapy there was a modest survival advantage for the use of paclitaxel in a multivariate analysis (median survival 17.3 v 13.9 months, P = 0.025). One RCT (392 women with anthracycline resistant metastatic disease) compared taxane docetaxel (100 mg/m^2 intravenously every 3 weeks) versus a standard relapse treatment of mitomycin C 12 mg/m^2 plus vinblastine 6 mg/m^2.[62] Docetaxel was associated with a significantly higher response rate (30% v 11.6%, P < 0.001), longer time to progression (median 19 weeks v 11 weeks, P = 0.001), and longer overall survival (11.4 v 8.7 months, P = 0.0097). Another RCT (283 women with anthracycline resistant metastatic disease) comparing docetaxel versus methotrexate and 5-fluorouracil found a similar improvement for docetaxel both in response rate (42% v 19%, P < 0.001) and time to progression (median 6 months v 3 months, P = 0.006).[63] In a separate RCT (326 women who had not responded to an alkylating regimen [CMF] either in the adjuvant setting or as first line treatment) docetaxel was associated with a significantly higher response rate than single drug doxorubicin (43% v 21%, P = 0.003).[64] **Semisynthetic vinca alkaloids:** We found no RCTs comparing vinorelbine versus a taxane for second line treatment. One RCT (303 women, first or second line treatment, no previous vinca alkaloid or anthracycline) compared doxorubicin combined with vinorelbine versus doxorubicin alone. The response rates, quality of life scores, and overall survival were not significantly improved with combined chemotherapy in this setting.[65] Vinorelbine has single agent antitumour activity with response rates of 20–33%, including in women with anthracycline resistant metastatic disease.[59] An RCT (183 women with anthracycline resistant disease) found improved time to progression and survival with vinorelbine 30 mg/m^2 weekly compared with intravenous melphalan (median survival 35 v 31 weeks, P < 0.001).[66] **Capecitabine:** We found one published systematic review of the use of the oral fluoropyrimidene capecitabine in metastatic breast cancer.[67] One RCT comparing capecitabine versus paclitaxel as second or third line therapy following anthracycline failure found no significant difference in response rate or time to disease progression.

Harms: **Taxanes:** Paclitaxel was better tolerated than doxorubicin with a lower incidence of febrile neutropenia (7% v 20%, P < 0.001) and grade 3/4 vomiting (2% v 13%, P < 0.001), although there was a higher incidence of sensory neurotoxicity (5% v 0%, P < 0.001).[60] Likewise compared with CMF based chemotherapy, paclitaxel was associated with significantly less febrile neutropenia/infection (10% v 27%, P = 0.001), and nausea/vomiting, but significantly more alopecia, sensory neuropathy, and myalgia/arthralgia (P < 0.0001).[61] Docetaxel is associated with moderate to severe haematological toxicity; 89% of women experienced grade 3/4 neutropenia in the phase III study compared with 69% given mitomycin plus vinblastine,[62] although the incidence of febrile neutropenia with docetaxel was only 9%. Other specific toxicities associated with docetaxel include alopecia, neurotoxicity, arthralgia, and occasionally fluid retention. Hypersensitivity reactions can be avoided by premedication with corticosteroids and histamine H_2 receptor antagonists. **Semisynthetic vinca alkaloids:** Vinorelbine is associated with minimal toxicity compared with anthracycline based chemotherapy (FAC/FEC), with considerably lower rates of nausea (8% v 16%, P = 0.03) and grade 3 alopecia (7% v 30%, P = 0.0001), although haematological toxicity that delayed treatment was more frequent (27% v 17%).[68] **Capecitabine:** The most commonly reported grade 3/4 toxicities were hand-foot syndrome (13%), diarrhoea (12%), and stomatitis (4%).[67]

Comment: The taxanes paclitaxel and docetaxel have an established role as second line therapy in advanced breast cancer, especially in people with disease progression despite a previous anthracycline based regimen, with evidence in some RCTs for a survival advantage over other available options. Trials are in progress to determine the efficacy and tolerability of taxanes in combination with anthracyclines as first line treatment, although there are concerns about cardiac toxicity. At present the indication for docetaxel remains as a single drug for second line treatment, especially in anthracycline resistant disease, although definitive data on improvement in quality of life are awaited. Vinorelbine seems to have a favourable toxicity profile, but data from phase III trials are awaited. Promising activity has been seen with capecitabine in paclitaxel–refractory heavily pretreated people,[69] and the low toxicity profile together with evidence of efficacy all warrant further investigation of this drug as an alternative to more toxic second or third line chemotherapy schedules. Vinorelbine associated with protracted infusional 5-fluorouracil is an active and well tolerated regimen (overall response rate OR 61.4, 95% CI 50.9 to 70.9), and further trials are under way.[70]

QUESTION **What are the effects of treatments for bone metastases?**

OPTION **BISPHOSPHONATES**

The American Society of Clinical Oncology released recent guidelines on the use of bisphosphonates,[71] stating that this therapy reduces the rate of bone complications (though not mortality) in women with lytic bone disease who may or may not also be receiving systemic therapy (chemotherapy of endocrine therapy). It remains unclear exactly when to start or stop therapy, which may impact on the costs involved.[72] Although these effects are likely to improve quality of life, this outcome has not been formally evaluated. We found no evidence that bisphosphonates improve survival.

Benefits: We found no systematic review. **Versus placebo:** Three double blind RCTs in women with metastatic breast cancer who had bone involvement compared bisphosphonates with placebo given in conjunction with standard treatment (either chemotherapy or hormonal treatment).[73–75] The first RCT (380 women with at least one lytic bone lesion who also received chemotherapy) found that intravenous pamidronate (90 mg as a 2 hour infusion every month for 12 cycles) significantly prolonged the median time to the first skeletal complication (13.1 months v 7.0 months, $P = 0.005$).[73] Significantly fewer women taking pamidronate developed skeletal complications (43% v 56%, $P = 0.008$), and there was a significantly reduced requirement for radiotherapy to treat painful sites of bone disease (19% v 33%, $P = 0.01$). In an updated analysis in women who completed 2 years of treatment, those taking placebo were more than twice as likely to suffer a fracture than those taking pamidronate (OR 2.3, 95% CI 1.5 to 3.5).[76] The second RCT (173 women with bone metastases who may also have received either chemotherapy or hormonal treatment) found that the addition of oral clodronate 1600 mg daily significantly reduced the number of hypercalcaemic episodes (23% v 35%, $P < 0.01$) and the incidence of vertebral fractures (84 v 124 per 100 person years, $P < 0.025$).[74] The third RCT (372 women with at least one lytic bone lesion who also received hormonal treatment) significantly prolonged the median time to the first skeletal complication (10.4 months v 6.9 months, $P = 0.049$).[75] Significantly fewer women taking pamidronate developed skeletal complications (2.4 v 3.8 events per year, $P = 0.008$), and there was significantly reduced requirement for radiotherapy to treat painful sites of bone disease (25% v 34%, $P = 0.042$). None of the three trials found an impact on overall survival. **Versus radiotherapy:** We found no RCTs.

Harms: In the first RCT, intravenous pamidronate was well tolerated, with no serious adverse events in women treated for up to 2 years.[76] One of the 185 women taking pamidronate developed symptomatic hypocalcaemia. Myalgia and arthralgia were more common in women taking pamidronate. Oral clodronate can be associated with minor gastrointestinal disturbance, but the RCT reported this in fewer than 5% of women.[74]

Comment: Large RCTs are in progress in the adjuvant setting to see whether these agents may delay or prevent the development of bone metastases.

OPTION   **RADIOTHERAPY**

We found limited evidence from non-randomised studies that persistent and localised bone pain can be successfully treated with radiotherapy in over 80% of cases. Longer courses and wide fields are rarely required, and adverse effects are minimal.

Benefits: We found no systematic review and no RCTs comparing radiotherapy versus no treatment or versus bisphosphonates (see comment below). **Pain control:** Questionnaire studies found that control of pain was successful in over 80% of women who received radiotherapy for bone metastases, with concomitant use of appropriate analgesia according to the World Health Organization ladder,[77] which moves upwards from non-steroidal anti-inflammatory drugs and paracetamol to opiate containing analgesia (codeine based products) through to morphine and its derivatives (diamorphine, hydromorphone). **Cranial nerve compression:** In people with skull base metastases causing cranial nerve involvement, retrospective data suggest that radiotherapy leads to improvement in 50–80% of women, which is usually maintained.[78] **Different radiotherapy regimens:** We found two RCTs comparing different radiotherapy regimens. These found no significant differences between short courses (8 Gy as a single fraction) and longer courses (e.g. 20 Gy/5 fractions or 30 Gy/10 fractions).[79,80] Studies of accelerated fractionation schedules (e.g. twice daily treatments for 5 days) have failed to show any benefit over conventional regimens in the control of disease secondary to metastatic breast cancer.[81]

Harms: Adverse effects of radiotherapy for bone metastases include nausea and vomiting.[81] Higher dose fractions per day produce more toxic effects.

Comment: RCTs are notoriously difficult to perform in the field of palliative care. Randomised comparisons against no treatment or placebo would be considered unethical in palliative care, and even RCTs comparing one treatment versus another are difficult to undertake since it is reasonable to try many different options in order to make a person comfortable. Rating of success of end of life care is difficult. Usual outcomes, such as response rates and survival duration, do not apply.[82] The prevention of nausea and vomiting caused by chemotherapy has been studied in one RCT (619 women). It compared placebo versus dexamethasone versus dexamethesone plus ondansetron following chemotherapy. In people who did not have acute nausea and vomiting with chemotherapy, dexamethasone alone was found to provide adequate protection against delayed nausea and vomiting.[83]

QUESTION What are the effects of treatments for spinal cord, cerebral, and choroidal metastases?

OPTION SPINAL CORD COMPRESSION

Spinal cord compression is an emergency. Retrospective studies suggest that early radiotherapy preserves function. One small RCT suggests that adding high dose steroids improves the chances of walking 6 months after radiotherapy for spinal cord compression.

Benefits: We found no systematic review. **Radiotherapy:** Retrospective analyses found an improvement with early radiotherapy, but that fewer than 10% of people walked again if severe deterioration of motor function occurred before radiotherapy.[84] **Addition of high dose steroids:** One blinded RCT (57 women) evaluated addition of high dose steroids to radiotherapy. It found that more people were walking 6 months after receiving intravenous dexamethasone 96 mg bolus followed by 96 mg orally for 3 days, compared with those who received no steroids (59% v 33%).[85]

Harms: In the RCT of high dose steroids,[85] significant adverse effects caused withdrawal from treatment in 11% of people. Use of lower doses of glucocorticoids in the control of symptoms from cerebral metastases may result in short term agitation and the longer term development of Cushingoid facies.

Comment: See comment under radiotherapy, p 1210.

OPTION CEREBRAL METASTASES

Non-randomised evidence suggests that symptoms from cerebral metastases can be successfully controlled with radiotherapy.

Benefits: We found no systematic review and no RCTs comparing one form of treatment with another. **Radiotherapy:** Retrospective data suggest that whole brain radiation produces general improvement in neurological function in 40–70% of women with brain metastases secondary to breast cancer.[86] **Different radiotherapy regimens:** An RCT of 544 symptomatic people comparing two whole brain radiotherapy schedules (30 Gy/10 fractions v 12 Gy/2 fractions) found no evidence that the response rate or duration of response in people with multiple brain metastases were improved with higher doses of radiation compared with the shorter regimen.[81] **Surgical resection:** This is rarely indicated, although may be beneficial in a small subgroup of people.[87] **Intrathecal chemotherapy:** We found no evidence that meningeal infiltration responds to intrathecal chemotherapy.

Harms: Adverse effects of radiotherapy in the treatment of cerebral metastases include hair loss and somnolence.[81] Higher dose fractions per day produce more toxic effects.

Comment: See comment under radiotherapy, p 1210. Dexamethasone should be given immediately for raised intracranial pressure and anticonvulsants to control seizures if necessary.

OPTION CHOROIDAL METASTASES

Non-randomised evidence suggests that symptoms from choroidal metastases can be successfully controlled with radiotherapy.

Benefits: We found no systematic review and no RCTs. External beam radiotherapy prevents functional loss and doses of approximately 40 Gy in total are used.[88] Retrospective data suggest that radiotherapy benefits 70% of people.[89]

Harms: People with choroidal metastases who are treated with radiotherapy may lose the sight in that eye. Optic atrophy and proliferative radiation retinopathy are possible late complications.

Comment: See comment under radiotherapy, p 1210. People with deteriorating vision should be treated as an emergency. Generally, choroidal metastases occur later than metastases to other organs. Choroidal metastasis is considered a poor prognostic sign; most people die within 6 months of diagnosis. Systemic chemotherapy can induce partial or complete remission of metastatic choroidal breast carcinoma.[90]

GLOSSARY

Adjuvant treatment This usually refers to systemic chemotherapy or hormonal treatment, or both, taken after removal of a primary tumour (in this case, surgery for early breast cancer), with the aim of killing any remaining micrometastatic tumour cells and thus preventing recurrence.

Anthracycline resistance This applies to people who have received at least one chemotherapeutic regimen with anthracyclines (doxorubicin or epirubicin) in either an adjuvant setting or for metastatic disease. Primary resistance to an anthracycline is defined as progressive disease during or within 6 months after completion of adjuvant anthracycline. People without any documented tumour response to first line chemotherapy that included anthracyclines for metastatic disease are also classified as having primary resistance. Secondary resistance is defined as disease progression after a documented clinical response to first line chemotherapy with anthracyclines for metastatic disease. Secondary resistance can be further divided into three categories as follows: (1) absolute resistance, or disease progression during treatment with regimens that contained anthracycline after a period of response; (2) relative resistance, or disease progression within 6 months after completion of the chemotherapy; and (3) sensitive regrowth, or disease progression more than 6 months after completion of the chemotherapy.[91]

Aromatase inhibitors Block the conversion of androgens into oestrogens. Aminoglutethimide, anastrozole and letrozole are non-steroidal aromatase inhibitors. Formestane and exemestane are steroidal aromatase inhibitors. Anastrozole, formestane, exemestane, and letrozole are selective inhibitors of oestrogen synthetase, which is a part of the aromatase enzyme system. Aminoglutethimide also inhibits adrenal steroid production. These drugs cause oestrogen suppression in postmenopausal women.

Bisphosphonates (pamidronate, clodronate) Bone specific palliative drugs that inhibit osteoclast induced bone resorption associated with breast cancer metastases.

Chemotherapy Therapy with cytotoxic drugs.

Colony stimulating growth factors Naturally occurring cytokines that stimulate development of different cell lines.

Combination chemotherapy regimens Use of different combinations of cytotoxic drugs.

Classical CMF Cyclophosphamide (100 mg/m^2 orally days 1–14), methotrexate (40 mg/m^2 intravenously (iv) day 1 + 8), and 5-fluoruracil 600 mg/m^2 iv day 1 + 8, every 4 weeks for up to six cycles of treatment given dependency on response.

CAF Cyclophosphamide (500 mg/m^2 iv), doxorubicin (50 mg/m^2 iv), and 5-fluoruracil (500 mg/m^2 iv), every 3 weeks for up to six cycles of treatment given dependency on response.

FEC 5-Fluorouracil, epirubicin, and cyclophosphamide every 3 weeks for up to six cycles of treatment given dependency on response.

FAC 5-Fluorouracil, doxorubicin (adriamycin), and cyclophosphamide every 3 weeks for up to six cycles of treatment given dependency on response.

Complete response Disappearance of all known lesions on two separate measurements at least 4 weeks apart.

Disease free interval Time between surgery for early breast cancer (see below) and developing metastatic breast cancer.

Early breast cancer Operable disease, restricted to the breast and sometimes to local lymph nodes.

First line treatment Initial treatment for a particular condition that has previously not been treated. For example, first line treatment for metastatic breast cancer may include chemotherapy or hormonal treatment, or both.

Hormonal therapy Includes treatment with antioestrogens such as tamoxifen, aromotase inhibitors and progestins.

Gonadorelin analogues (also called LHRH agonists) These are synthetic peptides that occupy the receptors for LHRH in the pituitary gland. Continuous administration of LHRH agonists may initially increase the release of luteinizing hormone, but continuous administration blocks the physiological pulsatile luteinizing hormone release and this causes a fall in oestrogen levels.

Overall objective response rate The proportion of treated people in whom a complete (see above) or partial response (see below) is observed.

Partial response More than a 50% reduction in the size of lesions.

Progestins (medroxyprogesterone acetate, megestrol acetate) The antitumour effects of progestins may be mediated by a direct action on tumour cells, or an indirect effect on the pituitary–ovarian/adrenal axes.

Progression free survival (or time to progression) Interval between diagnosis of metastatic disease and diagnosis of progression (see below).

Progressive disease More than a 25% increase in the size of lesions or the appearance of new lesions.

Second line treatment Treatment given after relapse following first line treatment (see above).

Tamoxifen An oral, non-steroidal, competitive oestrogen receptor antagonist.

Taxanes Drugs derived from the Pacific yew tree *Taxus brevifolia*, such as paclitaxel and docetaxel.

Substantive changes since last issue

Aromatase inhibitors in postmenopausal women Exemestane added.[34]

Second line chemotherapy Two RCTs added;[60,61] conclusions unchanged.

Second line chemotherapy Capecitabine added.[67]

REFERENCES

1. Pisani P, Parkin DM, Ferlay J. Estimates of the worldwide mortality from eighteen major cancers in 1985. Implications for prevention and projections of future burden. *Int J Cancer* 1993; 55:891–903.

2. Early Breast Cancer Trialists' Collaborative Group. Polychemotherapy for early breast cancer: an overview of the randomised trials. *Lancet* 1998; 352:30–42. Search date 1995; studies were identified using lists prepared by three international cancer research groups; by searching the international Cancer Research Data Bank, meeting abstracts, and references of published trials; and by consulting experts.

3. Slamon DJ, Clark GM, Wong SG, Levin WJ, Ullrich A, McGuire WL. Human breast cancer: correlation of relapse and survival with amplification of the HER-2/neu oncogene. *Science* 1987;235:177–182.

4. Rubens RD, Bajetta E, Bonneterre J, Kljin JGM, Lonning PE, Paridaens R. Treatment of relapse of breast cancer after adjuvant systemic therapy. *Eur J Cancer* 1994;30A:106–111.

5. Cold S, Jensen NV, Brincker H, et al. The influence of chemotherapy on survival after recurrence in breast cancer: a population based study of patients treated in the 1950s, 1960s, and 1970s. *Eur J Cancer* 1993;29:1146–1152.

6. Jackson IM, Litherland S, Wakeling AE. Tamoxifen and other antioestrogens. In: Powels TJ, Smith IE, eds. *Medical management of breast cancer.* London: Martin Dunitz, 1991:51–59.

7. Arafah BM, Pearson OH. Endocrine treatment of advanced breast cancer. In: Jordan VC, ed. *Estrogen/antiestrogen action and breast cancer therapy.* Madison: University of Wisconsin Press, 1986:417–429.

8. McGuire WL. Hormone receptors: their role in predicting prognosis and response to endocrine therapy. *Semin Oncol* 1978;5:428–443.

9. Kuss JT, Muss HB, Hoen H, Case LD. Tamoxifen as initial endocrine therapy for metastatic breast cancer: long term follow-up of two Piedmont Oncology Association (POA) trials. *Breast Cancer Res Treat* 1997;42:265–274.

10. Coates A, Gebski V, Signori D. Prognostic value of quality-of-life scores during chemotherapy for advanced breast cancer. *J Clin Oncol* 1992;10: 1833–1838.

11. European Organisation for Research and Treatment of Cancer (EORTC). A practical guide to EORTC studies. Brussels, Belgium: EORTC Data Center, 1996:126.

12. Miller AB, Hoogstraten B, Staquet M, Winkler A. Reporting results of cancer treatment. *Cancer* 1981;47:207–214.

13. Baum M, Priestman T, West RR, Jones EM. A comparison of subjective responses in a trial

comparing endocrine with cytotoxic treatment in advanced carcinoma of the breast. In: Mouridsen HT, Palshof T, eds. *Breast cancer - experimental and clinical methods*. London: Pergamon Press, 1980:223–228.

14. Bernhard J, Thurlimann B, Schmitz SF, et al. Defining clinical benefit in postmenopausal patients with breast cancer under second-line endocrine treatment: Does quality of life matter? *J Clin Oncol* 1999;17:1672–1679.

15. Greenberg PA, Hortobagyi GN, Smith TL, Ziegler LD, Frye DK, Buzdar AU. Long-term follow-up of patients with complete remission following combination chemotherapy for metastatic breast cancer. *J Clin Oncol* 1997;14:2197–2205.

16. Geels P, Eisenhauer E, Bezjak A, et al. Palliative effect of chemotherapy: objective tumor response is associated with symptom improvement in patients with metastatic breast cancer. *J Clin Oncol* 2000;18:2395–2405.

17. Fossati R, Confalonieri C, Torri V, et al. Cytotoxic and hormonal treatment for metastatic breast cancer: a systematic review of published randomised trials involving 31 510 women. *J Clin Oncol* 1998;16:3439–3460. Search date 1997; primary sources Medline, Embase, and search of reference lists from retrieved articles and lists from relevant meetings.

18. Litherland S, Jackson IM. Antioestrogens in the management of hormone-dependent cancer. *Cancer Treat Rev* 1988;15:183–194.

19. Johnston SRD. Acquired tamoxifen resistance in human breast cancer – potential mechanisms and clinical implications. *Anti Cancer Drugs* 1997;8:911–930.

20. Hayes DF, Van Zyl JA, Goedhals L, et al. Randomised comparison of tamoxifen and two separate doses of toremifene in postmenopausal patients with metastatic breast cancer. *J Clin Oncol* 1995;13:2556–2566.

21. Early Breast Cancer Trialists' Collaborative Group. Tamoxifen for early breast cancer: an overview of the randomised trials. *Lancet* 1998;351:1451–1467. Search date 1995; studies were identified using lists prepared by three international cancer research groups; by searching the international Cancer Research Data Bank, meeting abstracts, and references of published trials; and by consulting experts.

22. Parazzini F, Colli E, Scatigna M, Tozzi L. Treatment with tamoxifen and progestins for metastatic breast cancer in postmenopausal women: a quantitative review of published randomised clinical trials. *Oncology* 1993;50:483–489. Search date 1991; primary sources Medline, handsearching, and reference lists of articles identified.

23. Pannuti F, Martoni A, Murari G, et al. Analgesic activity of medroxyprogesterone acetate in cancer patients: an anti-inflammatory mediated activity? *Int J Tissue React* 1985;7:505–508.

24. Muss HB, Case DL, Atkins JN, Bearden JD, Cooper MR, Cruz JM. Tamoxifen versus high-dose oral medroxyprogesterone acetate as initial endocrine therapy for patients with metastatic breast cancer: a Piedmont Oncology Association study. *J Clin Oncol* 1994;12:1630–1638.

25. Ingle JN, Ahmann DL, Green SJ. Randomised clinical trial of megesterol acetate versus tamoxifen in paramenopausal or castrated women with advanced breast cancer. *Am J Clin Oncol* 1982;5:155–160.

26. Panutti F, Martoni A, Zamagni C, Melotti B. Progestins. In: Powles TJ, Smith IE, eds. *Medical management of breast cancer*. London: Martin Dunitz, 1991:95–107.

27. Crump M, Sawka CA, DeBoer G, et al. An individual patient-based meta-analysis of tamoxifen versus ovarian ablation as first-line endocrine therapy for premenopausal women with metastatic breast cancer. *Breast Cancer Res Treat* 1997;44:201–210. Search date not stated; primary sources Medline, Cancerlit, hand searches of bibliographies of related publications, and personal contact with principal investigators of unpublished trials.

28. Sawka CA, Pritchard KI, Shelley W, et al. A randomised crossover trial of tamoxifen versus ovarian ablation for metastatic breast cancer in premenopausal women: a report of the National Cancer Institute of Canada clinical trials group trial MA1. *Breast Cancer Res Treat* 1997;44:211–215.

29. Taylor CW, Green S, Dalton WS, et al. Multicenter randomised clinical trial of goserelin versus surgical ovariectomy in premenopausal patients with receptor-positive metastatic breast cancer: an intergroup study. *J Clin Oncol* 1998;16:994–999.

30. Boccardo F, Rubagotti A, Perotta A, et al. Ovarian ablation versus goserelin with or without tamoxifen in pre-perimenopausal patients with advanced breast cancer: results of a multicentric Italian study. *Ann Oncol* 1994;5:337–342.

31. Klijn JGN, Blamey RW, Boccardo F, et al. Combined tamoxifen and luteinising hormone-releasing hormone (LHRH) agonist versus LHRH agonist alone in premenopausal advanced breast cancer; a meta-analysis of four randomised trials. *J Clin Oncol* 2001;19:343–353.

32. Bonneterre J, Thurlimann B, Robertson JFR, et al. Anastrozole versus tamoxifen as first-line therapy for advanced breast cancer in 668 postmenopausal women: results of the tamoxifen or arimidex randomised group efficacy and tolerability study. *J Clin Oncol* 2000;18:3748–3757.

33. Nabholtz JM, Buzdar A, Pollak M, et al. Anastrozole is superior to tamoxifen as first-line therapy for advanced breast cancer in postmenopausal women: results of a North American multicentre randomised trial. *J Clin Oncol* 2000;18:3758–3767.

34. Buzdar A, Jonat W, Howell A, et al. Anastrozole, a potent and selective aromatase inhibitor, versus megestrol acetate in post-menopausal women with advanced breast cancer; results of overview analysis of two phase III trials. *J Clin Oncol* 1996;14:2000–2011.

35. Buzdar A, Jonat W, Howell A, et al. Significant improved survival with Arimidex (anastrozole) versus megesterol acetate in postmenopausal advanced breast cancer; updated results of two randomised trials. *Proc Am Soc Clin Oncol* 1997;16:A545.

36. Jones S, Vogel C, Arkhipov A, et al. Multicenter phase II trial of exemestane as third-line hormonal therapy of postmenopausal women with metastatic breast cancer. *J Clin Oncol* 1999;17:3418–3425.

37. Kaufman M, Bajetta E, Dirix LY, et al. Exemestane is superior to megestrol acetate after tamoxifen failure in postmenopausal women with advanced breast cancer: results of a phase III randomised double-blind trial. *J Clin Oncol* 2000;18:1399–1411.

38. Dombernowsky P, Smith IE, Falkson G, et al. Letrozole, a new oral aromatase inhibitor for advanced breast cancer: double-blind randomised trial showing a dose effect and improved efficacy and tolerability compared with megesterol acetate. *J Clin Oncol* 1998;16:453–461.

39. Gershanovich M, Chaudri HA, Campos D, et al. Letrozole, a new oral aromatase inhibitor:

randomised trial comparing 2.5 mg daily, 0.5 mg daily and aminoglutethimide in postmenopausal women with advanced breast cancer. *Ann Oncol* 1998;9:639–645.

40. Lønning PE, Bajetta E, Murray R, et al. Activity of exemestane in metastatic breast cancer after failure of nonsteroidal aromatase inhibitors: a phase II trial. *J Clin Oncol* 2000;18:2234–2244.

41. Engelsman E, Klijn JCM, Rubens RD, et al. "Classical" CMF versus a 3-weekly intravenous CMF schedule in postmenopausal patients with advanced breast cancer. *Eur J Cancer* 1991;27: 966–970.

42. Tannock IF, Boyd NF, DeBoer G, et al. A randomised trial of two dose levels of cyclophosphamide, methotrexate and fluorouracil chemotherapy for patients with metastatic breast cancer. *J Clin Oncol* 1988;6:1377–1387.

43. A'Hern RP, Smith IE, Ebbs SR. Chemotherapy and survival in advanced breast cancer: the inclusion of doxorubicin in Cooper type regimens. *Br J Cancer* 1993;67:801–805. Search date not given; primary sources CancerLit, and communication with colleagues.

44. Cummings FJ, Gelman R, Horton J. Comparison of CAF versus CMFP in metastatic breast cancer: analysis of prognostic factors. *J Clin Oncol* 1985; 3:932–940.

45. Smalley RV, Lefante J, Bartolucci A, Carpenter J, Vogel C, Krauss S. A comparison of cyclophosphamide, adriamycin, and 5-fluorouracil (CAF) versus cyclophosphamide, methotrexate, 5-fluorouracil, vincristine, and prednisolone (CMFVP) in patients with advanced breast cancer. *Breast Cancer Res Treat* 1983;3: 209–220.

46. French Epirubicin Study Group. A prospective randomised phase III trial comparing combination chemotherapy with cyclophosphamide, fluorouracil, and either doxorubicin or epirubicin. *J Clin Oncol* 1988;6:679–688.

47. Italian Multicentre Breast Study with Epirubicin. Randomised phase III study of fluorouracil, doxorubicin, and cyclophosphamide in advanced breast cancer: an Italian multicentre trial. *J Clin Oncol* 1988;6:976–982.

48. Stewart DJ, Evans WK, Shepherd FA, et al. Cyclophosphamide and fluorouracil combined with mitozanrone versus doxorubicin for breast cancer: superiority of doxorubicin. *J Clin Oncol* 1997;15: 1897–1905.

49. Stockler M, Wilcken NR, Ghersi D, Simwa RJ. Systematic reviews of chemotherapy and endocrine therapy in metastatic breast cancer. *Cancer Treat Rev* 2000; 26:151–168.

50. Sledge GW, Hu P, Torney D, et al. Comparison of chemotherapy with chemohormonal therapy as first-line therapy for metastatic, hormone sensitive breast cancer. An Eastern Cooperative Oncology Group Study. *J Clin Oncol* 2000;18:262–66.

51. Ross MB, Buzdar AU, Smith TL, et al. Improved survival of patients with metastatic breast cancer receiving combination chemotherapy. *Cancer* 1985;55:341–346.

52. Goldhirsch A, Glick JH, Gelber RD, Senn H-J. International consensus panel on the treatment of primary breast cancer. *J Natl Cancer Inst* 1998; 90:1601–1608.

53. Coates AS, Hurny C, Peterson HF, et al. Quality of life scores predict outcome in metastatic but not early breast cancer. *J Clin Oncol* 2000;18:3768–3774.

54. Hakamies-Blomquist L, Luoma M, Sjostrom J, et al. Quality of life in patients with metastatic breast cancer receiving either docetaxel or sequential methotrexate and 5-fluorouracil. A multicenter

randomised phase III trial by the Scandinavian breast group. *J Clin Oncol* 2000;36:1411–1417.

55. Houston SJ, Richards MA, Bentley AE, Smith P, Rubens RD. The influence of adjuvant chemotherapy on outcome after relapse for patients with breast cancer. *Eur J Cancer* 1993; 29A:1513–1518.

56. Stadtmauer E, O'Neill A, Goldstein L. Conventional-dose chemotherapy compared with high-dose chemotherapy plus autologous hematopoietic stem-cell transplantation for metastatic breast cancer. *N Engl J Med* 2000 (13 April) (http www/nejm.org/content/stadmauer/ 1.asp).

57. Hortobagyi GN, Bodey GP, Buzdar AU, Frye D, Legha SS, Malik R, et al. Evaluation of high-dose versus standard FAC chemotherapy for advanced breast cancer in protected environment units; a prospective randomised trial. *J Clin Oncol* 1987;5: 354–364.

58. Bastholt L, Dalmark M, Gjedde S, Pfeiffer P, Pedersen D, Sandberg E, et al. Dose-response relationship of epirubicin in the treatment of post-menopausal patients with metastatic breast cancer: a randomised study of epirubicin at four different dose-levels performed by the Danish Breast Cancer Co-operative Group. *J Clin Oncol* 1996;14:1146–1155.

59. Vermoken JB, Ten Bokkel Huinick WW. Chemotherapy for advanced breast cancer: the place of active new drugs. *Breast* 1996;5:304–311.

60. Paridaens R, Bignazoli L, Bruning P, et al. Paclitaxel versus doxorubicin as first-line single agent chemotherapy for metastatic breast cancer; an EORTC randomised study with cross-over. *J Clin Oncol* 2000;18:724–733.

61. Bishop JF, Dewar J, Toner GC, et al. Initial paclitaxel improves outcome compared with CMFP combination chemotherapy as front-line therapy in untreated metastatic breast cancer. *J Clin Oncol* 1999;17:2355–2364.

62. Nabholtz JM, Senn HJ, Bezwoda WR, et al. Prospective randomised trial of docetaxel vs mitomycin plus vinblastine in patients with metastatic breast cancer progressing despite previous anthracycline-containing chemotherapy. *J Clin Oncol* 1999;17:1434–1424.

63. Sjosrom J, Blomqvist C, Mouridsen H, et al. Docetaxel compared with sequential methotrexate and 5-fluorouracil in patients with advanced breast cancer after anthracycline failure; a randomised phase III study with cross-over on progression by the Scandinavian Breast Group. *Eur J Cancer* 1999;35:1194–1201.

64. Chan S, Friedrichs K, Noel D, et al. Prospective randomised trial of docetaxel versus doxorubicin in patients with metastatic breast cancer. *J Clin Oncol* 1999;35:2341–2354.

65. Norris B, Pritchard KI, James K, et al. Phase III comparative study of vinorelbine combined with doxorubicin versus doxorubicin alone in disseminated metastatic/recurrent breast cancer: National Cancer Institute of Canada Clinical Trials Group Study MA8. *J Clin Oncol* 2000;18:2385–2394.

66. Jones S, Winer E, Vogel C, Laufman L, et al. Randomised comparison of vinorelbine and melphalan in anthracycline-refractory advanced breast cancer. *J Clin Oncol* 1995;13:2567–2574.

67. Tomiak E, Verma S, Levine M, et al. Use of capecitabine in stage IV breast cancer: an evidence summary. *Curr Oncol* 2000;7:84–90.

68. Namer M, Soler-Michel P, Mefti F, et al. Is the combination FAC/FEC always the best regimen in advanced breast cancer? Utility of mitoxantrone and vinorelbine association as an alternative:

results from a randomised trial [abstract]. *Breast Cancer Res Treat* 1997;46:94(A406).

69. Blum JL, Jones SE, Buzdar AU, et al. Multicenter phase II study of capecitabine in paclitaxel-refractory metastatic breast cancer. *J Clin Oncol* 1999;17:485–493.

70. Berruti A, Sperone P, Bottini A. Phase II study of vinorelbine with protracted fluorouracil infusion as a second or third line approach for advanced breast cancer patients previously treated with anthracyclines. *J Clin Oncol* 2000;19:3370–3377.

71. Hillner BE, Ingle JN, Berenson JR, et al. American Society of Clinical Oncology guideline on the role of bisphosphonates in breast cancer: American Society of Oncology Bisphophonates Expert Panel. *J Clin Oncol* 2000;18:1378–1391.

72. Hillner BE, Weeks JC, Desch CE, Smith TJ. Pamidronate in prevention of bone complications in metastatic breast cancer; a cost-effectiveness analysis. *J Clin Oncol* 2000;18:72–79.

73. Hortobagyi GN, Theriault RL, Porter L, et al. Efficacy of pamidronate in reducing skeletal complications in patients with breast cancer and lytic bone metastases. *N Engl J Med* 1996;335: 1785–1791.

74. Paterson AHG, Powles TJ, Kanis JA, McCloskey E, Hanson J, Ashley S. Double-blind controlled trial of oral clodronate in patients with bone metastases from breast cancer. *J Clin Oncol* 1993;11:59–65.

75. Theriault RL, Lipton A, Hortobagyi GN. Pamidronate reduces skeletal morbidity in women with advanced breast cancer and lytic bone lesions; a randomised placebo controlled trial. *J Clin Oncol* 1999;17:846–854.

76. Hortobagyi GN, Theriault RL, Lipton A, et al. Long-term prevention of skeletal complications of metastatic breast cancer with pamidronate. *J Clin Oncol* 1998;16:2038–2044.

77. World Health Organization. *Cancer pain relief.* Geneva: WHO, 1996.

78. Hall SM, Budzar AV, Blumenschein GR. Cranial nerve palsies in metastatic breast cancer due to osseous metastasis without intracranial involvement. *Cancer* 1983;52:180–184.

79. Bone Trial Working Party. 8 Gy single fraction radiotherapy for the treatment of metastatic skeletal pain: randomised comparison with a multifraction schedule over 12 months of patient follow-up. *Radiother Oncol* 1999;52:111–121.

80. Price P, Hoskin PJ, Easton D, Austin D, Palmer SG, Yarnold JR. Prospective randomised trial of single and multifraction radiotherapy schedules in treatment of painful bony metastases. *Radiother Oncol* 1986;6:247–255.

81. Priestman TJ, Dunn J, Brada M, Rampling R, Baker PG. Final results of the Royal College of Radiologists' trial comparing two different radiotherapy schedules in the treatment of brain metastases. *Clin Oncol* 1996;8:308–815.

82. Bretscher N. Care for dying patients: what is right? *J Clin Oncol* 2000;18:233–2334.

83. The Italian Group for antiemetic research. Dexamethasone alone or in combination with ondansetron for the prevention of delayed nausea and vomiting induced by chemotherapy. *N Engl J Med* 2000;342:1554–1559.

84. Rades D, Blach M, Nerreter V, Bremer M, Karstens JH. Metastatic spinal cord compression. Influence of time between onset of motor deficits and start of irradiation on therapeutic effect. *Strahlenther Onkol* 1999;175:378–381.

85. Sorensen S, Helweg-Larsen S, Mouridsen H, Hansen HH. Effect of high-dose dexamethasone in carcinomatous metastatic spinal cord compression treated with radiotherapy: a randomised trial. *Eur J Cancer* 1994;30A:22–27.

86. Cancer Guidance Subgroup of the Clinical Outcomes Group. *Improving outcomes in breast cancer. The research evidence.* London: NHS Executive, 1996.

87. Diener-West M, Dobbins TW, Phillips TL, Nelson DF. Identification of an optimal subgroup for treatment evaluation of patients with brain metastases using RTOG study 7916. *Int J Radiat Oncol Biol Phys* 1989;16:669–673.

88. Ratanatharathorn V, Powers WE, Grimm J, Steverson N, Han I, Ahmad K. Eye metastasis from carcinoma of the breast: radiation treatment and results. *Cancer Treat Rev* 1991;18:261–276.

89. Piccone MR, Maguire AM, Fox KC, et al. Choroidal metastases. Case 1: breast cancer. *J Clin Oncol* 1999;17:3356–2258.

90. Hortobagyi GN. Treatment of breast cancer. *N Engl J Med* 1998;339:974–84.

91. Ando M, Watanabe T, Nagata K, et al. Efficacy of docetaxel 60 mg/m2 in patients with metastatic breast cancer according to the status of anthracycline resistance. *J Clin Oncol* 2001;19: 336–342.

Stephen Johnston
Senior Lecturer
in Medical Oncology

Justin Stebbing
Specialist Registrar
in Medical Oncology

The Royal Marsden NHS Trust
London
UK

Competing interests: None declared.

| TABLE 1 | Clinical factors that predict response to hormonal treatment in metastatic breast cancer, based on results of RCTs (see text, p 1198, p 1199, p 1205).[6-9,91] |

Factors predictive of good response to hormonal treatment

Postmenopausal status

Disease limited to soft tissue sites (skin, nodes)

Oestrogen receptor positive tumour

Long disease free interval since primary treatment for early breast cancer (> 18–24 months).

Factors making initial hormonal treatment less appropriate

Symptomatic visceral metastases (e.g. lymphangitis carcinomatosis or progressive liver metastases)

Oestrogen receptor negative tumour

Short disease free interval (12–18 months)

Relapse on adjuvant tamoxifen (unless oestrogen receptor positive tumour and other features predictive of good response).

Search date October 2000: expanded this issue

J Michael Dixon, Alan Rodger, Stephen Johnston and Kate Gregory

INTERVENTIONS

Key Messages

Ductal carcinoma in situ

- Two RCTs have found that radiotherapy is associated with a reduced risk of local recurrence and invasive carcinoma, but we found no evidence of a difference in survival.

- One RCT found that adjuvant tamoxifen reduced breast cancer events in women who had undergone wide excision and radiotherapy, but with no evidence of an effect on survival.

Neoadjuvant chemotherapy in primary operable carcinoma of the breast

- RCTs have found a reduction in mastectomy rates in people treated with neoadjuvant chemotherapy, but found no survival difference associated with chemotherapy given in the neoadjuvant rather than adjuvant setting.

Extent of surgery in operable breast cancer

- Systematic reviews have found that, providing all local disease is excised, more extensive surgery is not associated with better outcomes in early invasive breast cancer. More extensive local resection in breast conserving surgery gives worse cosmetic results.

Radiotherapy in operable breast cancer

- One systematic review has found that radiotherapy reduces the risk of isolated local recurrence, and loss of a breast but does not increase 10 year survival compared with breast conserving surgery alone. Similar rates of survival and local recurrence are achieved with breast conserving surgery plus radiotherapy as with mastectomy.

- One systematic review has found that radiotherapy to the chest wall after mastectomy reduces the risk of local recurrence by about two thirds and the risk of death from breast cancer at 10 years, but found no evidence of effect on overall 10 year survival.

- We found no direct evidence that radiotherapy to the internal mammary chain improves overall survival or breast cancer specific survival. Treatment may increase radiation induced cardiac morbidity.

- We found insufficient evidence to assess the impact on survival of irradiation of the ipsilateral supraclavicular fossa. RCTs have found that radiotherapy is associated with reduced risk of supraclavicular fossa nodal recurrence. Morbidity associated with irradiation of the supraclavicular fossa is rare and, where it occurs, is mild and temporary.

■ Three RCTs have found that total nodal irradiation improves survival in high risk disease. Earlier RCTs found reduced locoregional recurrence, but no evidence of improved survival.

Adjuvant systemic treatment in operable breast cancer

■ One systematic review has found that adjuvant chemotherapy reduces rates of recurrence and improves survival for women with early breast cancer. The benefit seems to be independent of nodal or menopausal status, although the absolute improvements are greater in those with node positive disease, and probably greater in younger women. It found no evidence of a survival advantage from either longer duration or dosage adjustment of polychemotherapy (two or more drugs).

■ Regimens containing an anthracycline modestly improve survival compared with the standard CMF regimen (see glossary, p 1240 and table 1, p 1245).

■ One RCT found that adding chemotherapy (CMF) to tamoxifen improves survival.

■ One systematic review has found that adjuvant tamoxifen taken for up to 5 years reduces the chance of recurrence and death in women with oestrogen receptor positive tumours irrespective of age, menopausal status, nodal involvement, or the addition of chemotherapy. Tamoxifen slightly increases the risk of endometrial cancer, but we found no evidence of an overall adverse effect on non-breast cancer mortality.

■ One systematic review has found that ovarian ablation significantly improves long term survival in women aged under 50 years with early breast cancer.

Management of the axilla in operable breast cancer

■ RCTs found no evidence that axillary clearance is associated with improved survival compared with axillary sampling, axillary radiotherapy, or sampling plus radiotherapy combined. One systematic review of mainly poor quality evidence found that the risk of arm lymphoedema was highest with axillary clearance plus radiotherapy, lower with axillary sampling plus radiotherapy, and lowest with sampling alone.

Locally advanced breast cancer (Stage III B)

■ For locally advanced breast cancer that is rendered operable, seven small RCTs have found that radiotherapy or surgery as sole local treatments have similar effects on response rates, duration of response and, overall survival.

■ One RCT found weak evidence that radiotherapy after attempted curative surgery can reduce local, regional recurrence, or both.

■ We found no evidence that the cytotoxic, multidrug chemotherapy regimen (CMF) improves survival, disease free survival, or long term locoregional control in locally advanced breast cancer.

■ One RCT found evidence that hormone treatment plus radiotherapy versus radiotherapy alone improves survival in locally advanced breast cancer.

DEFINITION **Ductal carcinoma in situ (DCIS)** is a non-invasive tumour characterised by the presence of malignant cells in the breast ducts but
with no evidence that they breach the basement membrane and
invade into periductal connective tissues. **Invasive breast cancer**
can be separated into three main groups: early or operable breast
cancer, locally advanced disease, and metastatic breast cancer
(see metastatic breast cancer, p 1196). Women with early or
operable breast cancer have disease that is apparently restricted to
the breast and sometimes to local lymph nodes and can be
surgically removed. Although these women do not have overt
metastases at the time of staging, they remain at risk of local
recurrence and of metastatic spread. They can be divided into those
with tumours greater than 4 cm (multifocal cancers) that can be
treated by mastectomy, and those with tumours less than 4 cm
(unifocal cancers) that can be treated by breast conserving surgery
(see glossary, p 1240). **Locally advanced breast cancer** is
defined according to the TNM staging system of the UICC TNM
system (see glossary, p 1241)[1] as Stage III B (includes T4 a–d; N2
disease, but absence of metastases). It is disease presentation with
evidence (clinical or histopathological) of skin and/or chest wall
involvement and/or axillary nodes matted together by tumour extension. **Operable primary breast cancer** is the presence of malignant disease that is confined to the breast (and or axillary nodes),
and which is of a size and in a position to render a potentially
curative surgical procedure possible. This does not include locally
advanced disease or inflammatory breast cancers.

INCIDENCE/ Breast cancer affects one in 12 women in the UK and causes about
PREVALENCE 21 000 deaths per year. Prevalence is about five times higher, with
over 100 000 women living with breast cancer at any one time. Of
the 15 000 new cases of breast cancer per annum in the UK, the
majority will present with primary operable disease.[2]

AETIOLOGY/ The risk of breast cancer increases with age, doubling every 10
RISK FACTORS years up to the menopause. Risk factors include an early age at
menarche, older age at menopause, older age at birth of first child,
family history, atypical hyperplasia, excess alcohol intake, radiation
exposure to developing breast tissue, oral contraceptive use, postmenopausal hormone replacement therapy, and obesity. Risk in
different countries varies fivefold. The cause of breast cancer in
most women is unknown. About 5% of breast cancers can be
attributed to mutations in the genes BRCA1 and BRCA2.[3]

PROGNOSIS **Primary carcinoma** of the breast is potentially curable. The risk of
relapse depends on various clinico-pathological features, including
axillary node involvement, oestrogen receptor status, and tumour
size. Tumour size, axillary node status, histological grade, and
oestrogen receptor status provide the most significant prognostic
information. Seventy per cent of women with operable disease are
alive 5 years after diagnosis and treatment (adjuvant drug treatment is given to most women after surgery). Risk of recurrence is
highest during the first 5 years, but the risk remains even 15–20
years after surgery. Those with node positive disease have a
50–60% chance of recurrence within 5 years, compared with
30–35% for node negative disease. Recurrence occurred in

60–70% of node positive women compared with 25–30% of node negative women within 10 years in one large systematic review.[4] The prognosis for a disease free survival (DFS) (see glossary, p 1240) at 5 years is worse for stage III B (33%) than that for stage III A (71%). Five year overall survival is 44% and 84%, respectively.[5] Poor survival and high rates of local recurrence characterise locally advanced breast cancer.

AIMS	To improve survival; to prevent local or regional node recurrence; to obtain prognostic information on the type and extent of tumour and the status of the axillary lymph nodes; to optimise cosmetic results and minimise psychosocial impact; to minimise adverse effects of treatment; and to maximise quality of life.
OUTCOMES	Survival; rates of local and regional recurrence; rates of mastectomy after breast conserving treatment; rates of development of metastases; cosmetic outcomes; quality of life; incidence of adverse effects of treatment, including upper limb lymphoedema.
METHODS	*Clinical Evidence* update search and appraisal October 2000.

QUESTION What are the effects of interventions after breast conserving surgery for ductal carcinoma in situ?

OPTION RADIOTHERAPY

Alan Rodger and Mike Dixon

Two RCTs have found that radiotherapy (see glossary, p 1241) is associated with a reduced risk of local recurrence and invasive carcinoma, but with no evidence of an effect on survival.

Benefits:	We found no systematic review. We found two RCTs comparing radiotherapy with no radiotherapy after surgery for ductal carcinoma in situ (DCIS). The first RCT (814 people) found no significant difference in survival at 8 years with radiotherapy, but a significant reduction in risk of local recurrence (survival 95% v 94%; local recurrence 12.1% v 26.8%, P = < 0.000005; risk of recurrent DCIS 8.2% v 13.4%, P = 0.007; risk of invasive carcinoma 3.9% v 13.4%, P < 0.0001).[6] The second RCT (102 people) found, at median follow up of 4.25 years, significantly lower recurrence of DCIS in women given radiotherapy.[7] At 4 years, local relapse free survival was more likely with radiotherapy than with surgery alone (84% v 91%, P = 0.005, HR 0.62, 95% CI 0.44 to 0.87). More women were free of DCIS recurrence after 4 years with radiotherapy but the difference was not significant (92% v 95%, HR 0.65, 95% CI 0.43 to 1.03). There was a significant reduction in invasive recurrence (92% v 96%, HR 0.60, 95% CI 0.37 to 0.97).
Harms:	One RCT found an increase in contralateral breast cancer associated with radiotherapy at 4 years (3% v 1%; HR 2.57, 95% CI 1.24 to 5.33).[7]
Comment:	Ongoing trials are evaluating radiotherapy in all grades of DCIS. Subset analyses may be required to identify subgroups of women who benefit most from radiotherapy after breast conserving surgery.

| OPTION | TAMOXIFEN PLUS RADIOTHERAPY |

Mike Dixon and Alan Rodger

One RCT has found that adjuvant tamoxifen (see glossary, p 1241) reduces breast cancer events in women who have undergone wide excision and radiotherapy, but found no evidence of an effect on survival.

Benefits: We found no systematic review. We found one RCT in women with DCIS treated with wide excision and radiotherapy, which compared adjuvant tamoxifen 20 mg daily (902 women) with placebo (902 women) for 5 years.[8] At median follow up of 74 months, there were fewer breast cancer events with tamoxifen than placebo (OR 0.63, 95% CI 0.47 to 0.83), and fewer invasive ipsilateral or contralateral breast cancers (OR 0.57, 95% CI 0.38 to 0.85). However, there was no significant difference in overall survival (RR 0.88, 95% CI 0.33 to 2.28).

Harms: One RCT found a higher, but non-significant rate of endometrial cancers associated with tamoxifen (RR 3.4, 95% CI 0.6 to 33.4).[8]

Comment: RCTs of tamoxifen in DCIS are underway (M Dixon, personal communication, 2000).

| QUESTION | What are the effects of neoadjuvant chemotherapy in the management of primary operable carcinoma of the breast? New |

Stephen Johnston and Kate Gregory

Four RCTs found no difference in survival with neoadjuvant versus adjuvant chemotherapy.

Benefits: We found no systematic review. We found four RCTs of neoadjuvant versus adjuvant chemotherapy. In the first RCT, 272 women (with tumours > 3 cm in whom mastectomy was indicated) were randomised to either preoperative (neoadjuvant) EVMTV (epirubicin, vincristine, mitomycin-C, thiotepa, vindesine) chemotherapy or mastectomy followed by EVMTV regimen. At an initial median follow up of 34 months, a statistically significant survival difference was reported in favour of neoadjuvant chemotherapy (see glossary, p 1240) (85% v 95%: P = 0.04).[9] However, the final analysis at 124 months showed that the survival improvement was no longer significant, with survival of about 55% in both groups (not significant).[10] The second RCT randomised 414 women to receive four cycles of FAC chemotherapy (see glossary, p 1240) either pre or postoperatively. At 54 months follow up, the primary (neoadjuvant) chemotherapy group had a better overall survival (86% v 68%, P = 0.039);[11] however, a subsequent analysis at 105 months did not demonstrate a long term survival benefit.[12] The third RCT randomised 309 women to either four cycles of MM (mitoxantrone, methotrexate) chemotherapy, then surgery, then four cycles of MM or to surgery then eight cycles of MM. At 48 months follow up, there was no difference in survival between the neoadjuvant and adjuvant groups (84% v 82%, not significant).[13] The largest RCT (NSABP-18), in which 1523 women were randomised to four cycles of AC (adriamycin, cyclophosphamide) either pre or postoperatively, found identical survival rates (67%) in the two groups at 60 months.[14]

Harms: We found no evidence that neoadjuvant chemotherapy has a negative impact on survival.

Comment: We found no evidence to support the use of neoadjuvant chemotherapy to improve the chances of survival for operable breast cancers outside the context of a clinical trial.

QUESTION What is the effect of neoadjuvant chemotherapy on mastectomy rates? New

Several RCTs have found that neoadjuvant chemotherapy leads to a marked reduction in the mastectomy rate.

Benefits: **Neoadjuvant versus adjuvant chemotherapy:** We found no systematic review. Three RCTs found a lower rate of mastectomy in women who had received neoadjuvant chemotherapy compared with women receiving adjuvant chemotherapy. **MM regimen:** In a UK study (309 women receiving MM chemotherapy), the mastectomy rate was 28% in the adjuvant arm compared with 13% in the neoadjuvant arm (P < 0.005).[15] **AC regimen:** In the NSABP-18 study (1523 women), breast conservation rates were lower in the adjuvant arm (60% v 67%), although this was not statistically significant.[14] **FAC regimen:** One RCT assessed 272 women at diagnosis in terms of the recommended surgical procedure, and two of three women who were initially advised to have mastectomy were able to have breast conserving surgery after neoadjuvant chemotherapy.[16]

Harms: None of the RCTs reported a significantly higher local recurrence rate with neoadjuvant chemotherapy compared with adjuvant chemotherapy.[9,13,14]

Comment: With an increased number of conservative operations being performed after downstaging by neoadjuvant chemotherapy for large primary tumours, there are theoretical concerns that this may result in an increased rate of local recurrence. Neoadjuvant chemotherapy can lead to a reduction in the requirement for mastectomy, and as such an increase in breast conservation surgery. In the three RCTs of women with operable breast cancer receiving breast conserving surgery, this has not been associated with a significant increase in the rate of local recurrence.[14–16]

QUESTION What are the effects of different regimens used in the neoadjuvant setting? New

We found no evidence that any one of the commonly used chemotherapy regimens is superior in the neoadjuvant setting.

Benefits: We found no systematic review. We found one non-systematic review and five RCTs comparing adjuvant to neoadjuvant chemotherapy using a variety of regimens.[13,14,17–20] Most studies used anthracycline based regimens, which are of proven benefit in the adjuvant setting.[17] **AC regimen:** The NSABP-18 trial treated women with AC and found an objective response rate (complete or partial clinical response) of 79%.[14] **MM regimen:** MM in the UK trial gave an overall response rate (see glossary, p 1240) of 85%.[13] Three RCTs compared different neoadjuvant regimens. **FAC regimen v paclitaxel:** A US trial (174 women) compared conventional FAC (see glossary, p 1240) with single agent paclitaxel, and found similar response rates in both groups; FAC 79%, paclitaxel 80%, with no significant difference in survival rates.[18] **Comparison between MPEMi, MPEpiE and MPEpiV regimens:** A European RCT (101 women treated with three different combinations: MPEMi [methotrexate, cisplatin, etoposide, mitomycin-C], MPEpiE [methotrexate, cisplatin, epirubicin, etoposide], and MPEpiV [methotrexate, cisplatin, epirubicin, vincristine] found the response to be 89%, with no significant differences between the groups.[19] **Comparison between routes of administration:** We found one study comparing routes of administration.[20] This Japanese study randomised women to either no neoadjuvant treatment, neoadjuvant intravenous epirubicin, or intra-arterial epirubicin. Response rates were higher in women receiving intra-arterial epirubicin (68% compared with 36%, $P < 0.05$); however, this was not associated with a survival benefit.

Harms: **FAC versus paclitaxel:** In the US RCT comparing FAC with paclitaxel, rates of septic neutropaenia (53% v 21%) and granulocyte colony stimulating factor usage (56% v 25%) were higher in the paclitaxel arm.[18]

Comment: More work is needed to determine the optimal regimen for neoadjuvant treatment. We found little evidence in the literature comparing different combinations, but anthracycline based combinations probably remain the treatment of choice. Ongoing RCTs are investigating the role of taxane sequencing after anthracycline based therapy (NSABP-27), and anthracycline in combination with infusional 5-FU.

QUESTION   **Is the extent of surgery related to outcome in early invasive breast cancer?**

Mike Dixon and Alan Rodger

Two systematic reviews have found that more extensive surgery is not associated with better outcomes, providing that all local disease is excised. The more extensive the local resection in breast conserving surgery, the worse the cosmetic result.

Benefits: **Comparisons between supraradical, radical, and total mastectomy:** We found one systematic review (search date 1990, 5 RCTs 2090 women with operable breast cancer) comparing supraradical mastectomy with radical mastectomy, radical with total mastectomy, and supraradical with total mastectomy (see glossary, p 1241).[21] It found no significant difference in risk of death over 10 years (ARR of more extensive v less extensive surgery 0.02, 95% CI −0.04 to +0.08). **Comparisons between radical, total, and simple mastectomy:** The same review included four RCTs comparing radical with simple mastectomy (3 trials) and total with simple mastectomy (1 trial) in 1296 women with operable breast cancer.[21] Meta-analysis found no significant difference in risk of death over 10 years (ARR for more extensive v less extensive surgery 2%, 95% CI –5% to +9%). **Mastectomy versus breast conservation:** We found two systematic reviews. One review (search date 1995)[22] analysed data on 10 year survival from six RCTs comparing breast conservation with mastectomy. Meta-analysis of data from five of the trials (3006 women) found no significant difference in the risk of death at 10 years (OR v mastectomy 0.91, 95% CI 0.78 to 1.05). The sixth trial used different protocols. Where more than half of node positive women in both mastectomy and breast conservation groups received adjuvant nodal radiotherapy, both groups had similar survival rates. Where fewer than half of node positive women in both groups received adjuvant nodal radiotherapy, survival was better with breast conservation (OR v with mastectomy 0.69, 95% CI 0.49 to 0.97). The second review (search date 1990)[21] identified nine RCTs in 4981 women potentially suitable for breast conserving surgery. All participants received postoperative radiotherapy. Meta-analysis found no significant difference in risk of death over 10 years (RRR for breast conservation compared with mastectomy 0.02, 95% CI –0.05 to +0.09). It also found no significant difference in rates of local recurrence (6 trials in 3107 women; RRR mastectomy v breast conservation 0.04, 95% CI –0.04 to +0.12). **Different extents of local excision in breast conservation:** We found no systematic review. We found one RCT (705 women) comparing lumpectomy with quadrantectomy (see glossary, p 1241).[23] There were significantly more local recurrences with lumpectomy than with quadrantectomy (7% v 2%), but a major factor associated with local recurrence in the lumpectomy group was incomplete excision (see comment below).[24] We found no RCTs comparing wide local excision (complete excision microscopically) with quadrantectomy.

Harms: More extensive surgery results in greater mutilation. Between 60–90% of women having breast conservation have an excellent or good cosmetic result (median 83%, 95% CI 67% to 87%).[23,25-33] The single most important factor influencing cosmetic outcome is the volume of tissue excised; the larger the amount of tissue excised the worse the cosmetic result.[23] The trial of different extents of local excision in breast conservation found that, in a subset of 148 women, there was a significantly higher rate of poor cosmetic outcome with quadrantectomy (RR v lumpectomy 3.11, 95% CI 1.2 to 8.1).[23] Only isolated small studies have shown no correlation between extent of surgical excision and cosmesis.[31]

Comment: The link between completeness of excision and local recurrence after breast conservation has been evaluated in 16 centres. In 13 of these, incomplete excision was associated with an increased relative risk of local recurrence compared with complete excision (estimated median RRI 3.4, 95% CI 2.6% to 4.6%).[24] The three centres not reporting increased rates of local recurrence after incomplete excision gave much higher doses of local radiotherapy (65–72 Gy). Two centres also used re-excision, and women with involved margins had only focal margin involvement.

Alan Rodger

OPTION RADIOTHERAPY AFTER BREAST CONSERVING SURGERY

One systematic review has found that radiotherapy reduces the risk of isolated local recurrence and loss of a breast, but does not increase 10 year survival compared with breast conserving surgery alone. Similar rates of survival and local recurrence are achieved with breast conserving surgery plus radiotherapy as with mastectomy.

Benefits: **Versus breast conserving surgery alone:** We found one systematic review (search date 1990, 4 RCTs, 382–1450 people),[21] comparing surgery plus radiotherapy with surgery alone. All four trials began before 1985 and used megavoltage X-rays. Pooled data from trials reporting sites of local recurrence (781 people) found that women with isolated local recurrence were less likely to have received radiotherapy (OR 0.25, 95% CI 0.16 to 0.34). Even a trial limited to "good prognosis disease" (tumour ≤ 2 cm, node negative, 381 people) found a significantly lower local relapse rate with radiotherapy at 5 and 10 years (5 years: relapse rate with radiotherapy 2.3%, 95% CI 1% to 4.3% v no radiotherapy 18.4%, 95% CI 12.5% to 24.2%).[34] Ten year data found that radiotherapy was associated with lower local recurrence rates (8.5%, 95% CI 3.9% to 13.1% v 24%, 95% CI 17.6% to 30.4%, P = 0.0001) but no difference in overall survival (77.5% v 78%).[35] One subsequent RCT (585 people) also found that after 6 years the proportion of women free of locoregional disease and with breast conservation was higher with radiotherapy (93.8% v 81.3%).[36] Pooled data from all four trials found no significant difference in 10 year survival (80.1% v 78.9%). **Versus mastectomy:** The systematic review identified nine RCTs (4891 people) comparing breast radiotherapy after breast conserving surgery with simple or modified radical mastectomy in women with invasive breast cancer.[21] It found no difference in survival rates at 10 years (22.9% v 22.9%; no CIs available) or in local recurrence (6.2% v 5.9% from pooled data from 6 trials, 3107 people).[21]

Harms: The RCTs and systematic review included in a consensus document published in 1998 (mainly of women undergoing breast conserving surgery or mastectomy with variation in radiotherapy techniques, doses, and fractionation) reported two severe adverse effects of radiotherapy: acute pneumonitis (0.7% to 7.0%) and pericarditis (0% to 0.3%); and the following long term adverse effects: significant arm oedema (1% without axillary dissection), radionecrotic rib fracture (1.1% to 1.5%), and brachial plexopathy (0% to 1.8%).[37] The risk and severity of adverse effects increased with volume irradiated, total dose received, dose per fraction, previous surgery (e.g. axillary dissection), and radiotherapy techniques that caused overlap in irradiated tissues. The review found an increased risk of non-breast cancer death (OR 1.24, 95% CI 1.09 to 1.43).[21] One systematic review (search date not given) of 10 RCTs found that the excess of non-breast cancer deaths after chest wall radiotherapy was caused by cardiac deaths resulting from the radiotherapy, but recent trials with data beyond 10 years did not find an excess of cardiac deaths.[38–41] A more recent systematic review of 40 RCTs in early breast cancer with meta-analysis of 10 and 20 year results confirms a reduction in local recurrence of two thirds, a reduction in breast cancer mortality, but an increase in other, particularly vascular, mortality.[42] Overall, 20 year survival was 37.1% with radiotherapy versus 35.9% for controls (two sided P value = 0.06). Studies assessing cosmetic results have mainly been retrospective using poorly validated outcomes. The effects of social, psychological, and financial disruptions from attending for 5–6 weeks of radiotherapy have not been clearly addressed. There is an extremely low reported incidence of radiation induced malignancy, usually soft tissue sarcomas, in the irradiated breast.

Comment: The four RCTs comparing breast conserving surgery with and without radiotherapy, as well as retrospective case series, found that prognostic factors for local recurrence after breast conserving surgery include positive tumour margins, an extensive intraduct component, younger age, lymphovascular invasion, histological grade, and systemic treatment. The only consistent independent risk factor is avoiding radiotherapy. Although the published data have reported no difference in survival rates at 10 years, data recently released following the 5th Early Breast Cancer Trialists' Group meeting, have shown that among 6100 women randomised between breast conservation surgery with radiotherapy and the same breast conservation surgery without radiotherapy, there was a significant 3.9% (SE 1.2) increase in survival in women receiving radiotherapy when mortality from breast cancer was considered in absence of other causes of death (M Dixon, personal communication, 2001).

| OPTION | RADIOTHERAPY AFTER MASTECTOMY |

RCTs have found that radiotherapy to the chest wall after mastectomy reduces the risk of local recurrence by about two thirds, and reduces the risk of death from breast cancer at 10 years compared with mastectomy alone.

Benefits: We found one systematic review (search date 1995, 32 RCTs) comparing mastectomy with mastectomy followed by radiotherapy to the chest wall.[21] Five trials were of mastectomy alone (4541 people); four of mastectomy and axillary sampling (see glossary, p 1240) (3286 people); and 23 of mastectomy and axillary clearance (6699 people). The review found that radiotherapy reduced local recurrence by two thirds and slightly reduced breast cancer mortality (OR 0.94, 95% CI 0.88 to 1.00), but found no significant difference in overall survival (OR 0.98, 95% CI 0.93 to 1.03).[21] **Versus mastectomy plus adjuvant chemotherapy or tamoxifen alone:** Two subsequent trials in high risk women receiving adjuvant chemotherapy (CMF) after mastectomy compared irradiation to the chest wall and peripheral lymphatics with no radiotherapy.[39,40] One found radiotherapy reduced relative locoregional relapse rates by 56% (RR 0.44, 95% CI 0.26 to 0.77) and the other by 76% (AR

58% v 14%).[39,40] One RCT found that survival at 10 years was higher with radiotherapy (54%, 95% CI 51% to 58% v 45%, 95% CI 42% to 48%).[40] The other, smaller trial found a 29% reduction in mortality at 15 years with radiotherapy (RR 0.71, CI 0.51 to 0.99), although when these results were pooled with the results of the review, no significant difference in overall mortality was detected (OR 0.96, 95% CI 0.91 to 1.01).[21,39,43,44] Another RCT in high risk postmenopausal women who underwent mastectomy and received tamoxifen 30 mg daily for 1 year, compared irradiation of the chest wall and peripheral lymphatics with no radiotherapy. It found that radiotherapy was associated with reduction in local or regional recurrence (as first site of recurrence) from 35% to 8%. Overall survival at 10 years was higher with radiotherapy (45%, 95% CI 41% to 49% v 36%, 95% CI 33% to 40%).[43] We found no evidence that reduction in relative risk of local recurrence was affected by age, nodal status, receptor status, tumour grade, or tumour size, nor that the effect of radiotherapy on mortality varied significantly with extent of surgery, type of radiotherapy (megavoltage or ortho-voltage), years the trials commenced or completed recruitment, or whether systemic treatment was given.[44]

Harms: See harms of radiotherapy after breast conserving surgery, p 1227. Three trials of postmastectomy total nodal irradiation in high risk disease found no significant increase in cardiac mortality.[39,40,41,43]

Comment: The trials in the large systematic review were heterogeneous, in part because they began when trial methods were less developed.[21] They varied in randomisation processes, areas irradiated, use of systemic treatment, radiotherapy doses, fractionation, and treatment schedules. We found little good evidence to identify which women should have post mastectomy radiotherapy to prevent local recurrence. One review of retrospective data found that extent of axillary node involvement, larger tumour size, higher histological grade, presence of lymphovascular invasion, and involvement of tumour margins reduced the chance of successful treatment.[44–47]

| OPTION | RADIOTHERAPY TO THE INTERNAL MAMMARY CHAIN |

We found no direct evidence that radiotherapy to the internal mammary chain improves overall survival or breast cancer specific survival. Treatment may increase radiation induced cardiac morbidity.

Benefits: We found no systematic review. We found one RCT (270 women treated with breast conserving surgery and radiotherapy), which compared internal mammary chain irradiation with no internal mammary chain irradiation.[48] At median follow up of 2.7 years there was no significant difference in relapse or survival (figures not provided).

Harms: See harms of radiotherapy after breast conserving surgery, p 1227. Radiotherapy to the internal mammary chain is more likely to affect the heart compared with other types of radiotherapy.

Comment: The risk of internal mammary chain node involvement is related to the location and size of the primary tumour and, most importantly, histopathological axillary nodal status. Up to 30% of women with axillary involvement will also exhibit internal mammary chain nodal metastases. Central or medial breast cancers are more likely to metastasise to the internal mammary chain, as are larger tumours.[49,50] The risk of internal mammary chain recurrence is low, and after modified radical mastectomy alone is 2%.[51] Modern radiotherapy planning and delivery should involve an assessment of the position and depth of the internal mammary chain nodes to be treated (using computerised tomography or ultrasound) and computer assisted placement, arrangement, and determination of dose distribution, technologies unavailable at the time of most RCTs included in the reviews.[21,38] Recent indirect evidence from RCTs suggests improved survival from nodal irradiation (including radiation to the internal mammary chain) after modified radical mastectomy combined with systemic treatment.[39,40,43] Another trial of internal mammary chain irradiation has recently started (sponsored by the EORTC).

OPTION	RADIOTHERAPY TO THE IPSILATERAL SUPRACLAVICULAR FOSSA

We found insufficient evidence to assess the impact on survival of irradiation of the ipsilateral supraclavicular fossa. RCTs have found that radiotherapy is associated with reduced risk of supraclavicular fossa nodal recurrence. Morbidity associated with irradiation of the supraclavicular fossa is rare and, where it occurs, is mild and temporary.

Benefits: We found no systematic review or RCTs on radiotherapy to the ipsilateral supraclavicular fossa. One systematic review (search date 1990) found that postoperative radiotherapy was associated with reduced locoregional recurrence: see radiotherapy after breast conserving surgery, p 1227; radiotherapy after mastectomy, p 1228, and radiotherapy to internal mammary chain irradiation, p 1229.[21] RCTs indicate reduced recurrence in the supraclavicular fossa. One trial in postmenopausal women at high risk of local recurrence who received tamoxifen after mastectomy found that radiotherapy was associated with lower recurrence in the supraclavicular fossa (37/686 [5.4%] v 9/689 [1.3%]) at median follow up of 123 months.[43]

Harms: The acute morbidity of irradiation to the supraclavicular fossa is mild and includes temporary upper oesophagitis in nearly all women. The risk of radiation pneumonitis increases with the volume of lung irradiated. Treatment irradiates the lung apex in addition to any lung included in the breast or chest wall fields. Possible late morbidity includes brachial plexopathy but this should not exceed 1.8% if attention is paid to limiting total dose to 50 Gy, the limiting the dose per fraction to 2 Gy or less, and avoiding field junction overlaps.[37,52] Late apical lung fibrosis is common and usually of no clinical importance. Demyelination of the cervical cord is an extremely rare complication of supraclavicular fossa radiotherapy.

Comment: None.

OPTION   TOTAL NODAL RADIOTHERAPY

Three RCTs have found that total nodal irradiation (see glossary, p 1241) improves survival in high risk disease. Earlier RCTs found reduced locoregional recurrence, but no evidence of improved survival.

Benefits: One systematic review (search date 1990) included RCTs of total regional nodal irradiation (to the internal mammary chain, supraclavicular fossa, and axilla).[21] It found that postoperative radiotherapy was associated with reduced locoregional recurrence, but no evidence of improved 10 year survival.[21] However, three recent RCTs found improved overall survival in women with high risk disease who underwent mastectomy, axillary dissection, and systemic adjuvant therapy, if total nodal postoperative radiotherapy was given.[39,40,43]

Harms: See radiotherapy to the internal mammary chain, p 1229, supraclavicular fossa, p 1230, and axilla, p 1235. The three RCTs found increase in cardiac mortality due to radiotherapy.[39–41,43]

Comment: None.

QUESTION   What are the effects of adjuvant systemic treatment?

Stephen Johnston

OPTION   ADJUVANT COMBINATION CHEMOTHERAPY

One systematic review of RCTs has found that adjuvant chemotherapy reduces rates of recurrence and improves survival for women with early breast cancer. The benefit seems to be independent of nodal or menopausal status, although the absolute improvements are greater in those with node positive disease, and probably greater in younger women. The review found no evidence of a survival advantage from additional months of polychemotherapy (two or more drugs), nor did RCTs find survival advantage from increased or reduced dosages of polychemotherapy. Regimens containing anthracycline may modestly improve outcomes compared with the standard CMF regimen (see glossary, p 1240 and table 1, p 1245).

Benefits: **Versus no chemotherapy:** We found one systematic review (search date 1995, 47 RCTs, 18 000 women) comparing prolonged combination chemotherapy (see glossary, p 1240) with no chemotherapy.[53] Chemotherapy was associated with significantly lower rates of any kind of recurrence (women aged under 50 years, OR 0.65, 95% CI 0.61 to 0.69; women aged 50 to 69 years, OR 0.80, 95% 0.72 to 0.88) and death from all causes (women aged under 50 years, OR 0.73, 95% CI 0.68 to 0.78; women aged 50 to 69 years, OR 0.89, 95% CI 0.86 to 0.92). Rates of recurrence were similar for women with node negative and node positive disease. Ten year survival according to nodal and age group is summarised in table 1 (see table 1, p 1245). **Duration of treatment:** The same review identified 11 RCTs (6104 people), which compared longer regimens (doubling duration of chemotherapy from between 4 and 6 months to 8 to 12 months) with shorter regimens.[53] It found no additional benefit from longer treatment duration. **Different doses:** Several RCTs found no significant improvement from enhanced dose regimens, whereas others found little difference from untreated controls when suboptimal doses were used.[54,55] **Anthracycline regimens versus standard CMF regimen:** The systematic review identified 11 RCTs (5942 people) comparing regimens containing anthracycline (including the drugs doxorubicin or 4-epidoxorubicin) with standard CMF regimens.[53] It found a significant reduction in recurrence rates in those on anthracycline regimens ($P = 0.006$), and a modest but significant improvement in 5 year survival (69% v 72%; $P = 0.02$).

Harms: **Acute adverse effects:** Adverse effects include nausea and vomiting, hair loss, bone marrow suppression, fatigue, and gastrointestinal disturbance. Prolonged chemotherapy is more likely to be associated with lethargy and haematological toxicity (anaemia and neutropenia), and anthracycline regimens cause complete hair loss. **Long term adverse effects:** Fertility and ovarian function may be permanently affected by chemotherapy, especially in women aged over 40 years, although for some women with hormone dependent cancer, reduced ovarian function may contribute to the benefit of adjuvant treatment (see glossary, p 1240). Other potential long term risks include induction of second cancers (especially haematological malignancies, although the risk is very low) and cardiac impairment with cumulative anthracycline dosages. Provided the cumulative dose of doxorubicin does not exceed $300–350 \, mg/m^2$, the risk of congestive heart failure is less than 1%.

Comment: The absolute benefits of these regimens need to be balanced against their toxicity for different women. Trials are underway of high dose chemotherapy with haematological support (bone marrow transplantation or peripheral stem cell support) in women with high risk disease (at least 10 positive lymph nodes), although a recent RCT did not find survival advantage for high dose treatment.[56,57] New and highly active cytotoxic agents such as the taxanes are being examined with anthracyclines (see glossary, p 1240) either in combination or sequence. Alternating sequences of cytotoxic agents may prove an effective way of circumventing acquired drug resistance and thus enhancing the efficacy of a regimen, such as the Milan regimen (see glossary, p 1240) of single agent anthracycline followed by standard CMF chemotherapy.[58]

OPTION **ADJUVANT TAMOXIFEN**

One systematic review has found that adjuvant tamoxifen taken for up to 5 years reduces the chance of recurrence and death in postmenopausal women, and in women with oestrogen receptor positive tumours irrespective of age, menopausal status, nodal involvement, or the addition of chemotherapy. Five years of treatment seems better than shorter durations, but available evidence does not find benefit associated with prolongation beyond 5 years. Tamoxifen carries a slightly increased risk of endometrial cancer, but we found no evidence of an overall adverse effect on non-breast cancer mortality (see table 2, p 1246).

Benefits: **Versus placebo:** We found one systematic review (search date 1995, 55 RCTs, 37 000 women), which compared adjuvant tamoxifen with placebo.[59] It found that 5 years of adjuvant tamoxifen had similar effect on recurrence and long term survival in all age groups, irrespective of menopausal status or age. For women over 50 years (usually postmenopausal), tamoxifen reduced the annual risk of recurrence by 29%, and of death from any cause by 20%. **Oestrogen receptor status:** Five years of tamoxifen treatment was associated with a greater reduction in the recurrence rate for women with oestrogen receptor positive rather than negative tumours (RRR 50% v 6%), and with a slightly greater reduction in the risk of 10 year recurrence in women with node positive compared with node negative disease (ARR 14.9% v 15.2%). **Duration of treatment:** The review found significantly greater reductions in recurrence with increasing duration of adjuvant tamoxifen (RRR 26% for 5 years of tamoxifen use v 12% for 1 year, P < 0.00001).[59] Table 2, p 1246, shows the absolute improvement in 10 year survival from 5 years of tamoxifen. One RCT (3887 women) comparing 2 and 5 years of treatment found similar results.[60] The effects of prolonged treatment beyond 5 years are unclear. In the largest trial in the systematic review, 1153 women who had completed 5 years of tamoxifen were randomised to either placebo or 5 more years of tamoxifen.[59,61] Disease free survival after 4 years of further follow up was greater for those who switched to placebo rather than continued tamoxifen (92% v 86%, P = 0.003), although there was no significant difference in overall survival. Other studies found no detrimental effect or improvement in continuing tamoxifen beyond 5 years.[62]

Harms:
One systematic review found an increased hazard ratio for endometrial cancer with tamoxifen (average HR 2.58, 95% CI 2.23 to 2.93).[59] For 5 years of tamoxifen treatment, this resulted in a cumulative risk over 10 years of two deaths (95% CI 0 to 4) per 1000 women. There was no evidence of an increased incidence of other cancers, nor of non-breast cancer related deaths (i.e. cardiac or vascular), although one extra death per 5000 women years of tamoxifen was attributed to pulmonary embolus. Bone loss was found in premenopausal women (1.4% bone loss per annum) but not in postmenopausal women, because of tamoxifen's partial agonist effects.[63] There were mixed effects on cardiovascular risk, with significant reductions in low density lipoprotein cholesterol associated with a reduced incidence of myocardial infarction in some studies, but an increased risk of thrombosis. Overall, no effect has been found on non-breast cancer mortality (HR 0.99 95% CI 0.88 to 1.16).[59]

Comment:
The risk to benefit ratio may vary between women, with oestrogen receptor negative women deriving little benefit. Even in oestrogen receptor positive women, any benefit on breast cancer could be offset with prolonged treatment (beyond 5 years), by drug resistance, and by adverse effects on the endometrium. Two multicentre trials of tamoxifen duration are in progress (Cancer Research Campaign, personal communication, 2000); however, because of concerns about long term toxicity with tamoxifen (see above), and in the absence of further definitive data, current clinical practice has been to recommend tamoxifen for 5 years.[64] For women with completely oestrogen receptor negative disease, the overall benefit of adjuvant tamoxifen needs further research.

| OPTION | COMBINED CHEMOTHERAPY PLUS TAMOXIFEN |

One RCT has found that adding chemotherapy to tamoxifen improves survival.

Benefits: We found no systematic review. We found one RCT (2306 women with lymph node negative, oestrogen receptor positive early breast cancer), which compared tamoxifen alone with tamoxifen plus CMF chemotherapy.[65] It found that adding chemotherapy to tamoxifen caused a further absolute improvement in disease free survival (at 5 years' follow up 90% v 85%, P = 0.006) and in overall survival (97% v 94%, P = 0.03).

Harms: Adding CMF chemotherapy to tamoxifen was associated with a greater incidence of grade 3/4 neutropenia (9% v 0%), greater than or equal to grade 2 nausea (35% v 4%), moderate/severe alopecia (35.6% v 0.4%), and thromboembolism/phlebitis (7.5% v 2.1%).[66]

Comment: None.

| OPTION | OVARIAN ABLATION |

One systematic review has found that ovarian ablation (see glossary, p 1240) significantly improves long term survival in women aged under 50 years with early breast cancer.

Benefits: We found one systematic review (search date 1995, 12 RCTs with at least 15 years' follow up, 2102 premenopausal women) comparing ovarian ablation by irradiation or surgery with no ablation.[66] Significantly more women with ovarian ablation survived (52% v 46%, P = 0.001) and survived recurrence free (45% v 39%, P = 0.0007). Benefit was independent of nodal status.

Harms: We found no good evidence on long term adverse effects. Concerns exist about late sequelae of ovarian ablation, especially effects on bone mineral density and cardiovascular risk. Acute adverse effects are likely to be menopausal symptoms.

Comment: Five of the RCTs compared ovarian ablation plus chemotherapy with chemotherapy alone.[66] In these, the absolute benefit of ablation was smaller than in trials of ovarian ablation alone. It may be that cytotoxic chemotherapy itself suppresses ovarian function, making the effect of ablation difficult to detect in combined trials. When only premenopausal women were considered in the absence of chemotherapy, there was a 27% improvement in the odds of recurrence free survival. Trials are under way of reversible oophorectomy using gonadotrophin releasing hormone analogues, which would allow preservation of fertility in younger women with oestrogen receptor positive tumours.

QUESTION What are the effects of axillary clearance, sampling, or radiotherapy in women with operable primary breast cancer?

Mike Dixon and Alan Rodger

RCTs found no evidence that axillary clearance (see glossary, p 1240) is associated with improved survival compared with axillary node sampling, axillary radiotherapy, or sampling plus radiotherapy (see glossary, p 1241) combined. One systematic review of mainly poor quality evidence found that the risk of arm lymphoedema was highest with axillary clearance plus radiotherapy, lower with axillary sampling plus radiotherapy, and lowest with sampling alone.

Benefits: **Versus axillary sampling:** We found no systematic review. One RCT (466 women) in women undergoing breast conserving surgery found that sampling was associated with improved survival compared with axillary clearance, but the difference was not significant (estimated 5 year survival 88.6% v 82.1%).[67] Similar rates of node positivity were found in both groups. **Versus axillary radiotherapy:** We found one systematic review (search date 1990, 8 RCTs, 4370 women) comparing axillary clearance (level I, II, and III dissection) with axillary radiotherapy (see glossary, p 1240). It found no significant difference in mortality at 10 years (54.7% v 54.9%) or in rates of recurrence (OR 1.01). Radiotherapy was associated with fewer isolated local recurrences (odds reduction 15%, 95% CI 7% to 22%).[21] **Versus sampling plus radiotherapy:** We found no systematic review. Two RCTs compared axillary clearance (level I, II, and III dissection) with sampling followed by radiotherapy in women with involved axillary nodes. They found no significant difference in local, axillary, or distant recurrence.[67,68] **Axillary clearance plus radiotherapy:** We found no evidence that radiotherapy in addition to axillary clearance (level I and II, or level I, II, and III dissection) improves regional control of disease.

Harms: **Axillary clearance:** Adverse effects of axillary surgery include seroma formation, arm swelling, damage to the intercostobrachial nerve, and shoulder stiffness. We found one RCT comparing the morbidity of different axillary procedures.[67] It compared complete axillary clearance (levels I, II, and III dissection) with four node axillary sampling followed by radiotherapy if the nodes were involved. The rate of arm swelling was higher after clearance than after sampling whether or not women received postoperative radiotherapy (at 3 years, forearm girth was significantly greater, P = 0.005). After removal of axillary drains, between a quarter and half of women who had undergone a level I and II, or levels I, II, and III axillary dissection developed seromas requiring aspiration. **Axillary radiotherapy:** One RCT comparing clearance with sampling plus radiotherapy for node positive disease found significantly reduced shoulder movement with radiotherapy, even though the shoulder joint was not irradiated.[67] At 6 months, both groups had significantly reduced shoulder movement compared with women receiving axillary sampling alone (P < 0.004).[67] However, by 3 years, the axillary clearance group had improved and was not significantly different from the sampling group. **Arm lymphoedema:** One Australian systematic review of lymphoedema prevalence, risks, and management found that, although current information is of poor quality, the combination of axillary dissection (to or beyond level II) and axillary radiotherapy was associated with a risk of lymphoedema of between 12% and 60%, with most studies suggesting that at least a third of women are affected.[69] Studies of axillary sampling followed by irradiation found lower rates (between 6% and 32%), and for axillary sampling alone, lower still (between 0% and 21%). Studies of dissection beyond level I found rates between 0% to 42%, with most studies reporting a rate of 20–30% 1 year after operation.[69] In women who receive axillary radiotherapy without axillary surgery, the overall lymphoedema rate is about 8%.

Comment: **Axillary staging:** Both clearance and sampling provide important prognostic information on which decisions on local and systemic treatment can be based. Further RCTs of less invasive and potentially less morbid staging procedures such as sentinel node biopsy are under way. A decision on axillary management should be based on the risk of involvement of axillary nodes (which varies according to tumour size, grade, and the presence of vascular/lymphatic invasion) and potential treatment related morbidity. Two retrospective cohort studies found that level I dissection accurately assessed axillary lymph node status, providing that at least 10 nodes were removed.[70,71] One RCT found that a sample of four nodes provided sufficient information to categorise an axilla as histologically positive or negative.[72] Removal of nodes at level I and level II, or removal of all nodes below the axillary vein (level I, II, and III), accurately stages the axilla.[70,71] RCTs comparing sentinel node biopsy with axillary node clearance and sampling are currently under way, and results of these will be incorporated in future issues of *Clinical Evidence* (JM Dixon, personal communication, 2000).

| QUESTION | What are the effects of interventions in locally advanced breast cancer (Stage III B)? | New |

Alan Rodger

| OPTION | LOCAL THERAPY FOR LOCALLY ADVANCED BREAST CANCER |

Seven small RCTs have found that, for locally advanced breast cancer that is rendered operable, radiotherapy or surgery as sole local treatments have similar effects on response rates, duration of response, and overall survival. One RCT found weak evidence that, if surgery is possible and is carried out, postoperative radiotherapy will reduce local/regional recurrence. Local skin toxicity (acute and late) after radiotherapy is greater in locally advanced breast cancer than after treatment for less advanced disease, because of the need for a higher radiation dose to skin.

Benefits: We found no systematic review of the role of radiotherapy in locally advanced (stage III B) breast cancer. We found seven RCTs, including women with stage III B, which compared radiotherapy versus no radiotherapy.[40,43,73–77] Other management options varied across these RCTs. Most RCTs were small, but included more than stage III

B women. **Postoperative radiotherapy versus no further local therapy after surgery:** We found two RCTs.[73,76] In one of these RCTs[73] pre and postoperative chemo-endocrine therapy was administered to all women who also underwent mastectomy while half the women were randomised to post mastectomy radiotherapy to the chest wall and regional lymphatics (45–50 Gy in 5 weeks). However, 43% of the 184 women were excluded with more exclusions in the radiotherapy group, and it is impossible to ascertain what percentage of women were stage III B. There were numerous chemotherapy complications, including one death. The RCT found no statistical difference in local or distant failures, but found an overall crude survival of 28.7 months for the non-radiotherapy group compared with 21.7 for the irradiated group ($P < 0.05$). Conclusions cannot be drawn from this trial. The second RCT of operable locally advanced breast cancer (332 women who were recurrence free after modified radical mastectomy and six cycles of chemo-hormone therapy; 38% stage T_4 and 14% N_2)[76] compared postoperative radiotherapy versus no further treatment. It found no significant difference in time to relapse (4.7 years for radiotherapy v 5.2 years for no further treatment) and median overall survival (8.3 years v 8.1 years). Radiotherapy reduced locoregional sites as first recurrence by 9%. **Postmastectomy radiotherapy in women having systemic therapy after surgery:** Two RCTs of "high risk breast cancer" (including women with stage III B disease) studied post mastectomy radiotherapy in women having systemic therapy after surgery.[40,34] The post menopausal trial separated some T_4 tumours by skin invasion (14%).[43] For those receiving postmastectomy radiotherapy with tamoxifen, 8% developed local recurrence versus 34% receiving tamoxifen alone (5 year disease free survival: 41% v 37%; 10 year disease free survival: 23% v 22%; 5 year survivals: 51% v 61%; 10 year survivals: 31% v 27%. However, the studies used small and retrospective subgroups, making conclusions uncertain. **Surgery alone versus radiotherapy alone:** Two RCTs compared surgery alone versus radiotherapy alone as local therapy.[74,75] In one RCT,[74] 113 women with stage III breast cancer (67% stage III B) were given chemotherapy and 81% became operable; 87 women were randomised to surgery or to radiotherapy. After local therapy, a further 2 years of chemotherapy was given. Both groups had similar duration of disease control (29.2 months with surgery v 24.4 months with radiation; $P = 0.5$), similar overall median survival (39.3 v 39 months), and similar sites of first relapse. In the other RCT (132 women, 91% stage III B, 9% stage III A) all women received chemotherapy before randomisation to either surgery or radiotherapy.[75] Total response rate was 75% in each group. Duration of remission was not significantly different (15 months with surgery v 22 months with radiotherapy; $P = 0.58$). Survival was similar at 4 years (52 months with radiotherapy v 49.1 months with surgery). **Low dose radiotherapy versus tamoxifen:** A small RCT (143 women)[77] compared low dose radiotherapy (40 Gy in 15 fractions) versus tamoxifen (20 mg twice daily). Women were given the alternative treatment on relapse. The RCT found no significant difference in response rates ($P = 0.34$), duration of response ($P = 0.76$), or survival ($P = 0.38$).

Harms: The type of harms from radiotherapy for locally advanced breast cancer were similar to those from radiotherapy after mastectomy or breast conserving surgery. However, in stage III B disease with skin involvement (T4 b, c, d), the skin is usually given a higher dose of radiotherapy. In addition, a higher dose (60 Gy) is often given to more of the breast volume. Acute skin toxicity (including moist desquamation) and late skin toxicity (pigmentation and telangiectasia) are also more likely than in women without skin involvement.

Comment: The lack of good quality, large trials addressing directly stage III B breast cancer and the role of radiotherapy render it difficult to draw firm conclusions on its value. Such trials are small and have varying approaches to management. From the results of two trials,[74,75] it can be concluded that in terms of overall response (which includes the response from local therapies such as surgery radiotherapy, or both, and the effects of any initial systemic therapy), duration of that response, and overall survival, there is no advantage of either surgery alone or radiotherapy alone as sole local treatment over the other. It is more difficult to detail the possible benefits of postoperative radiotherapy in women whose locally advanced breast cancers have been rendered operable by systemic therapy and who have undergone surgery, usually modified radical mastectomy. It is likely that such postoperative radiotherapy will reduce the risk of local (and regional if nodal areas are irradiated) recurrence. It is not possible to conclude that it will affect survival.

OPTION	SYSTEMIC THERAPY FOR LOCALLY ADVANCED BREAST CANCER

We found no evidence that cytotoxic chemotherapy of cyclophosphamide, methotrexate and 5-FU or an anthracycline based multidrug regimen improves survival, disease free survival, or long term locoregional control in locally advanced breast cancer. One RCT found evidence that hormone treatment plus radiotherapy versus radiotherapy alone improves survival in locally advanced breast cancer.

Benefits: We found no systematic review. **Radiotherapy versus radiotherapy plus systemic chemotherapy:** We found three RCTs,[78–80] which compared radiotherapy versus radiotherapy plus systemic therapy (hormone therapy, chemotherapy, or both). One RCT (410 women, most stage III B)[78] compared radiotherapy versus radiotherapy plus chemotherapy [CMF] for 12 cycles) versus radiotherapy plus hormone therapy (ovarian irradiation for premenopausal women, tamoxifen for postmenopausal women) versus radiotherapy plus both chemotherapy and hormone therapy. Both chemotherapy (P = 0.0002) and hormone therapy (P = 0.0007) significantly delayed locoregional recurrence. Combined chemotherapy and hormone therapy had the largest effect (P = 0.0001). Locoregional recurrence at 6 years was reduced (59% to 48% with chemotherapy v 61% to 47% with hormone therapy). The effect on distant metastases was similar but less marked. Significantly increased median survival was found only with hormone therapy (4.3 years with hormone therapy v 3.3 years without hormone therapy, after 8 years HR death 0.75, 95% CI 0.59 to 0.96; median survival 3.8 years with chemotherapy v 3.6 years without, HR 0.84,

95% CI 0.66 to 1.08). Another RCT (118 women with stage III B breast cancer)[79] compared radiotherapy versus radiotherapy plus chemotherapy (cyclophosphamide, methrotrexate and 5-FU–CMF for 12 cycles) plus tamoxifen versus chemotherapy (CMF alternating with adriamycin and vincristine–AV) followed by radiotherapy and then further similar chemotherapy and tamoxifen. (The radiotherapy in the third arm delivered a lower dose to the skin and a lower total dose). After a minimum follow up of 14 years, the RCT found no significant difference in survival, disease free survival, or locoregional control. The 10 year survival rates were 13% with radiotherapy alone, 21% with radiotherapy, CMF, and tamoxifen, and 28% for radiotherapy plus CMF/AV/tamoxifen. Differences in 10 year survival were 8% (95% CI 9% to 25%) for radiotherapy versus radiotherapy, CMF, and tamoxifen; and 15% (95% CI 3% to 33%) for radiotherapy versus radiotherapy plus CMF/AV/tamoxifen. There was no significant difference between the two arms with chemotherapy. The disease free survival at 10 years for radiotherapy alone was 4%; 15% for radiotherapy plus CMF/tamoxifen; and 15% for radiotherapy plus CMF/AV/tamoxifen. The difference in this at 10 years was 12% (95% CI 1% to 25%) between radiotherapy and radiotherapy plus CMF; and 12% (95% CI 1.4% to 25.4%) for radiotherapy versus the third arm. Local recurrence was similar in the three arms (42% v 45% v 49%). The third RCT (52 women with T_4 breast cancer)[80] compared an anthracycline chemotherapy regimen before radiotherapy versus similar radiotherapy alone. The combined therapy arm achieved a higher initial locoregional control rate (complete response 78.6% v 45.8%, P = 0.03). However, the number of women free of locoregional spread at death or last follow up was similar (57% combined v 50% radiotherapy alone). Overall survival and time to distant recurrence were not significantly different. **Multimodal treatment versus hormone treatment:** One RCT (108 women)[81] compared multimodal therapy (preoperative chemotherapy, surgery, radiotherapy, and tamoxifen) versus initial hormone treatment plus subsequent salvage therapies upon tumor progression. The objective remission after 6 months was higher with multimodal treatment than with tamoxifen alone (31/54 [57%] v 19/53 [36%]; OR 2.4, 95% CI 1.1 to 5.0; P = 0.03). However, at a median follow up of 30 months, there was no significant difference in survival or the development of metastases or uncontrolled local disease.

Harms: In many RCTs harms of treatment were not reported (see harms of adjuvant combination chemotherapy, p 1232).

Comment: The lack of large RCTs and the less frequent inclusion of less locally advanced disease (T3) with locally advanced breast cancer defined here as (stage III B) make it difficult to draw conclusions. There is, however, no evidence from the studies using CMF chemotherapy or various regimens incorporating anthracyclines that cytotoxic chemotherapy improves survival, disease free survival, or long term locoregional control in stage III B breast cancer. One RCT found evidence of improved survival with hormone therapy.

GLOSSARY

Adjuvant treatment This usually refers to systemic chemotherapy or hormonal treatment, or both, taken by people after removal of a primary tumour (in this case, surgery for early breast cancer), with the aim of killing any remaining micrometastatic tumour cells and thus preventing recurrence.

Anthracyclines Are also known as cytotoxic antibiotics, and are used as adjuvant therapy with radiotherapy. Examples of anthracyclines are aclarubicin, daunorubicin, doxorubicin, epirubicin and idarubicin

Axillary clearance Clearance of level I, II, and usually level III axillary lymph nodes. Level I nodes are lateral to the pectoralis minor muscle, level II nodes are under it, and level III nodes are medial to it at the apex of the axilla.

Axillary radiotherapy This usually includes irradiation of the supraclavicular fossa. Irradiation of this area incorporates some underlying lung that increases the risk of radiation pneumonitis. By increasing the volume of the lung irradiated, compared with chest wall or breast radiotherapy alone, the risk of acute pneumonitis is increased.

Axillary sampling Aims to remove the four largest, most easily palpable axillary lymph nodes, for histological examination.

Breast conserving surgery Surgery that consists of lumpectomy (minimal free margins), wide local excision (wider free margins), or segmental or quadrant resection (usually with very wide free margins).

CMF (classical) Chemotherapy regimen containing cyclophosphamide, methotrexate, and 5-fluoruracil.

Combination chemotherapy Two or more cytotoxic drugs given intravenously every 3–4 weeks for 4–6 months.

Disease free survival (DFS) Means being alive with no local or distant recurrence or contralateral disease.

FAC Chemotherapy regimen containing 5-fluorouracil, doxorubicin (adriamycin), and cyclophosphamide

Lumpectomy Gross tumour excision.

Milan regimen A sequential regimen of single agent anthracycline followed by CMF.

Non-invasive breast cancer (stage 0) is T_{is} (carcinoma *in situ*, intraductal carcinoma, lobular carcinoma *in situ*, or Paget's disease of the nipple with no associated tumor); N_0 (no axillary nodal involvement); and M_0 (no metastases).

Early invasive breast cancer (stage I or II) is M_0 with: T_1 or T_2 (tumour diameter 5 cm or less, no involvement of skin or chest wall) and N_0 or N_1 (mobile axillary nodes); or M_0 with T_3 (tumour diameter over 5 cm, no skin or chest wall involvement) but only N_0. **Advanced breast cancer** *Operable locally advanced breast cancer (stage IIIA)* i.e. T_3 (tumours greater than 5 cm) and N_1 (non-matted involved axillary nodes). *Locally advanced breast cancer (stage III B)* is M_0 with T_4 (skin or chest wall infiltration by tumour) and/or N_2 (matted axillary nodes)/N_3 (internal mammary node involvement) disease, not classified as non-invasive or early invasive breast cancer. *Metastatic breast cancer (stage IV)* is M1 (any supraclavicular fossa node involvement or distant metastases to bone, lung, liver etc.) with any combination of tumour and node parameters.

Neoadjuvant chemotherapy (Also known as primary medical therapy) involves the use of chemotherapy to treat breast cancer before locoregional therapy (surgery and or radiotherapy) to the breast to downstage large primary cancers that would require mastectomy to improve chances of survival.

Ovarian ablation Surgical, medical, or radiation induced suppression of ovarian function in premenopausal women.

Overall objective response rate The proportion of treated people in whom a complete response (disappearance of all known lesions on two separate measurements at least 4 weeks apart) or partial response (more than a 50% reduction in the size of lesions) is observed.

Quadrantectomy Tumour excised with at least 2 cm of normal surrounding breast tissue and with a segment of breast tissue from the periphery of the breast to the nipple.

Radical mastectomy Removal of breast and pectoralis major and minor muscles and axillary contents.

Radiotherapy Part of initial local and regional treatment. In early stage disease it may be an adjunct to surgery; in locally advanced disease (T4;N2) it may be the sole locoregional treatment. Radiotherapy may be delivered to the breast or postmastectomy chest wall, as well as to the lymphatic areas of the axilla, supraclavicular fossa or internal mammary node chain.

Staging of breast cancer A detailed description by tumour, nodal, and metastatic parameters at a particular time (TNM).[1]These are amalgamated into broader categories called stages (0 to IV). Stages can be aggregated into even broader categories (non-invasive, early invasive, and advanced breast cancer) (see table 3, p 1246).

Supraradical mastectomy Removal of breast, pectoralis major and minor muscles, axillary contents and internal mammary chain of nodes.

Tamoxifen A non-steroidal antioestrogen taken as daily oral tablets, usually for between 2–5 years.

TNM staging system See "staging of breast cancer" (above)

Total mastectomy Removal of breast.

Total nodal irradiation Radiotherapy to the regional lymph nodes, including supraclavicular, infraclavicular, axillary nodes, and internal mammary nodes in the upper intercostal spaces.

UICC system International Union against Cancer.

REFERENCES

1. UICC International Union Against Cancer. *TNM classification of malignant tumours* 5th ed. Sobin LH, Wittekind Ch, eds. New York: Wiley–Liss Inc, 1997.

2. CRC. Breast Cancer Factsheet. 1996.

3. Easton D, Ford D. Breast and ovarian cancer incidence in BRCA-1 mutation carriers. *Am J Hum Genet* 1995;56:265–271.

4. Relation of tumour size, lymph node status and survival in 24 740 breast cancer cases. *Cancer* 1989;63:181–187.

5. Hortobagyi GN, Ames FC, Buzdar AU, et al. Management of stage III primary breast cancer with primary chemotherapy, surgery and radiation therapy. *Cancer* 1988;62:2507–2516.

6. Fisher B, Dignam J, Wolmark N, et al. Lumpectomy and radiation therapy for the treatment of intraductal breast cancer: findings of the National Surgical Adjuvant Breast and Bowel Project B-17. *J Clin Oncol* 1998;16:441–452.

7. Julien JP, Bijker N, Fentiman IS, Peterse JL, et al. Radiotherapy in breast-conserving treatment for ductal carcinoma *in situ*; first results of EORTC randomised phase III trial 10853. *Lancet* 2000; 355:528–533.

8. Fisher B, Dignam J, Wolmark N, et al. Tamoxifen in treatment of intraductal breast cancer: National Surgical Adjuvant Breast and Bowel Project B-24 randomised controlled trial. *Lancet* 1999;353: 1993–2000.

9. Mauriac L, Durand M, Avril A, et al. Effects of primary chemotherapy in conservative treatment of breast cancer patients with operable tumours larger than 3 cm: results of a randomised trial in a single centre. *Ann Oncol* 1991;2:347–354.

10. Mauriac L, MacGrogan G, Avril A, et al.

Neoadjuvant chemotherapy for operable breast carcinoma larger than 3 cm: a unicentre randomized trial with a 124-month median follow-up. Institut Bergonie Bordeaux Groupe Sein (IBBGS). *Ann Oncol* 1999;10:47–52.

11. Scholl SM, Fourquet A, Asselain B, et al. Neoadjuvant versus adjuvant chemotherapy in premenopausal patients with tumours considered too large for breast conserving surgery: preliminary results of a randomised trial. *Eur J Cancer* 1994 30A:645–652.

12. Broet P, Scholl S, De La Rochrfordiere A, et al. Short and long term effects on survival in breast cancer patients treated by primary chemotherapy: an updated analysis of a randomised trial. *Breast Cancer Res Treat* 1999;58:151–156.

13. Powles TJ, Hickish TF, Makris A, et al. Randomized trial of chemoendocrine therapy started before or after surgery for treatment of primary breast cancer. *J Clin Oncol* 1995;13:547–552.

14. Fisher B, Bryant J, Wolmark N, et al. Effect of preoperative chemotherapy on the outcome of women with operable breast cancer. *J Clin Oncol* 1998;16:2672–2685.

15. Makris A, Powles TJ, Ashley SE, et al. A reduction in the requirements for mastectomy in a randomized trial of neoadjuvant chemoendocrine therapy in primary breast cancer. *Ann Oncol* 1998; 9:1179–1184.

16. Avril A, Faucher A, Bussieres E, et al. Resultats a 10 ans d'un essai randomise de chimiotherapie neo-adjuvante dans les cancers du sein de plus de 3 cm. *Chirurgie* 1998;123:247–256.

17. Early Breast Cancer Trialists Collaborative Group. Polychemotherapy for early breast cancer: an

overview of the randomised trials. Lancet 1998; 352:930–942

18. Buzdar AU, Singletary SE, Theriault RL, et al. Prospective evaluation of paclitaxel versus combination chemotherapy with fluorouracil, doxorubicin, and cyclophosphamide as neoadjuvant therapy in patients with operable breast cancer. J Clin Oncol 1999;17:3412–3417.

19. Cocconi G, Bisagni G, Ceci G, et al. Three new active cisplatin-containing combinations in the neoadjuvant treatment of locally advanced and locally recurrent breast carcinoma: a randomized phase II trial. Breast Canc Res Treat 1999;56: 125–132.

20. Takatsuka Y, Yayoi E, Kobayashi T, Aikawa T, Kotsuma Y. Neoadjuvant intra-arterial chemotherapy in locally advanced breast cancer: a prospective randomised study. Jpn J Clin Oncol 1994;24:20–25.

21. Early Breast Cancer Trialists' Collaborative Group. Effects of radiotherapy and surgery in early breast cancer: an overview of the randomised trials. N Engl J Med 1995;333:1444–1455. Search date not stated; the author sought information worldwide from investigators who conducted trials that began before 1985.

22. Morris AD, Morris RD, Wilson JF, et al. Breast conserving therapy versus mastectomy in early stage breast cancer: a meta-analysis of 10 year survival. Cancer J Sci Am 1997;3:6–12. Search date 1995, primary source Medline.

23. Sacchini V, Luini A, Tana S, et al. Quantitative and qualitative cosmetic evaluation after conservative treatment for breast cancer. Eur J Cancer 1991; 27:1395–1400.

24. Smitt NC, Nowels KW, Zdeblick MJ, et al. The importance of the lumpectomy surgical margin status in long-term results of breast conservation. Cancer 1995;76:259–267.

25. Wazer DE, DiPetrillo T, Schmidt-Ullrich R, et al. Factors influencing cosmetic outcome and complication risk after conservative surgery and radiotherapy for early-stage breast carcinoma. J Clin Oncol 1992;10:356–363.

26. Abner AL, Recht A, Vicini FA, et al. Cosmetic results after surgery, chemotherapy and radiation therapy for early breast cancer. Int J Radiat Oncol Biol Phys 1991;21:331–338.

27. Dewar JA, Benhamou S, Benhamou E, et al. Cosmetic results following lumpectomy axillary dissection and radiotherapy for small breast cancers. Radiother Oncol 1988;12:273–280.

28. Rochefordiere A, Abner A, Silver B, et al. Are cosmetic results following conservative surgery and radiation therapy for early breast cancer dependent on technique? Int J Radiat Oncol Biol Phys 1992;23:925–931.

29. Sneeuw KA, Aaronson N, Yarnold J, et al. Cosmetic and functional outcomes of breast conserving treatment for early stage breast cancer 1: comparison of patients' ratings, observers' ratings and objective assessments. Radiother Oncol 1992;25:153–159.

30. Ash DV, Benson EA, Sainsbury JR, et al. Seven year follow-up on 334 patients treated by breast conserving surgery and short course radical postoperative radiotherapy: a report of the Yorkshire breast cancer group. Clin Oncol 1995;7: 93–96.

31. Lindsey I, Serpell JW, Johnson WR, Rodger A. Cosmesis following complete local excision of breast cancer. Aust N Z J Surg 1997;67:428–432.

32. Touboul E, Belkacemi Y, Lefranc JP, et al. Early breast cancer: influence of type of boost (electrons vs iridium-192 implant) on local control and cosmesis after conservative surgery and radiation therapy. Radiother Oncol 1995;34:105–113.

33. Halyard MY, Grado GL, Schomber PJ, et al. Conservative therapy of breast cancer: the Mayo Clinic experience. Am J Clin Oncol 1996;19:445–450.

34. Liljegren G, Holmberg L, Adami HO, Westman G, Graffman S, Bergh J for the Uppsala–örebro Breast Cancer Study Group. Sector resection with or without postoperative radiotherapy for stage I breast cancer: five year results of a randomised trial. J Natl Cancer Inst 1994;86:717–722.

35. Liljegren G, Holmberg J, Bergh, J, et al and the Uppsala–örebro Breast Cancer Study Group. 10-year results after sector resection with or without postoperative radiotherapy for stage I breast cancer: a randomized trial. J Clin Oncol 1999;17:2326–2333.

36. Forrest AP, Stewart HJ, Everington D, et al on behalf of the Scottish Cancer Trials Breast Group. Randomised controlled trial of conservation therapy in breast cancer: 6 year analysis of the Scottish trial. Lancet 1996;348:708–713.

37. Steering Committee on Clinical Practice Guidelines for the Care and Treatment of Breast Cancer. A Canadian consensus document. Can Med Assoc J 1998;158(suppl 3):1–84.

38. Cuzick J, Stewart H, Rutqvist L, et al. Cause-specific mortality in long term survivors of breast cancer who participated in trials of radiotherapy. J Clin Oncol 1994;12:447–453. Search date not given. Includes trials that started before 1975.

39. Ragaz J, Jackson SM, Le N, et al. Adjuvant radiotherapy and chemotherapy in node-positive premenopausal women with breast cancer. N Engl J Med 1997;337:956–962.

40. Overgaard M, Hansen PS, Overgaard J, et al. Postoperative radiotherapy in high-risk premenopausal women with breast cancer who receive adjuvant chemotherapy. N Engl J Med 1997;337:949–955.

41. Hojris I, Overgaard M, Christensen JJ, Overgaard J. Morbidity and mortality of ischaemic heart disease in high-risk breast-cancer patients after adjuvant postmastectomy systemic treatment with or without radiotherapy: analysis of DBCG 82b and 82c randomised trials. Radiotherapy Committee of the Danish Breast Cancer Cooperative Group. Lancet 1999;354:1425–1430.

42. Early Breast Cancer Trialists Collaborative Group. Favourable and unfavourable effects on long-term survival of radiotherapy for early breast cancer: an overview of the randomised trials. Early Breast Cancer Trialists' Collaborative Group. Lancet 2000;355:1757–1770.

43. Overgaard M, Jensen MB, Overgaard J, et al. Postoperative radiotherapy in high risk postmenopausal breast cancer patients given adjuvant tamoxifen: Danish Breast Cancer Cooperative Group DBCG 82c randomised trial. Lancet 1999;353:1641–1648.

44. Ghersi D, Simes J. Draft report of effectiveness of postmastectomy radiotherapy and risk factors for local recurrence in early breast cancer. Report to NHMRC National Breast Cancer Centre, Sydney, 1998.

45. O'Rourke S, Gaba MH, Morgan D, et al. Local recurrence after simple mastectomy. Br J Surg 1994;81:386–389.

46. Fowble B, Gray R, Gilchrist K, Goodman RL, Taylor S, Tormey D. Identification of a subset of patients with breast cancer and histologically positive nodes who may benefit from postoperative radiotherapy. J Clin Oncol 1988;6:1107–1117.

47. Houghton J, Baum M, Haybittle JL. Role of radiotherapy following total mastectomy in patients with early breast cancer: the closed trials

working party of the CRC breast cancer trials group. *World J Surg* 1994;18:117–122.

48. Kaija H, Maunu P. Tangential breast irradiation with or without internal mammary chain irradiation: results of a randomised trial. *Radiother Oncol* 1995;36:172–176.

49. Handley R. Carcinoma of the breast. *Ann R Coll Surg Engl* 1975;57:59–66.

50. Veronesi U, Cascinelli NM, Bufalino R, et al. Risk of internal mammary lymph node metastases and its relevance on prognosis in breast cancer patients. *Ann Surg* 1983;198:681–684.

51. Veronesi U, Valagussa P. Inefficacy of internal mammary node dissection in breast cancer surgery. *Cancer* 1981;47:170–175.

52. Bates T, Evans RGB. Report of the Independent Review commissioned by The Royal College of Radiologists into brachial plexus neuropathy following radiotherapy for breast cancer. London: Royal College of Radiologists, 1995.

53. Early Breast Cancer Trialists' Collaborative Group. Polychemotherapy for early breast cancer: an overview of the randomised trials. *Lancet* 1998; 352:930–942. Search date 1995; the authors sought information on each woman in any randomised trial that began before 1990.

54. Fisher B, Anderson S, Wickerham DL, et al. Increased intensification and total dose of cyclophosphamide in a doxorubicin-cyclophosphamide regimen for the treatment of primary breast cancer: findings from national surgical adjuvant breast and bowel project B-22. *J Clin Oncol* 1997;15:1858–1869.

55. Wood WC, Budman DR, Korzun AH. Dose and dose intensity of adjuvant chemotherapy for stage II, node-positive breast carcinoma. *N Engl J Med* 1994;330:1253–1259.

56. Peters WP, Ross M, Vredenburgh JJ, et al. High-dose chemotherapy and autologous bone marrow support as consolidation after standard-dose adjuvant chemotherapy for high-risk primary breast cancer. *J Clin Oncol* 1993;11:1132–1143.

57. Rodenhuis S, Richel DJ, van der Wall E, et al. Randomised trial of high-dose chemotherapy and haemopoietic progenitor-cell support in operable breast cancer with extensive axillary lymph-node involvement. *Lancet* 1998;352:515–521.

58. Bonadonna G, Zambeti M, Valagussa P. Sequential or alternating doxorubicin and CMF regimens in breast cancer with more than three positive nodes. *JAMA* 1995;273:542–547.

59. Early Breast Cancer Trialists' Collaborative Group. Tamoxifen for early breast cancer: an overview of the randomised trials. *Lancet* 1998;351:1451–1467. Search date 1995, includes trials started before 1990. The authors sought data on each woman in any randomised trial that began before 1990.

60. Swedish Breast Cancer Cooperative Group. Randomised trial of two versus five years of adjuvant tamoxifen for post-menopausal early stage breast cancer. *J Natl Cancer Inst* 1996;88: 1543–1549.

61. Fisher B, Dignam J, Bryant J, et al. Five versus more than five years of tamoxifen therapy for breast cancer patients with negative lymph nodes and estrogen receptor-positive tumours. *J Natl Cancer Inst* 1996;88:1529–1542.

62. Stewart HJ, Forrest AP, Everington D, et al. Randomised comparison of 5 years of adjuvant tamoxifen with continuous therapy for operable breast cancer. *Br J Cancer* 1996;74:297–299.

63. Powles TJ, Hickish T, Kanis JA, Tidy A, Ashley S. Effect of tamoxifen on bone mineral density measured by dual-energy x-ray absorptiometry in healthy premenopausal and postmenopausal women. *J Clin Oncol* 1996;14:78–84.

64. Swain SM. Tamoxifen: the long and short of it. *J Natl Cancer Inst* 1996;88:1510–1512.

65. Fisher B, Dignam J, Wolmark N, et al. Tamoxifen and chemotherapy for lymph node-negative, estrogen receptor-positive breast cancer. *J Natl Cancer Inst* 1997;89:1673–1682.

66. Early Breast Cancer Trialists' Group. Ovarian ablation in early breast cancer: overview of the randomised trials. *Lancet* 1996;348:1189–1196. Search date 1995; the authors sought information on each patient in any randomised trial that began before 1990.

67. Chetty U, Jack W, Prescott RJ, Tyler C, Rodger A. Management of the axilla in operable breast cancer treated by breast conservation: a randomised controlled trial. *Br J Surg* 2000;87: 163–169.

68. Stelle RJC, Forrest APM, Gibson R, Stuart HJ, Chetty U. The efficacy of lower axillary sampling in obtaining lymph node status in breast cancer: a controlled randomised trial. *Br J Surg* 1985;72: 368–369.

69. Browning C, Thomas and Associates; Redman S, Pillar C, Turner J, Boyle F. NHMRC National Breast Cancer Centre, Sydney 1998. Lymphoedema: prevalence risk factors and management: a review of research. Search date 1996; primary sources Medline 1985 to 1996, hand searches of article references, and personal contact with key resources.

70. Axelsson CK, Mouridzsen HT, Zedeler K. Axillary dissection at level I and II lymph nodes is important in breast cancer classification. *Eur J Cancer* 1992;28A:1415–1418.

71. Kiricuta CI, Tausch J. A mathematical model of axillary lymph node involvement based on 1446 complete axillary dissections in patients with breast carcinoma. *Cancer* 1992;69:2496–2501.

72. Steele RJC, Forrest APM, Givson T, Stuart HJ, Chetty U. The efficacy of lower axillary sampling in obtaining lymph node status in breast cancer: a controlled randomised trial. *Br J Surg* 1985;72: 368–369.

73. Papaioannou A, Lissaios B, Vasilaros S, et al. Pre – and post-operative chemoendocrine treatment with or without post-operative radiotherapy for locally advanced breast cancer. *Cancer* 1983;51:1284–1290.

74. Perloff M, Lesnick G J, Korzun A, et al. Combination chemotherapy with mastectomy or radiotherapy for stage III breast carcinoma : a Cancer and Leukaemia Group B Study. *J Clin Oncol* 1988;6:261–269.

75. De Lena M, Varini M, Zucali R, et al. Multimodal treatment for locally advanced breast cancer. Results of chemotherapy–radiotherapy versus chemotherapy–surgery. *Cancer Clin Trials* 1981;4: 229–236.

76. Olson JE, Neuberg D, Pandya KJ, et al. The role of radiotherapy in the management of operable locally advanced breast carcinoma : results of a randomised trial by the Eastern Co-operative Oncology Group. *Cancer* 1997;79:1138–1149.

77. Willsher PC, Robertson JF, Armitage NC, et al. Locally advanced breast cancer: long term results of a randomised trial comparing primary treatment with tamoxifen or radiotherapy in post-menopausal women. *Eur J Surg Oncol* 1996;22:34–37.

78. Bartelink H, Rubens RD, van der Schueren E, et al. Hormonal therapy prolongs survival in irradiated locally advanced breast cancer: a European Organisation for Research and Treatment of Cancer randomised phase III trial. *J Clin Oncol* 1997;15:207–215.

79. Koning C, Hart G. Long term follow up of a randomised trial on adjuvant chemotherapy and hormonal therapy in locally advanced breast

cancer. *Int J Rad Oncol Biol Phys* 1998; 41:397–400.

80. Rodger A, Jack WJL, Hardman PDJ, et al. Locally advanced breast cancer: report of a phase II study and subsequent phase III trial. *Br J Cancer* 1992; 65:761–765.

81. Willsher PC, Robertson JF, Chan SY, et al. Locally advanced breast cancer: early results of a randomised trial of multimodal therapy versus initial hormone therapy. *Eur J Cancer* 1997;33: 45–49.

J Michael Dixon
Senior Lecturer in Surgery
Western General Hospital
Edinburgh
UK

Alan Rodger
Professor of Radiation Oncology
William Buckland Radiotherapy Centre
The Alfred Hospital, Monash University
Melbourne
Australia

Stephen Johnston
Senior Lecturer in Medical Oncology
The Royal Marsden NHS Trust
London
UK

Kate Gregory
Consultant Medical Oncologist
Royal Southants Hospital
Southampton
UK

Competing interests: None declared.

TABLE 1 Ten year survival with combination chemotherapy versus placebo, according to nodal and age/menopausal status: results of a systematic review of RCTs (see text, p 1231).[53]

	Control (%)	Chemotherapy (%)	Absolute benefit (%)	SD (%)	Significance (two sided)
Age < 50 years					
Node +ve	41.4	53.8	+12.4	2.4	P < 0.00001
Node −ve	71.9	77.6	+5.7	2.1	P = 0.01
Age 50–69 years					
Node +ve	46.3	48.6	+2.3	1.3	P = 0.001
Node −ve	64.8	71.2	+6.4	2.3	P = 0.0025

SD, standard deviation.

TABLE 2 Ten year survival in women treated with tamoxifen for 5 years compared with control treatment (no tamoxifen): results of a systematic review of RCTs (see text, p 1232).[59]

	Control (%)	Chemotherapy (%)	Absolute benefit (%)	SD (%)	Significance (two sided)
Node +ve	50.5	61.4	+10.9	2.5	$P < 0.00001$
Node −ve	73.3	78.9	+5.6	1.3	$P < 0.00001$

SD, standard deviation.

TABLE 3 Staging of breast cancer (the individual terms are explained in the glossary, p 1240).[1]

		TNM		Stage
Non−invasive	T_{is}	N_0	M_0	0
Early invasive	T_{1-2}	N_{0-1}	M_0	I, II A or B
	T_3	N_0	M_0	II B
Advanced				
Locally advanced	T_{any}	N_2	M_0	III A
	T_3	N_{1-2}	M_0	III A
	T_4	N_{0-3}	M_0	III B
	T_{any}	N_3	M_0	III B
Metastatic	T_{any}	N_{any}	M_1	IV

Search date November 2000

Nigel Bundred

QUESTIONS

INTERVENTIONS

Key Messages

- We found limited evidence from RCTs suggesting that:
  - Advice to follow a low fat, high carbohydrate diet versus general dietary advice reduces breast pain and tenderness.
  - Danazol versus placebo reduces pain after 12 months but with increased adverse effects.
  - Tamoxifen versus placebo reduces breast pain. There is no significant difference between danazol and tamoxifen.
  - Bromocriptine versus placebo relieves breast pain but with a high incidence of adverse effects.
  - Gestrinone versus placebo reduces breast pain but with increased adverse effects. Tibolone is more effective than hormone replacement therapy (HRT).
- We found no good evidence from RCTs on the effects of evening primrose oil, luteinising hormone releasing hormone agonists, progestogen cream, pyridoxine, diuretics, antibiotics, or vitamin E.

Breast pain

DEFINITION	Breast pain can be differentiated into cyclical mastalgia (worse before a menstrual period) or non-cyclical mastalgia (unrelated to the menstrual cycle).[1,2] Cyclical pain is often bilateral, usually most severe in the upper outer quadrants of the breast, and may refer to the medial aspect of the upper arm.[1–3] Non-cyclical pain may be caused by true breast pain or chest wall pain located over the costal cartilages.[1,2,4] Specific breast pathology and referred pain unrelated to the breasts are not included in this definition.
INCIDENCE/ PREVALENCE	Up to 70% of women develop breast pain in their lifetime.[1,2] Of 1171 US women attending a gynaecology clinic, 69% suffered regular discomfort, which was judged as severe in 11% of women, and 36% had consulted a doctor about breast pain.[2]
AETIOLOGY/ RISK FACTORS	The cause is multifactorial. Breast pain is more common in women aged 30–50 years.[1,2]
PROGNOSIS	Cyclical breast pain resolves spontaneously within 3 months of onset in 20–30% of women.[5] The pain tends to relapse and remit, and up to 60% of women develop recurrent symptoms 2 years after treatment.[1] Non-cyclical pain responds poorly to treatment but may resolve spontaneously in about 50% of women.[1]
AIMS	To reduce breast pain and improve quality of life.
OUTCOMES	Breast pain score based on the number of days of severe (score 2) or moderate (score 1) pain experienced in each menstrual cycle; visual analogue score of breast pain, heaviness, or breast tenderness; questionnaires.
METHODS	*Clinical Evidence* update search and appraisal November 2000 using the following key words: breast tenderness, discomfort, pain, mastalgia, mastodynia. Overall the evidence was poor and some studies with weaker methods were included when higher quality evidence was not found, as indicated in the text. Studies were included whatever the definition of breast pain, as indicated in the text.

QUESTION What are the effects of treatments for breast pain?

OPTION LOW FAT, HIGH CARBOHYDRATE DIET

One small RCT has found that advice to follow a low fat, high carbohydrate diet reduces breast pain and tenderness more than general dietary advice.

Benefits: We found no systematic review. We found one RCT (21 women with cyclical mastalgia for at least 5 years), which compared instruction to reduce fat content of the diet to 15% of total versus general dietary advice for 6 months.[6] One woman in each group withdrew and was excluded from the analysis. Over 6 months the severity of self reported breast swelling (P = 0.04) and tenderness (P = 0.0001) was significantly reduced in women receiving low fat dietary advice compared with those receiving general dietary advice. However, no significant difference in breast swelling, tenderness, and nodularity was found on physical examination after 6 months (6/10 [60%] of women with diet, 2/9 [22%] of women with control; RR 2.7, 95% CI 0.75 to 4.13).

Harms: The small trial reported no ill effects.

Comment: Diets can be difficult to sustain in the long term.

OPTION	EVENING PRIMROSE OIL

We found insufficient evidence on the effects of evening primrose oil.

Benefits: We found no systematic review and no good quality RCTs.

Harms: Poor quality RCTs found that adverse effects causing treatment discontinuation were similar with evening primrose oil and placebo (3%), and largely caused by abdominal bloating.[5,7]

Comment: In one partially blinded RCT, 72 women received evening primrose oil or placebo for 3 months, followed by 3 months of evening primrose oil.[7] It reported that pain, tenderness, and lumpiness improved in cyclical but not non-cyclical breast pain. However, the methodology of the trial was poor, and included post hoc revision of the inclusion criteria, subgroup analysis, exclusion of withdrawals, and the use of baseline comparisons (with the best response seen in women who were symptomatically worse at baseline). We found one survey of randomised and open studies, but data were reported as overall summary figures, making specific data extraction impossible.[5]

OPTION	DANAZOL

One RCT found that danazol reduced cyclical breast pain compared with placebo after 12 months, but with increased adverse effects. It found no significant difference between danazol and tamoxifen.

Benefits: We found no systematic review. We found one good quality three arm outpatient based RCT in 93 women with severe cyclical mastalgia.[8] **Versus placebo:** It compared danazol 200 mg/day versus tamoxifen 10 mg/day versus placebo over 6 months. It found that significantly more women achieved greater than 50% pain relief at the end of treatment with danazol versus placebo (pain relief AR 21/32 [66%] v 11/29 [38%]; RR 1.73, 95% CI 1.02 to 2.94; NNT 3, 95% CI 2 to 37). After 12 months of treatment the difference remained significant (pain relief AR 12/32 [38%] with danazol v 0/29 [0%] with placebo; RR 22, 95% CI 1.26 to 55). **Versus other drugs:** See tamoxifen, p 1251. The same RCT found no significant difference in pain relief after treatment with danazol compared with tamoxifen (AR 21/32 [66%] with danazol v 23/32 [72%] with tamoxifen; ARR 6%; RR 0.91, 95% CI 0.65 to 1.27).[8]

Harms: Adverse effects were reported in more women taking danazol than placebo.[8] These included weight gain (10 v 1), deepening of the voice (4 v 0), menorrhagia (4 v 0), and muscle cramps (3 v 0). The results were not assessed for significance.

Comment: Although we found no direct evidence, there is consensus that once a response is achieved, adverse effects can be avoided by reducing the dose of danazol to 100 mg daily, and confining treatment to the fortnight preceding menstruation.[8,9] Non-hormonal contraception is essential with danazol when given in 200 mg doses.[10]

Breast pain

| OPTION | BROMOCRIPTINE |

Two RCTs found limited evidence that bromocriptine versus placebo relieves breast pain. One RCT found a high incidence of adverse effects.

Benefits: We found no systematic review but found two RCTs. The first outpatient based, European RCT (272 premenopausal women with diffuse fibrocystic disease of the breast) compared bromocriptine 2.5 mg twice daily with placebo. After 3 and 6 months it found that bromocriptine versus placebo improved symptoms on self assessed visual analogue scoring of breast pain, tenderness, and heaviness. Analysis did not use intention to treat, and 49 women (35%) withdrew on bromocriptine compared with 36 women (26%) on placebo.[11] The second RCT (10 women) used a crossover design, and also found that bromocriptine reduced pain compared with placebo (P < 0.02).[12]

Harms: The larger RCT found that with bromocriptine treatment 61/135 (45%) of women complained of adverse events versus 41/137 (30%) on placebo (ARI 15%, 95% CI 3% to 28%; RR 1.51, 95% CI 1.11 to 1.92; NNH 7, 95% CI 4 to 29). Adverse effects caused 15/135 women (11%) to withdraw on active treatment compared with 8/137 women (6%) on placebo. The adverse reactions included nausea (32% v 13%), dizziness (12% v 7%), postural hypertension, and constipation.[11] The small RCT found that nausea and dizziness occurred in eight of 10 women (80%) on bromocriptine compared with none of the 10 on placebo.[12] Strokes and death have been reported after use of bromocriptine to inhibit lactation, and the US Food and Drug Administration has withdrawn its license for this indication.[13]

Comment: Bromocriptine is now rarely used because frequent and intolerable adverse effects at the therapeutic dose outweigh the benefits for this indication.

| OPTION | HORMONE REPLACEMENT THERAPY IN BREAST PAIN |

One small RCT has found that HRT reduces pain less than tibolone.

Benefits: We found no systematic review. **Versus placebo:** We found no RCTs. **Versus tibolone:** One RCT (44 postmenopausal women) compared tibolone 2.5 mg daily versus HRT (transdermal oestrogen patches 50 µg, twice weekly for 3 weeks per month, plus progestogen 5 mg daily for 12 days/month per cycle) versus no treatment. After 1 year it found that breast pain was significantly increased in women on HRT compared with those on tibolone (total increase in breast pain was 53% v 5%, P < 0.02).[14]

Harms: The RCT did not report on adverse effects.[14] See harms of HRT under secondary prevention of ischaemic cardiac events, p 95.

Comment: Tibolone is a synthetic steroid reported to have oestrogenic, progestogenic, and weak androgenic properties, which may be used as a form of HRT.[15]

| OPTION | TAMOXIFEN |

Two RCTs found limited evidence that tamoxifen is more effective than placebo. One RCT found no significant difference between tamoxifen and danazol.

Benefits: We found no systematic review. **Versus placebo:** We found two RCTs. One double blind crossover RCT (60 premenopausal women with cyclical breast pain) compared tamoxifen with placebo.[16] It found that more women experienced pain relief (visual analogue scale over 3 months) with tamoxifen than placebo (71% v 38%; RR 1.87, 95% CI 1.20 to 1.87; NNT 3, 95% CI 2 to 13). The second RCT (93 women) compared tamoxifen versus danazol versus placebo.[8] It found that significantly more women taking tamoxifen versus placebo achieved a good outcome (greater than 50% reduction in mean pain score) at the end of treatment, 6 months later, and 12 months later (pain relief after treatment: AR 23/32 [72%] v 11/29 [38%] with placebo; ARI 34%; RR 1.89, 95 CI 1.13 to 2.37). **Dose response:** One RCT (301 women with cyclical breast pain for more than 6 months) compared 10 mg versus 20 mg of tamoxifen daily from days 15–25 in the menstrual cycle for 3 months. It found no significant difference in pain relief or nodularity (pain relief: 127/155 [82%] v 107/142 [75%]; ARR 7%, 95% CI –3% to +13%; RR 1.09, 95% CI 0.96 to 1.18; nodularity: 41/155 [26%] v 52/142 [36%]; ARR –9%, 95% CI –18.6% to +0.4%; RR 0.72, 95% CI 0.49 to 1.01).[17] Another RCT (60 women) compared 10 mg versus 20 mg daily doses of tamoxifen for 3 and 6 months in cyclical and non-cyclical mastalgia.[18] Three month response rates were similar (12/14 [86%] had pain relief with 10 mg v 14/15 [93%] with 20 mg; ARR 8%, 95% CI 5% to 61%; RR 0.92, 95% CI 0.35 to 1.06). **Versus other treatments:** One RCT found no significant difference in pain relief between tamoxifen and danazol[8] (see versus other drugs in benefits section of danazol, p 1249).

Harms: One RCT found more women experienced hot flushes (26% v 10%; ARI 16%; RRI 1.49, 95% CI –0.34 to +3.33) and vaginal discharge (16% v 7%; ARI 9.2%; RRI 1.34, 95% CI –0.97 to +3.64) in women taking tamoxifen compared with placebo.[16] Two RCTs found that fewer adverse effects occurred with a daily dose of 10 mg than 20 mg.[17,18] The largest RCT found that adverse effects were reported in 66% of women taking 20 mg daily versus 52% on 10 mg daily (ARI 15%, 95% CI 3% to 26%; RR 0.78, 95% CI 0.60 to 0.95).[17] Adverse effects were primarily hot flushes (AR 54/142 [38%] with 20 mg dose of tamoxifen v 33/155 [21%] with the 10 mg dose; RR 1.79, 95% CI 1.24 to 2.58; NNH 6, 95% CI 3 to 16) and gastrointestinal disturbances (AR 54/142 [38%] with 20 mg v 30/155 [19%] with 10 mg tamoxifen; RR 1.97, 95% CI 1.34 to 2.88; NNH 6, 95% CI 4 to 12). See adverse effects of tamoxifen under treatment of breast cancer, p 1218.

Comment: Tamoxifen is not licensed for mastalgia in the UK or the USA. There is consensus that it should not be used for more than 6 months at a time, and because of the high incidence of adverse effects it should be used only under expert supervision and with appropriate non-hormonal contraception. Tamoxifen is contraindicated in pregnancy because of potential teratogenicity.[19]

Breast pain

| OPTION | LUTEINISING HORMONE RELEASING HORMONE AGONISTS |

We found no good evidence on the effects of luteinising hormone releasing hormone agonists (e.g. goserelin) in women with breast pain.

Benefits: We found no systematic review or good quality RCTs.

Harms: Adverse effects of goserelin may include hot flushes, headaches, nausea, depression, loss of libido, and amenorrhoea.

Comment: None.

| OPTION | SYNTHETIC STEROIDS (GESTRINONE, TIBOLONE) |

One RCT has found that gestrinone relieves breast pain more than placebo. One small RCT has found that tibolone reduces breast pain more than HRT.

Benefits: We found no systematic review. **Versus placebo:** We found one double blinded outpatient based RCT (145 premenopausal women with cyclical breast pain) comparing gestrinone 2.4 mg twice weekly with placebo.[20] It found that gestrinone reduced breast pain more than placebo after 3 months (using visual analogue score 0 to 100 where 0 = no pain, 100 = worst pain: pain score reduced from 59.5 to 11.0 with gestrinone compared with 58.2 to 36.7 with placebo, $P < 0.0001$) **Versus HRT:** See HRT versus tibolone, p 1250.[14]

Harms: **Versus placebo:** The RCT found that significantly more women taking gestrinone versus placebo had androgenic effects, including greasy skin, hirsutism, acne, reduction in breast size, headache, and depression (41% v 14%; ARI 0.27; RR 2.96, 95% CI 1.70 to 4.40).[20] **Versus HRT:** The RCT comparing tibolone versus HRT did not report on adverse effects.[14]

Comment: Gestrinone is a synthetic steroid, reported to have androgenic, anti-oestrogenic, and anti-progestogenic properties, which may be used for the treatment of endometriosis.[15]

| OPTION | PROGESTOGENS |

We found no good evidence on the effects of progestogens in women with breast pain.

Benefits: We found no systematic review or good quality RCTs.

Harms: We found no good evidence.

Comment: None.

| OPTION | OTHER AGENTS |

We found no evidence that pyridoxine, diuretics, antibiotics, or vitamin E, are effective compared with placebo for the treatment of breast pain.

Benefits: We found no systematic review or good quality RCTs.

Harms: We found no good evidence.

Comment: None.

REFERENCES

1. Gateley CA, Mansel RE. Management of the painful and nodular breast. *Br Med Bull* 1991;47: 284–294.

2. Ader DN, Shriver CD. Cyclical mastalgia: prevalence and impact in an outpatient breast clinic sample. *J Am Coll Surg* 1997;185:466–470.

3. Harding C, Osundeko O, Tetlow L, Faragher EB, Howell A, Bundred NJ. Hormonally-regulated proteins in breast secretions are markers of target organ sensitivity. *Br J Cancer* 2000;2:354–360.

4. Maddox PR, Harrison BJ, Mansel RE, Hughes LE. Non-cyclical mastalgia: improved classification and treatment. *Br J Surg* 1989;76:901–904.

5. Pye JK, Mansel RE, Hughes LE. Clinical experience of drug treatments for mastalgia. *Lancet* 1985;1: 373–377.

6. Boyd NF, McGuire V, Shannon P, et al. Effect of a low-fat high-carbohydrate diet on symptoms of cyclical mastopathy. *Lancet* 1988;2:128–132.

7. Preece PE, Hanslip JI, Gilbert L, et al. Evening primrose oil (Efamol) for mastalgia. In: Horrobin D, ed. *Clinical uses of essential fatty acids.* Montreal: Eden Press Inc, 1982:147–154.

8. Kontostolis E, Stefanidis K, Navrozoglou I, Lolis D. Comparison of tamoxifen with danazol for treatment of cyclical mastalgia. *Gynecol Endocrinol* 1997;11:393–397.

9. Maddox PR, Harrison BJ, Mansel RE. Low-dose danazol for mastalgia. *Br J Clin Pract* 1989;68: 43–47.

10. Anonymous. Danazol. In: *The ABPI Compendium of Data Sheets and Summaries of Product Characteristics.* London: Datapharm Publications Ltd, 1999–2000:1395.

11. Mansel RE, Dogliotti L. European multicentre trial of bromocriptine in cyclical mastalgia. *Lancet* 1990;335:190–193.

12. Blichert-Toft M, Anderson AN, Henrikson OB, Mygind T. Treatment of mastalgia with bromocriptine: a double blind crossover study. *BMJ* 1979;1:237.

13. Arrowsmith-Lowe T. Bromocriptine indications withdrawn. *FDA Med Bull* 1994;24:2.

14. Colacurci V, Mele D, De Franciscis P, Costa V, Fortunato N, De Seta L. Effects of tibolone on the breast. *Eur J Obs Gynae Rep Bio* 1998;80:235–238.

15. Parfitt K, ed. *Martindale. The complete drug reference,* 32nd ed. London: Pharmaceutical Press, 1999:1447–1448.

16. Fentiman IS, Caleffi M, Brame K, Choudary A, Hayward JL. Double blind controlled trial of tamoxifen therapy for mastalgia. *Lancet* 1986;1: 287–288.

17. GEMB Group. Tamoxifen therapy for cyclical mastalgia: dose randomised trial. *Breast* 1997;5: 212–213.

18. Fentiman IS, Hamed H, Caleffi M, Choudary MA. Dosage and duration of tamoxifen treatment for mastalgia: a controlled trial. *Br J Surg* 1988;845–846.

19. Anonymous. Nolvadex. In: *The ABPI Compendium of Data Sheets and Summaries of Product Characteristics.* London: Datapharm Publications Ltd, 1999–2000:1799.

20. Peters F. Multicentre study of gestinone in cyclical breast pain. *Lancet* 1992;339:205–208.

N Bundred
Reader in Surgical Oncology/Consultant Surgeon
University of Manchester Department of Surgery/South Manchester University Hospital
Manchester
UK

Competing interests: The author has received reimbursement by AstraZeneca, the maker of Tamoxifen, for attending several conferences and running education programmes. The author has also received support by Searle Pharmaceuticals for attending and speaking at symposia.

Dysmenorrhoea

Search date March 2000

Michelle Wilson and Cynthia Farquhar

INTERVENTIONS

Key Messages

- One systematic review of RCTs has found that aspirin is more effective for pain relief than placebo but less effective than naproxen and ibuprofen. One RCT found limited evidence that paracetamol/dextropropoxyphene (DPH) is more effective than placebo.

- One systematic review of RCTs found strong evidence that naproxen, ibuprofen, and mefenamic acid are more effective than placebo for pain relief. The review found some evidence of increased adverse effects with naproxen.

- Three small RCTs found insufficient evidence that oral contraceptives are effective for pain relief.

- One small RCT found limited evidence suggesting that laparoscopic uterine nerve ablation (LUNA) was more effective than diagnostic laparoscopy. A second RCT compared LUNA and laparoscopic presacral neurectomy (LPSN) and found no significant difference in pain relief in the short term. However, LPSN was significantly more effective in the long term.

- Small RCTs found that high frequency transcutaneous electrical nerve stimulation and acupuncture achieved more effective pain relief than placebo.

- We found insufficient evidence to determine the effectiveness of behavioural interventions, spinal manipulation, or herbal remedies.

- One large RCT found that vitamin B_1 was more effective than placebo. RCTs evaluating other dietary interventions were too small to provide adequate evidence of effectiveness.

© *Clinical Evidence* 2001;5:1254–1266.

DEFINITION	Dysmenorrhoea comprises painful menstrual cramps of uterine origin. It is commonly divided into primary dysmenorrhoea (pain without organic pathology) and secondary dysmenorrhoea (pelvic pain associated with an identifiable pathological condition, such as endometriosis or ovarian cysts). The initial onset of primary dysmenorrhoea is usually shortly after menarche (6–12 months) when ovulatory cycles are established. The pain duration is commonly 8–72 hours and is usually associated with the onset of the menstrual flow. Secondary dysmenorrhoea may arise as a new symptom during a woman's fourth and fifth decades.[1]
INCIDENCE/ PREVALENCE	Variations in the definition of dysmenorrhoea make it difficult to determine the precise prevalence. Various types of studies nonetheless consistently demonstrate a high prevalence in women of different ages and nationalities. A recent systematic review of the prevalence of chronic pelvic pain summarising both community and hospital surveys (search date December 1996) estimated the prevalence at 45–95%.[2] Reports focus on adolescent girls and generally include only primary dysmenorrhoea, although this is not always specified. Studies of prevalence are summarised in table 1, p 1265.
AETIOLOGY/ RISK FACTORS	A longitudinal study of a representative sample of women born in 1962 found that severity of dysmenorrhoea was significantly associated with duration of menstrual flow (average duration of menstrual flow was 5 days for women with no dysmenorrhoea and 5.8 days for women with severe dysmenorrhoea, $P < 0.001$, WMD –0.8, 95% CI –1.36 to –0.24); younger average menarcheal age (13.1 in women without dysmenorrhoea v 12.6 in women with severe dysmenorrhoea, $P < 0.01$, WMD 0.5, 95% CI 0.09 to 0.91); and cigarette smoking (41% of smokers and 26% of non-smokers experienced moderate or severe dysmenorrhoea).[9]
PROGNOSIS	Primary dysmenorrhoea is a chronic recurring condition that affects most young women. Studies of the natural history of this condition are sparse. One longitudinal study in Scandinavia found that primary dysmenorrhoea often improves in the third decade of a woman's reproductive life, and is also reduced following childbirth.[9]
AIMS	To relieve pain from dysmenorrhoea, with minimal adverse effects.
OUTCOMES	Pain relief, measured either by visual analogue scale, other pain scales, or as a dichotomous outcome (pain relief achieved yes/no); overall improvement in dysmenorrhoea measured by change in dysmenorrhoeic symptoms either self-reported or observed, quality of life scales, or other similar measures such as the Menstrual Distress or Menstrual Symptom questionnaire; adverse effects of treatment (incidence and type of adverse effects); proportion of women requiring analgesics in addition to their assigned treatment; proportion of women reporting activity restriction or absences from work or school, and hours or days of absence as a more selective measure.
METHODS	*Clinical Evidence* search and appraisal March 2000.

Dysmenorrhoea

| QUESTION | What are the effects of treatments? |

| OPTION | ASPIRIN, PARACETAMOL, AND COMPOUND ANALGESICS |

One systematic review of RCTs has found that aspirin is more effective for pain relief than placebo but less effective than naproxen and ibuprofen. One RCT found limited evidence that paracetamol/dextropropoxyphene (DPH) is more effective than placebo.

Benefits: We found one systematic review (see table 2, p 1266) of the effects analgesics in primary dysmenorrhoea (search date 1997, 13 RCTs), which compared analgesics with placebo, each other, or common non-steroidal anti-inflammatory drugs (NSAIDs).[10] **Aspirin versus placebo:** The review identified eight RCTs comparing aspirin with placebo (n = 486, 650 mg four times daily). For the outcome of pain relief, aspirin was significantly better than placebo (5 RCTs, RR 1.60, 95% CI 1.12 to 2.29). There was no significant difference between aspirin and placebo in the need for additional medication (3 RCTs, RR 0.79, 95% CI 0.58 to 1.08), or restriction of daily activity and absence from work (3 RCTs, RR 0.82, 95% CI 0.64 to 1.04; 1 RCT, RR 1.28, 95% CI 0.24 to 6.76). Overall, 10 women need to be treated with aspirin to achieve pain relief in one additional women (NNT 10, 95% CI 5 to 50). **Paracetamol versus placebo:** One RCT comparing paracetamol 500 mg four times daily with placebo found no significant difference in pain relief (n = 35, RR 1.00, 95% CI 0.28 to 3.63). **Paracetamol/DPH versus placebo:** The review identified one placebo controlled RCT, which found that paracetamol/DPH was significantly more effective in achieving marked or moderate pain relief than placebo (n = 72, 650 mg/65 mg four times daily, RR 3.72, 95% CI 2.13 to 6.52). **Paracetamol versus aspirin:** One RCT comparing aspirin and paracetamol (n = 35) found that pain relief from paracetamol was not significantly different from aspirin (using visual analogue scale, the median change from baseline was 1.6, 95% CI 0.4 to 3.3 with paracetamol v 1.2, 95% CI 0 to 2.7 with aspirin). **Aspirin or paracetamol versus NSAIDs:** There were six comparisons of aspirin or paracetamol versus NSAIDs (n = 313). Aspirin 650 mg four times daily was found to be less effective for pain relief than both naproxen 275 mg four times daily (one RCT, RR 2.29, 95% CI 1.16 to 4.29) and ibuprofen 400 mg four times daily (one RCT, RR 1.9, 95% CI 1.13 to 2.78). One RCT found no significant difference in pain relief (defined as at least moderate relief) between paracetamol 1000 mg three times daily and ibuprofen 400 mg three times daily (one RCT, RR 0.86, 95% CI 0.68 to 1.10). **Paracetamol/DPH versus NSAIDs:** The review identified one RCT that compared paracetamol/DPH 650 mg/65 mg three times daily with mefenamic acid 500 mg three times daily. The RCT found that mefenamic acid was significantly better for relief of all dysmenorrhoea related symptoms (P < 0.01). The need for additional medication was also lower in the mefenamic acid group (a mean of 2.6 v 6.8, no P value reported). There was no significant difference between treatments in terms of absence from work or school. Two RCTs (n = 98) compared paracetamol/DPH with naproxen 275 mg three times daily. Neither found a significant difference in pain severity (P > 0.05), but naproxen achieved better pain control on some of the days measured (P < 0.05).

Harms: The most commonly experienced adverse effects were nausea or abdominal discomfort, headaches, and dizziness. Adverse effects occurred in 7–17% of women taking aspirin and 3–17% of those taking placebo. Aspirin and paracetamol were not significantly different from placebo in terms of adverse effects (RR 1.31, 95% CI 0.79 to 2.17; RR 1.00, 95% CI 0.36 to 2.75). More women taking paracetamol/DPH experienced adverse effects than those taking naproxen (23–58% v 15–25%; RR 1.94, 95% CI 1.11 to 3.41).[10]

Comment: Most RCTs included in the systematic review were short (usually only one menstrual cycle on each treatment), small, and used a crossover design without a washout period. All of the RCTs, except one of paracetamol/DPH versus naproxen, used double blinding. All the RCTs used oral administration of treatment in the form of tablets or capsules.

OPTION   NON-STEROIDAL ANTI-INFLAMMATORY DRUGS

One systematic review of RCTs has found strong evidence that naproxen, ibuprofen, and mefenamic acid are all more effective than placebo for pain relief. The RCT found some evidence of increased adverse effects with naproxen.

Benefits: We found one recent systematic review of the effects of NSAIDs in primary dysmenorrhoea (search date March 1997), which included 23 RCTs of naproxen (n = 1728), 18 of ibuprofen (n = 748) and five of mefenamic acid (n = 257).[10] **NSAIDs versus placebo:** The systematic review found that all three NSAIDs provided significant pain relief compared with placebo (naproxen: 13 RCTs, RR 3.17, 95% CI 2.72 to 3.67, NNT 2.6, 95% CI 2 to 3.4; ibuprofen: 9 RCTs, RR 2.41, 95% CI 1.58 to 3.68, NNT 2.4, 95% CI 1.7 to 3.8; mefenamic acid: 3 RCTs, RR 2.03, 95% CI 1.65 to 2.48, NNT 2.4, 95% CI 1.6 to 4.5). The need for additional analgesics was significantly reduced for all NSAIDs when compared with placebo. Women taking naproxen were 60% less likely to require additional analgesics (10 RCTs; RR 0.4, 95% CI 0.3 to 0.4); those taking ibuprofen were 70% less likely (2 RCTs; RR 0.2, 95% CI 0.1 to 0.4); and those on mefenamic acid were 35% less likely (1 RCT; RR 0.7, 95% CI 0.5 to 0.8). Restriction of daily life was significantly less for naproxen (7 RCTs; RR 0.71, 95% CI 0.60 to 0.85) and ibuprofen (3 RCTs; RR 0.82, 95% CI 0.64 to 1.04). Absence from work or school was reduced significantly with naproxen (7 RCTs; RR 0.29, 95% CI 0.13 to 0.66) but not with ibuprofen (1 RCT; RR 0.14, 95% CI 0.02 to 1.10). **Comparison of NSAIDs:** The review identified five comparative RCTs. Three found no significant difference in pain relief between naproxen and ibuprofen (RR 1.1, 95% CI 0.8 to 1.5). One RCT found that naproxen provided more pain relief than mefenamic acid (RR 2.4, 95% CI 1.4 to 4.1), and a comparison of ibuprofen and mefenamic acid found no significant difference between the two treatments (no RR or P values reported).

Harms: The most commonly reported adverse effects were nausea, dizziness, and headaches. Naproxen caused significantly more adverse effects than placebo (RR 1.45, 95% CI 1.03 to 2.04). There was no significant difference in adverse effects with ibuprofen and mefenamic acid compared with placebo (RR 1.12, 95% CI 0.85 to 1.47; RR 0.59, 95% CI 0.28 to 1.23).[10]

Comment: All the RCTs used oral treatment. NSAIDs can be administered as suppositories, which have been shown to have a similar effect on overall pain relief but are less effective than tablets for spasmodic pain (P < 0.05).[11] The majority of the RCTs included in this systematic review used a crossover design without a washout period and were of short duration, usually only one menstrual cycle on each treatment. Nine of the included trials were only single blind. Many of the trials on NSAIDs were sponsored by industry. Pain relief figures used above refer to RCTs that include women with primary dysmenorrhoea only. However, some of the other figures regarding use of additional medication included data from women with undefined dysmenorrhoea. A systematic review with stricter inclusion criteria and methodological quality assessment is in progress (ML Wilson, personal communication, 2000).

OPTION   **COMBINED ORAL CONTRACEPTIVES**

Three small RCTs found insufficient evidence that oral contraceptives are effective for pain relief.

Benefits: We found no systematic review. We found three placebo controlled RCTs evaluating high dose oestrogen combined oral contraceptives for treatment of primary dysmenorrhoea.[12–14] The first double blind RCT evaluated Norinyl (norethisterone 2 mg and mestranol 0.1 mg). Primary dysmenorrhoea was diagnosed by physical examination and 35/44 women completed the study. Complete or partial pain relief was achieved in 14/17 (82%) receiving treatment compared with 3/18 (17%) on placebo.[12] The second RCT evaluated Sequens (mestranol 0.08 mg taken from day 5 to day 25, and chlormadinone acetate 2 mg added for the last 5 days). Only 29 women completed the trial. Pain relief was significantly higher with treatment compared with placebo (P < 0.02; further data extraction was not possible as the data were presented in graphic form).[13] The third RCT (n = 28) evaluated an oral contraceptive pill (OCP) comprising 0.05 mg ethinyl oestradiol and 0.5 mg norgestrel taken from day 5 to day 25 of the cycle, for 3–6 months. This RCT found pain relief was much better in the OCP group when the number of menstrual cycles with relief across the entire trial was compared (22/44 treated menstrual cycles with complete pain relief versus 1/31 placebo treated menstrual cycles, P < 0.05).[13] However, if the average number of women with pain relief was reported, there was no significant difference due to the small number of women in the trial (5/11 v 0/7; OR 12.69, 95% CI 0.58 to 27).

Harms: No adverse effects were reported, although in the third trial 2/18 women receiving the OCP reported breakthrough bleeding.[13]

Comment: All three RCTs evaluated oral contraceptives that are either banned or no longer commonly prescribed. All the RCTs were of poor methodological quality. A Cochrane systematic review is currently in progress (ML Wilson, personal communication, 2000).

One small RCT found limited evidence suggesting that laparoscopic uterine nerve ablation (LUNA) was more effective than diagnostic laparoscopy. A second RCT compared LUNA and laparoscopic presacral neurectomy (LPSN) and found no significant difference in pain relief in the short term. However, LPSN was significantly more effective in the long term.

Benefits: We found one systematic review of surgical pelvic nerve interruption for primary and secondary dysmenorrhoea (6 RCTs, search date December 1998).[15] Only two of the six RCTs included women with primary dysmenorrhoea. Meta-analysis was not possible because of trial heterogeneity. One trial (21 women) compared LUNA with diagnostic laparoscopy as a control. There was a significant difference in pain relief in favour of LUNA at 3 months (OR 15.5, 95% CI 2.91 to 82.7) and at 12 months (OR 10.9, 95% CI 1.5 to 77.4). The other trial (68 women) compared LUNA with LPSN. There was no significant difference in pain relief between the two treatments at 3 months follow up (OR 0.7, 95% CI 0.2 to 2.7). However, at 12 months follow up, the LPSN group had significantly better pain relief scores (OR 0.26, 95% CI 0.10 to 0.71).

Harms: Adverse effects were more common with LPSN than with LUNA. Constipation occurred in 94% of women receiving LPSN compared with 0% receiving LUNA (OR 0.02, 95% CI 0.01 to 0.06).

Comment: Two larger trials of LUNA are currently in progress, and data will be included in an update of the systematic review. We found a second relevant systematic review, but have not included it in this chapter because it includes lower levels of evidence, such as case studies.[16]

Two small RCTs found that high frequency transcutaneous electrical nerve stimulation (TENS) (see glossary, p 1263) was more effective than placebo for pain relief.

Benefits: We found no systematic review but found three small RCTs with a total of 71 participants.[17–19] **High frequency TENS versus placebo:** For pain relief, high frequency TENS was found to be more effective than placebo in two RCTs.[18,19] In one double blind trial, 14/32 women experienced at least moderate pain relief in the TENS group compared with 1/32 in the placebo group (OR 24, 95% CI 2.9 to 199). A single blind trial had nine women in each group: the mean decrease in pain was 72% with treatment and 26% with placebo (WMD 45, 95% CI 23 to 67). **Low frequency TENS versus placebo:** The third RCT (n = 18) found no significant benefit from low frequency TENS compared with placebo (WMD 24, 95% CI −2.9 to +51).[18] **High frequency TENS versus low frequency TENS:** One RCT found no significant difference between high frequency and low frequency TENS for pain relief (WMD 21, 95% CI

4.4 to 46).[18] **High frequency TENS versus NSAIDs:** One unblinded RCT found that high frequency TENS was less effective than ibuprofen, with 14/32 women experiencing pain relief compared with 24/32 using ibuprofen (OR 0.26, 95% CI 0.09 to 0.75).[17] Naproxen and high frequency/high intensity TENS were both shown to significantly reduce pain in a unblinded crossover trial of 12 women (P < 0.001), but were not significantly different from each other (data were presented in graphic form but no OR or P values were reported).[19]

Harms: Adverse effects of muscle vibrations, tightness, headaches, and slight burning or redness after use were experienced by four women on treatment and none on placebo (OR 10, 95% CI 0.5 to 199, P = 0.12).[17] In the unblinded crossover trial, 10/12 women considered TENS to be temporarily painful but were prepared to accept this effect for the pain relief achieved. None of the 12 women reported any adverse effects during treatment with naproxen.[19]

Comment: A systematic review is currently underway (ML Wilson, personal communication, 2000).

OPTION   ACUPUNCTURE

One small RCT found that acupuncture achieved more effective pain relief than placebo.

Benefits: We found no systematic review. We found one RCT (n = 48) comparing acupuncture, placebo acupuncture (see glossary, p 1263), and two no-treatment control groups, one of which had extra visits with a physician.[20] Treatment was for 30–40 minutes once a week for 3 weeks a month, for a total of 3 months. The proportion of women showing improvement in pain was significantly higher in the acupuncture group compared with all other groups ($\chi^2 = 13.6$, P < 0.001). Acupuncture was significantly more effective than placebo acupuncture in achieving pain relief (OR 17.5, 95% CI 1.6 to 192).

Harms: The trial did not report on adverse effects.

Comment: A systematic review is currently underway (ML Wilson, personal communication, 2000).

OPTION   BEHAVIOURAL INTERVENTIONS

We found insufficient evidence of the effectiveness of behavioural interventions (see glossary, p 1263).

Benefits: We found no systematic review. We found two small RCTs on behaviour therapy. One involved relaxation and imagery,[21] the other aerobic exercise.[22] **Relaxation therapy:** The first trial included 69 women divided into three groups. The treatment group used muscle relaxation combined with positive imagery regarding menstruation. A pseudo treatment group included self-directed group discussion about menstruation, and the third group was a waiting list control group. The groups were also divided into women with spasmodic or congestive dysmenorrhoea using the Menstrual Symptom Questionnaire. Spasmodic dysmenorrhoea was defined as spasms of pain mainly around the abdomen, and congestive dysmenorrhoea was defined as a dull aching pain in the lower abdomen and other areas of the body. The muscle relaxation group had significantly more pain and symptom relief than the waiting list controls (P < 0.01). However, only the women with spasmodic dysmenorrhoea had significantly more relief with relaxation than with all treatments (P < 0.001).[21] **Aerobic exercise:** The second trial had a training group that participated in 30 minutes of exercise 3 days a week and a sedentary control group. Results for the 26 women who completed the study showed that during the menstrual phase, the training group had significantly lower Menstrual Distress Questionnaire scores than controls (P < 0.05). Data were presented in a graph, making further data extraction impossible.

Harms: The trials did not report on adverse effects.

Comment: Both RCTs were small and of poor methodological quality. The classification of dysmenorrhoea into spasmodic and congestive categories is no longer commonly used and has little meaning. A systematic review is in progress (ML Wilson, personal communication, 2000).

OPTION   SPINAL MANIPULATION

One RCT found no evidence that spinal manipulation was effective in pain relief.

Benefits: We found no systematic review. We found one RCT in 138 women randomised either to spinal manipulative therapy or a low-force mimic manoeuvre used as a control.[23] The RCT found no significant differences in visual analogue pain scores between the two groups after two treatment cycles. The mean change in pain score from baseline in treatment group was 10.1 (95% CI 6.5 to 13.7) v 8.01 (95% CI 4.17 to 11.85) in the control group. There was also no significant difference between pre- and post-intervention pain scores after four treatment cycles (P = 0.29).

Harms: Soreness in the lower back region within 48 hours of the intervention occurred in 2/69 women in the control group and 3/69 in the treatment group. Soreness resolved within 24 hours. No other adverse effects were reported.

Comment: The RCT's overall methodological quality was good; low withdrawal rate (2%), adequate randomisation method, blinding of the outcome assessor, and potential blinding of the participants as the control procedure was very similar to the treatment.

OPTION   HERBAL REMEDIES

We found insufficient evidence to determine the effectiveness of herbal remedies.

Benefits: We found no systematic review. We found one trial (n = 40) comparing the Japanese herbal remedy toki-shakuyaku-san (taken three times daily for 6 months) versus a placebo remedy.[24] Pain relief using a visual analogue scale was significantly better in the treatment group (P < 0.005). The requirement for additional medication (diclofenac sodium) was also significantly less in the treatment group (P < 0.01). The data were presented in a graph, making further data extraction impossible.

Harms: The trials did not report on adverse affects.

Comment: Toki-shakuyaku-san is a mixture of six herbs, including angelica and peony root.

OPTION	DIETARY SUPPLEMENTS

One large RCT found vitamin B_1 to be more effective than placebo. RCTs of other dietary remedies were too small to provide evidence of effectiveness.

Benefits: We found no systematic review. We found four RCTs on four different treatments: magnesium, vitamin B_1, vitamin E/ibuprofen, and fish oil (an omega-3 fatty acid comprised of vitamin E, eicosapantaenoic acid, and docosapantaenoic acid). **Magnesium versus placebo:** One RCT (n = 50) evaluated magnesium aspartate taken three times daily.[25] After 6 months magnesium was significantly better than placebo in achieving pain relief (no pain in 21/25 on magnesium v no pain in 7/25 on placebo, RR 3.0, 95% CI 1.6 to 5.8, NNT 1.8). **Vitamin B versus placebo:** One RCT (n = 556) evaluated thiamine hydrochloride 100 mg daily for 3 months.[26] After 60 days, prior to crossover, the treatment group had significantly more pain relief than the placebo group (no pain in 142/277 on treatment v no pain in 0/279 on placebo; RR 287, CI 95% 18 to 4589; NNT 2). After completion of the trial, 87% of all participants experienced no pain. **Vitamin E plus ibuprofen versus ibuprofen:** One crossover RCT in 50 women evaluated vitamin E 100 mg daily for 20 days prior to menses, then ibuprofen 400 mg at the outset of painful menstruation. The comparison was ibuprofen 400 mg at the onset of pain.[27] Women were treated over two cycles, with treatments crossed over after one cycle. Pain relief was more effective with combined vitamin E/ibuprofen, but the confidence intervals were wide (cycle 1: no pain in 23/26 women on combined treatment v 17/24 on ibuprofen alone, OR 3.2, 95% CI 0.7 to 14; cycle 2: no pain in 17/20 women on combined treatment v 16/22 women on ibuprofen alone, OR 2.1, 95% CI 0.5 to 10). **Fish oil versus placebo:** One RCT in 42 women compared taking fish oil capsules twice daily versus placebo for 1 month.[28] Menstrual symptom scores were significantly lower with fish oil than placebo (44 v 70, P < 0.001). Less additional medication (ibuprofen 200 mg) was consumed in the fish oil group (mean 4.7 tablets with treatment v 10.1 with placebo, P = 0.015).

Harms: Circulation problems and intestinal discomfort were experienced by 5/25 women taking magnesium compared with 0/25 taking placebo, although relief of these symptoms occurred when the dose was reduced from three to two tablets daily. In the fish oil group, 2/42 women reported nausea and 1/42 participants reported acne.

Comment: The trial of vitamin B_1 used double blinding and was of good methodological quality.

GLOSSARY

Behavioural interventions Treatments that attempt modification of thought and beliefs (cognition) about symptoms and pain and/or modification of behavioural or physiological responses to symptoms and pain.

Placebo acupuncture Also known as sham acupuncture, a commonly used control intervention involving the use of acupuncture needles to stimulate non-acupuncture points not located on Chinese meridians. These points can be identified by a point detector as areas of the skin that do not have skin electrical activity similar to acupuncture points. There is some disagreement over correct needle placement, as placement of a needle in any position may elicit some biological response that can complicate interpretation of results.

Transcutaneous electrical nerve stimulation Electrodes are placed on the skin and different electrical pulse rates and intensities are used to stimulate the areas. Low frequency TENS (also referred to as acupuncture-like TENS) usually consists of pulses delivered at 1–4 Hz at high intensity so they evoke visible muscle fibre contractions. High frequency TENS (conventional TENS) usually consists of pulses delivered at 50–120 Hz at a low intensity, so there are no muscle contractions.

REFERENCES

1. Fraser I. Prostaglandins, prostaglandin inhibitors and their roles in gynaecological disorders. *Bailliere's Clinical Obstet Gynaecol* 1992;6:829–857.

2. Zondervan KT, Yudkin PL, Vessey MP, et al. The prevalence of chronic pelvic pain in the United Kingdom: a systematic review. *Br J Obstet Gynaecol* 1998;105:93–99. Search date December 1996; primary sources Medline from 1966, Embase from 1980, Psychlit from 1974.

3. Harlow SD, Park M. A longitudinal study of risk factors for the occurrence, duration and severity of menstrual cramps in a cohort of college women. *Br J Obstet Gynaecol* 1996;103:1134–1142.

4. Campbell MA, McGrath PJ. Use of medication by adolescents for the management of menstrual discomfort. *Arch Pediatr Adolesc Med* 1997;151:905–913.

5. Robinson JC, Plichta S, Weisman CS, et al. Dysmenorrhoea and the use of oral contraceptives in adolescent women attending a family planning clinic. *Am J Obstet Gynecol* 1992;166:578–583.

6. Andersch B, Milsom I. An epidemiologic study of young women with dysmenorrhea. *Am J Obstet Gynecol* 1982;144:655–660.

7. Pedron Neuvo N, Gonzalez-Unzaga LN, De Celis-Carrillo R, et al. Incidence of dysmenorrhoea and associated symptoms in women aged 12–24 years. *Ginecología y Obstetrica de Mexico* 1998;66:492–494.

8. Klein JR, Litt IF. Epidemiology of adolescent dysmenorrhea. *Pediatrics* 1981;68(5):661–664.

9. Sundell G, Milsom I, Andersch B. Factors influencing the prevalence and severity of dysmenorrhoea in young women. *Br J Obstet Gynaecol* 1990;97:588–594.

10. Zhang WY, LiWanPo A. Efficacy of minor analgesics in primary dysmenorrhoea: a systematic review. *Br J Obstet Gynaecol* 1998;105:780–789. Search date March 1997; primary sources Medline, Embase and Science Citation Index 1966–1997.

11. Ylikorkala O, Puolakka J, Kauppila A. Comparison between naproxen tablets and suppositories in primary dysmenorrhea. *Prostaglandins* 1980;20:463–438.

12. Kremser E, Mitchell GM. Treatment of primary dysmenorrhoea with a combined type oral contraceptive — a double blind study. *J Am Coll Health* 1971;19:195–196.

13. Nakano R, Takemura H. Treatment of function dysmenorrhoea: a double-blind study. *Acta Obstet Gynaecol Jpn* 1971;18:41–44.

14. Matthews AE, Clarke JE. Double-blind trial of a sequential oral contraceptive (Sequens) in the treatment of dysmenorrhoea. *J Obstet Gynaecol Br Commonw* 1968;75:1117–1122.

15. Wilson ML, Farquhar CM, Sinclair OJ, et al. Surgical interruption of pelvic nerve pathways for primary and secondary dysmenorrhoea. In: The Cochrane Library, Issue 1, 2000. Oxford: Update Software. Search date December 1998; primary sources Medline 1966–December 1998, Embase 1980–December 1998, Cochrane Controlled Trials Register 1966–December 1998, hand-searched citation lists and conference proceedings.

16. Khan KS, Khan SF, Nwosu CR, et al. Laparoscopic uterosacral nerve ablation in chronic pelvic pain: an overview. *Gynaecol Endosc* 1999;8:257–265. Search date 1997; primary sources Medline 1966–1997; Embase 1980–1997, Science Citation Index.

17. Dawood MY, Ramos J. Transcutaneous electrical nerve stimulation (TENS) for the treatment of primary dysmenorrhea: a randomized crossover comparison with placebo TENS and ibuprofen. *Obstet Gynecol* 1990;75:656–660.

18. Mannheimer JS, Whalen EC. The efficacy of transcutaneous electrical nerve stimulation in dysmenorrhea. *Clin J Pain* 1985;1:75–83.

19. Hedner N, Milsom I, Eliasson T, et al. Tens bra vid smatsam mens. [TENS is effective in painful menstruation.] *Lakartidningen* 1996;93:1219–1222 (in Swedish).

20. Helms JM. Acupuncture for the management of primary dysmenorrhea. *Obstet Gynecol* 1987;69:51–56.

21. Chesney MA, Tasto DL. The effectiveness of behavior modification with spasmodic and congestive dysmenorrhea. *Behav Res Ther* 1975;13:245–253.

22. Israel RG, Sutton M, O'Brien KF. Effects of aerobic training on primary dysmenorrhea symptomatology in college females. *J Am Coll Health* 1985;33:241–244.

23. Hondras MA, Long CR, Brennan PC. Spinal manipulation therapy versus a low force mimic maneuver for women with primary dysmenorrhea: a randomized, observer-blinded clinical trial. *Pain* 1999;81:105–114.

24. Kotani N, Oyama T, Sakai I, et al. Analgesic effect of a herbal medicine for treatment of primary dysmenorrhoea — a double-blind study. *Am J Chin Med* 1997;25s:205–212.

25. Seifert B, Wagler P, Dartsch S, et al. Magnesium — a new therapeutic alternative in primary dysmenorrhea. *Zentralbl Gynakol* 1989;111:755–60 (in German).

26. Gokhale LB. Curative treatment of primary (spasmodic) dysmenorrhoea. *Indian J Med Res* 1996;103:227–231.

27. De Roldan MES, Ruiz-Castro S. Primary dysmenorrhea treatment with ibuprofen and vitamin E. *Rev Obstet Ginecol Venez* 1993;53:35–37 (in Spanish).

28. Harel Z, Biro FM, Kottenhahn RK, et al. Supplementation with omega-3 polyunsaturated fatty acids in the management of dysmenorrhea in adolescents. *Am J Obstet Gynecol* 1996;174(4):1335–1338.

Michelle Wilson

Cynthia Farquhar
Associate Professor

School of Medicine
University of Auckland
Auckland
New Zealand

Competing interests: None declared.

TABLE 1 Prevalence of dysmenorrhoea: results of community and hospital surveys (see text, p 1255).[3-8]

Study population	Population size	Location	Year	Prevalence
College students aged 17–19 years[3]	165	USA	1996	72% (13% severe)
High school students aged 14–21 years[4]	291	Canada	1997	93% (5% severe)
Adolescents attending an inner city family planning clinic[5]	308	USA	1992	80% (18% severe)
Women from an urban population aged 19 years[6]	596	Sweden	1982	73% (15% severe)
Students aged 12–24 years[7]	1066	Mexico	1998	52–64%
Adolescents aged 12–17 years[8]	2699	USA	1981	60% (14% severe)

TABLE 2   Effects of aspirin, paracetamol, and compound analgesics for dysmenorrhoea: results of a systematic review of RCTs (see text, p 1256).[10]

Comparison	Usual dosage	Number of RCTs	Number of women	Pain relief	Adverse effects	Conclusion
Aspirin v placebo	650 mg four times daily	8	486	RR 1.60 (95% CI 1.12 to 2.29)	More frequent on aspirin (7–17% v 3–17% on placebo, RR 1.3, 95% CI 0.79 to 2.17)	Aspirin more effective than placebo (NNT 10, 95% CI 5 to 50)
Aspirin v paracetamol	650 mg v 500 mg four times daily	1	35	Median pain relief: paracetamol 1.6 (95% CI 0.4 to 3.3), aspirin 1.2 (95% CI 0 to 2.7)		No significant difference
Aspirin v naproxen	650 mg v 275 mg four times daily	1	32	RR 2.29 (95% CI 1.16 to 4.29)		Naproxen more effective than aspirin
Aspirin v ibuprofen	650 mg v 400 mg four times daily	1	56	RR 1.9 (95% CI 1.13 to 2.78)		Ibuprofen more effective than placebo
Paracetamol v placebo	500 mg four times daily	1	35	RR 1.00 (95% CI 0.28 to 3.63)	No significant difference (RR 1.00, 95% CI 0.36 to 2.75)	No significant difference
Paracetamol v ibuprofen	1000 mg v 400 mg three times daily	1	67	RR 0.86 (95% CI 0.68 to 1.10)		No significant difference
Paracetamol/DPH v placebo	650 mg/65 mg four times daily	1	72	RR 3.72 (95% CI 2.13 to 6.52)		Paracetamol/DPH more effective than placebo
Paracetamol/DPH v naproxen	650 mg/65 mg v 275 mg three times daily	2	98	P > 0.05 (no other data could be obtained from the report)	More frequent on paracetamol/DPH (23–58% v 15–25% on naproxen, RR 1.94, 95% CI 1.11 to 3.41)	No significant difference
Paracetamol/DPH v mefenamic acid	650 mg/65 mg v 500 mg three times daily	1	30	P < 0.01 (no other evidence can be obtained from the trial)		Mefenamic acid more effective than paracetamol/DPH

DPH: dextropropoxyphene.

INTERVENTIONS

IN WOMEN WITH PAIN ATTRIBUTED TO ENDOMETRIOSIS

Beneficial
Hormonal treatment at diagnosis (danazol, medroxyprogesterone, gestrinone, GnRH analogues) 1269

Likely to be beneficial
Oral contraceptive pill 1269
Combined ablation of endometrial deposits and uterine nerve .1271
Postoperative hormonal treatment 1272
Cystectomy for ovarian endometrioma (better than drainage) 1273

Unknown effectiveness
Dydrogesterone. 1269
Laparoscopic uterine nerve ablation (LUNA) 1271

Laparoscopic ablation of endometrial deposits without ablation of the uterine nerve 1271
Preoperative hormonal treatment 1273

IN WOMEN WITH SUBFERTILITY ATTRIBUTED TO ENDOMETRIOSIS

Likely to be beneficial
Laparoscopic ablation/excision of endometrial deposits 1271
Cystectomy for ovarian endometrioma (better than drainage) 1273

Unlikely to be beneficial
Hormonal treatment at diagnosis 1269
Postoperative hormonal treatment 1272

Key Messages

Hormonal treatment at diagnosis

- Four small systematic reviews found that all hormonal treatments, except for dydrogesterone, reduced pain attributed to endometriosis compared with placebo, and were equally effective. One systematic review of small RCTs found no evidence that hormonal treatments improved fertility. Adverse effects of hormonal treatment were common.

Surgical treatment

- We found insufficient evidence on the effects of laparoscopic uterine nerve ablation (LUNA) in women with pain attributed to endometriosis.

- We found insufficient evidence on the effects of laparoscopic ablation of deposits on its own. One RCT found that combined treatment with ablation of deposits plus LUNA reduced pain more than diagnostic laparoscopy at 6 months. One RCT found that laparoscopic surgery increased fertility compared with diagnostic laparoscopy, a subsequent smaller RCT found no significant difference.

- We found no RCTs comparing medical and surgical treatments.

Postoperative hormonal treatment

- RCTs have found that 6 months of postoperative hormonal treatment significantly reduces pain and delays the recurrence of pain compared with placebo; treatment for 3 months did not seem to be effective. RCTs found no evidence of an effect of postoperative hormonal treatment on fertility. Adverse effects of hormonal treatment were common.

Preoperative treatment

- One RCT found no evidence that preoperative treatment with GnRH analogues facilitated surgery.

Endometrioma

- One RCT found that cystectomy versus drainage significantly improved pain and subfertility caused by ovarian endometrioma. Complication rates were similar.

DEFINITION   Endometriosis is characterised by ectopic endometrial tissue, which can cause dysmenorrhoea, dyspareunia, non-cyclical pelvic pain, and subfertility. Diagnosis is made by laparoscopy. Most endometrial deposits are found in the pelvis (ovaries, peritoneum, uterosacral ligaments, pouch of Douglas, and rectovaginal septum). Extrapelvic deposits, including those in the umbilicus and diaphragm, are rare. Severity of endometriosis is defined by the American Fertility Society: this review uses the terms mild (stage I and II), moderate (stage III), and severe (stage IV).[1] Endometriomas are cysts of endometriosis within the ovary.

INCIDENCE/   In asymptomatic women, the prevalence of endometriosis ranges
PREVALENCE   from 2–22%, depending on the diagnostic criteria used and the populations studied.[2–5] In women with dysmenorrhoea, the incidence of endometriosis ranges from 40–60%, and in women with subfertility from 20–30%.[3,6,7] The severity of symptoms and the probability of diagnosis increase with age.[8] Incidence peaks at about age 40 years.[9] Symptoms and laparoscopic appearance do not always correlate.[10]

AETIOLOGY/   The cause of endometriosis is unknown. Risk factors include early
RISK FACTORS   menarche and late menopause. Embryonic cells may give rise to deposits in the umbilicus, whereas retrograde menstruation may deposit endometrial cells in the diaphragm.[11,12] Use of oral contraceptives reduces the risk of endometriosis, and this protective effect persists for up to 1 year after their discontinuation.[9]

PROGNOSIS   We found two RCTs in which laparoscopy was repeated in the women treated with placebo. Over 6–12 months, endometrial deposits resolved spontaneously in up to a third of women, deteriorated in nearly half, and were unchanged in the remainder.[13,14]

AIMS   To relieve pain (dysmenorrhoea, dyspareunia, and other pelvic pain) and to improve fertility, with minimal adverse effects.

OUTCOMES American Fertility Society scores for size and number of deposits;[1] recurrence rates; time between stopping treatment and recurrence; rate of adverse effects of treatment. **In women with pain:** Relief of pain, assessed by Visual Analogue Scale ranging from 0–10, and subjective improvement. **In women with subfertility:** Cumulative pregnancy rate, live birth rate. **In women undergoing surgery:** Ease of surgical intervention (rated as easy, average, difficult, or very difficult).[15]

METHODS *Clinical Evidence* update search and appraisal November 2000. The authors also sought RCTs by electronic searching of databases, hand searching of 30 key journals, searching the reference lists of other RCTs, and identifying unpublished studies from abstracts, proceedings, and pharmaceutical companies. They used the search strategy and database of the Cochrane Menstrual Disorders and Subfertility Group to identify RCTs on Medline and Embase. They included RCTs that used adequate diagnostic criteria for inclusion of participants (endometriosis diagnosed either by laparoscopy or laparotomy in association with dysmenorrhoea, dyspareunia, other pelvic pain, or infertility) and clinical outcomes (see outcomes above). Studies of assisted reproductive technologies were not included. Trials comparing different hormonal treatments of the same class were not included.

QUESTION **What are the effects of hormonal treatments at diagnosis?**

Four small systematic reviews found that all different hormonal treatments, except for dydrogesterone, reduced pain attributed to endometriosis compared with placebo, and were equally effective. One systematic review of small RCTs found no evidence that hormonal treatments improved fertility. Adverse effects of hormonal treatments were common.

Benefits: **In women with pain attributed to endometriosis:** We found four systematic reviews (search dates 1998, 1996, 1997, 1997), and one subsequent RCT evaluating 6 months of continuous ovulation suppression using danazol, gestrinone, depot medroxyprogesterone acetate (DMPA), dydrogesterone, oral contraceptives, or GnRH analogues.[16–20] The systematic reviews reported that all treatments were equally effective at reducing severe and moderate pain at 6 months, except dydrogesterone, which, given at two different dosages in the luteal phase, showed no evidence of effect. The first systematic review (search date 1998, 7 RCTs, nearly 400 women) compared danazol versus GnRH analogues. It found no significant difference in reduction of pain or in resolution of endometrial deposits after 6 months of treatment.[16] The second systematic review (search date 1996, 1 RCT, 269 women) compared danazol (200 mg/day) versus gestrinone (2.5 mg twice/week).[17] It found no significant difference in pain reduction.[21] The first systematic review[16] included one RCT (49 women), which compared combined oral contraceptives (COC) with GnRH analogues.[22] It found no significant difference in rate of relief for all types of pain except menstrual pain, for which oral contraceptives were better. A subsequent RCT (102 women) compared 12 months of COC versus

4 months of COC versus 8 months of GnRH analogues. At 12 months, no difference was found in pain reduction (either menstrual or non-menstrual).[20] The second systematic review included two RCTs of DMPA (140 women).[17] The larger RCT (80 women) compared DMPA (150 mg every 3 months) with COC plus danazol (50 mg/day). It found that DMPA was more effective at reducing dysmenorrhoea but not for any other outcomes. Long term follow up of one RCT (201 women), of 12 months treatment with GnRH agonist noresthisterone versus intermittent oestrogen for management of painful symptoms, found that maintenance of pain relief was significantly better with noresthisterone.[23] **In women with subfertility attributed to endometriosis:** We found one systematic review (search date 1996, 4 RCTs, 244 women with "visually diagnosed" endometriosis attempting conception for more than 12 months),[24] and one subsequent RCT.[14] The trials evaluated 6 months' treatment with danazol, medroxyprogesterone, or GnRH analogues versus placebo. The review found no significant effect on the likelihood of pregnancy with danazol (likelihood of pregnancy, danazol v placebo, RR 0.90, 95% CI 0.66 to 1.21). The subsequent RCT (100 infertile women) found no significant difference in pregnancy rates between medroxyprogesterone (50 mg/day) and placebo.[14]

Harms: **GnRH analogues:** The first systematic review found that GnRH analogues were associated with more hot flushes than placebo (about 80% v 30%, RR 2.7, 95% CI 1.5 to 4.8) and more headaches (33% v 10%, RR 3.6, 95% CI 1.1 to 11.5).[16] GnRH analogues are associated with hypo-oestrogenic symptoms, such as hot flushes and vaginal dryness. RCTs have found that adding oestrogen, progesterone, or tibolone significantly relieves hot flushes caused by GnRH analogues (reducing symptom scores by 50% or more).[15,25,26] **Danazol:** In one trial of 6 months' postoperative danazol (100 mg/day) versus no treatment, more adverse effects were associated with danazol: spotting (12% v 7%), bloating (16% v 9%), headache (21% v 13%), and weight gain (22% v 14%) (see postoperative hormonal treatment, p 1272).[27] **Gestrinone:** One trial found a significantly higher frequency of hot flushes versus GnRH analogues; other trials found greater frequency of greasy skin and hirsutism compared with danazol, but less reduction in breast size, muscle cramps, and hunger.[17] **Medroxyprogesterone:** The trials gave no information on adverse effects of medroxyprogesterone. One trial found more adverse events with DMPA versus danazol plus COC: amenorrhoea (20% v 0%); breakthrough bleeding (15% v 0%); spotting (65% v 10%); bloating (63% v 28%); and weight gain (53% v 30%).[28]

Comment: The trials were mainly small with no long term follow up. No summary statistics could be calculated because the trials compared different drugs versus placebo or no treatment. Trials comparing different hormonal treatments of the same class were not included.

QUESTION   **What are the effects of surgical treatments?**

OPTION   LAPAROSCOPIC UTERINE NERVE ABLATION (LUNA)

We found insufficient evidence on the effects of LUNA in women with pain attributed to endometriosis.

Benefits: We found one systematic review (search date 1998, 2 RCTs, 132 women with endometriosis, stages I–III, age range 18–40 years).[29] It found no significant difference in pain relief between LUNA versus laparoscopic treatment without LUNA. The largest trial (81 women) found that satisfaction with treatment was high in both groups (73% control v 68% LUNA).

Harms: The trials gave no information on adverse effects. Potential harms include denervation of pelvic structures and uterine prolapse.[29]

Comment: The trials may have been too small to exclude a significant effect.[29]

OPTION   LAPAROSCOPIC ABLATION OF ENDOMETRIAL DEPOSITS

We found insufficient evidence on the effects of laparoscopic ablation of deposits alone. One RCT found that combined treatment with ablation of deposits plus LUNA reduced pain more than diagnostic laparoscopy at 6 months. One RCT found that laparoscopic surgery increased fertility compared with diagnostic laparoscopy; another smaller RCT found no significant difference.

Benefits: We found no systematic review. **In women with pain attributed to endometriosis:** We found no RCTs evaluating laparoscopic ablation of deposits alone. We found one RCT (63 women with mild to moderate endometriosis) comparing ablation of deposits plus LUNA versus diagnostic laparoscopy.[30,31] It found that ablation plus LUNA reduced pain at 6 months (median decrease in pain score 2.85 for ablation v 0.05 for diagnostic laparoscopy; P = 0.01). **In women with subfertility attributed to endometriosis:** We found two RCTs (in women with subfertility attributed to mild or moderate endometriosis) of laparoscopic ablation/excision of mild to moderate endometriotic deposits versus diagnostic laparoscopy.[32,33] In the larger trial (341 women) laparoscopic surgery significantly increased cumulative pregnancy rates (RR of pregnancy after 36 weeks 1.7, 95% CI 1.2 to 2.6; NNT 8). A more recent RCT (101 women) found no significant difference in pregnancy rates at the end of 12 months' follow up (OR 0.75, 95% CI 0.31 to 1.88).[30] When the results of the studies were combined, the difference was significant (OR 1.56, 95% CI 1.01 to 2.43), but the studies did have different lengths of follow up.[33] **Laser versus diathermy ablation:** We found no RCTs.

Harms: The trials gave no information on adverse effects.[30–33] Potential harms include adhesions, reduced fertility, and damage to other pelvic structures.

Comment: Further RCTs of ablation alone versus ablation plus LUNA are underway (C Sutton, R Dover, personal communication, 1998). A systematic review of laser versus diathermy ablation is planned (C Farquhar, N Johnson, personal communication, 1999).

QUESTION	What are the effects of postoperative hormonal treatment?

RCTs have found that 6 months of postoperative hormonal treatment versus placebo significantly reduces pain and delays the recurrence of pain; treatment for 3 months did not seem to be effective. RCTs found no evidence of an effect of postoperative hormonal treatment on fertility. Adverse effects of hormonal treatment were common.

Benefits: We found no systematic review. We found six placebo controlled RCTs and one versus expectant management of medical treatment in women who had undergone surgery for endometriosis (GnRH analogues in 3 trials; danazol in 2 trials; 1 trial of COC; and 1 trial comparing danazol versus DMPA versus expectant management).[27,34–39] **In women with pain attributed to endometriosis:** One RCT (77 women with moderate to severe endometriosis) compared postoperative danazol (600 mg/day) versus placebo for 3 months after surgery. It found no significant difference in pain relief 6 months after finishing treatment.[35] A second RCT (28 women with moderate endometriosis who had undergone conservative surgery followed by monthly injections of decapeptyl for 6 months) compared danazol (100 mg/day) for 6 months versus expectant management.[27] It found danazol significantly reduced pain at both 12 months (P < 0.01) and 24 months (P < 0.05). Overall recurrence at 24 months was 44% with danazol versus 67% with expectant management (P < 0.05). A third RCT (60 women with mild to severe endometriosis) found that postoperative danazol (600 mg/day) or medroxyprogesterone (100 mg/day) for 180 days reduced pain more than placebo at 6 months.[36] Three trials assessed GnRH analogues. The smallest RCT (75 women with endometriosis stages I and II) evaluated 3 months' treatment and found no difference in pain relief at follow up.[34] The two larger trials (109 women and 269 women with mild to moderate symptomatic endometriosis) evaluated 6 months' treatment and found that GnRH analogues significantly reduced pain scores (P = 0.008) and delayed the recurrence of pain by more than 12 months.[37,38] One small RCT (70 women) compared the combined oral contraceptive pill versus placebo postoperatively for 6 months.[39] It found no benefit in recurrence of pain associated with endometriosis. **In women with subfertility attributed to endometriosis:** Three of the trials (28, 75, and 269 women, all stages of endometriosis) looked at effects of postoperative hormonal treatment on fertility and found no difference in pregnancy rates or time to conception compared with placebo.[27,34,38]

Harms: See harms of hormonal treatments, p 1270.

Comment: The trials were mainly small with no long term follow up. No summary statistics could be calculated because the trials compared different drugs with placebo or no treatment.

What are the effects of preoperative hormonal treatment?

One RCT found no evidence that preoperative treatment with GnRH analogues facilitated surgery.

Benefits: We found no systematic review. We found one RCT (75 women with moderate or severe endometriosis) comparing 3 months' preoperative treatment with a GnRH analogue versus no treatment.[40] It found no significant difference in ease of surgery, although more women with preoperative hormonal treatment were appraised as easy to treat by the surgeon (56% v 36%).

Harms: See harms of hormonal treatments, p 1270.

Comment: The trial may have been too small to exclude a clinically significant effect.

QUESTION   **What are the effects of treatments for ovarian endometrioma?**

OPTION   **LAPAROSCOPIC DRAINAGE VERSUS LAPAROSCOPIC CYSTECTOMY**

One RCT found that pain and fertility improved more with cystectomy versus drainage, but there was no evidence of a difference in complication rates.

Benefits: We found no systematic review. We found one RCT (64 women) comparing laparoscopic cystectomy versus laparoscopic drainage.[41] **In women with pain attributed to endometrioma:** Cystectomy versus drainage reduced recurrence of pain at 2 years (OR 0.2, 95% CI 0.05 to 0.77) and increased the pain free interval after operation (median interval 19 months v 9.5 months, $P < 0.05$). **In women with subfertility attributed to endometrioma:** Compared with drainage, cystectomy significantly increased the pregnancy rate (67% v 24%; OR 8.25, 95% CI 1.15 to 59).

Harms: The trial reported no intraoperative or postoperative complications in either group.

Comment: None.

Substantive changes since last issue

Hormonal treatments at diagnosis New RCT;[14] conclusions unchanged.
Hormonal treatments at diagnosis Follow up to RCT found that at 12 months maintenance of pain was significantly better with noresthisterone versus intermittent oestrogen.[23]
Postoperative hormones New RCT;[39] conclusions unchanged.

REFERENCES

1. American Fertility Society. Revised American Fertility Society (RAFS) classification of endometriosis. *Fertil Steril* 1985;43:351–352.

2. Mahmood TA, Templeton A. Prevalence and genesis of endometriosis. *Hum Reprod* 1991;6: 544–549.

3. Gruppo Italiano per lo studio dell'endometriosi. Prevalence and anatomical distribution of endometriosis in women with selected gynaecological conditions: results from a multicentric Italian study. *Hum Reprod* 1994;9: 1158–1162.

4. Moen MH, Schei B. Epidemiology of endometriosis in a Norwegian County. *Acta Obstet Gynecol Scand* 1997;76:559–562.

5. Eskenazi B, Warner ML. Epidemiology of endometriosis. *Obstet Gynecol Clin North Am* 1997;24:235–258.

6. Ajossa S, Mais V, Guerriero S, et al. The prevalence of endometriosis in premenopausal women undergoing gynecological surgery. *Clin Exp Obstet Gynecol* 1994;21:195–197.

7. Waller KG, Lindsay P, Curtis P, et al. The prevalence of endometriosis in women with infertile partners. *Eur J Obstet Gynecol Reprod Biol* 1993;48:135–139.

8. Berube S, Marcoux S, Maheux R. Characteristics related to the prevalence of minimal or mild endometriosis in infertile women. Canadian Collaborative Group on Endometriosis. *Epidemiology* 1998;9:504–510.

9. Vessey MP, Villard-Mackintosh L, Painter R. Epidemiology of endometriosis in women attending family planning clinics. *BMJ* 1993;306:182–184.

10. Vercellini P, Trespidi L, DeGiorgi O, et al. Endometriosis and pelvic pain: relation to disease stage and localization. *Fertil Steril* 1996;65:299–304.

11. Rock JA, Markham SM. Pathogenesis of endometriosis. *Lancet* 1992;340:1264–1267.

12. McLaren J, Prentice A. New aspects of pathogenesis of endometriosis. *Curr Obstet Gynaecol* 1996;6:85–91.

13. Cooke ID, Thomas EJ. The medical treatment of mild endometriosis. *Acta Obstet Gynecol Scand Suppl* 1989;150:27–30.

14. Harrison RF, Barry-Kinsella C. Efficacy of medroxyprogesterone treatment in infertile women with endometriosis: a prospective, randomized, placebo-controlled study. *Fertil Steril* 2000;74:24–30.

15. Compston JE, Yamaguchi K, Croucher PI, et al. The effects of gonadotrophin-releasing hormone agonists on iliac crest cancellous bone structure in women with endometriosis. *Bone* 1995;16:261–267.

16. Prentice A, Deary AJ, Goldbeck-Wood S, et al. Gonadotrophin releasing hormone analogues (GnRHAs) for painful symptoms associated with endometriosis. In: The Cochrane Library, Issue 1, 2001. Oxford: Update Software. Search date December 1998; primary sources Medline 1966 to August 1998; Embase 1987 to August 1998; Cochrane Controlled Trials Register 1966 to August 1999; plus unpublished trials by UK distributors of GnRHAs.

17. Prentice A, Deary AJ, Goldbeck-Wood S, et al. Progestogens and antiprogestogens for painful symptoms associated with symptomatic endometriosis. In: The Cochrane Library, Issue 1, 2001. Oxford: Update Software. Search date January 2000; primary sources Medline 1966 to September 1996; Embase 1987 to September 1996; Cochrane Controlled Trials Register 1966 to September 1996.

18. Selak V, Farquhar C, Prentice A, et al. Danazol versus placebo for the treatment of endometriosis. In: The Cochrane Library, Issue 1, 2001. Oxford: Update Software. Search date February 1997; primary sources Medline 1966 to February 1997; Embase 1987 to February 1997; Cochrane Controlled Trials Register 1966 to February 1997; and hand searched journals and conference proceedings.

19. Moore J, Kennedy S, Prentice A. Modern combined oral contraceptives for the treatment of painful symptoms associated with endometriosis. In: The Cochrane Library, Issue 1, 2001. Oxford: Update Software. Search date August 1997; primary sources Medline 1966 to August 1997; Embase 1987 to August 1997; Cochrane Controlled Trials Register 1966 to August 1997.

20. Parazzini F, Di Cintio E, Chatenoud L, et al. Estroprogestin vs. gonadotrophin agonists plus estroprogestin in the treatment of endometriosis-related pelvic pain: a randomized trial. Gruppo Italiano per lo Studio dell'Endometriosis. *Eur J Obstet Gynecol Reprod Biol* 2000;88:11–14.

21. Bromham DR, Bookere MW, Rose R, et al. Updating the clinical experience in endometriosis: the European perspective. *B J Obstet Gynaecol* 1995(suppl);102:12–16.

22. Vercellini P, Trespidi L, Colombo A, et al. A gonadotropin-releasing hormone agonist versus a low-dose oral contraceptive for pelvic pain associated with endometriosis. *Fertil Steril* 1993;60:75–79.

23. Surrey E, Hornstein M. Prolonged GNRH agonist add-back therapy for symptomatic endometriosis patients: Long term follow-up of a 12 month clinical trial. *Futil Steril* 1999;72:S80.

24. Hughes E, Fedorkow D, Collins J, et al. Ovulation suppression versus placebo in the treatment of endometriosis. In: The Cochrane Library, Issue 1, 2001. Oxford: Update Software. Search date February 1996; primary sources Medline 1966 to February 1996; Embase 1987 to February 1996; Cochrane Controlled Trials Register 1966 to February 1996; hand searched journals and conference proceedings.

25. Gregoriou O, Konidaris S, Vitoratos N, et al. Gonadotropin-releasing hormone analogue plus hormone replacement therapy for the treatment of endometriosis: a randomized controlled trial. *Int J Fertil Womens Med* 1997;42:406–411.

26. Taskin O, Yalcinoglu AI, Kucuk S. Effectiveness of tibolone on hypoestrogenic symptoms induced by goserelin treatment in patients with endometriosis. *Fertil Steril* 1997;67:40–45.

27. Morgante G. Low-dose danazol after combined surgical and medical therapy reduces the incidence of pelvic pain in women with moderate and severe endometriosis. *Hum Reprod* 1999;14:2371–2374.

28. Vercellini P, De-Giorgi O. Depot medroxyprogesterone acetate versus an oral contraceptive combined with very-low-dose danazol for long-term treatment of pelvic pain associated with endometriosis. *Am J Obstet Gynecol* 1996;175:396–401.

29. Wilson M, Farquhar CM, Sinclair O, et al. Surgical interruption of pelvic nerve pathways for primary and secondary dysmenorrhoea. In: The Cochrane Library, Issue 1, 2001. Oxford: Update Software. Search date 1998; primary sources Medline 1966 to 1998; Embase 1974 to 1998; Cochrane Controlled Trials Register 1966 to 1998, and hand searched journals, conference proceedings and references.

30. Sutton CJG, Ewen SP, Whitelaw N, et al. A prospective, randomised, double-blind, controlled trial of laser laparoscopy in the treatment of pelvic pain associated with minimal, mild and moderate endometriosis. *Fertil Steril* 1994;62:696–700.

31. Sutton CJG, Pooley AS, Ewen SP. Follow-up report on a randomised, controlled trial of laser laparoscopy in the treatment of pelvic pain associated with minimal to moderate endometriosis. *Fertil Steril* 1997;68:170–174.

32. Marcoux S, Maheux R, Berube S, et al. Laparoscopic surgery in infertile women with minimal or mild endometriosis. Canadian Collaborative Group on Endometriosis. *N Engl J Med* 1997;337:217–222.

33. Parazzini F. Ablation of lesions or no treatment in minimal-mild endometriosis in infertile women: a randomized trial. Gruppo Italiano per lo Studio dell'Endometriosis. *Hum Reprod* 1999;14:1332–1334.

34. Parazzini F, Fedele L, Busacca M, et al. Postsurgical medical treatment of advanced endometriosis: results of a randomized clinical trial. *Am J Obstet Gynecol* 1994;171:1205–1207.

35. Bianchi S, Busacca M, Agnoli B, et al. Effects of 3 month therapy with danazol after laparoscopic surgery for stage III/IV endometriosis: a randomized study. *Hum Reprod* 1999;14:1335–1337.

36. Telimaa S, Ronnberg L, Kauppila A. Placebo-controlled comparison of danazol and high-dose medroxyprogesterone acetate in the treatment of endometriosis after conservative surgery. *Gynecol Endocrinol* 1987;1:363–371.

37. Hornstein MD, Hemmings R, Yuzpe AA, et al. Use of nafarelin versus placebo after reductive laparoscopic surgery for endometriosis. *Fertil Steril* 1997;68:860–864.

38. Vercellini P, Crosignani PG, Fadini R, et al. A gonadotrophin-releasing hormone agonist compared with expectant management after conservative surgery for symptomatic endometriosis. *Br J Obstet Gynaecol* 1999;106: 672–677.

39. Muzii L, Marana R, Caruana P, et al. Postoperative administration of monophasic combined oral contraceptives after laparoscopic treatment of ovarian endometriosis: a prospective, randomized trial. *Am J Obstet Gynecol* 2000;183:588–592.

40. Audebert A, Descampes P, Marret H, et al. Pre or post operative medical treatment with nafarelin in Stage III–IV endometriosis: a French multicentered study. *Eur J Obstet Gynecol Reprod Biol* 1998;79: 145–148.

41. Beretta P, Franchi M, Ghezzi F, et al. Randomised clinical trial of two laparoscopic treatments of endometriomas: cystectomy versus drainage and coagulation. *Fertil Steril* 1998;709:1176–1180.

Cynthia Farquhar
Associate Professor
School of Medicine
University of Auckland
Auckland
New Zealand

Competing interests: None declared.

Essential vulvodynia (vulval pain)

Search date May 2000

Earlando Thomas, Damian Murphy and Charles Redman

QUESTIONS

INTERVENTIONS

Unknown effectiveness

To be covered in future issues of
Clinical Evidence
Topical steroids

Key Messages

- We found no randomised evidence on the effects of amitriptyline or pudendal nerve decompression in women with essential vulvodynia.

DEFINITION	Essential vulvodynia is characterised by a diffuse, unremitting burning of the vulva, which may extend to the perineum, thigh or buttock, and is often associated with urethral or rectal discomfort. Hyperaesthesia over a wide area is usually the only abnormal finding on physical examination. It is found primarily in postmenopausal women.
INCIDENCE/ PREVALENCE	We found no data on the prevalence of essential vulvodynia.
AETIOLOGY/ RISK FACTORS	The cause is unknown. Similar symptoms may be caused by pudendal nerve damage.[1–3]
PROGNOSIS	Without treatment, the unremitting symptoms of essential vulvodynia may reduce the quality of life. Frequency of micturition, stress incontinence, and chronic constipation may also rarely develop.[1–3]
AIMS	To control symptoms and improve quality of life with minimal adverse effects.
OUTCOMES	Symptom scores for itching, burning, pain, and dyspareunia; range from 0–3 (3 represents the most severe).
METHODS	*Clinical Evidence* search and appraisal May 2000. Where we found no good RCTs, we used the best available observational studies.

QUESTION   What are the effects of treatments?

OPTION   AMITRIPTYLINE

We found no randomised evidence on the effects of amitriptyline in women with essential vulvodynia.

Benefits:	We found no systematic review or RCTs.
Harms:	In one retrospective cohort study, adverse effects, mostly drowsiness and dry mouth, occurred in 45% (9/20) of women. Weight gain occurred in 10–15%. Tinnitus and palpitation were each reported by one women.[3]
Comment:	None.

OPTION   PUDENDAL NERVE DECOMPRESSION

We found no randomised evidence on the effects of pudendal nerve decompression in women with essential vulvodynia.

Benefits:	We found no systematic review or RCTs.
Harms:	No adverse effects were found during follow up.
Comment:	Pudendal nerve decompression may be technically challenging. Experience suggests that success depends on selection of suitable patients for surgical or medical management.

Women's health

Essential vulvodynia (vulval pain)

REFERENCES

1. Turner MLC, Marinoff SC. Pudendal neuralgia. *Am J Obstet Gynecol* 1991;165:1233–1236.
2. Shafik A. Pudendal canal syndrome as a cause of vulvodynia and its treatment by pudendal nerve decompression. *Eur J Obstet Gynecol* 1998;80: 215–220.
3. McKay M. Dysesthetic ("essential") vulvodynia. Treatment with amitriptyline. *J Reprod Med* 1993; 38:9–13.

Earlando Thomas
Senior Specialist Registrar
Department of Obstetrics and
Gynecology
Rochester General Hospital
Rochester, NY
USA

Damian Murphy
Consultant Obstetrician and
Gynaecologist
Department of Obstetrics and
Gynaecology
New Cross Hospital
Wolverhampton
UK

Charles Redman
Consultant Obstetrician and
Gynaecologist
Department of Obstetrics and
Gynaecology
City General Hospital
Stoke-on-Trent
UK
Competing interests: None declared.

Search date October 2000: expanded this issue

Kirsten Duckitt

INTERVENTIONS

INFERTILITY CAUSED BY OVULATION DISORDERS
Likely to be beneficial
Clomiphene 1282
Laparoscopic ovarian drilling .1285

Unknown effectiveness
Cyclofenil New 1283
Gonadotrophins 1283
Pulsatile gonadotrophin releasing
    hormone 1285

TUBAL INFERTILITY
Likely to be beneficial
In vitro fertilisation (IVF) 1287

Unknown effectiveness
Selective salpingography and
    tubal recanalisation 1286
Tubal surgery 1286

INFERTILITY ASSOCIATED WITH ENDOMETRIOSIS
Beneficial
Intrauterine insemination
    with ovarian
    stimulation New 1289

Likely to be beneficial
Surgical treatment 1290

Unknown effectiveness
IVF .1291

Likely to be ineffective or harmful
Drug-induced ovarian
    suppression 1289

MALE INFERTILITY
Beneficial
Intrauterine insemination 1291
Donor insemination 1293
Fallopian tube sperm
    perfusion 1296

Unknown effectiveness
Intracytoplasmic sperm injection
    plus IVF 1292
IVF versus gamete intrafallopian
    transfer 1293

UNEXPLAINED INFERTILITY
Beneficial
Intrauterine insemination 1295

Unknown effectiveness
Clomiphene 1294
Gamete intrafallopian
    transfer 1297
IVF .1297

To be covered in future issues of Clinical Evidence
Counselling

Covered elsewhere in this issue
See erectile dysfunction, p 605
See endometriosis, p 1267
See pelvic inflammatory disease,
    p 1123

See glossary, p 1298

Key Messages

In women with infertility caused by ovulation disorders

- One systematic review of randomised crossover trials has found that clomiphene increases the chances of becoming pregnant. We found no trials that compared clomiphene with other interventions in women with ovulation disorders.
- One RCT found no difference in pregnancy rates between cyclofenil and placebo.
- RCTs have compared follicle stimulating hormone (FSH), human menopausal gonadotrophin, and laparoscopic ovarian drilling. They found no difference in pregnancy rates. None of these interventions has been directly compared with placebo in women with ovulation disorders.
- One systematic review of RCTs found insufficient evidence to assess the value of pulsatile gonadotrophin releasing hormone (GnRH) in polycystic ovary syndrome. A large case series demonstrated clinically significant ovulation and pregnancy rates when used as replacement therapy in anovulatory women with hypogonadotrophic hypogonadism.

In women with tubal infertility

- Two RCTs have found improved pregnancy and live birth rates with immediate in vitro fertilisation (IVF) rather than delayed IVF.
- One systematic review found insufficient evidence on the effect of routine use of hydrotubation or second look laparoscopy following tubal surgery.

In women with infertility caused by endometriosis

- Two RCTs have found that intrauterine insemination with ovarian stimulation achieves higher birth rates than no treatment or intrauterine insemination alone in subfertile women with minimal or mild endometriosis.
- A systematic review has found that medical treatment to induce ovarian suppression does not increase pregnancy rates compared with placebo and removes the chance of spontaneous conception during pregnancy.
- Systematic reviews of cohort studies have found that pregnancy rates are higher with surgical than medical treatment.
- We found insufficient evidence on IVF.

In couples with male factor infertility

- One systematic review of RCTs has found that intrauterine insemination achieves higher pregnancy rates than intracervical insemination or natural intercourse.
- We found insufficient evidence on intracytoplasmic sperm injection plus IVF and on gamete intrafallopian transfer.
- Donor insemination achieves live birth rates of about 10% per cycle in women with no evidence of reduced fertility or in whom problems with fertility have been corrected. This compares to rates of about 30% in normal fertile couples and 0–1% if the man has no sperm or severely impaired semen quality.

In couples with unexplained infertility

- One systematic review of RCTs has found that in couples with unexplained infertility clomiphene doubles the rate of pregnancy, although the low background pregnancy rate means that benefits are unlikely to be clinically important. Another systematic review found no evidence of benefit from clomiphene use in such couples.

Infertility and subfertility
1281
Women's health

- Three systematic reviews of RCTs have found that intrauterine insemination achieves higher pregnancy rates than timed intercourse, especially when ovarian stimulation with gonadotrophins is also used.

- We found no RCTs of gamete intrafallopian transfer in couples with unexplained infertility. Limited data from RCTs found no difference in pregnancy rates between ovarian hyperstimulation and IVF.

- One systematic review of RCTs has found that fallopian tube sperm perfusion almost doubles the pregnancy rate compared with intrauterine insemination.

Interventions involving ovarian stimulation

- These carry the risk of multiple pregnancy and ovarian hyperstimulation syndrome. The risk of each varies with the type of ovarian stimulation used. Moderate to severe ovarian hyperstimulation complicates 4% of ovulation induction cycles and up to 10% of all IVF cycles. Multiple pregnancy occurs in 29% of women with polycystic ovaries when conventional (as opposed to low dose) regimens of gonadotrophins are used.

DEFINITION   Normal fertility has been defined as achieving a pregnancy within 2 years by regular sexual intercourse.[1] However, many define infertility as the failure to conceive after 1 year of unprotected intercourse. Infertility can be primary, in couples who have never conceived, or secondary, in couples who have previously conceived. Infertile couples include those who are sterile (who will never achieve a natural pregnancy) and those who are subfertile (who should eventually achieve a pregnancy).

INCIDENCE/   Although there is no evidence of a major change in prevalence of
PREVALENCE   infertility, many more couples are seeking help than previously. Currently, about one in seven couples in industrialised countries will seek medical advice for infertility.[2] Rates of primary infertility vary widely between countries, ranging from 10% in Africa to about 6% in North America and Europe.[1] Reported rates of secondary infertility are less reliable.

AETIOLOGY/   In the UK nearly a third of cases of infertility are unexplained. The
RISK FACTORS rest are caused by ovulatory failure (27%), low sperm count or quality (19%), tubal damage (14%), endometriosis (5%), and other causes (5%).[3]

PROGNOSIS   In developed countries, 80–90% of couples attempting to conceive are successful after 1 year, and 95% after 2 years.[3] The chances of becoming pregnant vary with the cause and duration of infertility, the woman's age, the couple's previous pregnancy history, and the availability of different treatment options.[4,5] For the first 2–3 years of unexplained infertility, cumulative conception rates remain high (27–46%) but decrease with increasing age of the woman and duration of infertility. The background rates of spontaneous pregnancy in infertile couples can be calculated from longitudinal studies of infertile couples who have been observed without treatment.[4]

AIMS   To achieve the delivery of one healthy baby; to reduce the distress associated with infertility; to help people come to terms with childlessness if treatments fail or are unavailable.

OUTCOMES   Rates of pregnancy, live birth, miscarriage, and multiple pregnancy; incidence of ovarian hyperstimulation syndrome; satisfaction with services and treatments; acceptance of childlessness if treatment is unsuccessful. Ovulation is an intermediate outcome. Pregnancy rate is an intermediate outcome, but one that is important in itself to many people. A large number of pregnancies in infertile couples will occur spontaneously without treatment.[4] Effectiveness of treatments for infertility should be assessed on the basis of pregnancy rates over and above the spontaneous pregnancy rates. Otherwise the impacts of treatments will be overestimated.

METHODS *Clinical Evidence* update search and appraisal October 2000. **Crossover design:** For infertility, RCTs with a crossover design may overestimate the treatment effect, because pregnancies occurring in the first half of the trial will remove couples from the second half.[6] Crossover trials were included in some systematic reviews where no or very few RCTs using a parallel group design were available. Ideally, only data from the first half of the trial, before crossover, should be used. However, a study that used a computer model to compare the results of crossover and parallel designed trials suggests that any overestimation may be clinically irrelevant.[7]

QUESTION What are the effects of treatments for infertility caused by ovulation disorders?

OPTION CLOMIPHENE

One systematic review of RCTs has found that clomiphene increases the likelihood of pregnancy in women who ovulate infrequently. We found insufficient evidence that prolonged use of clomiphene increases the risk of ovarian cancer. The incidence of multiple pregnancy (mostly with twins) is increased.

Benefits: **Versus placebo:** See table 1, p 1302. One systematic review (search date not stated) identified three double blind, crossover RCTs comparing clomiphene 50–200 mg versus placebo in 217 cycles in women who ovulate infrequently.[13] Pregnancy was over three times more likely per treatment cycle with clomiphene than placebo (OR 3.4, 95% CI 1.2 to 9.5). **Versus tamoxifen:** We found no systematic review. We found three studies comparing clomiphene versus tamoxifen in 102 anovulatory or infrequently ovulating women. One RCT used a parallel group design, one used alternate cycles design, and one was an observational study.[35–37] Two of the studies based estimates of pregnancy rates on fewer than 30 pregnancies.[35,37]

Harms: **Ovarian cancer:** Eleven women with ovarian cancer were detected in a cohort of 3837 infertile women.[38] In 135 women that were randomly selected as a subcohort from these 3837 women, there was an 11-fold increase in risk of ovarian cancer in women using clomiphene citrate for 12 or more cycles (RR 11.1, 95% CI 1.5 to 82.3). The association was present for both gravid and nulligravid women and for infertile women both with ovulatory disorders and with infertility from other causes. Subsequent studies have found no association between clomiphene and ovarian cancer.[14,39–41] **Multiple pregnancy:** Multiple pregnancy occurs in 2–13% of women with all causes of infertility taking clomiphene, compared with a spontaneous multiple pregnancy rate of about 1–2% of women in North American and European populations.[42,43] In a 1 year survey in the UK, 25 of the 44 triplet pregnancies reported were attributable to clomiphene.[44] Clomiphene was also implicated in two of the eight sets of quads and quins reported. **Ovarian hyperstimulation syndrome:** See glossary, p 1298. Clomiphene tends to cause only mild ovarian hyperstimulation that does not require treatment.

Comment: Clomiphene was first introduced in the 1960s and all the trials took place in the 1970s, before more recent quality standards for RCTs were established. With regard to the case-cohort study above,[38] five of the 11 ovarian cancers were borderline epithelial tumours that have low malignant potential, and two were granulosa cell tumours that have different embryological, pathological, and epidemiological features from epithelial tumours. Borderline and malignant tumours pose different risks that are not easy to combine and removing the two granulosa cell tumours from the small number of cases found diminishes the increased risk atrributed to clomiphene treatment.

| OPTION | CYCLOFENIL | New |

One RCT found no difference in pregnancy rates between cyclofenil and placebo.

Benefits: **Versus placebo:** One double blind RCT (213 women with either ovulatory disorders or unexplained infertility) compared three cycles of 800 mg cyclofenil a day versus placebo from days 4 to 8 of the cycle.[45] There was no significant difference in cumulative pregnancy rates after three cycles (26/114 [23%] with cyclofenil v 21/99 [21%] with placebo; RR 1.1, 95% CI 0.7 to 1.8).

Harms: No adverse effects were reported in this trial.

Comment: Only 123 of the 213 women in this RCT had ovulatory disorders and the results for these women were not presented separately. Such a trial does not exclude a possible benefit of cyclofenil.

| OPTION | GONADOTROPHINS |

One systematic review of RCTs found no evidence of a difference in pregnancy rates between human menopausal gonadotrophin and urinary FSH or laparoscopic ovarian drilling. However, compared with human menopausal gonadotrophin, FSH carried a lower risk of ovarian hyperstimulation syndrome (see glossary, p 1298), although this was only the case in cycles where GnRH analogues were not used. Gonadotrophins have not been compared with placebo or with clomiphene. We found insufficient evidence of an increased risk of ovarian cancer from using gonadotrophins.

Benefits: **Versus placebo:** We found no RCTs. **Versus clomiphene:** We found no RCTs. **Human menopausal gonadotrophin versus FSH:** One systematic review (search date not stated) identified six RCTs, three of which used crossover designs.[15] The RCTs (182 women with clomiphene resistant polycystic ovary syndrome) compared human menopausal gonadotrophin versus purified urinary FSH (see table 1, p 1302).[15] There was no significant difference in pregnancy rates (37% v 27%; OR for pregnancy v FSH 0.7, 95% CI

0.4 to 1.2). A further systematic review (search date not stated) identified 14 RCTs comparing human menopausal gonadotrophin with urinary derived FSH in subfertility associated with polycystic ovarian syndrome.[46] There was no significant difference in pregnancy rates (OR 0.8, 95 % CI 0.4 to 1.5). **Urinary versus recombinant FSH:** We found no systematic review for women with anovulation. We found two RCTs (223 women with clomiphene resistant, normogonadotrophic anovulation) comparing recombinant versus urinary FSH.[47,48] No significant differences in pregnancy rates were found between either group in either trial. However, in one trial, a significantly lower total dose and shorter duration of recombinant FSH achieved ovulation.[47] One systematic review (search date 1999) identified 12 RCTs that compared recombinant FSH versus urinary FSH in cycles using either IVF or intracytoplasmic sperm injection (ICSI) cycles.[49] There was a 20% increase in clinical pregnancy rates per started cycle when recombinant FSH was used compared with baseline (OR 1.2, 95% CI 1.0 to 1.4). The absolute risk difference represented an increase in clinical pregnancy rate per cycle started with recombinant FSH rather than urinary FSH of 3.7% (95% CI 0.5% to 6.9%). One subsequent assessor blind RCT (110 women undergoing pituitary downregulation prior to undergoing IVF) compared live birth rates in two types of recombinant FSH and two types of urinary FSH.[50] It found no significant difference between any of the groups, and no difference in birth rates when recombinant FSH was compared with urinary FSH (12/75 [16%] with recombinant FSH v 4/35 [11%] with urinary FSH; RR 1.4, 95% CI 0.5 to 4.0). **Versus laparoscopic ovarian drilling:** See option, p 1285.

Harms: **Ovarian cancer:** One case control study (200 women with ovarian cancer and 408 area matched controls) found that women with non-invasive ovarian tumours were over three times more likely to have been exposed to any ovulation induction agents (adjusted OR 3.5, 95% CI 1.2 to 10.1), particularly to human menopausal gonadotrophin (adjusted OR 9.4, 95% CI 1.7 to 52.1).[41] Women with invasive ovarian tumours were no more likely to have been exposed to any ovulation induction agents. **Multiple pregnancy:** Multiple pregnancy occurs in 29% of women with polycystic ovaries when conventional regimens of gonadotrophins are used to induce ovulation.[16] **Ovarian hyperstimulation:** In one systematic review, there was a significant reduction in the risk of ovarian hyperstimulation with urinary FSH in the seven RCTs that reported this outcome (OR versus human menopausal gonadotrophin 0.3, 95% CI 0.2 to 0.7).[46] However, the beneficial effect of FSH was only present where no concomitant GnRH analogue was used (5 RCTs, OR 0.2, 95% CI 0.1 to 0.5). Concomitant use of a GnRH analogue increased the risk of ovarian hyperstimulation (2 RCTs, OR 3.2, 95% CI 1.5 to 6.7). **Urinary versus recombinant FSH:** One large RCT found no significant difference in the risk of multiple pregnancy or ovarian hyperstimulation syndrome.[47]

Comment: Despite not being placebo controlled, trials of gonadotrophins often included women who were not ovulating and, therefore, provide some evidence that treatment is effective. The avoidance of gonadotrophins may reduce the risk of multiple pregnancy and ovarian hyperstimulation syndrome. Recombinant FSH is not derived from human tissues.

LAPAROSCOPIC OVARIAN DRILLING

One systematic review of RCTs has found no evidence of a significant difference in pregnancy rates between laparoscopic ovarian drilling and gonadotrophins.

Benefits: We found one systematic review (search date not stated), which identified two RCTs (one using a crossover design; 112 women with anovulatory, clomiphene resistant polycystic ovary syndrome), comparing laparoscopic ovarian drilling (see glossary, p 1298) versus gonadotrophins (see table 1, p 1302).[17] They found no significant difference in pregnancy rates (OR 0.72, 95% CI 0.3 to 1.8).

Harms: Laparoscopic drilling incurs the risks and morbidity of the laparoscopy under general anaesthetic and postoperative adhesion formation. We found no evidence to support the suggestion that laparoscopic drilling increases the long term risk of premature ovarian failure. However, it carried no increased risk of multiple pregnancy.

Comment: The trials of laparoscopic drilling included women who were not ovulating and therefore provide some evidence that treatment is effective despite the lack of placebo controls. However, the systematic review only included a relatively small number of women, hence the broad confidence interval. Two more RCTs are in progress (N Bayran and C Farquhar, personal communication, 2000).

PULSATILE GONADOTROPHIN RELEASING HORMONE

We found insufficient evidence on the effects of GnRH on infertility caused by ovulation disorders.

Benefits: We found one systematic review (search date not stated), which identified three RCTs and one non-randomised comparative trial comparing pulsatile GnRH versus another treatment to induce ovulation in subfertile women with clomiphene resistant polycystic ovary syndrome.[51] The trials describing four different comparisons, were small (each reporting between 1 and 4 pregnancies), and of short duration (1–3 cycles), and so provided insufficient evidence to assess the value of pulsatile GnRH in polycystic ovary syndrome. Case series in 256 anovulatory women with hypogonadotrophic hypogonadism undergoing 1043 treatment cycles found cumulative pregnancy rates of 59–73% at 6 months and 81–92% at 12 months.[52-54] Only one series reported the live birth rate; this was 65% after 12 treatment cycles.[52]

Harms: One retrospective analysis (229 cycles in 71 women) compared pulsatile GnRH versus gonadotrophins alone, and found no significant difference in multiple pregnancy rates after six cycles.[55] However, 75% of the multiple pregnancies in the gonadotrophin group were triplets or higher order multiple pregnancies, whereas all multiple pregnancies in the GnRH group were twins.

Comment: Pulsatile GnRH is used in women with anovulation caused by low serum gonadotrophins and oestrogen concentrations. It is a well defined condition so the evidence, although only from case series, should be generalisable to all women with hypogonadotrophic hypogonadism.

Women's health

OPTION   SELECTIVE SALPINGOGRAPHY/TUBAL CATHETERISATION

We found no RCTs of selective salpingography and tubal catheterisation. Non-randomised studies found that, if used in isolated proximal tubal obstruction, these procedures reduced the need for tubal surgery or IVF in some women.

Benefits: We found no RCTs. One recent systematic review (search date not stated) combined the raw data from 10 cohort and other observational studies of selective salpingography and tubal cannulation (482 women), and four studies from hysteroscopic cannulation for proximal tubal blockage (133 women).[56] The ongoing pregnancy rate (> 20 weeks' gestation) for the radiographic series was 23% versus 49% for the hysteroscopic series. One prospective cohort study followed 43 women with bilateral proximal tubal obstruction and 33 control women undergoing reversal of tubal sterilisation.[57] Those in whom tubal catheterisation was unsuccessful went on to have microsurgical resection and anastomosis. Cumulative pregnancy rates at 12 months were 68% with successful tubal catheterisation, 56% with microsurgery, and 29% in the control group.

Harms: Tubal perforation, which does not seem to be clinically important, occurred in 2%, and ectopic pregnancy in 3–9.4% of women undergoing selective salpingography and tubal catheterisation.[56,58]

Comment: None of the published studies included an untreated group, so it is not possible to give the treatment related pregnancy rate over and above the spontaneous pregnancy rate. Tubal patency and pregnancy without treatment have been reported in women diagnosed with bilateral proximal tube obstruction.[59]

OPTION   TUBAL SURGERY

We found limited evidence that surgical division of tubal adhesions improves pregnancy rates, and that laparoscopic techniques offer no benefit over open microsurgical techniques. We found no RCTs comparing tubal surgery with IVF. One systematic review found insufficient evidence to support the routine use of hydrotubation or second look laparoscopy following tubal surgery.

Benefits: **Versus IVF:** We found no systematic review or RCTs. Case series of tubal surgery have been compared with large databases of couples undergoing IVF. These found that tubal surgery was as effective as IVF in women with filmy adhesions, mild distal tubal occlusion, or proximal obstruction.[19,60–64] Success rates with tubal surgery depend on the severity and site of disease. The best figures from surgery in women with distal tubal occlusion are live birth rates of 20%–30% with rates of up to 60% reported for the less common proximal occlusion.[19–23] **Different types of tubal surgery:** We found two systematic reviews.[65,66] The first (search date not stated) identified eight RCTs and 14 non-randomised trials looking at all aspects of infertility surgery.[65] It found that pregnancy rates were higher with microsurgery for adhesiolysis plus salpingostomy than with macrosurgery (full term rates 36.8% v 20.0%; RR 1.9, 95% CI 1.2 to 3.3). Pregnancy rates were higher with adhesiolysis compared with no treatment. Pregnancy rates were no different with laparoscopic than with open microsurgical adhesiolysis (total pregnancy rates 85.2% v 75.0%; RR 1.1, 95% CI 0.8 to 1.6). The review found no difference in pregnancy rates between carbon dioxide laser for adhesiolysis, salpingostomy, or reversal of sterilisation than with standard techniques. Total and intrauterine pregnancy rates were lower with laparoscopic than with open microsurgical salpingostomy. However, the last conclusion was based on four trials reported between 1987 and 1991. The second systematic review (search date not stated, 5 RCTs) concluded that all the studies were either poor quality or underpowered. It found insufficient evidence to support the routine practice of hydrotubation or second look laparoscopy following tubal surgery.[66] **Proximal tubal blockage:** We found no RCTs. One recent systematic review (search date not stated) evaluated the raw data from five cohort and other observational studies (175 women) that used microsurgical techniques for proximal tubal blockage, and from two studies (104 women) that used macrosurgical techniques.[56] The overall pregnancy rate after microsurgery was 59%, with ongoing pregnancy rates of 47% and an ectopic rate of 7.4%. For macrosurgery the overall pregnancy rate was 42%, the ongoing pregnancy rate was 16%, and the ectopic rate was 16%. Ongoing pregnancy rates after microsurgery were significantly higher than those after macrosurgery (RR 2.2, 95% CI 1.5 to 3.2).

Harms: Tubal surgery involves general anaesthesia and admission to hospital, although the laparoscopic approach reduces hospital stay and recovery time. There is a risk of ectopic pregnancy caused by pre-existing tubal damage; rates of 7–9% have been reported compared with 1–3% with IVF.[9,10] IVF carries the risk of multiple pregnancy and ovarian hyperstimulation syndrome (see harms of IVF, p 1288).

Comment: These data precede recent improvements in case selection and laparoscopic training. If successful, tubal surgery allows women to have more pregnancies without further medical intervention and without the risks associated with IVF.[67]

| OPTION | IN VITRO FERTILISATION |

Two RCTs have found improved pregnancy and live birth rates with immediate compared with delayed IVF. Data from IVF databases suggest higher pregnancy rates compared with expected spontaneous pregnancy rates without treatment.

Benefits: We found no systematic review. We found two RCTs (598 infertile couples with all causes of infertility) comparing immediate versus delayed IVF.[68,69] The delayed group served as untreated controls for at least 6 months. One RCT found increased rates of live birth in the immediate compared with the delayed group (AR for live births, 11.6% for the immediate group v 4.9% for the delayed group; RR of live birth 2.4, 95% CI 1.0 to 5.7).[68] The other RCT found an increase in crude and cumulative pregnancy rates in the immediate

Women's health

compared with the delayed group, but the effect was significant only in women with severe bilateral tubal disease.[69] **Versus tubal surgery:** See option, p 1286. In all causes of infertility, IVF produced live birth rates per cycle of 15% in the UK and 20% in the USA.[5] If 3–5 cycles of IVF were possible, 59–77% of women with tubal infertility became pregnant, better than the best outcomes from tubal surgery.[8] **Versus IVF plus ICSI:** One RCT found no evidence of a benefit from adding ICSI to IVF for tubal infertility if the semen analysis is normal (live birth rates AR 7/38 [18%] with ICSI v 6/38 [16%] with IVF; RR 1.17, 95% CI 0.43 to 1.15) (see option, p 1292).[70]

Harms:
Multiple pregnancy: Multiple pregnancy rates were not reported in the RCTs mentioned above. However, of the 5538 live births following IVF in the UK in 1995–1996, 32% were multiple, including 230 (4.2%) sets of triplets and five sets of quads.[30] In the UK, the number of embryos that can be replaced is restricted to three. In the USA, where there are no such restrictions, 7939 deliveries included 36.6% multiple births, 7% of which were triplets and above. **Ovarian hyperstimulation syndrome:** Severe ovarian hyperstimulation syndrome occurs in 0.5–2% of all IVF cycles.[71] Ovarian hyperstimulation syndrome rates were not reported in the RCTs above.

Comment:
Similar clinics, ostensibly using the same methods, report different success rates. In the UK, the live birth rates per cycle vary from 0–28% with an average of 15%.[30] The equivalent average figure in the USA is nearly 20%, but again results vary widely.[72,73] In the UK, larger centres (200 or more cycles per year) report slightly higher live birth rates than smaller centres (15.7% per cycle started compared with 12.7%).[5] Such a difference has not been consistently reported in the USA. The success of IVF is influenced by age, duration of infertility, and previous pregnancy history. Pregnancy rates are highest between the ages of 25 and 35 years and decline steeply after 35 years.[5] A systematic review of nine retrospective comparative series and five abstracts found that the presence of a hydrosalpinx during an IVF cycle reduced pregnancy rates (14 retrospective comparative series AR 323/1642 [20%] with hydrosalpinx v 2203/7061 [31%] without hydrosalpinx; RR 0.63, 95% CI 0.57 to 0.70; NNH 8, 95% CI 7 to 10), implantation (14 retrospective comparative series AR 335/3929 [9%] with hydrosalpinx v 2414/17647 [14%] without hydrosalpinx; RR 0.62, 95% CI 0.56 to 0.70; NNH 19, 95% CI 16 to 24), and live birth rates (14 retrospective comparative series AR 190/1418 [13%] with hydrosalpinx v 1579/6735 [23%] without hydrosalpinx; RR 0.57, 95% CI 0.50 to 0.66; NNH 10, 95% 8 to 12), and increased rates of early pregnancy loss (14 retrospective comparative series AR 158/362 [44%] with hydrosalpinx v 728/2340 [31%] without hydrosalpinx; RR 1.4, 95% CI 1.23 to 1.60; NNH 8, 95% CI 5 to 14).[74] However, we found insufficient evidence to establish whether routine salpingectomy in these women would be beneficial prior to IVF.

OPTION   DRUG-INDUCED OVARIAN SUPPRESSION

One systematic review of RCTs found no evidence of a significant difference in pregnancy rates between drugs that induce ovarian suppression and either placebo or danazol in women with endometriosis. Ovarian suppression is less effective than surgical treatment.

Benefits: We found one systematic review (search date not stated), which identified 13 RCTs.[75] **Versus placebo:** Five RCTs (244 women with visually diagnosed endometriosis who had been attempting conception for over 12 months) compared ovulation suppression agents (medroxyprogesterone acetate, gestrinone, combined oral contraceptive pills, and GnRH analogues) versus placebo. Ovulation suppression agents versus placebo did not significantly increase the pregnancy rate (OR 0.8, 95% CI 0.5 to 1.4). **Versus danazol:** Eight RCTs compared ovulation suppression versus danazol in 658 similar women. They found no significant difference in pregnancy rates (OR compared with danazol 1.2, 95% CI 0.9 to 1.7). **Versus surgery:** See option, p 1290.

Harms: Drugs that suppress ovulation had important adverse effects that included weight gain, hot flushes, and osteoporosis.[75] Adverse effects of danazol were dose related. An average weight gain of 2–4 kg was common with 3 months of treatment. Other adverse effects included androgenic effects such as acne, seborrhoea, hirsutism, voice changes, and general complaints, including irritability, musculoskeletal pains, and tiredness. Hot flushes and breast atrophy were sometimes observed. Most of these adverse effects were reversible on stopping treatment.[76]

Comment: None of the RCTs in the systematic review used a crossover design. Combination of clomiphene with other infertility drugs was used in three of the trials. Treatment using ovulation suppression could waste valuable time for women who are trying to get pregnant, as the opportunity for spontaneous conceptions is lost during treatment.[75]

OPTION   INTRAUTERINE INSEMINATION   New

Two RCTs have found that intrauterine insemination with ovarian stimulation achieves higher birth rates than no treatment or intrauterine insemination alone in subfertile women with minimal or mild endometriosis.

Benefits: We found no systematic review. We found two RCTs. One RCT compared intrauterine insemination and gonadotrophins (53 couples, 127 cycles) with no treatment (50 couples, 184 cycles).[77] It found that live birth rates were significantly higher in the treated group (14/53 [26%] with intrauterine insemination v 4/50 [8%] with no treatment; RR 3.3, 95% CI 1.2 to 9.4; NNT 6, 95% CI 3 to 28). Another RCT (49 women with minimal or mild endometriosis) compared three cycles of pituitary downregulation, gonadotrophins, and intrauterine insemination with 6 months of expectant management.[78] There was no significant difference in the birth rates between the groups (7/24 [29%] with intrauterine insemination v 5/25 [20%] with expectant management; RR 1.5, 95% CI 0.5 to 4.0). When combined, these two trials show an overall twofold increase in live birth rates in the intrauterine insemination and gonadotrophin group compared to the no treatment group over a similar time period (RR versus no treatment 2.3, 95% CI 1.1 to 4.6). One further study randomised 119 couples with longstanding infertility (mean 3.7 years) to alternate cycles of gonadotrophins plus intrauterine insemination or intrauterine insemination alone.[79] After the first treatment cycle, the pregnancy rate was significantly higher in the group treated with gonadotrophins plus intrauterine insemination (19% with gonadotrophins plus intrauterine insemination v 0% with intrauterine insemination alone). Pregnancy rates were not presented according to diagnostic group. The 119 couples were subsequently followed up longitudinally and it was found that in the 57 couples with a diagnosis of endometriosis, gonadotrophins plus intrauterine insemination significantly increased the probability of pregnancy (RR 5.1, 95% CI 1.1 to 22.5).

Harms: No cases of severe ovarian hyperstimulation or hospital admission were reported in two RCTs.[77,79] In a third RCT, one severe case (1/24), one moderate case (1/24), and three mild cases (3/24) of ovarian hyperstimulation syndrome were reported.[78]

Comment: None.

OPTION   SURGICAL TREATMENT

Systematic reviews of cohort studies have found that surgery is more effective than ovarian suppression in women with infertility related to endometriosis, and that there is no significant difference in pregnancy rates between open and laparoscopic surgery. We found no RCTs that compared surgery with IVF in women with endometriosis.

Benefits: **Versus placebo or ovarian suppression:** We found one systematic review (search date not stated) and one non-systemic review (search date not stated), which together identified 21 cohort studies and one quasi randomised trial in a total of 3879 women with all stages of endometriosis.[25,26] Interventions were laparoscopic or open surgery versus medical treatment or no treatment. Surgical treatment produced a two fifths increase in pregnancy rate compared with medical treatment or no treatment (RR 1.4, 95% CI 1.3 to 1.5), but there was no significant difference between laparoscopic and open surgery (RR 0.9, 95% CI 0.8 to 1.0).[26] In women with mild or minimal endometriosis, analysis of pooled data found that laparoscopic surgery achieved higher pregnancy rates than danazol or no treatment (OR 2.7, 95% CI 2.1 to 3.5).[24] **Versus diagnostic laparoscopy:** We found two RCTs with conflicting results published since the reviews.[27,80] Both compared laparoscopic surgery (ablation or resection of endometriosis) versus diagnostic laparoscopy in a total of 452 infertile women with minimal or mild endometriosis. In the larger trial (341 women), the women undergoing laparoscopic surgery had a 13% absolute increase in the probability of a pregnancy occurring within 36 weeks and lasting longer than 20 weeks (RR 1.7, 95% CI 1.2 to 2.6; NNT 8).[27] However, the smaller trial (which was powered to detect a relative risk > 2.5 in pregnancy rates between the groups) found no difference between the groups either in conception rates (24% v 29%) or birth rates at 1 year (20% v 22%).[80]

Harms: The risks and morbidity of surgery under general anaesthesia, and of postoperative adhesion formation, should be balanced against the adverse effects of treatments involving ovarian suppression or stimulation. One multicentre series of 29 966 diagnostic and operative gynaecological laparoscopies found a mortality of 3.3 of 100 000 laparoscopies, and a complication rate of 3.2 of 1000 laporoscopies.[28]

Comment: In the RCT described above, 14% of the 341 women who received surgery for their endometriosis also had periadnexal adhesions lysed, which may have affected their fecundity.[27]

OPTION   IN VITRO FERTILISATION

Retrospective studies suggest that IVF achieves similar rates of pregnancy in women with endometriosis as in those with other causes of infertility. We found no evidence comparing IVF with drug-induced ovarian suppression or with surgery for women with moderate or severe endometriosis.

Benefits: We found no systematic review or RCTs. We found two retrospective cohort studies of women undergoing IVF.[29,81] They compared pregnancy rates in those with endometriosis and those with other causes of infertility. There were no significant differences in pregnancy rates for different stages of endometriosis or for endometriosis compared with other causes of infertility.

Harms: See harms of IVF for tubal fertility, p 1288.

Comment: There is a need for properly controlled prospective studies that present their results for different stages of endometriosis using a validated classification system. Comparisons with assisted reproductive techniques are also required.

QUESTION   What are the effects of treatments for male infertility?

OPTION   INTRAUTERINE INSEMINATION

One systematic review of RCTs has found that intrauterine insemination more than doubles the chance of pregnancy compared with intracervical insemination or natural intercourse in couples with male infertility.

Benefits: We found two systematic reviews (search date not stated,[33] search date 1996/1997[82]), the earliest of which identified 10 RCTs (2082 treatment cycles) comparing intrauterine insemination versus intracervical insemination or natural intercourse.[32] In couples reported as having male infertility, intrauterine insemination more than doubled the pregnancy rate compared with intracervical insemination or timed natural intercourse (OR 2.2, 95% CI 1.4 to

3.4). Pregnancy rate per cycle was 6.5% with intrauterine insemination versus 3.1% with intracervical insemination or timed natural intercourse. The more recent review identified 17 RCTs (3662 completed treatment cycles) comparing intrauterine insemination with timed intercourse in either natural or stimulated cycles in couples with male subfertility.[82] Intrauterine insemination more than doubled the pregnancy rate compared with timed intercourse, both in natural cycles (OR 2.4, 95% CI 1.5 to 3.8) and in cycles where controlled ovarian hyperstimulation was also used (OR 2.1, 95% CI 1.3 to 3.5). Intrauterine insemination in cycles with controlled ovarian hyperstimulation improved the probability of conception compared with intrauterine insemination in natural cycles, but did not reach significance (OR 1.8, 95% CI 1.0 to 3.3). When intrauterine insemination in controlled ovarian hyperstimulation cycles was compared with timed intercourse in natural cycles, the probability of conception was significantly increased (OR 6.2, 95% CI 2.4 to 16.5).

Harms: Apart from the risks of ovarian hyperstimulation syndrome and multiple pregnancy associated with ovarian stimulation, intrauterine insemination may increase the likelihood of infection and may be associated with some discomfort.[83] However, data from RCTs are scarce.

Comment: We found three RCTs that addressed the optimum number of inseminations in controlled ovarian stimulation cycles. Two trials found that two inseminations performed in the pre-ovulatory and peri-ovulatory periods produced significantly higher pregnancy rates than one peri-ovulatory insemination.[84,85] The other trial found a non-significant increase in pregnancy rates with two similarly timed inseminations.[86] One small crossover RCT addressed the timing of insemination in clomiphene stimulated cycles. It found similar pregnancy rates per cycle whether insemination was timed with a urinary luteinising hormone (LH) kit or whether ultrasound monitoring with human chorionic gonadotrophin (hCG) induction of ovulation was used.[87]

| OPTION | INTRACYTOPLASMIC SPERM INJECTION PLUS IVF |

We found insufficient evidence on the effect of ICSI plus IVF compared with no treatment.

Benefits: **Versus IVF alone:** We found one systematic review (search date not stated)[88] and one subsequent RCT.[70] The systematic review identified 10 RCTs (total 437 couples) comparing ICSI plus IVF versus IVF alone (eight compared ICSI with conventional IVF, one compared ICSI with subzonal sperm injection, and one compared ICSI with additional IVF).[88] For couples with normal semen, no evidence of a difference was found in fertilisation rates per retrieved oocyte or pregnancy rates between IVF alone and ICSI. However, there seemed to be a slight benefit of ICSI over IVF alone if fertilisation rate per inseminated oocytes was considered (combined OR 1.4, 95% CI 1.2 to 1.7). For couples with borderline semen (concentration 10–20 million/ml, motility 30–50%, morphology 4–14% normal forms), ICSI resulted in higher fertilisation rates compared with conventional IVF both for fertilisations per oocyte retrieved (OR 3.79, 95% CI 2.97 to 4.85) and for fertilisations per oocyte inseminated (OR 3.9, 95% CI 3.0 to 5.2). For couples with very poor semen (concentration < 10 million/ml, motility < 30%, morphology < 4% normal forms) two RCTs found better fertilisation outcomes with ICSI than with subzonal sperm injection or additional IVF. The subsequent RCT randomised 76 couples with tubal factor infertility but normal semen analysis to either ICSI plus IVF or IVF alone. No significant difference was found in clinical pregnancy rates per cycle (21.0% v 21.1%) or take home baby rates (18.4% v 15.8%).[70]

Harms: We found conflicting reports of congenital abnormality in children born after intracytoplasmic sperm injection. Some found no increase over background rates of abnormality. Others found that major birth defects may be twice as likely and minor defects 50% more likely.[12,89] There has also been a suggestion that sex chromosomal defects may be more likely in children born as a result of ICSI.[90,91]

Comment: Many couples have a strong preference for a child genetically related to both partners.[92] The data on congenital and chromosome abnormalities with intracytoplasmic sperm injection are constantly being revised as experience increases.

OPTION   **IVF VERSUS GAMETE INTRAFALLOPIAN TRANSFER**

We found insufficient evidence to compare IVF and gamete intrafallopian transfer in male infertility.

Benefits: We found no systematic review. We found one RCT in 14 couples with male infertility.[93] This RCT found no evidence of a difference in pregnancy rates.

Harms: See harms of IVF, p 1288.

Comment: None.

OPTION   **DONOR INSEMINATION**

Analysis of data from large databases has found live birth rates of about 10% per cycle with donor insemination in women without evidence of reduced fertility or in whom problems with fertility have been corrected. This compares to rates of about 30% in normal fertile couples and 0–1% if the man has no sperm or severely impaired semen quality. No RCTs have compared donor insemination with other treatments for male infertility. One systematic review has found that intrauterine insemination of frozen donor sperm leads to higher pregnancy rates than intracervical insemination (ICI) in centres where pregnancy rates per cycle for ICI were under 6%.

Benefits: **Versus no treatment:** We found no systematic reviews or RCTs that compared donor insemination with no treatment or other interventions for male infertility. **Type of insemination:** One systematic review (search date not stated, 12 RCTs, 2215 treatment cycles) found that intrauterine insemination of frozen donor sperm led to higher pregnancy rates than ICI in centres where pregnancy rates per cycle for ICI were under 6%.[83]

Infertility and subfertility

Harms: Few adverse effects are reported if ovarian stimulation is not used. The fact that the child is not the man's genetic offspring may be difficult for couples to come to terms with.

Comment: Data are available from large databases, but it is sometimes unclear whether ovarian stimulation was also used. The live birth rate per cycle in the UK Human Fertilisation and Embryology Authority database (based on 7136 women) was 9%.[30] Similar rates are reported from the French donor insemination database (23 700 women over 4 years), with a mean pregnancy rate of 10.3% per cycle, and the Sheffield database (343 women, 980 treatment cycles), with an 11.3% overall live birth rate.[31,32] Comparisons of donor insemination versus no treatment or other interventions may be inappropriate as, for many couples, donor insemination is not an acceptable option. RCTs have tended to concentrate on comparisons between different techniques of donor insemination.

QUESTION What are the effects of treatment for unexplained infertility?

OPTION CLOMIPHENE

One systematic review of RCTs has found that in couples with unexplained infertility clomiphene doubles the rate of pregnancy. However, this is unlikely to result in appreciable clinical benefits as the background pregnancy rate is low. Another systematic review has found no evidence of benefit from clomiphene use in such couples.

Benefits: We found two systematic reviews.[94,95] The first (search date not stated) identified five placebo controlled trials, four using crossover designs, in women with unexplained infertility (458 cycles).[94] It found that clomiphene versus placebo significantly increased pregnancy rates per cycle (OR 2.5, 95% CI 1.4 to 4.6). When only cycles before crossover were included (which was only possible with the data from three of these trials), the positive effect increased (OR 5.0, 95% CI 1.8 to 14.3). A recent RCT was excluded from their analysis because of the risk of selection bias with a pseudo-random allocation method based on odd or even chart numbers.[96] Had this RCT been included, the OR for pregnancy per patient would have decreased to 1.7 (95% CI 1.0 to 2.7). The other systematic review (search date not stated, 22 RCTs in couples with persistent infertility) found no independent effect of clomiphene compared with no ovarian stimulation.[95]

Harms: See harms of clomiphene, p 1282.

Comment: The RCTs were generally of poor quality and it is possible that, if one further medium sized RCT was performed, the direction of the overall effect found with meta-analysis could change again. The reviews highlighted important differences between the trials: two RCTs included women with surgically treated endometriosis, one included only couples with primary infertility, and one included couples with a short duration of infertility (median of 28 months). Three of the trials included co-intervention with intrauterine insemination or cervicovaginal insemination. The trials also differed in their design (4 were crossover trials) and in the quality of randomisation (only 1 used properly concealed randomisation). The authors of the first systematic review comment that as the baseline cycle fecundity of the women included in these trials would only be about 1–2%, even with clomiphene their cycle fecundity is unlikely to exceed 5%.[94]

OPTION	INTRAUTERINE INSEMINATION

Systematic reviews have found that, in couples with unexplained infertility receiving FSH, intrauterine insemination increases the rate of pregnancy compared with timed intercourse. Two reviews have found that intrauterine insemination doubles the rate of pregnancy, although a third found that the apparent benefit disappears when intrauterine insemination is compared with intercourse timed favourably rather than late. One systematic review of RCTs has found that fallopian tube sperm perfusion almost doubles the pregnancy rate compared with intrauterine insemination.

Benefits: We found three systematic reviews.[33,34,95] The first (search date not stated) identified eight RCTs (number of treatment cycles not stated) comparing intrauterine insemination versus timed intercourse in couples with unexplained infertility receiving FSH.[95] In stimulated cycles, intrauterine insemination more than doubled the likelihood of pregnancy compared with timed intercourse (OR 2.4, 95% CI 1.4 to 3.9). The review also assessed the independent effects of FSH, clomiphene, and intrauterine insemination across 22 trials in couples with all causes of infertility. The likelihood of pregnancy was more than doubled with FSH (OR 2.4, 95% CI 1.9 to 2.9), and nearly trebled with intrauterine insemination (OR 2.8, 95% CI 2.2 to 3.7). Clomiphene did not increase the chances of pregnancy compared with no ovarian stimulation. The second review (search date 1997) identified seven RCTs (980 treatment cycles) comparing intrauterine insemination versus timed intercourse in couples with unexplained infertility (both interventions in addition to ovarian stimulation with gonadotrophins).[34] In stimulated cycles, intrauterine insemination achieved nearly twice the rate of pregnancy compared with timed intercourse (AR 10/549 cycles [20%] with intrauterine insemination v 49/431 cycles [11%] with timed intercourse; OR 1.8, 95% CI 1.3 to 2.6). The third systematic review (search date not stated) identified seven RCTs comparing intrauterine insemination versus timed intercourse or intracervical insemination in couples with unexplained infertility (934 treatment cycles).[33] Four RCTs used gonadotrophins, two used clomiphene, and three used no ovarian stimulation. There was no significant difference in pregnancy rates with intrauterine insemination versus intracervical insemination or timed intercourse (OR 1.5, 95% CI 1.0 to 2.2). The addition of ovarian stimulation with gonadotrophins to any of the three interventions increased the overall pregnancy rates (AR 45/249 [18%] with intrauterine insemination or favourable timed intracervical insemination or natural intercourse and gonadotrophin stimulation v 9/108 [8%] with unstimulated intrauterine insemination or favourable timed ICI/natural intercourse; RR 2.17, 95% CI 1.10 to 4.28; NNT 11, 95% CI 7 to 58). One RCT (932 couples with unexplained infertility), published after the reviews, compared intracervical insemination, intrauterine insemination, ovarian stimulation plus intracervical insemination, and ovarian stimulation plus intrauterine stimulation for four cycles or until pregnancy was achieved. It found pregnancy rates of 14 of 233 (6%) with intracervical insemination, 35 of 234 (15%) with intrauterine insemination, 26 of 234 (11%) with ovarian stimulation plus intracervical insemination, and 54 of 231 (23%) with ovarian stimulation plus intrauterine insemination.[97] Women treated with ovarian stimulation and intrauterine insemination were more likely to become pregnant than those in the intracervical insemination group (OR 3.2, 95% CI 2.0 to 5.3), and more likely than those in the intrauterine insemination group (OR 1.7, 95% CI 1.2 to 2.6). One small RCT (58 women, 174 cycles) suggests ovarian stimulation with clomiphene (50–100 mg, day 3–7 of cycle) was at least as effective as ovarian stimulation with human menopausal gonadotrophin (150 IU days 4, 6, 8, and 9) before intrauterine insemination for either unexplained, male factor or female factor infertility in terms of clinical pregnancy rate and live birth rate.[98] **Versus fallopian tube sperm perfusion:** Fallopian tube sperm perfusion is based on a pressure injection of 4 ml sperm suspension with an attempt to seal the cervix to prevent semen reflux. It ensures a sperm flushing of the fallopian tubes and an overflowing of the inseminate into the pouch of Douglas. We found one RCT (with a review and meta-analysis of previous trials), which identified five RCTs comparing fallopian tube sperm perfusion versus intrauterine insemination in couples with unexplained infertility.[99] All five studies used gonadotrophins or gonadotrophins in combination with clomiphene citrate. In total, 293 cycles of intrauterine insemination and 317 cycles of fallopian sperm perfusion were evaluated. Fallopian sperm perfusion almost doubled the pregnancy rate when compared with intrauterine insemination (AR 70/317 [22%] cycles with fallopian sperm perfusion v 38/293 [13%] with intrauterine insemination; RR 1.7, 95% CI 1.19 to 2.44; NNT 11, 95% CI 7 to 33). **Versus gamete intrafallopian transfer:** See option, p 1297. **Versus IVF:** One RCT randomised 258 couples with either unexplained infertility or male subfertility to six cycles of intrauterine insemination in natural cycles, to intrauterine insemination in stimulated cycles, or to IVF. Pregnancy rates per started treatment cycle were similar in all groups (7.4%, 8.7%, and 12.2%, respectively) with no differences between the different diagnostic groups. More couples in the IVF group failed to complete their six cycles of treatment, and cumulative pregnancy rates after six cycles did not differ significantly between treatment groups. Multiple pregnancy rates were 4%, 29%, and 21%, respectively. Mild ovarian hyperstimulation syndrome occurred in two women in the stimulated intrauterine insemination group, and severe ovarian hyperstimulation syndrome occurred in three women in the IVF group.[100]

Harms: Apart from the risks of ovarian hyperstimulation syndrome and multiple pregnancy associated with the ovarian stimulation (see harms of gonadotrophins, p 1284), intrauterine insemination may increase the likelihood of infection and may be associated with some discomfort. However, data from RCTs are scarce. A recent RCT (97 couples with unexplained infertility) compared low dose, step up FSH versus a conventional FSH regimen combined with intrauterine insemination.[101] There was no significant difference in pregnancy rates (AR 7/49 [14%] with low dose FSH and intrauterine insemination v 7/48 [15%] with conventional FSH and intrauterine insemination; RR 0.98, 95% CI 0.37 to 2.58), but the low dose group had significantly reduced incidence of ovarian hyperstimulation syndrome

(AR 4/49 [8%] with low dose FSH v 13/48 [27%] with conventional FSH; RR 0.3, 95% CI 0.11 to 0.86; NNT 6, 95% 3 to 28) and ovarian hyperstimulation syndrome requiring hospitalisation (0% v 16.7%). However, the low dose regimen did not completely prevent multiple pregnancies.

Comment: Only three of the RCTs were common to all three systematic reviews. One of the reviews scored the included studies for validity.[34] They scored from 49–70% when 100% was taken as the ideal study. The evidence from RCTs for timing and the optimum number of inseminations per cycle is conflicting (see intrauterine insemination, p 1295).

OPTION   GAMETE INTRAFALLOPIAN TRANSFER

We found limited evidence suggesting that gamete intrafallopian transfer is more effective than no treatment in couples with unexplained infertility. RCTs comparing it with other treatments (intrauterine insemination, timed intercourse, and IVF) found no evidence of a difference.

Benefits: **Versus no treatment:** We found no systematic review or RCTs. One prospective cohort study (99 treatment cycles, 53 couples) reported pregnancy rates in couples with unexplained infertility before and after gamete intrafallopian transfer. It found that treatment with gamete intrafallopian transfer resulted in more pregnancies compared with no treatment.[102] **Versus intrauterine insemination or timed intercourse:** We found no systematic review. We found three RCTs in 283 couples with unexplained infertility. The first compared gamete intrafallopian transfer versus ovarian stimulation plus either timed intercourse or timed cervical donor insemination[103] and found no significant difference. Of the other two RCTs, one found higher pregnancy rates with gamete intrafallopian transfer than with ovarian stimulation plus intrauterine insemination, and the other found no significant difference.[104,105] **Versus IVF:** See option below.

Harms: Potential harms include the risks attributable to general anaesthesia and laparoscopy. Multiple pregnancy rates vary with the number of oocytes transferred.

Comment: Gamete intrafallopian transfer, unlike IVF, gives no diagnostic information regarding fertilisation, and involves a laparoscopy and general anaesthetic, both of which are usually avoided with IVF. Success rates decrease with increasing age.[106,107]

OPTION   IN VITRO FERTILISATION

Limited data provide no evidence of a difference in pregnancy rates between IVF and gamete intrafallopian transfer in unexplained infertility.

Benefits: We found no systematic review. We found two RCTs in 155 couples with unexplained infertility.[93,108] Neither found a significant difference between gamete intrafallopian transfer and IVF.

Harms: See harms of IVF, p 1288.

Comment: The RCTs were too small to rule out a beneficial effect.

GLOSSARY

Laparoscopic ovarian drilling Ovarian drilling can be performed laparoscopically by either cautery or laser vaporisation (using CO_2, argon, or Nd:YAG lasers), which are used to create multiple perforations (about 10 holes/ovary) of the ovarian surface and stroma (inner area of the ovary). This is thought to cause ovulation by restoring the intraovarian hormonal environment to normal, which in turn beneficially affects the hypothalamic–pituitary–ovarian axis.

Ovarian hyperstimulation syndrome Can occur in mild, moderate, and severe forms. Mild ovarian hyperstimulation syndrome is characterised by fluid accumulation, as shown by weight gain, abdominal distension, and discomfort. Moderate ovarian hyperstimulation syndrome is associated with the development of nausea and vomiting in addition to ovarian enlargement, abdominal distension, discomfort, and dyspnoea. Severe ovarian hyperstimulation syndrome is a life-threatening condition in which there is contraction of the intravascular volume, tense ascites, pleural and pericardial effusions, severe haemoconcentration, and the development of hepatorenal failure. Deaths have occurred caused usually by cerebrovascular thrombosis, renal failure, or cardiac tamponade.

Substantive changes since last issue

Gonadotrophins for ovulation disorders New systematic review[46] found no difference in pregnancy rates, with subfertility associated with polycystic ovarian syndrome, between treatment with human menopausal gonadotrophin and urinary derived FSH. Lack of placebo controlled trials or trials against a known effective treatment. Reclassified as "unknown effectiveness".

Gonadotrophins for ovulation disorders New RCT[50] found no difference in birth rates between treatment with recombinant FSH and urinary FSH.

Clomiphene for unexplained fertility Updated systematic review[94] found that clomiphene doubled the pregnancy rate in couples with unexplained infertility.

REFERENCES

1. European Society for Human Reproduction and Embryology. Guidelines to the prevalence, diagnosis, treatment and management of infertility, 1996. *Hum Reprod* 1996;11:1775–1807.
2. Schmidt L, Munster K. Infertility, involuntary infecundity, and the seeking of medical advice in industrialized countries 1970–1992: a review of concepts, measurements and results. *Hum Reprod* 1995;10:1407–1418.
3. Effective Health Care. The management of subfertility. *Effective Health Care Bulletin* 1992;3: 13. Search date and primary sources not stated.
4. Collins JA, Burrows EA, Willan AR. The prognosis for live birth among untreated infertile couples. *Fertil Steril* 1995;64:22–28.
5. Templeton A, Morris JK. — factors affecting outcome. In: Templeton A, Cooke ID, O'Brien PMS, eds. *35th RCOG study group evidence-based fertility treatment*. London: RCOG Press, 1998.
6. Khan KS, Daya S, Collins JA, Walter SD. Empirical evidence of bias in infertility research: overestimation of treatment effect in crossover trials using pregnancy as the outcome measure. *Fertil Steril* 1996;65:939–945.
7. Cohlen BJ, te Velde ER, Looman CW, Eijckemans R, Habbema JD. Crossover or parallel design in infertility trials? The discussion continues. *Fertil Steril* 1998;70:40–45.
8. Benadiva CA, Kligman I, Davis O, Rosenwaks Z. In vitro fertilization versus tubal surgery: is pelvic reconstructive surgery obsolete? *Fertil Steril* 1995; 64:1051–1061.
9. Holst N, Maltau JM, Forsdahl F, Hansen LJ. Handling of tubal infertility after introduction of in vitro fertilization: changes and consequences.

Fertil Steril 1991;55:140–143.
10. Vilos GA, Verhoest CR, Martin JS, Botz C. Economic evaluation of in vitro fertilization-embryo transfer and neosalpingostomy for bilateral tubal obstruction. *J Soc Obstet Gynecol Can* 1998;20: 139–147.
11. Meirow D, Schenker JG. Appraisal of Gift. *Eur J Obstet Gynecol Reprod* 1995;58:59–65.
12. Kurinczuk J, Bower C. Birth defects in infants conceived by intracytoplasmic sperm injection: an alternative interpretation. *BMJ* 1997;315:1260–1265.
13. Hughes E, Collins J, Vandekerckhove P. Clomiphene citrate vs placebo for ovulation induction in oligo-amenorrhoiec women. In: The Cochrane Library, Issue 4, 1999. Oxford: Update Software. Search date not stated; primary source Cochrane Subfertility Group Register of Controlled Trials.
14. Venn A, Watson L, Lumley J, Giles G, King C, Healy D. Breast and ovarian cancer incidence after infertility and IVF. *Lancet* 1995;346:995–1000.
15. Hughes E, Collins J, Vandekerckhove P. Ovulation induction with urinary follicle stimulating hormone vs human menopausal gonadotrophin for clomiphene-resistant polycystic ovary syndrome. In: The Cochrane Library, Issue 4, 1999. Oxford: Update Software. Search date not stated; primary source Cochrane Subfertility Group Register of Controlled Trials.
16. Wang CF, Gemzell C. The use of human gonadotrophins for the induction of ovulation in women with polycystic ovarian disease. *Fertil Steril* 1980;33:479–486.
17. Farquhar C, Vandekerckhove P, Arnot M, Lilford R. Polycystic ovary syndrome: laparoscopic "drilling"

by diathermy or laser for ovulation induction in patients with anovulatory polycystic ovarian syndrome. In: The Cochrane Library, Issue 4, 1999. Oxford: Update Software. Search date not stated; primary source Cochrane Menstrual Disorders and Subfertility Group Register of Controlled Trials.

18. RCOG Infertility Guideline Group. *The management of infertility in secondary care.* London: RCOG, 1998. Primary Sources Medline, Embase, Cochrane Library, hand searching major journals.

19. Winston RM, Margara RA. Microsurgical salpingostomy is not an obsolete procedure. *Br J Obstet Gynaecol* 1991;98:637–642.

20. Singhal V, Li TC, Cooke ID. An analysis of factors influencing the outcome of 232 consecutive tubal microsurgery cases. *Br J Obstet Gynaecol* 1991; 98:628–636.

21. Marana R, Quagliarello J. Distal tubal occlusion: microsurgery versus in vitro fertilization: a review. *Int J Fertil* 1988;33:107–115.

22. Marana R, Quagliarello J. Proximal tubal occlusion: microsurgery versus IVF: a review. *Int J Fertil* 1988;33:338–340.

23. Patton PE, Williams TJ, Coulam CB. Results of microsurgical reconstruction in patients with combined proximal and distal occlusion: double obstruction. *Fertil Steril* 1987;47:670–674.

24. Wahab M, Li TC, Cooke ID. Reversal of sterilization versus IVF. *J Obstet Gynaecol* 1997;17:180–185.

25. Hughes EG, Fedorkow DM, Collins J. A quantitative overview of controlled trials in endometriosis-associated infertility. *Fertil Steril* 1993;59:963–970. Search date not stated; primary sources Medline 1966 to 1992; Science Citation Index January 1986 to December 1989; abstracts from scientific meetings 1986 to 1992; and hand searches of relevant trials and personal contacts.

26. Adamson GD, Pasta DJ. Surgical treatment of endometriosis-associated infertility: meta-analysis compared with survival analysis. *Am J Obstet Gynecol* 1994;171:1488–1504.

27. Marcoux S, Maheux R, Berube S. Laparoscopic surgery in infertile women with minimal or mild endometriosis. *N Engl J Med* 1997;337:217–222.

28. Chapron C, Querleu D, Bruhat M, et al. Surgical complications of diagnostic and operative gynaecological laparoscopy: a series of 29 966 cases. *Hum Reprod* 1998;13:867–872.

29. Geber S, Paraschos T, Atkinson G, Margara M, Winston RML. Results of IVF in patients with endometriosis: the severity of the disease does not affect outcome or the incidence of miscarriage. *Hum Reprod* 1995;10:1507–1511.

30. Human Fertilisation and Embryology Authority. Sixth Annual Report 1997. London: HFEA, 1998.

31. Le Lannou D, Lansac J. Artificial procreation with frozen donor sperm: the French experience of CECOS. In: Barratt CLR, Cooke ID, eds. *Donor insemination.* Cambridge: Cambridge University Press, 1993;152–169.

32. Cooke ID. Donor insemination – timing and insemination method. In: Templeton A, Cooke ID, O'Brien PMS, eds. *35th RCOG Study Group evidence-based fertility treatment.* London: RCOG Press, 1998.

33. Ford WCL, Mathur RS, Hull MGR. Intrauterine insemination: is it an effective treatment for male factor infertility? *Balliere Clin Obstet Gynecol* 1997;11:691–710. Search date not stated; primary sources Medline; BIDS; and manual scanning of leading reproductive journals.

34. Zeyneloglu HB, Arici A, Olive DL, Duleba AJ. Comparison of intrauterine insemination with timed intercourse in superovulated cycles with gonadotrophins: a meta-analysis. *Fertil Steril* 1998; 69:486–491. Search date 1997; primary sources Medline and hand searches of bibliographies of relevant publications and review articles.

35. Buvat J, Buvat-Herbaut M, Marcolin G, Ardaens-Boulier K. Antiestrogens as treatment of female and male infertilities. *Horm Res* 1987;28:219–229.

36. Messinis IE, Nillius SJ. Comparison between tamoxifen and clomiphene for induction of ovulation. *Acta Obstet Gynecol Scand* 1982;61: 377–379.

37. Gerhard I, Runnebaum B. Comparison between tamoxifen and clomiphene therapy in women with anovulation. *Arch Gynecol* 1979;227:279–288.

38. Rossing MA, Daling JR, Weiss NS, Moore DE, Self SG. Ovarian tumours in a cohort of infertile women. *N Engl J Med* 1994;331:771–776.

39. Parazzini F, Negri E, La Vecchia C, Moroni S, Franceschi S, Crosignani PG. Treatment for infertility and risk of invasive epithelial ovarian cancer. *Hum Reprod* 1997;12:2159–2161.

40. Mosgaard BJ, Lidegaard O, Kjaer SK, Schou G, Andersen AN. Infertility, fertility drugs, and invasive ovarian cancer: a case-control study. *Fertil Steril* 1997;67:1005–1012.

41. Shushan A, Paltiel O, Iscovich J, Elchalal U, Peretz T, Schenker JG. Human menopausal gonadotrophin and the risk of epithelial ovarian cancer. *Fertil Steril* 1996;65:13–18.

42. Dunn A, Macfarlane A. Recent trends in the incidence of multiple births and associated mortality in England and Wales. *Arch Dis Child Fetal Neonatal Ed* 1996;75:F10–19.

43. State-specific variation in rates of twin births — United States, 1992–1994. *MMWR Morb Mortal Wkly Rep* 1997;46:121–125.

44. Levene MI, Wild J, Steer P. Higher multiple births and the modern management of infertility in Britain. British Association of Perinatal Medicine. *Br J Obstet Gynaecol* 1992;99:607–613.

45. Cabau A, Krulik DR. Sterilites de cause hormonale et sterilites inexpliquees. Traitement par le cyclofenil. Etude controlee a double insu. *J Gynecol Obstet Biol Reprod* 1990;19:96–101.

46. Nugent D, Vandekerckhove P, Hughes E, Arnot M, Lilford R. Gonadotrophin therapy for ovulation induction in subfertility associated with polycystic ovarian syndrome. In: The Cochrane Library, Issue 4, 2000. Oxford: Update Software.

47. Coelingh-Bennink HJ, Fauser BC, Out HJ. Recombinant follicle-stimulating hormone (FSH; Puregon) is more efficient than urinary follicle stimulating hormone (Metrodin) in women with clomiphene-resistant, normogonadotrophic, chronic anovulation: a prospective, multicenter, assessor-blind, randomized, clinical trial. European Puregon collaborative anovulation study group. *Fertil Steril* 1998;69:19–25.

48. Yarali H, Bukulmez O, Gurgan T. Urinary follicle stimulating hormone (FSH) versus recombinant FSH in clomiphene citrate resistant normogonadotropic, chronic anovulation: a prospective randomised study. *Fertil Steril* 1999; 72:276–281.

49. Daya S, Gunby J. Recombinant versus urinary follicle stimulating hormone for ovarian stimulation in assisted reproduction. *Hum Reprod* 1999;14: 2207–2215. Search date 1999; primary sources Medline; Excerpta Medica Fertility Database; and hand searches of article bibliographies and meeting abstracts.

50. Nardo LG, Bellanca SA, Messina K, Nardo F. Efficacy of recombinant follicle stimulating hormone versus urinary follicle stimulating hormone in in-vitro fertilization: A prospective, randomized, assessor-blind study. *Ital J Gynaecol Obstet* 2000;12:49–53.

51. Bayram N, van Wely M, Vandekerckhove P, Lilford R, van der Veen F. Pulsatile luteinising hormone

releasing hormone for ovulation induction in subfertility associated with polycystic ovary syndrome. In: The Cochrane Library, Issue 4, 1999. Oxford: Update Software. Search date not stated; primary sources Cochrane Menstrual Disorders and Subfertility Group Register of Controlled Trials, and hand searches of reference lists of included trials.

52. Balen AH, Braat DD, West C, Patel A, Jacobs HS. Cumulative conception and live birth rates after the treatment of anovulatory infertility: safety and efficacy of ovulation induction in 200 patients. Hum Reprod 1994;9:1563–1570.

53. Braat DD, Schoemaker R, Schoemaker J. Life table analysis of fecundity in intravenously gonadotropin-releasing hormone-treated patients with normogonadotropic and hypogonadotropic amenorrhea. Fertil Steril 1991;55:266–271.

54. Filicori M, Flamigni C, Dellai P, et al. Treatment of anovulation with pulsatile gonadotropin-releasing hormone: prognostic factors and clinical results in 600 cycles. J Clin Endocrinol Metab 1994;79:1215–1220.

55. Martin KA, Hall JE, Adams JM, Crowley WF Jr. Comparison of exogenous gonadotropins and pulsatile gonadotropin-releasing hormone for induction of ovulation in hypogonadotropic amenorrhea. J Clin Endocrinol Metab 1993;77:125–129.

56. Honore GM, Holden AE, Schenken RS. Pathophysiology and management of proximal tubal blockage. Fertil Steril 1999;71:785–795. Search date not stated; primary sources Medline, Science Citation Index.

57. Ransom MX, Garcia AJ. Surgical management of cornual-isthmic tubal obstruction. Fertil Steril 1997;68:887–891.

58. Thurmond AS. Pregnancies after selective salpingography and tubal recanalization. Radiology 1994;190:11–13.

59. Marana R. Proximal tubal obstruction: are we overdiagnosing and overtreating? Gynaecol Endoscopy 1992;1:99–101.

60. Filippini F, Darai E, Benifla JL, et al. Distal tubal surgery: a critical review of 104 laparoscopic distal tuboplasties. J Gynecol Obstet Biol Reprod 1996;25:471–478.

61. Donnez J, Casanas-Roux F. Prognostic factors of fimbrial microsurgery. Fertil Steril 1986;46:200–204.

62. Tomazevic T, Ribic-Pucelj M, Omahen A, Colja B. Microsurgery and in vitro fertilization and embryo transfer for infertility resulting from pathological proximal tubal blockage. Hum Reprod 1996;11:2613–2617.

63. Wu CH, Gocial B. A pelvic scoring system for infertility surgery. Int J Fertil 1988;33:341–346.

64. Oelsner G, Sivan E, Goldenberg M, Carp HJ, Admon D, Mashiach S. Should lysis of adhesions be performed when in vitro fertilization and embryo transfer are available? Hum Reprod 1994;9:2339–2341.

65. Watson A, Vandekerchove P, Lilford R. Techniques for tubal surgery. In: The Cochrane Library, Issue 4, 1999. Oxford: Update Software. Search date not stated; primary source Cochrane Menstrual Disorders and Subfertility Group Register of Controlled Trials.

66. Johnson NP, Watson A. Postoperative procedures for improving fertility following pelvic reproductive surgery. In: The Cochrane Library, Issue 1, 2000. Oxford: Update Software. Search date not stated; primary source Cochrane Menstrual Disorders and Subfertility Group Register of Controlled trials.

67. Gillett WR, Clarke RH, Herbison GP. First and subsequent pregnancies after tubal surgery:

evaluation of the fertility index. Fertil Steril 1998;68:1033–1042.

68. Jarrell J, Labelle R, Goeree R, Milner R, Collins J. In vitro fertilization and embryo transfer: a randomized controlled trial. Online J Curr Clin Trials 1993;2:Doc 73

69. Soliman S, Daya S, Collins J, Jarrell J. A randomized trial of in vitro fertilization versus conventional treatment for infertility. Fertil Steril 1993;59:1239–1244.

70. Bukulmez O, Yarali H, Yucel A, Sari T, Gurgan T. Intracytoplasmic sperm injection versus in vitro fertilization for patients with a tubal factor as their sole cause of infertility: a prospective, randomized trial. Fertil Steril 2000;73:38–42.

71. Brinsden PR, Wada I, Tan SL, Balen A, Jacobs HS. Diagnosis, prevention and management of ovarian hyperstimulation syndrome. Br J Obstet Gynaecol 1995;102:767–772.

72. Centers for Disease Control and Prevention. US Department of Health and Human Services. 1995 Assisted Reproductive Technology Success Rates. National Summary and Fertility Clinic Reports 1997;1–23.

73. Chapko KM, Weaver MR, Chapko MK, Pasta D, Adamson GD. Stability of in vitro fertilization-embryo transfer success rates from the 1989,1990, and 1991 clinic-specific outcome assessments. Fertil Steril 1995;64:757–763.

74. Camus E, Poncelet C, Goffinet F, et al. Pregnancy rates after in vitro fertilization in cases of tubal infertility with and without hydrosalpinx: a meta-analysis of published comparative studies. Hum Reprod 1999;14:1243–1249. Search date not stated; primary sources Medline and Cochrane Database of Systematic Reviews.

75. Hughes E, Fedorkow D, Collins J, Vandekerckhove P. Ovulation suppression for endometriosis. In: The Cochrane Library, Issue 3, 2000. Oxford: Update Software. Search date not stated; primary source Cochrane Subfertility Group Register of Controlled Trials.

76. Dockeray CJ, Sheppard BL, Bonnar J. Comparison between mefenamic acid and danazol in the treatment of established menorrhagia. Br J Obstet Gynaecol 1989;96:840–844.

77. Tummon IS, Asher LJ, Martin JSB, Tulandi T. Randomized controlled trial of superovulation and insemination for infertility associated with minimal or mild endometriosis. Fertil Steril 1997;68:8–12.

78. Fedele L, Bianchi S, Marchini M, Villa L, Brioschi D, Parazzini F. Superovulation with human menopausal gonadotrophins in the treatment of infertility associated with endometriosis: a controlled randomised study. Fertil Steril 1992;58:28–31.

79. Nulsen JC, Walsh S, Dumez S. A randomised and longitudinal study of human menopausal gonadotrophin with intrauterine insemination in the treatment of infertility. Obstet Gynaecol 1993;82:780–786.

80. Parazzini F. Ablation of lesions or no treatment in minimal-mild endometriosis in infertile women: a randomized trial. Gruppo Italiano per lo Studio dell'Endometriosi. Hum Reprod 1999;14:1332–1334.

81. Olivennes F, Feldberg D, Liu H-C, Cohen J, Moy F, Rosenwaks Z. Endometriosis: a stage by stage analysis — the role of in vitro fertilization. Fertil Steril 1995;64:392–398.

82. Cohlen BJ, Vandekerckhove P, te Velde ER, Habbema JDF. Timed intercourse versus intra-uterine insemination with or without ovarian hyperstimulation for subfertility in men. In: The Cochrane Library, Issue 4, 1999. Oxford: Update Software. Search date 1996/1997; primary sources Medline; Embase; DDFU; Biosis; SciSearch; handsearching; and conference abstracts.

83. O'Brien P, Vandekerckhove P. Intra-uterine versus cervical insemination of donor sperm for subfertility. In: The Cochrane Library, Issue 3, 2000. Oxford: Update Software. Search date not stated; primary source Cochrane Subfertility Group Specialist Register of Controlled Trials.

84. Ragni G, Maggioni P, Guermandi E, et al. Efficacy of double intrauterine insemination in controlled ovarian hyperstimulation cycles. Fertil Steril 1999; 72:619–622.

85. Silverberg KM, Johnson JV, Olive DL, Burns WN, Schenken RS. A prospective, randomized trial comparing two different intrauterine insemination regimens in controlled ovarian hyperstimulation cycles. Fertil Steril 1992;576:357–361.

86. Ransom MX, Blotner MB, Bohrer M, Corsan G, Kemmann E. Does increasing frequency of intrauterine insemination improve pregnancy rates significantly during superovulation cycles? Fertil Steril 1994;61:303–307.

87. Zreik TG, Garcia-Velasco JA, Habboosh MS, Olive DL, Arici A. Prospective, randomized, crossover study to evaluate the benefit of human chorionic gonadotrophin-timed versus urinary luteinising hormone-timed intrauterine inseminations in clomiphene citrate-stimulated treatment cycles. Fertil Steril 1998;71:1070–1074.

88. van Rumste MME, Evers JLH, Farquhar CM, Blake DA. Intra-cytoplasmic sperm injection versus partial zona dissection, subzonal insemination and conventional techniques for oocyte insemination during IVF. In: The Cochrane Library, Issue 4, 1999. Oxford: Update Software. Search date not stated; primary source Cochrane Menstrual Disorders and Subfertility Group Specialised Register of Controlled Trials.

89. Bonduelle M, Legein J, Buyesse A, Van Assche E, Wisanto A, Devroey P. Prospective follow-up study of 423 children born after intracytoplasmic sperm injection. Hum Reprod 1996;11:1558–1564.

90. Bonduelle M, Legein J, Derde M, et al. Comparative follow-up study of 130 children born after ICSI and 130 children born after IVF. Hum Reprod 1995;10:3327–3331.

91. Velde E, van Baar R, van Kooije R. Concerns about assisted reproduction. Lancet 1998;351: 1524–1525.

92. de Wert G. Ethics of intracytoplasmic sperm injection: proceed with care. Hum Reprod 1998; 13(suppl 1):219–227.

93. Leeton J, Healy D, Rogers P. A controlled study between the use game intrafallopian transfer (GIFT) and in vitro fertilization and embryo transfer in the management of idiopathic and male infertility. Fertil Steril 1987;48:605–607.

94. Hughes E, Collins J, Vandekerckhove P. Clomiphene citrate for unexplained subfertility in women. In: The Cochrane Library, Issue 4, 2000. Oxford: Update Software. Search date May 2000; primary sources Cochrane Menstrual Disorders and Subfertility Review Group specialised register of controlled trials; Medline; Embase; and CINAHL.

95. Hughes EG. The effectiveness of ovulation induction and intrauterine insemination in the treatment of persistent infertility: a meta-analysis. Hum Reprod 1997;12:1865–1872. Search date not stated; primary source Cochrane Menstrual Disorders and Subfertility Group's register of controlled trials.

96. Fujii S, Fukui A, Fukushi Y, Kagiya A, Saito Y. The effects of clomiphene citrate on normally ovulatory women. Fertil Steril 1997;68:997–999.

97. Guzick DS, Carson SA, Coutifaris C, et al. Efficacy of superovulation and intrauterine insemination in the treatment of infertility. National Cooperative Reproductive Medicine Network. N Engl J Med 1999;340:177–183.

98. Ecochard R, Mathieu C, Royere D, Blache G, Rabilloud M, Czyba JC. A randomized prospective study comparing pregnancy rates after clomiphene citrate and human menopausal gonadotrophin before intrauterine insemination. Fertil Steril 2000;73:90–93.

99. Trout SW, Kemmann E. Fallopian sperm perfusion versus intrauterine insemination: a randomized controlled trial and meta-analysis of the literature. Fertil Steril 1999;71:881–885. Search date not stated; primary source Medline.

100. Goverde AJ, McDonnell J, Vermeiden JPW, Schats R, Rutten FFH, Schoemaker J. Intrauterine insemination or in vitro fertilisation in idiopathic subfertility and male subfertility: a randomised trial and cost-effectiveness analysis. Lancet 2000;355:13–18.

101. Sengoku K, Tamate K, Takaoka Y, et al. The clinical efficacy of low-dose step-up follicle stimulating hormone administration for treatment of unexplained infertility. Hum Reprod 1999;14: 349–353.

102. Murdoch AP, Harris M, Mahroo M, Williams M, Dunlop W. Is GIFT (gamete intrafallopian transfer) the best treatment for unexplained infertility. Br J Obstet Gynaecol 1991;98:643–647.

103. Hogerzeil HV, Spiekerman JCM, de Vries JWA, de Schepper G. A randomized trial between GIFT and ovarian stimulation for the treatment of unexplained infertility and failed artificial insemination by donor. Hum Reprod 1992;7: 1235–1239.

104. Murdoch AP, Harris M, Mahroo M, Williams M, Dunlop W. Gamete intrafallopian transfer (GIFT) compared with intrauterine insemination in the treatment of unexplained infertility. Br J Obstet Gynaecol 1991;98:1107–1111.

105. Wessels PHX, Cronje HS, Oosthuizen AP, Trumpelmann MD, Grobler S, Hamlett DK. Cost-effectiveness of gamete intrafallopian transfer in comparison with induction of ovulation with gonadotrophins in the treatment of female infertility: a clinical trial. Fertil Steril 1992;57: 163–167.

106. Rombauts L, Dear M, Breheny S, Healy DL. Cumulative pregnancy rates and live birth rates after gamete intra-fallopian transfer. Hum Reprod 1997;12:1338–1342.

107. Society for Assisted Reproductive Technology and the American Society for Reproductive Medicine. Assisted reproductive technology in the United States and Canada: 1995 results generated from the American Society for Reproductive Medicine/ Society for Assisted Reproductive Technology Registry. Fertil Steril 1998;69:389–398.

108. Ranieri M, Beckett VA, Marchant S, Kinis A, Serhal P. Gamete intra-fallopian transfer or in vitro fertilization after failed ovarian stimulation and intrauterine insemination in unexplained infertility. Hum Reprod 1995;10:2023–2026.

Kirsten Duckitt
Clinical Lecturer
John Radcliffe Hospital
Oxford, UK

Competing interests: None declared.

TABLE 1 Comparative success rates of treatments for infertility: evidence from RCTs and analysis of database data (see text, p 1283, p 1285).

Treatment	Live birth rates	Pregnancy rates	Adverse effects
All causes of infertility			
IVF (per treated cycle)	UK 15%; US 20%[5]	59–77% (with 3–5 treatment cycles)[8]	Ectopic pregnancy: 1–3%[9,10]
GIFT (per cycle) (not including tubal infertility)	23%[11]	–	23%[12]
Infertility caused by ovulation disorders			
Clomiphene to induce ovulation in amenorrhoeic women (cumulative rate after 11 cycles of treatment)		90% 33 times more likely than with placebo[13]	Risk of ovarian cancer, unproved.[14] MP: 2–13%, mostly twins. OHSS: infrequent and mild
Gonadotrophins to induce ovulation in clomiphene resistant women (cumulative rate after four months of treatment)		27–40%[3,15]	Risk of ovarian cancer, unproved.[14] MP: 29%[16] OHSS: 4%
PCOS (cumulative rate after four months of treatment)		FSH 27%[15]	
Laparoscopic drilling (cumulative rate 1–2 years after treatment)		48%[17,18]	Risks of laparoscopy, general anaesthesia, and adhesions. Risk of premature ovarian failure unproved
Tubal infertility			
Tubal surgery for distal occlusion (cumulative rate 2 years after surgery)	20–30%[19-21]		Risks of general anaesthesia. Ectopic pregnancy: 7–9%[9,10]
Tubal surgery for proximal occlusion (cumulative rate)	40–60%[22,23]		
Reversal of female sterilisation (cumulative live birth rate 1–2 years after surgery)	50–90%[24] depending on method used for sterilisation		
Infertility associated with endometriosis			
Surgery (per cycle)		13–38%†[25-27,29]	Risks of surgery and general anaesthesia (for laparoscopic surgery). Mortality 3.33/100 000; complication rate 3.2/1000[28]
Male infertility			
IUI ± ovarian stimulation (per cycle)			
ICSI plus IVF (per cycle)	20%[5]	6.5%[33]	
Donor insemination* (per cycle)	9–12%[30-32]		No adverse effects if no ovarian stimulation is given, but child is not male partner's genetic offspring
Unexplained infertility			
IUI ± ovarian stimulation (per cycle)		9–12% without stimulation; 19–20% with stimulation[33,34]	

*Using frozen donor sperm in women without female factor or with corrected female factor infertility; †over spontaneous rate; MP, multiple pregnancy; GIFT, gamete intrafallopian transfer; ICSI, intracytoplasmic sperm injection; IVF, in vitro fertilisation; IUI, intrauterine insemination; OHSS, ovarian hyperstimulsyndrome; PCOS, polycystic ovary syndrome.

Search date October 2000

Janice Rymer and Edward Morris

QUESTIONS

INTERVENTIONS

Key Messages

- Systematic reviews of RCTs have found that oestrogen relieves symptoms of urogenital atrophy and vasomotor symptoms. RCTs have found that oestrogen improves quality of life in the short term.
- Pooled estimates from observational studies have found that long term use of oestrogen is associated with an increased risk of thromboembolic disease, and endometrial and breast cancers.
- RCTs have found that:
  - Progestogens relieve vasomotor symptoms when used in high doses.
  - Tibolone relieves vasomotor symptoms and improves sexual symptoms.
  - Clonidine reduces hot flushes.
- Limited evidence from small RCTs suggests that soy flour, which contains phyto-oestrogens, might relieve vasomotor menopausal symptoms.
- We found insufficient evidence on the effects of testosterone and antidepressants on menopausal symptoms.

DEFINITION Menopause is defined as the end of the last menstrual period. A woman is deemed to be postmenopausal 1 year after her last period. For practical purposes most women are diagnosed as menopausal after 1 year of amenorrhoea. Menopausal symptoms often begin in the perimenopausal years.

INCIDENCE/ PREVALENCE In the UK, the mean age for the start of the menopause is 50 years and 9 months. The median onset of the perimenopause is between 45.5 and 47.5 years. One Scottish survey (6096 women aged 45–54 years) found that 84% of women had experienced at least one of the classic menopausal symptoms, with 45% finding one or more symptoms a problem.[1]

AETIOLOGY/ RISK FACTORS Urogenital symptoms of menopause are caused by decreased oestrogen concentrations, but the cause of vasomotor symptoms and psychological effects is complex and remains unclear.

PROGNOSIS Menopause is a physiological event. Its timing may be determined genetically. Although endocrine changes are permanent, menopausal symptoms such as hot flushes, which are experienced by about 70% of women, usually resolve with time.[2] However, some symptoms may remain the same or worsen, for example genital atrophy.

AIMS To reduce or prevent menopausal symptoms; and to improve quality of life, with minimum adverse effects.

OUTCOMES Frequency and severity of vasomotor, urogenital, and psychological symptoms; quality of life.

METHODS *Clinical Evidence* update search and appraisal October 2000. We included only RCTs and systematic reviews that met *Clinical Evidence* quality criteria.

QUESTION What are the effects of medical treatments?

OPTION OESTROGENS

Over 50 RCTs have found that oestrogen improves vasomotor symptoms. Systematic reviews of RCTs have found that oestrogen improves urogenital symptoms and depressed mood. Important adverse effects include venous thromboembolic disease, breast cancer, and endometrial cancer.

Benefits: **Vasomotor symptoms:** We found no systematic review. We found over 50 RCTs comparing oestrogen versus placebo and versus each other. Most found that oestrogen reduced vasomotor symptoms (data from one five arm RCT in 875 women, oral conjugated equine estrogen versus placebo: OR 0.53, 95% CI 0.31 to 0.93).[3] Two RCTs found that transdermal oestrogen at a low dose of 25 µg daily reduced severity of vasomotor symptoms compared with placebo.[4,5] **Urogenital system:** We found one systematic review (search date 1995)[6] and four subsequent RCTs.[4,7–9] The review pooled data from six RCTs. It found that oestrogen improved urogenital symptoms regardless of the route of administration (no figures available). One subsequent RCT (136 women) found that low dose transdermal oestrogen (25 µg daily) plus norethisterone acetate significantly reduced vaginal dryness and dyspareunia compared with placebo over 6 months.[4] The second subsequent RCT (145 women) found that low dose 17 β-oestradiol (1 mg or 0.5 mg daily) versus placebo was associated with a higher number of days without vaginal dryness (at weeks 9–12, 1 mg β-oestradiol 86.1% v 0.5 mg β-oestradiol 76.1% v placebo 73.8%), but significance was not tested.[9] Two other RCTs (192 women) found that local administration of oestrogen using a silicone oestradiol releasing vaginal ring over 24–36 weeks improved vaginal oestrogenisation and pH compared with placebo.[7,8] One of these trials also found a significant reduction in incidence of urinary tract infection in treated women (P = 0.008).[7] **Psychological symptoms:** We found one systematic review (search date 1995, 14 RCTs, 12 cohort studies), which found that oestrogen reduced depressed mood among menopausal women.[10] Duration of treatment ranged from 1 month to 2 years. Data pooling for oestrogen versus placebo (10 studies) found that oestrogen reduced depressive symptoms (no figures available). We found no RCTs of oestrogen treatment in women with clinically proven depression. We found one systematic review (search date 1996, 10 controlled trials and 9 observational studies) of the effects of oestrogen on cognitive function in postmenopausal women and women with Alzheimer's disease.[11] Studies were too weak to allow reliable conclusions. An additional crossover RCT (62 women) found a beneficial effect of oestrogen on sleep quality compared with placebo over 7 months.[12] **Quality of life:** We found no systematic review. We found four RCTs (639 women, 3 placebo controlled RCTs, 3 v progestogen), which found significant improvement in quality of life in women treated with oestrogen compared with baseline or placebo.[13–16] The largest RCT (242 women) found that oestrogen improved quality of life (P = 0.0003) and wellbeing (P = 0.003) compared with placebo over 12 weeks.[13]

Harms: Many RCTs have found that oestrogen causes weight gain and breast tenderness in the short term. Although many women report an increase in weight when starting oestrogen, we found no evidence from RCTs that oestrogen causes significant weight gain in the long term. The most important long term adverse effects are increased risk of venous thromboembolic disease (see hormone replacement therapy [HRT] under prevention of ischaemic cardiac events, p 95), endometrial cancer, and breast cancer.[17–20] One systematic review (search date not stated) reanalysed 51 studies of more than 160 000 women of the relation between oestrogen (as HRT) and breast cancer. It found that the risk of breast cancer increased by 2.3% (95% CI 1.1% to 3.6%) each year in women using HRT.[21] Five or more years after HRT was stopped, there was no significant excess of breast cancer.[21] One systematic review of the effects of HRT (18 RCTs, 5247 women) found significant risks of endometrial hyperplasia in women taking unopposed oestrogen (OR 5.4, 95% CI 1.4 to 20.9 for 6 months' treatment; OR 16.0, 95% CI 9.3 to 27.5, for 36 months' treatment).[20] The review also found significant reductions in the incidence of hyperplasia when women are given progestogens, either cyclically or continuously, with continuous combined HRT having the greatest effect (OR 0.3, 95% CI

0.09 to 0.97). One recent systematic review (search date 1998) of 22 studies has found no effect of either unopposed or combined HRT on body weight.[17]

Comment: Many studies used selected populations, such as women attending hospital clinics, who may be different in their behaviour, personality, and symptom profile to women of the same age seen in primary care or those who do not seek medical advice.

OPTION   PROGESTOGENS

We found good evidence from RCTs that progestogens reduce vasomotor symptoms. We found no good quality evidence on other outcomes, including quality of life.

Benefits: We found no systematic review. **Vasomotor symptoms:** We found five RCTs (257 women, all trials less than a year in duration), which found that women taking progestogens experienced a significant reduction in vasomotor symptoms compared with placebo.[22–26] One RCT comparing oestrogen alone versus progesterone (150 mg of depot medroxyprogesterone for 25 days a month) found that over 3 months, 18% of women taking oestrogen and 33% taking progestogen reported no vasomotor symptoms.[23] One RCT (102 women) found that transdermal progesterone cream 20 mg daily improved vasomotor symptoms compared with placebo ($P < 0.001$).[27] **Urogenital system:** We found no RCTs evaluating the effects of progestogens alone on urinary incontinence, the lower genital tract, or sex life. **Psychological symptoms:** We found no RCTs. **Quality of life:** One RCT of cyclical progestogen plus oestrogen versus oestrogen alone for 6 months found no evidence of an effect on quality of life.[28] We found no studies of progestogen alone on quality of life.

Harms: We found two RCTs that evaluated harms of progestogens. The first compared continuous progestogen (norgestrel) versus placebo in 321 women who had undergone hysterectomy and were already taking conjugated oestrogen. The trial found no difference in symptoms (including weight gain and bloating).[29] The second RCT (875 women) compared various oestrogen/progestogen combinations over 3 years.[3] It found that additional progestogen increased breast discomfort (OR 1.92, 95% CI 1.16 to 3.09). Neither trial found evidence of an effect on cardiovascular events.

Comment: Progestogen is seldom given alone, which makes it hard to isolate its effects. When given without oestrogen, doses of progestogens were high, the lowest dose being 20 mg medroxyprogesterone acetate a day.

OPTION   TIBOLONE

RCTs have found that tibolone significantly improve vasomotor symptoms, libido, and vaginal lubrication.

Benefits: We found no systematic review. **Vasomotor symptoms:** We found three RCTs, two of tibolone versus continuous combined oestrogen/progestogen treatment over 48 and 52 weeks (672 women with menopausal symptoms)[30,31] and one versus placebo over 16 weeks (82 women with menopausal symptoms).[32] The first RCT found that the combined regimen versus tibolone reduced hot flushes over 48 weeks (P = 0.01). The second trial found no significant difference in vasomotor symptoms between HRT and tibolone (58/68 [85%] women on tibolone v 67/72 [86%] women on HRT; RR 0.99, 95% CI 0.87 to 1.13), but both groups improved from baseline. The third trial found tibolone versus placebo significantly reduced vasomotor symptoms (39% reduction in mean score, P = 0.001).[32] **Urogenital system:** We found three RCTs.[30,33,34] The first RCT found no significant difference between tibolone and combined hormonal treatment in terms of subjective reports of vaginal lubrication; both interventions improved lubrication compared with baseline.[30] The second RCT (437 women) found that tibolone improved sexual satisfaction compared with oestradiol plus norethisterone (P < 0.05).[33] One small additional RCT of tibolone versus conjugated estrogen found tibolone significantly improved sexual desire and coital frequency.[34] We found no RCTs examining effects on urinary incontinence. **Psychological symptoms:** We found no RCTs. **Quality of life:** We found no RCTs.

Harms: We found no evidence on adverse effects from RCTs. One non-randomised controlled trial found that the main adverse effect of tibolone was breakthrough bleeding, which occurred in about 10% of users.[35] We found no good evidence of androgenic adverse effects, such as hair growth and greasiness of the skin. Two RCTs of short term use found a 33% reduction in plasma high density lipoproteins with tibolone,[36,37] although the long term effects on cardiovascular disease are unknown.

Comment: None.

OPTION   PHYTO-OESTROGENS

Limited evidence from small RCTs suggests that soy flour, which contains phyto-oestrogens, may relieve vasomotor menopausal symptoms.

Benefits: We found no systematic review. **Vasomotor symptoms:** We found four placebo controlled RCTs. Two double blind RCTs evaluated soy supplements (which contain phyto-oestrogen); the other, which was not blinded, evaluated isoflavone. The first RCT (58 postmenopausal women) compared soy flour with wheat flour for 12 weeks. It found no significant difference in reduction of hot flushes between soy flour and wheat flour (40% reduction with soy v 25% with wheat), although both groups were significantly reduced from baseline.[38] The second RCT used a crossover design to evaluate 6 weeks' administration of soy protein 34 mg daily. The trial found reduced severity but not frequency of vasomotor symptoms.[39] The third crossover RCT (51 women) compared isoflavone 40 mg daily versus placebo. It found no significant difference between isoflavone and placebo.[40] The fourth RCT (39 women) found that soy flour reduced mean flushes per week more than placebo (45% reduction with soy v 25% with placebo, P < 0.01).[41] **Urogenital system:** We found no RCTs. **Psychological symptoms:** We found no RCTs. **Beneficial effects of treatment on quality of life:** We found no RCTs.

Menopausal symptoms

Harms: We found no evidence of significant adverse effects.

Comment: None.

OPTION   CLONIDINE

Two RCTs found that clonidine reduced vasomotor symptoms.

Benefits: We found no systematic review. **Vasomotor symptoms:** We found two RCTs.[42,43] One crossover RCT (66 women) found that clonidine reduced the mean number of flushing attacks in the 14 days after crossover compared with placebo (56.8 v 64.3, P < 0.05).[30] The second RCT (30 women) found that more women taking clonidine reported reduced mean number of flushes at 8 weeks (12/15 [80%] with clonidine v 5/14 [35%] with placebo, RR 2.4, 95% CI 1.1 to 4.7; NNT 3, 95% CI 2 to 12).[43] **Psychological symptoms:** We found no RCTs. **Quality of life:** We found no RCTs.

Harms: The two RCTs found no significant difference in the incidence of unwanted effects between placebo and active treatment groups.[42,43]

Comment: None.

OPTION   TESTOSTERONE

We found evidence from RCTs that testosterone improves sexual enjoyment and libido. We found no studies evaluating effects on other commonly experienced menopausal symptoms.

Benefits: We found no systematic review. **Vasomotor symptoms:** We found no RCTs evaluating testosterone alone in women with menopausal symptoms. We found one RCT (93 postmenopausal women) comparing oestrogen alone versus oestrogen plus methyltestosterone. It found that the addition of a small dose of methyltestosterone reduced the dose of oestrogen needed to control menopausal symptoms.[44] **Urogenital system:** We found two RCTs, one in 40 women and one crossover study in 53 women. Both found benefit from exogenous testosterone on self-reported sexual enjoyment, desire, and arousal.[45,46] **Psychological symptoms:** We found no RCTs. **Beneficial effects of treatment on quality of life:** We found no RCTs.

Harms: We found no evidence from RCTs or other controlled studies on the incidence of androgenic adverse effects with testosterone.

Comment: None.

OPTION   ANTIDEPRESSANTS

We found insufficient evidence on the effects of antidepressants on menopausal symptoms.

Benefits: We found no systematic review or RCTs that specifically addressed the effects of antidepressants on menopausal symptoms or quality of life in menopausal women.

Harms: We found no evidence on adverse effects in postmenopausal women. Antidepressants as a group can cause many central nervous system adverse effects, including sedation and agitation, as well as urinary and vision problems, liver dysfunction, and cardiac dysrhythmias (see antidepressants under depressive disorders, p 652).

Comment: None.

Substantive changes since last issue

Oestrogens at diagnosis New RCT;[9] conclusion unchanged.
Oestrogens at diagnosis New systematic review;[20] conclusion unchanged.
Tibolone New RCT;[34] conclusion unchanged.

REFERENCES

1. Porter M, Penney G, Russell D, Russell E, Templeton A. A population based survey of women's experience of the menopause. *Br J Obstet Gynaecol* 1996;103:1025–1028.

2. Hagsta TA, Janson PO. The epidemiology of climacteric symptoms. *Acta Obstet Gynecol Scand* 1986;134(suppl):59.

3. Greendale GA, Reboussin BA, Hogan P, et al. Symptom relief and side effects of postmenopausal hormones: results from the postmenopausal estrogen/progestin interventions trial. *Obstet Gynecol* 1998;92:982–988.

4. Mattsson L A. Clinical experience with continuous combined transdermal hormone replacement therapy. *J Menopause* 1999;6:25–29.

5. Utian WH, Burry KA, Archer DF, et al. Efficacy and safety of low, standard, and high dosages of an estradiol transdermal system (Esclim) compared with placebo on vasomotor symptoms in highly symptomatic menopausal patients. The Esclim Study Group. *Am J Obstet Gynecol* 1999;181:71–79.

6. Cardozo L, Bachmann G, McClish D, Fonda D. Meta-analysis of estrogen therapy in the management of urogenital atrophy in postmenopausal women: second report of the hormones and urogenital therapy committee. *Obstet Gynecol* 1998;2:722–727. Search date April 1995; primary sources Medline, Excerpta Medica, Biosis, and hand searched journals.

7. Eriksen B. A randomized, open, parallel-group study on the preventive effect of an estradiol-releasing vaginal ring (Estring) on recurrent urinary tract infections in postmenopausal women. *Am J Obstet Gynecol* 1999;180:1072–1079.

8. Casper F, Petri E. Local treatment of urogenital atrophy with an estradiol-releasing vaginal ring: a comparative and a placebo-controlled multicenter study. Vaginal Ring Study Group. *Int Urogynecol J Pelvic Floor Dysfunct* 1999;10:171–176.

9. Notelovitz M, Mattox JH. Suppression of vasomotor and vulvovaginal symptoms with continuous oral 17β-estradiol. *Menopause* 2000; 7:310–317.

10. Zweifel JE, O'Brien WH. A meta-analysis of the effect of HRT upon depressed mood. *Psychoneuroendocrinology* 1997;22:189–212. Search date 1995; primary sources Psychological Abstracts, Medline, and hand searches of Dissertation Abstracts International.

11. Haskell SG, Richardson ED, Horwitz RI. The effect of ORT on cognitive function in women: a critical review of the literature. *J Clin Epidemiol* 1997;50: 1249–1264. Search date 1996; primary sources Medline, and hand searches of reference lists.

12. Polo-Kantola P, Erkkola R, Irjala K, Pullinen S, Virtanen I, Polo O. Effect of short-term transdermal estrogen replacement therapy on sleep: a randomized, double-blind crossover trial in postmenopausal women. *Fertil Steril* 1999;71: 873–880.

13. Wiklund I, Karlberg J, Mattsson L. Quality of life of postmenopausal women on a regimen of transdermal estradiol therapy: a double-blind placebo-controlled study. *Am J Obstet Gynecol* 1993;168:824–830.

14. Karlberg J, Mattsson L, Wiklund I. A quality of life perspective on who benefits from estradiol replacement therapy. *Acta Obstet Gynecol Scand* 1995;74:367–372.

15. Derman RJ, Dawood MY, Stone S. Quality of life during sequential hormonal replacement therapy – a placebo-controlled study. *Int J Fertil Menopausal Stud* 1995;40:73–78.

16. Hilditch JR, Lewis J, Ross AH, et al. A comparison of the effects of oral conjugated equine estrogen and transdermal estradiol-17 β combined with an oral progestin on quality of life in postmenopausal women. *Maturitas* 1996;24:177–184.

17. Norman RJ, Flight IHK, Rees MCP. Oestrogen and progestogen hormone replacement therapy for peri-menopausal and post-menopausal women: weight and body fat distribution. In: The Cochrane Library, Issue 1, 2001. Search date 1998; primary sources Medline, Embase, Current Contents, Biological Abstracts, Cinahl, citation lists, and contact with authors of eligible trials retrieved.

18. Grady D, Sawaya G. Postmenopausal hormone therapy increases risk of deep vein thrombosis and pulmonary embolism. *Am J Med* 1998;105: 41–43.

19. Barrett-Connor E. Fortnightly review: hormone replacement therapy. *BMJ* 1998;317:457–461.

20. Lethaby A, Farquhar C, Sarkis A, Roberts H, Jepson R, Barlow D. Hormone replacement therapy in postmenopausal women: endometrial hyperplasia and irregular bleeding. In: The Cochrane Library, Issue 4, 2000. Oxford: Update Software. Search date not stated; primary sources Cochrane Menstrual Disorders and Subfertility Group Trials Register, Medline, Embase, Current Contents, Biological Abstracts, Social Sciences Index, Psychlit, Cinahl, and hand searched of citation lists and contact with drug companies and trials authors.

21. Collaborative Group on Hormonal Factors in Breast Cancer. Breast cancer and hormone replacement therapy: collaborative reanalysis of data from 51 epidemiological studies of 52 705 women with breast cancer and 108 411 women without breast cancer. *Lancet* 1997;350:1047–1059. Search date and primary sources not stated; the authors collected epidemiological data on 52 705 women with breast cancer and 108 411 women without

breast cancer from 51 studies identified from literature searches, review articles, and discussions with colleagues.

22. Loprinzi CL, Michalak JC, Quella SK, et al. Megestrol acetate for the prevention of hot flashes. N Engl J Med 1994;331:347–352.

23. Lobo RA, McCormick W, Singer F, Roy S. DMPA compared with conjugated oestrogens for the treatment of postmenopausal women. Obstet Gynecol 1984;63:1–5.

24. Aslaksen K, Frankendal B. Effect of oral MPA on menopausal symptoms on patients with endometrial carcinoma. Acta Obstet Gynecol Scand 1982;61:423–428.

25. Schiff I, Tulchinsky D, Cramer D, Ryan KJ. Oral MPA in the treatment of postmenopausal symptoms. JAMA 1980;244:1443–1445.

26. Bullock JL, Massey FM, Gambrell RD. Use of MPA to prevent menopausal symptoms. Obstet Gynecol 1975;46:165–168.

27. Leonetti HB, Longo S, Anasti JN. Transdermal progesterone cream for vasomotor symptoms and postmenopausal bone loss. Obstet Gynecol 1999; 94:225–228.

28. Reginster JY, Zartarian M, Colau JC. Influence of nomogestrel acetate on the improvement of the quality of life induced by estrogen therapy in menopausal women. Contracep Fertil Sex 1996; 24:847–851.

29. Medical Research Council's General Practice Research Framework. Randomised comparison of oestrogen versus oestrogen plus progestagen hormone replacement therapy in women with hysterectomy. BMJ 1996;312:473–478.

30. Hammar M, Christau S, Nathorst-Boos J, Rud T, Garre K. A double-blind, randomised trial comparing the effects of tibolone and continuous combined hormone replacement therapy in postmenopausal women with menopausal symptoms. Br J Obstet Gynaecol 1998;105:904–911.

31. Al Azzawi F, Wahab M, Habiba M, Akkad A, Mason T. Continuous combined hormone replacement therapy compared with tibolone. Obstet Gynecol 1999;93:258–264.

32. Kicovic PM, Cortes-Prieto J, Luisi M, Milojevic S, Franchi F. Placebo-controlled cross-over study of effects of Org OD14 in menopausal women. Reproducion 1982;6:81–91.

33. Nathorst-Boos J, Hammar M. Effect on sexual life – a comparison between tibolone and a continuous estradiol-norethisterone acetate regimen. Maturitas 1997;26:15–20.

34. Kokcu A, Cetinkaya MB, Yanik F, Alper T, Malatyalioglu E. The comparison of effects of tibolone and conjugated estrogen-medroxyprogesterone acetate therapy on sexual performance in postmenopausal women. Maturitas 2000;36:75–80.

35. Morris EP, Wilson POG, Robinson J, Rymer JM. Long term effects of tibolone on the genital tract in postmenopausal women. Br J Obstet Gynaecol 1999;106:954–959.

36. Benedek-Jaszmann LJ. Long-term placebo-controlled efficacy and safety study of Org OD14 in climacteric women. Maturitas 1987;1:25–33.

37. Walker ID, Davidson JF, Richards A, Yates R, McEwan HP. The effect of the synthetic steroid Org OD14 on fibrinolysis and blood lipids in postmenopausal women. Thromb Haemost 1985; 53:303–305.

38. Murkies AL, Lombard C, Stauss BJ, Wilcox G, Burger HG, Morton MS. Dietary flour supplementation decreases postmenopausal hot flushes: effect of soy and wheat. Maturitas 1995; 21:189–195.

39. Washburn S, Burke GL, Morgan T, Anthony M. Effect of soy protein supplementation on serum lipoproteins, blood pressure, and menopausal symptoms in perimenopausal women. Menopause 1999;6:7–13.

40. Baber RJ, Templeman C, Morton T, Kelly GE, West L. Randomized placebo-controlled trial of an isoflavone supplement and menopausal symptoms in women. Climacteric 1999;2:85–92.

41. Scambia G, Mango D, Signorile PG, et al. Clinical effects of a standardized soy extract in postmenopausal women: a pilot study. Menopause 2000;7:105–111.

42. Edington RF, Chagnon JP. Clonidine (Dixarit) for menopausal flushing. Can Med Assoc J 1980; 123:23–26.

43. Nagamani M, Kelver ME, Smith ER. Treatment of menopausal hot flashes with transdermal administration of clonidine. Am J Obstet Gynecol 1987;156:561–565.

44. Simon J, Klaiber E, Wiita B, Bowen A, Yang HM. Differential effects of estrogen-androgen and estrogen-only therapy on vasomotor symptoms, gonadotropin secretion, and endogenous androgen bioavailability in postmenopausal women. Menopause 1999;6:138–146.

45. Dow MG, Hart DM, Forrest CA. Hormonal treatments of sexual unresponsiveness in postmenopausal women: a comparative study. Br J Obstet Gynaecol 1983;90:361–366.

46. Sherwin BB, Gelfand MM, Brender W. Androgen enhances sexual motivation in females: a prospective crossover study of sex steroid administration in the surgical menopause. Psychosom Med 1985;47:339–351.

Janice Rymer
Senior Lecturer/Consultant in
Obstetrics and Gynaecology
Guys, Kings, and St Thomas'
Medical School, London, UK

Edward Morris
Senior Registrar/Honorary Lecturer
HRT Research Unit
Guys Hospital
London, UK

Competing interests: JR has been sponsored to attend conferences by Organon, Solvay Healthcare Ltd, Wyeth Novon, Janssen-Cilag, and Servier. JR has also received research funding from Organon and consultancy fees from Organon, Wyeth, Janssen-Cilag, and Pfizer. EM has been sponsored to attend conferences and has received speakers fees from Eli Lilly, Organon, and Astra Zeneca.

QUESTIONS

INTERVENTIONS

Beneficial

Trade off between benefits and harms

Unknown effectiveness

Unlikely to be beneficial

See glossary, p 1323

Key Messages

Medical treatments

- Systematic reviews of RCTs have found that non-steroidal anti-inflammatory drugs (NSAIDs) and tranexamic acid reduce menstrual blood loss. NSAIDs also alleviate dysmenorrhoea. Systematic reviews of RCTs have found danazol to be effective, but unacceptable adverse effects occur in two fifths of women.

- One systematic review of RCTs on ethamsylate has found conflicting results that suggest at most a small reduction in menstrual blood flow.

- We found no placebo controlled RCTs of oral or intrauterine progestogens. Two systematic reviews of comparative RCTs have found little benefit from oral progestogens given in the luteal phase, although oral progestogen treatment for 21 days of the cycle significantly reduces menstrual blood loss from baseline. We found one systematic review of the levonorgestrel releasing intrauterine device (IUD), which identified four small RCTs. It found no evidence of a difference compared with norethisterone and found it less effective than endometrial resection.

- We found no good evidence on the effects of oral contraceptives or gonadotrophin releasing hormone (GnRH) analogues in women with menorrhagia.

Surgical treatments

- Hysterectomy and endometrial destruction are suitable only for women who have completed childbearing. One systematic review of RCTs has found high levels of patient satisfaction after both procedures but significantly higher levels after hysterectomy. It found that 30–90% of women who had undergone endometrial destruction experienced continued bleeding, although in most cases this was light.

■ One prospective cohort study found that hysterectomy caused major and minor complications in about one third of women. One RCT found that by 4 years, 38% of women who had undergone endometrial destruction required repeat surgery.

■ RCTs have found no evidence of a difference in effectiveness between different methods of endometrial destruction.

■ We found no good quality evidence on the effects of dilatation and curettage or myomectomy in women with menorrhagia.

■ RCTs comparing resection versus medical treatments found conflicting results.

■ One systematic review of RCTs has found that medical treatment to thin the endometrium before hysteroscopic surgery facilitates and reduces the duration of surgery and increases the rate of postoperative amenorrhoea.

DEFINITION	Menorrhagia is defined as heavy but regular menstrual bleeding. Idiopathic ovulatory menorrhagia is regular heavy bleeding in the absence of recognisable pelvic pathology or a general bleeding disorder. Objective menorrhagia is taken to be a total menstrual blood loss of 80 ml or more each menstruation.[1] Subjectively, menorrhagia may be defined as a complaint of regular excessive menstrual blood loss occurring over several consecutive cycles in a woman of reproductive years.
INCIDENCE/ PREVALENCE	In the UK, 5% of women, aged 30–49 years, consult their general practitioner each year with menorrhagia.[2]
AETIOLOGY/ RISK FACTORS	Idiopathic ovulatory menorrhagia is thought to be caused by disordered prostaglandin production within the endometrium.[3] Prostaglandins may also be implicated in menorrhagia associated with uterine fibroids, adenomyosis, or the presence of an IUD. Fibroids have been reported in 10% of women with menorrhagia (80–100 ml/cycle) and 40% of those with severe menorrhagia (≥ 200 ml/cycle).[4]
PROGNOSIS	Menorrhagia limits normal activities and causes iron deficiency anaemia in two thirds of women proved to have objective menorrhagia.[1,5,6] One in five women in the UK and one in three women in the USA will have a hysterectomy before the age of 60 years; menorrhagia is the main presenting problem in at least half of these women.[7–9] About half of the women who have a hysterectomy for menorrhagia have a normal uterus removed.[10]
AIMS	To reduce menstrual bleeding, improve quality of life, and prevent or correct iron deficiency anaemia with minimum adverse effects.
OUTCOMES	Menstrual blood flow (assessed objectively [ml/cycle] or subjectively), haemoglobin concentration, quality of life, patient satisfaction, incidence of adverse drug effects, and incidence of postoperative complications. Whether a particular percentage reduction in menstrual blood loss is considered clinically important will depend on pretreatment menstrual loss and the individual woman's perception of acceptable menstrual loss.
METHODS	*Clinical Evidence* search and appraisal May 2000. We also hand searched reference lists of non-systematic reviews and studies

obtained from the initial search, and recent issues of key journals. We did not systematically search the "grey literature" (conference abstracts, theses, unpublished trials).

QUESTION   What are the effects of medical treatments?

OPTION   NON-STEROIDAL ANTI-INFLAMMATORY DRUGS

One systematic review of RCTs has found that NSAIDs, with the exception of ibuprofen, significantly reduce menstrual blood loss compared with placebo. Another systematic review of RCTs found no evidence of a difference in effectiveness between mefenamic acid and naproxen. One systematic review of a few small RCTs found no evidence of a difference between NSAIDs and other medical treatments. NSAIDs have the additional advantage of relieving dysmenorrhoea in three quarters of women.

Benefits: **Versus placebo:** We found one systematic review comparing NSAIDs (mefenamic acid, naproxen, meclofenamic acid, ibuprofen, and diclofenac) versus placebo (search date 1996, 12 RCTs, n = 313).[11] All the NSAIDs tested, except ibuprofen, reduced menstrual blood loss compared with placebo. Treatment was taken only during menstruation, but doses varied depending on the specific drug. The mean reduction in menstrual blood loss compared with placebo ranged from 23 ml (mefenamic acid) to 74 ml (diclofenac). When all the NSAIDs were combined, the difference compared with placebo was a reduced blood loss of 35 ml (WMD −35 ml, 95% CI −43 ml to −27 ml). **Versus other NSAIDs and other drugs:** We found one systematic review comparing different NSAIDs, and NSAIDs versus other drugs (search date not given, 16 RCTs).[12] It found no important difference between mefenamic acid and naproxen. In the few small studies suitable for evaluation it also found no important difference between NSAIDs and oral progestogens given in the luteal phase, the combined oral contraceptive, or a progesterone releasing IUD.

Harms: Commonly reported adverse effects were headaches and gastrointestinal disturbances, including indigestion, nausea, vomiting, and diarrhoea. These occurred in at least half of women taking NSAIDs in the RCTs that reported data on adverse effects, but similar levels of adverse effects were found in placebo cycles.[11,12]

Comment: NSAIDs have the additional benefit of relieving dysmenorrhoea. One systematic review (search date 1983, 51 RCTs) found that three quarters of women with dysmenorrhoea reported significant pain relief with NSAIDs.[13] A more recent systematic review (search date 1997, 56 RCTs) found that naproxen, ibuprofen, and mefenamic acid were all significantly better than placebo in relieving dysmenorrhoea (RR for relief of dysmenorrhoea versus placebo: 3.17, 95% CI 2.72 to 3.65 with naproxen; 2.41, 95% CI 1.58 to 3.68 with ibuprofen; and 2.03, 95% CI 1.65 to 2.48 with mefanamic acid).[14]

Menorrhagia

OPTION	TRANEXAMIC ACID

Two systematic reviews of RCTs have found that tranexamic acid significantly reduces menstrual blood loss compared with placebo. One of these reviews has also found that tranexamic acid significantly reduces menstrual blood loss compared with luteal phase oral progestogens, mefenamic acid, and ethamsylate. Small individual RCTs found that tranexamic acid was significantly more effective than mefenamic acid, ethamsylate, flurbiprofen, diclofenac, and norethisterone. Leg cramps occurred in one third of women. Long term follow up studies have found no evidence to confirm the possibility of an increased risk of thromboembolism.

Benefits:
Versus placebo: We found two systematic reviews. The first review (search date 1996, 5 RCTs, n = 153) found a significant reduction in mean menstrual blood loss with tranexamic acid (250–500 mg 4 times a day during menstruation) compared with placebo (WMD –52 ml, graph in published report shows significant difference).[11] Few studies measured patient satisfaction. The second systematic review (search date 1997, 7 RCTs) identified two RCTs that compared tranexamic acid (1 g 4 times a day) or a pro-drug of tranexamic acid (Kabi 2161, 1.2 g twice a day) versus placebo.[15] It found a significant reduction in mean blood loss compared with placebo (WMD –94 ml, 95% CI –151 ml to –37 ml). **Versus other drugs:** We found two systematic reviews.[11,15] One review (search date 1997) found a significant reduction in mean menstrual blood loss compared with luteal phase oral progestogens (WMD –111 ml, 95% CI –179 ml to –44 ml) and mefenamic acid (WMD –73 ml, 95% CI –123 ml to –23 ml).[15] The other review (search date 1996) identified but did not pool data from several RCTs comparing tranexamic acid versus other drugs.[11] The trials consistently found that tranexamic acid was significantly more effective than mefenamic acid, ethamsylate, flurbiprofen, diclofenac, and norethisterone. One of the RCTs that looked at quality of life (n = 46) found that tranexamic acid reduced limitations on social activities and sex life significantly more than norethisterone.[16]

Harms:
Nausea and leg cramps occur in a third of women taking tranexamic acid. One systematic review (search date not given) found no increase in gastrointestinal adverse effects compared with either placebo or other drugs.[15] Isolated case reports have suggested a risk of thromboembolism, but a large population based study over 19 years found no evidence that this was higher than expected in the normal population.[17]

Comment:
Unlike NSAIDs, tranexamic acid has no effect on dysmenorrhoea.

OPTION	ETHAMSYLATE

One systematic review of RCTs has found a small reduction in menstrual blood loss compared with baseline, with minimal adverse effects. We found limited evidence from RCTs suggesting that ethamsylate is less effective than tranexamic acid, mefenamic acid, and aminocaproic acid.

Benefits:
We found one systematic review (search date not given, 4 RCTs) comparing ethamsylate versus placebo (one trial), mefenamic acid

(one trial), aminocaproic acid (one trial), and mefenamic acid plus tranexamic acid (one trial).[18] Most results were presented as comparison with baseline. The review concluded that ethamsylate achieved an overall reduction in menstrual blood loss compared with baseline of 13.1% (95% CI 10.9% to 15.3%), which may not be clinically significant. The individual trials reported conflicting results. One RCT (n = 23) found a 7% reduction in blood loss with ethamsylate and a 56% reduction with aminocaproic acid. A second RCT (n = 34) found a 20% reduction in blood loss with ethamsylate and a 24% reduction with mefenamic acid. A third RCT (n = 82) was the only one of the four to give direct comparative results rather than comparison with baseline.[19] It found that both tranexamic acid and mefenamic acid were significantly more effective than ethamsylate (WMD tranexamic acid v ethamsylate –97 ml, 95% CI –140 ml to –54 ml, and mefenamic acid v ethamsylate –51 ml, 95% CI –96 ml to –6 ml). The only placebo controlled trial (n = 22) found that ethamsylate reduced menstrual blood loss by 50% compared with baseline in women with "primary menorrhagia" and by 19% in women who were using IUDs.

Harms: The review found no significant difference between different regimens, in the rate of adverse effects such as nausea, headaches, and dizziness, and these seldom caused women to withdraw from studies.[18]

Comment: The individual trials differed in their methods. Two included women who were using IUDs as well as women with "idiopathic" menorrhagia and did not require a menstrual blood loss of more than 80 ml before entry. The other two studies looked only at women with a pretreatment menstrual blood loss greater than 80 ml. The placebo controlled trial may not be comparable with the other trials because it did not use the normally accepted alkaline haematin method to determine menstrual blood loss, and the women started ethamsylate 5 days before the expected start of their period instead of on day one as in the other trials.[18]

OPTION   DANAZOL

One systematic review of RCTs has found that danazol reduces menstrual blood flow more than placebo. Individual RCTs found that danazol was as or more effective than luteal phase oral progestogens, mefenamic acid, naproxen, or oral contraceptives. Unacceptable adverse effects occurred in 40% of women.

Benefits: **Versus placebo:** We found one systematic review comparing danazol (200 mg/day continuously for 2–3 months) versus placebo (search date 1996, 3 RCTs, n = 127).[11] It found a significant reduction in menstrual blood loss compared with placebo (WMD –108 ml, 95% CIs presented graphically). **Versus other drugs:** Several RCTs have found no difference or greater effectiveness with danazol compared with luteal phase oral progestogens, mefenamic acid, naproxen, and oral contraceptives.[20–23]

Harms: In one RCT (n = 40) adverse effects occurred in three quarters of those given danazol (200 mg daily) compared with one third of those given mefenamic acid; 40% of these adverse effects were deemed unacceptable.[20] An average weight gain of 2–4 kg occured in about a quarter of women after 3 months' treatment. Other adverse effects, which together occur in about half of women, include androgenic effects such as acne, seborrhoea, hirsutism, voice changes, and general complaints, including irritability, musculoskeletal pains, and tiredness. Hot flushes and breast atrophy can sometimes occur. Most of these adverse effects are reversible on cessation of treatment.

Comment: Women must be advised to use barrier methods of contraception because of potential virilisation of the fetus if pregnancy occurs during treatment.

OPTION COMBINED ORAL CONTRACEPTIVES

We found insufficient evidence on the effects of oral contraceptives in the treatment of menorrhagia.

Benefits: We found one systematic review (search date 1997), which identified one small RCT (n = 38) comparing the combined oral contraceptive versus danazol, mefenamic acid, or naproxen.[24] It found no significant difference between any of the interventions but was too small to rule out a clinically important difference.

Harms: Minor adverse effects are common and include nausea, headache, breast tenderness, changes in body weight, hypertension, changes in libido, and depression.

Comment: One non-randomised controlled trial (n = 164) found that a 50 mg oral contraceptive pill led to a 53% reduction in menstrual blood loss compared with baseline. Aminocaproic acid (n = 85) led to a 54% reduction, and tranexamic acid (n = 172) led to a 47% reduction.[25] Two longitudinal case control studies found that women taking the pill were less likely than those not taking the pill to experience heavy menstrual bleeding or anaemia.[26,27] The oral contraceptive has the advantage of reducing symptoms of dysmenorrhoea and providing effective contraception. See oral contraceptives under dysmenorrhoea, p 1258.

OPTION ORAL PROGESTOGENS

We found no placebo controlled RCTs. Two systematic reviews of comparative RCTs have found little benefit from oral progestogens given in the luteal phase, although oral progestogen treatment for 21 days of the cycle significantly reduces menstrual blood loss from baseline.

Benefits: **Versus placebo:** We found no placebo controlled RCTs. **Versus other drugs:** We found two systematic reviews (search dates not given).[18,28] The earlier systematic review identified four comparative RCTs.[18] Results were presented as comparison with baseline. The review found that norethisterone (taken on days 15–26 or 19–26) was associated with a small significant increase in menstrual loss from baseline (WMD in percentage reduction −3.6%, 95% CI −6.1% to −1.1%). Only two of the RCTs gave direct comparative data. One found a 16% reduction in blood loss with norethisterone (n = 15) and a 34% reduction with mefenamic acid (n = 17). The other found a 4% increase in blood flow with nore-thisterone (n = 18) and a 40% reduction with danazol (n = 19). The later systematic review identified seven comparative RCTs, including three RCTs not in the earlier review.[28] Mean menstrual blood loss was significantly greater with luteal progestogen than with danazol (WMD −56 ml, 95% CI −96 ml to −15 ml), tranexamic acid (WMD −111 ml, 95% CI −179 ml to −43.5 ml), and the progesterone releasing IUD (WMD −51 ml, 95% CI −84 ml to −18 ml). Luteal progestogens were associated with a significantly greater self assessed blood loss than danazol (OR 4.2, 95% CI 1.5 to 12.0). **Longer treatment cycle:** One RCT included in the review evaluated a longer regimen of progestogen (21 days/cycle) in 48 women.[28] It found no significant difference in the reduction in menstrual blood loss between norethisterone and the levonorgestrel releasing IUD (94 ml v 104 ml). There was a large and significant reduction from baseline with both treatments (P < 0.001), but a higher proportion of women who were using the levonorgestrel releasing IUD had menstruation reduced to "normal" (< 80 ml/cycle) compared with women taking oral progestogens.

Harms: Adverse effects were reported in one third to half of the women but were not usually serious. They consisted mainly of headache, breast tenderness, premenstrual symptoms, and gastrointestinal distur-bances.[18,28] In the trial of the longer treatment cycle, only 44% of women said they liked the treatment "well" or "very well", and only 22% elected to continue with treatment after the 3 months of the study.

Comment: The large number of withdrawals (27%) from the norethisterone group of one RCT may make the findings less valid.

OPTION	INTRAUTERINE PROGESTOGENS

We found one systematic review evaluating the levonorgestrel releasing IUD, which identified four small RCTs. It found no evidence of a difference compared with norethisterone and found the IUD less effective than endometrial resection.

Benefits: We found one systematic review of progesterone/progestogen releasing IUDs in menorrhagia (search date not given).[29] **Progest-erone releasing IUD:** The systematic review found one RCT that examined effects of a progesterone releasing IUD (65 µg/day), danazol, mefenamic acid, or norethisterone in women with menor-rhagia.[29] The review found that all treatments reduced menstrual blood loss from baseline, but did not compare treatments. **Levonorgestrel releasing IUD:** The review found four RCTs that examined effects of levonorgestrel releasing IUDs (20 µg/day).[29] Two trials (n = 60 and n = 70) compared levonorgestrel releasing IUDs versus transcervical endometrial resection (see glossary, p 1324), using the pictorial blood loss assessment chart. A system-atic review of these trials found that at 1 year follow up, resection reduced blood loss from baseline more than levonorgestrel releas-ing IUDs (WMD for reduction in blood loss, resection v IUD 27, 95% CI 17 to 38).[29] However, mean blood loss and satisfaction rates were not significantly different between groups (WMD for mean blood loss, resection v IUD 12.2, 95% CI –1.9 to +26.3; satisfaction rate 85% with IUD, 94% with resection, P = NS).[29] The third RCT (n = 44) found no significant difference in reduction of blood loss or rates of satisfaction between norethisterone (15 ml/day, day 5 to day 26 of cycle) and levonorgestrel releasing IUDs (median reduction from baseline for norethisterone 6 ml/cycle v 20 ml/cycle for levonorgestrel; satisfaction data not given).[29] The fourth RCT (n = 56) found that levonorgestrel releasing IUDs improved all the quality of life scores that were assessed when compared with medical treatment (details of medical treatment and results not given). After 6 months of treatment, women using levonorgestrel releasing IUDs were more likely to cancel their hysterectomy than women using medical treatment (levonorgestrel releasing IUDs, AR of cancellation 64%, 95% CI 44% to 81%, v medical treatment, 14%, 95% CI 4% to 33%).[29]

Harms: Progesterone releasing IUDs were withdrawn in the UK because of concerns about increased rates of ectopic pregnancy. We found no evidence of this adverse effect. The systematic review found that most adverse effects in women using a levonorgestrel releasing IUD were typical of progestogens (bloating, weight gain, breast tenderness). One included trial found that 56% of women had at least one adverse event with the IUD, compared with 26% for transcervical endometrial resection (RR 2.17, 95% CI 1.2 to 3.0).[30] One further trial found that a greater proportion of women were amenorrhoeic after 3 months of treatment with levonorgestrel releasing IUDs compared with norethisterone (32% v 0%).[31] The other main adverse effect was irregular (although not usually heavy) menstrual bleeding. RCTs looking at the contraceptive effect of levonorgestrel releasing IUDs in younger women found that during the first few months of use, the total number of bleeding days (including menstrual bleeding, intermenstrual bleeding, and spotting) increased in most women.[32] However, by 12 months most women bled lightly for only 1 day a month and about 15% were amenorrhoeic.[33]

Comment: None of the trials included in the systematic review compared progestogen-releasing IUDs versus placebo.[29] Long term follow up on women with menorrhagia is required to assess continuation rates, satisfaction, and whether surgical treatment is avoided or just postponed. The trials that considered long term bleeding patterns were mainly in women aged under 40. It is not yet known whether these data can be extrapolated to older women with menorrhagia.

OPTION **GONADOTROPHIN RELEASING HORMONE (GNRH) ANALOGUES**

We found insufficient evidence on the effects of GnRH analogues in women with menorrhagia.

Benefits: We found no systematic review or RCTs. A few small nonrandomised studies have looked at GnRH analogues in menorrhagia. Others have looked at their effects in women with fibroids or on thinning the endometrium before ablation or resection.

Harms: Adverse effects are mainly caused by reduced oestrogens. Hormone replacement to counteract hypo-oestrogenism has been tried with limited success to reduce hot flushes.[34] Bone demineralisation occurs in most women after 6 months of treatment but is reversible after treatment is stopped.[35]

Comment: Contraception is not guaranteed.[36]

QUESTION **If medical treatments fail, what are the effects of surgical treatments?**

OPTION **DILATATION AND CURETTAGE**

We found insufficient evidence on the effects of dilatation and curettage in women with menorrhagia.

Benefits: We found no systematic review or RCTs.

Harms: The procedure has small risks of serious morbidity, including uterine perforation and cervical laceration as well as the usual risks of general anaesthesia.[37]

Comment: Dilatation and curettage still plays a part in the investigation of menorrhagia. We found one uncontrolled cohort study (n = 50) that measured blood loss before and after dilatation and curettage. It found a reduction in menstrual blood loss immediately after the procedure, but losses returned to previous levels or higher by the second menstrual period.[38]

OPTION **HYSTERECTOMY**

Hysterectomy is the only certain way to stop all menstrual loss. One systematic review of RCTs has found that patient satisfaction is significantly higher after hysterectomy than after endometrial destruction. One large cohort study reported major and minor complications in about a third of women.

Benefits: **Versus endometrial resection or laser ablation:** We found two systematic reviews (search dates 1996 and not stated).[11,39] Both identified the same five RCTs (708 premenopausal women) comparing either transcervical endometrial resection or laser ablation (see glossary, p 1323) versus hysterectomy. Two of the authors were common to both reviews, and the conclusions were essentially the same. Follow up ranged from 1–4 years. The five RCTs consistently found a significantly greater reduction in menstrual blood loss with hysterectomy. Fewer women experienced reduction in blood loss with endometrial destruction compared with hysterectomy (RR for improvement 0.87, 95% CI 0.82 to 0.91). After longer follow up, the differences in improvement in blood loss between the groups seemed to narrow, possibly because of retreatment in the endometrial ablation group or women reaching the menopause. The reviews found that between 30–90% of women continued bleeding after endometrial destruction, although blood loss was usually light. The proportion of women who were very or moderately satisfied was significantly lower after endometrial ablation, both at 1 and 2 years (1 year: RR 0.93, 95% CI 0.89 to 0.99; 2 years: RR 0.87, 95% CI 0.81 to 0.94).[11,39] Two studies included in the review found no significant difference between satisfaction rates at longer follow up

(3 and 4 years). However, the duration of surgery, hospital stay, and time to return to work were all significantly shorter with endometrial destruction than with hysterectomy (reduced by a mean of 23 minutes, 5 days, and 4.5 weeks, respectively). Risk of repeat surgery was significantly higher at all follow up periods after endometrial destruction than after hysterectomy (first year: OR 7.3, 95% CI 4.2 to 12.9; second year: OR 7.5, 95% CI 4.2 to 13.4; third year: OR 4.5, 95% CI 1.8 to 11.2; fourth year: OR 9.8, 95% CI 4.9 to 19.7). One RCT found that by 4 years, 38% of women who had undergone endometrial destruction required repeat surgery for menstrual problems compared with 1% of those who had undergone hysterectomy.[40] **Different techniques:** We found no systematic review. A few small RCTs (total 334 women) compared abdominal, vaginal, or laparoscopic hysterectomy.[41–45] They found no evidence of a difference in effectiveness or complication rates. However, operating and recovery times varied.

Harms:　Large population based analyses stratified by age have found a mortality after hysterectomy for non-malignant conditions of 1/2000 women aged under 50.[46] When compared with endometrial destruction, hysterectomy had a greater risk of sepsis, blood transfusion, urinary retention, anaemia, pyrexia, vault and wound haematoma, and cautery of hypergranulation before hospital discharge. One large, prospective cohort study of hysterectomy for non-malignant conditions found combined major and minor complication rates (mainly fever) of 25% for vaginal hysterectomy and 43% for abdominal hysterectomy.[47]

Comment:　None.

| OPTION | ENDOMETRIAL DESTRUCTION (RESECTION OR ABLATION) |

One systematic review of RCTs has found that, although patient satisfaction is high after endometrial destruction, it is significantly lower than after hysterectomy. Endometrial destruction has several short term advantages over hysterectomy: shorter operating time, fewer complications, faster recovery, and less need for analgesia. Between 30–90% of women treated with endometrial destruction will experience continued bleeding, although in most cases this is light. One RCT found that about 40% of women required repeat surgery within 4 years. RCTs have found no evidence of a difference in effectiveness between different methods of endometrial destruction. RCTs comparing medical treatment and endometrial destruction found conflicting results.

Benefits:　**Endometrial destruction versus hysterectomy:** See hysterectomy, p 1319. **Resection versus laser ablation:** We found no systematic review. We found one RCT (n = 372) comparing transcervical endometrial resection versus laser ablation.[48] It found no significant differences in operative complications (23% v 19.5%), satisfaction rates (90.3% v 89%), or need for further treatment (20% v 16%). It also found no significant difference in recovery times or symptom relief. **Rollerball ablation versus electrosurgical ablation:** We found no systematic review. One recent RCT (n = 276) comparing rollerball ablation (see glossary, p 1323) versus electrosurgical ablation (see glossary, p 1323) found no significant difference in reduction of blood loss assessed at 12 months by pictorial blood loss assessment charts (91% v 94%), and no significant difference in the proportion of women reporting amenorrhoea (39.6% v 31.8%).[49] **Resection versus microwave ablation:** We found no systematic review. One RCT (n = 263) comparing transcervical endometrial resection with microwave endometrial ablation (see glossary, p 1323) found no significant difference in patient satisfaction at 12 months, the same rates of amenorrhoea at 6 months, and a similar proportion of both groups requiring further surgery at 12 months. Satisfaction rates 75% with resection versus 77% with microwave ablation. Rates of amenorrhoea in both groups 40%. Proportion requiring further surgery 7.8% with ablation versus 9.7% with resection.[49] The mean operating time was significantly shorter for ablation compared with resection (11.4 minutes v 15 minutes).[50] **Rollerball ablation versus thermal balloon therapy:** We found no systematic review. One multicentre RCT (n = 255) comparing thermal uterine balloon therapy (see glossary, p 1324) versus hysteroscopic rollerball ablation, found no significant difference in mean menstrual blood loss at 12 months (85.5% v 91.7%).[51] Significantly more women were amenorrhoeic after rollerball ablation than after thermal balloon therapy (27.2% v 15.2%). However, 85.6% of women after balloon therapy and 86.7% of women after rollerball ablation were highly satisfied with the results 12 months after their ablative procedure (measured by quality of life questionnaires). **Resection versus medical treatment:** We found no systematic review. We found two RCTs, which reported conflicting results.[52] One RCT (n = 70) found no significant difference in menstrual blood loss or patient satisfaction between a levonorgestrel releasing IUD and transcervical endometrial resection. The other RCT (n = 197) found that satisfaction was significantly lower among women treated with one of a variety of medical treatments (not including a levonorgestrel releasing IUD) other than with transcervical endometrial resection (27% v 76%).[52] However, the women in this trial had already found no benefit from medical management and may differ from women newly presenting with menorrhagia. A 2 year follow up study on these women has recently been published.[51] It found increased average satisfaction for all women but higher satisfaction with transcervical endometrial resection than medical management. Satisfaction after resection was 79% compared with 55% after medical management (95% CI for the difference 9% to 36%). Bleeding and pain had also improved with medical management at 2 years and were comparable to levels in women who had undergone resection. These results could have arisen because 59% of women in the medical group had gone on to either transcervical endometrial resection or hysterectomy. However, 20% of women continued to take medical treatment and 41% of women avoided surgery.

Harms: Intraoperative complications include uterine perforation, haemorrhage, and fluid overload from the distension medium. Immediate postoperative complications include infection, haemorrhage and, rarely, bowel injury. Complication rates in the five RCTs described above ranged from 0–15%.[48–51,53] One large prospective survey of 10 686 women undergoing endometrial destructive procedures in the UK found an immediate complication rate of 4.4%.[54]

Intraoperative emergency procedures were performed in 1.26%, and two procedure related deaths occurred. Newer methods of endometrial destruction, such as thermal balloon therapy have been evaluated only in small numbers of women and, although complications in the RCTs seem minimal, safety data for routine use are awaited.

Comment: These were good quality RCTs with results that should be widely generalisable. The prospective survey gave a good indication of what happened when the procedure was used in clinical practice.[54] RCTs of other methods of endometrial destruction are in progress.

OPTION   MYOMECTOMY

We found insufficient evidence on the effects of myomectomy in women with menorrhagia.

Benefits: We found no systematic review. **Open versus laparoscopic myomectomy:** We found no RCTs or other studies in women with menorrhagia that measured menstrual blood loss. **Hysteroscopic myomectomy:** We found no RCTs. One uncontrolled study (15 women, 10 with additional symptoms) reported objective measures of menstrual blood loss.[55] Mean menstrual blood loss, assessed preoperatively and at 3 and 6 months postoperatively, was significantly reduced (261 ml at baseline; 76 ml at 3 months, and 57 ml at 6 months). The study found a significant reduction in pain scores and menstrual duration, despite the fibroids removed measuring only 1–4 cm.

Harms: Intraoperative complications for hysteroscopic myomectomy are similar to those with endometrial destructive procedures that use a hysteroscope. The main complication of open myomectomy is haemorrhage, making a hysterectomy necessary.

Comment: RCTs are needed that use objective assessment of menstrual blood loss. This is especially important in the evaluation of surgical procedures because of the greater difficulty in blinding.

QUESTION   What are the effects of endometrial thinning before hysteroscopic surgery?

OPTION   ENDOMETRIAL THINNING BEFORE SURGERY

One systematic review of RCTs has found that use of GnRH analogues to thin the endometrium before hysteroscopic surgery facilitates and reduces the duration of surgery, and increases the rate of postoperative amenorrhoea. The review found that danazol was also effective but less so than GnRH analogues. There was insufficient evidence on the use of progestogens in this context.

Benefits: We found one systematic review evaluating medical treatment to thin the endometrium before hysteroscopic surgery for menorrhagia (search date not given, 8 RCTs, n = 946).[56] **GnRH analogues:** Four RCTs (n = 566) compared the GnRH analogue goserelin versus placebo or no treatment, with 6–12 months' follow up. Goserelin was associated with significant reductions in endometrial thickness on ultrasound (n = 358, 1.61 mm *v* 3.53 mm); weight of endometrium removed (n = 60, 2.4 g *v* 7.8 g, P < 0.01); duration of surgery (time difference ranging from 2–14 minutes, WMD –4.7 minutes, 95% CI –6.1 minutes to –3.2 minutes); volume of distension medium absorbed (no statistical analysis given); and operative difficulty (RR of encountering difficulty during procedure compared with placebo or no treatment 0.32, 95% CI 0.22 to 0.46). Goserelin was also associated with a significant increase in the rate of postoperative amenorrhoea (RR compared with placebo or no treatment 1.73, 95% CI 0.13 to 0.25, NNT for one additional case of postoperative amenorrhoea 5.3), and lighter menstrual periods (RR of continuing to have moderate or heavy periods 0.74, 95% CI 0.59 to 0.92). The data did not suggest any major difference in intraoperative complications, (uterine perforations were reported in 2/266 on goserelin and in 1/275 on no treatment or placebo), patient satisfaction, or the likelihood of undergoing further surgery. **GnRH analogue versus danazol:** Three RCTs (n = 340) compared danazol versus GnRH analogues (goserelin or decapeptyl). GnRH analogues were associated with significant reductions in endometrial thickness, greater uterine atrophy (RR of atrophic or inactive glands compared with danazol 1.42, 95% CI 1.11 to 1.82), and a significant increase in the rate of postoperative amenorrhoea (RR 1.57, 95% CI 1.06 to 2.33, NNT for 2 months 5.9). However, there was no significant difference in operative difficulty (RR 0.68, 95% CI 0.31 to 1.51). On the basis of data from two RCTs, duration of surgery seemed to be less with GnRH analogues (WMD –3.9 minutes, 95% CI –6.1 minutes to –1.7 minutes). None of the trials reported any intraoperative complications. **Progestogens:** One RCT (n = 40) compared progestogens versus GnRH analogues versus danazol versus no treatment. The trial was too small to allow firm conclusions to be drawn.

Harms: Hot flushes, reduced libido, depression, and vaginal dryness were significantly more common with goserelin than danazol. Oily skin, hirsutism, and weight gain were significantly more common with danazol. Withdrawals from trials because of adverse effects occurred in 1/566 women receiving goserelin (headache) and 11/139 receiving danazol.

Comment: None of the trials used objective measures of postoperative menstrual blood loss. One used allocation concealment and one used intention to treat analysis. Rates of withdrawal or loss to follow up were low in all studies.

GLOSSARY

Electrosurgical ablation A procedure in which an inflatable device with electrodes on the outside is inserted into the uterine cavity via the cervix. The electrodes make contact with the endometrium and cause necrosis.

Laser ablation A hysteroscopic procedure in which endometrium is destroyed under direct vision by a laser beam.

Microwave endometrial ablation A procedure in which a microwave probe is passed through the cervix into the uterine cavity. When activated it is moved slowly from side to side over the whole surface of the uterine cavity in order to destroy the endometrium.

Rollerball ablation A hysteroscopic procedure in which endometrium is destroyed under direct vision by the use of diathermy applied by a rollerball.

Thermal uterine balloon therapy A procedure in which a balloon catheter is passed through the cervix into the uterine cavity. The balloon is then filled with fluid which is heated to about 87°C, and left for 8 minutes. This causes necrosis of the endometrium.

Transcervical endometrial resection A hysteroscopic procedure in which endometrium is removed under direct vision by using an electrosurgical loop.

REFERENCES

1. Hallberg L, Hogdahl A, Nilsson L, et al. Menstrual blood loss – a population study: variation at different ages and attempts to define normality. *Acta Obstet Gynecol Scand* 1966;45:320–351.

2. Vessey MP, Villard-Mackintosh L, McPherson K, et al. The epidemiology of hysterectomy: findings in a large cohort study. *Br J Obstet Gynaecol* 1992;99:402–407.

3. Smith SK, Abel MH, Kelly RW, et al. A role for prostacyclin (PGI₂) in excessive menstrual bleeding. *Lancet* 1981;i:522–524.

4. Rybo G, Leman J, Tibblin R. Epidemiology of menstrual blood loss. In: Baird DT, Michie EA, eds. *Mechanisms of menstrual bleeding*. New York: Raven Press, 1985:181–193.

5. Alexander DA, Naji AA, Pinion SB, et al. Randomised trial comparing hysterectomy with endometrial ablation for dysfunctional uterine bleeding: psychiatric and psychosocial aspects. *BMJ* 1996;312:280–284.

6. Coulter A, Peto V, Jenkinson C. Quality of life and patient satisfaction following treatment for menorrhagia. *Fam Pract* 1994;11:394–401.

7. Coulter A, McPherson K, Vessey M. Do British women undergo too many or too few hysterectomies? *Soc Sci Med* 1988;27:987–994.

8. Pokras R, Hufnagel VG. *Hysterectomy in the United States, 1965–84*. Washington, DC: Public Health Service, 1987:87–1753.

9. Coulter A, Kelland J, Long A. The management of menorrhagia. *Effective Health Care Bull* 1995;9:1–14.

10. Clarke A, Black N, Rowe P, et al. Indications for and outcome of total abdominal hysterectomy for benign disease: a prospective cohort study. *Br J Obstet Gynaecol* 1995;102:611–620.

11. Working Party of the National Health Committee New Zealand. *Guidelines for the management of heavy menstrual bleeding*. Wellington: Ministry of Health, 1998. (Available from The Ministry of Health, 133 Molesworth Street, PO Box 5013, Wellington, New Zealand.) Search date 1996; primary sources Medline, Embase, Current Contents, Biological Abstracts, Social Sciences Index, Psychlit, Cinahl.

12. Lethaby A, Augood C, Duckitt K. Nonsteroidal anti-inflammatory drugs vs either placebo or any other medical treatment for heavy menstrual bleeding (menorrhagia). In: The Cochrane Library, Issue 2, 2000. Oxford: Update Software. Search date not given; primary sources Cochrane Menstrual Disorders and Subfertility Group trials register, Medline, Embase, Psychlit, Current Contents, Biological Abstracts, Social Sciences Index, Cinahl, reference lists and drug companies.

13. Owen PR. Prostaglandin synthetase inhibitors in the treatment of primary dysmenorrhoea. *Am J Obstet Gynecol* 1984;148:96–103. Search date January 1982; primary sources Medline 1974–1982.

14. Zhang WY, Li Wan Po A. Efficacy of minor analgesics in primary dysmenorrhoea: a systematic review. *Br J Obstet Gynaecol* 1998;105:780–789. Search date 1997; primary sources Medline, Embase, Science Citation Index, reference lists of retrieved RCTs, review articles, communication with the manufacturers.

15. Cooke I, Lethaby A, Farquhar C. Antifibrinolytics for heavy menstrual bleeding. In: The Cochrane Library, Issue 2, 2000. Oxford: Update Software. Search date 1999; primary sources Cochrane Menstrual Disorders and Subfertility Group trials register, Medline, Embase and hand searches of reference lists from experts and drug companies.

16. Preston JT, Cameron IT, Adams EJ, et al. Comparative study of tranexamic acid and norethisterone in the treatment of ovulatory menorrhagia. *Br J Obstet Gynaecol* 1995;102:401–406.

17. Rybo G. Tranexamic acid therapy is effective treatment in heavy menstrual bleeding: clinical update on safety. *Ther Adv* 1991;4:1–8.

18. Coulter A, Kelland J, Peto V, et al. Treating menorrhagia in primary care. An overview of drug trials and a survey of prescribing practice. *Int J Technol Assess Health Care* 1995;11:456–471. Search date not given; primary sources Medline, Embase.

19. Bonnar J, Sheppard BL. Treatment of menorrhagia during menstruation: randomised controlled trial of ethamsylate, mefenamic acid, and tranexamic acid. *BMJ* 1996;313:579–582.

20. Dockeray CJ, Sheppard BL, Bonnar J. Comparison between mefenamic acid and danazol in the treatment of established menorrhagia. *Br J Obstet Gynaecol* 1989;96:840–844.

21. Higham JM, Shaw RW. A comparative study of danazol, a regimen of decreasing doses of danazol, and norethindrone in the treatment of objectively proven unexplained menorrhagia. *Am J Obstet Gynecol* 1993;169:1134–1139.

22. Fraser IS, McCarron G. Randomized trial of 2 hormonal and 2 prostaglandin-inhibiting agents in women with a complaint of menorrhagia. *Aust NZ J Obstet Gynaecol* 1991;31:66–70.

23. Dunphy BC, Goerzen J, Greene CA, et al. A double-blind randomised study comparing danazol and medroxyprogesterone acetate in the management of menorrhagia. *J Obstet Gynaecol* 1998;18:553–555.

24. Iyer V, Farquhar C, Jepson R. The effectiveness of oral contraceptive pills versus placebo or any other medical treatment for menorrhagia. In: The Cochrane Library, Issue 2, 2000. Oxford: Update Software. Search date 1997; primary sources Cochrane Register of Controlled Trials.

25. Nilsson L, Rybo G. Treatment of menorrhagia. *Am J Obstet Gynecol* 1971;5:713–720.

26. Ramcharan S, Pellegrin FA, Ray MR, et al. The Walnut Creek contraceptive drug study – a prospective study of the side effects of oral contraceptives. Vol III. An interim report: a comparison of disease occurrence leading to hospitalization or death in users and nonusers of oral contraceptives. *J Reprod Med* 1980;25:345–372.

27. Royal College of General Practitioners. *Oral contraceptives and health*. London: Pitman Medical, 1974.

28. Lethaby A, Irvine G, Cameron I. Cyclical progestogens for heavy menstrual bleeding. In: The Cochrane Library, Issue 2, 2000. Oxford: Update Software. Search date not given; primary sources Cochrane Menstrual Disorders and Subfertility Group trials register, Medline, Embase,

Psychlit, Current Contents, Biological Abstracts, Social Sciences Index, Cinahl, reference lists.

29. Lethaby AE, Cooke I, Rees M. Progesterone/progestogen releasing intrauterine systems versus either placebo or any other medication for heavy menstrual bleeding. In: The Cochrane Library, Issue 2, 2000. Oxford: Update Software. Search date 1999; primary sources Medline, Embase, Cochrane Library, and experts contacted.

30. Crosignani PG, Vercellini P, Mosconi P, et al. Levonorgestrel-releasing intrauterine device versus hysteroscopic endometrial resection in the treatment of dysfunctional uterine bleeding. Obstet Gynecol 1997;90:257–263.

31. Irvine GA, Campbell-Brown MB, Lumsden MA, et al. Randomised comparative study of the levonorgestrel intrauterine system and norethisterone for the treatment of idiopathic menorrhagia. Br J Obstet Gynaecol 1998;105:592–598.

32. Long-acting progestogen-only contraception. Drug Ther Bull 1996;34:93–96.

33. Luukkainen T. The levonorgestrel-releasing IUD. Br J Fam Plann 1993;19:221–224.

34. Thomas EJ, Okuda KJ, Thomas NM. The combination of a depot gonadotrophin releasing hormone agonist and cyclical hormone replacement therapy for dysfunctional uterine bleeding. Br J Obstet Gynaecol 1991;98:1155–1159.

35. Eldred JM, Haynes PJ, Thomas EJ. A randomized double blind placebo controlled trial of the effects on bone metabolism of the combination of nafarelin acetate and norethisterone. Clin Endocrinol 1992;37:354–359.

36. Pickersgill A, Kingsland CR, Garden AS, et al. Multiple gestation following gonadotrophin releasing hormone therapy for the treatment of minimal endometriosis. Br J Obstet Gynaecol 1998;101:260–262.

37. Smith JJ, Schulman H. Current dilatation and curettage practice: a need for revision. Obstet Gynecol 1985;65:516–518.

38. Haynes PJ, Hodgson H, Anderson AB, et al. Measurement of menstrual blood loss in patients complaining of menorrhagia. Br J Obstet Gynaecol 1977;84:763–768.

39. Lethaby A, Shepperd S, Cooke I, et al. Endometrial resection and ablation versus hysterectomy for heavy menstrual bleeding. In: The Cochrane Library, Issue 2, 2000. Oxford: Update Software. Search date not stated; primary sources Cochrane Menstrual Disorders and Subfertility Group Register of Trials, Medline, Embase, Psychlit, Current Contents, Biological Abstracts, Social Sciences Index, and Cinahl.

40. Aberdeen Endometrial Ablation Trials Group. A randomised trial of endometrial ablation versus hysterectomy for the treatment of dysfunction uterine bleeding: outcome at four years. Br J Obstet Gynaecol 1999;106:360–366.

41. Phipps JH, John M, Nayak S. Comparison of laparoscopically assisted vaginal hysterectomy and bilateral salpingo-oophorectomy with conventional abdominal hysterectomy and bilateral salpingo-oophorectomy. Br J Obstet Gynaecol 1993;100: 698–700.

42. Raju KS, Auld BJ. A randomised prospective study of laparoscopic vaginal hysterectomy versus abdominal hysterectomy each with bilateral salpingo-oophorectomy. Br J Obstet Gynaecol 1994;101:1068–1071.

43. Richardson RE, Bournas N, Magos AL. Is laparoscopic hysterectomy a waste of time? Lancet 1995;345:36–41.

44. Summitt RL Jr, Stovall TG, Lipscomb GH, et al. Randomized comparison of laparoscopy-assisted vaginal hysterectomy with standard vaginal hysterectomy in an outpatient setting. Obstet Gynecol 1992;80:895–901.

45. Langebrekke A, Eraker R, Nesheim B, et al. Abdominal hysterectomy should not be considered as primary method for uterine removal. Acta Obstet Gynecol Scand 1996;75:404–407.

46. Carlson KJ. Outcomes of hysterectomy. Clin Obstet Gynecol 1997;40:939–946.

47. Dicker RC, Greenspan JR, Strauss LT, et al. Complications of abdominal and vaginal hysterectomy among women of reproductive age in the United States—the Collaborative Review of Sterilization. Am J Obstet Gynecol 1982;144:841–848.

48. Bhattacharya S, Cameron IM, Parkin DE, et al. A pragmatic randomised comparison of transcervical resection of the endometrium with endometrial laser ablation for the treatment of menorrhagia. Br J Obstet Gynaecol 1997;104:601–607.

49. Corson SL, Brill AI, Brooks PG, et al. Interim results of the American Vesta trial of endometrial ablation. J Am Assoc Gynecol Laparosc 1999;6:45–49.

50. B. Cooper KG, Bain C, Parkin DE. Comparison of microwave endometrial ablation and transcervical resection of the endometrium for treatment of heavy menstrual loss: a randomised trial. Lancet 1999;354:1859–1863.

51. Meyer WR, Walsh BW, Grainger DA, et al. Thermal balloon and rollerball ablation to treat menorrhagia: a multicenter comparison. Obstet Gynecol 1998;92:98–103.

52. Cooper KG, Parkin DE, Garratt AM, et al. A randomised comparison of medical versus hysteroscopic management in women consulting a gynaecologist for treatment of heavy menstrual loss. Br J Obstet Gynaecol 1997;104:1360–1366.

53. Cooper KG, Parkin DE, Garratt AM, et al. Two-year follow up of women randomised to medical management or transcervical resection of the endometrium for heavy menstrual loss: clinical and quality of life outcomes. Br J Obstet Gynaecol 1999;106:258–265.

54. Overton C, Hargreaves J, Maresh M. A national survey of the complications of endometrial destruction for menstrual disorders: the MISTLETOE study. Minimally invasive surgical techniques — laser, endothermal or endoresection. Br J Obstet Gynaecol 1997;104:1351–1359.

55. Broadbent JAM, Magos AL. Menstrual blood loss after hysteroscopic myomectomy. Gynaecol Endoscop 1995;4:41–44.

56. Sowter MC, Singla AA, Lethaby A. Pre-operative endometrial thinning agents before hysteroscopic surgery for heavy menstrual bleeding. In: The Cochrane Library, Issue 2, 2000. Oxford: Update Software. Search date not stated; primary sources Medline, Embase, Psychlit, Cinahl, biological abstracts, reference lists, authors of conference abstracts, Zeneca Pharmaceuticals and Sanofi Winthrop.

Kirsten Duckitt

Clinical Lecturer

John Radcliffe Hospital

Oxford

UK

Competing interests: None declared.

Premalignant vulval disorders

Search date May 2000

Earlando Thomas, Damian Murphy and Charles Redman

INTERVENTIONS

LICHEN SCLEROSUS

Likely to be beneficial

Trade off between benefits and harms

Likely to be ineffective or harmful

VULVAL INTRAEPITHELIAL NEOPLASIA

Unknown effectiveness

To be covered in future issues of *Clinical Evidence*

Lichen sclerosus: effects of topical lignocaine

VIN: effects of 5-fluorouracil

Petroleum jelly

See glossary, p 1330

Key Messages

Lichen sclerosus

- Limited evidence from three small RCTs suggests that topical clobetasol propionate is the most effective treatment for lichen sclerosus. Good quality prospective observational studies reported minimal adverse effects when clobetasol was used as required for maintenance treatment.

- Small RCTs found no evidence that testosterone was more effective than petroleum jelly, either as initial treatment or as maintenance treatment after treatment with clobetasol propionate. Testosterone is associated with virilisation.

- One small RCT found acitretin significantly reduced symptoms compared with placebo, but was associated with hair loss and severe skin peeling.

- We found insufficient evidence on the effects of surgery in women with lichen sclerosus.

Vulval intraepithelial neoplasia

- We found insufficient evidence on the effects of surgical or topical treatments in women with vulval intraepithelial neoplasia (VIN).

DEFINITION There are two recognised premalignant conditions of the vulva. **Lichen sclerosus** is characterised by epithelial thinning, inflammation, and distinctive histological changes in the dermis. It affects all age groups but is typically found in the anogenital region in postmenopausal women. The most common presentation is severe intractable itching (pruritus vulvae) and vaginal soreness with dyspareunia. **Vulval intraepithelial neoplasia (VIN)** is dysplasia of the vulval epithelium, categorised as mild (VIN I), moderate (VIN II), or severe (VIN III). The vulval lesions are often multifocal and are usually associated with itching and pain.

INCIDENCE/ We found no data on the prevalence of lichen sclerosus. The true
PREVALENCE incidence of VIN is unknown, but it is being diagnosed with increased frequency in the UK and the USA. This may be because of increased recognition of the disease or a true increase in incidence.[1–3]

AETIOLOGY/ The cause is unknown. VIN is associated with human papilloma
RISK FACTORS virus 16.[1]

PROGNOSIS There is currently no cure for lichen sclerosus, but the risk of progression to vulval carcinoma ranges from 0% to 9%.[4] People with concomitant squamous cell hyperplasia are at increased risk of malignancy.[5] Malignant transformation appears to be low in women with VIN I and II, but has been reported in 2–4% of women with VIN III.[2,6] About 30% of vulval carcinomas are associated with VIN.[1]

AIMS To control symptoms, to reduce the risk of malignant transformation, and to improve quality of life, with minimal adverse effects.

OUTCOMES Scores for symptoms (itching, burning, pain, and dyspareunia), gross appearance (relating to severity of lesions and extent of vulval involvement), and histological stage. Scores range from 0 to 3, where 3 represents the most severe. Other outcomes are rates of histological regression, recurrence, malignant transformation, and adverse effects of treatment.

METHODS *Clinical Evidence* search and appraisal May 2000. We included all RCTs that were appropriately randomised and double blinded with follow up of 80% or more participants, and with a minimum of 15 people in each study arm. Where confidence intervals were not reported but adequate information was provided, we calculated them using the software Statsdirect.[7] Where we found no good RCTs, we used the best available observational studies.

QUESTION What are the effects of treatments for lichen sclerosus?

OPTION TOPICAL CORTICOSTEROIDS AND TOPICAL TESTOSTERONE

We found limited evidence from three small RCTs suggesting that topical clobetasol propionate is more effective than topical testosterone propionate or petroleum jelly. We found no evidence that topical testosterone is more effective than petroleum jelly. Testosterone is associated with virilisation and pain.

Benefits: We found no systematic review. **Short term treatment:** We found two placebo- or vehicle- (petroleum jelly) controlled RCTs. One RCT compared clobetasol propionate 0.05% (n = 20), testosterone propionate (n = 20), and petroleum jelly (n = 19) for 3 months, with follow up of 3 months.[8] Clobetasol propionate was associated with significantly higher rates of symptom control and reversal of histological changes (AR for symptom control 75% on clobetasol, 20% on testosterone, and 10.5% on petroleum jelly). A significant difference in both gross and histological changes occurred only in the clobetasol group.[8] A second RCT compared testosterone propionate in petroleum jelly (n = 30) versus petroleum jelly alone (n = 28) for 12 months with at least 12 months' follow up. There was no significant difference in response rates (75% v 66.6%; AR difference 8.3%, 95% CI −31.1% to +15.5%, calculated from data reported).[9] **Maintenance treatment:** Recurrence of symptoms on maintenance treatment was more common with topical testosterone than with petroleum jelly (AR 9/16 [56%] with testosterone, 3/16 [19%] with petroleum jelly; ARI [38%], 95% CI 2% to 67%; NNH 3, 95% CI 1 to 53). There was no significant difference in control of gross features between testosterone and petroleum jelly.[10]

Harms: One RCT found no evidence that topical clobetasol propionate was associated with adverse effects,[8] and good prospective observational studies reported minimal adverse effects when clobetasol propionate was used as required for maintenance treatment for 1–3 years (see glossary, p 1330).[11,12] Topical testosterone was associated with virilisation (4/20 women),[8] hypertrichosis (1/30),[9] pruritus and pain (3/30),[9] and burning (4/16).[10] No harmful effects were reported with petroleum jelly.[8–10,13]

Comment: None of the RCTs was double-blinded and none included a power calculation to justify sample size. All had follow up rates of > 80% for assessment of treatment efficacy. The high response rate to petroleum jelly may have been more than a placebo effect: petroleum jelly has a soothing effect on the vulvar skin.

| OPTION | ORAL RETINOIDS (ACITRETIN) |

One small RCT found that acitretin was more effective than placebo. Acitretin is associated with severe peeling of palms and soles, and with hair loss.

Benefits: We found no systematic review. We found one RCT comparing acitretin versus placebo for 12–16 weeks with 4–6 weeks' follow up in 46 eligible patients.[13] Compared to placebo, acitretin reduced the incidence of pruritus, atrophic features, hyperkeratosis, burning, and large lesions (8/22 v 18/24; ARR: 38.6%, 95% CI 9.8% to 61.1%; NNT 3, 95% CI 2 to 10).

Harms: Adverse effects were reported in 100% of people taking acitretin and 56% of those taking placebo.[13] Acitretin was associated with severe peeling of the palms and soles (11/39 people) and increased rates of hair loss (23/39 v 2/39 on placebo).[13] Acitretin was associated with congenital abnormalities in women exposed during the first trimester of pregnancy,[14,15] and is therefore contraindicated in pregnancy. Contraception has been recommended for use during treatment and for 2 years afterwards.[16]

Comment: The RCT was double-blinded. Follow up rates were > 80% for assessment of treatment efficacy.

OPTION   **SURGICAL TREATMENTS**

We found insufficient evidence on the effects of surgery in lichen sclerosus.

Benefits: We found no systematic review, RCTs, or good quality observational studies.

Harms: Three cohort studies reported reoperation rates after vulvectomy (33%, 23%, and 50%). The reasons for reoperating were recurrence, progression to vulval cancer, and constricted vaginal outlet.[4]

Comment: We found one non-systematic review, which identified uncontrolled cohort studies of vulvectomy, cryosurgery and laser treatment.[4] **Vulvectomy:** Five studies were reviewed. Four evaluated simple, partial, or complete vulvectomy (44–120 women, follow up 3–23 years, recurrence rates 39–59%). One study evaluated skinning vulvectomy (see glossary, p 1330) and skin graft (n = 4, follow up 4–8 years, recurrence rate 50%). **Cryosurgery:** One study was reviewed (n = 12, follow up 3 years, two women lost to follow up, rate of recurrence/failed treatment 42%). Complete healing took up to 3 months. **Laser treatment:** Four studies were reviewed. The largest (n = 62, follow up 0.3–7 years) found a 16% recurrence rate. The other studies were small (5–7 women, follow up 1–6 years, recurrence rates 0–14%). Complete healing took up to 6 weeks.

QUESTION   **What are the effects of treatments for vulval intraepithelial neoplasia?**

OPTION   **SURGICAL TREATMENTS**

We found insufficient evidence on the effects of surgical treatments in women with vulval intraepithelial neoplasia (VIN).

Benefits: We found no systematic review or RCTs.

Harms: Laser skinning vulvectomy may be associated with labial fusion (14%), and in 5% of cases laser treatment of perianal lesions caused an incomplete anal sphincter. Moderate to severe postoperative pain is also common after laser vaporisation.[3,17] Vaporisation using carbon dioxide produces a plume containing carcinogenic substances, and the radiant energy can cause thermal burns, fires, and eye injuries in the operator. The risk of aerosol produced during ultrasound surgical aspiration is unclear, and precautions to protect surgeons from patients' body fluids may be required.[18,19] Cryosurgery may be associated with oedema, pain, and ulceration. Difficulties with precision and control may also result in vulval scarring and distortion.[18]

Premalignant vulval disorders

Comment: A minimum of 5 years' follow up would be necessary to assess properly the effects of treatment on rates of recurrence and malignant transformation in women with VIN. One retrospective cohort study in women with VIN I, II, or III reported on rates of recurrence or persistence, at a mean of 31 months, after local excision (n = 61, recurrence 25%), primary surgery including local excision, simple vulvectomy, and knife skinning vulvectomy with grafting (n = 103, recurrence 39%) and laser vaporisation (n = 30, recurrence 67%). The difference between laser vaporisation and local excision was significant (P ≤ 0.001). By 10 years, histological recurrence was seen in 79% of women treated with laser compared with 36% treated with local excision. Progression to malignant disease occurred after surgical intervention in nine women (7%).[2] A smaller cohort study found recurrence or persistence in 21% of women after simple vulvectomy (n = 9, median follow up 74 months), 44% after local excision (n = 14, median follow up 74 months), and 52% after laser skinning vulvectomy (n = 21, median follow up 38 months).[3] Other small, uncontrolled studies found recurrence rates of 8.6% with laser vaporisation (n = 35, follow up 12–36 months),[17] 22% with ultrasound surgical aspiration (n = 9, median follow up 12 months),[20] and 90% with cryosurgery (n = 10, mean follow up 12 months).[6]

OPTION **TOPICAL α INTERFERON**

We found insufficient evidence on the effects of topical α interferon in women with VIN.

Benefits: We found no systematic review and no placebo controlled or comparative RCTs. We found one small blinded crossover RCT (n = 18) evaluating topical α interferon with and without 1% nonoxinol-9. Outcomes were symptom control (itching, burning, and pain), reversal of histological changes, and adverse effects of treatment. Overall, 14/18 (67%) of participants had some response to α interferon (no P values or CIs reported). The addition of 1% nonoxinol-9 made no significant difference to the number of complete responders (complete response occurred in 3/10 treatment episodes with 1% nonoxinol-9 and 6/14 without).[21]

Harms: Topical α interferon was associated with transitory adverse effects, including fever (8%), mild discomfort, and mild pruritus (17%).[21]

Comment: None.

GLOSSARY

Skinning vulvectomy The epidermis and the underlying dermis of the vulva are removed by knife or laser. Split thickness skin graft is usually employed to cover the defect following knife excision.

REFERENCES

1. Crum CP, McLachlin CM, Tate JE, Mutter GL. Pathobiology of vulvar squamous neoplasia. *Curr Opin Obstet Gynecol* 1997;9:63–69.

2. Herod JJO, Shafi MI, Rollason TP, et al. Vulvar intraepithelial neoplasia: long term follow up treated and untreated. *Br J Obstet Gynaecol* 1996;103:446–452.

3. Shafi MI, Luesley DM, Byrne P, et al. Vulval

intraepithelial neoplasia – management and outcome. *Br J Obstet Gynaecol* 1989;96:1339–1344.

4. Abramov Y, Elchalal U, Abramov D, Goldfarb A, Schenker JG. Surgical treatment of vulvar lichen sclerosus: a review. *Obstet Gynecol Surv* 1996;51:193–199.

5. Elchalal U, Gilead L, Vardy DA, et al. Treatment of

vulvar lichen sclerosus in the elderly: an update. *Obstet Gynecol Surv* 1995;50:155–162.

6. Marren P, Dawber R, Wojnarowska F, et al. Failure of cryosurgery to eradicate vulval intraepithelial neoplasia: a pilot study. *J Eur Acad Dermatol Venereol* 1993;2:247–252.

7. Buchan IE. Statsdirect http://www.statsdirect.com. Cambridge (England) CamCode 2000.

8. Bracco GL, Carli P, Sonni L, et al. Clinical and histologic effects of topical treatments of vulval lichen sclerosus. *J Reproductive Med* 1993;38: 37–40.

9. Sideri M, Origoni L, Spinaci L, Ferrari A. Topical testosterone in the treatment of vulvar lichen sclerosus. *Int J Gynaecol Obstet* 1994;46:53–56.

10. Cattaneo A, Carli P, De Marco A, et al. Testosterone maintenance therapy. Effects on vulval lichen sclerosus treated with clobetasol propionate. *J Reprod Med* 1996;41:99–102.

11. Dalziel KL, Wojnarowska F. Long-term control of vulval lichen sclerosus after treatment with a potent topical steroid cream. *J Reprod Med* 1993; 38:25–27.

12. Bornstein J, Heifetz S, Kellner Y, et al. Clobetasol dipropionate 0.05% versus testosterone propionate 2% topical application for severe vulval lichen sclerosus. *Am J Obstet Gynecol* 1998;178: 80–84.

13. Bousema MT, Romppanen U, Geiger J-M, et al. Acitretin in the treatment of severe lichen sclerosus or atrophicus of the vulva: a double-blind, placebo-controlled study. *J Am Acad Dermatol* 1994;30:225–231.

14. De Die-Smulders CE, Sturkenboom MC, Veraart J, van Katwijk C, Sastrowijoto P, van der Linden E. Severe limb defects and craniofacial anomalies in a fetus conceived during acitretin therapy. *Teratology* 1995;52:215–219.

15. Geiger JM, Baudin M, Saurat JH. Teratogenic risk with etretinate and acitretin treatment. *Dermatology* 1994;89:109–116.

16. *British National Formulary*. London: British Medical Association/Royal Pharmaceutical Society of Great Britain, September 1999;38:504.

17. Baggish MS, Dorsey JH. CO2 laser for the treatment of vulvar carcinoma in situ. *Obstet Gynecol* 1981;57:371–374.

18. Townsend DE, Levine RU, Richart RM, et al. Management of vulvar intraepithelial neoplasia by carbon dioxide laser. *Obstet Gynecol* 1982;60:49–51.

19. Adelson MD. Ultrasonic surgical aspiration in the treatment of vulvar disease. *Obstet Gynecol* 1991; 78:477–479.

20. Rader JS, Leake JF, Dillon MB, et al. Ultrasound surgical aspiration in the treatment of vulvar disease. *Obstet Gynecol* 1991;77:573–576.

21. Spirtos NM, Smith LH, Teng NNH. Prospective randomised trial of α-interferon (α-interferon gels) for the treatment of vulvar intraepithelial neoplasia III. *Gynecol Oncol* 1990;37:34–38.

Earlando Thomas
Senior Specialist Registrar
Department of Obstetrics and
Gynecology
Rochester, New York
USA

Damian Murphy
Consultant Obstetrician and
Gynaecologist
Department of Obstetrics and
Gynaecology
New Cross Hospital
Wolverhampton
UK

Charles Redman
Consultant Obstetrician and
Gynaecologist
Department of Obstetrics and
Gynaecology
City General Hospital
Stoke on Trent
UK
Competing interests: None declared.

Women's health

Pyelonephritis in non-pregnant women

Search date October 2000

Bruce Cooper

QUESTIONS

INTERVENTIONS

Key Messages

- We found no RCTs of antibiotics versus no antibiotics for the treatment of acute pyelonephritis.

- One systematic review of RCTs found no consistent differences in the bacteriological and clinical cure rates between oral co-trimoxazole, co-amoxiclav, or a fluoroquinolone (ciprofloxacin, norfloxacin, levofloxacin, or lomefloxacin) in healthy, non-pregnant women with acute pyelonephritis who are able to take oral treatment and lack signs of sepsis.

- One RCT found no significant difference between oral or intravenous ciprofloxacin in the duration of fever or symptoms.

- One RCT found that intravenous co-trimoxazole or ampicillin plus gentamicin were effective and well tolerated in non-pregnant women admitted to hospital with acute uncomplicated pyelonephritis.

- We found no well designed trials comparing newer intravenous antibiotics with older regimens.

- We found no direct evidence comparing inpatient and outpatient management of acute, uncomplicated pyelonephritis in non-pregnant women.

DEFINITION Acute pyelonephritis, or upper urinary tract infection, is an infection of the kidney, characterised by dysuria, fever, flank pain, nausea, and vomiting. Pyuria is almost always present, and occasionally white blood cell casts are seen on urine microscopy. Uncomplicated infection occurs in an otherwise healthy person without underlying comorbidity. Complicated infection occurs in people with structural or functional urinary tract abnormalities or comorbid diseases. People with acute pyelonephritis can be divided into those able to take oral antibiotics and without signs of sepsis who may be managed at home, and those requiring parenteral treatment in hospital.

INCIDENCE/ In the USA, there are 250 000 cases of acute pyelonephritis a **PREVALENCE** year.[1] Worldwide prevalence and incidence are unknown.

AETIOLOGY/ Pyelonephritis is most commonly caused when bacteria in the **RISK FACTORS** bladder ascend the ureters and invade the renal parenchyma. In some cases, this results in bacteraemia.

PROGNOSIS With prompt diagnosis and treatment, the prognosis is good. Complications include sepsis, metastatic infection, renal impairment, and renal abscess. Comorbidity such as renal disease, diabetes mellitus, and immunosuppression may worsen prognosis, with a potential increase in risk of sepsis and death, but we found no good long term evidence about such people.

AIMS To reduce the duration and severity of symptoms; to prevent or minimise potential complications, with minimum adverse effects.

OUTCOMES Urine culture after treatment; signs and symptoms of infection; rates of complications of infection; and adverse effects of treatment.

METHODS *Clinical Evidence* update search and appraisal October 2000, using the MeSH terms pyelonephritis, upper urinary tract infection, hospitalisation, outpatient therapy, and oral antibiotics. We included RCTs and systematic reviews that focused on the inpatient and outpatient management of acute uncomplicated pyelonephritis in non-pregnant women. We excluded studies that were primarily in men, pregnant women, and people with complicated infections.

QUESTION What are the effects of treatments for acute pyelonephritis?

OPTION ORAL ANTIBIOTICS

We found no RCTs comparing oral antibiotics with placebo. One systematic review of RCTs found no consistent differences in the bacteriological and clinical cure rates between oral co-trimoxazole, co-amoxiclav, or a fluoroquinolone (ciprofloxacin, norfloxacin, levofloxacin, or lomefloxacin) in healthy, non-pregnant women with acute pyelonephritis who are able to take oral treatment and lack signs of sepsis. One RCT found no significant difference between oral or intravenous ciprofloxacin in the duration of fever or symptoms.

Benefits: **Versus placebo:** We found no systematic review or RCTs. **Versus other oral antibiotics:** We found one systematic review (search date 1991, 9 RCTs, 470 men and non-pregnant women) and two subsequent RCTs comparing different oral antibiotics in acute pyelonephritis (see table 1, p 1337).[2] Five RCTs were conducted with people outside hospital and four in people admitted to hospital. The studies were conducted in the USA, Europe, and Peru. All included more women than men. Most studies excluded people with complicating factors such as structural abnormalities of the urinary tract, comorbid illnesses, pregnancy, or signs of possible sepsis. All except one found no significant difference in rates of early cure (negative urine culture within 7–10 days), and six of the nine studies found no significant difference in rates of late cure (negative urine culture 2–4 weeks or more after stopping treatment). However, several of the individual studies were too small to rule out a difference between antibiotic regimens. One subsequent RCT (multicentre, 47 people with acute uncomplicated pyelonephritis admitted to hospital) compared oral lomefloxacin 400 mg daily versus oral co-trimoxazole 160 mg/800 mg twice daily, both for 14 days.[3] At 5–9 days, there was a significantly higher rate of bacteriological eradication on lomefloxacin compared with co-trimoxazole (100% v 89%, P = 0.05), but no significant difference in clinical cure rates. At 4–6 weeks, there were no significant differences. The other subsequent RCT (186 outpatients, 162 women, with acute uncomplicated pyelonephritis) compared 10 days of levofloxacin 250 mg daily versus 10 days of ciprofloxacin 500 mg twice daily or 14 days of lomefloxacin 400 mg daily.[4] It found no significant difference in rates of early cure (negative urine culture 5–9 days after treatment, which occurred in 94% of people on each of the 3 drugs) or microbiological relapse at long term follow up. **Oral versus intravenous antibiotics:** We found no systematic review but found one Swiss based multicentre RCT in 163 people admitted to hospital with pyelonephritis or complicated urinary tract infection (infection associated with a structural or functional abnormality of the urinary tract or nosocomially acquired), which compared oral ciprofloxacin 500 mg every 12 hours versus intravenous ciprofloxacin 200 mg every 12 hours. The analysis included 83 non-pregnant women. It found no significant difference between oral and intravenous ciprofloxacin in the duration of symptoms (1.7 days, 95% CI 1.5 to 1.9 with oral v 1.9 days, 95% CI 1.7 to 2.2 with intravenous; P = 0.15) or fever (1.8 days, 95% CI 1.4 to 2.2 v 1.8 days, 95% CI 1.4 to 2.2; P = 0.85), the number of people with persistent infection after 3–5 days of treatment (2 v 1, P = 0.95), or the median duration of hospitalisation (7 days, 95% CI 2 to 35 v 8 days, 95% CI 2 to 32; P = 0.15). There were no infection related deaths.[5]

Harms: Adverse effects were reported in 12% of people taking lomefloxacin and 17% taking co-trimoxazole.[3] The most frequent adverse effects were skin reactions. Three people taking co-trimoxazole withdrew from treatment, one because of dermatitis and one because of hepatocellular damage. There were no withdrawals because of adverse events in people taking lomefloxacin.[3] Adverse effects were reported in 2% of people on levofloxacin, 8% on ciprofloxacin, and 5% on lomefloxacin.[4] Gastrointestinal symptoms were common with both ciprofloxacin and levofloxacin, whereas rash was the most common adverse effect with lomefloxacin. One of the 186 people discontinued treatment (lomefloxacin) because of adverse effects.[4] In the RCT that compared oral and intravenous ciprofloxacin, one person on oral ciprofloxacin discontinued treatment because of the development of mental confusion. Another person on intravenous ciprofloxacin developed pruritus, but treatment was continued until completed. No other adverse affects were reported.[5]

Comment: Calculated cure rates from the systematic review are likely to overestimate rates that would be achieved in clinical practice because many people were excluded, including those who experienced adverse effects, had growth of resistant bacteria on initial culture, or did not adhere to treatment. The high rate of ampicillin resistance found in laboratory tests has led to a consensus view that ampicillin and amoxicillin are not recommended in pyelonephritis. We found no direct evidence to confirm or refute this view. Ampicillin and amoxicillin were found in the trials to have cure rates comparable with other antibiotics, but the studies were too small to exclude a clinically important difference. The RCT comparing oral and intravenous ciprofloxacin included people with underlying structural or functional urinary abnormalities.

OPTION   **INTRAVENOUS ANTIBIOTICS**

One RCT found that intravenous co-trimoxazole or ampicillin plus gentamicin were effective and well tolerated in non-pregnant women admitted to hospital with acute uncomplicated pyelonephritis. We found no well designed trials comparing newer intravenous antibiotics with these standard regimens.

Benefits: **Versus placebo:** We found no systematic review and no RCTs.
Versus other intravenous antibiotics: We found no systematic review but found one RCT (85 women admitted to hospital for acute uncomplicated pyelonephritis), which compared intravenous ampicillin 1 g every 6 hours versus intravenous co-trimoxazole 160 mg/ 800 mg every 12 hours, initiated before culture results were known.[6] Both regimens were combined with gentamicin and followed by oral treatment with either ampicillin or co-trimoxazole. *Escherichia coli* was the sole micro-organism isolated from the urine in 91% of women. Fourteen of the 42 women (32%) treated with ampicillin and gentamicin were infected with ampicillin resistant isolates and were withdrawn from the study. No women allocated to co-trimoxazole required a change of treatment, and there were no other treatment failures in either group. We found no other adequately designed RCTs comparing treatments that included intravenous quinolones, cephalosporins, broad spectrum β lactams, or co-trimoxazole. **Versus oral antibiotics:** See oral antibiotics, p 1334.

Harms: Adverse effects varied by agent. In the RCT,[6] adverse effects that may have been a result of treatment were reported equally in the two groups (33% ampicillin v 32% co-trimoxazole) but the nature of these adverse effects was not reported. One person from each group discontinued treatment because of adverse effects.[6] Common adverse effects with ampicillin include rash, diarrhoea, and vaginitis, and with co-trimoxazole include nausea, vomiting, and vaginitis.

Pyelonephritis in non-pregnant women

Comment: There is a consensus view that the choice of empirical antibiotics should take into account the setting, medical history of the patient, Gram stain of the urine, previous infecting organism, and local antibiotic sensitivities.

OPTION   INPATIENT VERSUS OUTPATIENT MANAGEMENT

We found no direct evidence comparing inpatient and outpatient management of acute, uncomplicated pyelonephritis in non-pregnant women.

Benefits: We found no systematic review and no RCTs comparing inpatient with outpatient management of acute uncomplicated pyelonephritis in non-pregnant women.

Harms: We found no evidence.

Comment: Hospitals may be able to provide closer monitoring and supervision of people with pyelonephritis than can be provided outside hospital. However, it is not clear whether treatment in hospital delivers any benefit in terms of outcomes or whether there is an increased risk of harm from hospital treatment.

REFERENCES

1. Stamm WE, Hooton TM, Johnson JR. Urinary tract infection: from pathogenesis to treatment. *J Infect Dis* 1989;15:400–406.
2. Pinson AG, Philbrick JT, Lindbeck GH, et al. Oral antibiotic therapy for acute pyelonephritis: a methodologic review of the literature. *J Gen Intern Med* 1992;7:544–553. Search date 1991; primary sources Medline 1965 to 1990, Current Contents 1990 to 1991.
3. Mouton Y, Ajana F, Chidiac C, et al. A multicenter study of lomefloxacin and trimethoprim/sulfamethoxazole in the treatment of uncomplicated acute pyelonephritis. *Am J Med* 1992;92(suppl):87–90.
4. Richard GA, Klimberg IN, Fowler CL, et al. Levofloxacin versus ciprofloxacin versus lomefloxacin in acute pyelonephritis. *Urology* 1998;52:51–55.
5. Mombelli G, Pezzoli R, Pinoja-Lutz G, et al. Oral vs intravenous ciprofloxacin in the initial empirical management of severe pyelonephritis or complicated urinary tract infections: a prospective randomized clinical trial. *Arch Intern Med* 1999;159:53–58.
6. Johnson JR, Lyons MF, Pearce W, et al. Therapy for women hospitalized with acute pyelonephritis: a randomized trial of ampicillin versus trimethoprim-sulfamethoxazole for 14 days. *J Infect Dis* 1991; 163:325–330.

Bruce Cooper
Renal Research Fellow
University of Sydney
Royal North Shore Hospital
St Leonards
Sydney
Australia

Competing interests: None declared.

TABLE 1 Oral antibiotic treatment for acute pyelonephritis: results of RCTs (see text, p 1334).[2]

Study number	Oral antibiotic regimens	Total number of patients	Early cure* rates %	Late cure* rates %	P value
1	Amoxicillin 500 mg three times daily for 14 days	16	–	94	NS
	Co-trimoxazole (160 mg/800 mg) twice daily for 14 days	12	–	92	
2	Norfloxacin 400 mg twice daily for 10 days	14	100	86	NS
	Co-trimoxazole (160 mg/800 mg) twice daily for 10 days	10	100	90	
3	Ampicillin 500 mg four times daily for 10 days	8	88	–	NS
	Cefaclor 250 mg twice daily for 10 days	6	67	–	
4	Norfloxacin 400 mg twice daily for 7 days or longer	3	67	–	NS
	Co-trimoxazole (160 mg/800 mg) twice daily for 7 days or longer	12	92	–	
5	Co-amoxiclav 250 mg/125 mg three times daily for 10 days	54	94	85	P = 0.02 for late cure; NS for early cure
6	Co-trimoxazole (160 mg/800 mg) twice daily for 10 days	50	82	64	P = 0.004 for late cure; NS for early cure
	Ampicillin 500 mg four times daily for 2 or 6 weeks	17	100	47	
7	Co-trimoxazole (160 mg/800 mg) twice daily for 2 or 6 weeks	22	100	91	NS
	Amoxicillin 2000 mg one time dose then 1000 mg twice daily for 9 days	22	100	100	
8	Amoxicillin 750 mg three times daily for 12 days	23	96	87	NS
	Cefetamet 2000 mg daily or 1000 mg twice daily for 10–15 days	28	93	79	
9	Cefadroxil 1000 mg twice daily for 10–15 days	22	73	52	P < 0.0001 for both early and late cures
	Norfloxacin 400 mg twice daily for 14 days	76	91	82	
	Cefadroxil 1000 mg twice daily for 14 days	75	59	44	

Table adapted with permission.[2] NS, not significant. *Early cure: negative urine culture within 7–10 days of starting treatment; late cure: negative urine culture 2–4 weeks or more after stopping treatment.

Recurrent cystitis in non-pregnant women

Search date November 2000

Bruce Cooper and Ruth Jepson

INTERVENTIONS

Key Messages

- Consistent evidence from RCTs has found that medium term antibiotic prophylaxis (either continuous or postcoital), using nitrofurantoin, a quinolone, trimethoprim, or co-trimoxazole (trimethoprim-sulfamethoxazole, TMP-SMZ) reduces infection rates in women with high rates of recurrent urinary tract infections (at least two a year).

- One RCT has found that intermittent, single dose, self administered treatment taken at the onset of symptoms is an effective alternative management strategy to continuous antibiotic prophylaxis in women with high rates of recurrent infection.

- Evidence from one cohort study suggests that long term continuous prophylaxis (longer than 12 months) is likely to benefit women with a baseline rate of more than two infections a year over many years.

- We found insufficient evidence of the effects of cranberry juice and other cranberry products on the prevention of recurrent urinary tract infections.

- In women who experience recurrent, uncomplicated urinary tract infections, we found no good evidence to support routine investigation of the urinary tract with excretory urography, ultrasonography, cystoscopy, or voiding cystourethrography. No subgroups of women who would clearly benefit from investigation have yet been adequately defined.

DEFINITION	Cystitis is an infection of the lower urinary tract causing dysuria, frequency, urgency, haematuria, or suprapubic pain. Pyuria and bacteriuria are almost always present. The presence of fever, flank pain, nausea, or vomiting suggests pyelonephritis (see pyelonephritis in non-pregnant women, p 1332). Recurrent cystitis may be either a reinfection (after successful eradication of infection) or a relapse after inadequate treatment.
INCIDENCE/ PREVALENCE	The incidence of cystitis among premenopausal sexually active women is 0.5–0.7 infections per person year,[1] and 20–40% of women will experience cystitis during their lifetime. Of those, 20% will develop recurrence, almost always (90% of cases) because of reinfection rather than relapse. Rates of infection fall during the winter months.[2]
AETIOLOGY/ RISK FACTORS	Cystitis is caused by uropathogenic bacteria in the faecal flora that colonise the vaginal and periurethral introitus, and ascend the urethra into the bladder. Prior infection, sexual intercourse, and exposure to vaginal spermicide are risk factors for developing cystitis.[3,4]
PROGNOSIS	We found little evidence on the long term effects of untreated cystitis. One study found that progression to upper urinary tract infection was infrequent, and that most cases of cystitis regressed spontaneously, although symptoms sometimes persisted for several months.[5] Women with a baseline rate of more than two infections a year, over many years, are likely to continue to suffer from recurrent infections.[6]
AIMS	To prevent recurrent infection in women predisposed to frequent infections, with minimal adverse effects.
OUTCOMES	Rate of infection based on urine culture and symptoms.
METHODS	*Clinical Evidence* update search and appraisal November 2000. We reviewed all systematic reviews and RCTs comparing different forms of prophylaxis, or comparing prophylaxis versus placebo in non-pregnant women with a history of recurrent urinary tract infection. We excluded studies in populations consisting mainly of men or pregnant women.

QUESTION   Which interventions prevent further recurrence in women experiencing at least two infections per year?

OPTION   MEDIUM TERM CONTINUOUS ANTIBIOTIC PROPHYLAXIS

RCTs have found that continuous antibiotic prophylaxis using trimethoprim, co-trimoxazole, nitrofurantoin, cefaclor, or a quinolone reduces rates of recurrent urinary tract infection in non-pregnant women. We found no good evidence of any difference between different continuous regimens, nor between continuous and postcoital regimens.

Benefits:	We found no systematic review. We found seven RCTs comparing different regimens for continuous antibiotic prophylaxis lasting 6–12 months in women with high rates of recurrent urinary tract infection (at least two episodes a year) (see table 1, p 1344).[7-13] Three of the RCTs included a placebo or no treatment arm.[7-9] All

found significantly lower rates of infection with active treatment (nitrofurantoin, ciprofloxacin, norfloxacin, or co-trimoxazole), but confidence intervals were not given. **Versus each other:** Five RCTs compared different antibiotic regimens.[7,10–13] One RCT (72 women) found significantly fewer infections ($P < 0.05$) in women taking a nocturnal dose of nitrofurantoin compared with those using a nocturnal dose of trimethoprim.[10] In the other larger studies comparing different regimens over 6–12 months, no significant differences were found.[7,11–13] Most of the reported rates of infection in these studies were much less than 0.6 per person year, suggesting that they were all as effective in reducing the rate of infection in people with a history of recurrent cystitis. However, these studies were not powered to exclude a clinically important difference between treatments. **Versus postcoital prophylaxis:** One RCT (135 women) compared daily versus postcoital treatment with ciprofloxacin. It found no significant difference in rates of infection, but no confidence interval was given.[8]

Harms: Rates of adverse effects in these studies ranged from 7–40% for trimethoprim; 0–40% for nitrofurantoin; 5% for cefaclor; 7–21% for norfloxacin; and 13% for ciprofloxacin.[7–9,11–13] The most common adverse effects for all agents were gastrointestinal symptoms, rash, and yeast vaginitis.

Comment: Many of the studies were not placebo controlled or blinded, and had small study populations. However, despite the small study sizes, infection rates were significantly less in women using continuous prophylactic antibiotics compared to those without antibiotics. Adjustments were not made for confounding factors such as frequency of sexual intercourse.

OPTION   POSTCOITAL ANTIBIOTIC PROPHYLAXIS

RCTs have found that taking nitrofurantoin, a quinolone, trimethoprim, or co-trimoxazole within 2 hours after sexual intercourse significantly reduces the rates of infection in women with recurrent urinary tract infection. One RCT found no evidence of any difference between postcoital and continuous daily antibiotic regimens.

Benefits: We found no systematic review. We found four RCTs of postcoital antibiotic regimens (treatment taken within 2 hours of sexual intercourse), evaluated over 6–14 months, in women with high rates of recurrent urinary tract infection (at least two episodes a year) (see table 2, p 1345).[8,14–16] **Versus placebo or no treatment:** All RCTs found a significant reduction in rates of infection with active treatment (co-trimoxazole, nitrofurantoin, or a quinolone). **Versus continuous daily prophylaxis:** One RCT (135 women) compared continuous daily versus postcoital treatment with ciprofloxacin.[8] It found no significant difference in rates of infection.

Harms: Rates of adverse effects were as follows: co-trimoxazole 18%; ciprofloxacin 6%; and nitrofurantoin less than 1%.[8,14–16] The most common adverse effects for all agents were gastrointestinal symptoms, rash, and yeast vaginitis.

Comment: Only one of the studies was placebo controlled and blinded.[14] Adjustments were not made for confounding factors such as frequency of sexual intercourse.

OPTION   SELF TREATMENT WITH ANTIBIOTICS

Limited evidence from one small RCT suggests that self treatment with a single dose of co-trimoxazole is an effective alternative management strategy to continuous antibiotic prophylaxis in women with high rates of infection.

Benefits: We found no systematic review. We found one RCT using a cross-over design in 38 non-pregnant women with two or more culture documented urinary tract infections in the previous 12 months.[17] This compared continuous antibiotic prophylaxis with co-trimoxazole (40 mg/200 mg) versus a self administered single dose of co-trimoxazole (40 mg/200 mg) to be taken at the onset of symptoms of cystitis. The self treatment group was given enough tablets for four single treatments. Although infection rates were higher in the self treatment group (2.2 per person year compared with 0.22 per person year with continuous prophylaxis; P < 0.001, see comment below), 85% of infections responded to a single dose. We found no evidence relating to effects on quality of life.

Harms: The trial found no evidence of significant differences in adverse effects between continuous antibiotic prophylaxis and self administered treatment.

Comment: The trial found that the women were almost always able to diagnose their own infections from symptoms (positive predictive value 92%).[17] The higher rate of infections in the self treatment group is to be expected since self treatment was only administered after the onset of symptoms.

OPTION   LONG TERM CONTINUOUS ANTIBIOTIC PROPHYLAXIS

Evidence from one cohort study suggests that long term prophylaxis (longer than 12 months) is likely to benefit women with a baseline rate of more than two infections a year over many years.

Benefits: We found no systematic review or RCTs. We found one cohort study[2] (see comment below).

Harms: The cohort study reported no significant adverse effects, even when treatment continued for as long as 5 years. The development of bacterial resistance from continuous antibiotic prophylaxis was rare. However, the number of co-trimoxazole resistant organisms increased during the latter part of the study.[2]

Comment: The cohort study followed 51 non-pregnant women treated for over 112 person years with continuous trimethoprim, co-trimoxazole, or nitrofurantoin, and found that this intervention was effective in preventing cystitis and pyelonephritis.[2]

One systematic review found insufficient evidence of the effects of cranberry juice and other cranberry products on the prevention of recurrent urinary tract infections.

Benefits: We found one systematic review (search date 1998, 2 RCTs, 211 women) comparing cranberry juice and other cranberry products with placebo in the prevention of urinary tract infections in susceptible populations.[18] One was a crossover trial (19 women with recurrent infections) comparing cranberry capsules versus placebo. The withdrawal rate was 47%. It found 21 infections among the 10 remaining women, of which six infections occurred while taking cranberry capsules. The other RCT (192 elderly women) compared cranberry juice versus placebo. The withdrawal rate was 20%. It found that cranberry juice versus placebo significantly reduced the rate of infection (defined as $\geq 100\,000$ organisms per ml plus pyuria; OR 0.42, P = 0.004).

Harms: No data on adverse effects were reported.

Comment: These studies were small, with high withdrawal rates, and the lack of intention to treat analyses in either trial may mean that they overestimated the effectiveness of cranberry juice and products. High withdrawal rates suggest that long term adherence may be difficult to achieve.

We found limited evidence suggesting that routine investigation is unlikely to be beneficial. Subgroups of women who would clearly benefit from investigation have not yet been adequately defined.

Benefits: We found no systematic review or RCTs.

Harms: We found two cross sectional studies[19,20] and one prospective study[21] of routine excretory urography (see comment below). The studies had insufficient power to report on harms. Excretory urography with iodinated dye can cause anaphylactoid reactions and renal dysfunction. Cystoscopy can cause bleeding and other complications depending upon the type of procedure and anaesthesia used. Ultrasonography has no known adverse effects.

Comment: Two older, cross sectional studies[19,20] and one prospective study[21] examined the yield of routine excretory urography in women with recurrent urinary tract infections. Among the 421 women studied, urography was normal in 88%, showed anatomic variants in about 6%, and was abnormal in about 5%. None of the abnormalities detected were correctable or thought to be causally related to infection. Two of the studies found no evidence that cystoscopy detected clinically important abnormalities.[20,21] In a more recent cross sectional study, 186 women were non-randomly selected from a larger group of 475 women with recurrent urinary tract infections because the referring physician suspected an underlying problem.[22] Of these, 21% had an abnormality reported on cystoscopy, excretory urography, ultrasonography, or voiding cystourethrography. The reported rates of detection of abnormalities in these observational studies[19-21] are likely to be overestimates because the studies took place in specialist urology units. Results from the more recent cross sectional study are difficult to interpret because there was no standard protocol for evaluation and results were collected retrospectively.[22]

REFERENCES

1. Hooton TM, Scholes D, Hughes JP, et al. A prospective study of risk factors for symptomatic urinary tract infection in young women. *N Engl J Med* 1996;335:468–474.

2. Stamm WE, McKevitt M, Roberts PL, White NJ. Natural history of recurrent urinary tract infections in women. *Rev Infect Dis* 1991;13:77–84.

3. Fihn SD, Latham RH, Roberts P, Running K, Stamm WE. Association between diaphragm use and urinary tract infection. *JAMA* 1985;254:240–245.

4. Fihn SD, Boyko EJ, Normand EH, et al. Association between use of spermicide-coated condoms and *Escherichia coli* urinary tract infection in young women. *Am J Epidemiol* 1996;144:512–520.

5. Mabeck CE. Treatment of uncomplicated urinary tract infection in non-pregnant women. *Postgrad Med J* 1972;48:69–75.

6. Stamm WE, Counts GW, McKevitt M, Turck M, Holmes KK. Urinary prophylaxis with trimethoprim and trimethoprim-sulfamethoxazole: efficacy, influence on the natural history of recurrent bacteriuria and cost control. *Rev Infect Dis* 1982;4:450–455.

7. Stamm WE, Counts GW, Wagner KF, et al. Antimicrobial prophylaxis of recurrent urinary tract infections: a double-blind placebo-controlled trial. *Ann Intern Med* 1980;92:770–775.

8. Melekos MD, Asbach HW, Gerharz E, Zarakovitis IE, Weingaertner K, Naber KG. Post-intercourse versus daily ciprofloxacin prophylaxis for recurrent urinary tract infections in premenopausal women. *J Urol* 1997;157:935–939.

9. Nicolle LE, Harding GKM, Thompson M, Kennedy J, Urias B, Ronald AR. Prospective, randomized, placebo-controlled trial of norfloxacin for the prophylaxis of recurrent urinary tract infection in women. *Antimicrob Agents Chemother* 1989;33:1032–1035.

10. Brumfitt W, Smith GW, Hamilton-Miller JMT, Gargan RA. A clinical comparison between macrodantin and trimethoprim for prophylaxis in women with recurrent urinary infection. *J Antimicrob Chemother* 1985;16:111–120.

11. Raz R, Boger S. Long-term prophylaxis with norfloxacin versus nitrofurantoin in women with recurrent urinary tract infection. *Antimicrob Agents Chemother* 1991;35:1241–1242.

12. Brumfitt W, Hamilton-Miller JMT, Smith GW Al-Wali W. Comparative trial of norfloxacin and macrocrystalline nitrofurantoin (Macrodantin) in the prophylaxis of recurrent urinary tract infection in women. *Q J Med* 1991;81:811–820.

13. Brumfitt W, Hamilton-Miller JMT. A comparative trial of low-dose cefaclor and macrocrystalline nitrofurantoin in the prevention of recurrent urinary tract infection. *Infection* 1995;23:98–102.

14. Stapleton A, Latham RH, Johnson C, Stamm WE. Postcoital antimicrobial prophylaxis for recurrent urinary tract infection: a randomized, double-blind placebo-controlled trial. *JAMA* 1990;264:703–706.

15. Pfau A, Sacks TG. Effective postcoital quinolone prophylaxis of recurrent urinary tract infection in women. *J Urol* 1994;152:136–138.

16. Pfau A, Sacks T, Englestein D. Recurrent urinary tract infections in premenopausal women: prophylaxis based on an understanding of the pathogenesis. *J Urol* 1983;129:1153–1156.

17. Wong ES, McKevitt M, Running K, Counts GW, Turck M, Stamm WE. Management of recurrent urinary tract infections with patient-administered single-dose therapy. *Ann Intern Med* 1985;102:302–307.

18. Jepson RG, Mihaljevic L, Craig J. Cranberries for preventing urinary tract infections. In: The Cochrane Library, Issue 3, 2000. Oxford: Update Software. Search date 1998; primary sources Medline; Embase; Psychlit; LILACS; Cinahl; Biological Abstracts; Current Contents; Cochrane Controlled Trials Register; Cochrane Renal Group; The Internet; Conference Proceedings; and hand searched references.

19. Fair WR, McClennan BL, Jost RG. Are excretory urograms necessary in evaluating women with urinary tract infection? *J Urol* 1979;121:313–315.

20. Engle G, Schaeffer AJ, Grayhack JT, Wendel EF. The role of excretory urography and cystoscopy in the evaluation and management of women with recurrent urinary tract infection. *J Urol* 1980;123:190–191.

21. Fowler JE Jr, Pulaski ET. Excretory urography, cystography, and cystoscopy in the evaluation of women with urinary tract infection: a prospective study. *N Engl J Med* 1981;304:462–465.

22. Nickel JC, Wilson J, Morales A, Heaton J. Value of urologic investigation in a targeted group of women with recurrent urinary tract infections. *Can J Surg* 1991;34:591–594.

Bruce Cooper
Renal Research Fellow
University of Sydney Royal North
Shore Hospital
St Leonards
Australia

Ruth Jepson
Research Fellow
NHS Centre for Reviews and
Dissemination
University of York
York, UK

Competing interests: None declared.

TABLE 1 Continuous antimicrobial prophylactic regimens for recurrent urinary tract infections: results of RCTs (see text, p 1339).

Study	Total number of people	Regimen	Duration of prophylaxis (months)	Infections per patient year	P value
Stamm et al[7] (placebo controlled RCT) 1980	60	Placebo	6	2.80	< 0.001 (placebo v drug treatment)
		Co-trimonazole (40 mg/200 mg) at bedtime		0.15	
		Nitrofurantoin 100 mg at bedtime		0.14	
		Nitrofurantoin 100 mg at bedtime		0	
Melekos et al[8] (open RCT) 1997	135	Without prophylaxis	12	3.62–3.66	< 0.001
		Ciprofloxacin 125 mg postcoital		0.043	
		Ciprofloxacin 125 mg daily		0.031	
Nicolle et al[9] (placebo controlled RCT) 1989	30	Placebo	12	1.6	< 0.001
		Norfloxacin 200 mg at bedtime		0	
Brumfitt et al[10] (open RCT) 1985	72	Trimethoprim 100 mg at bedtime	12	1.00	< 0.05
		Nitrofurantoin 100 mg bedtime		0.17	
Raz et al[11] (open RCT) 1991	94	Norfloxacin 200 mg at bedtime	6	0.04	= 0.05
		Nitrofurantoin 50 mg at bedtime		0.60	
Brumfitt et al[12] (open RCT) 1991	88	Norfloxacin 200 mg at bedtime	12	0.002	Not reported
		Nitrofurantoin 100 mg at bedtime		0.003	
Brumfitt et al[13] (open RCT) 1995	97	Cefaclor 250 mg at bedtime	12	0.006	Not reported
		Nitrofurantoin 50 mg at bedtime		0.006	

TABLE 2 Postcoital regimens for recurrent urinary tract infections: results of RCTs (see text, p 1340).

Study	Total number of people	Regimen	Duration of prophylaxis (months)	Infections per patient year	P value
Stapleton et al[14] (placebo controlled RCT) 1990	27	Placebo	6	3.6	= 0.0001
		Postcoital Co-trimonazole (40 mg/20 mg)		0.3	
Pfau et al[15] (open RCT) 1994	33	Without prophylaxis	14	6.13	= 0.0000
		Postcoital prophylaxis with either ofloxacin 100 mg, norfloxacin 200 mg, or ciprofloxacin 125 mg		0.02	
Melekos et al[8] (open RCT) 1997	135	Without prophylaxis	12	3.62–3.66	< 0.0001
		Ciprofloxacin 125 mg daily		0.031	
		Ciprofloxacin 125 mg postcoital		0.043	
Pfau et al[16] (open RCT) 1983	56	Without prophylaxis	12	4.6	< 0.001
		Postcoital prophylaxis with either Co-trimonazole 80 mg/400 mg		0	
		Nitrofurantoin 50–100 mg		0.1	

Stress incontinence

Search date May 2000

Jason Coop and Ash Monga

INTERVENTIONS

PREVENTION
Likely to be beneficial
Postnatal pelvic floor muscle
  exercises. 1348

Unknown effectiveness
Antenatal pelvic floor muscle
  exercises. 1348

TREATMENT
Beneficial
Pelvic floor muscle exercises .1348
α Adrenergic agonists
  (phenylpropanolamine). . . .1351
Open colposuspension 1352

Likely to be beneficial
Biofeedback 1349
Slings. 1352
Tension free vaginal tape 1353

Unknown effectiveness
Bladder training 1349
Weighted vaginal cones 1351
Weight loss. 1351
Control of fluid intake 1351
Marshall-Marchetti-Krantz
  urethropexy 1352

Implantable devices 1353
Artificial sphincters 1353

Unlikely to be beneficial
Addition to pelvic floor muscle
  exercises of intravaginal
  resistance devices, or
  biofeedback 1348
Electrical stimulation of pelvic floor
  (less effective than pelvic floor
  muscle exercises, and causes
  adverse effects) 1350
Oestrogen 1350
Endoscopic colposuspension (less
  effective then open
  colposuspension) 1353

Likely to be ineffective or harmful
Anterior colporrhaphy 1352

To be covered in future issues of
  Clinical Evidence
Treatment of women in whom
  primary surgery has failed

See glossary, p 1354

Key Messages

- One RCT has found that postpartum pelvic floor muscle exercises reduce the risk of developing stress incontinence in the short term. The effect of antenatal exercises in preventing stress incontinence has not been assessed in good quality RCTs.

- One systematic review of RCTs has found that pelvic floor muscle exercises and electrical stimulation of the pelvic floor improve objective measures of stress incontinence.

- Meta-analysis of a systematic review of RCTs has found that biofeedback is associated with a higher cure rate compared with pelvic floor exercises. The difference was not quite significant.

- RCTs found no evidence of benefit from oestrogen in postmenopausal women.
- One RCT found no evidence of a difference between pelvic floor muscle exercises and α adrenergic agonists.
- RCTs comparing different surgical procedures found that colposuspension and slings were the most effective approach, both in the short and long term.
- We found limited evidence suggesting that endoscopic procedures are currently less effective than open procedures.

DEFINITION Urinary incontinence is defined as involuntary loss of urine that is objectively demonstrable and is a social or hygienic problem.[1] There are two main types of urinary incontinence: stress incontinence (see glossary, p 1354) and detrusor instability (see glossary, p 1354), together account for more than 80% of all cases of urinary incontinence. Urinary incontinence is eight times more common in women than in men. This review deals specifically with stress incontinence.

INCIDENCE/ PREVALENCE Prevalence is increasing as the population ages. In 1990, the number of women in the UK suffering from urinary incontinence was estimated at 2.5 million (see table 1, p 1356).[2,3] A community based study in the USA found that the self reported, age adjusted prevalence of female urinary incontinence was 48% (95% CI 45% to 52%).[4] A questionnaire based study in Sweden estimated the prevalence of urinary incontinence to be 3% in women aged 20–29 years old, increasing to 32% in women > 80 years old.[5]

AETIOLOGY/ RISK FACTORS Stress incontinence is made more likely with some genetic alterations in connective tissue, pregnancy and childbirth, menopause, aging, obesity, some races, chronic constipation, other causes of chronic raised intra-abdominal pressure, and pelvic surgery.[6] Psychological factors, bladder neck surgery, caffeine, and smoking may aggravate the condition. Other causes of urinary incontinence include urinary tract infection, immobility, loss of physical function and dexterity, dementia, and other conditions causing impaired mental state.

PROGNOSIS Urinary incontinence affects physical, psychological, and social wellbeing, and impairs quality of life. We found no good studies of its natural history. Prognosis after treatment is probably better for stress incontinence than for most other forms of urinary incontinence.

AIMS To improve or cure urinary incontinence, and to restore normal social functioning and confidence, with minimal adverse effects.

OUTCOMES Objective demonstration of urinary loss by urodynamic investigation; subjective improvement in urinary loss; improvement in quality of life indicators; adverse effects of drug treatment; complications of surgical treatment.

METHODS *Clinical Evidence* search and appraisal May 2000.

QUESTION What are the effects of preventive interventions?

OPTION PELVIC FLOOR MUSCLE EXERCISES

We found no evidence of sufficient quality on the effectiveness of antenatal pelvic floor exercises in the prevention of postpartum stress incontinence. One RCT has found that postnatal pelvic floor exercises significantly reduce stress incontinence in the short term.

Benefits: We found no systematic review. **Antenatal pelvic floor exercises:** We found one RCT (72 primigravidas) which found pelvic floor exercise training starting at 20 weeks gestation versus routine care reduced urinary incontinence symptoms during late pregnancy and up to 6 months postpartum. The RCT had methodological problems (see comment below).[7] **Postnatal pelvic floor exercises:** We found one RCT published in abstract form, which compared instructed pelvic floor exercises plus bladder retraining versus routine postnatal exercises. Nearly 8000 women responded to a questionnaire survey 3 months after delivery. Of these, 749 who reported incontinence were randomised. At 12 months postpartum, the intervention group showed a significant reduction in stress incontinence (rates of stress incontinence 58% v 68%, P = 0.02).[8]

Harms: None reported.

Comment: The RCT of pelvic muscle exercises versus normal care[7] recruited 72 people but reported results for only 46 (63%) of them; dropouts were due to conceiving the second child within 1 year of the first birth (5 women), no data collection (eight women), and partial data collection (7 women). Overall, 13 of the 72 women had caesarean deliveries; more women had caesarean deliveries in the treatment group than in the control group. A subgroup analysis of 37 women who had vaginal delivery found no significant effect of training for pelvic floor exercises versus control treatment.

QUESTION What are the effects of non-surgical treatments?

OPTION PELVIC FLOOR MUSCLE EXERCISES

One systematic review and additional RCTs have found that pelvic floor muscle exercises reduce symptoms of stress incontinence, and that high intensity exercise is more effective than low intensity. RCTs have found that pelvic floor muscle exercises are more effective than electrical stimulation of the pelvic floor or vaginal cones. Meta-analysis of three RCTs found biofeedback to be significantly more effective than pelvic floor muscle exercises.

Benefits: We found one systematic review (search date 1997), which identified 11 RCTs of conservative treatments for stress incontinence in women.[9] Included trials had at least 50 participants in each group, appropriate randomisation and blinding, less than 10% withdrawal rate, and relevant baseline and outcome measurements. **Versus no treatment:** The review identified two RCTs comparing pelvic floor muscle exercises versus no treatment. One found that women in the pelvic floor muscle exercise group were more likely to be dry or mildly incontinent than the no treatment group (61% v 3%). After 3 months, the mean weekly frequency of incontinent episodes fell from 17.3 to 4.8 in the treatment group, whereas in the controls it increased from 23.1 to 25.3. The second RCT found major decreases in frequency of incontinence episodes in the pelvic floor muscle exercise group, with no significant change in the control group (reduction in frequency 54% v 6%).[9] **High versus low intensity exercises:** The review identified one RCT comparing high and low intensity home based pelvic floor muscle exercise programmes and found a greater rate of "cure or almost cure" for high intensity exercise (60% v 17%). It also found improved social and urodynamic parameters.[9] **Plus intravaginal resistance devices or biofeedback:** The systematic review[9] identified three RCTs of sufficient quality comparing pelvic floor muscle exercises alone and in combination with an intravaginal resistance device (one RCT) or biofeedback (two RCTs). These found no significant difference in the frequency of incontinent episodes per week. **Versus biofeedback:** The systematic review identified five RCTs comparing biofeedback versus pelvic floor muscle exercises.[9] One trial found a significant difference in favour of biofeedback and four trials found no significant difference. Meta-analysis of the three trials with a common outcome measure (published separately) found no significant increase in the proportion of women cured after biofeedback (OR 2.1, 95% CI 0.99 to 4.4).[10] **Versus electrical stimulation or vaginal cones:** One RCT (107 women) compared pelvic floor muscle exercises versus electrical stimulation, vaginal cones, or no treatment.[11] It found no significant difference between electrical stimulation, resistance devices, and no treatment. However, pelvic floor muscle exercises versus other interventions or no treatment increased muscle strength and social activity index, and decreased leakage over 3 days (P < 0.01). Significantly more women reported being continent or almost continent in the exercise group than in other groups (control 1/30, exercise 12/25, electrical stimulation 3/25, cones 5/27; P < 0.001 for exercise compared with other groups). **Versus or combined with bladder training:** One RCT (145 women) compared pelvic floor muscle training versus bladder training or the two treatments combined.[12] Combined treatment was associated with greater satisfaction immediately after treatment began, but at 3 months, there were no significant differences between groups. Reduction of incontinence episodes by 50% or more was reported by 59% with combination treatment, 56% with pelvic muscle exercises alone, and 41% with bladder training alone.

Harms: None reported.

Comment: The RCT that compared pelvic floor muscle training versus bladder training or the two treatments combined found that outcomes improved with increased contact between women in the trial and the intervention team.[12] The authors speculated that specific treatment may not be as important as having a structured intervention programme with education, counselling, and frequent patient contact.

| OPTION | ELECTRICAL PELVIC FLOOR STIMULATION |

Two systematic reviews of RCTs have found conflicting evidence on the effects of electrical stimulation of the pelvic floor in women with stress incontinence. RCTs have found it to be less effective than pelvic floor muscle exercises.

Benefits: We found two systematic reviews. The first review (search date 1997) identified two RCTs of sufficient quality comparing electrical and sham stimulation of the pelvic floor in women with stress incontinence.[9] Electrical stimulation was associated with improvements in daily and weekly leakage episodes, pelvic floor muscle strength, and pad tests. In the first RCT (35 women), voiding diaries indicated a 50% or greater improvement in 48% of participants in the active group compared with 13% in the sham group. The second RCT, in 14 women, also compared active versus sham electrical stimulation, but all participants were also treated with pelvic floor muscle exercises. It found improvements in pelvic floor muscle strength and endurance and significantly reduced episodes of incontinence in the women receiving electrical stimulation. None of the women receiving electrical stimulation required further treatment, compared with a third of those receiving sham treatment. The second review (search date 1996) identified two additional RCTs and excluded the smaller of the two RCTs identified in the first review.[13] Neither of the two additional RCTs found significant benefit compared with controls. **Versus pelvic floor muscle exercises:** See pelvic floor muscle exercises, p 1348. **Versus pelvic floor muscle exercises plus biofeedback:** One RCT (70 people) compared electrical stimulation versus pelvic floor muscle exercises plus biofeedback. There was no significant difference in outcomes between groups.[14]

Harms: Adverse effects included vaginal irritation and infection, pain, and urinary tract infection.

Comment: There were considerable variations in the methods used for delivering the electrical stimulation. Further trials are needed that compare electrical stimulation alone versus no treatment, using adequate sample sizes and sufficiently long treatment periods.

| OPTION | OESTROGEN SUPPLEMENTATION IN POSTMENOPAUSAL WOMEN |

RCTs have found no evidence that oestrogen supplementation improves stress incontinence. The combination of oestrogen plus an α adrenergic agonist may improve objective measures.

Benefits: **Oestrogen alone:** We found one systematic review (published in 1994, 6 RCTs: 1 vaginal oestrogen, 5 oral oestrogen), and 17 uncontrolled trials of oestrogen on the treatment of urinary incontinence in women.[15] It concluded that, although the uncontrolled trials (5 vaginal, 9 oral, 3 intramuscular oestrogen found there was subjective improvement in symptoms of incontinence, 3 RCTs (84 women with genuine stress incontinence) found no objective improvement assessed from various measures of urine loss. The two subsequent RCTs (135 postmenopausal women with genuine stress incontinence) found no significant difference between treated and placebo groups in the number of incontinent episodes at 3–6 months follow up.[16–17] **Combined with an α adrenergic agonist:** See benefits of α adrenergic agonists below.

Harms: Adverse effects of long term hormone replacement therapy include increased risk of breast cancer and thromboembolic disease.

Comment: The studies included clinically heterogeneous groups, and used a range of diagnostic criteria, therapeutic interventions, and outcome assessments.

OPTION   α ADRENERGIC AGONISTS (PHENYLPROPANOLAMINE)

One RCT found no evidence of a difference in effectiveness between phenylpropanolamine and pelvic floor muscle exercises. Limited evidence suggests that combination of phenylpropanolamine with oestrogen in postmenopausal women improves objective measures of urinary incontinence more than oestrogen alone.

Benefits: **Versus placebo:** We found no RCTs. **Versus pelvic floor muscle exercises:** We found one systematic review,[9] which identified one RCT of sufficient quality. The RCT found no significant difference between pelvic floor muscle exercises and phenylpropanolamine (77% v 84% improvement from baseline). **Combined with oestrogen:** A non-systematic review of combined oestrogen and phenylpropanolamine (published in 1995) reviewed two trials of combination therapy in 84 postmenopausal women, and concluded that frequency and nocturia improved more with combined treatment than with oestrogen alone.[18] Levels of significance were not given in the review. Stress incontinence improved subjectively in all groups but objectively only in the combined group.

Harms: We found no evidence from RCTs.

Comment: Limited data are available, which limits generaliseability. A consensus view exists that α adrenergic agonists should be used with care or not at all in women with hypertension, hyperthyroidism, or coronary heart disease, or in those taking monoamine oxidase inhibitors.

OPTION   OTHER CONSERVATIVE INTERVENTIONS

One RCT found that vaginal cones were less effective than pelvic floor muscle exercises but not significantly different compared with electrical stimulation of the pelvic floor or no treatment. We found insufficient evidence on the effects of regulation of fluid intake and weight loss in women with stress incontinence.

Benefits: **Vaginal cones versus pelvic floor muscle exercises or electrical stimulation:** See pelvic floor muscle exercises, p 1348. **Fluid intake and weight loss:** We found no systematic review or adequate RCTs.

Harms: Insufficient data.

Comment: None.

QUESTION	How do the main surgical treatments for stress incontinence compare?

OPTION	COLPOSUSPENSION, ANTERIOR COLPORRHAPHY, NEEDLE SUSPENSION, SLINGS, AND IMPLANTABLE DEVICES

From limited data, colposuspension seems to be the most successful surgical procedures for stress incontinence. We found limited and conflicting evidence that sling procedures (see glossary, p 1354) may have a similar cure rate as colposuspension. We found no evidence to support the use of anterior colporrhaphy or needle suspension. Newer treatments such as injectable devices and artificial slings (see glossary, p 1354) have not been adequately evaluated in RCTs. One RCT found that tension free vaginal tape had similar effectiveness as colposuspension at 6 months follow up. One small RCT found that the Marshall-Marchetti-Krantz urethropexy (see glossary, p 1354) compared with colposuspension increases the 1 year subjective cure rate. We found no good comparative data on the harms of different procedures.

Benefits: We found two systematic reviews of surgery for stress incontinence in women (first review published in 1996; 11 RCTs, 20 non-randomised trials/prospective cohort studies, and 45 retrospective cohort studies).[19] The second review will be appraised in the next issue.[20] **Colposuspension versus anterior colporrhaphy:** The review identified four RCTs and 11 non-randomised prospective studies. The studies were small and most were not able to exclude a clinically important effect. Overall, they found that colposuspension cured or improved stress incontinence after 1 year more than anterior colporrhaphy (see table 2, p 1356). The benefits of colposuspension were sustained for at least 5 years whereas those of anterior colporrhaphy seemed to diminish rapidly.[19] Three RCTs published since the review compared open colposuspension versus anterior colporrhaphy. One (35 woman) found significantly greater improvement 1 year after surgery with colposuspension than with colporrhaphy (16/18 v 5/16; RR 0.15, 95% CI 0.04 to 0.59).[21] The second RCT (81 women) found no difference at 2 months, but significantly greater cure rate with colposuspension at 3 years' follow up (88% v 57%; P < 0.001).[22] The third RCT (68 women) found that 14 years after surgery colposuspension versus anterior colporrhaphy improved both the objective cure rate (26/35 [74%] v 14/33 [42%]; OR 3.9, 95% CI 1.3 to 12.5) and the subjective cure rate (30/35 [86%] v 17/33 [52%]; OR 5.6, 95% CI 1.6 to 21.6).[23] **Colposuspension versus needle suspension:** The review identified three RCTs and 10 non-randomised studies comparing colposuspension versus needle suspension procedures.[19] Two RCTs and two non-randomised studies found a higher success rate with colposuspension, whereas one RCT and eight non-randomised studies found no significant difference. **Colposuspension versus slings:** The review[19] identified no RCTs and we found two subsequent small RCTs.[24,25] The first RCT found that colposuspension versus paravaginal repair increased the number of women with subjective cure at follow up of 1 to 3 years (18/18 [100%] v 13/18 [72%], P = 0.02).[24] The second RCT (36 women) found a similar cure rate 3 months after both colposuspension and suburethral sling.[25] **Colposuspension versus tension free vaginal tape:** One RCT (344 women) found that colposuspension versus tension free vaginal tape had no significant effect on subjective cure rates after 6 months (71% v 66%) or on objective cure rate (66% v 68%).[26] **Colposuspension versus Marshall-Marchetti-Krantz urethropexy:** One RCT in 30 women found that more were subjectively cured at 1 year after Marshall-Marchetti-Krantz urethropexy versus colposuspension (subjective cure rate 100% v 66%; P = 0.02).[27] **Anterior colporrhaphy versus needle suspension:** The review identified three RCTs and five non-randomised prospective studies, which found no difference in the effectiveness of anterior colporrhaphy and needle suspension procedures.[19] **Implantable devices and artificial sphincters:** We found no RCTs.

Harms: Reported complications of surgery include urinary retention, frequency, and urgency. However, we found no good data on the frequency of complications.

Comment: A review published in 1997 identified 282 articles with acceptable outcome data (as determined by an expert panel, rejection encompassing such points as being published only in abstract form, lack of original data, or inadequate follow up).[28] Combined data from the 282 included articles gave cure rates of 84% for retropubic suspensions, 65–79% for transvaginal suspensions, 61–85% for anterior repairs, and 82–83% for paravaginal sling procedures. The authors concluded that at 48 months' follow up, retropubic suspensions (colposuspension) and slings were more effective than anterior colporrhaphy or needle suspension. No differentiation was made between primary and secondary procedures. Studies suffered from lack of standardisation on definition, severity, and diagnosis of stress incontinence. Information on detrusor instability, prior surgery, quality of life measurements, surgical technique, length of follow up, and external validity were often not available. One cohort study of 259 women who underwent the Stamey endoscopic bladder neck suspension found a 6% success rate at 10 year follow up.

QUESTION How do endoscopic and open colposuspension compare?

We found limited evidence suggesting that open colposuspension procedures are currently superior to endoscopic colposuspension.

Benefits: We found one systematic review (search date 1996)[29] and one subsequent RCT.[30] The review identified one RCT (60 women), comparing open versus laparoscopic colposuspension. At both 1 year and in a follow up study at 3 years, open colposuspension was significantly more effective as judged by visual analogue scores and pad tests (P = 0.03).[31,32] The subsequent RCT (minimum follow up 1 year, 92 women) also found that open colposuspension was significantly more effective than laparoscopic. Based on objective outcome measures, success rate for the open procedure was 96% (95% CI 90% to 100%) compared with 80% (95% CI 69% to 92%) for laparoscopic.[30]

Harms: The review also identified four non-randomised comparisons and 10 case series.[29] Rates of postoperative complication in these studies were low. Other studies have reported postoperative complications including bladder injuries, postoperative urinary retention, haematuria, urinary tract infection, ureteric injury, and detrusor instability.[33] We also found two reported cases of transmural bladder sutures.[34] The subsequent RCT found that rates of postoperative complication were higher with open than with laparoscopic colposuspension.[30]

Comment: None.

GLOSSARY

Artificial sling There are many different types of sling procedure that differ in the type of material, sutures, and points of anchoring. Many artificial materials have been used in the construction of slings (e.g. polyester, polytetrafluoroethylene [Gore-Tex]).

Detrusor instability Diagnosed when the detrusor muscle contracts, spontaneously or on provocation, during the filling phase, while the woman is attempting to inhibit micturition.[1]

Marshall-Marchetti-Krantz urethropexy A surgical procedure through an incision in the lower abdomen in which the bladder neck and urethra are elevated by suturing tissues around the urethra and bladder to the periosteum on the rear of the symphysis pubis. The aim is to create a valve mechanism at the bladder neck. The procedure has been modified in various ways (e.g. Burch colposuspension, Stamey urethropexy, Pereyra procedure, paravaginal repair).

Sling procedure Typically a piece of fascia placed under the bladder neck and then secured to either bone, abdominal wall, or ligament. This sling then support the urethra where it connects to the bladder and may restore the valve mechanism at the bladder neck. It is performed through the vagina or the abdomen.

Stress incontinence Diagnosed when, in the absence of a detrusor contraction, the pressure inside the bladder exceeds the pressure in the urethra.

REFERENCES

1. Abrams P, Blaivas JG, Stanton SL, et al. Standardisation of terminology of lower urinary tract function. *Scand J Urol Nephrol* 1988; 114(suppl):5–19.

2. MORI Health Survey Questionnaire 1990. London: Market and Opinion Research International (MORI).

3. Royal College of Physicians. *Incontinence: causes, management and provision of services. Report of a working party.* London: Royal College of Physicians,1995.

4. Roberts RO, Jacobsen SA, Reilly WT, et al. Prevalence of combined fecal and urinary incontinence: A community–based study. *J Am Geriatr Soc* 1999;47:837–841.

5. Simeonova Z, Milsom I, Kullendorff A-E, et al. The prevalence of urinary incontinence and its influence on the quality of life in women from an urban Swedish population. *Acta Obstet Gynecol Scand* 1999;78:546–551.

6. Handa VL, Harris TA, Ostergard DR. Protecting the pelvic floor: obstetric management to prevent incontinence and pelvic organ prolapse. *Obstet Gynecol* 1996;88:470–478.

7. Sampselle CM, Miller JM, Mims BL, et al. Effect on pelvic muscle exercise on transient incontinence during pregnancy and after birth. *Obstet Gynecol* 1998;91:406–412.

8. Gladzener CMA, Lang G, Wilson PD, et al. Postnatal incontinence: a multicentre randomised controlled trial of conservative treatment. *Br J Obstet Gynaecol* 1998;105(suppl 117):47.

9. Berghmans LCM, Hendriks HJM, Bo K, et al. Conservative treatment of stress urinary incontinence in women: a systematic review of randomised controlled trials. *Br J Urol* 1998;82: 181–191. Search date 1997; primary sources Medline, Excerpta Medica, Cochrane Field in Therapies and Rehabilitation database, Dutch National Institute of Allied Professions database.

10. Weatherall M. Biofeedback or pelvic floor muscle exercises for female genuine stress incontinence: a meta-analysis of trials identified in a systematic review. *BJU Int* 1999;83:1015–1016.

11. Bo K, Talseth T, Holme I. Single blind randomised controlled trial of pelvic floor exercises, electronical stimulation, vaginal cones, and no treatment in management of genuine stress incontinence. *BMJ* 1999;318:487–493.

12. Wyman JF, Fantl JA, McClish DK, et al. Comparative efficacy of behavioural interventions in the management of female urinary incontinence. *Am J Obstet Gynecol* 1998;179: 999–1007.

13. Bo K, Effect of electronic stimulation on stress and urge incontinence. *Acta Obstet Gynaecol Scand* 1998;77(suppl 168):3–11. Search date 1996; primary source Medline, and hand searches of relevant journals.

14. Knight S, Laycock J, Naylor D. Evaluation of neuromuscular electronical stimulation in the treatment of genuine stress incontinence. *Physiotherapy* 1998;84:61–71.

15. Fantl JA, Cardozo LD, Ekberg J, et al. Estrogen therapy in the management of urinary

incontinence in post-menopausal women: a meta-analysis. *Obstet Gynecol* 1994;83:12–18. Search date 1992; primary sources English language articles found in Excerpta Medica, Biosis, and Medline.

16. Fantl JA, Bump RC, Robinson D, et al. and the Continence Program for Women Research Group. Efficacy of oestrogen supplementation in the treatment of urinary incontinence. *Obstet Gynecol* 1996;88:745–749.

17. Jackson S, Shepherd A, Brookes S, et al. The effect of oestrogen supplementation on post-menopausal urinary stress incontinence: A double blind placebo controlled trial. *Br J Obstet Gynaecol* 1999; 106:711–718.

18. Cardozo LD, Kelleher CJ. Sex hormones, the menopause and urinary problems. *Gynecol Endocrinol* 1995;9:75–84.

19. Black NA, Downs SH. The effectiveness of surgery for stress incontinence in women: a systematic review. *Br J Urol* 1996;78:497–510. Search dates and primary sources: English and non-English articles found in Medline (1966 to June 1995), Embase (1980 to June 1995), Science Citation Index (1980 to June 1995), British Library Information Index (1995), together with information from experts.

20. Anterior vaginal repair for unrinary incontinence in women. In: The Cochrane Library. Issue 1, 2000. Oxford: Update Software. Search date 1999; primary sources Cochrane Incontinence Group's trials register and reference lists of relevant articles.

21. Kammerer-Doak DN, Dorin MH, Rogers RG, et al. A randomised trial of Burch retropubic urethropexy and anterior colporrhaphy for stress urinary incontinence. *Obstet Gynaecol* 1999;93:75–78.

22. Liapis A, Pyrgiotis E, Kontoravdis A, et al. Genuine stress incontinence: prospective randomised comparison of two operative methods. *Eur J Obstet Gynaecol Reprod Biol* 1996;64:69–72.

23. Colombo M, Vitobello D, Proietti F, et al. Randomized comparison of Burch colposuspension versus anterior colporrhaphy in women with stress urinary incontinence and anterior vaginal wall prolapse. *Br J Obstet Gynaecol* 2000;107:544–551.

24. Colombo M, Milani R, Vitobello P, et al. A randomised comparison of Burch colposuspension and abdominal paravaginal defect repair for female stress urinary incontinence. *Am J Obstet Gynecol* 1996;175:78–84.

25. Sand PK, Winkler H, Blackhurst DW, et al. A prospective randomized study comparing modified Burch retropubic urethropexy and suburethral sling for treatment of genuine stress incontinence. *Am J Obstet Gynecol* 2000;182:30–34.

26. Ward KL, Hilton P, Browning J. A randomised trial of colposuspension and tension free vaginal tape for primary genuine stress incontinence (abstract) *Neurourol Urodynam* 2000;19:386–388.

27. Quadri G, Magatti F, Belloni C, et al. Marshall-Marchetti-Krantz urethropexy and Burch colposuspension for stress urinary incontinence in women with low pressure and hypermobility of the urethra: early results of a prospective randomized clinical trial. *Am J Obstet Gynecol* 1999; 181:12–18.

28. Leach GE, Dmochowski RR, Appell RA, et al. Female stress urinary incontinence clinical guidelines panel summary report on surgical management of female stress urinary incontinence. *J Urol* 1997;158:875–880.

29. Lose G. Laparoscopic Burch colposuspension. *Acta Obstet Gynaecol Scand* 1998;88(suppl 168): 29–33. Search date 1991–1996, primary sources Medline search of English language articles, and search of references cited in all identified studies.

30. Su T-H, Wang D-G, Hsu C-Y, et al. Prospective comparison of laparoscopic and traditional colposuspensions in the treatment of genuine stress incontinence. *Acta Obstet Gynecol Scand* 1997;76:576–582.

31. Burton GA. A randomised comparison of laparoscopic and open colposuspension. *Neurol Urodyn* 1994;88:29–33.

32. Burton G. A three year prospective randomised urodynamic study comparing open and laparoscopic colposuspension. *Neurourol Urodyn* 1997;16:353–354.

33. Aslan P, Woo HH. Ureteric injury following laparoscopic colposuspension. *Br J Obstet Gynaecol* 1997;104:266–268.

34. Flax S. The gasless laparoscopic Burch bladderneck suspension; early experience. *J Urol* 1996;156:1105–1107.

Jason Cooper
Consultant Gynaecologist
City General Hospital
Stoke-on-Trent
UK

Ash Monga
Consultant Urogynaecologist
Princess Anne Hospital
Southampton
UK

Competing interests: None declared.

Women's health

Women living at home	%
15–44 years	5–7
45–64 years	8–15
> 65 years	10–20

Institutionalised women	
Residential homes	25
Nursing homes	40
Hospitals: long stay care	50–70

TABLE 2 Results of RCTs in the systematic review comparing colposuspension versus anterior colporrhaphy and needle suspension (see text, p 1352).[19]

Study	Follow up (years)	Anterior colporrhaphy		Colposuspension	
		cured	total (%)	cured	total (%)
34	1	88/101	87	70/99	70
35	1	5/19	25	0/15	0
36	1	34/38	89	23/35	65
37	5	27/33	82	11/30	37

Study	Follow up (years)	Anterior colporrhaphy		Needle suspension	
		cured	total (%)	cured	total (%)
34	1	88/101	87	66/98	67
35	1–3.7	17/24	71	15/26	58
37	5	27/33	82	13/30	43

*In some cases the numbers of people cured has been calculated from the information provided in the papers.

Search date October 2000

Nicky Cullum, E Andrea Nelson and Jane Nixon

QUESTIONS

INTERVENTIONS

PREVENTION

Beneficial

Likely to be beneficial

Unknown effectiveness

Likely to be ineffective or harmful

TREATMENT

Likely to be beneficial

Unknown effectiveness

See glossary, p 1363

Key Messages

Prevention

- One systematic review of RCTs has found that foam alternatives to the standard hospital foam mattress reduce the incidence of pressure sores in people at high risk.

- The relative merits of alternating and constant low pressure, and of the different alternating pressure devices, are unclear.

- One systematic review of RCTs has found that pressure relieving overlays on operating tables reduce the incidence of pressure sores.

- We found insufficient evidence on the effects of seat cushions, constant low pressure devices, regular repositioning ("turning"), sheepskins, topical lotions, or dressings.

- One RCT has found that air filled vinyl boots with foot cradles are associated with more rapid development of pressure sores.

Treatment

- One systematic review of RCTs has found that air fluidised supports improve healing rates.
- We found insufficient evidence on the effects of other types of beds and mattresses, seat cushions, becaplermin, dressings, debridement, surgery, nutritional supplementation, electrotherapy, ultrasound, or low level laser therapy on healing rates of pressure sores.

DEFINITION	Pressure sores (also known as pressure ulcers, bed sores, and decubitus ulcers) may present as persistently hyperaemic, blistered, broken, or necrotic skin, and may extend to underlying structures, including muscle and bone. Whether blanching and non-blanching erythema constitute pressure sores remains controversial.
INCIDENCE/ PREVALENCE	The most comprehensive data on prevalence and incidence come from hospital populations. Studies have found prevalences of 6.6–10.1% in National Health Service hospitals in the UK[1] and 8.7% in a teaching hospital in the USA.[2]
AETIOLOGY/ RISK FACTORS	Pressure sores are caused by unrelieved pressure, shear, or friction, and are most common below the waist and at bony prominences such as the sacrum, heels, and hips. They occur in all healthcare settings. Increased age, reduced mobility, and impaired nutrition emerge consistently as risk factors. However, the relative importance of these and other factors is uncertain.[3]
PROGNOSIS	The presence of pressure sores has been associated with a two- to fourfold increased risk of death in elderly people in intensive care.[4,5] However, pressure sores are a marker for underlying disease severity and other comorbidities rather than an independent predictor of mortality.[4] Pressure sores vary considerably in size and severity.
AIMS	To prevent pressure sore formation; to heal existing pressure sores; and to improve quality of life.
OUTCOMES	Incidence and severity of pressure sores, rate of change of area and volume, and time to heal. Interface pressure recorded at various anatomical sites is a surrogate outcome sometimes used in studies of preventive interventions; it has not yet been linked to clinical outcomes.
METHODS	*Clinical Evidence* update search and appraisal October 2000. We searched the Specialist Trials Register of the Cochrane Wounds Group in June 2000. The register is compiled by searching 19 electronic databases, including Medline (1966 to March 2000), Cinahl, BIDS, and Embase, and hand searching journals and conference proceedings. We reviewed all RCTs that used objective clinical outcome measures. For many trials, we could not be sure that pressure sore size was evenly distributed between groups at baseline. Unequal distribution of wound size at baseline will impact on all measures of wound healing. Ideally, studies of treatment should stratify randomisation by initial wound area and be of sufficient size to ensure even distribution of baseline wound size.

Many of the studies performed by manufacturers were in healthy people who are not representative of clinical subjects, and these studies have been excluded.

OPTION   PRESSURE RELIEVING SURFACES

One systematic review of RCTs has found that foam alternatives to the standard hospital foam mattress reduce the incidence of pressure sores in people at high risk. There is no obvious "best" foam alternative. The relative merits of alternating and constant low pressure therapy, and of the different devices used in alternating pressure therapy, are unclear. We found insufficient evidence on the effects of seat cushions and low tech constant low pressure supports. The systematic review has found that the use of pressure relieving overlays on operating tables reduces the incidence of pressure sores. One RCT has found that air filled vinyl boots with foot cradles are associated with more rapid development of pressure sores.

Benefits: We found one systematic review (search date February 1999).[6] **Foam alternatives versus standard hospital mattress:** The systematic review identified four RCTs.[6] The RCTs found that using various foam alternatives to the standard hospital mattress reduced the risk of sores (RRR 71%, 95% CI 57% to 81%; NNT for 10–14 days treatment to prevent one additional sore 4, 95% CI 3 to 6). **Different foam alternatives:** The systematic review identified four RCTs comparing different foam alternatives.[6] One reported a reduction in the risk of pressure sores associated with using a five section foam and fibre replacement compared with a 4 inch (10 cm) thick dimpled foam overlay (RR 0.42%, 95% CI 0.18 to 0.90; NNT for 10–21 days treatment 3, 95% CI 2 to 25). The other trials were too small to distinguish between the foam alternatives. **Cushions:** The systematic review identified two RCTs (194 people) comparing different types of seat cushion for preventing pressure sores.[6] They found no significant difference. **Low tech constant low pressure supports:** See glossary, p 1363. The systematic review identified eight RCTs.[6] Most were too small or flawed to allow conclusions. **Low air loss beds:** See glossary, p 1363. The systematic review identified one RCT (98 people in intensive care), and we found one subsequent RCT.[6,7] The intensive care RCT found a reduction in the risk of developing a new sore on low air loss beds compared with a standard intensive care unit bed (RR 0.24, 95% CI 0.09 to 0.55; NNT 3, 95% CI 2 to 5).[6] The second RCT (incontinent people admitted to acute and long stay hospital wards) found a non-significant increased risk of developing a sore in the low air loss hydrotherapy bed (RR 2.67, 95% CI 0.91 to 7.90) compared with a range of support surfaces.[7] **Alternating pressure therapy:** See glossary, p 1363. The systematic review identified eight comparisons of standard foam or constant low pressure with alternating pressure devices in the prevention of pressure sores,[6] and we found one subsequent RCT.[8] Most trials were too small to rule out a clinically important difference. One trial reported a significant reduction in the incidence of pressure sores in people on an alternating pressure device versus a standard foam mattress (RRR 68%, 95% CI 28% to 86%; NNT for 10 days treatment 11, 95% CI 6 to 34). Another trial compared a range of constant low pressure supports with a range of alternating pressure devices and reported that the incidence of pressure sores was significantly reduced with alternating pressure. The other seven comparisons found no significant difference between alternating pressure devices and constant low pressure supports. The relative merits of the different alternating pressure devices are unclear. **Pressure relieving overlays on the operating table:** The systematic review identified three RCTs.[6] The first compared a viscoelastic polymer pad versus a standard table in people undergoing elective major general, gynaecological, or vascular surgery. It found a significant reduction in the incidence of postoperative pressure sores with the polymer pad (RRR 48%, 95% CI 17% to 68%; NNT 11, 95% CI 6 to 36). The other two RCTs compared an alternating system used both during and after surgery versus a gel pad during surgery and a standard mattress after surgery for 7 days. Meta-analysis of these two trials gave a significant reduction in the incidence of pressure sores with the alternating system (RRR 80%, 95% CI 35% to 94%; NNT 16, 95% CI 9 to 48). **Air filled vinyl boot with foot cradle:** We found one small RCT comparing hospital pillows versus a vinyl, air filled boot with a built-in foot cradle for the prevention of heel pressure sores in hospitalised people.[9] Sores developed significantly more quickly in the people wearing the boot (mean time to skin breakdown 10 days v 13 days; P < 0.036 log rank test).

Harms: Hypothermia has been reported in a small number of people using low air loss hydrotherapy beds.[7]

Comment: Trials have tended to be small, of poor quality, and few comparisons have been undertaken more than once. Foam alternatives use foam of varying densities, often within the same mattress, and are sometimes sculptured.

OPTION   **OTHER PREVENTIVE INTERVENTIONS**

We found no good evidence that regular repositioning ("turning"), sheepskins, topical lotions, or dressings are effective. However, this may represent a lack of evidence rather than a lack of benefit from these interventions.

Benefits: **Repositioning/turning:** We found one systematic review (search date February 1995), which identified three RCTs of regular manual repositioning.[10] These were small and found no significant difference between experimental and control groups. We found no RCTs that evaluated the impact of positioning patients in different ways. **Sheepskin:** We found one systematic review (search date February 1999), which identified one small trial of sheepskin overlays.[10] This was inconclusive and of poor quality. **Topical lotions and dressings:** We found one RCT (120 people), which compared a lotion containing hexachlorophene versus one containing cetrimide; it found no significant difference in skin condition.[11]

Harms: We found no direct or indirect evidence of harm arising from repositioning, sheepskins, topical applications, or dressings.

Comment: The RCTs were small, of poor quality, and few comparisons have been undertaken more than once.

OPTION PRESSURE RELIEVING SURFACES

One systematic review of RCTs has found that air fluidised supports improve healing rates. We found insufficient evidence on the effects of seat cushions or other types of bed or mattress.

Benefits: We found one systematic review (search date February 1999)[6] and two further RCTs.[12,13] **Constant low pressure supports:** See glossary, p 1363. One trial found no difference in healing rates between a layered foam replacement mattress and a water mattress in elderly people in a nursing home who had existing pressure sores.[12] **Air fluidised support:** See glossary, p 1363. The systematic review identified four RCTs comparing air fluidised support versus standard care.[6] In two RCTs of people in hospital, standard care involved use of pressure relieving surfaces such as alternating pressure mattresses, regular changes of position, sheepskin or gel pads, and limb protectors. Both RCTs found that air fluidised support was more effective in healing established sores. A third RCT (97 people being cared for at home) found no significant difference. However, this trial had a high withdrawal rate. The fourth RCT was small and involved people who had undergone plastic surgery to repair pressure sores. It found no significant difference between air fluidised support and dry flotation. **Low air loss beds:** See glossary, p 1363. The systematic review identified one RCT comparing low air loss with foam beds and one has been identified subsequently.[6,13] There was no significant difference in the number of sores healed in these trials. We found no RCTs comparing low air loss beds versus alternating pressure or air fluidised supports. **Seat cushions:** The systematic review identified one RCT in 25 people.[6] This found no significant difference between seat cushions using dry flotation compared with alternating pressure.

Harms: Hypothermia has been reported in a small number of people using low air loss hydrotherapy beds.[7]

Comment: **Air fluidised support:** People are unable to move into and out of bed independently while using an air fluidised bed, and this limits the type of people for whom it is suitable. Air fluidised support has been evaluated in a range of settings, including surgical and medical wards and home care. Thus, the evidence could be viewed as generally applicable to people with pressure sores. The trials were of varying quality. **Low air loss beds:** These have been evaluated in a range of acute and elderly care settings.

OPTION OTHER TREATMENTS

Evidence on the effects of dressings is unclear. A meta-analysis of trials comparing hydrocolloids and gauze dressings found no significant difference. We found insufficient evidence on the effects of other types of dressings, debridement, surgery, nutritional supplementation,

electrotherapy, therapeutic ultrasound (see glossary, p 1363), or low level laser therapy on healing rates of pressure sores.

Benefits: **Hydrocolloid and gauze dressings:** We found one systematic review (28 RCTs)[14] and one subsequent RCT.[15] Most RCTs were small, of poor quality, and did not find significant results. Both the meta-analysis within the review and the subsequent RCT found a significant effect. However, a subsequent meta-analysis (Cullum N, Nelson EA, personal communication, 2001) using preferred statistical techniques found no significant difference (RR 1.63, 95% CI 0.97 to 2.75).[15–20] The wide confidence intervals only just crossing the line of no effect suggests this may represent a lack of evidence of benefit rather than evidence of no benefit. **Other dressings:** Twelve of the RCTs identified in the systematic review compared hydrocolloid versus other dressings, 11 RCTs compared other dressing types such as foam and alginate, and two (one using hydrocolloid versus saline-gauze dressings and the other using becaplermin gel versus placebo) have been published subsequently.[21,22] All were too small and most were too flawed to allow conclusions to be drawn. **Debridement:** One systematic review (search date 1998) found no RCTs comparing debridement versus no debridement.[23] It identified 32 RCTs comparing different debriding agents, but these were small, included a range of wounds, and few comparisons were undertaken more than once. The authors concluded that there was insufficient evidence to promote the use of any particular debriding agent over another. One subsequent RCT (43 people) comparing collagenase with hydrocolloid found no significant difference in healing (3 people in each group healed, no denominator given).[24] A further RCT (23 people with 30 ulcers) of dextranomer paste (see glossary, p 1363) with saline soaked gauze found no difference in proportion of sores prepared for skin grafting within 15 days (AR 5/15 [33%] with dextranomer v 4/15 [27%] with saline; ARI 7%, 95% CI –26% to 38%).[25] **Surgery:** We found no RCTs evaluating surgical treatments for pressure sores. **Nutritional supplements:** We found two RCTs of ascorbic acid supplementation for healing pressure sores. One small RCT in people undergoing surgery who had pressure sores found that ascorbic acid supplementation (500 mg twice daily versus placebo) improved healing rates.[26] A larger trial (88 people) found no significant difference in healing rates between those receiving ascorbic acid 500 mg twice daily and those receiving 10 mg twice daily.[27] We found no RCTs of the effects of parenteral nutrition or hyperalimentation on wound healing. **Electrotherapy:** See glossary, p 1363. We found four RCTs comparing electrotherapy versus sham treatment.[28–31] They were of varying quality. Overall, they suggested that electrotherapy improved healing of pressure sores, but confirmatory studies are needed. **Ultrasound:** We found three RCTs comparing ultrasound versus sham or standard treatment.[32–34] All found no difference. **Low level laser therapy:** We found one systematic review (search date 1998, 1 RCT, 18 people) of low level laser therapy in pressure sores. It found no evidence of benefit in this trial.[35]

Harms: We found no reports of harms with these treatments.

Comment: Overall, the evidence relating to these treatments is poor.

GLOSSARY

Air fluidised support A membrane covering a layer of particles, which are fluidised by having air forced through them. The air flow can be turned off, making the surface solid again, to allow the person to be moved. It is difficult for people to get in and out of these beds independently; therefore, they are usually reserved for people who spend most of the day in bed.

Alternating pressure therapy Mattresses or overlays made of one or two layers of parallel air sacs. Alternate sacs are inflated and deflated, providing alternating pressure and then release for each area of skin.

Constant low pressure supports Mattresses, overlays, and cushions made of high density or contoured foam, or filled with fibre, gel, water, beads, or air. They increase the area of contact between the person and the support surface, and therefore reduce the interface pressure.

Dextranomer paste Anhydrous, porous beads 0.1–0.3 mm diameter. These beads are hydrophilic and absorb/adsorb exudate, wound debris, and bacteria depending on particle size.

Electrotherapy The application of electrical fields by placing electrodes near a wound. Treatments include pulsed electromagnetic therapy, low intensity direct current, negative polarity and positive polarity electrotherapy, and alternating polarity electrotherapy.

Low air loss beds A mattress comprising inflatable upright sacs made of semi-permeable fabric. Inflating the sacs increases the area of contact between the individual and the support surface, and reduces the pressure on the skin. It is difficult for people to get in and out of these beds independently; therefore, they are usually reserved for people who spend most of the day in bed.

Therapeutic ultrasound The application of ultrasound to a wound, using a transducer and a water based gel. The power of ultrasound waves used in wound healing is low in order to avoid heating the tissues.

Substantive changes since last issue

Debridement Two additonal RCTs[24,25] found no significant benefit in healing of pressure sores for collagenase or dextranomer paste.

REFERENCES

1. O'Dea K. Prevalence of pressure damage in hospital patients in the UK. *J Wound Care* 1993; 2:221–225.
2. Granick MS, Solomon MP, Wind S, Goldberg M. Wound management and wound care. *Adv Plastic Reconstruct Surg* 1996;12:99–121.
3. Allman RM. Pressure ulcer prevalence, incidence, risk factors, and impact. *Clin Geriatr Med* 1997; 13:421–436.
4. Thomas DR, Goode PS, Tarquine PH, Allman RM. Hospital acquired pressure ulcers and risk of death. *J Am Geriatr Soc* 1996;44:1435–1440.
5. Clough NP. The cost of pressure area management in an intensive care unit. *J Wound Care* 1994;3: 33–35.
6. Cullum N, Deeks J, Sheldon TA, Song F, Fletcher AW. Beds, mattresses and cushions for pressure sore prevention and treatment. In: The Cochrane Library, Issue 3, 2000. Oxford. Update Software. Search date 1999; primary sources 19 electronic databases and hand searches of journals, conference proceedings, and bibliographies.
7. Bennett RG, Baran PJ, DeVone L, et al. Low airloss hydrotherapy versus standard care for incontinent hospitalized patients. *J Am Geriatr Soc* 1998;46:569–576.
8. Price P, Bale S, Newcombe R, Harding K. Challenging the pressure sore paradigm. *J Wound Care* 1999;8:187–190.
9. Tymec AC, Pieper B, Vollman K. A comparison of two pressure relieving devices in the prevention of heel pressure ulcers. *Adv Wound Care* 1997;10: 39–44.
10. Cullum N, Deeks JJ, Fletcher AW, Sheldon TA, Song F. Preventing and treating pressure sores. *Qual Health Care* 1995;4:289–297. Search date February 1995; primary sources Medline (1966 to February 1995); Cinahl (February 1995); hand searching of five journals.
11. Van der Cammen TJ, O'Callaghan U, Whitefield M. Prevention of pressure sores. A comparison of new and old pressure sore treatments. *Br J Clin Pract* 1987;41:1009–1011.
12. Groen HW, Groenier KH, Schuling J. Comparative study of a foam mattress and a water mattress. *J Wound Care* 1999;8:333–335.
13. Mulder GD, Taro N, Seeley JE, Andrews K. A study of pressure sore response to low air loss beds versus conventional treatment. *J Geriatr Dermatol* 1994;2:87–91.
14. Bradley M, Cullum N, Nelson EA, Petticrew M, Sheldon T, Torgerson D. Systematic reviews of wound care management: (2) Dressings and topical agents used in the healing of chronic wounds. *Health Technol Assess* 1999;3(17 pt 2). Search date 1997; primary source Medline.
15. Matzen S, Peschardt A, Alsbjørn B. A new amorphous hydrocolloid for the treatment of

pressure sores: a randomised controlled study. *Scand J Plast Reconstr Surg Hand Surg* 1999;33: 13–15.

16. Barrois B. Comparison of Granuflex and medicated paraffin gauze in pressure sores. *Proceedings of the 2nd European Conference on Advances in Wound Management*. London: Macmillan, 1993: 209.

17. Alm A, Hornmark AM, Fall PA, et al. Care of pressure sores: a controlled study of the use of a hydrocolloid dressing compared with wet saline gauze compresses. *Acta Derm Venereol Suppl (Stockh)* 1989;149:1–10.

18. Colwell JC, Foreman MD, Trotter JP. A comparison of the efficacy and cost-effectiveness of two methods of managing pressure ulcers. *Decubitus* 1993;6:28–36.

19. Xakellis GC, Chrischilles EA. Hydrocolloid versus saline-gauze dressings in treating pressure ulcers: a cost-effectiveness analysis. *Arch Phys Med Rehabil* 1992;73:463–469.

20. Gorse GJ, Messner RL. Improved pressure sore healing with hydrocolloid dressings. *Arch Dermatol* 1987;123:766–771.

21. Thomas DR, Goode PS, LaMaster K, Tennyson T. Acemann hydrogel dressing versus saline dressing for pressure ulcers. A randomized, controlled trial. *Adv Wound Care* 1998;11:273–276.

22. Rees RS, Robson MC, Smiell JM, et al. Becaplermin gel in the treatment of pressure ulcers: a phase II randomized, double-blind, placebo controlled study. *Wound Repair Regen* 1999;7:141–147.

23. Bradley M, Cullum N, Sheldon T. The debridement of chronic wounds: a systematic review. *Health Technol Assess* 1999;3(17 pt 1). Search date June 1998; primary sources 19 electronic databases, including Medline and Embase.

24. Burgos A, Gimenez J, Moreno E, et al. Cost, efficacy, efficiency and tolerability of collagenase ointment versus hydrocolloid occlusive dressing in the treatment of pressure sores. A comparative, randomised, multicentre study. *Clin Drug Invest* 2000;19:357–365.

25. Ljunberg S. Comparison of dextranomer paste and saline dressings for the management of decubital ulcers. *Clin Ther* 1998;20:737–743.

26. Taylor TV, Rimmer S, Day B, Butcher J, Dymock IW. Ascorbic acid supplementation in the treatment of pressure sores. *Lancet* 1974;2:544–546.

27. Ter Riet G, Kessels AG, Knipschild PG. Randomized clinical trial of ascorbic acid in the treatment of pressure ulcers. *J Clin Epidemiol* 1995;48:1453–1460.

28. Salzberg CA, Cooper Vastola SA, Perez F, Viehbeck MG, Byrne DW. The effects of non-thermal pulsed electromagnetic energy on wound healing of pressure ulcers in spinal cord-injured patients: a randomized, double-blind study. *Ostomy Wound Manage* 1995;41:42–48.

29. Wood JM, Evans PE 3rd, Schallreuter KU, et al. A multicenter study on the use of pulsed low-intensity direct current for healing chronic stage II and stage III decubitus ulcers. *Arch Dermatol* 1993;129:999–1009.

30. El-Zeky F. Efficacy of high voltage pulsed current for healing of pressure ulcers in patients with spinal cord injury. *Phys Ther* 1991;71:433–442.

31. Kloth LC, Feedar JA. Acceleration of wound healing with high voltage, monophasic, pulsed current. *Phys Ther* 1988;68:503–508.

32. McDiarmid T. Ultrasound in the treatment of pressure sores. *Physiotherapy* 1985;February:66–70.

33. Ter Riet G, Kessels AG, Knipschild P. Randomised clinical trial of ultrasound treatment for pressure ulcers. *BMJ* 1995;310:1040–1041.

34. Nussbaum EL, Biemann I, Mustard B. Comparison of ultrasound/ultraviolet-C and laser for treatment of pressure ulcers in patients with spinal cord injury. *Phys Ther* 1994;74:812–823.

35. Lucas C, Stanborough RW, Freeman CL, De Haan RJ. Efficacy of low level laser therapy on wound healing in human subjects. A systematic review. *Lasers Med Sci* 2000;15:84–93. Search date 1998; primary sources Medline, Embase, Cinahl.

Nicky Cullum
Reader

E Andrea Nelson
Research Fellow

Jane Nixon
Research Fellow

Centre for Evidence Based Nursing
Department of Health Studies
University of York
York
UK

Competing interests: EAN and NC are applicants on a trial of compression bandages for which Beiersdorf UK Ltd is providing trial related education; JN, none declared.

E Andrea Nelson, Nicky Cullum and June Jones

QUESTIONS

INTERVENTIONS

Key Messages

- RCTs have found that compression heals venous leg ulcers more effectively than no compression.

- One systematic review has found that oral oxpentifylline versus placebo increases the proportion of ulcers that heal completely.

- One systematic review has found that, in the presence of compression, hydrocolloid dressings do not heal venous leg ulcers more effectively than simple, non-adherent dressings.

- We found insufficient evidence to determine whether any particular occlusive or non-occlusive dressing increases healing or reduces the pain of venous leg ulcers.

- We found limited evidence that human skin equivalent or peri-ulcer injection of granulocyte–macrophage colony stimulating factor may accelerate healing.

- Two RCTs have found that flavonoids increase the rate of healing of venous leg ulcers, but we found no evidence that either stanozolol or rutoside decrease recurrence rates.

Venous leg ulcers

- We found insufficient evidence on the effects of aspirin, intermittent pneumatic compression, oral zinc supplements, ultrasound, low level laser therapy, skin grafting, or vein surgery.
- We found limited evidence that compression prevents recurrence of venous leg ulcers.

DEFINITION Definitions of leg ulcers vary, but the following is widely used: loss of skin on the leg or foot that takes more than 6 weeks to heal. Some definitions exclude ulcers confined to the foot, whereas others include ulcers on the whole of the lower limb. This review deals with ulcers of venous origin in people without concurrent diabetes mellitus, arterial insufficiency, or rheumatoid arthritis.

INCIDENCE/ Between 1.5 and 3 people per 1000 have active leg ulcers.
PREVALENCE Prevalence increases with age to around 20 per 1000 in people aged over 80 years.[1]

AETIOLOGY/ Leg ulceration is strongly associated with venous disease. However,
RISK FACTORS about a fifth of people with leg ulceration have arterial disease, either alone or in combination with venous problems, which may require specialist referral.[1] Venous ulcers (also known as varicose or stasis ulcers) are caused by venous reflux or obstruction, both of which lead to poor venous return and venous hypertension.

PROGNOSIS People with leg ulcers have a poorer quality of life than age matched controls because of pain, odour, and reduced mobility.[2] In the UK, audits have found wide variation in the types of care (hospital inpatient care, hospital clinics, outpatient clinics, home visits), in the treatments used (topical agents, dressings, bandages, stockings), in healing rates, and in recurrence rates (26–69% in 1 year).[3,4]

AIMS To promote healing; to reduce recurrence; to improve quality of life, with minimal adverse effects.

OUTCOMES Ulcer area; number of ulcers healed; number of ulcer free limbs; recurrence rates; number of new ulcer episodes; number of ulcer free weeks or months; number of people who are ulcer free; frequency of dressing/bandage changes; quality of life; adverse effects of treatment.

METHODS *Clinical Evidence* update search and appraisal October 2000. We included RCTs with clinically important and objective outcomes: proportion of wounds healed, healing rates, incidence of new or recurring wounds, infection, and quality of life.

QUESTION What are the effects of treatments?

OPTION COMPRESSION

One systematic review of RCTs has found that compression heals venous leg ulcers more effectively than no compression. Elastomeric multilayer, high compression bandages, Unna's boot, high compression hosiery, and European short stretch bandages are all effective. We found insufficient evidence to compare different methods of compression.

Benefits: **Compression versus no compression:** We found one recent systematic review (search date 2000, 6 RCTs, 260 people) comparing compression versus no compression.[5] The review found that compression (e.g. short stretch bandages, double layer bandage, and Unna's boot — see glossary, p 1374) healed venous leg ulcers more effectively than no compression (e.g. dressing alone). The trials were heterogeneous, using different forms of compression in different settings and populations. The results were not pooled. The results of individual RCTs consistently favoured compression. **Elastomeric versus non-elastomeric multilayer compression:** See glossary, p 1373. The systematic review identified three RCTs (273 people) comparing elastomeric multilayer high compression bandages versus non-elastomeric multilayer compression.[5] Meta-analysis found an increase in the proportion of people whose ulcers healed with 12–15 weeks of high compression treatment versus controls (RRI for healing 54%, 95% CI 19% to 100%; NNT 5, 95% CI 3 to 12)[5] (see table 1, p 1375). **Multilayer high compression versus short stretch regimens:** The systematic review identified four small RCTs (164 people), which found no significant difference between multilayer high compression and short stretch regimens (RRI for healing 10%, 95% CI −22% to +55%).[5] The lack of power in these small studies means that a clinically important difference cannot be excluded. **Multilayer high compression versus single layer bandage:** The systematic review identified four RCTs (280 people) comparing multilayer high compression versus a single layer of bandage.[5] Meta-analysis found an increase in the proportion of ulcers healing with multilayered compression versus controls (RRI 41%, 95% CI 11% to 80%; NNT 6, 95% CI 4 to 18) (see table 1, p 1375).

Harms: High levels of compression applied to limbs with insufficient arterial supply, or inexpert application of bandages, can lead to tissue damage and, at worst, amputation.[10] Complication rates were rarely reported in trials.

Comment: People suitable for high compression were those with clinical signs of venous disease (ulcer in the gaiter region, from the upper margin of the malleolus to the bulge of the gastrocnemius; staining of the skin around an ulcer; or eczema), no concurrent diabetes mellitus or rheumatoid arthritis, and adequate arterial supply to the foot as determined by ankle/brachial pressure index. The precise ankle/brachial pressure index below which compression is contraindicated is often quoted as 0.8; however, many trials used the higher cut off of 0.9.[5] Effectiveness is likely to be influenced by the ability of those applying the bandage to generate safe levels of compression. Bandages may be applied by the person with the leg ulcer, their carer, nurse, or doctor. We found no comparisons of healing rates between specialist and non-specialist application of compression. Training improves bandaging technique among nurses.[11] Bandages containing elastomeric fibres can be applied weekly as they maintain their tension over time. Bandages made of wool or cotton, or both, such as short stretch bandages, may need to be reapplied more frequently as they do not maintain their tension.

Three small RCTs found no evidence of improved healing with intermittent pneumatic compression plus compression bandages versus compression bandages alone.

Benefits: We found one systematic review (search date 1997, 2 RCTs, 67 people) comparing intermittent pneumatic compression (see glossary, p 1373) in conjunction with compression (bandages or hosiery) versus compression alone.[9] We found one subsequent RCT (53 people).[12] These trials were all different in design. Pooling of results, using a random effects model, found no difference in healing rates.

Harms: No harmful effects have been reported.

Comment: Availability may vary widely between healthcare settings. Treatment can be delivered in the home, in outpatient clinics, or in the hospital ward. Clinical trials have evaluated the use of intermittent pneumatic pressure for 1 hour twice a week and 3–4 hours a day. Treatment requires resting for 1–4 hours daily, which may reduce quality of life.

One RCT has found that bilayer skin replacement versus simple dressings significantly increases complete ulcer healing. Another small RCT has found that infections of granulocyte– macrophage colony stimulating factors versus placebo significantly increased complete healing. We found insufficient evidence that any of the following dressings are more effective in healing ulcers than any other: occlusive or semi-occlusive dressings, simple primary dressings, other topical agents, or antimicrobial agents.

Benefits: **Simple low adherent dressings versus occlusive or semi-occlusive dressings:** We found one systematic review (search date 1997, 16 RCTs) comparing occlusive (hydrocolloids) or semi-occlusive dressings (foam, film, alginates) versus simple dressings (such as paraffin-tulle, knitted viscose dressings).[13] Nine of the RCTs compared hydrocolloid dressings versus simple dressings in the presence of compression. A pooled analysis of seven RCTs (714 people) found no evidence of benefit. Two comparisons of foam dressings versus simple dressings; two of film dressings versus simple dressings; and one comparing an alginate versus a simple dressing found no evidence of benefit. However, the RCTs, were too small (10–132 people, median 60) to detect anything but a very large difference in effectiveness. **Comparisons between occlusive or semi-occlusive dressings:** The same systematic review identified 12 small RCTs comparing different occlusive or semi-occlusive dressings.[13] There was no significant difference in healing rates between dressings, or insufficient data were provided to calculate their signficance. We found one subsequent RCT comparing hydrocolloid and hydrocellular dressings, and this found no difference in healing rates.[14] **Topical agents versus inert comparators:** The same systematic review identified 16 RCTs comparing topical agents (such as growth factors, cell suspensions, oxygen free-radical scavengers) versus either placebo preparations or standard care in the treatment of venous leg ulcers.[13] There was insufficient evidence to recommend any topical agent. The studies were small (9–233 people, median 45) and heterogeneous, and therefore results could not be pooled. Four RCTs of topical agents have been published since the systematic review search. One RCT (66 people) of calcitonin gene related peptide and vasoactive intestinal polypeptide administered by iontophoresis (see glossary, p 1373) versus electrical stimulation, found no evidence of benefit.[15] One RCT (60 people) compared a 13 week course of injections around the ulcer of granulocyte– macrophage colony stimulating factor 400 µg versus placebo and found an increased proportion of ulcers completely healed (RRI 236%, 95% CI 13% to 1134%; NNT 2, 95% CI 1 to 19) (see table 1, p 1375).[7] One RCT (293 people) comparing a cultured allogenic bilayer skin (see glossary, p 1373) replacement, which contained both epidermal and dermal components with a non-adherent dressing, found a greater proportion of ulcers healed completely in 6 months with the skin replacement (RRI for the proportion of ulcers healed 29%, 95% CI 4% to 61%; NNT 7, 95% CI 4 to 41) (see table 1, p 1375).[8] One RCT (40 people) of topically applied mesoglycan, a profibrinolytic agent, found no evidence of benefit.[16] **Antimicrobial agents versus placebo or standard care:** We found one systematic review (search date 1997, 14 RCTs) comparing antimicrobial agents versus either placebo agents or standard care.[17] The RCTs were small (25–153 participants, median 56), of poor quality, and no firm conclusions could be drawn.

Harms: It is unlikely that low adherent primary wound dressings cause harm, although dressings containing iodine may affect thyroid function if used over large surface areas for extended periods.[18] Many people (50–85%) with venous leg ulcers have contact sensitivity to preservatives, perfumes, or dyes.[19]

Comment: Simple primary dressings maintain a moist environment beneath compression bandages by preventing loss of moisture from the wound.[20]

OPTION   THERAPEUTIC ULTRASOUND

We found insufficient evidence of the effects of therapeutic ultrasound in the treatment of venous leg ulcers.

Benefits: We found one systematic review (search date 1999, 7 RCTs, 470 people) comparing therapeutic ultrasound (see glossary, p 1374) versus no ultrasound or sham ultrasound for venous leg ulcers.[21] Ultrasound improved ulcer healing in all studies, but a significant difference was found in only four of the seven RCTs.

Harms: Mild erythema, local pain, and small areas of bleeding have been reported in some trials.

Comment: None.

Wounds

OPTION   DRUG TREATMENTS

One systematic review has found good evidence that oral oxpentifylline versus placebo accelerates the healing of venous leg ulcers. Two RCTs found that flavonoids increase the rate of healing of venous leg ulcers. We found limited evidence from one RCT that sulodexide accelerates the healing of venous leg ulcers. We found no good evidence on the effects of aspirin or oral zinc supplements.

Benefits:	**Oxpentifylline:** We found one systematic review (search date 1999, 9 RCTs).[6] Eight RCTs compared oxpentifylline (1200 mg or 2400 mg a day) versus placebo in venous leg ulcers. The review pooled results from five RCTs, in which compression was standard therapy, and found that more ulcers healed with oxpentifylline than placebo (RRI for healing 30%, 95% CI 10% to 54%; NNT for 6 months' treatment 6, 95% CI 4 to 14). One RCT found no evidence of benefit for oxpentifylline compared with defibrotide (see table 1, p 1375). **Flavonoids:** We found two RCTs (245 people) comparing flavonoid 1000 mg daily (900 mg diosmin and 100 mg hesperidin) versus placebo or standard care.[22,23] These RCTs had different lengths of follow up but were similar in other respects. When pooled in a random effects model, flavonoids healed more ulcers than placebo (RRI 80%, 95% CI 20% to 170%). **Thromboxane α_2 antagonists:** We found one RCT (165 people) of an oral thromboxane α_2 antagonist versus placebo for venous leg ulcers. It found no significant difference in the proportion of ulcers healed (54% v 55%).[24] **Oral zinc:** We found one systematic review (search date 1997, 5 RCTs, 151 people) comparing daily doses of 440–660 mg oral zinc sulphate with placebo. The review found no evidence of benefit for oral zinc.[25] **Aspirin:** We found one small RCT of aspirin (300 mg a day, enteric coated) versus placebo. It found that more ulcers healed with aspirin (38% v 0%), but the trial had several weaknesses.[26] **Sulodexide:** We found one RCT (94 people). It found that more ulcers healed after 60 days treatment with sulodexide (daily intramuscular injection for 30 days and then orally for 30 days) in addition to compression therapy than with compression alone (35% v 58%; RRI 61%, 95% CI 3.5% to 163%; NNT 4, 95% CI 2 to 64).[27]
Harms:	The systematic review found more adverse effects with oxpentifylline than with placebo, although this was not significant (RR 1.25, 95% CI 0.87 to 1.80). Nearly half of the adverse effects were gastrointestinal (dyspepsia, vomiting, or diarrhoea).[21] Adverse effects of flavonoids, such as gastrointestinal disturbance, were reported in 10% of people.
Comment:	Sulodexide is not widely available and daily injections may be unacceptable to some people. Pentoxifylline is also referred to as oxpentifylline.

| OPTION | VEIN SURGERY |

We found insufficient evidence of the effects of vein surgery on ulcer healing.

Benefits: We found no systematic review. We found one RCT (47 people) comparing vein surgery (perforator ligation) versus no surgery or surgery plus skin grafting.[28] There was no difference in the proportion of ulcers healed after 1 year or the rate of ulcer healing. The trial was too small to rule out a beneficial effect.

Harms: Vein surgery carries the usual risks of surgery and anaesthesia.

Comment: Several operative approaches are commonly used, including perforator ligation, saphenous vein stripping, and a combination of both procedures.

| OPTION | SKIN GRAFTING |

We found insufficient evidence of the effects of skin grafting on ulcer healing.

Benefits: We found one systematic review (search date 1999, 6 RCTs, 197 people) of skin grafts (autografts or allografts) for venous leg ulcers. In five RCTs people also received compression bandaging; two RCTs (98 people) evaluated split thickness autografts; three RCTs (92 people) evaluated cultured keratinocyte allografts; and one RCT (7 people, 13 ulcers) compared tissue engineered skin (artificial skin) with split thickness skin grafts. We found insufficient evidence to determine whether skin grafting increased the healing of venous ulcers.[29]

Harms: Taking a skin graft leaves a wound that itself requires management and may cause pain. We found no evidence of harm from tissue engineered skin.

Comment: None.

| OPTION | LOW LEVEL LASER THERAPY |

We found insufficient evidence of the effects of low level laser therapy on ulcer healing.

Benefits: We found two systematic reviews.[30,31] The larger review (search date 1998, 4 RCTs) of laser therapy for venous leg ulcers included the only two RCTs identified by the smaller review. Two RCTs compared low level laser therapy (see glossary, p 1373) with sham; one RCT compared laser with ultraviolet therapy; and one RCT with non-coherent, unpolarised red light. Neither of the two RCTs of laser versus sham found a significant difference in healing rates. There was no significant difference in healing rates with laser when the trials were pooled. A three arm study (30 people) compared laser therapy with laser therapy plus infrared light and with non-coherent, unpolarised red light. Significantly more ulcers healed completely after 9 months' treatment in the group receiving a combination of laser and infrared light compared with non-coherent, unpolarised red light (RRI 140%, 95% CI 22% to 442%; NNT 2, 95% CI 1 to 9). A fourth RCT compared laser and ultraviolet light and found no significant difference.[30]

Harms: Eye protection is required when using some types of laser as the high energy beam may lead to damage of the retina.

Comment: The laser power, wavelength, frequency, duration, and follow up of treatment were different for all the studies.

QUESTION **What are the effects of interventions to prevent recurrence?**

OPTION **COMPRESSION**

We found limited evidence that compression reduces recurrence but non-compliance with compression is a risk factor for recurrence.

Benefits: We found one systematic review (search date 1997), which identified no RCTs comparing compression hosiery versus no compression.[9] The review identified two RCTs comparing different types of compression. One RCT (166 people) compared two brands of UK Class 2 stockings (see comment below) and found no difference in recurrence. The larger RCT (300 people) compared Class 2 and Class 3 stockings (see comment below) (see table 1, p 1375). With intention to treat analysis, the RCT found no significant reduction in recurrence after 5 years with high compression hosiery (UK Class 3) compared with moderate compression hosiery (UK Class 2). This analysis may underestimate the effectiveness of the Class 3 hosiery because a significant proportion of people changed from Class 3 to Class 2. Both RCTs found that non-compliance with compression hosiery was associated with recurrence.

Harms: The application of high compression to limbs with reduced arterial supply may result in ischaemic tissue damage and, at worst, amputation.[10]

Comment: Compression hosiery is classified according to the magnitude of pressure exerted at the ankle; the UK classification states that Class 2 hosiery is capable of applying 18–24 mm Hg pressure, and Class 3 is capable of applying 25–35 mm Hg pressure at the ankle. Other countries use different classification systems. Hosiery reduces venous reflux by locally increasing venous pressure in the legs relative to the rest of the body. This effect only takes place while hosiery is worn. The association between non-compliance with compression and recurrence of venous ulceration provides some indirect evidence of the benefit of compression in prevention. People are advised to wear compression hosiery for life and may be at risk of pressure necrosis from their compression hosiery if they subsequently develop arterial disease. Regular reassessment of the arterial supply is considered good practice, but we found no evidence about the optimal frequency of assessment. Other measures designed to reduce leg oedema, such as resting with the leg elevated, may be useful.

OPTION	SYSTEMIC DRUGS

We found insufficient evidence on the effects of systemic drugs on ulcer recurrence.

Benefits: We found one systematic review (search date 1997, 2 RCTs, 198 people) of drugs in the prevention of leg ulcer recurrence.[9] The review concluded that there was no evidence that stanozolol or rutoside decreased recurrence rates. One RCT (60 people) of stanozolol versus placebo found no significant difference in recurrence (17% v 20%). The other RCT (139 people) of rutoside versus placebo found no significant difference in recurrence (32% v 34%).

Harms: Stanozolol is an anabolic steroid; adverse effects included acne, hirsutism, amenorrhoea, oedema, headache, dyspepsia, rash, hair loss, depression, jaundice, and changes in liver enzymes. Tolerance of rutoside was reported to be good; adverse effects included headache, flushing, rashes, and mild gastrointestinal disturbances.[32]

Comment: None.

OPTION	VEIN SURGERY

We found insufficient evidence on the effects of vein surgery on ulcer recurrence.

Benefits: We found one systematic review (search date 1997, 1 RCT, 30 people).[9] The identified RCT, which was poorly controlled, compared surgery plus compression hosiery versus compression hosiery alone for prevention of recurrence. It found a reduced rate of recurrence when surgery was carried out in addition to the use of elastic stockings (5% v 24%; RRR 0.79, 95% CI 0.20 to 0.97).

Harms: Vein surgery has the usual risks of surgery and anaesthesia.

Comment: The results of this trial should be interpreted with caution because it was small and poorly controlled.

GLOSSARY

Cultured allogenic bilayer skin equivalent Also called human skin equivalent. This is made of a lower (dermal) layer of bovine collagen containing living human dermal fibroblasts, and an upper (epidermal) layer of living human keratinocytes.

Elastomeric multilayer high compression bandages Usually a layer of padding material followed by one to three additional layers of elastomeric bandages.

Intermittent pneumatic compression External compression applied by inflatable leggings or boots either over, or instead of, compression hosiery or bandages. A pump successively inflates and deflates the boots to promote the return of blood from the tissues. Newer systems have separate compartments in the boots so that the foot is inflated before the ankle, which is inflated before the calf.

Iontophoresis The delivery of an ionic substance by application of an electrical current.

Low level laser therapy Application of treatment energy ($< 10 \text{ J/cm}^2$) using lasers of 50 mW or less.

Short stretch bandages Minimally extensible bandages usually made of cotton with few or no elastomeric fibres. They are applied at near full extension to form a semi-rigid bandage.

Therapeutic ultrasound Application of ultrasound to a wound, using a transducer and a water based gel. Prolonged application can lead to heating of the tissues, but when used in wound healing the power used is low and the transducer is constantly moved by the therapist so that the tissue is not significantly heated.

Unna's boot An inner layer of zinc oxide impregnated bandage, which hardens as it dries to form a semi-rigid layer against which the calf muscle can contract. It is usually covered in an elastomeric bandage.

Substantive changes since last issue

Dressings and topical agents New RCT comparing hydrocolloid and hydrocellular dressings;[14] conclusion unchanged.

Drug treatments: flavonoids New RCT;[23] conclusion unchanged.

REFERENCES

1. Callam MJ, Ruckley CV, Harper DR, et al. Chronic ulceration of the leg: extent of the problem and provision of care. BMJ 1985;290:1855–1856.
2. Roe B, Cullum N, Hamer C. Patients' perceptions of chronic leg ulceration. In: Cullum N, Roe B, eds. Leg ulcers: nursing management. Harrow: Scutari, 1995:125–134.
3. Roe B, Cullum N. The management of leg ulcers: current nursing practice. In: Cullum N, Roe B, eds. Leg ulcers: nursing management. Harrow: Scutari, 1995:113–124.
4. Vowden KR, Barker A, Vowden P. Leg ulcer management in a nurse-led, hospital-based clinic. J Wound Care 1997;6:233–236.
5. Cullum N, Nelson EA, Fletcher AW, et al. Compression bandages and stockings in the treatment of venous leg ulcers. In: The Cochrane Library, Issue 3, 2000. Oxford: Update Software. Search date May 2000; primary sources 19 electronic databases, hand searches, and personal contacts.
6. Jull AB, Waters J, Arroll B. Oral pentoxifylline for treatment of venous leg ulcers. In: The Cochrane Library, Issue 3, 2000. Oxford: Update Software. Search date 1999; primary sources Cochrane Peripheral Vascular Diseases and Wounds Group, specialised registers, hand searches of reference lists, relevant journals and conference proceedings, personal contact with Hoechst, manufacturers of pentoxifylline, and experts in the field.
7. Da Costa RM, Ribeiro Jesus FM, Aniceto C, et al. Randomized, double-blind, placebo-controlled, dose-ranging study of granulocyte–macrophage colony stimulating factor in patients with chronic venous leg ulcers. Wound Repair Regen 1999;7:17–25.
8. Falanga V, Margolis D, Alvarez O, et al. Rapid healing of venous ulcers and lack of clinical rejection with an allogeneic cultured human skin equivalent. Human Skin Equivalent Investigators Group. Arch Dermatol 1998;134:293–300.
9. Cullum N, Fletcher A, Semlyen A, et al. Compression therapy for venous leg ulcers. Qual Health Care 1997;6:226–231. Search date April 1997; primary sources 18 databases, including Medline, Embase and Cinahl with no restriction on date, hand search of relevant journals, conference proceedings, and correspondence with experts to obtain unpublished papers.
10. Callam MJ, Ruckley CV, Dale JJ, et al. Hazards of compression treatment of the leg: an estimate from Scottish surgeons. BMJ 1987;295:1382.
11. Nelson EA, Ruckley CV, Barbenel J. Improvements in bandaging technique following training. J Wound Care 1995;4:181–184.
12. Schuler JJ, Maibenco T, Megerman J, et al. Treatment of chronic venous leg ulcers using sequential gradient intermittent pneumatic compression. Phlebology 1996;11:111–116.
13. Bradley M, Cullum N, Nelson EA, et al. Dressings and topical agents for healing of chronic wounds: a systematic review. Health Technol Assess 1999;3 No17(Pt2). Search date October 1997; primary sources Cochrane Library, Medline, Embase, Cinahl.
14. Seeley J, Jensen JL, Hutcherson J. A randomised clinical study comparing a hydrocellular dressing to a hydrocolloid dressing in the management of pressure ulcers. Ostomy Wound Manage 1999;45:39–47.
15. Gherardini G, Gurlek A, Evans GRD, et al. Venous ulcers: improved healing by iontophoretic administration of calcitonin gene-related peptide and vasoactive intestinal polypeptide. Plast Reconstr Surg 1998;101:90–93.
16. La Marc G, Pumilia G, Martino A. Effectiveness of mesoglycan topical treatment of leg ulcers in subjects with chronic venous insufficiency. Minerva Cardioangiol 1999;47:315–319.
17. O'Meara S, Cullum N, Majid M, et al. Systematic reviews of wound care management: (3) antimicrobial agents for chronic wounds. Health Technol Assess 2000;4(No 21):1–237. Search date October 1997; primary sources Cochrane Library, Medline, Embase, Cinahl.
18. Thomas S. Wound management and dressings. London: Pharmaceutical Press, 1990.
19. Cameron J, Wilson C, Powell S, et al. Contact dermatitis in leg ulcer patients. Ostomy Wound Manage 1992;38:10–11.
20. Wu P, Nelson EA, Reid WH, et al. Water vapour transmission rates in burns and chronic leg ulcers: influence of wound dressings and comparison with in vitro evaluation. Biomaterials 1996;17:1373–1377.
21. Flemming K, Cullum N. Therapeutic ultrasound for venous leg ulcers. In: The Cochrane Library, Issue 3, 2000. Oxford: Update Software. Search date 1999; primary sources Cochrane Wounds Group Specialised Trials Register, and hand searches of citation lists.
22. Guilhou JJ, Dereure O, Marzin L, et al. Efficacy of Daflon 500 mg in venous leg ulcer healing: a double-blind, randomized, controlled versus placebo trial in 107 patients. Angiology 1997;48:77–85.
23. Glinski W, Chodynicka B, Roszkiewicz J, et al. The beneficial augmentative effect of micronised purified flavonoid fraction (MPFF) on the healing of leg ulcers: an open, multicentre, controlled randomised study. Phlebology 1999;14:151–157.
24. Lyon RT, Veith FJ, Bolton L, et al. Clinical benchmark for healing of chronic venous ulcers. Venous Ulcer Study Collaborators. Am J Surgery 1998;176:172–175.

25. Wilkinson EAJ, Hawke CI. Does oral zinc aid the healing of chronic leg ulcers? A systematic literature review. *Arch Dermatol* 1998;134:1556–1560. Search date 1997; primary sources Medline, Embase, Cinahl, Science Citation Index, Biosis, British Diabetic Association Database, Ciscom, Cochrane Controlled Register of Clinical Trials, Dissertation Abstracts, Royal College of Nursing Database, electronic databases of ongoing research, hand searches of wound care journals and conference proceedings, and contact with manufacturer of zinc sulphate tablets.

26. Layton AM, Ibbotson SH, Davies JA, et al. Randomised trial of oral aspirin for chronic venous leg ulcers. *Lancet* 1994;344:164–165.

27. Scondotto G, Aloisi D, Ferrari P, et al. Treatment of venous leg ulcers with sulodexide. *Angiology* 99;50:883–889.

28. Warburg FE, Danielsen L, Madsen SM, et al. Vein surgery with or without skin grafting versus conservative treatment for leg ulcers. *Acta Dermatol Vereol* 1994;74:307–309.

29. Jones JE, Nelson EA. Skin grafting for venous leg ulcers. In: The Cochrane Library, Issue 3, 2000. Oxford: Update Software. Search date 1999; primary sources Cochrane Wounds Group Specialised Register, hand searches of reference lists, relevant journals, conference proceedings, and personal contact with experts in the field.

30. Flemming K, Cullum N. Laser therapy for venous leg ulcers. In: The Cochrane Library, Issue 3, 2000. Oxford: Update Software. Search date 1998; primary sources 19 electronic databases, hand searches of journals, conference proceedings, and bibliographies.

31. Lucas C, Stanborough RW, Freeman CL, et al. Efficacy of low level laser therapy on wound healing in human subjects: a systematic review. *Lasers Med Sci* 2000;15:84–93. Search date 1998; primary sources Medline, Embase, Cinahl, Cochrane Rehabilitation, and Related Therapies Register of Trials.

32. Taylor HM, Rose KE, Twycross RG. A double-blind clinical trial of hydroxyethylrutosides in obstructive arm lymphoedema. *Phlebology* 1993;8(suppl 1):22–28.

E Andrea Nelson
Research Fellow

Nicky Cullum
Reader

Centre for Evidence Based Nursing
University of York
York
UK

June Jones
Clinical Nurse Specialist
North Sefton and West Lancashire
Community Services NHS Trust
Southport
UK

Competing interests: EAN has been reimbursed for attending symposia by Smith and Nephew, Huntleigh Healthcare Ltd, and Convatec. EAN and NC are applicants on a trial of compression bandages for which Beiersdorf UK Ltd is providing trial related education. JJ has been reimbursed for attending symposia by 3M and Convatec.

TABLE 1	NNTs for healing of leg ulcers (see text, p 1367).

Intervention	NNT (95% CI)
Elastomeric multilayer compression v non-elastomeric multilayer compression bandages	5 (3 to 12)[5]
Multilayer high compression v single layer compression bandages	6 (4 to 18)[5]
Oxpentifylline 400 mg three times a day v placebo (concurrent use of compression)	6 (4 to 14)[6]
Peri-ulcer injection of GM-CSF* (400 µg) v placebo	2 (1 to 19)[7]
Cultured allogenic bilayer skin equivalent v non-adherent dressing	7 (4 to 41)[8]
Sulodexide plus compression v compression alone	4 (2 to 64)[27]

*GM–CSF, granulocyte–macrophage colony stimulating factor.

INDEX

Estimating cardiovascular risk and treatment benefit

Adapted from the New Zealand guidelines on management of dyslipidaemia[1] and raised blood pressure [2] by Rod Jackson

Appendix 1

How to use these colour charts

The charts help the estimation of a person's absolute risk of a cardiovascular event and the likely benefit of drug treatment to lower cholesterol or blood pressure. For these charts cardiovascular events include: new angina, myocardial infarction, coronary death, stroke or transient ischaemic attack (TIA), onset of congestive cardiac failure or peripheral vascular syndrome.

There is a group of patients in whom risk can be assumed to be high (>20% in 5 years) without using the charts. They include those with symptomatic cardiovascular disease (angina, myocardial infarction, congestive heart failure, stroke, TIA, and peripheral vascular disease), or left ventricular hypertrophy on ECG.

To estimate a person's absolute five-year risk:
■ Find the table relating to their sex, diabetic status (on insulin, oral hypoglycaemics or fasting blood glucose over 8 mmol/l), smoking status and age. The age shown in the charts is the mean for that category, i.e. age 60 = 55 to 65 years.
■ Within the table find the cell nearest to the person's blood pressure and total cholesterol : HDL ratio. For risk assessment it is enough to use a mean blood pressure based on two readings on each of two occasions, and cholesterol measurements based on one laboratory or two non-fasting Reflotron measurements. More readings are needed to establish the pre-treatment baseline.
■ The colour of the box indicates the person's five-year cardiovascular disease risk (see below).

Notes: (1) People with a strong history of CVD (first degree male relatives with CVD before 55 years, female relatives before 65 years) or obesity (body mass index above 30 kg/m^2) are likely to be at greater risk than the tables indicate. The magnitude of the independent predictive value of these risk factors remains unclear—their presence should influence treatment decisions for patients at borderline treatment levels. (2) If total cholesterol or total cholesterol:HDL ratio is greater than 8 then the risk is at least 15%. (3) Nearly all people aged 75 years or over also have an absolute cardiovascular risk over 15%.

Charts reproduced with permission from The National Heart Foundation of New Zealand. Also available on http://www.nzgg.org.nz/library/gl_complete/bloodpressure/table1.cfm

REFERENCES

1. Dyslipidaemia Advisory Group. 1996 National Heart Foundation clinical guidelines for the assessment and management of dyslipidaemia. *NZ Med J* 1996;109:224–232.
2. National Health Committee. Guidelines for the management of mildly raised blood pressure in New Zealand: Ministry of Health National Health Committee Report, Wellington, 1995.

RISK LEVEL Five-year CVD risk (non-fatal and fatal)		BENEFIT (1) CVD events prevented per 100 treated for five years*	BENEFIT (2) Number needed to treat for five years to prevent one event*
Very High	>30%	>10 per 100	<10
Very High	25–30%	9 per 100	11
Very High	20–25%	7.5 per 100	13
High	15–20%	6 per 100	16
Moderate	10–15%	4 per 100	25
Mild	5–10%	2.5 per 100	40
Mild	2.5–5%	1.25 per 100	80
Mild	<2.5%	<0.8 per 100	>120

*Based on a 20% reduction in total cholesterol or a reduction in blood pressure of 10–15 mmHg systolic or 5–10 mmHg diastolic, which is estimated to reduce CVD risk by about one third over 5 years.

Estimating cardiovascular risk and treatment benefit

Appendix 1

RISK LEVEL: MEN

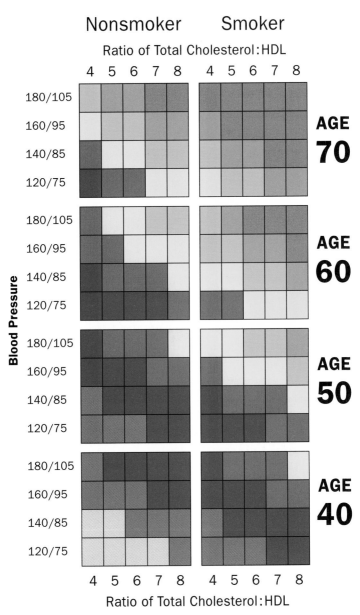

Estimating cardiovascular risk and treatment benefit

DIABETES

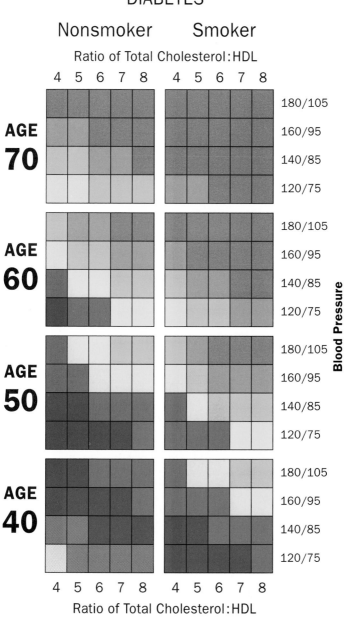

Nonsmoker   Smoker

Ratio of Total Cholesterol:HDL

Blood Pressure

Ratio of Total Cholesterol:HDL

RISK LEVEL: WOMEN

NO DIABETES

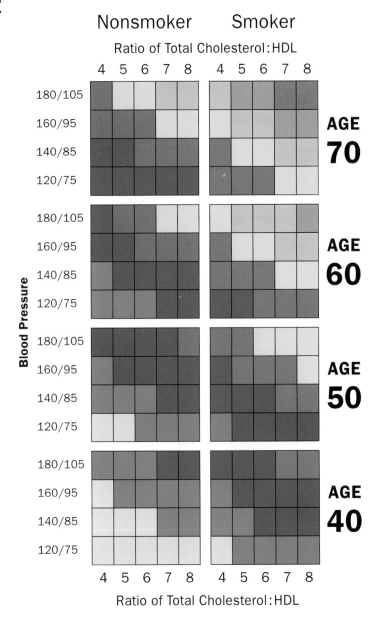

Nonsmoker   Smoker

Ratio of Total Cholesterol : HDL

AGE 70

AGE 60

AGE 50

AGE 40

Blood Pressure

Ratio of Total Cholesterol : HDL

Estimating cardiovascular risk and treatment benefit

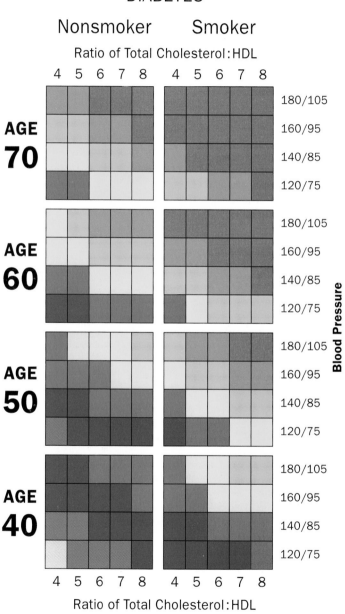

DIABETES

Nonsmoker   Smoker

Ratio of Total Cholesterol:HDL

The number needed to treat: adjusting for baseline risk

Adapted with permission from Chatellier et al, 1996[1]

BACKGROUND

The number needed to treat (NNT) to avoid a single additional adverse outcome is a meaningful way of expressing the benefit of an active treatment over a control. It can be used both to summarise the results of a therapeutic trial or series of trials and to help medical decision making about an individual patient.

If the absolute risk of adverse outcomes in a therapeutic trial is ARC in the control group and ART in the treatment group, then the absolute risk reduction (ARR) is defined as (ARC − ART). The NNT is defined as the inverse of the ARR:

$$NNT = 1/(ARC - ART)$$

Since the Relative Risk Reduction (RRR) is defined as (ARC − ART)/ARC, it follows that NNT, RRR and ARC are related by their definitions in the following way:

$$NNT \times RRR \times ARC = 1$$

This relationship can be used to estimate the likely benefits of a treatment in populations with different levels of baseline risk (that is different levels of ARC). This allows extrapolation of the results of a trial or meta-analysis to people with different baseline risks. Ideally, there should be experimental evidence of the RRR in each population. However in many trials, subgroup analyses show that the RRR is approximately constant in groups of patients with different characteristics. Cook and Sackett therefore proposed that decisions about individual patients could be made by using the NNT calculated from the RRR measured in trials and the baseline risk in the absence of treatment estimated for the individual patient.[2]

The method may not apply to periods of time different to that studied in the original trials.

USING THE NOMOGRAM

The nomogram shown on the next page allows the NNT to be found directly without any calculation: a straight line should be drawn from the point corresponding to the estimated absolute risk for the patient on the left hand scale to the point corresponding to the relative risk reduction stated in a trial or meta-analysis on the central scale. The intercept of this line with the right hand scale gives the NNT. By taking the upper and lower limits of the confidence interval of the RRR, the upper and lower limits of the NNT can be estimated.

REFERENCES

1. Chatellier G, Zapletal E, Lemaitre D, Menard J, Degoulet P. The number needed to treat: a clinically useful nomogram in its proper context. *BMJ* 1996;321:426–429.
2. Cook RJ, Sackett DL. The number needed to treat: a clinically useful measure of treatment effect. *BMJ* 1995;310:452–454.

The number needed to treat

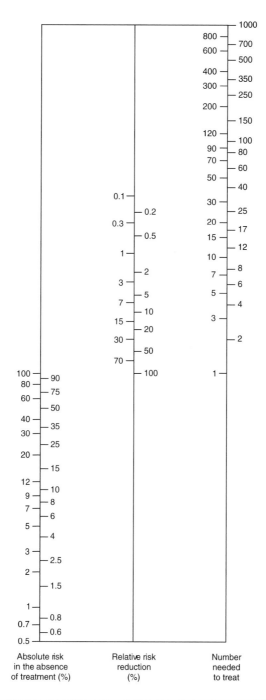

Absolute risk in the absence of treatment (%)	Relative risk reduction (%)	Number needed to treat

FIGURE Nomogram for calculating the number needed to treat. Published with permission[1]

Abbreviations

AR	Absolute risk	**NS**	Not significant
ARR	Absolute risk reduction	**OR**	Odds ratio
ARI	Absolute risk increase	**P**	P value
CI	Confidence interval	**RCT**	Randomised controlled trial
CCT	Controlled clinical trial	**RR**	Relative risk
HR	Hazard ratio	**RRI**	Relative risk increase
NNH	Number needed to harm	**RRR**	Relative risk reduction
NNT	Number needed to treat	**WMD**	Weighted mean difference

How to calculate risk

AR = # events (good or bad) in treated or control groups/ # people in that group

ARC = AR of events in the control group

ART = AR of events in the treatment group

ARR = ARC − ART

RR = ART/ARC = 1 − RRR

RRR = (ARC − ART)/ARC = 1 − RR

NNT = 1/ARR

To express decimals as percentages, multiply by 100.

If:

the RR (or OR) = 1, or the CI includes 1, there is no significant difference between treatment and control groups

the RR > 1 and the CI does not include 1, events are significantly more likely in the treatment than the control group

the RR < 1 and the CI does not include 1, events are significantly less likely in the treatment than the control group

RR of 0.8 means a RRR of 20% (meaning a 20% reduction in the relative risk of the specified outcome in the treatment group compared with the control group).

RRR is usually constant across a range of absolute risks. But the ARR is higher and the NNT lower in people with higher absolute risks.

Example: If a person's AR of stroke, estimated from his age and other risk factors (see appendix 1), is 0.25 without treatment but falls to 0.20 with treatment, the ARR is 25% − 20% = 5%; the RRR is (25% − 20%)/25% = 20%; and the NNT is 1/0.05 = 20. In a person with an AR of stroke of only 0.025 without treatment, the same treatment will still produce a 20% RRR, but treatment will reduce her AR of stroke to 0.2, giving a much smaller ARR of 2.5% − 2% = 0.5%, and a NNT of 200.

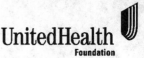

UnitedHealth Foundation
MN008-T500 P.O. Box 1459 Minneapolis, MN 55440-1459

July, 2001

Dear Colleague:

The UnitedHealth Foundation is pleased to provide you with a complimentary copy of *Clinical Evidence*, Issue 5.

We at UnitedHealth Foundation share in the belief that the practice of science and evidence-based medicine is an essential requirement for quality and safe health outcomes. We also share in the understanding that physicians, other health care professionals, and their patients should be free to make the best possible health care decisions and that those decisions should be supported by the best possible clinical information. Because the science of medicine is continuously enhanced, reviewed and updated, so too is *Clinical Evidence*. In February you received a copy of Issue 4 and now we are pleased that we can provide you with this fifth edition.

We have noticed that busy physicians are increasingly making use of the internet as a source for clinical information. As such we are particularly excited that UnitedHealth Foundation recipients of *Clinical Evidence* are eligible for free access to *Clinical Evidence* Online, which provides full text and fully searchable access to *Clinical Evidence*. To make use of this feature go to www.clinicalevidence.org. Once there, click on "CE-On-line" and follow the instructions to register.

Clinical Evidence is an international resource that provides easy access to the most up-to-date information on what is proven to work in medicine. Produced and published under the strict editorial leadership of the 160-year old British Medical Journal, it is the result of the best efforts of internationally recognized leaders in a variety of medical disciplines. *Clinical Evidence* has been proven to be an important aid to clinical decision making when used in conjunction with other credible medical information. The BMJ Publishing Group is solely responsible for the content of all issues of *Clinical Evidence* and is continually revising *Clinical Evidence* based on feedback from practicing physicians and clinical experts. I encourage you to provide them with comments via CEfeedback@bmjgroup.com.

If you would like to receive a copy of *Clinical Evidence*, Issue 6, upon its' release in January 2002, please visit our website at www.unitedhealthfoundation.org or complete the postcard included with this issue. Either will ensure you are on the mailing list for Issue 6. You may also write us at UnitedHealth Foundation, *Clinical Evidence*, MN008-T500, P.O. Box 1459, Minneapolis, Minnesota 55429.

All of us at the Foundation look forward to supporting you in your efforts to provide the best possible health and medical care to your patients. We are convinced that providing you with this edition of *Clinical Evidence* will go a long way to accomplishing our shared objectives.

Sincerely,

William W. McGuire, M.D.
Chairman
UnitedHealth Foundation

Sincerely,

William W. McGuire, M.D.
Chairman
UnitedHealth Foundation